W 50 ENG £125

MONKLAND

Medical Ethics Today
The BMA's Handbook of Ethics and Law

Third Edition

Information about major developments since the publication of this book may be obtained from the BMA's website or by contacting:

Medical Ethics Department
British Medical Association
BMA House
Tavistock Square
London WC1H 9JP
Tel: 020 7383 6286
Email: ethics@bma.org.uk
Website: www.bma.org.uk/ethics

Medical Ethics Today
The BMA's Handbook
of Ethics and Law

Third Edition

Project Manager

Veronica English

Head of Medical Ethics

Ann Sommerville

Written by

Sophie Brannan
Eleanor Chrispin
Martin Davies
Veronica English
Rebecca Mussell
Julian Sheather
Ann Sommerville

Director of Professional Activities

Vivienne Nathanson

BMA

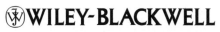**WILEY-BLACKWELL**
A John Wiley & Sons, Ltd., Publication

BMJ|Books

This edition first published 2012 © 2012 by BMA Medical Ethics Department.

BMJ Books is an imprint of BMJ Publishing Group Limited, used under licence by Blackwell Publishing Ltd which was acquired by John Wiley & Sons in February 2007. Blackwell's publishing programme has been merged with Wiley's global Scientific, Technical and Medical business to form Wiley-Blackwell.

Registered Office
John Wiley & Sons, Ltd, The Atrium, Southern Gate, Chichester, West Sussex, PO19 8SQ, UK

Editorial Offices
9600 Garsington Road, Oxford, OX4 2DQ, UK
The Atrium, Southern Gate, Chichester, West Sussex, PO19 8SQ, UK
111 River Street, Hoboken, NJ 07030-5774, USA

For details of our global editorial offices, for customer services and for information about how to apply for permission to reuse the copyright material in this book please see our website at www.wiley.com/wiley-blackwell

Library of Congress Cataloging-in-Publication Data
Medical ethics today : the BMAs handbook of ethics and law / project manager, Veronica English ; head of medical ethics, Ann Sommerville ; written by Sophie Brannan . . . [et al.]. – 3rd ed.
    p. ; cm.
  Includes bibliographical references and index.
  ISBN 978-1-4443-3708-2 (cloth)
  I. English, Veronica.   II. Sommerville, Ann.   III. Brannan, Sophie.   IV. British Medical Association.
  [DNLM: 1. Ethics, Medical–Great Britain.   2. Jurisprudence–Great Britain. W 50]
  LC-classification not assigned
  174.2–dc23   2011033670

A catalogue record for this book is available from the British Library.

Wiley also publishes its books in a variety of electronic formats. Some content that appears in print may not be available in electronic books.

Set in 9.5/11.5pt Garamond by Aptara Inc., New Delhi, India.
Printed and bound in Great Britain by TJ International Ltd, Padstow, Cornwall.

1   2012

Contents

List of statues and regulations   *xiii*

Directives and conventions   *xvii*

List of cases   *xix*

Where to find legal references online   *xxiii*

Medical Ethics Committee   *xxv*

Acknowledgements   *xxvii*

Preface to the third edition   *xxix*

Bridging the gap between theory and practice: the BMA's approach to
medical ethics   1

    What is medical ethics?   1
    The framework of good practice   6
    The theoretical and philosophical background   9
    The BMA's approach   13
    A hypothetical case on refusal of life-prolonging treatment 17

1 The doctor–patient relationship   21

    General principles   21
    Changing expectations of the doctor–patient relationship   22
    Types of relationships in modern medicine   27
    Choice and duty   28
    Maintaining a balanced relationship   31
    Importance of good communication   33
    Trust and reciprocity   39
    Breakdown of the doctor–patient relationship   43
    Recognising responsibilities and boundaries   45
    Patients' responsibilities   54

2 Consent, choice and refusal: adults with capacity   59

    The nature and purpose of consent   59
    General principles   60
    Standards and good practice guidance   60
    The process of seeking consent   61
    The scope of consent   73
    Pressures on consent   74
    Refusal of treatment   75
    Are there limits to an individual's choices?   80

3 Treating adults who lack capacity   93

    Consent and the alternatives   93
    General principles   97

Assessing an individual's decision-making capacity   98
Research and innovative treatment involving adults lacking the
capacity to consent   102
Providing treatment to adults lacking capacity – England and Wales   102
Providing treatment to adults lacking capacity – Scotland   122
Providing treatment to adults lacking capacity – Northern Ireland   134

4   Children and young people   145

Combining respect for autonomy with best interests   145
Has human rights legislation changed things for children?   146
Scope of this chapter   147
General principles   147
Emergencies   154
Consent and refusal by competent young people   154
Consent and refusal by people with parental responsibility   160
The courts   165
Refusal of blood products by Jehovah's Witnesses   166
Providing treatment against a child or young person's wishes   168
Cultural practices   170
Conjoined twins   173
Child protection   174

5   Confidentiality   183

The duty of confidentiality   184
General principles   184
What data are confidential?   185
Contacting patients   186
Implied consent for disclosure of information as part of the direct
provision of healthcare   187
The law   189
GMC guidance   192
NHS Care Record Guarantee   192
Anonymous information   193
Pseudonymised data   194
Statutory and legal disclosures   194
Statutory restrictions on disclosure   198
Disclosures in the public interest   199
Secondary uses of patient information   207
Adults who lack capacity to consent   218
Children and young people   220
Deceased patients   221

6   Health records   229

The importance of health information   229
Records and record keeping   230
General principles   230
Content of health records   231
Omitting information from health records   235

Removing information from health records 235
Tagging records 238
Electronic records 239
Security 243
Transmission 246
Recordings 247
Ownership 253
Retention of records 253
Disposal 255
Private records 255
Access to health records 255
Access to medical reports 260
Looking towards the future 261

7   Contraception, abortion and birth 267

The nature of reproductive ethics 267
General principles 268
Autonomy, rights and duties 268
Contraception 271
Sterilisation 277
Abortion 281
Prenatal screening and diagnosis 294
Pregnancy 298
Childbirth 301
Reproductive ethics: a continuing dilemma 306

8   Assisted reproduction 311

New reproductive technologies, new dilemmas? 311
General principles 312
Regulation of assisted reproduction 312
Monitoring the outcome of fertility treatment 314
What, if any duties, are owed to 'hypothetical' people? 316
Access to treatment 316
Consent to the storage and use of gametes and embryos 324
Use of donated gametes or embryos 327
Preimplantation genetic testing 337
Sex selection 345
Surrogacy 348
Seeking treatment in other countries 355
A law for the twenty-first century? 357

9   Genetics 365

The impact of developments in genetics 365
General principles 366
Does genetics raise different ethical issues? 366
Genetic testing of those with a family history of genetic disease 368
Consent for genetic testing 369
Confidentiality within families 374

Diagnostic testing   378
Carrier testing for recessive or X-linked disorders   378
Predictive or presymptomatic testing   383
Susceptibility testing   388
Incidental findings   389
Population genetic screening   390
Genetic tests supplied direct to consumers   393
Controversial uses of genetic information   396
Other developments   404
Law and regulation   408

10   Caring for patients at the end of life   415

Issues covered in this chapter   415
General principles   417
Communication when patients are approaching death   418
Diagnosing the dying patient and preparing for death   426
Decisions to withhold or withdraw life-prolonging treatment   440
Cardio-pulmonary resuscitation   447
Caring for children and young people   450
After the patient's death   455
Training   456

11   Euthanasia and physician assisted suicide   463

General principles   464
Terms and definitions   464
Public and professional views on assisted dying   467
The law   469
Moral, legal and pragmatic arguments   476

12   Responsibilities after a patient's death   489

Scope of this chapter   489
General principles   490
Terminology   490
Society's and individuals' attitudes to deceased people   491
The impetus for law reform   494
Duties and responsibilities after death   496
Confidentiality after death   498
Certifying and confirming death   501
Post-mortem examinations   506
Organ and tissue transplantation   512
Organ and tissue donation for research and teaching   515
Anatomical examination   516
Use of bodies or body parts for public display   516
Use of skeletons for private study   517
Testing for communicable diseases   517
Post-mortem DNA testing   518
Practising procedures on newly deceased people   519
Dealing with unusual requests   520

Ownership and trade in human bodies, body parts and tissue   521
The law   522

13   Prescribing and administering medication   533

The challenges and dilemmas   533
General principles   534
Responsibility for prescribing   534
Providing information to patients about medication   539
Prescribing for different patient groups   541
Pressure from patients   545
Pressure from employers   549
Clinical freedom and official guidance   552
Conflicts of interest in prescribing matters   554
Shared prescribing   557
Referrals and discharge summaries   562
Doctors who prescribe complementary and alternative medicine   563
Prescribing placebos   564
Controlled drugs   565
Self-prescribing and prescribing for family members   567
Prescribing at a distance   567
Drug administration   572
Reporting adverse drug reactions   573
Generic prescribing   574
Supply of drugs into the UK   575
Pharmacogenetics   576

14   Research and innovative treatment   583

Definitions   583
General principles   587
People who cannot consent to research or innovative therapy   597
Confidentiality   604
Research governance   607
Law and regulation   612
Specialised areas of research   616
Fraud and misconduct in research and innovative treatment   621
Summary   623

15   Emergency situations   629

General principles   629
Consent and refusal   629
Confidentiality   633
Duties to families   634
Treating the victims or perpetrators of crime or abuse   637
Recognising skill and competence levels   641
Emergency care outside healthcare establishments   642

16	Doctors with dual obligations	649
	When do dual obligations arise?	649
	General principles	651
	Providing reports for third parties	651
	Medical reports for insurance	654
	Expert witnesses	661
	Refereeing firearms licences	663
	Doctors examining asylum seekers	667
	Pre-employment reports and testing	669
	Occupational health physicians	673
	Doctors in the armed forces	679
	Sports doctors	682
	Media doctors	684
	Doctors with business interests	685
17	Providing treatment and care in detention settings	689
	Doctors' duties in detention settings	689
	General principles	691
	General issues of consent, confidentiality and choice within detention settings	692
	Practical issues common to various detention settings	701
	Healthcare in prisons	716
	Facilities accommodating young adult offenders, children and young people	722
	Immigration removal centres (IRCs)	724
	Police stations and forensic physicians	728
18	Education and training	739
	The ethical practice of medicine	739
	General principles	739
	Medical education: the changing landscape	740
	The teaching of medical ethics and law	742
	Ethical issues raised in teaching medical students	752
	Particular dilemmas of medical students	760
	The teaching of ethics and the ethics of teaching	765
19	Teamwork, shared care, referral and delegation	771
	General principles	771
	Working in multi-disciplinary teams	772
	Coordination and information sharing among care providers	779
	Delegation, referral and second opinions	788
	Administrative issues in working with others	792
20	Public health dimensions of medical practice	799
	General principles	799
	The public health perspective	800
	Legal aspects of public health	807
	Public health threats – tackling diseases, changing lives	811
	Public health tools	819

Commissioning services – tackling inequities 835
Processing health data for public health management 847
Looking towards the future 848

21 Reducing risk, clinical error and poor performance 855

The duty to protect patients 855
General principles 857
Standard setting 857
Duties of doctors to monitor quality and performance 865
Poorly performing systems and poor management 872
Identifying and addressing doctors' health problems 879

Appendix a The Hippocratic Oath 887

Appendix b Declaration of Geneva 889

Appendix c Declaration of a new doctor, as devised by Imperial College
School of Medicine graduating year of 2001 891

Index *893*

List of statutes and regulations

Page numbers are shown in **bold**

United Kingdom

Abortion (Scotland) Regulations 1991 (SI 1991/460)   **225**
Abortion Act 1967   **276, 277, 290, 293**
Abortion Regulations 1991 (SI 1991/499)   **195**
Access to Health Records (Northern Ireland) Order 1993   **222, 256, 259, 527, 660**
Access to Health Records Act 1990   **222, 256, 259, 527, 660**
Access to Medical Reports Act 1988   **27, 256, 260, 653, 655**
Access to Personal Files and Medical Reports (Northern Ireland) Order 1991   **256, 260**
Adult Support and Protection (Scotland) Act 2007   **49**
Adults with Incapacity (Conditions and Circumstances Applicable to Three Year Medical Treatment Certificates) (Scotland) Regulations 2007 (SI 2007/100)   **142**
Adults with Incapacity (Requirements for Signing Medical Treatment Certificates) (Scotland) Regulations 2007 (SI 2007/105)   **126**
Adults with Incapacity (Scotland) Act 2000   **62, 122, 123, 124, 219, 371, 400, 442, 595, 614, 630, 660, 694, 783**
Adults with Incapacity (Specified Medical Treatments) (Scotland) Regulations 2002 (SI 2002/275)   **143**
Age of Legal Capacity (Scotland) Act 1991   **149, 159**
Age of Majority Act (Northern Ireland) 1969   **180**
Anatomy (Northern Ireland) Order 1992   **522**
Anatomy Act 1984   **522, 526**
Care Quality Commission (Registration) Regulations 2009 (SI 2009/3112)   **529**
Child Support (Pensions and Social Security) Act 2000   **412**
Child Support, Pensions and Social Security Act (Northern Ireland) 2000   **412**
Children (Northern Ireland) Order 1995   **145**
Children (Scotland) Act 1995   **145**
Children Act 1989   **145, 723**
Children Act 2004   **176, 784**
Civil Partnership Act 2004   **181**
Computer Misuse Act 1990   **192**
Congenital Disability (Civil Liability) Act 1976   **309**
Coroners (Amendment) Rules 2005 (SI 2005/420)   **529**
Coroners (Amendment) Rules 2008 (SI 2008/1652)   **528**
Coroners Act (Northern Ireland) 1959   **506**
Coroners Act 1988   **526**
Coroners and Justice Act 2009   **511, 526, 469, 470**
Cremation (England and Wales) Regulations 2008 (SI 2008/2841)   **528**
Cremation (Scotland) Regulations 1935   **506**
Cremation Act 1902   **506**
Cremation Act 1952   **506**
Crime and Disorder Act 1998   **197**
Criminal Attempts Act 1981   **469**
Criminal Justice (Northern Ireland) Act 1966   **470**

Criminal Justice (Northern Ireland) Order 1998 **737**

Criminal Justice (Northern Ireland) Order 2005 **638, 730, 731**

Criminal Justice Act 2003 **401, 467**

Criminal Justice and Police Act 2001 **401**

Criminal Procedure and Investigations Act 1996 **731**

Data Protection (Miscellaneous Subject Access Exemptions) Order 2000 (SI 2000/419) **264**

Data Protection (Processing of Sensitive Personal Data) (Elected Representatives) Order 2002 (SI 2002/2905) **215**

Data Protection (Processing of Sensitive Personal Data) Order 2000 (SI 2000/417) **191**

Data Protection Act 1998 **190, 214, 234, 239, 240, 245, 253, 256, 527, 604, 614, 655, 669, 728, 756**

Detention Centre Rules 2001 (SI 2001/238) **726, 727**

Environment Act 1995 **809**

Environmental Protection Act 1990 **809**

Family Law Reform (Northern Ireland) Order 1977 **412**

Family Law Reform Act 1969 **412**

Fatal Accidents and Sudden Deaths Inquiry (Scotland) Act 1976 **735**

Female Genital Mutilation Act 2003 **172**

Firearms (Northern Ireland) Order 1981 **686**

Firearms (Scotland) Rules 1989 (SI 1989/889) **686**

Firearms Acts 1968 to 1997 **665**

Firearms Rules 1998 (SI 1998/1941) **686**

Freedom of Information (Scotland) Act 2002 **222, 259**

Freedom of Information Act 2000 **221, 259, 660**

Gender Recognition Act 2004 **188, 198, 237**

Health and Social Care Act 2001 **53, 209, 848**

Health and Social Care Act 2008 **196, 871**

Health Protection (Notification) (Wales) Regulations 2010 (SI 2010/1546) **224**

Health Protection (Notification) Regulations 2010 (SI 2010/659) **224**

Health Service (Control of Patient Information) Regulations 2002 (SI 2002/1438) **185, 188, 195, 210, 604**

Human Fertilisation and Embryology (Deceased Fathers) Act 2003 **325**

Human Fertilisation and Embryology (Disclosure of Donor Information) Regulations 2004 (SI 2004/1511) **360**

Human Fertilisation and Embryology (Disclosure of Information for Research Purposes) Regulations 2010 (SI 2010/995) **199**

Human Fertilisation and Embryology (Parental Orders) Regulations 2010 (SI 2010/985) **360**

Human Fertilisation and Embryology (Quality and Standards) Regulations 2007 (SI 2007/1522) **360**

Human Fertilisation and Embryology (Research Purposes) Regulations 2001 (SI 2001/188) **626**

Human Fertilisation and Embryology (Statutory Storage Period for Embryos and Gametes) Regulations 2009 (SI 2009/1582) **359**

Human Fertilisation and Embryology Act 1990 **72, 199, 286, 312, 313, 616**

Human Fertilisation and Embryology Act 2008 **199, 290, 313, 325, 348, 619**

Human Organ and Tissue Live Transplants (Scotland) Regulations 2006 (SI 2006/390) **532**

Human Organ Transplants (Northern Ireland) Order 1989 **522**

Human Organ Transplants Act 1989   **84, 522**

Human Reproductive Cloning Act 2001   **407, 618**

Human Rights Act 1998   **8, 29, 132, 160, 676, 704, 750, 810, 842**

Human Tissue (Quality and Safety for Human Application) Regulations 2007 (SI 2007/ 1523)   **523**

Human Tissue (Scotland) Act 2006   **489**

Human Tissue Act (Northern Ireland) 1962   **522**

Human Tissue Act 1961   **522**

Human Tissue Act 2004   **522**

Human Tissue Act 2004 (Persons who lack capacity to consent and transplants) Regulations 2006 (SI 2006/1659)   **91**

Immigration and Asylum Act 1999   **727**

Infant Life (Preservation) Act 1929   **291**

Ionising Radiation Regulations 1999 (SI 1999/3232)   **686**

Joint Inspection of Children's Services and Inspections of Social Work Services (Scotland) Act 2006   **221**

Law Reform (Miscellaneous Provisions) (Scotland) Act 1990   **412**

Medical Act 1983   **196**

Medicines (Advertising) Regulations 1994 (SI 1994/1932)   **554**

Medicines (Marketing Authorisations etc.) Amendment Regulations 2005 (SI 2005/2759) Mental Capacity Act 2005   **554**

Medicines for Human Use (Clinical Trials) and Blood Safety and Quality (Amendment) Regulations 2008 (SI 2008/941)

Medicines for Human Use (Clinical Trials) Regulations 2004 (SI 2004/1031)   **599, 602**

Medicines for Human Use (Marketing Authorisations etc.) Regulations 1994 (SI 1994/ 3144)   **581**

Medicines for Human Use (Manufacturing, Wholesale Dealing and Miscellaneous Amendments) Regulations 2005 (SI 2005/2789)   **581**

Mental Capacity Act 2005 (Independent Mental Capacity Advocates) (General) Regulations 2006 (SI 2006/1832)   **142**

Mental Capacity Act 2005 (Loss of Capacity During Research Project) (England) Regulations 2007 (SI 2004/679)   **626**

Mental Capacity Act 2005 (Loss of Capacity During Research Project) (Wales) Regulations 2007 (SI 2007/837)   **626**

Mental Health (Care and Treatment) (Scotland) Act 2003   **130, 694, 717**

Mental Health (Northern Ireland) Order 1986   **694**

Mental Health (Scotland) Act 1984   **159**

Mental Health Act 1983   **117, 305, 502, 694, 714**

National Assistance Act 1947   **809**

National Health Service (General Medical Services Contracts) (Prescription of Drugs etc.) Regulations 2004 (SI 2004/629)   **579**

National Health Service (General Medical Services Contracts) Regulations 2004 (SI 2004/291)   **579**

National Health Service (Primary Medical Services) (Miscellaneous Amendments) Regulations 2010 (SI 2010/578)   **228**

National Health Service (Reimbursement of the Cost of EEA Treatment) Regulations 2010 (SI 2010/915)   **782**

National Health Service (Venereal Disease) Regulations 1974 (SI 1974/29)   **198**

National Health Service (Scotland) Act 1978   **808**

National Health Service Act 1977   **808**

National Health Service Act 2006   **188, 191, 209, 212, 216, 782, 848**
Offences Against the Person Act 1861   **277**
Police and Criminal Evidence (Northern Ireland) Order 1989   **738**
Police and Criminal Evidence Act 1984   **700**
Police Reform Act 2002   **730**
Prescription Only Medicines (Human Use) Amendment (No. 3) Order 2000 (SI 2000/
    3231)   **307**
Prohibition of Female Genital Mutilation Act 2005   **172**
Protection of Vulnerable Groups (Scotland) Act 2007   **49**
Public Health (Control of Disease) Act 1984   **850**
Public Health (Infectious Diseases) Regulations 1988 (SI 1988/1546)   **224**
Public Health Act (Northern Ireland) 1967   **850**
Public Health etc (Scotland) Act 2008   **850**
Public Interest Disclosure (Northern Ireland) Order 1998   **778**
Public Interest Disclosure Act 1998   **778**
Public Services Reform (Scotland) Act 2010   **221**
Registration of Births, Deaths and Marriages (Scotland) Act 1965   **506**
Regulation of Investigatory Powers (Scotland) Act 2000   **58**
Regulation of Investigatory Powers Act 2000   **41**
Reporting of Injuries, Diseases and Dangerous Occurrences Regulations 1995 (SI
    1995/3163)   **195**
Road Traffic Act 1988   **195**
Safeguarding Vulnerable Groups Act 2006   **49**
Sanitary Act 1866   **822**
Sexual Offences (Northern Ireland) Order 2008   **275**
Sexual Offences Act 2003   **198, 273**
Suicide Act 1961   **470, 473, 496**
Surrogacy Arrangements Act 1985   **313, 348, 349**
Telecommunications Act 1984   **251**
Terrorism Act 2000   **195**
Terrorism Act 2006   **732**
Water Industry Act 1991   **809**

Non-United Kingdom

Death with Dignity Act 1994 (Oregon)   **477**
Genetic Information Non-discrimination Act 2008 (USA)   **413**
Termination of Life on Request and Assisted Suicide (Review Procedures) Act 2001 (The
    Netherlands)   **480**

Directives and conventions

Page numbers are shown in **bold**

Directive 2001/20/EC of the European Parliament and of the Council of 4 April 2001 on the approximation of the laws, regulations and administrative provisions of the member states relating to the implementation of good clinical practice in the conduct of clinical trials on medicinal products for human use   **586, 607**

Directive 2001/83/EC of the European Parliament and of the Council of 6 November 2001 on the Community code relating to medicinal products for human use   **575, 787**

Directive 2003/88/EC of the European Parliament and of the Council of 4 November 2003 concerning certain aspects of the organisation of working time   **23, 864, 877**

Directive 2004/23/EC of the European Parliament and of the Council of 31 March 2004 on setting standards of quality and safety for the donation, procurement, testing, processing, preservation, storage and distribution of human tissues and cells   **313, 333**

Directive 2004/24/EC of the European Parliament and of the Council of 31 March 2004, amending, as regards traditional herbal medicinal products, Directive 2001/83/EC on the Community code relating to medicinal products for human use   **787**

Directive 2008/142/EC of the European Parliament and of the Council on the application of patients' rights in cross-border healthcare   **782, 840**

European Convention for the Protection of Human Rights and Fundamental Freedoms   **110, 112, 132, 146, 191, 197, 269, 273, 279, 280, 317, 318, 444, 470, 612, 671, 676, 698, 704, 706, 709, 831, 839**

United Nations Convention on the Rights of the Child 1989   **146, 726**

United Nations Convention on the Rights of Persons with Disabilities 2006   **95**

United Nations International Covenant on Civil and Political Rights 1966   **8, 650**

United Nations International Covenant on Economic, Social and Cultural Rights 1966   **8**

United Nations Universal Declaration of Human Rights 1948   **8**

List of cases

Page numbers are shown in **bold**

United Kingdom

A (children), Re, sub nom Re A (conjoined twins: medical treatment), sub nom Re A (children) (conjoined twins: surgical separation) [2000] 4 All ER 961   **181**

A (male sterilisation), Re [2000] 1 FLR 549   **308**

AB v Leeds Teaching Hospital NHS Trust [2005] Q.B. 506   **532**

Airedale NHS Trust v Bland [1993] 1 All ER 821   **90, 461**

Ashworth Security Hospital v MGN [2002] UKHL 29   **224**

Attorney General v Able and others [1984] 1 All ER 277   **486, 487**

B (a minor) (wardship: sterilisation), Re [1987] 2 All ER 206   **308**

B (adult: refusal of treatment), Re [2002] 2 All ER 449   **90**

B (wardship: abortion), Re [1991] 2 FLR 426   **309**

Barnett v Chelsea and Kensington Hospital Management Committee (1969) 1 QB 428   **30, 57**

Birch v UCL Hospital NHS Foundation Trust [2008] 104 BMLR 168   **884**

Bolam v Friern Hospital Management Committee [1957] 2 All ER 118   **89, 858, 859, 884**

Bolitho v City and Hackney Health Authority [1997] 4 All ER 771   **859, 884**

BPAS v Secretary of State for Health [2011] EWHC 235 (Admin)   **308**

C (a minor) (medical treatment), Re, sub nom Re C (a minor) (withdrawal of lifesaving treatment) [1998] 1 FLR 384   **181, 461**

C (adult: refusal of medical treatment), Re [1994] 1 All ER 819   **91, 141, 143**

C (welfare of child: immunisation), Re [2003] 2 FLR 1095 CA   **181**

Campbell v MGN [2004] UKHL 22   **223**

Chester v Afshar [2005] 1 AC 134   **89**

D (a minor), Re [1976] 1 All ER 326   **308**

D (medical treatment), Re [1998] 1 FLR 411   **461**

Dobson v North Tyneside Health Authority [1996] 4 All ER 741   **531**

Dundee City Council v M (2004) SLT 640   **180**

Evans v Amicus Healthcare Ltd and Others [2004] 1 FLR 67; [2004] 2 FLR 766   **359**

F (in utero), Re [1988] 2 All ER 193   **309**

F (mental patient: sterilisation), Re, sub nom F v West Berkshire Health Authority [1989] 2 All ER 545   **308**

Frenchay Healthcare NHS Trust v S [1994] 1 WLR 601   **461**

Froggatt v Chesterfield and North Derbyshire NHS Trust [2002] WL 31676323   **37, 57**

G (surrogacy: foreign domicile), Re [2007] EWHC 2814 (Fam)   **362**

Gillick v Wisbech and West Norfolk AHA [1985] 3 All ER 402   **180, 307**

H and A (children) (paternity: blood tests) [2002] 1 FLR 1145   **412**

Hartman v South Essex Mental Health and Community Care NHS Trust [2005] EWCA civ 6   **686**

Houston (applicant) (1996) 32 BMLR 93   **180, 181**

Hunter v Hanley [1955] SC 200; [1955], SLT 213   **858, 884**

J (a minor) (prohibited steps order: circumcision), Re, sub noms Re J (child's religious upbringing and circumcision); Re J (specific issue orders: Muslim upbringing and circumcision) [2000] 1 FLR 571   **181**

J (a minor) (wardship: medical treatment), Re [1992] 4 All ER 614   **852**

Janaway v Salford HA [1988] 3 All ER 1079   **309**

Jepson v The Chief Constable of West Mercia [2003] EWHC 3318   **308**

Kay's Tutor v Ayrshire & Arran Health Board [1987] 2 All ER 417; (1987) SC 145; (1987) SLT 588   **860, 861, 884**

L v Human Fertilisation and Embryology Authority and the Secretary of State for Health [2008] 2 FLR 1999   **359**

Law Hospital NHS Trust v Lord Advocate (1996) SLT 848   **461**

M (child: refusal of medical treatment), Re [1999] 2 FLR 1097   **180**

MB (medical treatment), Re [1997] 2 FLR 426   **89, 141, 307, 310**

N (a child), Re [2007] EWCA Civ 1053   **362**

NHS Trust A v M; NHS Trust B v H [2001] 1 All ER 801   **461**

NHS Trust and D (by her litigation friend The Official Solicitor) [2003] EWHC 2793 (fam)   **309**

NHS Trust v MB [2006] EWHC 507 (Fam)   **181, 410**

Nicholas Lewis (Claimant) v Secretary of State for Health (Defendant) and Michael Redfern QC (Interested Party) [2008] EWHC 2196 (QB)   **150**

O (a minor) (medical treatment), Re [1993] 2 FLR 149   **181**

P (a minor), Re [1986] 1 FLR 272   **309**

P (medical treatment: best interests), Re [2003] EWHC 2327 (Fam)   **181**

Palmer v Tees Health Authority & Anor [1999] Lloyd's Rep Med 351   **410**

Pamela Cornelius v Dr Nicola de Taranto [2002] 68 BMLR 62   **685**

Paton v British Pregnancy Advisory Service Trustees [1978] 2 All ER 987   **309**

Pearce v United Bristol Healthcare NHS Trust (1999) 48 BMLR 118   **89**

Portsmouth NHS Trust v Wyatt [2005] 1 FLR 21; [2005] 1 FLR 554; [2005] 2 FLR 480; [2005] EWHC 117; 21 October 2005 (unreported)   **181**

Quintavalle v Human Fertilisation and Embryology Authority [2003] 2 All ER 105; CA [2003] 3 All ER 257; [2005] 1 WLR 1061   **362**

R (on the application of ARGC and H) v HFEA [2003] 1 FCR 266   **358**

R (on the application of Axon) v Secretary of State for Health [2006] 2 WLR 1130   **180, 307**

R (on the application of Burke) v General Medical Council [2005] 2 FLR 1223   **91, 461**

R (on the application of Murphy) v Salford Primary Care Trust [2008] EWHC 1908 (Admin)   **852**

R (on the application of Pretty) v Director of Public Prosecutions (2001) UKHL 61   **486**

R (on the application of Quintavalle) v Secretary of State for Health [2001] 4 All ER 1013; CA [2002] 2 All ER 625; [2003] 2 All ER 113   **626**

R (on the application of S) v Chief Constable of South Yorkshire, R (on the application of Marper) v Chief Constable of South Yorkshire [2003] 1 All ER 148; [2004] UKHL 39   **308, 412**

R (on the application of Smeaton) v Secretary of State for Health [2002] 2 FLR 146   **308**

R (on the application of TB) v The Combined Court at Stafford [2006] EWHC 1645 (Admin)   **225**

R (on the application of the Howard League for Penal Reform) v Secretary of State for the Home Department (No.2) [2003] 1 FLR 484   **737**

R (on the application of Watts) v Bedford Primary Care Trust and another [2004] EWCA Civ 166   **852**

R v Bourne [1939] 1 KB 687   **309**

R v Brown [1993] 2 All ER 75   **91**

R v Collins, ex parte Ian Stewart Brady [2001] 58 BMLR 173   **736**

R v HS Dhingra – Birmingham Crown Court Judgment 24 January 1991 Daily Telegraph 1991 Jan 25   **308**

R v Human Fertilisation and Embryology Authority, ex parte Blood [1997] 2 All ER 687   **359**

R v Kelly [1998] 3 All ER 741   **521, 531, 632**

R v Misra [2004] EWCA Crim 2375   **863, 884**

R v North West Lancashire Health Authority, ex parte A and Others [2000] 1 WLR 977   **852**

R v Prentice [1993] 3 WLR 927   **852**

R v Secretary of State for the Home Department, ex parte Mellor [2001] 2 FLR 1158; [2001] 3WLR 533   **358, 735**

RB (A Child), Re [2009] EWHC 3269 (Fam)   **461**

Rose v Secretary of State for Health and Human Fertilisation and Embryology Authority [2002] 2 FLR 962   **360**

R v Department of Health (Respondent), ex parte Source Informatics Ltd (Appellant) and (1) Association Of The British Pharmaceutical Industry (2) General Medical Council (3) (4) National Pharmaceutical Association Ltd (Interveners) [2000] 1 All ER 786 Medical Research Council   **224**

S (a minor) (medical treatment), Re [1993] 1 FLR 377   **181**

S (sterilisation: patient's best interests), Re, sub noms Re SL (adult patient: medical treatment), SL v SL [2000] 1 FLR 465   **308**

S v McC; W v W [1970] 3 All ER 107   **412**

Savage v South Essex Partnership NHS Foundation Trust [2008] UKHL 74   **852**

Sidaway v Board of Governors of the Bethlem Royal Hospital [1985] AC 871   **89, 141**

Simms v Simms, A v A [2002] 2 WLR 1465; [2003]1 All ER 669   **597, 624**

Society for the Protection of Unborn Children v Department of Health, Social Services and Public Safety [2009] NIQB 92   **309**

South Glamorgan CC v B sub nom South Glamorgan CC v W and B [1993] FLR 574   **182**

St George's Healthcare NHS Trust v S, R v Collins and others, ex parte S [1998] 3 All ER 673 1 FLR 502, CA   **91, 310**

T (adult: refusal of medical treatment), Re [1992] 4 All ER 649   **90, 141**

W (a minor) (medical treatment: court's jurisdiction), Re [1992] 4 All ER 627   **180, 181**

W (adult: refusal of medical treatment), Re (2002) MHLR 411   **646, 734**

W v Egdell and Ors [1990] 1 All ER 835   **199, 225**

Wilsher v Essex AHA [1986] 3 All ER 801; [1987] 1 QB 730; [1988] AC 1074; [1988] 1 All ER 871, HL   **647**

X & Y (foreign surrogacy), Re [2009] 1 FLR 733   **362**

Non-United Kingdom

D v United Kingdom (1997) 24 EHRR 423   **735**

Dickson v United Kingdom (2008) 46 EHRR 41   **358, 735**

Evans v The United Kingdom (6339/05) [2006] ECHR 200 (7 March 2006); [2007] ECHR 264 (10 April 2007)   **359**

Glass v United Kingdom (61827/00) [2004] ECHR 103 (9 March 2004)   **165, 166, 181**

HL v United Kingdom (45508/99) [2004] 40 EHRR 761; 81 BLMR 131   **142**

I v Finland (20511/03) [2008] ECHR 623 (17 July 2008) **240, 263**

Paton v United Kingdom (1981) 3 EHRR 408 **309**

Pretty v UK (2346/02) (2002) 35 EHRR 1 **90, 486**

R (on the application of the Association of the British Pharmaceutical Industry) v Medicines and Healthcare Products Regulatory Agency [2010] EUECJ C-62/09_O **581**

R (on the application of Yvonne Watts) v Bedford Primary Care Trust and Secretary of State for Health [2006] EUECJ C-372/04 **796**

S and Marper v The United Kingdom (30562/04 and 30566/04) [2008] ECHR 1581 **412**

Shelley v United Kingdom (2008) 46 EHRR SE16 **735, 736**

Szuluk v United Kingdom (2010) 50 EHRR 10 **734**

Vo v France (2005) 40 EHRR 12 **90, 269, 307**

W v UK (1987) 10 EHRR 29 **180**

X v Austria (1980) 18 DR 154 **90**

X v Denmark (9974/82) (1983) 32 DR 282 **614, 626**

X v Germany (1985) 7 EHRR 152 **181**

X v The European Commission [1995] IRLR 320 **686**

YF v Turkey (2004) 39 ECHR 34 **90**

Where to find legal references online

All UK legislation since 1988, and some from before that date, is available on the Government's legislation website at: www.legislation.gov.uk. Some statutory instruments are also available on this site.

Selected judgments from UK Courts, the European Court of Human Rights and the European Court of Justice are available from the British and Irish Legal Information Institute at: www.bailii.org

Selected legal judgments, including Supreme Court judgments, are available on the Court Service website at: www.hmcourts-service.gov.uk

House of Lords' judgments delivered between 14 November 1996 and 31 July 2009 are available on the House of Lords website at: www.publications.parliament.uk (Thereafter see the Court Service website for judgments from the Supreme Court.)

In addition, a number of commercial companies provide online access to legal judgments.

Medical Ethics Committee

A publication from the BMA's Medical Ethics Committee (MEC). The following people were members of the MEC for one or both of the two committee sessions this book was in preparation.

Dr Anthony Calland, Chairman – *General practice (retired), Gwent*

Dr Kate Adams – *General practice, London*
Dr John Chisholm – *General practice, Bromley*
Dr Mary Church – *General practice, Glasgow*
Dr Peter Dangerfield – *Academic staff, Liverpool*
Mr Nicholas Deakin – *Medical student*
Professor Bobbie Farsides – *Medical law and ethics, Brighton*
Professor Ilora Finlay – *Palliative medicine, Cardiff*
Claire Foster – *Medical ethics, London*
Professor Robin Gill – *Theology, Canterbury*
Professor Raanan Gillon – *General practice (retired) and medical ethics, London*
Dr Evan Harris – *Former MP and hospital doctor, Oxford*
Professor Emily Jackson – *Medical law and ethics, London*
Professor David Katz (deputy) – *Academic staff, London*
Dr Rajesh Kumar – *Anaesthetics, Preston*
Dr Surendra Kumar – *General practice, Widnes*
Professor Graeme Laurie – *Medical law, Edinburgh*
Professor Sheila McLean – *Medical law, Glasgow*
Miss Louise McMenemy – *Medical student*
Dr Lewis Morrison – *General and geriatric medicine, Lothian*
Dr Kevin O'Kane (deputy) – *Acute medicine, London*
Dr Brian Patterson – *General practice, County Antrim*
Professor Wendy Savage – *Obstetrics and gynaecology, London*
Professor Julian Savulescu – *Practical ethics, Oxford*
Dr Jan Wise – *Psychiatry, London*

Ex-officio
Dr Hamish Meldrum, Chairman of BMA Council
Professor Averil Mansfield, President BMA (2009–2010)
Professor Sir Michael Marmot, President BMA (2010–2011)
Dr Peter Bennie, Chairman of the BMA Representative Body (until 2010)
Dr Steve Hajioff, Chairman of the BMA Representative Body (from 2010)
Dr David Pickersgill, BMA Treasurer

Thanks are due to other BMA committees and staff for providing information and comments on draft chapters.

Acknowledgements

Thanks are due to the many people and organisations who gave so generously of their time in commenting on earlier drafts and discussing the very difficult medical, legal and ethical issues with us. Although these contributions helped to inform the BMA's views, it should not be assumed that this guidance necessarily reflects the views of all those who contributed. Particular thanks are due to the following:

Professor Richard Ashcroft, Dr Marcus Bicknell, Dr Laura Bowater, Professor Peter Braude, Sir Kenneth Calman, Professor Angus Clarke, Dr John Coggon, Professor Sir Alan Craft, Dr Angus Dawson, Ms Jane Denton, Professor John Ellershaw, Ms Sarah Elliston, Professor Peter Furness, Dr Richard Hain, Dr Jake Hard, Ms Penny Letts, Professor Penney Lewis, Professor Anneke Lucassen, Mr Denzil Lush, Professor Derek Morgan, Ms Deborah Murphy, Dr Joseph Palmer, Professor Michael Parker, Dr Christine Patch, Dr Michael Peel, Dr Fiona Randall, Mr Harald Schmidt, Professor Gordon Stirrat, Ms Karen Thomson, Dr Howard Thomson, Dr Stephen Watkins, Dr Frank Wells, Dr James Welsh, Dr Mark Wilkinson.

Children and Family Court Advisory and Support Service, College of Emergency Medicine, Department of Health (Children, Families and Maternity; Health, Science and Bioethics; Research, Systems and Governance; Medicines, Pharmacy and Industry; Information Governance; Offender Health and Offender Partnerships), Faculty of Forensic and Legal Medicine, General Medical Council, Human Fertilisation and Embryology Authority, Infertility Network UK, National Prescribing Centre, NHS Blood and Transplant, Nursing and Midwifery Council, Resuscitation Council UK, Royal College of General Practitioners, Royal College of Nursing, Royal College of Obstetricians and Gynaecologists, Royal College of Paediatrics and Child Health, Royal College of Pathologists, The Patients Association.

Preface to the third edition

This is the BMA's handbook of ethical advice. It reflects the fact that doctors in England, Scotland, Wales and Northern Ireland work in separate healthcare systems with different administrative arrangements and, in some cases, different legislation. The period within which the book was drafted (2010–2011) saw proposals for considerable NHS change and, at the time of writing, it is not clear how these will develop. Our aim throughout is to provide advice which is practical and relevant to doctors' daily lives and so, while recognising this is a time of flux and some uncertainty, the book sets out the law and best practice at the time of drafting. It also flags up, where possible, the likely direction of future change. More information is available on the BMA's website and we have identified, in each chapter, other sources of ethical and medico-legal guidance.

The very first BMA ethics handbook appeared in 1949. Every subsequent version has increased the detail and practical orientation of the advice, including relevant aspects of law. This is the third update of the version called *Medical Ethics Today*, first published in 1993. Since then, much has changed within the profession and society. New challenges, or new twists on old dilemmas, have arisen. Some reflect developments within the health service, such as the challenge to ensure equity for patients as NHS services undergo radical change. Some echo the altered expectations of doctors and patients as healthcare is increasingly seen from a consumerist perspective, within which its role is partly about furthering patients' personal goals, through cosmetic and lifestyle aids. Other dilemmas highlight apparent differences of views between many doctors and their patients on issues such as students' reliance on drugs to enhance cognitive functioning or requests for assisted dying.

Most issues in this book are not entirely new but some broad attitudinal changes in society and the profession need to be reflected, as well as the practical changes since the last edition. Doctors now have to prove their competence in medicine and decision making through revalidation at more stages of their careers. They are exhorted to combine traditional professional values with an ability to meet expanding patient expectations. In the past, doctors based their decisions on conscience, intuition, received wisdom and codes of practice. Now they need to use reason, analysis and knowledge of the law. They should be able to explain and justify their decisions to patients, colleagues, the media, regulators and the courts. An awareness of ethics is central to this process and also important in doctors' appraisal and revalidation. This book is designed to provide that background knowledge.

Through its confidential advice service for its members, the BMA remains aware of the changing ethical dilemmas confronting the profession. BMA policy on controversial subjects is thrashed out in debate at the annual representatives meeting (ARM) by members' representatives. Briefings and background data to the discussions are provided by the BMA's Medical Ethics Committee (MEC): a multidisciplinary group combining clinical, legal, philosophical, ethical and theological expertise. All BMA ethics publications are reviewed by MEC members, other BMA committees and a supervisory Board of Professional Activities. These bodies supply expert analysis, practical experience and intellectual rigour. BMA guidance and discussion papers have been quoted approvingly by courts, Parliament and policy-making bodies.

Among general trends since the previous version of this book, the courts have continued to increase their role in resolving medical cases. Such precedent judgments provide useful guidance, much of which is included throughout the book. Devolution has introduced many variations in practice and guidance throughout the UK. Its impact on statute law and quasi-law, such as NHS circulars and executive letters, is also reflected here. Charting trends which develop differently in the devolved nations, however, inevitably leads to some repetition in sections of the book dealing with issues, such as mental capacity.

Patients and the public generally are better informed than in the past about their rights and choices in medicine. More sources of information are open to them. The emphasis on patient choice has continued to increase and more recognition is demanded for the views of marginalised populations. Older people are demographically more important and feature more in terms of resource allocation, service planning and research. Patient confidentiality – a staple of professional codes since Hippocrates – has frequently been revisited and redefined in recent years to meet the needs of the electronic age and the ever growing requirement for data for research and administrative purposes. There is more awareness of cultural and religious diversity – among patient populations and also among health professionals.

Issues of rationing and commercialisation of the health service are ever more challenging in the midst of organisational change. Public health ethics increasingly commands attention, including debate about whether patients should be penalised for rejecting immunisation, for example, or offered rewards for taking positive steps to improve their health. Cross-border healthcare is a growing phenomenon which can raise some difficult ethical and practical issues as some patients choose to bypass UK rules and travel abroad for services such as assisted dying or fertility treatment using anonymous or paid gamete donors.

Most of the ethical issues discussed in the following chapters have arisen in enquiries submitted to the BMA by its members. They need a prompt workable solution for an immediate case and so much of the book focuses on practical responses to common questions but reference to philosophy and law is essential as background. Abortion, embryo research and euthanasia, for example, raise weighty moral issues that should be explored even though the actual procedures are regulated by law so that most questions about what is permissible can be answered briefly. Even superficially simple queries, such as how much information to give a patient, or whether children can choose treatment for themselves, cannot be answered fully without mentioning how legal cases and ethical discussions influence medical practice and vice versa.

Although ethics is more firmly embedded now in medical education and today's doctors and students are probably more familiar than previous generations with the principles, applying them to changing circumstances can be challenging. In addition to the guidance provided here, the BMA provides an advice line for members who wish to talk through specific problems and a range of detailed guidance notes on law and ethics on its website at: www.bma.org.uk/ethics.

Bridging the gap between theory and practice: the BMA's approach to medical ethics

The questions covered in this chapter include the following.

- What is meant by medical ethics and what are the key principles?
- Why do interpretations of terms, such as 'harm' and 'benefit' change?
- How do ethics and law interact?
- How do concepts of professionalism fit in?
- What is the difference between moral rights and legal rights?

The British Medical Association (BMA) is a doctors' professional organisation. Its guidance is not binding but supplements the rules set out by the regulatory body, the General Medical Council (GMC) as well as summarising relevant legislation. This chapter sets out the background for the BMA's specific advice in following chapters. For readers who are particularly interested in the philosophy and theory that underpin the guidance, this chapter sketches out the main philosophical approaches to medical ethics and illustrates how they relate to modern day medical practice. Practical guidance is given on how to approach an ethical dilemma and a hypothetical case shows how different methodologies would approach the same issues.

What is medical ethics?

'Medical ethics' is one subset of the broader disciplines of 'healthcare ethics' and 'bioethics'. It overlaps with both but focuses on the duties of doctors. The original Greek and Latin expressions for 'ethics' and 'morals' conveyed the same idea of a code of conduct acceptable to a particular group. Nowadays, 'ethics' can either mean conforming to recognised standards of practice or describe the general study of morality. The distinction is important. Traditionally, professional ethics was what doctors defined for themselves, from their own perspective. Their duty was to work to the standards established by their peers and avoid any action that would bring the profession into disrepute. Ethics, in this sense, has always been a central concern of medicine. Doctors were expected to observe the duty to provide 'benefit' to the sick, respect confidentiality and demonstrate integrity. Such values, often labelled 'Hippocratic', are echoed in the writings of philosopher-physicians in all cultures. Through history, professional codes called on doctors to adhere to such virtues which, by constant repetition, became seen as part of what it is to be a doctor. Such traditional concepts remain relevant because doctors generally want solutions that not only make logical and legal sense, but also do not contravene their intuitions about the core purpose of medicine.

Medical Ethics Today: The BMA's Handbook of Ethics and Law, Third Edition. Sophie Brannan, Eleanor Chrispin, Martin Davies, Veronica English, Rebecca Mussell, Julian Sheather and Ann Sommerville.
© 2012 BMA Medical Ethics Department. Published 2012 by Blackwell Publishing Ltd.

The discipline of modern medical ethics is rather different. It involves adherence to similar values but they often need some interpretation. It does not attempt to provide ready-made answers but requires analysis and reasoning (see the discussion of the shift from 'traditional' to 'analytical' medical ethics on page 3). It requires critical reflection about 'norms or values, good or bad, right or wrong, and what ought or ought not to be done in the context of medical practice'.[1] The object of medicine continues to be the provision of net health benefit with minimal harm but modern ethical thinking insists that this must also be done in ways that respect patients' autonomy and that are just and fair. Modern ethics deals with everyday practice as well as with the unusual, dramatic and contentious. It involves a search for morally acceptable and reasoned answers in situations where different moral concerns, interests or priorities conflict. This involves critical scrutiny of the issues and careful consideration of various options. It is often as concerned with the process through which a decision is reached as with the decision itself.

Key concepts in medical ethics

Many of the most commonly used ethical terms are self-evident, others may require some interpretation.

Self-determination or autonomy: the ability to think, choose, decide and act for oneself constitutes self-determination or autonomy. There is a moral obligation to respect people's self-determination as long as that does not impinge on the rights or welfare of someone else. Respect for autonomy means that competent and informed individuals can accept or refuse treatment without having to explain why. They can choose things that are harmful or bad for themselves but they do not have the same liberty to choose things that would harm others.

Honesty or integrity: this is much broader than just truth-telling. Doctors must ensure that their actions are not intended to deceive or exploit the recipient. The skills necessary for communicating effectively are also a key part of ethical consideration. A failure to communicate effectively can invalidate patient consent if information the patient needs to know is left unsaid and it can undermine trust.

Confidentiality: all patients are entitled to confidentiality but their right is not absolute, especially if other people are at serious risk of harm as a result. Cases arise where an overriding public interest would justify a breach of confidentiality. Although this is one of the oldest values reiterated in ethical codes, it is increasingly difficult to define in practical terms as notions of public interest change.

Fairness and equity: the individual patient is the main focus of concern but doctors also have to consider the wider picture and whether the impact of treating one person will foreseeably and detrimentally affect others. These values are closely linked with the practicalities needed to prioritise and ration the use of scarce communal resources.

Harm and benefit: notions of maximising benefit and minimising harm can be among the most tricky aspects of modern medical ethics. These values have always been central to traditional medical ethics and are expressed in professional statements in all cultures and epochs. Keeping people alive and functioning has been what most doctors understood by the obligation to avoid 'harm' and promote 'benefit' but although the terminology easily crossed cultural and historical divides, the interpretations of the terms has not necessarily done so. Nowadays, the usual interpretation is that an action is only harmful if the person experiencing it believes it to be so. Patients choose for themselves what is a harm or benefit in their own circumstances. Among the controversies brewing in medical ethics, for example, is that concerning the status of male infant circumcision which some people classify as a non-therapeutic and therefore harmful assault on a child and others see as conferring a range of benefits, including social integration and cultural acceptance. Although they can be slippery, notions of 'harm' and 'benefit' continue to feature strongly in the BMA's problem-solving methodology and increasingly preoccupy the courts, even though there is no clear and universal definition. Interpretation of the terms depends in different contexts on a number of variables, including individuals' perceptions as well as legal and professional benchmarks.

Looking back: how medical ethics developed from inflexible rules to reasoned analysis

The history of doctors' professional ethics encompassed a radical shift in thinking within the profession and society in the mid-twentieth century. Prior to that, medical organisations set out brief principles of acceptable professional behaviour, codifying how doctors should respond in various circumstances. These were based on early instruction manuals, such as Thomas Percival's *Medical Ethics* (1803)[2] which expanded upon traditional Hippocratic precepts. The guidance encouraged a benignly paternalistic way of thinking that reflected contemporary societal expectations. Patients were to be protected from information and the burdens of decision making were doctors' duties, not patients' rights. Professional codes of behaviour and etiquette explained the accepted rules but without any analysis of the issues. Major upheavals in the twentieth century increasingly showed that traditional codes were outdated as developments such as organ transplantation and reproductive technologies raised moral questions far outside the scope of traditional professional codes. Medical ethics had to develop a more analytical approach and started to do so in the 1960s when public confidence in medical research, for example, was threatened by publicity about unethical experiments[3] and moral debate about the purpose of medicine was taken up by non-doctors: philosophers, lawyers and patient representatives. This led to guidance which was more analytical, less addressed to the routine practicalities of medicine and increasingly driven by notions of patient autonomy. In an influential series of broadcasts, Kennedy highlighted how doctors made moral as well as medical decisions and argued that medical ethics must be 'part of the general moral and ethical order by which we all live. Decisions as to what the doctor ought to do must therefore be tested against the ethical principles of society.'[4] Set rules and statements from medical organisations were superseded by patients and professionals expecting to have analysis and reasoned justifications. Patients were now seen as best placed to interpret what was in their own interests. For this, they needed truthful information which doctors had previously been taught was harmful to give. Looking back, among the most significant changes in medical ethics has been this transition from medical decision making to the recognition that healthcare works best as a doctor–patient partnership (see also Chapter 1, pages 22–26).

Looking ahead to new challenges

Each chapter of this book attempts to identify foreseeable areas where new dilemmas are likely to occur but providing advice for such future challenges is particularly difficult when the provision of health services faces significant reorganisation. This has been the situation at the time of drafting the book in 2010–2011 and, in all cases, the most recent BMA guidance on any ethical issues can be found on its website. Under plans for the NHS put forward by the Coalition Government[5] in 2010, it seems likely that dilemmas involving maintaining equity and managing conflicts of interest may become more prominent for some doctors (see also page 6). Good quality patient care and choice remain key aims but there is some anxiety that these may come into tension with commercial interests. The Government's proposed changes to the NHS in England constitute the most radical restructuring of the service since its foundation in 1948 and may also have an impact on the devolved nations. Proposed changes in NHS structure include:

- the abolition of Strategic Health Authorities and Primary Care Trusts

- transfer of their functions to a central Commissioning Board and local commissioning groups
- encouraging an 'any qualified provider' approach to provision of services
- increasing private sector provision of NHS services
- abolishing NHS Trusts in favour of NHS Foundation Trusts
- transferring local health improvement functions to Local Authorities
- abolishing a number of arm's-length bodies, including the Human Fertilisation and Embryology Authority and the Human Tissue Authority.

Despite the proposed reorganisation, core concepts and aspirations which had been accepted as central to NHS care were reiterated, including:

- the importance of the NHS remaining free, based fairly on patient need
- continuing commitment to evidence-based policy making
- continuing to give patients choice, personalised care and information as part of shared decision making
- keeping services patient-centred
- using valid Patient-Reported Outcome Measures and patient experience data
- focusing on clinical outcomes and clinically justified, evidence-based measures
- incentivising quality and inspecting against essential quality standards
- continuing to develop quality standards at national level
- making payment to providers reflect quality of care and outcomes, not just volume
- ensuring clinical values direct managerial activity
- aligning clinical decisions with the financial consequences of those decisions
- producing comparative information on safety, effectiveness and experience to support choice and accountability
- promoting integration and partnership working between the NHS, social care and public health
- developing coherent urgent care services including GP out-of-hours services
- empowering health professionals to use their clinical judgement
- devolving power and commissioning responsibility to local commissioning consortia
- focusing on general practice leadership
- promoting better self-care by patients.

Practical anxieties about the proposed structural changes focused on issues such as the possibility of greater inequality for patients, reflecting the priorities and expertise of the doctors who would be new to commissioning; greater conflicts of interest for GPs who would have to balance patient choice with scarce resources; financial competition within the NHS which might impact on the quality of care and fear the NHS would become increasingly privatised. The BMA produced a series of guidance notes for the profession, addressing issues such as the principles of GP commissioning and these can be found on the BMA website.

Professionalism and core values

From the time it was first established in the mid-nineteenth century, the BMA has been deeply concerned with maintaining the reputation of the profession but this was not always necessarily labelled as 'ethics'. Rather, it was seen as a facet of professionalism. Debates about the nature of 'professionalism' and core values re-emerged as topics of significant concern at the start of the twenty-first century at a time when the profession was under considerable scrutiny, following a series of medical controversies. The King's Fund published a report on professionalism in 2004,[6] followed by another from the Royal College of Physicians (RCP).[7] This defined professionalism as 'a set of values, behaviours and relationships that underpins the trust that the public has in doctors' and so closely mirrored what doctors perceived as their ethical duties. It focused on partnership with patients and with other disciplines but also reiterated many of the same core virtues that the traditional codes had listed centuries earlier. Qualities doctors should strive for included integrity, compassion, altruism, continuous improvement, excellence and multi-disciplinary working.

The BMA's Medical Ethics Committee (MEC) conducted its own discussions about professionalism and the core values of medicine. It recognised the need to preserve traditional values such as the service ethos and altruism which should be demonstrated by all doctors, regardless of whether they work in management, academic or public health roles, or caring for patients. It also highlighted the fundamental concept of professionals having special obligations as part of an implicit social contract whereby they corporately bind themselves to high standards of behaviour rather than focus on their own self-interest. In this sense, the concept of professionalism is closely allied to virtue ethics and traditional notions of ethical behaviour, corporate responsibility, 'professional conscience' and shared values such as compassion and non-discrimination. Crucial aspects are seen to be the notion of medicine serving and promoting the welfare and goals of society. In the MEC's view, the primary focus of all professional groups should be a sense of special commitment rather than just working to a contract. For doctors, the essential attributes they need to exhibit include commitment to vulnerable groups, awareness of their own and others' duty to provide competent care, compassion and active adherence to shared core values (see also the box below). This MEC discussion contained echoes of a previous BMA-wide debate about core values that had taken place in the 1990s when representatives of medical bodies debated how the core values of the profession were changing.[8] Over 800 doctors from a range of grades and disciplines helped to define, and rank in order of importance, the values they saw as most relevant to the profession. At that stage, the core values most doctors saw as enduring and relevant medical principles, combining both skills and virtues, were: competence, caring/compassion, commitment, integrity, responsibility, confidentiality, spirit of enquiry and advocacy.

Core elements of medical professionalism

There are numerous definitions of professionalism but most include the same elements.

- specialised knowledge
- specialised training
- self-regulation
- altruism and a service ideology
- a clear code of ethics
- a sense of vocation
- core values: integrity, caring, empathy, respect for others and trustworthiness
- accountability
- responsiveness to changing societal expectations
- an explicit recognition of duties to patients and to the community
- a discipline taught and evaluated.

In 2010, many doctors again expressed concerns about the impact on professionalism of the expansion into the UK of market models of healthcare delivery. Traditionally in the

NHS, the impact of direct monetary interests on the provision of care had been muted. Although NHS doctors have always had an ethical obligation to consider the impact of clinical decisions on resources, their personal remuneration was largely unlinked to clinical decisions about patient care. Increasingly, however, the use of more commercially oriented tools, including incentives and the adoption by some providers of commissioning responsibilities has led to concerns about how potential conflicts of interest should be managed. More generally, concerns have been expressed that a broader cultural shift towards a more consumer-led model of healthcare could undermine the core values of medical professionalism. Outside the medical profession, commentators suggested that 'the introduction of markets creates huge layers of bureaucracy and often brings a de-professionalising of the people who are at the heart of the service, teachers, doctors, nurses, social workers. [The] introduction of the market to services is . . . bringing about a shift in ethics.'[9] The traditional public service ethos that had long underpinned the professions was perceived to be eroded by an increasing focus on financial rewards. Key challenges for the future include looking at ways in which values such as compassion, beneficence and a strong obligation to promote the interests of patients can still guide the therapeutic encounter in a more commercially oriented and consumer-led health environment.

Summary – what is medical ethics?

- Medical ethics has evolved from sets of inflexible rules to an analytical exercise.
- The facts and context of a dilemma are crucial.
- Superficially similar dilemmas may have very different solutions, depending on context.
- Concepts of professionalism draw on traditional principles of doctors' codes.

The framework of good practice

The General Medical Council (GMC)

As well as reflecting traditional values and making reasoned judgements in specific cases, doctors must also work within the law and the rules of the GMC, which are binding on them. Failure to comply can result in a finding of serious professional misconduct with a range of sanctions including, ultimately, erasure from the medical register. It is essential that doctors familiarise themselves with GMC guidance which is also flagged up in the following chapters of this book.

GMC guidance on the duties of a doctor

'Patients must be able to trust doctors with their lives and health. To justify that trust, you must show respect for human life and you must:

- Make the care of your patient your first concern
- Protect and promote the health of patients and the public
- Provide a good standard of practice and care
  - keep your professional knowledge and skills up to date
  - recognise and work within the limits of your competence
  - work with colleagues in the ways that best serve patients' interests.
- Treat patients as individuals and respect their dignity
  - treat every patient politely and considerately
  - respect patients' right to confidentiality

- Work in partnership with patients
  - listen to patients and respond to their concerns and preferences
  - give patients the information they want or need in a way they can understand
  - respect patients' rights to reach decisions with you about their treatment and care
  - support patients in caring for themselves to improve and maintain their health
- Be honest and open and act with integrity
  - act without delay if you have good reason to believe that you or a colleague may be putting patients at risk
  - never discriminate unfairly against your patients or colleagues
  - never abuse your patients' trust in you or the public trust in the profession

You are personally accountable for your professional practice and must always be prepared to justify your decisions and actions.'[10]

The relationship between ethics and law

Problems referred to the BMA frequently involve both law and ethics and much guidance for doctors has evolved through court judgments. Therefore, case examples illustrating the law are included in the book. The judgments in these cases often contain a large amount of critical analysis. Some ponder fundamental moral questions such as what it means to be 'alive' and when 'human life' begins or begins to count morally. Increasingly, the issues addressed by medical law have important philosophical, ethical, sociological, religious and political dimensions as well as legal ones. The relationship between ethics and law has been a reciprocal one: 'law frames the setting within which ethical choices may be practically exercised, but ethics frames the limits within which law is voluntarily obeyed and respected as an expression of the values and aspirations of the society in which it applies'.[11] The two are, to a large extent, inseparable and it is difficult to disengage moral considerations from legal rules.

The medical profession is also often involved in debates about what the law is and whether it should be changed. In many past high profile medical cases, the role of the court was to issue a declaration about the lawfulness of a proposed action, taking into account the views of patients and doctors. In many instances, the courts issue guidance to doctors for future cases. In the chapters that follow, examples are given of the types of cases in which, if agreement cannot be reached between the parties involved or if the law is unclear, a court declaration may be required. Statute governs many contentious areas such as abortion, reproductive technology and the use of human tissue but much remains common (judge made) law. In these cases, judges note the precedents in previous cases and rules are extracted from those decisions. Recognising the difficulty for busy doctors of keeping up to date with changes in the law, this book draws attention to relevant legal provisions. Major developments following its publication will be included on the BMA's website. Where relevant, differences in the law applicable in England and Wales, Scotland and Northern Ireland are highlighted in the text.

Medical ethics and human rights

Guidance for doctors generally reflects and merges several sets of values: the traditional duties from professional codes, the analysis supplied by theorists and the concepts of 'rights' that are incorporated in modern culture. Any discussion of 'rights' needs to distinguish between 'moral' rights and legally enforceable ones. Many of the rights we recognise are essentially moral claims which we intuitively consider appropriate in the context of the case ('he had a right to know his child was ill'). Human rights, however, are more formal, legally enforceable and generally non-negotiable, although some legitimate interference with rights is permitted, as long as it is proportionate. In ethical analysis, the concept of a 'right' may be derived from statements of human rights or reflect them closely, even if couched in terms of a moral claim. Problems arise when the rights or moral claims of different individuals clash (A's right to confidentiality conflicts with B's right to know). Ethical analysis is a problem-solving tool that takes into account the context of the dilemma in order to balance out such conflicts of moral rights. Since they are set out in law (see below), human rights are not dependent upon context in the same way as moral rights. They are less flexible even though there is scope for interpretation in some contexts. Many aspects of the way in which concepts of human rights are reflected in law have implications for medicine.[12] The language of human rights and the underlying principle that all people have the same legal rights have affected medical ethics. The United Nations' Universal Declaration of Human Rights of 1948[13] ushered in an era in which ideas of personal autonomy and 'rights' came to be seen as central in many parts of the world, including Britain and Europe. The international and legal concepts about human dignity, self-determination, freedom from interference and welfare protection articulated in the UN Declaration were defined further in international covenants.[14] These detailed two broad categories of human rights: 'liberty' rights (freedom from certain things) and 'entitlement' or 'welfare' rights (to receive certain benefits). Freedom from torture or unfair punishment is a typical example of the former. Rights to education and the highest attainable standard of physical and mental health exemplify the latter. Some (but not all) of these basic notions of human rights were enacted in European and domestic legislation. The UK passed the Human Rights Act 1998 which focuses more on being free from interference than the right to receive specific benefits.

The Human Rights Act 1998

The Human Rights Act 1998, which came fully into force in October 2000, incorporated into UK law the bulk of the rights set out in the European Convention for the Protection of Human Rights and Fundamental Freedoms. This did not result in a major change in practice, however, since the requirements of the Act reflect pre-existing good practice. Doctors' decisions based on existing ethical standards, such as respect for patient dignity and good communication, were likely to be compliant with the Act. Nevertheless, doctors need to be generally aware of it and act in conformity with this legislation. This is not always straightforward as some of the human rights that are particularly relevant to medicine (see list below) do not necessarily appear so. Also, some which seem central to healthcare require some interpretation. The right to life, for example, does not mean that life must be prolonged by medical technology at all costs and the right to found a family does not imply a universal right to fertility treatment. Legal cases about withdrawing life-prolonging treatment have been argued under the right to freedom from torture and degrading treatment. The right to respect for privacy and family life is applied to cases about confidentiality and information sharing. The BMA has issued specific guidance on the impact of the Human Rights Act on medical decision making and throughout the following chapters reference is made, where appropriate, to areas of practice that could be open to challenge under the Act. In brief, when making decisions, doctors must consider whether an individual's human rights are affected and, if so, whether it is legitimate to interfere with those rights. Any interference with a right must be proportionate to the intended objective. This means that, even if there is a legitimate reason for interfering with a particular right, the desired outcome must be sufficient to justify the level of interference proposed. Where different rights come into conflict, doctors must be able to justify choosing one over the other in a particular case.

European Convention for the Protection of Human Rights and Fundamental Freedoms

The following articles are the most relevant to health professionals:

- right to life (Article 2)
- prohibition of torture, inhuman or degrading treatment or punishment (Article 3)
- right to liberty and security (Article 5)
- right to a fair trial (Article 6)
- right to respect for private and family life (Article 8)
- freedom of thought, conscience and religion (Article 9)
- freedom of expression (Article 10)
- right to marry and found a family (Article 12)
- prohibition of discrimination (Article 14).

Summary – the framework of good practice

- Doctors are bound by the GMC's guidance and need to be aware of it.
- Law and medical ethics are often very closely inter-related; some court judgments debate the ethical principles in detail and generally reflect current ethical guidance in medical cases.
- There is also considerable overlap between medical ethics and human rights; doctors need to be generally aware of how their practice is affected by the Human Rights Act 1998.

The theoretical and philosophical background

Part of the fascination of medical ethics derives from the interplay of different perspectives and principles in the search for morally coherent solutions to ethical dilemmas. Practical problem solving involves verifying the facts as accurately as possible before weighing up the different values and interests to reach an acceptable balance. Although there may be various ways of doing this, practical approaches tend to come up with fairly similar solutions as, despite cultural nuances, ethical decisions in medicine draw upon the same pool of established values. For the practical decision maker as opposed to the theoretician, legal boundaries and societal mores also increasingly delimit the range of choices that can be made even before we begin to examine the ethical arguments. Indeed, in some situations, the legally viable options are so clearly stated that it seems pointless to look beyond them when the aim is to provide practical advice. The obligation to look beyond statute and legal precedents, however, springs from the need to ensure that ethical advice is morally consistent and justifiable in different contexts, regardless of whether or not the law has pronounced upon all the relevant scenarios. Practical ethical advice must also be consistent with society's changing expectations, especially in areas where the law is open to interpretation.

For those who are interested in examining the theory underpinning the ethical discussion in the book, brief and simplified accounts of some of the main philosophies and methodologies used in medical ethics are given below.

Consequentialist ethics

Consequentalist arguments (such as utilitarianism) focus on consequences, with the basic aim of maximising welfare, or utility, or in some way achieving 'the greatest good for the greatest number'. It is clearly important for doctors to take account of the consequences of their decisions and to provide the maximum net benefit for their patients. Leaving aside some of the inherent difficulties of deciding what is meant by 'welfare' or 'happiness' and how it should be measured, a major criticism of a solely consequentialist approach is that it can result in morally counterintuitive outcomes. In theory, some people can be sacrificed, if the outcome benefits a much greater number. So moral principles that intuitively seem essential, such as respect for other people, can be dispensed with when greater overall welfare would derive from ignoring those principles. Some variations of consequentialism, such as rule utilitarianism, attempt to overcome this problem by weighing the consequences of acting according to general moral rules.

Communitarian ethics

Communitarianism focuses on the fact that people have responsibilities as well as rights. It advocates policies based on consensus rather than compromise. It asserts that individuals need to concentrate not only on their own rights, but also their responsibilities to people close to them and to community. Communitarian arguments expect a concern for others to be taken into account when decisions are made. This approach comes to the fore when considering the health of communities rather than individuals. It is particularly relevant to public health ethics, genetics and any situation in which an important factor is the interrelatedness of individuals and of their interests. Theories based on notions of community, however, tend to have difficulties explaining why practices such as female genital mutilation or sexual abuse would be wrong if a particular community approves of them. They also raise concerns about conflict and discrimination within the group and questions about the extent to which individuals may and should be sacrificed for the good of the community.

Deontological ethics

Deontology focuses primarily on duties ('deontology' comes from the Greek for 'duty' or 'what is due'). Such theories are based on principles, such as respect for other people. The philosopher Kant, the most significant exponent of this view, held that people should never be treated merely as means to an end but always as ends in themselves. He also said that people should act as if they were legislating for a kingdom of such individuals who are ends in themselves. Kant's views influenced the development of medical ethics because they fitted well with modern concepts of respect for individuals and their autonomy. Nevertheless, Kant's notion of autonomy is a highly demanding one in which people are only autonomous insofar as they act in the pursuit of their moral duty. Modern concepts of autonomy are broader than Kant's and rights to autonomy now are not seen as restricted to self-determination only in the pursuit of one's moral duty. Kantian notions of respect for individuals' autonomy also take into account the autonomy of all other potentially affected people in the 'kingdom of ends'. Many of the moral dilemmas that arise in medical practice are those in which doctors' duties to different people conflict.

The 'four principles approach' to ethics

This is not a philosophical approach but rather a methodology for ensuring that all facets of a dilemma have been considered. Many ethicists adopt this method of problem solving[15] or some modification of it. At its core are the principles of promoting benefit (beneficence) and avoiding or minimising harms (non-maleficence) which directly reflect Hippocratic values and traditional codes. Two more modern principles are respect for other people's choices (respect for autonomy) and fairness (the principle of justice). Assessing the relevance of each of these principles to a particular situation provides a mechanism for analysing it. Many doctors see the four principles as providing a very familiar moral language regarding the duty to produce net medical benefit with minimum harm, respect patients' choices and work in an unprejudiced way. Difficulties can arise because of the different ways that individual doctors interpret these duties or because the duties come into conflict. Also, although it may seem that only four factors need to be considered, the framework is more complex and can require consideration of other values, guidelines, codes and legislation. In very general terms, however, the principles approach prioritises respect for autonomy if the patient is informed, competent and not a risk to others. Beneficence comes more to the fore if the patient has impaired mental capacity. In both cases, there would generally be a strong resonance in the outcome between the BMA's methodology (discussed on pages 13–17) and the four principles, even though the approaches are different. This is not unexpected since most moral approaches draw on a set of common values but may categorise them under different headings. Differences between the BMA's methodology and the four principles approach, or indeed other practically viable approaches, may be largely semantic.

Narrative ethics

Another practical approach is to use narrative or storytelling in order to give the problem context and clarify the ethical crux of it. This has been described as 'the oldest way of exploring and expounding ethical issues' through myth, parable or biography.[16] It approaches problems by looking at the patient's situation as a whole rather than considering a particular facet in isolation. It can involve an overview of the patient's life, values and experiences of illness. Different health professionals and family members may present the picture from different angles and considering the same dilemma from such various viewpoints provides a way of ensuring that all relevant perspectives and perceptions are considered.

Virtue ethics

Virtue ethics is derived from Aristotelian ethics and embeds ethics in people's characters rather than in general principles. In medicine, it is concerned with the virtuous character traits of doctors rather than their actions. So doctors who are kind, caring, respectful of others, honest and compassionate comply with everything expected of a role model. Such traits clearly form an important part of what it means to be a good doctor and they are traits echoed in traditional codes and currently in the GMC's *Good Medical Practice*.[17] The benefit of virtue theories to those confronted by ethical dilemmas is that they question what a virtuous person would do in such circumstances. They also highlight what is expected of doctors by society and by their peers. Although theorists who concentrate on moral principles do not deny the importance of virtue and virtues, they argue that the very decision that a character trait is virtuous requires reference to some general moral principle or norm and that both principles and virtues are needed for moral life.

Why is it useful to have different approaches to ethical dilemmas?

While philosophical theories can appear remote from daily practice, in reality they underpin the decisions made in healthcare and some ethical frameworks seem particularly suited to certain areas of ethical debate. Despite the different approaches that individual doctors may adopt, their actions must be consistent with the law and with the expectations of the society in which they practise. In the UK, this means that greater emphasis is generally placed on autonomy relative to other values. Genetic knowledge, however, highlights the inter-connectedness of individuals who share the same DNA and can challenge notions of the primacy of personal choice and individual privacy. In this sphere, individuals' decisions are particularly likely to impinge on others and that fact differentiates them somewhat from other spheres of medicine where personal choice is the main determinant. For dilemmas about the confidentiality of genetic information or notions of inter-generational justice, an approach reflecting communitarian values and mutual responsibilities rather than autonomy alone might be helpful and also reflect how many patients do take account of people close to them when deciding. Other approaches and methodologies might be suited to particular spheres of medical, psychiatric, psychological or nursing care.

Although we have highlighted a few of the main approaches above, a range of other problem-solving frameworks can be used, such as feminist ethics, casuistry, contextualism, intuitionism, pragmatism, relativism and liberalism as well as rights and duties-based methodologies. To practising doctors and medical students, this range of philosophical and methodological approaches can be a daunting prospect. Arguably, however, having a range of approaches available can aid debate in the context of teaching or be helpful in clarifying the nub of a problem in particular contexts. Even when the law apparently gives a clear direction, a solution for one patient's case may not necessarily be applicable to another superficially similar case if the context and the patient's views are different. Although general rules and precedents are illuminating, the particular circumstances of the case are often crucial. As is discussed in the hypothetical case at the end of the chapter, general understanding of different moral theories can help to show how and why ethical problems in medicine are often formulated and resolved in different, and sometimes competing, ways.

Summary – the theoretical and philosophical background

- Different methods of analysing ethical dilemmas exist but the method used must also be consistent with the law and GMC guidance.
- It can be useful to apply different methods to clarify the nub of a problem.
- Despite their differences in approach most methods, when combined with awareness of the law and best practice guidance, produce similar conclusions.

The BMA's approach

Bridging the gap between theory and practice

In its guidance, the BMA takes a reasoned eclectic approach, combining practicality with moral theory and law. Ethical problems are addressed with an awareness of widely accepted general principles, professional guidelines and previously settled legal cases. Principles and virtues, duties and consequences, community-orientated perspectives and individual or patient-orientated perspectives are considered. To provide a very practical approach, the BMA uses the concepts and case examples familiar to practising doctors.

While much emphasis is placed on the virtues and qualities expected of doctors, it needs to be acknowledged that many work in far from ideal environments where discussion of abstract values can seem divorced from the raw reality of trying to maintain partnerships with violent or difficult patients. All discussion of medical ethics centres attention on doctors' *duties* rather than their rights or the practical limitations they face. Modern ethics focuses on the need for a well-balanced relationship between patients and doctors but rarely discusses if, and how, both sides of the relationship have obligations. Doctors must be truthful, respectful and willing to discuss various options but so ideally should their patients. (This is discussed in Chapter 1, page 38.) If there is a social contract which is at the centre of professional status, both sides have responsibilities and rights. Often, doctors' freedom to define matters such as standards of care is curtailed and they may have little opportunity to input into structural reorganisations that significantly affect the way they interact with patients. Ethically, they are urged to put individual patient interests first while simultaneously ensuring that limited resources are well used, patients' rights to access care and to exercise preferences are respected and futile measures avoided. Some of these expectations are in tension with each other. Part of the aim of this book is to help doctors find good answers to dilemmas, accompanied by an understanding of the pressures and limitations they often face in real life.

The way in which a dilemma is approached depends, in part, on the complexity of the question. Many decisions raise ethical issues but can nonetheless be easily and quickly resolved. This could be by reference to the general duties of a doctor, such as the duty of confidentiality, or by referral to relevant law or professional guidance, such as to determine who may give consent on behalf of a young child. In more complex cases, particularly where duties to different parties conflict, more detailed consideration is needed to ensure that the dilemma is given a thorough critical analysis and all relevant perspectives are considered. There are various ways of doing this. Over a number of years the BMA's ethics department has developed its own methodology for helping doctors to analyse and resolve ethical questions. This approach involves up to six separate stages.

Approaching an ethical dilemma

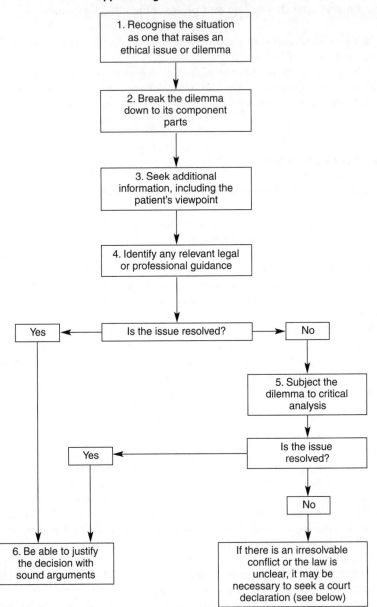

1. Recognise the situation as one that raises an ethical issue or dilemma

Although it sounds self-evident, many difficulties arise because professionals fail to recognise that there is an ethical issue or a conflict of interest at play, or they understand the principles but do not see their relevance to a particular case. Responding to a relative's enquiry about a patient's health, without the patient's consent, is a mundane example in which a breach of confidentiality can occur unintentionally. Doctors may not articulate the dilemma in the language of ethics, perceiving it as mainly a clinical problem, but complex issues of clinical judgement can also have ethical dimensions. The two categories of problems are not mutually exclusive but the complexity of the former may distract attention from the latter. Deciding whether to offer an expensive new treatment, for example, may require not only a clinical assessment of the patient, but also consideration of the opportunity costs for others when resources are limited. Ethical reflection is needed when the situation involves a conflict of interests, values, rights or civil liberties. If the general principles that would normally be relied upon for dealing with such issues are of no help or conflict with one another, an ethical dilemma arises. These are situations where there are good moral reasons to act in two or more different ways, each of which is also in some way morally flawed.

2. Break the dilemma down into its component parts

Many ethical enquiries to the BMA's ethics department are complex and detailed. Although it is necessary to consider the dilemma in context, it is also important mentally to clear away the excess information to identify the key issues raised by the dilemma. When various different rights and interests compete, it may still be clear which should take precedence, especially if a particularly vulnerable person is involved. When child protection concerns arise, for example, parents' preferences often take second place to the child's interests.

3. Seek additional information, including the patient's viewpoint

Having identified the key issues, the next stage is to analyse them. This needs clarity about the facts. If, for example, the issue is about the treatment or confidentiality of a child or young person, it is crucial to know whether that person is sufficiently mature to make a valid decision. If the child is competent, he or she should be involved. If the child is very young, it is important to know who has parental responsibility. In most cases, it is also essential to take the patient's viewpoint into account rather than relying on one's own assumptions. In the past, this was frequently overlooked. It was assumed, for example, that it was ethically acceptable to publish case studies, provided patients' names were removed although patients and their families could still recognise the facts of the case. The option of obtaining patient consent to publication was often overlooked, even though interesting cases in professional journals are sometimes picked up and publicised by mainstream media.

4. Identify any relevant legal or professional guidance

In each case, part of identifying the relevant factors includes the law and guidance issued by the GMC. With some ethical dilemmas, this information provides a straightforward answer. Others are more complex and require a careful balancing of the competing interests. Depending upon the complexity of the issue, information may be needed from a range of sources, including relevant:

- statute or case law about the subject
- guidance from the GMC
- guidance from professional bodies, such as the BMA or the Royal Colleges
- advice issued by authorities in England, Scotland, Wales and Northern Ireland
- guidance from organisations regulating the area of enquiry, such as the Human Fertilisation and Embryology Authority or the Human Tissue Authority
- advice from the medical defence organisations.

5. Subject the dilemma to critical analysis

When considering difficult ethical decisions, doctors may need to involve other members of the healthcare team who may have a different perspective, particularly if they have more contact with the individual or family. The key issues and facts that have been identified are analysed to balance the competing interests. Decisions often have to be made quickly and in stressful circumstances. In such cases, doctors are not expected to be omniscient but to act reasonably on the facts and to be able to justify their decisions. Knowing where to find professional guidance when it is needed can be good preparation for difficult dilemmas. (It was with this in mind that the BMA has published on its website a range of brief 'tool kits', summarising the main points of law and GMC guidance on a range of issues.)

Duties owed to different parties often conflict. A common enquiry, for example, concerns requests from the police for full access to patients' medical records. The duty of confidentiality has to be balanced against doctors' duty to protect others from foreseeable harm. The factors that need to be taken into account in deciding how to proceed are the following.

- Is it possible or desirable to obtain the patient's consent?
- Is the crime or threat sufficiently serious for the public interest to prevail?
- Is someone at risk of death or serious harm?
- Would a refusal to disclose seriously hinder the investigation?
- Is the information available elsewhere without a breach of confidentiality?
- Is any information on the medical record relevant to the crime?

Based on an assessment of these types of factors, the doctor needs to decide whether to accede to the request. In some cases disclosure to the police is justified; in others it is not. Sometimes the police will seek a court order if access is refused (see also Chapter 5, pages 196–197, where disclosure authorised by a court is discussed).

6. Be able to justify the decision with sound arguments

Sometimes it is helpful to discuss the dilemma, on an anonymous basis, with a colleague, the BMA or a defence body. Ultimately, however, the doctor who is responsible for the patient's care must make the decision about how to proceed, be prepared to justify it and explain his or her reasoning. For example, doctors who decide to withdraw treatment that is prolonging life should be able to demonstrate, from both a clinical and an ethical perspective, on what basis the decision was reached. Any discussions that took place with the patient should be noted in the medical record. If the patient lacked capacity and left no valid advance decision, the doctor needs to be able to explain why continuing treatment was not in the patient's best interests. Information should be recorded on the medical record about any guidance referred to or any advice sought. In some cases, it is not possible for the healthcare team and the patient to resolve the dilemma, either because there is an apparently irresolvable conflict or because the law is unclear. In such cases it may be necessary to seek a court declaration.

Summary – the BMA's approach

- In making decisions, there is a framework of factors that doctors need to take into account. These include the GMC's guidance, the law and advice from professional bodies. They need to be able to identify and analyse the morally important aspects of any situation and arrive at a reasonable conclusion.
- In providing guidance, the BMA considers and balances a range of philosophical approaches to address different situations. It takes account of duties and consequences, autonomy and the needs of the community, as well as reflecting the principles and virtues that make a good doctor. It provides information on the law and professional guidance.

A hypothetical case on refusal of life-prolonging treatment

Ms X, a 36-year-old mother of two, has a close-knit extended family. Paralysed from the neck down after a traffic accident, she is unable to breathe unaided. After extensive investigations, doctors tell her that she will remain ventilator-dependent for the rest of her life. Ms X has capacity, is articulate and able to interact with her family. Protracted discussions about her prognosis have taken place, involving the healthcare team, her family and, at her request, a priest. Now Ms X says she wants to have the ventilator disconnected, after she has said goodbye to her family, knowing that her death will result. The family is distressed by her decision, believing that she should continue with treatment at least until her children are old enough to understand. The family insists that treatment should continue contrary to her wishes but doctors explain that patients with capacity are legally entitled to make this decision and that treatment cannot be given without her consent. There is a clear legal answer but personal views in the healthcare team and the family are mixed about the ethical position.

Some doctors believe that they should focus on maximising the health and welfare of their patients, rather than following what they perceive to be the unwise and harmful wishes of an individual. A focus on the consequences of intervention may lead them to believe it morally wrong to comply with this patient's wishes. They think her decision unacceptably harmful because it would result in her death. Taking this approach of focusing on the consequences, the doctors are relying on one form of utilitarian moral reasoning. Despite knowing that continuing the treatment is unlawful, they feel unable to withdraw it because that offends their own moral views. It would be misleading, however, to imply that a consequentialist approach would inevitably be morally opposed to withdrawing treatment. Some doctors may focus on the consequences of ignoring individuals' wishes and argue, also on utilitarian grounds, that more satisfaction would be produced for more people by following individuals' wishes.

Other doctors place more moral emphasis on the autonomy right of patients. They recognise the right of Ms X to plan her own life and decide what represents a 'harm' and 'benefit' for herself, even if others disagree. To do otherwise than comply with her informed decision would be an affront to their values. Respecting her reasons and her choice is part of respecting her. Doctors who see their primary duty as being to respect the patient's views, despite the consequences for her, could be seen as taking a version of the deontological approach to ethics. They concentrate on their perceived duty rather than the consequences. Another doctor, however, might take the opposite view on deontological grounds. He might see that the primary duty of doctors is not to respect autonomy but to save human life.

Although personal autonomy and individual decision making generally take precedence in modern liberal democracies, this is not always the case. A more communitarian approach to ethics might focus less on the individual's wishes and more on the needs of others close to her. More weight might then be given to the family's views and the needs of her children, to whom she owes some duty. Ms X could be encouraged to consider her responsibility for the well-being of her family. She might be thought to have a moral obligation to continue treatment for their sake. The fact that individuals are perceived to have moral obligations, however, does not mean that they can be obliged to fulfil them.

Another important moral perspective focuses on the moral character of doctors, arguing that the virtues they exhibit in their professional lives are as important as their clinical competence. The ability to do what is 'right' (however defined) requires certain attitudes and personal skills. Decisions about how to break bad news to patients like Ms X, and explain the severity of the condition, are influenced by the degree to which doctors take seriously the rights of patients. Recognising that patients need such information, however, is not the same as having the courage and honesty to give it. Fear of distressing or burdening the patient might deter a doctor who wants to act virtuously. On the other hand, believing that Ms X needs accurate information might require another virtuous doctor to have the strength of character and compassion to tell her in a sensitive manner. Courage, prudence and compassion are examples of the virtues emphasised by those who argue that it is just as important to build moral character in medical students and young doctors as it is to teach them philosophical theories about the moral basis of good clinical practice.

The purpose of this hypothetical case is to illustrate that a particular philosophical approach may not lead inevitably to a particular outcome. By recognising the moral approach underpinning their views, however, doctors can be clearer about what their beliefs are and why. It may help them to articulate their reasons for advocating one course of moral action rather than another. Ultimately, however, doctors must be able to reconcile their own approach with both the expectations of society and the requirements of the law and their regulatory body.

References

1   Gillon R. (1985) *Philosophical Medical Ethics*, Wiley, Chichester, p.2.
2   Leake CD. (ed.) (1927) *Percival's Medical Ethics*, Williams & Wilkins, Baltimore.
3   British Medical Association (2001) *The Medical Profession and Human Rights: Handbook for a Changing Agenda*, Zed Books, London, Chapter 9.
4   Kennedy I. (1981) *The Unmasking of Medicine*, George, Allen & Unwin, London.
5   Department of Health (2010) *Equity and Excellence: Liberating the NHS*, The Stationery Office, London.
6   The King's Fund (2004) *On being a doctor: redefining medical professionalism for better patient care*, King's Fund, London.
7   Royal College of Physicians (2005) *Doctors in society: medical professionalism in a changing world*, Report of a Working Party of the Royal College of Physicians of London, RCP, London.

8   British Medical Association (1995) *Core values for the medical profession in the 21st century*, BMA, London.
9   Kennedy H. (2010) The Decline of Ethics in a Material World. Public lecture at St George's House, Windsor. Available at: www.stgeorges-windsor.org (accessed 10 January 2011).
10 General Medical Council (2006) *Good Medical Practice*, GMC, London.
11 Dickens B. (1977) Ethical issues in health. In: Shenfield F, Sureau C. (eds.) (1977) *Ethical Dilemmas in Assisted Reproduction*, Parthenon, Carnforth, p.77.
12 British Medical Association (2008) *The impact of the Human Rights Act 1998 on medical decision making*, BMA, London.
13 United Nations Universal Declaration of Human Rights 1948.
14 United Nations International Covenant on Economic, Social and Cultural Rights 1966 and International Covenant on Civil and Political Rights 1966.
15 Beauchamp T, Childress J. (2001) *Principles of Biomedical Ethics*, 5th edn, Oxford University Press, New York. See also: Gillon R. (1994) *Principles of Healthcare Ethics*, Wiley, Chichester. Ashcroft RE, Dawson A, Draper H. *et al*. (eds.) (2007) *Principles of Healthcare Ethics*, 2nd edn, Wiley, Chichester.
16 Boyd KM, Higgs R, Pinching AJ (eds.) (1997) *The New Dictionary of Medical Ethics*, Wiley, Chichester, p.166.
17 General Medical Council (2006) *Good Medical Practice*, GMC, London.

1: The doctor–patient relationship

The questions covered in this chapter include the following.

- Do doctors in different types of relationship with patients have different obligations?
- Can doctors choose their patients in the same way as patients choose their doctor?
- When does the 'duty of care' start and end?
- What, if any, responsibilities do patients have?
- Can patients choose not to have any information about their treatment?
- What happens when the doctor–patient relationship breaks down?

This chapter looks at how attitudes and some facets of the relationship between patients and their doctor have changed. It examines the rights and duties on both sides, while recognising that doctors have particular responsibilities to make the relationship work well. The emphasis is on doctors respecting patient autonomy, while doing more than providing a menu of options, but tensions arise when patients request treatments or procedures that doctors feel unable to provide. This may be due to the cost or the lack of evidence of efficacy. The likelihood of such problems becoming more prevalent for some doctors as the NHS undergoes significant change is among the factors flagged up here. Doctors are expected to be supportive of patients and offer them as holistic a type of care as possible, while ensuring that professional boundaries are maintained and that empathy does not result in inappropriate closeness or dependency. They should learn from their mistakes and those of colleagues so that services and patient safety are improved. They must not offer moral comment or make reference to their own personal views unless explicitly invited by patients to do that. Above all, they must act with integrity and be quick to spot any measure which might lessen their patients' trust in them.

General principles

General principles that all doctors must observe are listed in the previous chapter, where the General Medical Council's (GMC) guidance[1] on the duties of a doctor is set out (see pages 6–7). In this chapter we focus more closely on the practical implications of the requirement that doctors be honest, open and act with integrity, that they respect patients' dignity and treat them politely. Principles underpinning the doctor–patient relationship can be summarised as follows.

- Doctors owe special duties of care to their patients.
- All interactions involving doctors and patients should be characterised by honesty, politeness and respect on both sides.
- Effective communication requires both parties to listen, talk frankly and recognise uncertainties.

Medical Ethics Today: The BMA's Handbook of Ethics and Law, Third Edition. Sophie Brannan, Eleanor Chrispin, Martin Davies, Veronica English, Rebecca Mussell, Julian Sheather and Ann Sommerville.
© 2012 BMA Medical Ethics Department. Published 2012 by Blackwell Publishing Ltd.

- Doctors have the main duty to make the relationship work but patients also have responsibilities.
- Establishing and maintaining appropriate boundaries is essential.

Changing expectations of the doctor–patient relationship

Patients expect more and different things from medicine than they previously did. Along with the increased life expectancy for most people has come a greater focus on medicine's contribution to their quality of life (see the discussion of 'health' as an evolving concept in Chapter 20, pages 802–804). Through media such as the internet, patients tend to be better informed about what medicine can achieve. They rightly expect to share in deciding how different treatment options fit with their own preferences. Some use online technology to obtain advice, diagnoses or direct-to-consumer testing. They can switch between NHS and private providers and buy medicines over the internet, without discussion with their GP. (These issues are covered in detail in Chapter 19, pages 780–781.) Although this puts more tools within the grasp of patients, they still need professional expert advice when making treatment decisions. Part of the doctor's role is to help people make the decisions that best suit them, in a fair and well-informed way. Listening to patients' views and feedback about their experience is essential to the provision of a patient-centred service.

The strong emphasis on patient autonomy and choice, combined with the focus on doctors being trained to have good communication skills should ensure a better balance in the doctor–patient relationship than in the past, when access to information was more one-sided. Tensions arise, however, if there is a mismatch of expectations between what patients want and what doctors see as appropriate evidence-based solutions. Wider awareness of newly evolving treatments, including elective, cosmetic or alternative therapies, can also create tensions between differing interpretations of 'wants' and 'needs'. The use of consumerist language also raises patients' expectations. The growth of a range of 'lifestyle' drugs, for example, can contribute to misperceptions about the primary focus of medicine. Examples include patient demand for amphetamine-type appetite suppressants, steroids to improve sporting performance or cognitively enhancing drugs to aid concentration. (These are discussed in Chapter 13, pages 547–549.) Part of the doctor's role in maintaining a workable relationship is to try to ensure that patients are aware of any risks attached to the medicines or interventions they seek and also the limits on what doctors can provide. The NHS is a bureaucratic organisation through which patients can find it difficult to navigate. Doctors see themselves simultaneously as patient advocates, helping patients obtain appropriate and timely care, and custodians of NHS resources, with an important role in containing costs fairly.

Changing expectations about what medicine can provide coincide with some patients no longer having a sense of continuity of care, provided by a doctor with whom they have had a long relationship. Different doctors or other healthcare professionals probably deal with some aspects of their routine care and locums provide out-of-hours cover. Patients also obtain health advice from various other sources, such as telephone helplines and walk-in clinics. Doctors' expectations about some aspects of their role have also changed. Greater emphasis on medical appraisal, governance, audit and performance management can mean that they feel they have less scope for clinical discretion in individual cases. Health and social care are intended to be more joined up than in the past so that patient care is often provided by multi-disciplinary teams, which may include other professionals such as social workers. Proposed changes in how the commissioning of services will work in future is likely to mean that GPs face more conflicts of interest between trying to do the best for the individual and simultaneously trying to conserve NHS funds. Changes in hospital team structure mean that contact between individual clinicians and patients can be a more transitory experience, as opposed to the traditional model of one doctor having responsibility for continuity of the patient's care. Other changes to NHS organisation, such as shorter hospital stays, more shift working following the implementation of the European Working Time Directive, GPs relinquishing 'out-of-hours' responsibilities, and the tendency for multi-practitioner primary care surgeries, can mean that contact is fragmentary. Some doctors know their patients less well as individuals.

Ethical guidance continues to emphasise doctors' traditional duty to benefit patients and help them function well but what counts as 'benefit' has undergone significant reappraisal. Fundamental concepts of 'harm' and 'benefit' have changed greatly to reflect the wishes and values of the individual patient. Prolonging life at all costs was sometimes seen as a 'benefit' in the past whereas it is now recognised that 'benefit' and 'harm' must be judged in terms of what the individual patient would like. Imposing a treatment – even to save life – contrary to the wishes of an informed patient with capacity is now recognised as a 'harm' rather than a 'benefit'. Expectations have also changed in relation to issues such as patient satisfaction and dignity. Healthcare is not only about preventing disease and trying to make people well, but also about providing the right treatment environment. As well as prompt access to good quality care, clean and safe premises are a high priority for patients.[2] The focus on patient rights in ethical guidance, the law and in charters, such as the NHS Constitution, influences public perceptions about what doctors should provide and when.

Medicine is both an art and a science, although some think that the technological and scientific side has become more pre-eminent. While acknowledging the vital importance of technical competence, the British Medical Association (BMA) also emphasises the need to develop the personal characteristics of 'a good doctor' (see the introductory chapter, pages 4–6, and Chapter 18, pages 743–745). A former BMA President noted that:

> Two hundred years ago, when little effective treatment was possible, the ability to comfort and help a patient to accept illness and death – in other words the *art* of medicine – was paramount. Today, when many patients with previously fatal diseases can expect from medicine an almost normal life span, science is vital. Even now, however, common complaints cause much misery, there is no cure for many serious diseases and the death rate for us all is one hundred percent in the end. So the old art is still a vital characteristic of the good doctor.[3]

Telemedicine and other forms of care at a distance

Face-to-face interaction between patient and doctor is acknowledged to be the best in most circumstances but providing medical advice and treatment by video, telephone or internet can be a useful addition. Telemedicine involves consultations carried out at a distance, using tools such as videoconferencing, multi-media communications, internet and intranet for a range of clinical purposes such as diagnosis, treatment and clinical education. It includes both live and time-delayed consultations. Live telemedicine usually involves a combination of patients, primary care practitioners and specialists communicating by means of an audiovisual link. At its best, it can improve communication because the patient and the doctor who knows the patient's history can be present together when a specialist is consulted by videoconferencing. GPs can begin treatment following the advice of the specialist via the video link. Time-delayed telemedicine involves the electronic transmission of a previously recorded visual image of the patient, consisting either of a visual sequence, such as a video clip of an echocardiogram, or single pictures, for example of a skin abnormality. Among its advantages are cost reduction, the speeding up of referral for the patient, avoidance of unnecessary referrals, greater consistency in healthcare and improved contact between doctors. The number of broken appointments can be reduced and one specialist can provide services to a number of different locations.

Among the ethical considerations, principal concerns are accuracy of the image or text, security and confidentiality. Mistakes can be made and an erroneous diagnosis given by video link as in any other consultation, and teleconsultation cannot convey the same information as a physical examination. The accountability of doctors and their ethical duties remain the same. There are both advantages and drawbacks of consulting and prescribing electronically and over the internet (see Chapter 13, pages 567–569).

Routine telephone communications can also replace some consultations and provide rapid review of some patients. Such systematic monitoring of patients by telephone can be as effective as and less time consuming than face-to-face consultations as they can be more focused and more flexible in terms of time needed to talk to the patient than surgery consultations.

Background to changed expectations

Thomas Percival's 1803 influential text on medical ethics[4] set the benchmark for the traits of a good doctor which, he said, should be a balance of compassion and authority. He advised that doctors should be sensitive to patients' fears and anxieties by shielding them from disturbing information. Generations of doctors were taught to keep up patients' hopes and spirits by withholding bad news which would depress them. The duty of beneficence was interpreted as an obligation to be reassuring rather than honest. From the 1950s, this interpretation became discredited and, by the 1980s, paternalism was seen as completely outmoded. All current ethical guidance, including that from the BMA, sees patients themselves as the most suitable arbiters of their own best interests. This entails them being given all the relevant information about their condition. Throughout this book, we emphasise the key importance of patient autonomy and the need for health professionals to help patients to make the decisions that are best for them rather than assuming that they have similar goals or values as their doctor. In a multi-cultural society such as the UK, values and expectations can differ considerably. Most patients are willing and able to know about the options open to them. Some may have other expectations and do not want full information or a list of options. They may not want to feel that they alone are responsible for making decisions or they may want others to take the decision for them. (This is discussed in more detail in Chapter 2, pages 70–71.)

Changing expectations of the doctors' role led some to be concerned that they would be seen as mere technicians rather than real partners in relationships with patients. Terms such as 'cafeteria medicine' describe situations in which doctors are perceived as simply offering patients a menu of choices in a mechanistic approach to patient autonomy. A common enquiry to the BMA, for example, concerns whether there is a duty to discuss cardiopulmonary resuscitation (CPR) with all patients, including those who are terminally ill. Some think that they should automatically raise the issue of CPR even with dying patients because they have rights to such information, futile though it may be. Although there must be a presumption that patients are informed about decisions in relation to their treatment, the fear of being seen as paternalistic or disrespectful of patient autonomy should not mean that doctors automatically apply the same checklist in all cases. As is made clear in the discussion on caring for patients at the end of life (see Chapter 10, pages 447–450), the BMA does not see a duty to discuss treatments that would be futile in the sense that they would be incapable of improving the patient's condition and could confer no benefit to that individual. Rather, it emphasises the importance of looking at patients as individuals, listening to them to understand their needs and wishes. In deciding which issues to raise with patients, health professionals must not discriminate on factors such as the patient's age or medical condition but criteria such as the likelihood of success are relevant to whether or not an option is offered.

GMC guidance on the doctor–patient partnership

'Relationships based on openness, trust and good communication will enable you to work in partnership with your patients to address their individual needs.
    To fulfil your role in the doctor–patient partnership you must:

- be polite, considerate and honest
- treat patients with dignity
- treat each patient as an individual
- respect patients' privacy and right to confidentiality
- support patients in caring for themselves to improve and maintain their health
- encourage patients who have knowledge about their condition to use this when they are making decisions about their care.'[5]

Patient-centred and personalised care

Patient-centred or 'whole person' care takes account of individuals' values and circumstances as well as aspects of their health. It involves tailoring treatment, where possible, to reflect the patient's preferences.

Listening to patients' treatment preferences and helping to implement them is not always straightforward. Situations can arise when the individual's expressed wish is temporarily distorted by emotions such as fear, grief or denial. Such situations have to be approached carefully, on a case-by-case basis, with the aim of engaging the patient to reflect on the implications of his or her apparent choice. In some cases, it may be sufficient to make sure that the patient has enough information and knows there will be later options for a change of heart but, in others, delays will prejudice the chances of recovery. Ideally, the doctor who best knows the patient should try to explore the reasons for the decision but such discussions can be extremely difficult if the patient is unwilling to talk or if the timescale for choosing is very limited. This may be the case if the patient is approaching the end of life (see Chapter 10).

Patient-centred care can also involve gathering data about patients' responses to past treatment, information about their lifestyle, genetic profiles, environmental information and family history. 'Personalised' care has traditionally been seen as a benchmark of good medical practice but the term is also increasingly used to describe the effects of advances in medical profiling that permit new methods of disease prediction and prevention, as well as targeted drugs and interventions. 'Personalisation' is seen as an appropriate term 'because the new developments can be claimed to be conducive to a mode of healthcare more tailored to the particular genetic and physiological characteristics of each individual (as ascertained by testing, assessing and imaging) and thus likely to be more effective than the more blunderbuss methods of an earlier age.'[6] One facet of the growth of personalised medicine is that people can exercise choice and control by using services offering direct-to-consumer body imaging as part of a health check and genetic profiling to identify the individual's potential susceptibility to disease. This can have advantages for patients by providing reassurance but it also side-steps the usual doctor–patient relationship and can create confusion or anxiety for patients. The Nuffield Council on Bioethics urges caution in the use of such terms which imply approval and benefit to patients whereas some so-called personalised interventions 'are not necessarily an advantage to either individuals or healthcare systems'.[7]

Psychological, spiritual and practical support

'Whole person' care can also involve recognising the psychological, emotional, imaginative and symbolic elements of the patient's experience of disease. When people are sick or facing very serious life events, they often experience a range of physical, emotional, psychological and social needs. Supportive relationships with people close to them are important to patients facing physical or mental illness, loss, bereavement and death. If patients wish to do so, opportunities to discuss their anxieties with appropriate counsellors or other professionals can assist them to develop inner resources and make sense of their experience of serious or long-term illness. Psychological support can take various forms and 'spirituality' is a term sometimes applied to the way in which people develop coping mechanisms to deal with critical situations and try to find meaning in them. Not everyone wants to discuss their feelings but those who desire such support should have access to pastoral or support services from trained counsellors or relevant spiritual advisers. Attention should also be given to respecting patients' values on matters such as modesty, diet and ritual practices in healthcare settings. The main thing is to listen to patients rather than making assumptions. Although not limited to terminal care, one of the areas of medical treatment where psychological or spiritual support is often welcomed is at the end of patients' lives. (This is discussed in more detail in Chapter 10, pages 439–440.) The impetus for discussion about spiritual or emotional needs should be initiated by patients but doctors should create opportunities for patients to share information about their needs. The GMC[8] makes clear that doctors should not normally discuss their own personal beliefs and values at work or impose them on patients (see pages 32–33).

Some primary care practices engage in providing a range of other types of practical support for patients by liaising with other agencies in the community which can provide advice on issues such as work and housing. This is whole person care in the sense of looking at patients' overall environment and its impact on their health and well-being. Through a multi-disciplinary and multi-agency approach, only part of which is directly related to healthcare, patients may be supported to change unhealthy lifestyles and learn new skills as well as manage chronic illness. (An example of such a primary care facility is given in Chapter 19, page 774.)

Summary – changing expectations of the doctor–patient relationship

- Patients have increased expectations about the services available.
- Doctors must always offer to involve patients in any decisions concerning them.
- Doctors should provide information in a supportive way and not merely offer a menu of options.
- Efforts should be made to accommodate patients' preferences.

Types of relationships in modern medicine

All doctors have moral and legal duties for people in their care but the extent of those duties can vary, according to the type of professional relationship.

The therapeutic relationship and duties to the patient

Discussion of the 'doctor–patient partnership' has the therapeutic model in mind, whether it takes place in a primary care or hospital setting. The doctor has a commitment to the patient although other professionals may manage specific episodes of care. What distinguishes this from other models of care is that the doctor focuses on the best interests of that patient, even though the patient's wishes may have to be overridden in exceptional cases if they conflict seriously with other duties of the doctor, such as the need to use evidence-based therapies, manage NHS resources carefully or avoid putting other people's health at risk.

Independent assessors and duties to the commissioning agent

Doctors may act as impartial examiners accountable to a third party who commissions their services. Common examples include pre-employment or insurance examiners, doctors who examine patients who wish to claim state benefits and experts providing reports to the courts or immigration authorities. (These issues are discussed further in Chapter 16.) Patients often have no choice about which doctor is approached by the agency commissioning the report. Promoting patients' own health interests and protecting their confidentiality are not the goals of this interaction, as they are in therapeutic relationships. Therefore the exact nature of the doctor's role must be clearly explained to patients. Patients should be aware that any tests and the information derived from the examination are not for the purposes of healthcare. Reports such as those for insurance and employment are undertaken either by the patient's own GP acting temporarily in a non-therapeutic capacity or by a doctor who has no other relationship with the patient. In this context, the patient's own GP can be seen as temporarily having 'dual obligations', whereas other independent examiners have no continuing obligations to the patient and do not become involved in treatment. Acting in an independent capacity can create some dilemmas and a lack of openness. Patients may try to limit or conceal some information because the goal of examination is unrelated to their healthcare, or the party commissioning the report may instruct doctors to keep their findings secret from the patient. Despite such instructions, however, patients have some right of access to insurance, employment and pre-employment reports under the Access to Medical Reports Act 1988 (see Chapter 6, pages 260–261). Also, in the BMA's view, doctors who do not have a clinical relationship with such patients still have some responsibilities to them (see page X). If doctors discover information significant to the management of the patient's health, they should bring it to the attention of the patient and (if the patient agrees) to their GP. The patient, and the agency commissioning the report, should be advised in advance about how such eventualities will be handled.

Doctors with dual obligations

In addition to these two categories, there are also some doctors, such as those who work in prisons, who have a split responsibility to the patient and another party.

They have enhanced responsibilities to their employer but they also have duties to the detainees who are their patients and who may have no real choice of doctor. Unlike the independent medical assessor, doctors with this type of dual obligation have a therapeutic relationship with their patients but usually have to work within additional constraints in comparison with other doctors in the community. Ethical responsibilities and the duty of care are the same for all patients and are not diminished when the patient is a prisoner or a detained asylum seeker. (This is discussed in detail in Chapter 17.)

Summary – types of relationships in modern medicine

- All doctors have duties to the people they see but the extent of the duty varies with the relationship.
- The 'doctor–patient partnership' refers to the normal therapeutic model.
- Doctors acting as impartial examiners for a third party need to make their role clear to the patient.
- Doctors with dual obligations work with additional constraints but must still exercise a duty of care for patients.

Choice and duty

How can patients choose their doctor or hospital?

In NHS primary care, patients can generally choose their GP unless local lists are full, in which case they may be allocated to a practice with capacity to accept them. All asylum seekers have the right to be registered with a NHS general practice but GPs have discretion about whether they register refused asylum seekers. There is no obligation for GPs to check people's immigration status. (The BMA has specific guidance on its website on the rights of asylum seekers to healthcare.[9]) In custodial settings, patients have no choice of doctor but if they are already registered with a local doctor, remand prisoners and people held in police stations can request a visit from that GP. Whether or not the GP will agree to attend depends on the circumstances of the case. Once a person is in detention and has been convicted, the choice of calling his or her own GP is no longer available (see Chapter 17, page 700).

Patients often have increased expectations from the health service as a result of terminology which emphasises their right to choose. For NHS hospital treatment, the electronic 'choose and book' referral system allows patients to select from a choice of hospitals or alternative providers but they need accurate information about the options. Some patients may be able to request a named doctor but not all systems permit this and trusts may transfer patients from long waiting lists to another consultant's shorter list. Clearly, where it is feasible to do so, patient preferences should be respected, particularly in situations such as intimate examinations where the patient prefers a male or female doctor. Doctors cannot participate in marginalising some colleagues unfairly, simply on the basis of patient choice if, for example, the patient prefers only to see health professionals from a specific cultural or religious background. NHS bodies have obligations to provide competent, appropriately trained professionals but cannot use racist or unfairly discriminative judgements in their employment or referral policies. Informed patients with capacity have an absolute right to decline treatment for any reason, even if their choices appear irrational to others, but NHS patients do not have comparable rights to insist on being treated by specific health personnel. Although there is considerable emphasis on the concept of patient choice, it would be unacceptable if some doctors who are appropriately qualified are excluded from some patients' care.

Patients who choose to receive treatment privately can often exercise more choice if they have particular requirements. They can usually choose the specialist of their choice but, if their care is funded by their insurer, the latter may specify where treatment is provided and designate a consultant. The BMA occasionally receives enquiries about disagreements between private doctors concerning who should be providing care for a specific patient. In private facilities, a patient may be referred to one doctor but be seen initially by another, who begins treatment. In the past, when the concept of 'poaching' patients was current, doctors had a sense of ownership of 'their' patients in a way that is now outdated. In some cases, private patients may prefer to wait to see the specific doctor to whom they were referred and their choice should be respected, where feasible. Once an episode of care has begun, the doctor who initiated it has a responsibility to ensure that it is completed unless all agree to an alternative arrangement.

Can doctors choose their patients?

Within the NHS, GPs have an obligation to provide care on an equitable basis according to their capacity to take on new patients. They cannot exclude people whose condition requires a lot of resources (so-called 'uneconomic' patients) or older people who have multiple conditions and may need a lot of attention. They must take into consideration the GMC's advice as well as the Human Rights Act 1998 ban on discrimination (Article 14). While patients cannot be refused care without good reason, those with a history of threatening or violent behaviour are likely to have problems finding a GP. (Violent patients are discussed on pages 55–57.) Primary care practices sometimes ask if they have to register homeless people who have no address. If they have vacancies on their list, they must do so. Homeless patients can be registered by using the practice address. It is also unacceptable to discriminate unfairly by only registering English speakers or refusing all asylum seekers. As mentioned above, however, GPs do have discretion about whether they register refused asylum seekers. In the private sector, too, doctors should not act in an arbitrary or unfairly discriminatory manner in terms of taking on new patients. Similarly, in the hospital setting, doctors must treat all patients equitably and in a non-judgemental manner. It is not their role to verify the immigration status of patients presenting for care.

If the doctor–patient relationship has broken down, either the doctor or the patient can initiate a change in the provision of services. In some cases, based on their past experience of the patient, doctors know that they are unlikely to achieve a constructive relationship with that person. In such cases, hospital doctors should recommend that the patient be seen by a colleague.

Who has a duty of care?

It is usually obvious when a doctor–patient relationship exists but situations can arise where there is doubt. Doctors are not under an obligation to treat a 'stranger'. Exceptions arise in emergencies when no other health professional is available and where first aid is urgently needed (see Chapter 15, pages 642–643). The common law position is that the doctor has a legal duty of care once he or she assumes responsibility for the patient.[10] It usually occurs when the doctor knows of the patient's need for medical services and either accepts that patient or interacts with the person in a professional capacity. In hospitals, this can be the case as soon as the patient presents for treatment.

Barnett v Chelsea and Kensington Hospital Management Committee

This case clarified when a hospital doctor's duty of care begins. Three night watchmen drank tea which was later discovered to have contained arsenic. They began vomiting and went to the casualty department of the local hospital. A nurse telephoned the casualty officer, Dr Banerjee, who advised that the men should go home and call their own doctors. Dr Banerjee himself felt tired and unwell and did not see the men. They all died from arsenic poisoning. In the subsequent court case, the judge ruled that the doctor had undertaken to exercise reasonable care and that he owed the men who came to the hospital a duty of care which he had breached by failing to examine them.[11]

Doctors may question the duty owed to patients who continually transfer between the NHS and private practice, or the duty they have to patients who consult them by email or the internet. In the BMA's view, if a doctor accepts some aspect or episode of a patient's management, a duty of care exists. (Email prescribing issues are discussed in Chapter 13, pages 567–569 and shared care is covered in more detail in Chapter 19, pages 780–781.) When patients are simultaneously accessing NHS and private treatment, two or more health professionals may share a duty of care. Consultants have a duty to patients seen by them or by their team but within the NHS, they are unlikely to have information about – or a duty towards – patients referred to them but not yet seen. In secondary NHS care, triage of such patients referred by their GP is not usually carried out by the consultant who will provide treatment, but by nurses or junior doctors, or it can involve a referral management centre (RMC). In such cases, the BMA advises that the team or RMC has a responsibility to ensure that appropriate action is taken. Once a consultant has accepted a patient, however, either by examining that person or having studied the clinical details of an individual referred for treatment, a duty of care exists. Similar duties exist for specialists, such as radiologists or endoscopists, who are involved only with one aspect of a patient's investigation.

When a patient has been assessed as non-urgent and placed on a list, the case still needs periodic review by the person or group responsible for triage if that patient's condition is likely to deteriorate during the waiting time. If clinics are overbooked, the referring doctor should be informed so that an alternative arrangement can be made. Doctors may be asked by patients about waiting times and they obviously need to be accurate in replying.

Doctors working on a sessional basis in private clinics owned by non-medical managers may wish to take 'their' patients with them when they leave, although the patients have contracted with the clinic rather than the doctor. Clearly, employment contracts need to make clear at the outset the rights and responsibilities of such doctors, who need to assure themselves that adequate arrangements are in place for continuity of care. Doctors may also express concerns that confidential medical records should remain in medical ownership in the absence of any new incoming practitioner. Patients also need information about how transfer of care and of records will be handled. (Aspects of security, retention and disposal of medical records are discussed further in Chapter 6.)

Scope of the duty of care – is there a 'duty to pursue'?

Questions sometimes arise about when precisely the duty of care ends. Doctors question, for example, what responsibilities they have for patients who fail to return following an initial consultation on a serious matter or who discharge themselves from hospital contrary to medical advice. Adults with capacity are entitled to opt out of treatment or diagnostic tests (unless being treated compulsorily under mental health legislation) but ideally they should be aware of the likely consequences. (The rights of patients to refuse treatment are discussed in Chapter 2, pages 75–80.) A common question concerns the extent of doctors' duties to pursue patients who drop out of treatment but seem not to have realised the implications or they lack a vital piece of information, such as a test result. Doctors should try contacting the patient but if laboratory test results are particularly sensitive, an arrangement should be made in advance as to how they will be communicated (see Chapter 5, pages 186–187). Particular issues of confidentiality arise if the patient is a minor or a person who does not wish to be contacted at home. Teenagers awaiting the results of a test for pregnancy or a sexually transmitted infection, for example, should be asked in advance to specify how they wish to receive the results. When patients fail to attend for hospital appointments for which they have been referred, their GP should be informed. Some hospitals are reluctant to offer follow up appointments to patients who have previously not attended without explanation but the BMA's general stance is that they should not be penalised. Similarly, the BMA does not support the idea of fining patients who fail to attend appointments with their GP, but general information in hospitals or surgeries can make the public aware of the costs to the NHS of non-attendance. The extent to which doctors should attempt to encourage patients to persist with treatment or diagnosis depends on whether the patient's decision seems to be an informed choice. Ultimately, a balance must be sought between attempting to encourage them to protect their health, if they seem willing to do so, and respecting their rights to refuse. If it seems likely that patients have made a firm decision not to continue with treatment, that must be respected but they should know that they can change their mind. Other common situations raised with the BMA concern patients who repeatedly request extensions of their prescriptions but decline to attend for the examination that should accompany renewal. GPs need to make patients aware that for them to prescribe repeatedly without carrying out an examination may be considered negligent and contrary to their duty to ensure that their prescribing is appropriate and justifiable. (This is discussed further in Chapter 13, page 547.)

Summary – choice and duty

- Whenever feasible, patients' preferences in terms of doctor or hospital should be respected, without disadvantaging other patients.
- Doctors should not discriminate against patients who need a lot of attention.
- Asylum seekers have the right to be registered with a general practice but GPs have a measure of discretion in registering failed asylum seekers.
- In emergencies, the doctor should provide care when no other suitably qualified person is available, but otherwise there is no obligation to treat a 'stranger'.

Maintaining a balanced relationship

Doctor–patient contact is seen as special. Doctors often have access to considerable detail about patients' lives, dealing with social issues such as insurance applications, sick notes, housing-related problems, stress and child protection issues. Although often concerning mundane matters, healthcare also deals with the most intimate and basic aspects of life. 'Medicine means life and death, deliverance and despair, hope and fright, mystery and mechanics. It is a microscope trained upon life's fundamentals'.[12] Although patients are generally better informed and have many more means of accessing health information than in the past, they can still be at a disadvantage as doctors have the experience and influence. Ethical guidance attempts to bring balance into an inherently asymmetrical relationship.

The GMC sets out a series of ethical obligations that doctors must observe to create successful relationships with patients.[13] Doctors have particular responsibilities for making these relationships work, through partnership and collaboration. Ideally, decisions are made through frank discussion, in which clinical expertise seeks to match the available options to the patient's individual needs and preferences. Patients of all abilities are encouraged to be actively engaged in health decisions that affect them, even if they choose to decline some medical advice. Doctors should provide information, explain the implications of the patient's choice and address any misunderstandings. They may also need to explain the limitations on patients' options, making clear that treatment that is not clinically appropriate is not on offer. Medical advice should be evidence-based and reflect best practice guidelines. Wherever possible, a solution acceptable to the patient should be the goal.

Doctors' personal moral views

The need for frankness and openness with patients does not extend to doctors offering opinions about their own moral views. They are entitled to such opinions but should not share them unless explicitly asked by patients to do so. Doctors are particularly warned against making pejorative or judgemental comments about patients' values or behaviour. If doctors believe their personal moral views would affect their advice or treatment, the patient must be given the option of seeing a different doctor. Doctors who oppose contraception or the termination of pregnancy, for example, should inform patients who want those services how they can access them from another doctor. (This is discussed in Chapter 7, pages 277 and 288–290.)

Patients should be offered factual information about how to safeguard their health but the fact that their actions have sometimes contributed to their condition should not give rise to moralising or delaying treatment. In some cases, habits such as smoking, drug or alcohol addiction have clinical implications for the effectiveness of any proposed treatment. These need to be discussed candidly, in a non-judgemental manner, as part of informing patients. Doctors must avoid language or actions that imply discrimination, including gratuitous comments about patients' lifestyles. NHS guidance makes clear that such behaviour in a healthcare setting could be construed as harassment.[14] Some health professionals see prayer or religious comment as part of the routine provision of support to patients but such matters should not be raised unless the patient requests them. In 2008, a nurse was suspended on the basis of failing to demonstrate a professional commitment to equality and diversity, after offering to pray for a patient, who reported the comment.[15] She was reinstated but it was made clear that offering prayers is only acceptable when patients ask for them. The issue was discussed at the BMA's 2009 annual meeting, which recognised that the NHS is committed to providing spiritual care but that the initiative for it must rest with the patient.

Patients' rights to non-judgemental care and doctors' rights to conscientious objection

Patients have rights to high quality care, provided in a non-judgemental manner. Doctors have rights to opt out of some lawful procedures, as long as doing so would not endanger a patient's welfare. In an emergency situation, they must provide appropriate care despite any conscientious objection. In 2008, the GMC issued guidance, *Personal Beliefs and Medical Practice*,[16] which aims to balance doctors' rights to opt out of some procedures with the rights of patients to receive those interventions. It noted an increasing number of enquiries centred on the scope of doctors' conscientious objection in a range of circumstances not covered by the statutory opt-out clauses which only relate to abortion and fertility treatment. The BMA subsequently went on to pass policy at its annual meeting in 2008 that went beyond what the GMC says. Although not binding in the same way as the GMC's advice, the BMA argues that doctors should only claim a conscientious exemption to the procedures where statute recognises their right (abortion and fertility treatment) and to withdrawing life-prolonging treatment from a patient who lacks capacity. The BMA's policy is to support doctors' rights to conscientiously object to carrying out non-emergency procedures in these limited instances. Like the GMC, it emphasises that in urgent cases doctors must follow good practice guidance and provide appropriate care, regardless of their personal beliefs. The BMA also advises that, in the event of seeing a patient seeking advice on one of those procedures, doctors should immediately make clear if they have a conscientious objection and inform patients of their right to see another doctor. They should ensure that patients have sufficient information to exercise their right to receive advice elsewhere. If patients want to transfer but cannot readily make their own arrangements to see another doctor, the practitioner they have consulted must ensure that arrangements are made, without delay, for another doctor to take over their care. This should be done in as seamless a way as possible so that the patient is not disadvantaged.

Summary – maintaining a balanced relationship

- Doctors have special duties to maintain a successful and balanced relationship with their patients.
- Doctors should not mention their own moral views to patients unless explicitly asked.
- Doctors have rights to their own moral views and can opt out of some lawful procedures, if this would not endanger patients.

Importance of good communication

A large body of literature has developed about aspects of doctor–patient communication, particularly about how to communicate risks to patients and how to break bad news. (Giving bad news is covered on page 35. Chapter 10 deals in more detail with talking to patients who have a life-limiting condition.) Effective communication is about establishing positive interpersonal relationships, as well as exchanging information. When the BMA investigated the main aspects of primary care that patients most valued, effective communication and continuity of the relationship were identified as key issues.[17] In secondary care too, the importance of hearing and understanding patients' views is highly valued. One patient's experience of surgery, for example, was reported as much better when doctors listened and understood that he was the expert on his own body. 'The surgeon may have performed a thousand of these procedures,' he said, 'but I doubt if he'd ever had one'.[18]

The GMC also emphasises good communication as a prerequisite for valid patient consent. It tells doctors that they should do their best to understand patients' views and preferences but not make assumptions about patients' understanding of risk or the importance they attach to different outcomes.[19] Chronic diseases impact on patients' lives in various ways. People need information to manage their condition in ways compatible with their own wishes and lifestyle. Even though the balance of control in decision making increasingly passes to patients, doctors still need to offer more than simply a list of options. Much medical information is contested knowledge even if based on statistical probability. Patients generally need to know what is evidence-based advice and also an indication of the uncertainties and limitations of what is known.

The GMC has also drawn attention to the way in which aspects of personal choice, such as doctors' clothing, can alter the way in which patients relate to them. It has discussed, for example, the use of a veil, the *niqab*, by some doctors as part of their cultural identity. Ultimately, the GMC says, dress is a matter for employers but it does stress the importance of patients being able to build relationships of trust and communicate freely with their doctors. It notes that some patients find that a doctor's face veil presents an obstacle to effective communication and the development of trust.[20]

Communication and concordance

Giving patients the information they need to protect their health is one important means of supporting them to complete a course of treatment or comply with recommended activities. 'Concordance' is about patients understanding the advantages and disadvantages of specific treatment and why it is prescribed for them. It has been defined as 'shared decision making and arriving at an agreement that respects the wishes and beliefs of the patient'.[21] (This is discussed further in Chapter 13, pages 539–541.) One of the criticisms sometimes made by older patients is that the lack of candid information over a long period left them unready to cope with the eventual knowledge of their condition.[22] Had they been better informed at an earlier stage, they might have had opportunities to improve their health. Everyone has the right to refuse treatment if they understand the implications but this means that information needs to be continually presented to them in a way they can absorb it. Best practice entails offering patients information about why a medication or intervention is recommended and its effects. Pharmacists can be helpful in backing up the information supplied by doctors and explaining to patients how their medication works, why they need it and whether they should refrain from self-medicating with other products. In hospitals and care homes, patients often complain that they are not always told the reason for some medication, nor given a choice about it. Explaining the purpose of medicines or other interventions is an essential part of good practice. As a back-up to discussion, written information can be valuable because it generally increases patient satisfaction, reduces complaints and contributes to patient adherence to treatment. It can also assist self-management activity and help patients to cope better with their condition.[23] Patient input into such information sheets can also be helpful in providing insight into the actual daily experience of living with a particular condition.

Can patients refuse to receive information?

Most patients want to be closely involved in decisions. They may want more or less information at different stages of their treatment, especially as assimilating difficult or painful news takes time and appropriate support. If individuals make clear that they want very little information, it cannot be forced upon them but, in order for their consent to be valid, they should know the core facts about what is proposed (see Chapter 2). They may agree in general terms to a procedure whose purpose they understand but without wanting to know every aspect of it. Nevertheless, patients with capacity should be encouraged to know information that is essential to maintaining their own health, as well as that relevant to the treatment in question and its potential side effects, although they may opt out of receiving other details. Patients can also choose to delegate some decisions to others and the information needed to make these decisions then needs to be given to those nominated decision makers. Health teams need to be sensitive to individuals' wishes while ensuring that core information is communicated effectively. Relatives sometimes ask for information to be withheld from patients but the importance of listening to patients' own views about what they want to know cannot be over-emphasised. (This issue is discussed in Chapter 10, pages 418–424.)

Failing to offer sufficient information could invalidate the patient's consent. In particular, when innovative or risky procedures are proposed, patients need to be aware that there are risks involved. Nevertheless, effective communication about risks, their probability and magnitude, is often difficult even when patients are keen to understand. It is liable to be more so if patients are reluctant to acknowledge them. They should always be given a chance to ask questions, seek clarification and ask for more information and the necessary time slots need to be made available for this to happen. The kind of information patients need to make valid and informed decisions is discussed in detail in Chapter 2. The basic information includes:

- the evidence base for the diagnosis and prognosis, including the limits of what is known
- available treatment options, including those that may not be available on the NHS
- the implications, drawbacks and likely side effects of those treatments
- the main alternatives, including non-treatment, and their implications
- if possible, sources of further information and relevant patient support groups.

Truth telling by doctors

It is never easy to deliver or receive bad news, particularly when no cure is available and there is little that the patient or health team can do to alter the situation. The BMA strongly emphasises the importance of all health professionals being properly trained to communicate in an honest and supportive manner. Special additional training in communication and providing support is needed when caring for people with dementia or fluctuating mental capacity. The doctor's role is to ensure that decision making is returned as much as possible to the patient, rather than pre-empting the choice. Although in the past, doctors often fudged the issue because they feared that the truth might result in lost hopes, sadness, suffering and grief, patients now expect honest answers and support for the anxieties that may flow from them. They should be supported in dealing with the additional anxiety sometimes created by greater knowledge. They have their own goals and need as accurate information as possible about what is achievable. The clinical limitations need to be discussed but doctors also need to be open about any other factors that are likely to affect treatment decisions or their timing. The need to meet externally set targets for treatment, for example, may impinge on the scheduling of certain procedures. This should not be concealed from those affected by it. Health professionals provide information in order to empower patients to exercise informed choice and this is equally important when the options are limited. Obviously, difficult information has to be given with sensitivity. Traditionally, doctors were discouraged from confessing any doubts or uncertainties because this could undermine patients' morale. Now, it is recognised that patients can experience stress and anxiety precisely because information is concealed.

Telling patients about unfunded treatments

One area of enquiry to the BMA concerns the range of options that patients should be told about when there is little or no likelihood of those options being made available on the NHS. Patients can opt to have some investigations or treatment privately in addition to their NHS care but this does not resolve the situation of patients who cannot afford to pay for them. Although it is not doctors' place to make any assumptions about their patients' financial resources, they often feel embarrassed about telling patients about treatment only available privately. Although it might be argued that patients should be protected from the anxiety of receiving information about treatment options that are unfunded, this undermines the principle of partnership between patients and health professionals. Patients generally want to have the choice of making even difficult decisions for themselves. In the BMA's view, doctors should be as open and frank as possible about potentially beneficial procedures or drugs. Patients lose trust in their medical advisers if they discover belatedly that information about potential options has been withheld. (The movement of patients in and out of the NHS is discussed in more detail in Chapter 19, pages 780–781.)

Rationing decisions should be transparent, which means that when doctors are responsible for commissioning services or products, they need to explain to patients why some may be unaffordable within the NHS. The situation is complicated when there is no clinical agreement about the efficacy of the treatment or where only a small improvement can be expected but the financial cost is great. Some purchasers or commissioners may pay for innovative treatments for patients who are devoid of other options but this risks perpetuating a 'post code lottery'. Doctors have to make clinical decisions about which treatments are potentially beneficial to individual patients and which would be futile. There is no obligation to tell patients about treatments that would clearly be futile.

Patient choice and payments

NHS doctors have responsibilities to try and ensure that resources are used fairly, which means that they are likely to be unable to offer everything that patients want. This is different to situations where the doctor declines to provide a drug or treatment that is simply not clinically indicated. In some cases, a potential element of care cannot be NHS-funded because the cost is deemed disproportionate to the expected benefit. If it is available privately, some patients would want to purchase a drug, for example, even if it might only extend their life expectancy very slightly. They may purchase it privately and have it delivered separately to the NHS care.[24] They should not be influenced to think that they have to buy such top-up treatment but should be offered information, if they wish it, about what is available.

Doctors' duty to acknowledge mistakes

Doctors should be honest in acknowledging mistakes in treatment and diagnosis. Errors need to be acknowledged and learnt from so that appropriate changes can be implemented. (Monitoring one's own performance and learning from mistakes are also discussed throughout Chapter 21.) The GMC says that, when patients suffer harm or distress, doctors should act immediately to put matters right if that is possible.[25]

They should explain fully and promptly to the patient what has happened and the likely long-term and short-term implications. The BMA supports this advice. If the injured person is an incapacitated adult or a young child, an explanation needs to be given to the carer or parent. Where relevant, information should also be given about how to make a complaint. The GMC also reminds doctors[26] that when patients complain, they have the right to a prompt, honest and constructive response, and an apology where appropriate. A complaint must not be allowed to affect the care or treatment provided.

The BMA receives queries about the handling of very difficult and sensitive cases where clinicians believe that previous doctors have either missed important signs of a serious condition or laboratory tests have been misinterpreted. In any situation where it seems that substandard practice has occurred, there is an obligation to do something about it. An important consideration must also be whether the error was likely to have been a one-off occurrence or part of a pattern of mistakes that may mean an ongoing risk of harm. Whistleblowing involves drawing mistakes to the attention of the person or organisation who can remedy them as well as ensuring that those who have suffered from them are informed. (Whistleblowing is discussed in Chapter 21, pages 878–879.) Where there is a pattern of error in secondary care, it is usual for the hospital to set up a system for contacting patients and informing them. Audit and notification of significant events may expose incidents of substandard care but doctors should also monitor their own performance so that they can spot their errors and address the implications.

Froggatt v Chesterfield and North Derbyshire NHS

A patient's breast biopsy was confused with someone else's sample by the histopathologist, with the result that a healthy patient had a mastectomy and suffered distress, believing herself at risk of premature death. The mistake was suspected by a consultant oncologist who contacted the histopathologist and asked him to review the slides. This revealed normal tissue without evidence of malignancy. The patient's GP was informed and it was agreed that the situation should be explained to the patient at the hospital by the surgeon who had operated on her, with two nurses to provide support. Telling patients that they have undergone unwarranted distress and surgery is clearly difficult. The patient said it was easier to accept the mastectomy when she thought she had cancer but she felt worse knowing that it had been unnecessary. She became depressed, wept and thought constantly about the operation. The patient developed a serious psychiatric disorder which seemed unlikely to improve. In court, the patient was awarded £350,000 damages and lesser sums were awarded to her family for the trauma they had undergone.[27]

Mistakes are hard to acknowledge and traumatic for patients to learn about. Even when sensitively handled, the situation can seem worse rather than better by the disclosure, but grief or the expense of litigation are not good reasons for secrecy. Patients need support and counselling to cope with such information and also need to understand the difference between errors and legitimate differences of clinical opinion. Clearly, it is important not to impose knowledge gained by hindsight on the information available to the diagnosing clinician when the decision was made. When there is ambiguity, it is important for health professionals to obtain a clear view of the facts before talking to the patient. Clarifying what has occurred in the past is likely to involve contacting the previous clinician and reviewing samples taken and records made at the time of diagnosis. A specialist interpretation of the evidence may be needed. If it is obvious that an error was made, there should be discussion about how the patient can sensitively be prepared for that information and who should take responsibility for doing so.

When a mistake has been instrumental in causing a death, people close to the deceased need to be informed sensitively and the events investigated. If a child has died, the circumstances should be explained to parents or people with parental responsibility. If the cause of death is misadventure or is not fully known, the coroner or procurator fiscal must be involved. Even when there is no evidence of error, an elective (or hospital) post-mortem examination may be requested by the deceased's clinician to verify the diagnosis or assess the effect of treatment. (Chapter 12, pages 502–503 discuss which deaths must be referred to a coroner or procurator fiscal and pages 498–499 discuss the duty of confidentiality after the patient's death.)

Being open about employment disputes

When doctors are suspended by an employer or have restrictions placed on their practice, they need to inform any other organisations for whom they work so that cover arrangements can be made. Questions can also arise about what patients should be told when doctors are in dispute with employers. Any information they give to patients about a dispute should not cast aspersions on the standards of care provided by the unit or by colleagues. If there are concerns about care standards, these need to be raised through the appropriate channels (see the discussion of whistleblowing in Chapter 21, pages 878–879).

Truth telling by patients

The importance of doctors being truthful is well recognised but the concept of patients being equally frank is complex. Ideally, they should provide doctors with accurate information about their health and relevant aspects of lifestyle but are often reluctant to do so. Patients need to be aware that withholding relevant facts can affect treatment decisions or risk drug interaction. Some patients, for example, feel awkward about mentioning weight reduction drugs or medicines bought over the internet. They may worry some matters will be disclosed to employers, insurers or family members. Mental health problems, sexually transmitted infections, addiction and stress-related illnesses may be concealed. Some doctors consider that the best solution would be for health records to be used only for the provision of healthcare and related purposes such as clinical audit, with a prohibition on social functions that currently require medical records. Reports for insurance and employment would be carried out by independent medical examiners without access to the patient's health record. Although this might encourage patients to be more forthcoming with their own doctor, the BMA has argued that there are often advantages for patients in having reports written by a doctor who has an ongoing relationship with them and who can point out if test results appear inconsistent in relation to the overall health record. From the patient's perspective, this is also often the most convenient solution. (Reports for third parties are discussed further in Chapter 16, pages 651–654.)

Communication, interpretation and translation

In some cases, a third party is needed to aid communication. In many health facilities, information given in a range of languages encourages patients to give advance notice if they need language or signing assistance. Patients often come accompanied by people who they want to translate for them or, among some communities, patients may expect that another family member will actually make decisions for them as well as translate relevant information. This can pose problems for health professionals as they may be unsure how accurately information is being passed on to the patient and to what extent the individual can make a choice. (Consent and its validity are discussed further in Chapter 2.) Children should not be expected to interpret for adults, especially when sensitive subjects are discussed. In all cases, it needs to be made clear that individual patients are entitled to privacy, while recognising that not all patients wish to exercise that right. Interpretation and translation should be provided, wherever possible, by professionals rather than other staff such as hospital porters. Translators and interpreters, including those who provide sign language, can often be found through providers such as 'Language Line' or the National Register of Interpreters.

Summary – the importance of good communication

- Patients should be offered information but are not obliged to receive all the details.
- Efforts must be made to convey information in a manner in which patients can understand; this may include translation.
- Questions should be answered as honestly as possible.
- Frankness should extend to funding and rationing decisions as well as treatment.

Trust and reciprocity

Covert medication

Patients with capacity

Covert medication for a person with capacity is unacceptable but the BMA continues to receive queries about whether it is ever ethically permissible. As it involves deliberate deception, covert medication breaches the principle of informed consent. Refusal of treatment by an informed adult with capacity is legally and ethically binding; the exception is compulsory treatment authorised under mental health legislation when patients – sometimes despite retaining their mental capacity – are considered a danger to themselves or others (see Chapter 3).

Contexts in which this question arises commonly involve the residential care of older people, people with learning disabilities or patients with challenging behaviour. In some cases raised with the BMA, no formal assessment of patients' capacity has been undertaken but it is assumed that their age, diagnosis or medical condition necessarily means that they cannot, or need not, give consent. Despite their impairments, many of these patients have sufficient capacity to understand the purpose of medication and so must be asked to consent to it. In some cases, drugs are administered covertly to disguise the fact that they are intended to facilitate patient management rather than being necessary in the patients' interests.[28] Health professionals must seek consent from individuals with capacity and ensure that an assessment of capacity is carried out in cases of doubt. They must not mislead patients about the purpose of their medication, nor should they fail to answer patients' questions on the grounds of lack of time or difficulties in communicating.

Patients who lack mental capacity

Cases may arise in which covert medication is in the best interests of patients who lack mental capacity but it should not be routine. A decision to administer medication covertly in such circumstances should be taken by the clinician in overall charge of the incapacitated patient's medical care, in consultation with the multi-disciplinary care team. People close to incapacitated individuals should be involved in the decision. This includes proxy decision makers and independent mental capacity advocates where relevant (see Chapter 3 on the legal aspects of proxy consent for incapacitated adults.) The Mental Welfare Commission for Scotland also provides guidance on the use of covert medication in relation to adults lacking capacity.[29] The reasons for a decision to give drugs covertly should be recorded in the patient's care plan and regularly reviewed. In making the decision, consideration should be given to:

- whether the patient genuinely lacks capacity to consent to or refuse treatment
- why covert medication is proposed and whether it is in the patient's best interests
- whether there are feasible alternatives that are more respectful of the individual's choice.

Patients with fluctuating mental capacity

Some of the cases concerning covert medication raised with the BMA are far from straightforward if, for example, patients have fluctuating mental capacity. Some patients with a history of psychotic episodes progressively lose insight about their illness and, believing themselves well, decline the medication that would prevent a crisis occurring. Health professionals are then faced with the dilemma of either effectively allowing a mental health crisis by stopping the treatment that the patient declines, until the patient deteriorates to the extent that the compulsory treatment criteria are met, or risk breaching the law. The law is very clear that people who do not fall within the remit of mental health legislation and have sufficient capacity and understanding to make a valid decision should not be treated against their will. The BMA's advice is that when patients appear to meet the legal criteria to make valid decisions, health professionals can only offer support and counselling to try to restore voluntary adherence to the recommended regime. One mechanism occasionally proposed for such situations is a form of advance decision. Patients with such a history of illness can be asked, when at their most lucid and insightful, to agree in advance a treatment plan that would be triggered at the very start of a decline in mental capacity, rather than allowing the patient to reach crisis point and the need for compulsory treatment. Although such a mechanism appears more respectful of patient autonomy, it is fraught with practical difficulties. Not least of these is the fact that, legally and ethically, patients are not required to demonstrate profound insight, but rather need a grasp of the core information, in order to decline treatment and override their previously given consent. A patient's current decision, if backed by information and an understanding of the implications, effectively trumps any earlier agreement. Nevertheless, an agreed treatment plan that has involved the patient in advance planning may be the best option available (see Chapter 3 on issues of mental capacity and treatment without consent).

Recording of consultations

Patients sometimes ask to record the consultation. Doctors may feel that such a request is symptomatic of a lack of trust or an intention to bring a complaint later if any of the doctor's opinions subsequently prove to be erroneous. In the enquiries raised by doctors with the BMA, most anxiety is expressed about patients attempting to record the interview clandestinely, apparently for the purposes of potential litigation at a later stage. In the BMA's view, doctors should not seek to prohibit recording but should encourage patients to do it openly rather than secretly. Recording by either side can alter the nature of the consultation and may reduce doctors' willingness to admit to uncertainty. Fear of possible litigation could result in health professionals becoming overly cautious in their advice. On the other hand, audio recording has increasingly come to be seen as a way in which patients can remember important advice. Any mechanism likely to assist patients to remember and cooperate actively with medical advice should be supported.

Audio or video recording of consultations by doctors is sometimes undertaken for the purposes of training or audit as well as for the investigation or treatment of the patient's condition. Any recording of people with capacity for such purposes should have their consent or, for young children, the permission of parents. The GMC has published detailed guidance on this.[30] (Identifiable recording of patients for purposes such as training or audit is discussed in detail in Chapter 6, pages 249–250.)

Covert recording and surveillance

People using healthcare facilities should be made aware by notices if surveillance cameras are in use for purposes such as security. The GMC states that doctors must obtain consent to use any recording made for reasons other than the patient's treatment or assessment, unless the secondary purpose only requires anonymised material and uses recordings made as part of a treatment.[31] It acknowledges as an exception the use of covert surveillance to detect illness induced in children by carers (see below), noting that, in exceptional circumstances, doctors may consider that it is in the patient's best interests to make a recording without first seeking permission. Before proceeding, however, doctors should discuss this with an experienced colleague, follow national or local guidance and must be prepared to justify their decision.

There has been much debate about the use of covert video surveillance (CVS) in health settings where it is occasionally used as part of a formal child protection multi-agency strategy, to monitor children receiving inpatient care when there are grounds to suspect relatives or carers of causing injury to the child. Such surveillance without the knowledge and consent of families might occur in cases where the child would otherwise be placed at unacceptable risk of harm. When that is the case, it may be justified but can only be undertaken by the police acting under the Regulation of Investigatory Powers Act 2000,[32] which includes a requirement for the police to obtain authorisation from the chief constable. The BMA has expressed strong reservations about surveillance for other purposes, such as for gathering evidence for a legal case against an alleged perpetrator of abuse, and CVS is unlikely to be justified where there is already some compelling evidence of abuse. The Royal College of Paediatrics and Child Health (RCPCH) has issued detailed guidance[33] on when CVS may be used which says that if the child is likely to remain in the care of a suspected perpetrator, because there is insufficient evidence of abuse to ensure the child's protection, and a high risk of future harm, CVS might be acceptable as part of evidence gathering. Each case must be considered on its merits. The RCPCH guidance also sets out the steps that have to be taken first, including working with the police, involving the trust chief executive and detailed discussion with the staff caring for the child.

As any recording involving covert video surveillance of a patient is likely to be within the scope of the Regulation of Investigatory Powers Act 2000, doctors need to seek expert advice about any situation in which it is proposed. In connection with compensation claims for injury, covert monitoring may be proposed to verify whether patients are as disabled as they claim and identify those who may be acting fraudulently. The GMC says that, even when doctors are acting as expert witnesses or producing a medico-legal report and therefore have a primary duty to the court, this does not negate their duties owed to the individual being examined.[34] Both the GMC and the BMA advise that doctors should not collude with covert recordings other than very exceptional cases where it is in the patient's interest. Doctors should not arrange such secret surveillance on the premises where they work. They should take legal advice if they believe that filmed material that they have been asked to view or comment on is likely to have been improperly obtained.

Trust and declaring a financial interest

Patients trust that doctors will base their advice on an assessment of patients' best interests rather than on any other consideration, such as a possible advantage for the doctor in recommending one treatment, medical device or healthcare facility over another. Both the BMA and the GMC emphasise the importance of doctors being open with patients and families in situations where the doctor or people close to the doctor stand to benefit financially from the patient accepting a particular course of action. A common situation in which this is likely to occur is that in which a doctor has invested in a residential nursing home or similar facility and would like to refer some patients to it. Even if it is the doctor's spouse or partner that stands to benefit, rather than the doctor personally, it is best to be open about such investments and declare them to patients. Other cases brought to the BMA concern instances where doctors have substantial investments in a particular pharmaceutical company and wish, for clinical reasons, to change their patients' existing medication to one produced by that company. Despite the fact that the link may be relatively distant and the sums gained in terms of investment revenue relatively small, such practices can undermine patient trust. It is partly for this reason that the BMA generally advises doctors not to hold investments in such companies if they are likely to want to prescribe its products for their patients.

Receiving payment for referrals or recommendations

The GMC says that doctors must be open and honest in their financial arrangements and not accept or offer payment for a referral.[35] Accepting any inducement, gift or hospitality as a reward from another practitioner, agency or company for referring patients or arranging their care is unacceptable. Payment for endorsing other practitioners to patients is also unacceptable. Any measure that seems to be a variation on the concept of payment in exchange for recommendation or endorsement should be avoided. Payment for referral to solicitors or other non-health professionals is also unacceptable.

Patient requests for a second opinion

Patient requests for a second opinion can appear a sign of mistrust in a doctor's clinical judgement but the BMA emphasises that patients have a right to ask and, if reasonable, efforts should be made to meet such requests. This is not necessarily the same as saying that patients always have an automatic 'right' to obtain a second opinion, unless treatment is being provided within the private sector and financed by the patient. Such requests sometimes reflect a previous breakdown in communication and the fact that a patient is worried enough to request a second opinion may mean that more discussion is needed between the treating doctor and patient. In some cases, the doctor's willingness to listen and respond to the patient's anxiety may be sufficient but, if not, serious consideration needs to be given to whether it would be appropriate to refer the patient to another doctor. The GMC also says that doctors should respect the patient's right to seek a second opinion.[36] Where it is agreed that a second opinion would be useful, the responsibility for identifying a suitable doctor rests with the referring GP.

Summary – trust and reciprocity

- Informed adults with capacity can refuse treatment and it is unacceptable to administer medication to them covertly.
- In some situations, covert medication may be appropriate for patients lacking capacity. The reasons should be documented and regularly reviewed.
- Patient consent is needed for the recording of consultations and doctors should not prohibit patients from recording them, particularly if it would help the patient's recall of the advice.
- Covert surveillance falls within the scope of Regulation of Investigatory Powers legislation.
- Doctors should declare their financial interests when these might be perceived as influential in decision making.
- Patient requests for a second opinion should be met, when reasonable, and the reasons for the request may need discussion.

Breakdown of the doctor–patient relationship

When the doctor–patient relationship breaks down irretrievably, patients generally transfer to another practice or they may ask to be referred to another consultant. In cases other than violence and abuse, the BMA recommends that the decision to refer or transfer a patient elsewhere should be made only after careful consideration and not in the heat of the moment. Wherever possible, there should be some discussion with patients so that they have prior warning that their removal is being considered. Patients who are misusing services or failing to attend appointments may alter their behaviour if this is brought to their attention. If all else fails, however, the BMA believes that it is not in anyone's best interests for an unsatisfactory relationship to continue. It is obviously important for doctors to maintain a high standard of professionalism even in circumstances where patients are difficult. In secondary care, the clinician in overall charge of an inpatient's management needs to ensure that an appropriate colleague is able to take on care. The patient's primary care practice should also be kept informed if the practice itself has not arranged the new referral. In general practice, patients can apply direct to another practice or be allocated by the local primary care organisation. Practices should not remove patients from their list for reasons such as their treatment is costly or on grounds of age. Sometimes it is not the patients themselves but carers, including staff of nursing and residential homes, who can generate excessive demands for services from the practice. In these cases, the practice should attempt to resolve any problems through discussion.

If the behaviour of one member of a household has led to his or her removal from a practice list, this does not mean that the removal of other family members should automatically follow. Bearing in mind the need for patient confidentiality and prior discussion with the individual concerned, an explicit discussion with other family members about the problem can obviate the need for any further action. In rare cases, however, because of the possible need to visit patients at home, it may be necessary to terminate responsibility for other members of the family or the entire household. The prospect of visiting patients where a relative resides who is no longer a patient of the practice by virtue of this person's unacceptable behaviour, or being regularly confronted by such a patient, may make it too difficult for the practice to continue to look after the whole family. This is particularly likely when the patient has been removed from the list because of violence or threatening behaviour and continuing to treat the other family members could put doctors or their staff at risk. (Violent patients are discussed on pages 55–57.)

GMC guidance on ending a professional relationship with a patient

'In rare circumstances, the trust between you and a patient may break down, and you may find it necessary to end the professional relationship. For example, this may occur if a patient has been violent to you or a colleague, has stolen from the premises, or has persistently acted inconsiderately or unreasonably. You should not end a relationship with a patient solely because of a complaint the patient has made about you or your team, or because of the resource implications of the patient's care or treatment.

Before you end a professional relationship with a patient, you must be satisfied that your decision is fair . . . You must be prepared to justify your decision. You should inform the patient of your decision and your reasons for ending the professional relationship, wherever practical in writing.

You must take steps to ensure that arrangements are made promptly for the continuing care of the patient, and you must pass on the patient's records without delay.

If you charge fees, you may refuse further treatment for patients unable or unwilling to pay for services you have already provided.'[37]

Complaints

NHS practices and hospitals must make information available about their complaints procedure. Private practitioners should also ensure that their patients are aware of how to register a complaint. Such information should make clear that patients will not be disadvantaged simply for complaining. If made in a reasonable and constructive manner, complaints can help to improve services. Early notification of a possible problem in their relationship can give doctors and patients an opportunity to discuss ways of preventing future difficulties. Persistent or unfounded complaints, however, are usually indicative of a serious breakdown of the doctor–patient relationship. It is a breakdown of the relationship rather than a complaint *per se* that must form the basis of any decision to transfer the patient to a colleague. Doctors who experience such a situation may want to consult their defence organisation or trust lawyer.

Summary – breakdown of the doctor–patient relationship

- Patients should not be removed from the doctor's list solely because they have difficult or multiple health problems.
- If the relationship breaks down irretrievably, transferring the patient to another practitioner is in the interests of all.
- Patients should be made aware if their actions cause doctors to consider recommending a transfer, so that the patient has an opportunity to change.

Recognising responsibilities and boundaries

Self-diagnosis and treating people who are emotionally close

In medicine, there is an expectation that doctors do not take sick leave as that puts pressure on colleagues and patients. There has long been adherence to the notion of doctors 'working through illness' and either neglecting health problems or treating themselves. Traditionally, few doctors registered with a GP. Efforts are being made to change this culture but unease about adopting the role of a patient and worries about confidentiality still often lead to self-treatment. The hazards of self-diagnosis are many, but particular concerns include the temptation to extend oneself beyond one's competence and the possibility of denial in the face of serious illness. All doctors should be registered with a GP, rather than treating themselves or informally asking a colleague to do so. Nor should they become involved in treating their families, other than for very minor ailments. Although doctors must monitor their own health, especially in terms of whether they may pose any health risk to others, they should not self-treat. Where they suspect that they may have been exposed to a communicable disease, they must seek and follow professional advice without delay and must not rely on their own assessment of the risks they pose to patients. (General advice about sick doctors is given in Chapter 21, pages 879–883.)

GMC guidance on self-treatment and treatment of one's family

'Wherever possible, you should avoid providing medical care to anyone with whom you have a close personal relationship.'[38]

'You should be registered with a GP outside your family to ensure that you have access to independent and objective medical care. You should not treat yourself.

You should protect your patients, your colleagues and yourself by being immunised against common serious communicable diseases where vaccines are available.

If you know that you have, or think that you might have, a serious condition that you could pass on to patients, or if your judgement or performance could be affected by a condition or its treatment, you must consult a suitably qualified colleague. You must ask for and follow their advice about investigations, treatment and changes to your practice that they consider necessary. You must not rely on your own assessment of the risk you pose to patients.'[39]

Staff who are also patients

When selecting new staff, primary care practices should avoid discriminating against people who apply for the job but are already on their practice list as patients. In small communities, it is often unavoidable for staff to be patients but, where there are other options, it is not an ideal arrangement for either party. Conflicts and difficulties most often arise in relation to patient confidentiality. Some problems can be avoided by discussing them frankly in advance, or both sides may conclude that this is unlikely to be problematic, once thought has been given to potential difficulties, such as the management of situations where the patient/employee needs a lot of sick leave. Situations in which disciplinary procedures need to be invoked can be challenging as the patient/employee's health record may hold relevant information, known only to the employer by virtue of being the employee's doctor. As a general principle, patient records should not be used without consent for purposes other than the provision of care. Employees' permission is needed for them to be disclosed in the event of an employment dispute.

In some rare cases, patients have tried to use the opportunity of working in a surgery to look at friends' or relatives' records or to alter their own to remove information about sensitive topics such as depression, violence or termination of pregnancy. The computerisation of primary care records has made it harder to attempt to alter records without being detected. All staff must be trained about confidentiality issues and be made aware that it is a dismissible offence to look at the medical records of relatives, neighbours or friends. All information is confidential and available only to those working in the practice on a strict 'need to know' basis. If an employee's relatives are worried about the possibility of the employee having access to their records, they should be reassured about the strict confidentiality measures in place or, if feasible, they may choose to move to another practice. (Confidentiality is discussed in detail in Chapter 5.)

Managing patient expectations

It can be difficult to manage patients' expectations successfully, but providing them with explanations can help (see also the section on pressure from patients on prescribing decisions in Chapter 13, pages 545–549). Patients often expect their GP practice to assist them in a range of matters not directly related to their healthcare, such as providing references or signing passport applications. While some doctors are able to take on a range of tasks or direct the patient to another suitable agency, as part of a wider concept of care, many cannot. In all situations, doctors must act with honesty and integrity and so cannot agree to sign anything they do not know to be accurate. Sometimes the sheer volume of such requests for social reasons is unmanageable. The countersigning of documents related to health and the provision of reports, such as those supporting requests for special housing or assistance at home on health grounds, may well need to involve doctors. Again, it is important that they only put their signature to documents that they have verified as they will be open to complaint if they countersign something untrue.

Doctors as witnesses to wills and legal documents

Patients often ask doctors to be a witness to a will or a variety of other legal documents. A distinction can be made between documents that have little or no connection to the patient's healthcare and could, therefore, be witnessed by other appropriate agencies, and documents such as a patient's advance decision about treatment which are likely to have an important impact on the care provided. (Advance decisions are covered in detail in Chapter 3.) It is often seen as desirable that a doctor should witness legal documents in situations where the drafter's mental capacity may later be questioned. Doctors need to be aware that, by acting as signatory of legal documents, they may be assumed to have verified the patient's mental capacity. They should not presume that they are just witnessing the authenticity of the signature. The law assumes that people have capacity unless there is some evidence to the contrary and when doctors are confident that the patient has capacity to make the decision in question, it is not essential to carry out a formal assessment of that fact. Where there is any doubt about mental capacity, however, an assessment is needed. Doctors should be wary of witnessing documents for patients whom they suspect may be suffering some impairment, without considering whether an assessment of mental capacity is needed.

Chaperones and accompanying persons

Patients often want to have someone accompany them in a range of situations, such as where they expect to be given distressing news or complicated information or need physical assistance. People undergoing an examination in connection with an insurance or litigation claim may also want to bring a witness such as a lawyer or trade union representative to the consultation. The same applies to people being examined for forensic purposes by a forensic physician (formerly known as police surgeons). Doctors are sometimes uncomfortable about seeing children and young people without a parent or other adult present but, if an unaccompanied minor asks for an appointment alone, that wish should generally be respected. Exceptions can arise, however, when an advocate may need to be present when minors are examined in detention or in relation to a criminal offence. (Chaperones in child protection cases are mentioned below and Chapter 17 covers healthcare in custodial settings, including for minors.) Even if the medical examination is routine and does not involve particularly sensitive or controversial issues, patients may still want someone to accompany them, to provide moral support. Doctors may also want to have someone else present if there is a significant risk of a patient becoming violent. In addition, it is advisable to have an independent person present as chaperone – if the patient agrees – for situations in which patients have to undress. Complaints of indecent assault are made by patients of both sexes and are not restricted to allegations against a doctor of the opposite sex. The GMC and the BMA recommend chaperones for intimate examinations of patients of either gender. Chaperones should also be offered in situations where patients might feel uncomfortable about being alone with a doctor, such as when it is necessary to darken the room for retinoscopy. Ideally, the option of having a chaperone or accompanying person should be discussed with patients in advance, particularly if they need to think about bringing a relative or friend. Providing an appropriate male chaperone for men in clinics where most health staff are female can be difficult and in some situations there may be little option but to proceed without one, if the patient agrees. Wherever possible, the need should be foreseen and planned for. In primary care in the past, options such as leaving an intercom switched on or the surgery door ajar were adopted but these solutions are now seen as unacceptable.

The issue of chaperones became particularly prominent in 2004, when Dr Ayling, a GP, was found guilty of indecently assaulting female patients and put on the sex offenders' register. The role of chaperones was discussed in considerable detail by the Committee of Inquiry into his case, which recommended that chaperoning should only be undertaken by trained staff, although the GMC's advice is that a patient's relative or friend may be acceptable. The use of untrained administrative staff in primary care surgeries was considered unacceptable by the Inquiry but, again, the GMC's advice permits this. All NHS trusts were advised to have accredited training for chaperones, to make resource provision for this and to make their chaperoning policies explicit to patients. In 2005, guidance was issued on chaperoning in relation to children, in child protection cases and for people with learning difficulties. A chaperone is also recommended for patients whose religion or culture imposes strict limitations on how they may be physically examined. These matters are addressed in detail in NHS guidance.[40]

GMC guidance on chaperones

'Wherever possible, you should offer the patient the security of having an impartial observer (a "chaperone") present during an intimate examination. This applies whether or not you are the same gender as the patient. A chaperone does not have to be medically qualified but will ideally:

- be sensitive, and respectful of the patient's dignity and confidentiality
- be prepared to reassure the patient if they show signs of distress or discomfort
- be familiar with the procedures involved in a routine intimate examination
- be prepared to raise concerns about a doctor if misconduct occurs.

In some circumstances, a member of practice staff, or a relative or friend of the patient may be an acceptable chaperone.

If either you or the patient does not wish the examination to proceed without a chaperone present, or if either of you is uncomfortable with the choice of chaperone, you may offer to delay the examination to a later date when a chaperone (or an alternative chaperone) will be available, if this is compatible with the patients best interests. You should record any discussion about chaperones and its outcome. If a chaperone is present, you should record that fact and make a note of their identity. If the patient does not want a chaperone, you should record that the offer was made and declined.'[41]

Intimate examinations

The GMC and medical defence bodies have long recommended that a chaperone be offered for intimate examinations. In 1997 the Royal College of Obstetricians and Gynae-cologists (RCOG) published a detailed report specifically about intimate examinations, which emphasised the importance of having a chaperone, regardless of the gender of the doctor.[42]

GMC guidance on intimate examinations

'It is particularly important to maintain a professional boundary when examining patients: intimate examinations can be embarrassing or distressing for patients. Whenever you examine a patient you should be sensitive to what they may perceive as intimate. This is likely to include examinations of breasts, genitalia and rectum, but could also include any examination where it is necessary to touch or even be close to the patient.

Before conducting an intimate examination you should:

- explain to the patient why an examination is necessary and give the patient an opportunity to ask questions
- explain what the examination will involve, in a way the patient can understand, so that the patient has a clear idea of what to expect, including any potential pain or discomfort
- obtain the patient's permission before the examination and record that permission has been obtained
- give the patient privacy to undress and dress and keep the patient covered as much as possible to maintain their dignity. Do not assist the patient in removing clothing unless you have clarified with them that your assistance is required.

During the examination you should explain what you are going to do before you do it and, if this differs from what you have already outlined to the patient, explain why and seek the patient's permission; be prepared to discontinue the examination if the patient asks you to; keep discussion relevant and do not make unnecessary personal comments.'[43]

The importance of good communication both in advance and after an intimate examination cannot be overemphasised. It is also important for doctors to be aware about how remarks they perceive as innocuous can be offensive to patients. The GMC sometimes receives complaints from patients who feel that doctors have behaved or spoken inappropriately during intimate examinations when the root of the issue is very poor communication. Providing a full explanation of what is intended and why, and then gaining patient consent are obviously essential. Ideally, there should also be appropriate opportunities for patients to raise the issue promptly with the practice or clinic if they feel a doctor's behaviour has been untoward (see also page 44 on complaints).

Checking colleagues' reliability

Doctors have a responsibility for ensuring patient safety and should speak out if they consider that colleagues present a risk. Delays have sometimes occurred in preventing harm to patients because health professionals think that they need knowledge of more than one incident involving a colleague before action can be taken.[44] This is not the case (see also the section on whistleblowing in Chapter 21, pages 878–879). When doctors employ colleagues or other staff or accept volunteers to do specific tasks, they must take steps to ensure that these people are safe and reliable, especially those working with children or vulnerable adults. Traditionally, in the primary care setting, it was left to each practice to decide what checks to make. In 2002 in England and Wales, guidance was published regarding pre- and post-appointment checks for anyone working in the NHS, whether as an employee, volunteer or contracted service provider. This included the need to check with the Criminal Records Bureau.[45] In 2004, the Department of Health published guidance for England and Wales on the protection of vulnerable adults in care homes.[46] In 2006, the Safeguarding Vulnerable Groups Act (England, Wales and with some sections covering Northern Ireland) was passed as a result of the Bichard inquiry into the Soham murders of two schoolgirls by a school caretaker in 2002. It introduced a formal system of vetting and barring for all those working with vulnerable people, including health and social care workers. It placed a statutory duty on employers and regulators to provide information to an independent Barring Board. It is a criminal offence to employ someone who has been barred from working with vulnerable groups in that capacity. In Scotland, general guidance was published in 2005 by the Northern Constabulary on best practice in protecting vulnerable adults.[47] The Adult Support and Protection (Scotland) Act 2007 made provision for safeguarding adults deemed to be at risk of harm including those with impaired capacity. It set out principles on when intervening in the adult's affairs would be justifiable, set out a system of banning certain individuals from attending the adult and rules about notification to the sheriff of an adult thought to be at risk. This was backed up by the Protection of Vulnerable Groups (Scotland) Act 2007, which barred certain people from working with children or vulnerable adults and required Ministers to keep lists of such barred individuals.

In 2011, the Government announced new recommendations for the future of the Vetting and Barring Scheme and criminal records checks. The Protection of Freedoms Bill was introduced into Parliament in early 2011 with the expectation that it would be finalised by the end of the year. When implemented (which is scheduled to be in 2012), it will provide a new legislative framework. The BMA response[48] highlighted the implications of the regulatory function of the Independent Safeguarding Authority (ISA) and the need for repeated criminal records checks. Under the revised vetting scheme, doctors will no longer be required to register with the ISA. Other key recommendations included:

- portability of criminal records checks between jobs
- introduction of an online system to allow employers to check if updated information is held on an applicant
- merging of the Criminal Records Bureau (CRB) and the ISA
- large reduction of the number of positions requiring checks to just those working most closely and regularly with children and vulnerable adults.

When the new scheme is implemented, criminal records checks will include a check to find out whether an individual is on the adults' barred list, the children's barred list or both. Employers will be able to check the status of the potential employee's criminal record certificate online; a new CRB check will only be requested when changes are indicated. (The BMA has guidance on its website on vetting and barring[49] and this is also discussed in Chapter 19, pages 794–795.)

When offering employment, GP practices routinely check the colleague's indemnity and registration details. For other information, they generally rely heavily on references provided. The importance of providing accurate testimonials is paramount (see Chapter 21, page 872). Trusts carry out health screening and pre-employment checks on all staff and similar checks are made in relation to volunteer workers. In addition, all staff, volunteers, and people such as students doing work observation must be aware of the obligation to maintain patient confidentiality and should be asked to sign a declaration to that effect (see Chapter 18, pages 755–757).

Abusive behaviour by health professionals

Very high standards of behaviour are expected of all health professionals. Any action which exploits patients' vulnerability, financially, emotionally or sexually is subject to severe penalties. The 2004 Ayling Committee (mentioned above) urged changes in the way that patient complaints and staff concerns were handled. It called for guidance to be developed for employers and regulatory authorities about how to recognise 'sexualised behaviour' among NHS employees. This was picked up in 2006 by the GMC, which published guidance on sexualised behaviour by either health professionals or patients.

GMC guidance on sexualised behaviour

'You must never make a sexual advance towards a patient nor display 'sexualised behaviour'. Sexualised behaviour has been defined as 'acts, words or behaviour designed or intended to arouse or gratify sexual impulses and desires'. If you have grounds to believe that a colleague has, or may have demonstrated sexualised behaviour with a patient, you must take appropriate steps without delay so that your concerns are investigated and patients protected. Where there is a suspicion that a sexual assault or other criminal activity has taken place, it should be reported to the police. If you are not sure what to do, discuss your concerns with an impartial colleague or contact your defence body, a professional organisation or the GMC for advice. You should respect patient confidentiality wherever possible when reporting your concerns but the safety of patients must come first at all times and takes precedence over maintaining confidentiality. If you are satisfied that it is necessary to identify the patient, wherever practical you should seek the patient's consent to disclosure of any information and, if this is refused, inform the patient of your intention to disclose the information. In all cases where a patient reports a breach of sexual boundaries, appropriate support and assistance must be offered to the patient. All such reports must be properly investigated, whatever the apparent credibility of the patient. If a patient displays sexualised behaviour, wherever possible treat them politely and considerately and try to re-establish a professional boundary.'[50]

Any form of intimate personal contact between doctors and patients raises questions of professional misconduct. Such contact need not necessarily be sexual to be abusive or exploitative. The GMC tells doctors that they must not use their 'professional position to pursue a sexual or improper emotional relationship with a patient or someone close to them'.[51] Doctors who abuse or exploit patients are liable to disciplinary action by the GMC and prosecution under the criminal law. They are likely to be struck off the medical register if it is shown that they have used their position to establish an improper relationship with a patient or a patient's close relative. Health professionals who have grounds to suspect that a colleague is abusing or exploiting patients should take steps to have the matter promptly investigated. In January 2008, the Council for Healthcare Regulatory Excellence (CHRE) published guidance[52] on sexual boundaries in the doctor–patient relationship. It consists of three documents covering the following:

- the responsibilities of health professionals
- guidance for regulatory bodies' fitness to practise panels
- guidance for higher education institutions and training providers.

In 2009, CHRE published further information on sexual boundaries for patients and carers.[53]

GMC case example: abusive behaviour

A GP locum was found guilty by the GMC of serious professional misconduct for carrying out, without explanation, a breast examination on a patient complaining of earache and attempting to persuade her to consent to an internal examination. He asked the patient irrelevant questions of a sexual nature and refused her request for a chaperone.[54] In another case, a GP was struck off the register for carrying out an unnecessary breast examination on a pregnant 16-year-old patient. He carried out a rectal examination on another patient without explaining what it would involve or why it was necessary. He claimed that he did not discuss it with the patient as he thought she had a cancer phobia but agreed that he had failed to offer a chaperone when he should have done. He was also found guilty of embracing other patients, including an 11-year-old. The GMC Panel rejected his explanation that he was offering support and consolation and found him guilty of harming patients by touching them in ways they perceived as sexual, even if he did not.[55]

Managing personal relationships with patients

Boundaries may be inadvertently crossed, even when there is no intention to do so. Doctors sometimes enquire whether it is permissible to give apparently innocuous gifts, such as flowers or concert tickets, to patients who they know are having a difficult time but they need to be wary about how that might be interpreted by the patient. Personal gifts between doctors and patients can mean that professional boundaries cease to be seen as significant. Any emotional dependence between doctors and their patients, or the close relatives of patients, must be discouraged. Doctors have access to past health information about their patients and see them when they are feeling vulnerable, all of which puts patients at a disadvantage. Some circumstances need to be particularly carefully handled, such as when patients consult a doctor for emotional difficulties after a loss or bereavement. Any personal relationship in such circumstances is likely to be seen as a cause for disciplinary proceedings. Patients' relatives are also particularly vulnerable during the progress of a patient's acute or terminal illness. Doctors must ensure that inappropriate attachments or dependence are not allowed to develop. The BMA is occasionally contacted by doctors who, having acted completely properly, are concerned that during the progress of a long illness the spouse or close relative of a patient has become inappropriately dependent upon them. This can occur gradually over time if the doctor becomes the main focus for an otherwise isolated carer. Such situations are delicate and relatives may be particularly emotional, anticipating bereavement. Nevertheless, it is essential that an emotional distance is maintained. Wherever possible, other health and social care professionals should be involved and it may assist relatives to be put in touch with patient support groups. In the case of terminal illness, other members of the primary healthcare team and hospice outreach services may be able to share in providing support.

Although personal relationships can arise in good faith when doctors and patients meet in a purely social setting, it is essential that doctors take steps to establish and maintain clear boundaries. If they discover that a person with whom they are developing a relationship is also their patient, they should immediately cease the relationship or ensure that medical care is transferred to another doctor. In a secondary care setting, doctors must not embark on a personal relationship with a patient or a person close to a patient while they are responsible for an episode of care. Doctors sometimes ask for advice on how to handle a situation in which they feel attracted to a patient or the close relative of a patient and therefore need to ask that person to transfer to another doctor before it is clear whether or not a personal relationship is likely to grow. It can seem very presumptuous to ask patients to transfer, but this is advisable at an early stage if a personal relationship is intended.

Doctors' use of social media

Internet social media can blur the boundary between doctors' private and professional lives. Personal material uploaded onto social networking sites such as Facebook and Twitter intended only for friends may be accessible to a wider audience, such as patients and employers. In 2011, the BMA became concerned about the use of such media, as well as some blogs and internet fora aimed specifically at doctors and medical students.[56] It appeared that some health professionals were unknowingly exposing themselves to risk by uploading very personal material. Although such media provide them with opportunities to discuss aspects of clinical practice, great caution is required if mention is made of specific medical cases. Disclosing information about patients that could be identifiable, without consent, would breach GMC standards and could give rise to legal complaints. Informal discussion that mentions patients should be avoided. Even if cases are anonymised, any flippant or derogatory remarks could undermine public trust.

Doctors sometimes divulge personal information about themselves when talking to patients face-to-face but the potential disclosure via social media can go far beyond what they would normally allow. Examples have arisen of patients attempting to strike up a personal relationship after discovering information about their doctor through a social networking site.[57] Entering into informal relationships with patients on social media can increase the likelihood of inappropriate boundary transgressions and difficult ethical issues can arise if, for example, doctors acquire information about patients that has not been disclosed in a clinical consultation. Doctors and medical students who receive 'friend requests' from patients are advised to decline. Some sites have privacy settings that put restrictions on access but not all users activate these and not all content on the web can be protected in this way. Medical students need to be conscious about the image they present on social media. Guidance published jointly by the GMC and Medical Schools Council (MSC) reminds them that because they 'have certain privileges and responsibilities different from those of other students . . . different standards of professional behaviour are expected of them.'[58] American research into the material posted online by medical students found patient confidentiality violations; instances of discriminatory language and profanity; and depictions of intoxication and illicit substance use, which in some cases resulted in official warnings from medical schools and dismissal.[59]

Doctors and medical students should also be aware of their ethical obligations if they recommend or mention online any healthcare organisation or pharmaceutical product in which they have a financial interest. Even if they blog anonymously, such material may be viewed by the public as an objective recommendation. Failing to declare conflicts of interest could undermine public trust, compromise the professionalism of authors and risk referral to the GMC. People can often feel less inhibited when posting comments online and as a result may say things they would not express in other circumstances. Posting comments under a username does not guarantee anonymity as comments can be traced back to the original author. Doctors and medical students need to exercise sound judgement when posting online and avoid making gratuitous, unsubstantiated or unsustainable comments about individuals or organisations. Defamation law can apply to any comments posted on the web, irrespective of whether they are made in a personal or professional capacity. Defamation is the act of making an unjustified statement about a person or organisation that is considered to harm their reputation. If an individual makes a statement that is alleged to be defamatory, it could result in legal action against either the individual or the organisation they are representing.

Gifts and bequests

The GMC emphasises that doctors must not exploit patients, such as by encouraging them to make loans, gifts or donations to any organisation or individual.[60] NHS employees are prohibited from accepting substantial gifts from patients or other people. Inexpensive items, such as diaries or calendars, or small tokens of gratitude from patients or their relatives, can be accepted. Doctors who are not NHS employees, such as private doctors and GPs, can accept unsolicited gifts from patients but it would be a disciplinary offence to demand them or exert any pressure to obtain a donation. Doctors should make clear to patients that the quality of care is not influenced by the provision or absence of gifts. The BMA often receives enquiries from GPs who are aware that patients intend to leave them substantial amounts of money or property in their will. Again it is important that the patient knows that the care they receive is not contingent upon, or influenced in any way, by the promise of such gifts. The BMA also advises that in those cases, the GP who may benefit from the patient's will should not be involved in assessing that patient's capacity because that would involve a conflict of interests. If an assessment of testamentary capacity is needed, this should be undertaken by a doctor who has no financial interest in the outcome and the patient should be told why this is advisable. Transparency is important in the handling of donations. In England and Wales, the Health and Social Care Act 2001 made provision for a reporting and recording system for gifts, and Regulations concerning the acceptance by GPs of gifts from patients came into force in March 2004.[61] These specify that a register should be kept of gifts from patients or their relatives that have a value of £100 or more unless the gift is unconnected with the provision of services.

These regulations cover England; equivalent sets of rules operate in the other UK countries. The register of gifts should include the donor's name and the nature of the gift.

Summary – recognising responsibilities and boundaries

- Responsibility for maintaining boundaries lies with doctors.
- Doctors are responsible for taking steps to check if colleagues are a risk to patients and must speak out where that is the case.
- In cases where tensions are foreseeable, such as when staff are also patients, advance discussion of the problems should take place so that all are clear about their own rights and duties.
- Abuse by doctors – emotional, sexual or financial – is likely to result in erasure from the register.

Patients' responsibilities

'Responsibilisation'

'Responsibilisation' is a rather clumsy term that 'refers to a movement that arose initially out of criticisms of social welfare practices that were seen as destroying individual responsibility and encouraging dependency.'[62] By strongly supporting the concept of patient autonomy, providing public health information about lifestyle choices regarding smoking, diet and alcohol use and urging that patients have more say in treatment decisions, the BMA has long hoped that patients would be empowered and encouraged to exercise a greater role in maintaining their health. The converse is not true, however, and the Association has traditionally opposed the notion that patients should be penalised in some way if their behaviour has contributed to their illness or injury.

Most patients are generally aware of the importance of taking steps to remain healthy, including completing any course of treatment. They have choices about whether to accept medical advice and are more likely to do so when the risks and options have been clearly explained to them (see also the section on concordance in Chapter 13, pages 539–541). The doctor's role is to encourage and support patients in maintaining their health, without being judgemental about habits that potentially undermine it. As is stressed throughout this chapter, the main responsibility for making the doctor–patient relationship work well rests with doctors. For their part, patients should be willing to accept information about their health and respect the health professionals who provide it.

Patients' responsibilities within the health service

The BMA supports the provision of information to patients that not only clarifies their rights, but also mentions their responsibilities to use health services appropriately. They should keep appointments, continue treatment they have agreed to follow and provide doctors with relevant information. The NHS Constitution for England[63] set out what the Government considers to be patients' duties, including an obligation to take some personal responsibility for their health, register with a GP, provide accurate information about their health, follow agreed courses of treatment or discuss them with a doctor if unable to do so, and participate in public health programmes such as vaccination. These responsibilities are not binding. The BMA's Patient Liaison Group has produced brief web-based guidance for patients about how they can, for example, get involved in providing feedback on NHS services or express concerns and minimise risks of spreading infection.[64]

Sometimes patients make unreasonable demands, such as unjustified demands for home visits and misuse of emergency services, which waste resources. In some cases, the patients are mentally ill and lacking insight into the effects of their behaviour. In others, they regard the health facility as a general source of social support. Offering counselling or arranging for the patient to have an advocate can help to modify the excessive or inappropriate demands, as can providing information about other possible sources of support and advice. Alternatively, healthcare staff may arrange a meeting or case conference with the patient to establish a reasonable agreement about how the problems can be handled. Establishing clear boundaries about the regularity of contact, case review and the limits to what can be provided by the health service may be the only feasible way forward.

Can violent or aggressive people expect to receive medical care?

Aggression includes racist or abusive remarks, threats and physical assault. Inappropriate words or behaviour that cause distress, as well as the use of force to cause injury or discomfort come within the definition of violence. Such behaviour has been discussed in 'zero tolerance' campaigns since 2000. Whether or not doctors are obliged to treat violent people depends on the reason for the behaviour and the urgency of the patient's need. Sometimes the reasons are complex and the violence or passive aggression is a facet of the patient's distress and inability to cope with the situation in which they find themselves. Unexpectedly aggressive behaviour can also be caused by patients' medical condition or their medication. Identifying whether there is an organic cause is essential when patients appear to be acting out of character. In cases where violent behaviour is a facet of mental illness, the patient may have to be restrained and possibly admitted to hospital for assessment. In facilities providing care for people with mental illness, it is essential that all staff have appropriate training in conflict avoidance and management of aggression. It is also essential that physical restraint and sedation are limited to situations where they are necessary to prevent harm to the patient or to other people.

When it is not a symptom of their illness, patients who are threatening or racially abusive should not be denied urgent treatment or necessary immediate care, if this can be provided safely. In some health premises, however, it has proved necessary, as a last resort, to withhold treatment from some patients. Health facilities should be advised to develop their own local policies on withholding treatment in these circumstances. Withholding treatment is appropriate only when abusive behaviour is likely to:

- prejudice any benefit for the patient
- prejudice the safety of people providing treatment
- lead staff to believe that they cannot undertake their duties properly
- result in damage to property, or
- prejudice the safety of other patients.

If any violent patient does not need treatment urgently, or when treatment is impossible because of the patient's behaviour, the police can be called to remove the patient, either from hospital or primary care premises. If the patient is detained, a forensic physician may supervise him or her until appropriate treatment can be given. Doctors and health facility personnel may need to take legal advice if they intend to ban from medical premises some patients or their relatives (but see also the violent patient scheme mentioned below, in which the patient is forewarned that this is likely). In some cases, as a result of a previous assault or threatened assault, bail conditions may specify a prohibition on returning. Primary care practices can also request the immediate removal from their lists of any patient who is threatening or violent. In some premises, special segregated areas or after hours clinics deal with persistently aggressive patients in a secure environment with police or security officers on hand. Such patients should be allowed to return to normal surgeries if their behaviour improves.

Some health facilities use a 'violent patient scheme' (VPS) which sets out the framework within which patients identified as prone to violence receive treatment in a restricted manner. For some patients, being told that they are included in the scheme and being given an explanation about what they have to do in order to come out of it is a sobering experience. Clear criteria are set as to what constitutes unacceptable behaviour and the patient is made aware of these and the implications of continuing to be aggressive, which may include the inconvenience of having to travel further for treatment. If the patient's actions continue to meet the VPS criteria, a report is written and copied to the patient's record. A VPS review panel receives reports from doctors of all such instances and the patient may be instructed not to attend the usual health facility or attend only with a police escort. If the patient is removed from a primary care list, other relevant practices are notified that the patient is on the VPS scheme and should not be registered by them but registered for treatment with a specific VPS provider. The VPS provider sees the patient in a secure setting which may involve police escorts and completes a report after each appointment. Patient behaviour is reviewed periodically with the intention of allowing the patient to register again in the usual manner.

Patient confidentiality and violent patient markers

All healthcare premises should have clear policies on the handling of violent people and these can be publicised in leaflets or posters. Patients should be made aware that there are limits to their rights to treatment and to confidentiality. They should know that violent or threatening behaviour is unacceptable and can result in them being removed from healthcare premises, and information about them being passed on to other healthcare providers and possibly the police. In the past, violent patient markers were used in primary care and NHS trusts for tagging the paper health records of certain patients and alerting healthcare professionals who came into contact with them. With electronic records, other mechanisms exist as markers but need to be regularly reviewed. (This is discussed further in Chapter 6, pages 238–239.)

Advice from the Information Commissioner

To comply with the fairness element of the first data protection principle, as soon as the decision is made data controllers should inform individuals who are identified as being potentially violent that their records will indicate this. They should also be informed of the incident which led to them being so identified, to whom this information may be passed and when the decision to identify them as potentially violent will be removed or examined with a view to removal.[65]

In hospitals, senior staff and managers should be closely involved in establishing policies and making decisions about the treatment of aggressive individuals. Such decisions should not be left to unsupported junior doctors and nurses. In addition to advice from the Department of Health, a range of guidance covers aspects of conflict management and dealing with aggression.

Summary – patients' responsibilities

- The obligations of doctors to treat patients politely and considerately should be mirrored by patients.
- Patients are not obliged to receive information or follow medical advice but should be prepared to consider them.
- Patients should be aware that if they threaten or attack health professionals, this may affect their ability to access services and their actions may also be flagged up to other treatment providers.

References

1 General Medical Council (2006) *Good Medical Practice*, GMC, London.
2 Reeves R, Bruster S. (2009) *Better Together: Scotland's patient experience programme. Patient Priorities for Inpatient Care*, Scottish Government, Edinburgh. Available at: www.scotland.gov.uk (accessed 12 April 2011).
3 Paine C. (2002) Il dissoluto punito: medicine in the age of blame. *Med Leg J* **70**, 161–75, p.63.
4 Leake CD (ed.) (1927) *Percival's Medical Ethics*, Williams and Wilkins, Baltimore, p.71.
5 General Medical Council (2006) *Good Medical Practice*, GMC, London, paras 20–1.
6 Nuffield Council on Bioethics (2010) *Medical profiling and online medicine: the ethics of personalised healthcare in a consumer age*, Nuffield Council on Bioethics, London, p.28.
7 Nuffield Council on Bioethics (2010) *Medical profiling and online medicine: the ethics of personalised healthcare in a consumer age*, Nuffield Council on Bioethics, London, p.29.
8 General Medical Council (2008) *Personal Beliefs and Medical Practice*, GMC, London.
9 British Medical Association (2008) *Access to Healthcare for Asylum Seekers and Refused Asylum Seekers*, BMA, London.
10 Jackson E. (2010) *Medical Law: text, cases and materials*, 2nd edn, Oxford University Press, Oxford, p.104.
11 *Barnett v Chelsea and Kensington Hospital Management Committee* (1969) 1 QB 428.
12 Gordon R. (ed.) (1993) *The Literary Companion to Medicine*, Sinclair Stevenson, London, p.2.
13 General Medical Council (2006) *Good Medical Practice*, GMC, London.
14 Department of Health (2009) *Religion or Belief: a practical guide for the NHS*, DH, London.
15 Gledhill R (2009) Victory for suspended Christian nurse. *The Times* (February 7). Available at: www.timesonline.co.uk (accessed 12 April 2011).
16 General Medical Council (2008) *Personal Beliefs and Medical Practice*, GMC, London.
17 Mihill C. (2000) *Shaping Tomorrow: issues facing general practice in the new millennium*, BMA, London.
18 Macdonald S. (2003) Doctors are servants of patients, says chief medical officer. *BMJ* **326**, 569.
19 General Medical Council (2008) *Consent: patients and doctors making decisions together*, GMC, London, para 31.
20 General Medical Council (2008) *Personal Beliefs and Medical Practice*, GMC, London, paras 27–8.
21 Jones G. (2003) Prescribing and taking medicines: concordance is a fine theory but is mostly not being practised. *BMJ* **327**, 819–20.
22 British Medical Association (2009) *The Ethics of Caring for Older People*, Wiley, Chichester.
23 Payne SA. (2002) Balancing information needs: dilemmas in producing patient information leaflets. *Health Informatics J* **8**, 174–179, p.175.
24 British Medical Association (2009) *The Interface Between NHS and Private Treatment: a practical guide for doctors in England, Wales and Northern Ireland*, BMA, London.
25 General Medical Council (2006) *Good Medical Practice*, GMC, London, para 30.
26 General Medical Council (2006) *Good Medical Practice*, GMC, London, para 31.
27 *Froggatt v Chesterfield and North Derbyshire NHS Trust* [2002] All ER(D) 218; [2002] WL 31676323.
28 House of Commons Health Committee (2004) *Elder Abuse. Second Report of Session 2003–04. Volume 1*, The Stationery Office, London, para 65.

29 Mental Welfare Commission for Scotland (2006) *Covert Medication: legal and practical guidance*, MWCS, Edinburgh. Available at: www.mwcscot.org.uk (accessed 13 February 2011).

30 General Medical Council (2011) *Making and using visual and audio recordings of patients*, GMC, London.

31 General Medical Council (2011) *Making and using visual and audio recordings of patients*, GMC, London, paras 11–12.

32 The Regulation of Investigatory Powers Act 2000 covers England, Wales and Northren Ireland. Scotland is covered by the Regulation of Investigatory Powers (Scotland) Act 2000.

33 Royal College of Paediatrics and Child Health (2009) *Fabricated or Induced Illness by Carers (FII): a practical guide for paediatricians*, RCPCH, London, pp.27–8 and 50.

34 General Medical Council (2003) Covert video recording is unacceptable. *GMC News* **17**, 8.

35 General Medical Council (2006) *Good Medical Practice*, GMC, London, para 74.

36 General Medical Council (2006) *Good Medical Practice*, GMC, London, para 3 (e).

37 General Medical Council (2006) *Good Medical Practice*, GMC, London, paras 38–40.

38 General Medical Council (2006) *Good Medical Practice*, GMC, London, para 5.

39 General Medical Council (2006) *Good Medical Practice*, GMC, London, paras 77–9.

40 Department of Health Clinical Governance Support Team (2005) *Guidance on the Role and Effective Use of Chaperones in Primary and Community Care*. Available at: www.lmc.org.uk (accessed 12 April 2011).

41 General Medical Council (2006) *Maintaining Boundaries*, GMC, London, paras 10–13.

42 Royal College of Obstetricians and Gynaecologists (1997) *Intimate Examinations*, RCOG, London.

43 General Medical Council (2006) *Maintaining Boundaries*, GMC, London, paras 9, 14 and 15.

44 Anon. (2009) Sexual abuse allowed to carry on, report shows. *Health Care Risk Report*. Available at: www.healthcareriskreport.com (accessed 20 January 2010).

45 NHS Employment Policy Branch (2003) *Pre-employment checks for NHS staff [extract taken from HSG 98/064]*, NHS Employment Policy Branch, Leeds. National Assembly for Wales (2003) *Pre and post-employment checks for all persons working in the NHS in Wales*, National Assembly for Wales, Cardiff (WHC 007).

46 Department of Health (2004) *Protection of Vulnerable Adults Scheme in England and Wales: a practical guide*, DH, London.

47 Northern Constabulary (2005) *Protecting Vulnerable Adults: good practice guidance and procedures*, Highland Council, Inverness.

48 British Medical Association (2011) *Briefing on the Vetting and Barring Scheme: BMA position*, BMA, London.

49 British Medical Association (2010) *Vetting and Barring Scheme. ISA Regulations: guidance for doctors in secondary care*, BMA, London.

50 General Medical Council (2006) *Maintaining Boundaries*, GMC, London, paras 20–6.

51 General Medical Council (2006) *Good Medical Practice*, GMC, London, para 32.

52 Council for Healthcare Regulatory Excellence (CHRE) guidance documents can be accessed at: www.chre.org.uk.

53 Council for Healthcare Regulatory Excellence (2009) *Clear Sexual Boundaries Between Healthcare Professionals and Patients: information for patients and carers*, CHRE, London.

54 General Medical Council (2002) Conduct Committee hearing, 11–15 March.

55 General Medical Council (2009) Doctor crosses boundaries and abuses patient trust. *GMC Today*, May/June.

56 British Medical Association (2011) *Using Social Media: practical and ethical guidance for doctors and medical students*, BMA, London.

57 British Medical Association (2011) *Using Social Media: practical and ethical guidance for doctors and medical students*, BMA, London.

58 General Medical Council, Medical Schools Council (2009) *Medical Students: professional values and fitness to practise*, GMC, London, para 3.

59 Chretien KC, Greysen SR, Chretien JP, *et al.* (2009) Online posting of unprofessional content by medical students. *JAMA* **302**(12), 1309–15.

60 General Medical Council (2006) *Good Medical Practice*, GMC, London, para 72.

61 National Health Service (General Medical Services Contracts) Regulations 2004, SI 2004/291.

62 Nuffield Council on Bioethics (2010) *Medical Profiling and Online Medicine: the ethics of personalised healthcare in a consumer age*, Nuffield Council on Bioethics, London, p.38.

63 Department of Health (2009) The NHS Constitution. Available at: www.nhs.uk (accessed 30 March 2011).

64 British Medical Association (2011) *Working together for better health*. BMA, London. Available at: www.bma.org.uk (accessed 11 April 2011).

65 Information Commissioner (2002) *Data Protection Act 1998 compliance advice. Violent warning markers: use in the public sector*. Information Commissioner, Wilmslow, p.2.

2: Consent, choice and refusal: adults with capacity

The questions covered in this chapter include the following.

- What is the purpose of seeking consent from patients?
- Who should seek consent?
- What types of information should patients be given before consenting to treatment?
- When is a signed consent form needed?
- How long is consent valid for?
- When may patients refuse treatment?
- What are the limits to a patient's consent?

The nature and purpose of consent

Decisions about medical treatment are ideally made following discussion, with the doctor's clinical expertise and the patient's individual needs and preferences being shared in order to select the best treatment option. The patient's consent is then the trigger that allows treatment or examination to take place. Seeking consent from patients therefore forms a crucial part of the practice of almost every doctor. It is central to the partnership between doctor and patient, with each having a role in decisions about treatment or care. Patients should be listened to and their views respected in the course of discussion. This should involve the sharing of information required by patients in order for them to reach decisions for themselves (see the discussion in Chapter 1). Consent is central to good medical practice.

Legal and ethical requirements often overlap in medicine and this is particularly true with issues of consent. Many medical and surgical interventions could be harmful, but are acceptable because the expected benefits outweigh the harms. Patients agree to the invasive procedures of medicine, which, under any other circumstances, could lead to criminal charges. Doctors must be aware that if they fail to seek consent from patients who have capacity (patients who lack capacity are discussed in Chapter 3 and treatment in emergencies is covered in Chapter 15) they could be vulnerable to criminal prosecution for battery or assault, or a challenge in civil law for negligence or breach of the patient's human rights.

Consent is a legal requirement, clearly established in case law; the purpose of consent is not, however, purely or even primarily to protect doctors from legal challenge. Seeking consent is also a moral requirement, and the British Medical Association (BMA) believes that respect for others and their rights lies at the heart of this issue. Society values individuals and their dignity. Adult patients with capacity have both an ethical and a legal right to self-determination and to respect for their autonomy. This entails them having choice about what happens to their bodies. In addition to the moral importance of consent,

Medical Ethics Today: The BMA's Handbook of Ethics and Law, Third Edition. Sophie Brannan, Eleanor Chrispin, Martin Davies, Veronica English, Rebecca Mussell, Julian Sheather and Ann Sommerville.
© 2012 BMA Medical Ethics Department. Published 2012 by Blackwell Publishing Ltd.

the need for patient cooperation with examination and treatment is a very practical reason for seeking patient consent.

It would be wrong to assume that consent is relevant only when initiating an examination or treatment. Consent is a process and not a one-off event or box-ticking exercise that happens in isolation. It is important that there is continuing discussion to reflect the evolving nature of treatment. Clearly, the opportunity to consent to treatment is counterbalanced by a right to refuse it. This chapter therefore covers issues of the refusal of treatment by patients with capacity, as well as their consent (issues relating specifically to consent and children and young people are addressed in Chapter 4).

General principles

- A patient gives consent when he or she has capacity, is adequately informed and voluntarily agrees to treatment, examination or another aspect of healthcare.
- Before examining or treating adult patients with capacity, doctors must obtain patient consent,[1] except in emergencies where it is not possible to do so or where the law prescribes otherwise, for example where compulsory treatment is authorised by mental health legislation.[2]
- Adults are always presumed to have capacity unless demonstrated otherwise.
- Unexpected or apparently irrational decisions do not mean a patient lacks capacity, but may indicate a need for further information or explanation.
- For consent to be valid the patient must:
  - have capacity
  - be offered sufficient information to make an informed decision
  - be acting voluntarily and free from undue pressure
  - be aware that he or she can refuse.
- Patients may have capacity to make some healthcare decisions but not others. Their capacity may also fluctuate over time.
- Patients may give explicit or express consent orally, in writing or by other means of communication available to them. They may also imply consent non-verbally, for example by complying with the proposed examination or treatment.
- Adult patients with capacity are entitled to refuse treatment, even where treatment would clearly benefit their health. The only exception to this rule is where the treatment is for a mental disorder and the patient is detained under mental health legislation (see Chapter 3, pages 121–122).[3]

Standards and good practice guidance

There is a considerable amount of written guidance on consent, from regulatory, professional and indemnifying bodies, as well as from government departments in England, Wales, Scotland and Northern Ireland.[4] This guidance has not necessarily guaranteed that good practice is always followed when consent is sought in practice. In the past, the BMA has been concerned by the lack of emphasis placed on the initial explanation given to the patient and the provision of continuing opportunity for discussion in order that the patient can raise any questions or concerns.[5] Initiatives from the UK health departments have sought to raise standards and have contributed to a new context for healthcare providers' and health professionals' policy and processes on consent. Raising standards and embedding good practice cannot, however, be achieved through a directive, top-down approach. The Department of Health in England stresses that it is important for doctors and other healthcare professionals to have the freedom to develop local solutions to local issues, while ensuring that policies and practices on consent, developed within their own organisations, are in line with the law and available guidance.[6]

The process of seeking consent

Consent is not a one-off event, but involves a process of information giving and explanation that facilitates informed decision making. It is essential that informing and involving patients, in a way that they can understand, is not seen as 'additional' to medical practice, but as an integral part of it.

In much of healthcare, informed patients indicate their consent through actions, such as opening their mouth for examination, offering an arm for blood pressure to be taken or attending a doctor and giving information about an illness. Consent that is indicated in this way is often termed 'implied' consent and applies only to the immediate procedure, and not necessarily to subsequent tests or treatment that flow from it. However, acquiescence when a patient does not know what the intervention entails, or that there is an option of refusing, is not 'consent'.

Consent that is given orally, in writing or via other means of communication available to the patient, is known as 'explicit', or 'express', consent. A signed consent form is simply prima facie evidence that the process of information giving and explanation has taken place. It is the quality and clarity of the information provided, along with the capacity of the patient and the voluntariness of the consent given, which determine the validity of the consent, rather than a signature on a piece of paper (see pages 72–73).

Capacity to give valid consent

In order for patients to be able to make choices about care, they must have the mental capacity to make a decision. The terms mental 'capacity' and 'competence' are often used interchangeably, although the former is most often used in law and is used throughout this text when referring to adult patients. Adult patients (those 18 years old and over in England, Wales and Northern Ireland, and 16 years old and over in Scotland) are presumed to have the capacity to make treatment decisions unless there is evidence to the contrary. They can decide on whatever basis they wish, and decisions can still be valid even if they appear to others to be irrational or unjustified. Irrational decisions that are based on a misperception of reality, on the other hand, such as believing that blood is poisoned because it is red,[7] or that are clearly contrary to previously expressed wishes, may indicate a lack of capacity and it will be necessary to consider further whether the patient has the capacity to make a decision. A patient who has a mental disorder or impairment of mental functioning does not, necessarily, lack the capacity to consent to treatment. Similarly, a lack of capacity should not be simply assumed based on factors such as disability, appearance, behaviour or age. Older hospital patients and care home residents, for example, have the same rights as other patients and, where they have capacity, must not be subjected to medical procedures, treatment, protective measures or restraint, unless they consent.[8]

Where there are reasons to doubt an adult patient's capacity to make decisions, an individual assessment should be made. This assessment is a matter for clinical judgement, guided by professional practice and subject to legal requirements. The Mental Capacity Act 2005 in England and Wales sets out a statutory framework for making decisions for people who lack the capacity to make such decisions themselves. The 2005 Act establishes overarching statutory principles governing these decisions, setting out who can make them and when. It also sets out the legal requirements for assessing whether or not a person lacks the capacity to make a decision.[9] In Scotland, these issues are covered by the Adults with Incapacity (Scotland) Act 2000. At the time of writing, mental capacity legislation for Northern Ireland was being drafted (see Chapter 3, pages 140–141). Meanwhile, issues of capacity in Northern Ireland are governed by common law. Guidance on decision making for patients who lack capacity can be found in Chapter 3. The guidance on capacity set out below reflects both the legal requirements and good medical practice applicable throughout the UK.

In order to give valid consent, the patient must have capacity; to have capacity to make decisions about medical treatment, patients should be able to:

- understand (with the use of communication aids, if appropriate) in simple language what the medical treatment is, its nature and purpose, and why it is being proposed for them
- understand its principal benefits, risks and alternatives
- understand in broad terms what will be the consequences of not receiving the proposed treatment
- retain the information for long enough to make an effective decision
- weigh the information, balancing the risks and benefits, to arrive at a choice
- communicate their decision.

A patient can definitively lack capacity, for example when he or she is unconscious; likewise, many patients will definitely have capacity. However, the boundary will sometimes be uncertain. Patients who would otherwise have capacity may be temporarily incapable of giving valid consent (see, for example, the case of MB discussed in Chapter 3, pages 99–100). People's abilities fluctuate, often in response to temporary factors, such as confusion, shock, fatigue, pain, fear, drunkenness or the effects of medication,[10] and because capacity is judged according to the particular decision that has to be made, at the time it needs to be made, patients who are not able to make complex choices may be capable of making simpler decisions. Where a decision can be put off, in the case of temporary intoxication for example, it should be. It is important that health professionals give patients who need it practical assistance to maximise their decision-making capacity. Patients should not be regarded as incapable of making or communicating a decision unless all practical steps have been taken to maximise their ability to do so.[11] There is further advice on enhancing capacity for patients who have some impairment in Chapter 3 (see, for example, page 106).

Patients with capacity are able to make provision for a time in the future when they may lose decision-making capacity. They have the option to make advance decisions or to appoint a welfare attorney to make healthcare decisions on their behalf in the event that they lose capacity. (This is discussed in Chapter 3).

Summary – capacity to give valid consent

- Adult patients are presumed to have capacity to make treatment decisions unless there is evidence to the contrary.
- A patient's capacity should be assessed on an individual basis and should not be assumed on grounds of disability, age, appearance or the fact that the patient's decisions appear to others to be irrational or unjustified.

- Capacity is decision specific and patients' abilities can fluctuate over time.
- Patients should not be regarded as incapable of making or communicating a decision unless all practical steps have been taken to maximise their ability to do so.
- Patients with capacity can make advance decisions or appoint a welfare attorney to make healthcare decisions on their behalf in the event that they lose capacity.

Who should seek consent?

The BMA believes that ideally the doctor recommending the treatment or intervention should provide an explanation to the patient about what the procedure involves – including a discussion of the various treatment options, the alternatives available, the prognosis and the risks associated with the intervention – and obtain the patient's consent. In a hospital setting, this will normally be the senior clinician.

The doctor providing treatment also has responsibility for ensuring that the patient has been given sufficient time to make the decision about his or her treatment, and that consent is valid. Responsibility in law rests with the doctor who is in overall charge of the care, usually a consultant or GP. Once a GP has referred a patient to a specialist, responsibility passes to the specialist. Additionally, doctors who take responsibility for a particular aspect of care, for example anaesthesia, should ensure that they seek consent before proceeding. (For further guidance on the consent process for anaesthetic procedures see page 65.)

The General Medical Council (GMC) allows doctors to delegate explanation, discussion and seeking consent to their colleagues in certain circumstances, but it does not permit doctors to delegate the process of seeking consent to other doctors who are unfamiliar with the procedure. It states:

If you are the doctor undertaking an investigation or providing treatment, it is your responsibility to discuss it with the patient. If this is not practical, you can delegate the responsibility to someone else, provided you make sure that the person you delegate to:

- is suitably trained and qualified
- has sufficient knowledge of the proposed investigation or treatment, and understands the risks involved
- understands, and agrees to act in accordance with, the guidance in this booklet.

If you delegate, you are still responsible for making sure that the patient has been given enough time and information to make an informed decision, and has given their consent, before you start any investigation or treatment.[12]

Health professionals are also reminded that when they are providing information as part of seeking consent, they 'must be competent to do so: either because they themselves carry out the procedure, or because they have received specialist training in advising patients about this procedure, have been assessed, are aware of their own knowledge limitations and are subject to audit'.[13] This is vital if patients are to be provided with adequate information and given an ongoing opportunity to ask questions and raise concerns.

If there has been a significant time lapse between consent being given and the procedure being carried out, it is crucial to reaffirm the patient's agreement. Clinical circumstances may have changed by the time the patient is due to undergo the procedure and the risks associated with it could have altered significantly if, for example, the patient's condition has deteriorated. As with the initial process of seeking consent, this further discussion of the patient's wishes should ideally be undertaken either by the clinician who originally proposed the procedure or by the clinician who is due to undertake the intervention. However, it may, in the circumstances outlined by the GMC (see above), be delegated to another member of the healthcare team. The delegated person must possess the necessary communication skills and should know where to seek help if he or she is unable to respond to the patient's questions (good communication is discussed in Chapter 1).

In addition to the more formal part of the process of seeking consent, in which the patient indicates a decision about treatment, throughout the process other members of the healthcare team are involved. Patients often find it easier to communicate with nurses and junior doctors than with more senior clinicians, and these professionals can have an important role in clarifying the information the patient has been given and answering questions. Senior clinicians should provide information and support for their junior colleagues in this process (multi-disciplinary working is discussed in more detail in Chapter 19).

Summary – who should seek consent?

- The doctor recommending a treatment or intervention ideally should provide an explanation to the patient about what it involves, such as the risks and benefits, obtain the patient's consent and ensure that consent is valid.
- Doctors who take responsibility for a particular aspect of care, for example anaesthesia, should ensure that they seek consent before proceeding.
- Doctors may delegate explanation, discussion and seeking consent only where delegation is to a colleague who is suitably trained and qualified, and sufficiently familiar with the procedure to be undertaken.
- Where the process of seeking consent is delegated, the doctor who is in overall charge of care is still responsible for making sure that the patient has given valid consent before treatment begins.
- Other members of the healthcare team can have an important role in the consent process and should be supported by senior colleagues where they are asked by patients to clarify information or answer questions about treatment.

Providing information

Providing patients with sufficient information to enable them to make an informed choice is both an ethical and a legal requirement. Without the provision of information about the nature and purpose of a treatment or procedure, any 'consent' obtained is invalid. Information-giving and communication skills are crucial to the process of information provision (for a discussion of the doctor–patient relationship see Chapter 1). Improving the quality of information available to patients is a crucial aspect of improving patient care.

Accessibility of information

Information is useful only if it is provided in a manner that is accessible and intelligible to the patient, and is given at a pace at which the recipient can understand. The use of clear, well-written, accurate and up-to-date patient information leaflets and audiovisual materials can be a useful aid to discussion. It should not be seen as a substitute for a personal consultation but a supplement to it. The BMA and GMC recommend the provision of written material wherever practicable. An advantage of these types of information is that patients can refer to them in their own time and share them with friends and family. It is important that the patient has time to digest the information and reflect on it, before and after making a decision, especially if the information is complex or the proposed treatment involves significant risks. However, the patient must also be aware if there is a time limit on making the decision. The BMA recommends that high quality patient information materials covering common clinical problems, for patients to review when ready to do so, should be available wherever possible.

The practical circumstances in which consent is sought for certain procedures can limit opportunities for clinicians to provide patients with the time and space required to absorb information properly, maximise their ability to communicate their concerns and decisions, and ask further questions. As a general principle, patients should be given information about anaesthetic or other procedures relevant to their treatment prior to the day on which the procedure itself is due to take place. Surgeons are likely to mention anaesthesia to patients when seeking consent for surgical procedures, but this will inevitably be more general information than that given by the anaesthetist. An example of good practice here is for patients to be given specific information, including written information, on the anaesthetic procedure related to their surgery, at a pre-operative assessment clinic. Pre-operative clinics are particularly important in the provision of information about risk, allowing patients to absorb the details in their own time and then raise questions or concerns with the anaesthetist at a later stage. (For guidance on how much information patients should be given about risk see pages 66–70.) The Royal College of Anaesthetists produces a comprehensive range of patient information leaflets[14] and detailed guidance on pre-operative assessments has been published by the Association of Anaesthetists of Great Britain and Ireland.[15] Where consent for anaesthesia is sought immediately prior to a surgical procedure, patients have only a very limited opportunity to reflect on the information they are given and consider their decision. Clinicians should be aware that they may be potentially negligent in law if they only provide information to patients, for the purposes of gaining consent, immediately before a surgical or day procedure, as this is likely to deprive patients of the opportunity to fully absorb the information, understand the nature and purpose of the procedure, and ask questions. Consent obtained in such circumstances may not, therefore, be adequately informed and, as a consequence, may be invalid.

In certain types of case, for example where a patient is very ill, hard of hearing or has difficulty communicating, there is sometimes a tendency to discuss the patient's care primarily with relatives, simply because it is quicker and easier than doing so with the patient. Usually, however, patients can be helped to express their views by being given appropriate aids, such as hearing aids or communicators. Taking the patient to a quiet room and minimising distractions may also help him or her to concentrate and express what he or she wants. Patients may also respond better to the approaches of particular staff or relatives. Occasionally, when communication difficulties are so severe that only family members are able to communicate with the patient, this may be the only option. Where this is the case, doctors must be aware of their duty to respect patient confidentiality (see Chapter 5).

It is obviously very important that translation services are provided for patients who require them in order to access information before consenting to treatment.

Type of information to be given

The GMC provides helpful guidance on the type of information that patients want or ought to know before deciding about treatment. Doctors must give patients the information they want or need about:

- the diagnosis and prognosis
- any uncertainties about the diagnosis or prognosis, including options for further investigations
- options for treating or managing the condition, including the option not to treat
- the purpose of a proposed investigation or treatment and what it will involve
- the potential benefits, risks and burdens, and the likelihood of success, for each option; this should include information, if available, about whether the benefits or risks are affected by which organisation or doctor is chosen to provide care
- whether a proposed investigation or treatment is part of a research programme or is an innovative treatment designed specifically for their benefit; information should include how the proposed treatment differs from the usual methods, why it is being offered, and if there are any risks or uncertainties
- the people who will be mainly responsible for and involved in their care, what their roles are, and to what extent students may be involved
- their right to refuse to take part in teaching or research
- their right to seek a second opinion
- any bills they will have to pay
- any conflicts of interest that the doctor, or healthcare organisation, may have
- any treatments that the doctor believes have greater potential benefit for the patient than those that the doctor, or his or her healthcare organisation, can offer.[16]

It is not sufficient for doctors simply to provide patients with a list of alternatives from which to select their preferred option. In seeking treatment, patients are generally looking for their doctor's advice about which procedure is likely to be the most effective or appropriate for them from a clinical perspective. Failing to give this advice can be as unhelpful as failing to offer any information about possible alternatives to the treatment proposed.

Amount of information to be given

Providing information, as part of the process of obtaining consent, is an integral aspect of the duty of care owed by the doctor to the patient.[17] Open access to, for example, web-based information resources and direct-to-consumer medical testing, can mean that patients expect an increasing amount of detailed information in order to feel sufficiently informed about a condition or proposed treatment. Patients do, however, vary in how much information they want about their diagnosis, prognosis and care. Doctors should presume that patients want to be well informed, and should volunteer information of the type that is necessary for patients to make informed choices. In addition, doctors are legally required to answer patients' questions truthfully and as fully as patients wish.[18] This may include responding to questions about treatments that are not funded on the National Health Service (NHS) (see Chapter 1, page 36 and Chapter 20, page 843), or referring patients to other sources of specialist advice if necessary. At times, however, information may need to be given with great care and sensitivity over a period of time (see, for example, Chapter 10 on the care of patients at the end of life).

Effective communication skills are key to obtaining valid consent; the clinician should deploy these skills in order to identify what the individual patient wants to know, and to convey the relevant information in an appropriate manner.

The precise amount and nature of information doctors should provide to patients, and the specific type of risk factors they should mention, varies according to the individual circumstances of the patient. Although there must be clinical assessment of the significance of particular information, the patient should be as fully informed as possible so that he or she can reach a decision in the knowledge of all the relevant circumstances. A variety of factors affect the manner in which, and how much, information should be given. Doctors must take steps to find out what patients want to know about their condition and its treatment, while avoiding making assumptions about what a patient might need or want to know, or consider significant. A careful balance must be struck between listening to what patients want and providing enough information in order that their decisions are informed. The GMC advises that:

> In deciding how much information to share with your patients you should take account of their wishes. The information you share should be in proportion to the nature of their condition, the complexity of the proposed investigation or treatment, and the seriousness of any potential side effects, complications or other risks.[19]

The legal duty to inform patients, as part of the doctor's duty to exercise reasonable care and skill, was established by the House of Lords in 1985.[20] This classic judgment is still often quoted.

Duty to warn about risks

Mrs Sidaway had been suffering from a recurrent pain in her neck, right shoulder and arms. She had an operation in 1974, which was performed by a senior neurosurgeon at the Bethlem Royal Hospital. The operation, even if performed with proper care and skill, carried an inherent risk of about 2 per cent of damage to the nerve roots and a less than 1 per cent risk of damage to the spinal cord, which had more serious implications. The surgeon reportedly warned Mrs Sidaway of the risk of damage to the nerve root but not of the risk to the spinal cord (although the surgeon died before the case was taken to court and so was unable to confirm this). Mrs Sidaway had the operation, during which her spinal cord was damaged and as a result she was severely disabled. She claimed damages for negligence against the hospital and the estate of the deceased surgeon on the grounds that the surgeon had failed to disclose or explain to her the risks inherent in the operation he had recommended. The case was taken to the House of Lords. Mrs Sidaway's claim was rejected at all levels.[21]

Despite giving different reasons for rejecting Mrs Sidaway's claim that she should have been warned about the risk of damage to her spinal cord, there was a general reliance among the judges on the approach that had been taken in the earlier case of Bolam,[22] which had determined that a doctor would not be considered negligent if his or her practice conformed to that of a responsible body of medical opinion held by practitioners skilled in the field in question (see Chapter 21, pages 857–861).

Lord Scarman's reasoning for rejecting Mrs Sidaway's appeal is held by many to encapsulate the true ethical position. Although it was not shared by the other judges at the time, his opinion marked the beginning of a shift towards a more patient-centred, rather than a professionally focused, test. In Lord Scarman's view, the standard for the amount of information to be given is not what the medical profession thinks appropriate, but ideally what the individual patient requires and, failing that, what the average 'prudent patient' would want to know.

The prudent patient

'If one considers the scope of the doctor's duty by beginning with the right of the patient to make his own decision whether he will or will not undergo the treatment proposed, the right to be informed of significant risk and the doctor's corresponding duty are easy to understand: for the proper implementation of the right requires that the doctor be under a duty to inform his patient of the material risks inherent in the treatment. And it is plainly right that a doctor may avoid liability for failure to warn of a material risk if he can show that he reasonably believed that communication to the patient of the existence of the risk would be detrimental to the health (including, of course, the mental health) of his patient.

Ideally, the court should ask itself whether in the particular circumstances the risk was such that this particular patient would think it significant if he was told it existed. I would think that, as a matter of ethics, this is the test of the doctor's duty. The law, however, operates not in Utopia but in the world as it is: and such an inquiry would prove in practice to be frustrated by the subjectivity of its aim and purpose. The law can, however, do the next best thing, and require the court to answer the question, what would a reasonably prudent patient think significant if in the situation of this patient. The 'prudent patient' cannot, however, always provide the answer for the obvious reason that he is a norm (like the man on the Clapham omnibus), not a real person: and certainly not the patient himself.'[23]

Since the Sidaway case there has been considerable debate about how much information should be routinely given about very exceptional risks, especially in the context of a growing recognition of the importance of patient autonomy. In *Pearce v United Bristol Healthcare NHS Trust*, an action was brought by a couple whose child died *in utero* when almost 3 weeks overdue. The mother had pleaded with the consultant either to induce the birth or carry out a caesarean section. He advised against both procedures, citing the high risks associated with induction and the long recovery time from caesarean section, but at the same time failed to disclose the risks of fetal death in the womb as a result of delay in delivery. In the Court of Appeal, Lord Woolf held that:

> if there is a significant risk which would affect the judgement of a reasonable patient, then in the normal course it is the responsibility of a doctor to inform the patient of that significant risk, if the information is needed so that the patient can determine for him or herself as to what course he or she should adopt.[24]

This judgment indicated a shift in emphasis, from what the 'reasonably prudent medical man' would see as a significant risk, towards the measure of significant risk as perceived by a 'reasonable patient'. The degree of information needed for informed consent was later considered by the House of Lords in 2004, in a case concerning a surgeon's omission to forewarn a patient of a risk that a back operation could cause paralysis even though the patient had specifically asked about the risk.

Failure to warn of the risks of surgery

Ms Chester suffered from severe back pain and was referred to a consultant neurosurgeon who advised her to undergo surgery on her spine. Three days later, with her consent, the surgeon carried out the operation. The surgery resulted in significant nerve damage which left Ms Chester partially paralysed. Although the procedure carried a small (1–2 per cent) but foreseeable risk that the patient would sustain such damage, the surgeon had failed to advise her of the risks that were inherent in the operation, even though she had specifically asked about those risks.

Both the court of first instance and Court of Appeal found that there had been no question of the surgery being negligently performed, as the operation had been skilfully carried out and the patient would probably have eventually gone ahead with the operation even if she had been informed of the risk. Nevertheless, the surgeon was found to have failed in his duty to mention it and to obtain properly informed consent, thereby resulting in negligence. The original ruling against the surgeon was upheld by the House of Lords.[25]

The majority of judges in the Chester case focused on the purpose of warning patients about risks. The duty of a doctor to warn of the dangers inherent in a particular procedure is intended to enable the patient to make an informed choice about whether to undergo the treatment recommended and, if so, under whose care and when. Although the failure to inform did not affect the level of risk to which Ms Chester was exposed, the surgeon was perceived as having denied her the right to choose for herself. Lord Steyn referred to ensuring that 'due respect is given to the autonomy and dignity of each patient'[26] and stated that, 'In modern law medical paternalism no longer rules and a patient has a *prima facie* right to be informed by a surgeon of a small, but well established, risk of serious injury as a result of surgery.'[27] By failing to give the patient information about the risks associated with the operation, the surgeon had deprived her of the opportunity to make an adequately informed choice by weighing up the risks.

The effect of the Chester case is that doctors who fail to warn patients about material risks associated with treatment may be open to negligence claims should those risks materialise, despite the exercise of all proper care and skill in carrying out the operation, and despite the fact that the patient admits that they would have been prepared to run the risk on a future occasion.

The GMC draws the following central conclusions from the ruling in the Chester case.

- Patients should be told of any possible significant adverse outcomes of a proposed treatment.
- In this case, a small but well-established risk of a serious adverse outcome was considered by the House of Lords to be 'significant'.[28]

Department of Health guidance states that: 'In considering what information to provide, the health practitioner should try to ensure that the person is able to make an informed judgment on whether to give or withhold consent . . . It is therefore advisable to inform the person of any 'material' or 'significant' risks or unavoidable risks, even if small, in the proposed treatment; any alternatives to it; and the risks incurred by doing nothing . . .'[29]

Doctors' actions are therefore likely to meet the legal and ethical requirements if they inform patients about any significant risks inherent in the treatment, and also any risks that may be particularly important to the individual patient. In this way, doctors are likely to satisfy both tests applied by the courts when considering the issue of information provision and consent to medical treatment: the 'professional standard', which looks to a responsible body of medical opinion to determine what patients should be told in order to give valid consent, and the 'patient standard', where the amount of information required by the individual patient determines how much information he or she needs in order for consent to be obtained.[30] The risks and benefits of alternatives and of non-treatment need also to be explained. More recent case law has suggested that unless the patient is informed of the comparative risk of different procedures, he or she will not be in a position to give fully valid consent to one procedure rather than another.[31] As patient choice can only be valid if it is based on adequate information, including about the range of choices and the consequences of making one choice over another, doctors should ensure that patients are informed of the comparative risks associated with any alternative treatments or procedures.

While failure to provide sufficient relevant information could result in doctors facing legal challenge, there is inevitably a degree of selectivity about the amount of information patients are given. It would be overly burdensome on both patients and health services for every detail to be explained, and patients are unlikely to want this. It is, however, important that patients can be confident that the information they will be given is that which is likely to be relevant to them, and understand that they may always ask for more details or explanation if they wish.

Withholding information

In the past, concern to avoid worrying or upsetting patients was seen as a reason for not telling them the full implications of either their condition or different options for treatment. Sometimes, only their relatives were told about the likely outcome of treatment (presenting problems of confidentiality as well as consent; see Chapter 5). Generally, however, patients do want to know and, even those who do not, need to have the option. Where the patient has capacity, doctors should take the lead from the patient. They should assume patients with capacity want information unless there are good reasons to think otherwise. Withholding relevant information in an effort to prevent patients from worrying is not a defensible reason for failing to provide them with all the material and relevant facts about their health and care. As Kennedy and Grubb argue:

> Despite all the anecdotes about patients who committed suicide, suffered heart attacks, or plunged into prolonged depression upon being told 'bad news', little documentation exists for claims that informing patients is more dangerous to their health than not informing them, particularly when the informing is done in a sensitive and tactful fashion . . . In light of the values at stake, the burden of justification should fall upon those who allege that the informing process is dangerous to patient health, and information should be withheld on therapeutic grounds only when the harm of its disclosure is both highly probable and seriously disproportionate to the affront to self-determination.[32]

The GMC advises that, in the rare event that a doctor decides to withhold information on the basis that providing it would have a deleterious effect on the patient's health, this view, and the reasons for it, should be recorded in the patient's notes and the doctor must be prepared to explain and justify that decision. Doctors withholding information for this reason are advised to keep the decision under regular review and to consider whether information could be given to the patient later without causing them serious harm.[33] The GMC[34] and health departments state that, in an individual case, the courts may accept such a justification, but would examine it with great care, and confirm that, '[t]he mere fact that the patient might become upset by hearing the information, or might refuse treatment, is not sufficient to act as a justification'.[35]

Refusing to receive information

In most cases, doctors and patients decide together which treatment option would be the most appropriate. Doctors contribute their clinical knowledge and experience and patients bring their personal needs, preferences and values to the decision-making process.

In some cases, however, patients do not want to know and ask their doctor to make the decision on their behalf. When this happens, doctors should try to find out why the patient feels this way, and explain the importance of knowing the options open to them and what the treatment will involve. Even if they continue to refuse, it is a legal requirement that basic information, such as what the treatment or procedure is intended to achieve and what it will involve, including any serious risks, be provided in order for consent to be valid.[36] If patients insist that they do not want even this basic information, the doctor must explain the potential consequences of not receiving it; for example, their consent to the treatment or procedure may not be valid. Doctors must record the fact that a patient has declined basic information and make it clear to patients that they can change their minds and have more information at any time.[37]

Without basic information, patients cannot make a valid choice to delegate responsibility for treatment decisions to the doctor. The amount of basic information needed depends upon the individual circumstances, the severity of the condition and the risks associated with the treatment. Doctors must seek to strike a balance between giving the patient sufficient information for a valid decision, while at the same time respecting the patient's wish not to know. Doctors may find it helpful to discuss the situation, on an anonymous basis, with colleagues.

When patients refuse to receive information, this should not be seen as total renunciation of choice or as relinquishing choice on other issues. Nevertheless, although information and uncertainties should not be forced upon patients at a time when they are particularly vulnerable and clearly unready, most people are able to deal with very difficult choices, despite their anxieties, if they are given support. It must be clear to patients that they may change their mind about how much information they want at any point.

Details that are not wanted by a patient at one stage of treatment may be sought at another. Patients must be in control, not only of the amount of information being given, but also of the speed and flow of that information. Busy doctors sometimes point out the apparent impracticality of attempting to give information in stages to suit the patient. Increasingly, written material or advice about specific patient support groups or voluntary organisations is seen as essential in helping patients to inform themselves at their own speed. The GMC explicitly states that doctors should consider what other sources of information and support are available for patients, including 'patient information leaflets, advocacy services, expert patient programmes, or support groups for people with specific conditions'.[38] Contact with group members can show how others in the same position have managed. Such solutions, however, are not a substitute for appropriate discussion between the doctor and patient.

Some doctors ask patients to sign a form confirming that they were offered information but declined it, both in order to emphasise the importance of the decision the patient is taking and to protect the doctor against future charges of failing to provide sufficient information. Others record each discussion that takes place in the medical notes. Either way, it is important to have thorough documentation of the refusal of information, and to do so in a form that is easily accessible to others providing care for the patient.

Summary – providing information

- Patients must be offered sufficient information, in an accessible format, that takes account of individual patients' needs, to allow them to make informed decisions about their treatment and care.
- Patients vary in how much information they want, but doctors should presume that patients want to be well informed, and should volunteer information of the type that is necessary for patients to make informed choices.
- When patients have additional questions about their treatment and care, including potential risks, these must be answered truthfully and as fully as patients wish.

- Doctors are under a legal duty to inform patients, as part of their duty to exercise reasonable care and skill, and are likely to fulfil this duty if they inform patients about any significant risks inherent in a treatment, and also any risks that may be particularly important to the individual patient.
- Information may only be withheld from a patient in exceptional circumstances, where providing it would have a deleterious effect on the patient's health.
- Patients may refuse information, but basic information about their condition and treatment must be provided in order for consent to be valid.
- Doctors should document patients' refusals to receive information.

Documenting consent

Doctors should make a note of the information provided in discussions they have with patients about the nature and purpose of more complex or ongoing procedures, or, for example, elective surgical interventions, when seeking consent.[39] This is usually by recording contemporaneously in the health record that information has been provided and a discussion has taken place.

In many cases, there is no need for patients to indicate their agreement in writing. Where complex procedures are proposed, or there are significant risks associated with the procedure, consent forms are used to document the patient's agreement. They are common, for example, in surgery. A signed consent form is prima facie evidence of a process, not the process itself. The form simply documents that some discussion about the procedure or investigation has taken place, but it is the quality and clarity of the information given, rather than a signature on a form, that is paramount.

The GMC recommends that written consent should be obtained in cases where:

- the investigation or treatment or procedure is complex or involves significant risks
- there may be significant consequences for the patient's employment, or social or personal life
- providing clinical care is not the primary purpose of the investigation or treatment
- the treatment is part of a research programme or is an innovative treatment designed specifically for the patient's benefit.[40]

The Royal Colleges also recommend that written consent is obtained for certain types of procedure. In this respect, doctors should familiarise themselves with guidance relevant to their area of practice. In addition, consent forms are a legal requirement under certain parts of the Human Fertilisation and Embryology Act 1990 (as amended).[41]

The Department of Health issued consent guidance in 2001, which included a reference guide, a good practice implementation guide and model consent forms, to help improve practice and raise standards.[42] The reference guide was updated in 2009 to reflect legislative changes,[43] and a qualitative review of consent practice in the NHS was undertaken in 2010. This showed that consent processes have generally improved since 2001, with more formalised systems in place, but awareness of Department of Health guidance varied considerably. The review also found that consent is now largely embedded in NHS practice, with local practices being developed to meet local needs. The Department will continue to make available consent form templates and a guide to good practice, alongside the reference guide.[44] The Department advises that these should be used in conjunction with the guidance available from professional bodies, such as the GMC and BMA.

Model consent forms have been issued by the health departments in Northern Ireland and Wales. All documentation is available online and, in many cases, in a number of languages.[45] The BMA does not publish any standard forms for consent to treatment.

Summary – documenting consent

- Doctors should make a note of discussions they have with patients when seeking consent for more complex or ongoing procedures.
- In most cases, there is no need for patients to indicate their agreement in writing.
- Written consent should be obtained where complex procedures are proposed, where there are significant risks associated with the procedure and in relation to other treatments as specified by the General Medical Council and the Human Fertilisation and Embryology Act 1990 (as amended).
- A signed consent form only documents that some discussion about the procedure or investigation has taken place; the quality and clarity of the information given is vital to ensuring the validity of the consent.

The scope of consent

Duration

Consent should be perceived as a continuing process rather than a one-off decision. Before beginning treatment, a member of the healthcare team should check that the patient still wants to go ahead. Doctors sometimes query the length of time for which consent is valid. In usual practice, this is not an issue because patients' continued participation in treatment is an indication that they have not changed their minds. Occasionally, however, if treatment involves a number of invasive or complex procedures over a period of time, for example successive surgical interventions, it may be appropriate to ask for explicit, or even written, consent for each intervention.

Sometimes there is a long period between the original consent being sought and the procedure being undertaken, during which time the patient's condition or wishes may have changed, or new information may have become available. It is then important to reaffirm that the patient still consents to the procedure going ahead, even if no new information or explanations are needed. It is important that the patient is given continuing opportunities to ask further questions and to review the decision.

Exceeding consent

Consent is valid only insofar as it applies to the treatment in question; so, for example, when a patient agrees to a surgical procedure, the surgeon cannot simply change his or her mind and perform a different or additional operation. If it becomes clear that the original proposed procedure is no longer indicated, patients generally need to have the opportunity to decide about alternatives. It follows that, when seeking consent, doctors should discuss beforehand with patients any foreseeable problems that could arise when the patient is unconscious, and ask in advance what the patient would like to do if such a problem occurs.[46] The purpose of such discussion is to ascertain the patient's views about additional or alternative procedures. The only time when doctors are justified in proceeding without prior authority is when it is essential to do so immediately in order to save life or prevent a serious deterioration in the patient's condition, and it is not possible to obtain that person's consent.[47] (For further information on emergency treatment, see Chapter 15, and for treating patients who lack capacity or under mental health legislation, see Chapter 3.)

Exceeding consent during surgery

In 2002, a consultant obstetrician and gynaecologist was found guilty of serious professional misconduct by the GMC for his management of a patient's total abdominal hysterectomy and bilateral salpingo-oophorectomy.

The GMC's Professional Conduct Committee found that, during the course of the operation, the doctor had cause to suspect that the patient may have been pregnant but nonetheless continued with the operation, without her consent, thereby terminating the pregnancy. This action was held to be inappropriate because the doctor knew, or should have known, that the patient had not given her consent for termination of pregnancy and yet he made no effort to consult her about it. The consultant was severely reprimanded. (For a further discussion of this case see Chapter 7, page 278).[48]

Summary – the scope of consent

- Consent generally remains valid unless the patient indicates otherwise, although consent should be reaffirmed if there has been a significant lapse of time between the initial agreement and the actual procedure, or if the situation has changed since consent was given.
- If treatment involves a number of invasive or complex procedures over a period of time, it may be necessary to obtain explicit, or written, consent for each intervention.
- Consent covers only those procedures to which the patient has actually agreed; where there are foreseeable complications that could arise, these should be discussed as part of the consent process.

Pressures on consent

Patients' choices are often influenced by their relationships with people who are close to them and this is normal, unless the patient seems to have been persuaded to disregard his or her own wishes. Patients may also be put under pressure by employers or insurers. Many people factor into their decision making the effects of their actions on others. There are particular situations in which patients may be vulnerable to other kinds of pressure, for example if they are resident in a care home, or are detained by the police or immigration services. Sometimes the pressures are so great as to bring into question the extent to which the patient is making a voluntary decision about his or her care, and doctors should be aware of this. (For a discussion of issues relevant to doctors working in detention settings see, for example, Chapter 17, pages 693–694.)

In order for consent to be valid, the patient must be able to make a choice free from undue pressure. In a case involving a 20-year-old woman who had been brought up as a Jehovah's Witness, the Court of Appeal did not uphold her refusal of a blood transfusion because she had been unduly influenced by her mother (see Chapter 3, page 101).[49] Doctors should be alert to the susceptibility of some patients to decide in a way that pleases others, sometimes even the medical staff. They must ensure that undue pressure is not put on patients to decide in a particular way. Giving patients the opportunity to decide when away from their family and friends, and making sure that they know they have a right to refuse treatment, can also help to ensure that the patient's decision is a true indication of his or her wishes.

Patients may also be influenced by the way that health professionals explain the treatment options available but doctors themselves must not put pressure on patients to accept their advice. Information should be given to patients in a balanced way, and if a particular treatment or course of action is being recommended, it should be explained to the patient why this is the case.[50]

Refusal of treatment

The right to refuse

Adult patients with capacity have the right to refuse any medical treatment (except where the law prescribes otherwise, for example where compulsory treatment is authorised under mental health legislation;[51] see below and Chapter 3), contemporaneously or in advance, even if that refusal results in their permanent physical injury or death.[52] (They do not generally have a concomitant right to request procedures that have the same result; see pages 85–88, and also Chapter 11.) The right to refuse also extends to decisions where a woman is carrying a viable fetus. The European Court of Human Rights has confirmed that the right to have one's life protected does not extend to the unborn.[53] (This issue is discussed in more detail in Chapter 7, pages 269–270.)

Despite finding some patients' decisions difficult, because medical care could prolong or improve life, or save the life of a fetus, doctors must respect a competent refusal. The courts have said that it is irrelevant that other people think it is in the patient's best interests to agree to the treatment.[54] Respect for patient choice is further reinforced by the Human Rights Act 1998, which is rooted in respect for the dignity of the person. Although there is a primary duty to protect life in Article 2, this must be balanced against the right to respect for private and family life in Article 8, which includes the right to bodily integrity,[55] and the right to freedom of expression, which includes the right to hold opinions and receive information, in Article 10.

When patients are experiencing mental illness, there are rare occasions on which treatment for mental disorder may be provided even in the face of a competent refusal of treatment (see Chapter 3, pages 121–122). If there is doubt about a person's capacity to refuse, it is important to resolve that doubt as quickly as possible, and meanwhile the patient must be cared for according to the treating doctors' judgement about best interests (see Chapter 3). In the event of continuing doubt or disagreement about capacity, legal advice should be sought.

Refusal of treatment by an adult with capacity

Ms B was a 43-year-old woman who, in the summer of 1999, suffered a haemorrhage of the spinal cord in her neck. She was admitted to hospital and a cavernoma was diagnosed, a condition caused by a malformation of blood vessels in the spinal cord. Shortly after her diagnosis she made an advance decision refusing treatment stating that, if she became unable to give instructions, she wished for treatment to be withdrawn if she was suffering from a life-threatening condition, permanent mental impairment or permanent unconsciousness.

After a few weeks her condition improved and she was able to leave hospital and return to work. In February 2001, Ms B sustained further damage to her spinal cord, as a result of which she became tetraplegic, suffering complete paralysis from the neck down. She was treated in an intensive care unit where, after experiencing respiratory problems, she was placed on a ventilator. In March 2001, Ms B asked for the first time for her ventilator to be switched off. This request was repeated on a number of occasions and in April formal instructions were given to the hospital by her solicitor to withdraw artificial ventilation. According to the medical evidence, without artificial ventilation Ms B would have a less than 1 per cent chance of breathing independently and death would almost certainly follow. The clinicians were not willing to switch off the ventilator but offered the option of a programme of weaning whereby ventilation would be gradually reduced over a period of time with the aim of allowing the body to breathe again on its own. Ms B rejected this on the grounds that it would lead to a painful death over a period of weeks. She had also rejected rehabilitation because it offered her no chance of recovery and because she had no guarantee that the ventilator would be removed in the future at her request.

Ms B was assessed by a number of consultant psychiatrists and in August an independent assessment was conducted, which concluded that she was not depressed and that she had the capacity to make the decision to discontinue treatment. Despite her refusal of treatment, ventilation was continued and Ms B applied to the High Court for a declaration that the artificial ventilation being provided represented unlawful trespass. The Trust argued that Ms B did not have the capacity to make the decision to stop treatment.

In clarifying her role in the case, the judge, Dame Elizabeth Butler-Sloss, said, 'I am not asked directly to decide whether Ms B lives or dies but whether she, herself, is legally competent to make that decision. It is also important to recognise that this case is not about the best interests of the patient but about her mental capacity'.[56] In his evidence, one of the doctors expressed the view that Ms B was: 'unable to give informed consent, not because of a lack of capacity in general but her specific lack of knowledge and experience of exposure to a spinal rehabilitation unit and thereafter to readjustment to life in the community. Without that opportunity ... Ms B did not have the requisite information to give informed consent.'[57]

The judge rejected this view, which, she said, was not the law.

The court held that Ms B had the capacity to make all relevant decisions about her medical treatment, including the decision whether to seek withdrawal of artificial ventilation. The judge also found that Ms B had been treated unlawfully by the Trust.

Ms B died in her sleep a month later when her ventilation was withdrawn.

In the case of Ms B, the hospital Trust had received clear legal advice that if Ms B had decision-making capacity she should not be treated against her wishes. When the case went to court, the Trust was criticised for not following that advice. In making some general comments about refusal of treatment, the judge reminded hospitals that they must take steps to resolve dilemmas of this nature and not allow the situation to continue without resolution. Ultimately, if there is doubt about the legality of complying with a refusal of treatment because the patient may lack capacity, it should be assessed as a matter of priority. If doubts about the patient's capacity still remain, legal advice should be sought. Such steps are unnecessary, however, if it is clear that the patient has the capacity to make the decision.

The BMA supports the widely accepted view that valid treatment refusal by a patient is not in itself suicide, even if that refusal results in his or her death. When considered by the House of Lords as part of its deliberations during the case of Tony Bland, Lord Goff said:

in cases of [advance decisions refusing treatment], there is no question of the patient having committed suicide, nor therefore of the doctor having aided or abetted him in doing so. It is simply that the patient has, as he is entitled to do, declined to consent to treatment which might or would have the effect of prolonging his life, and the doctor has, in accordance with his duty, complied with his patient's wishes.[58]

Of course, some patients with decision-making capacity who genuinely do attempt suicide may also refuse resuscitation or other forms of potentially life-prolonging treatment.

Refusal of treatment following a suicide attempt

In 2007, 26-year-old Kerrie Wooltorton was admitted to hospital after consuming a fatal quantity of antifreeze. Diagnosed with an 'emotionally unstable personality disorder' and depressed at her inability to have a child, she had repeatedly taken poisons in the previous year and had been treated in hospital. This time, on arrival at hospital, she presented the medical team with a written note refusing all treatment and expressing her wish not to die alone or in pain. After extensive consultation and a second opinion from a fellow consultant, the doctor in charge of her care deemed her to have decision-making capacity. Her refusal of treatment was respected and four days after admission she died.

The decision to accede to her refusal was controversial. In a subsequent letter to the Royal College of Psychiatrists, Louis Appleby, National Director for Mental Health, commenting not on the individual case but on points of principle, indicated that treatment can be provided to individuals for the consequences of a mental disorder, even where she or he retained capacity.[59] In September 2009, following an inquest, a coroner upheld the decision of the treating doctors.[60]

Media coverage of the decision was inaccurate and confusing, with several commentators suggesting that this was the first time that a 'living will' – an advance decision refusing treatment (see Chapter 3, page 96) – had been used by an individual wanting to commit suicide.[61] There were even suggestions that the Mental Capacity Act 2005, which placed advance decisions on a statutory footing, should be amended as a result.[62]

In fact, neither the advance decision refusing treatment, nor mental capacity legislation, other than in assessing Ms Wooltorton's capacity to refuse treatment, was applicable in this case. Ms Wooltorton made a contemporaneous decision to refuse treatment and was assessed as having the capacity to make such a decision. As the coroner stated in his verdict, 'She refused...treatment in full knowledge of the consequences and died as a result.'[63] Treatment by doctors in the face of a competent verbal refusal, unless mental health legislation was engaged, would have been unlawful.

Although a refusal of life-sustaining treatment from a patient with a history of serious mental disorder presents doctors with a significant ethical challenge, the presence of a mental disorder is not in itself synonymous with a lack of decision-making capacity.[64] Treatment of patients who have attempted suicide is discussed in Chapter 15 (pages 630–633).

Benefit to others

There are certain circumstances where the principal aim of a medical treatment or procedure is to provide significant benefit to others, with no or minimal harm to the patient; for example, taking and testing a blood sample from a patient to determine their infection status when a healthcare worker has sustained a needlestick injury or other occupational exposure to body fluids. Even where such a benefit is the aim of treatment, a patient's competent refusal must still be respected.

Informed refusal

Patients are not obliged to justify their decisions to refuse treatment, but the healthcare team should ensure that patients base their decisions on accurate information and that they have corrected any misunderstandings. Just as patients giving consent should have sufficient accurate information, those refusing should ideally have an awareness of their condition, the proposed treatment, any significant risks or side effects, the probability of a successful recovery, the consequences of not having the treatment and alternative forms of treatment. Doctors must not put pressure on patients to decide in a particular way, but should allow them time to consider a decision with potentially serious consequences.

Continuing care

A refusal of a particular treatment does not imply a refusal of all treatment or all facets of care. When a patient has refused treatment, alternative treatments and procedures intended to keep the patient comfortable and free from pain or discomfort should still be offered. (The general issue of patient choice at the end of life is discussed in more detail in Chapter 10 and advance decisions refusing treatment are discussed in Chapter 3.) In addition, patients are entitled to change their minds about a decision, including a refusal, at any time, so long as they have the capacity to do so. If there are circumstances in which not providing treatment at a given time would limit the options for providing treatment in the future, this should be made clear to patients from the outset. For example, a cancer may be operable at the time a patient presents for treatment; if the patient refuses and then changes his or her mind a month later, the cancer might have progressed to a stage that is inoperable.

Documenting refusal

Patients are sometimes asked to sign a declaration to document that they have refused a particular treatment and that they accept responsibility for declining medical advice. The courts have said that, for their own protection, hospital authorities should seek unequivocal assurances from the patient (to be recorded in writing) that the refusal represents an informed decision; that is, that the patient understands the nature of and the reasons for the proposed treatment, and the risks and likely prognosis involved in the decision to refuse or accept it. If the patient is unwilling to sign a written indication of this refusal, it is likely to be unhelpful, or even counterproductive, to force the issue. Instead, the fact should be noted in the health record. Like consent forms, this documentation can provide evidence that some discussion has taken place between the doctor and the patient about the implications of refusing treatment, but it does not constitute a disclaimer.[65] It is important that patients understand that they may still change their mind even after signing a form. (For guidance on documenting advance decisions refusing treatment see Chapter 3.)

Refusal of blood products by Jehovah's Witnesses

Most Jehovah's Witnesses have a conscientiously held religious opposition to the use of blood and blood products, and, as with other patients, adults' competent refusals of treatment must be respected. Witnesses are, however, generally very anxious to cooperate in every way with alternative options. Most do not accept their own blood donated in advance (predeposit), but many are willing to accept the use of blood salvage equipment that serves to recycle their blood in a continuous circuit. Patients refusing blood products should be given the opportunity to discuss all available treatment options, particularly as the use of 'bloodless' medical procedures becomes increasingly commonplace, including their successful use in organ transplants.

Doctors should not assume that a patient will refuse a particular treatment just because he or she is a Jehovah's Witness. There must be clear evidence of refusal and doctors should not simply rely on reports from others concerning a patient's purported views. A range of individual choice is displayed by patients who are Jehovah's Witnesses, especially in relation to blood derivatives, the use of which is seen as a matter of individual patient choice. It is therefore essential that doctors establish the personal views of individual patients regarding the use of blood, blood products and related procedures applicable to their treatment,[66] as well as being satisfied with the voluntariness of any decision (see pages 74–75).

Failure to respect a known refusal

In 2001, University Hospitals Birmingham NHS Trust paid £100,000 in damages to a patient who had been given a transfusion of blood products 6 years previously. Ms B was admitted to hospital with chest pain in October 1995. She had a history of myocardial infarction, diabetes and deep vein thrombosis, and was taking the anticoagulant, warfarin. On admission to hospital, she made it known to the admitting healthcare team that she declined the use of blood or blood products as a result of her religious beliefs.

After admission, Ms B's anticoagulant was reversed and, when asleep, she was given a transfusion of fresh frozen blood plasma. She awoke while the transfusion of the second bag of plasma was in progress and became agitated and distressed. Her psychological condition deteriorated from this point onwards.

The treating doctors admitted failing to obtain consent prior to administering two units of frozen blood plasma. Psychiatrists reported that, prior to the transfusion, Ms B had a long-standing phobic anxiety with intermittent depression. Following the transfusion she felt dirty, impure, humiliated and distressed. She was diagnosed with post-traumatic stress disorder and obsessive compulsive disorder, entirely due to the transfusion. Her previous depressive disorder was determined as having deteriorated by 30 per cent following the transfusion. As a result, Ms B relied heavily on her daughter for care and psychological support.[67]

Lists of centres of excellence in bloodless surgery and of doctors experienced in working constructively with Jehovah's Witnesses are held by the UK-wide network of Jehovah's Witness hospital liaison committees. The Hospital Information Service for Jehovah's Witnesses, a department of their coordinating body, the Watch Tower Society, holds contact information for these committees[68] and has published a summary of alternative therapies and references to supporting medical research.[69] Many hospitals produce their own guidelines on the clinical management of patients who refuse transfusion of blood or blood products.

Summary – refusal of treatment

- Adult patients with capacity have the right to refuse any medical treatment, with the exception of compulsory treatment authorised under mental health legislation, even if that refusal results in their permanent physical injury or death, or the permanent physical injury or death of a viable fetus.
- Patients should be offered information about the following on which to base their decisions:
  - the nature of their condition
  - the proposed treatment

- significant risks or side effects
- probability of a successful recovery
- consequences of not having the treatment
- alternative forms of treatment.
- Patients who refuse treatment may be prepared to accept alternatives and should be offered care and symptom management appropriate to their needs.
- Refusal should be documented in health records, and patients may be asked to sign a form or declaration confirming their refusal.

Are there limits to an individual's choices?

There are limits on patients' choices, not only because of legal constraints about what options are allowed, but also because of the professional judgement of doctors. Doctors provide treatment, not simply because it is requested, but because in their view it is clinically appropriate. They recommend the treatment that is best for an individual patient, having regard to that patient's needs and the treatments and resources available. The courts have recognised that doctors are under no legal or ethical obligation to agree to a patient's request for treatment if they consider the treatment is not clinically appropriate or in the patient's best interests.[70]

Difficult questions arise for doctors when patients reject low cost remedies in favour of costly alternatives that divert resources from others. Yet, if the patient is a Jehovah's Witness, for example, and the choice is between an expensive alternative to blood products or allowing the patient to die, doctors make every effort to accommodate the patient's choice. This example highlights the difficult question of whether greater weight should be given to patient choice based on strongly held religious convictions over those based on other values, or purely on personal preference. (For a discussion of resource allocation see Chapter 20.)

Occasionally, healthy people seek medical assistance to do something that leaves them less physically healthy or even disabled. Achieving well-being obviously takes different forms for different people and requests for procedures that do not appear to be for the direct benefit of the patient, even though the patient him or herself may believe there is a direct benefit to be gained, need careful consideration. Some requests of this nature aim to help others, such as donating bone marrow or a kidney. Others come from patients with body integrity identity disorder (BIID) who ask to have healthy limbs amputated. These specific issues, and the dilemmas to which they give rise, are explored in the remainder of this chapter.

Consent to procedures carried out for the benefit of others

Altruism is important to medicine; the UK health service depends heavily on the regular altruistic donation of blood. People are often moved by the plight of others to donate bone marrow, gametes or embryos. Consent for donating where there are no (or only minimal) risks or discomfort for the donor, as with blood for example, is unproblematic and the BMA supports the concept of the altruistic gift relationship. Increasing numbers of people are also offering to donate whole organs to others, which carries some risks. The BMA supports living organ donation with appropriate safeguards.

Organ donation from live donors

There are two different types of living donor. In the first, an organ becomes available as a result of a procedure carried out primarily for the benefit of the donor. The most common scenario is what is known as a 'domino' transplant, in which a patient needing new lungs has his or her heart and lungs removed and replaced by organs from a cadaveric donor. The patient's own heart is then available for transplantation to another person. Recipients are asked to consent both to the clinical procedure itself and to the donation of other organs removed in the course of the treatment.

The second type of live donation – altruistic donation from healthy donors – raises more issues around consent. Such donations have traditionally formed only a very small part of the overall transplant programme in the UK, but the numbers have increased considerably such that by 2009–2010 over half of all organ donors in the UK were living donors[71] and 38 per cent of all kidney transplants were from living donors.[72] It is also possible for living donors to donate segments of liver, lung or bowel, although the numbers doing so are small.

The main concern about living donation from healthy volunteers is that it exposes donors to the small[73] but significant risks of major surgery for no personal physical benefit. Living donation does, however, carry significant advantages for recipients. Donation from a healthy volunteer – both related and unrelated – carries a higher chance of success for the recipient compared with cadaveric donors.[74] Living donation has other advantages: it facilitates pre-emptive transplantation for someone with progressive renal failure, so avoiding the need for dialysis; it allows the transplant to proceed at the optimal time for the recipient; and it allows those with end-stage renal failure to escape the long wait for a kidney from a cadaveric donor. Although the physical benefit is all for the recipient, those who donate to people close to them may achieve psychological and practical benefits from the recipient's recovery, such as their ability to return to work or participate more in everyday activities.[75]

Many medical interventions carry a risk of harm, but this is outweighed by the anticipated benefit for the individual. In the examples discussed here, however, the risk is one of significant harm and the anticipated benefit for the individual undergoing it is solely (or mainly) psychological. Nevertheless, it has long been accepted that, with limited exceptions, adults with capacity are entitled to put themselves at risk to help other people. Bone marrow and oocyte donation, for example, are accepted even though they put the donor at some degree of risk with no personal physical benefit. The BMA has considered the arguments for and against live donation and believes that living donation is a morally acceptable practice that should be encouraged, provided that donors are properly informed and that safeguards are in place to ensure that they are not subjected to any pressure or coercion, whether financial or emotional.

Having accepted that, as a general principle, people may expose themselves to risk for the benefit of another person, are there limits to the extent of that risk?[76] If a surgeon removed, for donation, an individual's heart, resulting in the patient's inevitable death, 'any consent would be invalid since the surgeon would commit murder'.[77] Apart from such extremes, however, there is no legal restriction on the extent of risk to which individuals may expose themselves in the process of donating organs. Arguably, it is for the individual, who has capacity, sufficient information and is acting voluntarily, to establish what level of risk he or she is willing to take. Living organ donation is, however, subject to legal restrictions and a formal approval mechanism (see below). In addition, surgeons cannot be forced to act contrary to their clinical judgement and any surgeon asked to undertake the operation would need to be satisfied not only that the potential donor had capacity, was informed and acting voluntarily, but also that the overall benefits of carrying out the procedure outweighed the harms.

Surgeon's refusal to meet a patient's request

Mr P had two sons, aged 33 and 29 years. Both sons had Alport's syndrome, an inherited condition that causes kidney failure. Mr P successfully donated a kidney to his younger son. His older son, R, received a cadaveric kidney, but the transplant failed. As it had been a poor match, R developed antibodies that made him incompatible with 96 per cent of the population. Finding a suitable kidney was therefore extremely unlikely, unless his parents were suitable donors. Mrs P was told that she was not suitable. Mr P wanted to donate his second kidney to R.

Mr P argued it would be better for him to be on dialysis rather than his son. He was retired and prepared for the lifestyle change that dialysis would bring. Despite finding support from some doctors, Mr P's request was turned down by three transplant teams. Some of the deliberations of the third were filmed and shown on television.[78]

Members of the transplant team had mixed views about Mr P's request. Some understood and felt they would want to do the same for their own children. Although some believed that the benefits were one-sided, others agreed that there could be emotional benefits for Mr and Mrs P if the transplant was a success for R. There were also concerns about the impact on the family (the younger brother was opposed to the operation) and about how R, in particular, would feel about the effects on his father's length and quality of life. The resource implications of ending up with two people on dialysis rather than one if the transplant was not successful were also discussed.

The decision rested with the transplant surgeon. Although he knew that Mr P understood the nature and implications of his request, and that he could see ethical and rational justifications for the operation taking place, he knew that ultimately he would feel unable to perform the operation. Mr P was therefore turned down.

As a last resort, Mrs P was tested again to see if she might be a match. Although she had been rejected several times in the past, she was found to be a match.

The BMA believes it is right that the level of harm to which people can give consent is limited but, as in other areas, resists the imposition of inflexible rules. Each case needs to be considered individually and, if the health professionals concerned believe that the risks are too great, the decision and the reasons for it should be sensitively explained to both the potential donor and the recipient.

Safeguards for living organ donation

Any use of healthy living donors must be subject to strict safeguards to ensure that the fundamental principles of consent – capacity, information, and voluntariness – are met. Legislation introducing safeguards for living organ donation has been in place since 1989.[79] The area is currently regulated by the Human Tissue Act 2004 and Human Tissue (Scotland) Act 2006, which extended the need for prior approval to all living solid organ donation (previously only donation between individuals who were not genetically related needed approval). The Unrelated Live Transplants Regulatory Authority (ULTRA), which previously took on this role, has been abolished and the approval process (for the whole of the UK) now falls within the remit of the Human Tissue Authority (HTA). The BMA welcomed both of these changes, which acknowledged the risk of coercion or pressure to donate within families and also streamlined the approval procedure, making it quicker and more efficient. (At the time of writing, the Government was seeking to reallocate the functions of the HTA and abolish the regulatory body, as part of its plan to reduce the number of arm's-length bodies. Up-to-date information on this can be found on the BMA website.)

Under the new system an application to the HTA must be submitted and approved in advance of all solid organ donation from living donors. Before approval is given, the donor and recipient must be interviewed together and separately by an 'independent assessor', trained and accredited by the HTA, and a report submitted.[80] In cases of directed donation to a genetically or emotionally close recipient, the HTA also requires evidence of the claimed relationship to be provided.

Content of reports from independent assessors

A report from an independent assessor, following interviews with the donor and recipient, must include the following:[81]

- the information given to the potential donor (or other person giving consent) as to the nature of the medical procedure and the risk involved
- the full name of the person who gave that information to the potential donor (or other person giving consent) and their qualifications for giving it
- the capacity of the potential donor (or other person giving consent) to understand the nature of the medical procedure and the risks involved, and the fact that consent may be withdrawn at any time before the removal of the organ or part organ
- whether there is any evidence of duress or coercion affecting the decision to give consent
- whether there is any evidence of an offer of a reward
- whether there were any difficulties in communicating with the person interviewed (for example, language or hearing) and, if so, an explanation of how those difficulties were overcome.

In straightforward cases a decision to approve the application, on the recommendation of the independent assessor, will be made by the transplant approvals team within the HTA secretariat. Where either the independent assessor or the transplant approvals team have concerns, the case is referred to a panel of at least three members of the HTA for consideration. There are also some cases that raise specific concerns and where approval is always required by a panel of at least three members of the HTA; these include all cases where the donor is a child or an adult who lacks capacity to consent. (For general information on decision making in relation to adults lacking capacity and children and young people, see Chapters 3 and 4.)

Expanding the pool of donors

The Human Tissue Act 2004 and the Human Tissue (Scotland) Act 2006 also expanded the pool of potential living donors by specifically permitting two new types of living donation – 'paired and pooled donation' and 'altruistic non-directed donation'.

Paired and pooled donation

Under this system, where someone needs a donor organ and has a friend or relative willing to donate but the two are not compatible with each other, they can pair up with one or more other incompatible donor and recipient pairs in an organ exchange. In paired donation, donor A gives an organ to recipient B and donor B gives to recipient A. In pooled donation, more than two donor–recipient pairs take part in an organ exchange, coordinated by the HTA (so, for example, donor A's kidney goes to recipient B, donor B's kidney goes to recipient C and donor C's kidney goes to recipient A). These types of donation had been proposed prior to the new legislation but questions were raised about whether such arrangements entailed a 'benefit in kind' given that the donor's partner would be given priority for donation. Concern was expressed that this would be contrary to the prohibition on payment contained in the Human Organ Transplants Act 1989 (and replicated in the new human tissue legislation). This was clarified in the 2004 Act (and the 2006 Act in Scotland). The BMA supports this type of donation believing that, while the donation is made with the expectation of getting some benefit in return, the motivation for donation is purely altruistic and not driven by financial gain. Under the human tissue legislation, all cases of paired and pooled donation need to be considered by an independent assessor and approved by a panel of at least three members of the HTA. In 2009–2010 there were 32 paired living kidney donor transplants.[82]

Altruistic non-directed donation

Donation of blood, gametes or bone marrow by strangers is commonplace, and sometimes people offer to donate a kidney to a stranger. Under the 2004 and 2006 Acts, such donation is now permitted, subject to each case being considered by an independent assessor and approved by a panel of at least three members of the HTA.

The motives of such people are sometimes questioned. It is, of course, essential to consider whether the potential donor has the capacity to give consent, but it is equally important to recognise acts of genuine altruism. The lengths to which some people go in order to help others, even people they do not know, can be quite astounding. Some people are moved by the plight of others and genuinely want to do what they can to help. It is also increasingly recognised that donation can bring personal benefits to the donor in terms of improved self-esteem and personal satisfaction.

Altruistic donation to strangers

One of the first people in the UK to donate a kidney to a stranger was Barbara Ryder, a 59-year-old nurse from Cornwall. Her kidney was donated to 68-year-old Andy Loudon, a retired carpenter from Bedfordshire who had been receiving dialysis for 2 years as a result of polycystic kidney disease. Barbara Ryder said she wanted to give something back to society and, in interviews, described the great feeling of joy she received from donating her kidney. She said, 'It's better than Christmas. You get a lot more fun and happiness by giving something that can change a life.'[83]

The number of people offering to donate a kidney to a stranger is small but increasing. The HTA has reported that 10 cases were approved in 2007–2008, increasing to 15 in 2008–2009.[84] Many of those who initially volunteer may do so without realising the true nature of the procedure or the risks involved, and some may decide not to proceed once that information has been received. For those who are informed and have capacity, however, the BMA supports this option.

A 'special case' for priority

While the increase in living kidney donation has been widely hailed as a success, some commentators have noted a word of caution. Glannon, for example, suggests that studies may be underestimating the long-term risk in living kidney donation given the increasing incidence of hypertension and diabetes – a common cause of end-stage renal disease – in both developed and developing countries.[85] Although he uses this argument to question the extent to which people should be permitted to take risks for the benefit of others, the possibility of failure of the remaining kidney in altruistic living donors also raises another interesting question. Should those who find themselves in need of a transplant, as a direct result of their altruistic donation to others, be considered a special case and given priority in the competition for donated cadaveric organs? Under the policy of the United Network of Organ Sharing (UNOS) in the USA, those who have previously been living organ donors are given priority to receive a transplant from a deceased donor should they ever need one.[86] This could be seen as acting as an incentive to people to donate or it could be seen as removing a counter-incentive. If fear of failure of the remaining kidney deters people from acting as living donors, then assuring them that they would be given priority for an organ, should they need one in future, might increase the number of donors and therefore the number of lives saved and transformed by a transplant.

While it may seem reasonable to give priority to those whose need is directly related to their altruistic act, we do not generally adopt this approach in other areas of healthcare. For example, a fireman injured rescuing people from a burning building would not be given priority access to intensive care facilities over a driver injured while speeding, but rather resources would be allocated on the basis of clinical need. The BMA has also consistently argued that organs should be allocated to adults on the basis of clinical need and should not take account of social factors, such as occupation or perceived value to society. In practice, however, those who have only one remaining kidney are likely to have greater clinical need and therefore be given a higher priority in the allocation of organs without the need to introduce a priority system. The BMA has also rejected the notion that people should be given an incentive to donate – either during their lifetime or after death – such as that established in legislation in Israel, which came into effect in January 2010, whereby those who sign up to donate their organs after death, or act as living donors to a stranger, are given priority for organs during their lifetime.[87]

Requests for amputation of healthy limbs

Doctors sometimes ask the BMA for advice about patients requesting the amputation of a healthy limb or limbs. Although there are various psychological conditions linked to the desire for amputation, such as body dysmorphic disorder (BDD), where patients seek body modification in response to some perceived physical imperfection or defect, the phenomenon has been particularly associated with a rare condition known as body integrity identity disorder (BIID) (also referred to as amputee identity disorder).[88] Patients with BIID often have what they perceive to be an extraneous or 'alien' limb (or limbs) that they want removed.[89]

Understanding of the psychological conditions linked to the desire for amputation of healthy limbs, although still relatively limited, has increased; those with these conditions have become more outspoken about their desires for amputation.[90] There has been an increasing recognition, among experts, of BIID as a clinical condition and of surgery as an effective treatment for it. Many empirical questions surrounding BIID remain unanswered, however; for example, whether amputation actually cures the condition; and the potential for the condition to be managed effectively with non-surgical treatments is not yet known, beyond anecdotal reports that psychological therapy and pharmacotherapy do not help alleviate the distress it causes.

There was considerable public disquiet when, in 2000, it was announced that a surgeon in Scotland had removed healthy limbs from two such patients. The hospital subsequently withdrew its permission for any further operations of that nature to be undertaken on its premises.

Elective amputation of healthy limbs in the UK

In 1997, a surgeon in Scotland amputated the apparently healthy limbs of two patients, assessed as having capacity by psychiatrists, but experiencing a psychological condition that was at the time classed as BDD. Both patients reported having what they perceived to be an extraneous or 'alien' limb, in each case a leg, that they wanted removed.

Three years later, 55-year-old Gregg Furth, a psychoanalyst from New York, travelled to the UK to see psychiatrists and the surgeon who had carried out the 1997 amputations.[91] Since before he was 10 years old, Mr Furth could recall feeling that the lower part of his right leg was not part of his body; since then he constantly thought about being without that part of his leg and had searched for many years to find a surgeon willing to amputate it. Mr Furth had undergone many years of therapy but had not been able to repress the feelings he had about his leg. He was assessed by two psychiatrists in the UK, both of whom confirmed that he had capacity to make the decision and had BDD. Both psychiatrists recommended him for amputation and the surgeon agreed to carry out the procedure.[92]

When the story about the previous operations subsequently broke in the national media, it was met by widespread public outcry. Before Mr Furth's planned amputation could take place, the hospital withdrew its permission for any more operations of this type to be undertaken on its premises. [93]

The BMA has profound reservations about the ethical and legal acceptability of such operations. Having a psychiatric disorder does not, of itself, render a person unable to give valid consent, but it may affect the individual's decision-making capacity in relation to issues connected with the disorder. Similarly, an apparently irrational decision should not automatically lead to the presumption that a patient lacks decision-making capacity. Consent for amputation would, however, have to be carefully scrutinised.

Legal issues

There is debate about whether amputating a healthy limb in these circumstances is lawful. Discussion often focuses on the ancient common law offence of maim, which grew up in relation to the duty of all males to fight for their sovereign and country, if required. Maim is therefore defined as, 'bodily harm whereby a man is deprived of the use of any member of his body, or of any sense which he can use in fighting, or by the loss of which he is generally and permanently weakened'.[94] It has also been suggested that, 'were a patient to consent to having his limbs amputated, for no good reason, his consent would not prevent the amputation from amounting to the offence of battery'.[95] This invites the question of what would be 'good reason'.

Much discussion about the limits of consent followed the 1993 House of Lords' judgment in a case about men practising consensual sadomasochistic activities involving maltreatment of the genitals, ritualistic beating and branding.[96] The men were convicted and imprisoned, despite the fact that the 'victims' gave consent. Although the two scenarios are clearly different, the latter case highlighted the legal limits of consent as a defence when a person carries out a potentially harmful act at the request of another person. The Law Commission's subsequent consultation on consent in the criminal law considered the extent to which an individual's apparently valid consent to 'injury' removes the act from the remit of the criminal law. It recommended that, 'the intentional causing of seriously disabling injury [including injuries that involve the loss of a bodily member] to another person should continue to be criminal, even if the person injured consents to such injury or to the risk of such injury'.[97] It went on to make an exception for cases in which the injury is caused during the course of proper medical treatment, in which it included the surgical aspects of gender reassignment.

The Law Commission did not specifically consider amputation as treatment for a psychological condition and the legality of this practice remains untested in the courts. Extreme caution should therefore be exercised and it is essential to seek specific legal advice before proceeding in such a case.

Ethical issues

One of the goals of medicine is to enable patients to live as healthy and independent a life as possible. Mutilating surgical procedures are usually seen as a last resort in cases where a physical disease has been identified. Therefore, most doctors have an intuitive aversion to the notion of deliberately removing healthy tissue in the absence of physical disease, even at the patient's request. Part of this reluctance is due to the permanent disabling effect for the patient, which sets amputation apart from other, more conventional patient choices involving surgery and the destruction of healthy tissue for reasons of psychological well-being, such as cosmetic surgery. Some autonomy-based arguments draw no such distinction between elective amputation and other surgical procedures, and suggest that surgeons should be permitted to act, in the case of long-standing and informed requests for amputation from adult patients with decision-making capacity.[98] Yet the fact remains that, whereas doctors may disagree with patients' views about the need for interventions like cosmetic surgery, or find them irrational, at least ideally, patients are not deliberately or permanently disabled by them. Similarly, as a treatment for gender dysphoria, surgery is a major step but is not intrinsically disabling and the psychological benefits are recognised. Amputation, on the other hand, is disabling and in some cases may render the patient dependent upon lifelong support from society, raising questions about the burdens of patient choice and whether people have duties to society as well as rights.

Significant harms that follow from respecting other patient choices, such as refusals of life-saving treatments, can also be distinguished from amputation requests on similar grounds.[99] Acceding to such requests has the potential to divert medical resources away from other patients, thereby potentially placing them in danger. Even when no patient is endangered by respecting a request for amputation, a patient's right to refuse treatment, and the duty of doctors to respect that refusal, does not entail a right to demand treatment or a corresponding ethical or legal obligation on doctors to agree to a patient's request for treatment.[100]

Another potentially analogous situation here is the practice of allowing residential psychiatric patients the freedom to self-injure, as a method of harm minimisation in certain prescribed circumstances. As with the deliberate removal of healthy tissue in elective amputation, overseeing such practice may at first sight seem contrary to the doctor's duty of care. Health professionals working with a patient who wants to self-injure are confronted with a choice between prohibiting the self-injury by restricting the patient's freedom, and allowing self-injury, albeit in controlled and hygienic conditions, which allows the patient to harm him or herself. Like elective amputation, the issue remains legally untested and is not currently standard practice. Research has cautiously suggested that self-injury should be permitted with some patients whilst they undertake a programme of treatment to enhance their autonomy aimed at the reduction of self-injury and, ultimately, its avoidance.[101] It is on this point that a distinction can again be drawn between a harm minimisation programme of this kind and the amputation of healthy limbs on request; amputation remains an intrinsically disabling and irreversible procedure.

Although amputation of healthy limbs is not in a person's best medical interests in terms of physical health, amputation may be justified in terms of the benefit to the individual's psychological well-being, where no other treatment is effective.[102] Some argue that, in this sense, the accepted notion of harm does not apply in BIID cases, and that too much emphasis is placed on notions of physical health as distinct from mental well-being. Even where such an argument is rejected, meeting the requests of those with BIID could be justified on the grounds that surgical amputation prevents the patient resorting to dangerous self-injury in the pursuit of self-amputation, or seeking surgery overseas or on the black market, where the quality of practices cannot be guaranteed.[103] Methods of attempted self-amputation include gunshot or power tool wounds to the affected limb, or lying across rail tracks, to make amputation a medical necessity; others are reported to have committed suicide as a result of their inability to rid themselves of their obsession.[104] The argument follows that, by removing the need for those with this condition to seek more life-threatening alternatives, doctors performing elective amputations would be pursuing the principle of non-maleficence. Best interest considerations certainly invite the question of whether it is better in some circumstances to amputate rather than let the patient destroy the limb, often risking death in the process; consequentialist arguments contend that surgery can be carried out where the risk of self-harm outweighs the risks and disadvantages of the amputation. In order for this to be convincing, however, it would be necessary to be able to distinguish those patients for whom the desire for an amputation might be transient, from those who will persist in their desire. It would also have to be shown that all other, less invasive alternatives, had been exhausted and that the patient is expected to suffer even more serious harm if the procedure is not carried out. Clinical understanding of BIID is not yet sufficiently developed to allow such distinctions to be drawn.

Treating patients with body integrity identity disorder

Where a patient presents as a result of obvious self-injury and BIID is a suspected cause, questions are likely to be raised about the validity of the patient's consent to any surgical amputation procedure. Doctors should seek input from mental health professionals and other colleagues regarding the medical necessity of amputation if there is any doubt.

This condition can have extremely serious consequences and entails very real suffering for those patients affected. The needs of these patients certainly require further exploration, research and debate. Some researchers have campaigned for the inclusion of BIID as a distinct condition in future versions of the Diagnostic and Statistical Manual of Mental Disorders (DSM), which, they argue, would facilitate the development of further treatments and greater understanding of the causes of elective amputation requests.[105] Although the condition is extremely rare, as BIID becomes further recognised and understood as a clinical phenomenon, it seems at least possible that more patients will present with elective requests for surgery and, as with gender reassignment surgery, at some point in the future amputation may be recognised as an acceptable treatment.

Summary – are there limits to an individual's consent?

- Society imposes limits on what people with capacity are allowed to consent to – people cannot consent to being killed, for example.
- The BMA believes that procedures that are primarily for the physical benefit of another person are acceptable in some circumstances, but that there should be safeguards in place to ensure that consent is valid.
- When physically healthy patients seek procedures that are disabling, legal advice should be sought before proceeding.

References

1 General Medical Council (2006) *Good Medical Practice*, GMC, London, para 36.
2 Treatment must be under the direction of the approved clinician in charge of the treatment, which must be for the patient's mental disorder or the symptoms of it (Mental Health Act 1983, s 63), or in respect of certain treatments under the Mental Health Act 1983, s 62.
3 Based on: Department of Health (2001) *12 Key Points on Consent: the law in England*, DH, London.
4 See, for example: General Medical Council (2008) *Consent: patients and doctors making decisions together*, GMC, London; Department of Health (2009) *Reference Guide to Consent for Examination or Treatment*, 2nd edn. DH, London; Scottish Executive Health Department (2006) *A Good Practice Guide on Consent for Health Professionals in NHS Scotland*, SEHD, Edinburgh; Welsh Assembly Government (2009) *Reference Guide for Consent to Examination or Treatment*, WAG, Cardiff; Department of Health, Social Services and Public Safety (2003) *Reference Guide to Consent for Examination, Treatment or Care*, DHSSPS, Belfast; The Medical and Dental Defence Union of Scotland (2007) *Essential Guide to Consent*, MDDUS, Glasgow; The Medical Defence Union, *Advice centre: consent to treatment*, available at: www.the-mdu.com (accessed 7 February 2011).
5 British Medical Association (2001) *Report of the Consent Working Party: incorporating consent tool kit*, BMA, London, recommendation 2.
6 See, for example: Department of Health (2001) *Good Practice in Consent Implementation Guide: consent to examination or treatment*, DH, London; Department of Health (2009) *Reference guide to consent for examination or treatment*, 2nd edn. DH, London. Further documentation and guidance for clinicians can be found on the Department of Health website at www.dh.gov.uk (accessed 7 February 2011); Welsh Assembly Government (2009) *Reference Guide for Consent to Examination or Treatment*, WAG, Cardiff; Welsh Assembly Government (2002) *Good Practice in Consent Implementation Guide: consent to examination or treatment*, WAG, Cardiff; Scottish Executive Health Department (2006) *A Good Practice Guide on Consent for Health Professionals in NHSScotland*, SEHD, Edinburgh; Department of Health, Social Services and Public Safety (2003) *Reference Guide to Consent for Examination, Treatment or Care*, DHSSPS, Belfast; Department of Health, Social Services and Public Safety (2003) *Good Practice in Consent: Consent for Examination, Treatment or Care*, DHSSPS, Belfast.
7 *Re MB (medical treatment)* [1997] 2 FLR 426.
8 British Medical Association (2009) *The Ethics of Caring for Older People*, 2nd edn, Wiley-Blackwell, London, p.78.
9 Further guidance is available in: Department for Constitutional Affairs (2007) *Mental Capacity Act 2005 Code of Practice*, The Stationery Office, London.
10 *Re MB (medical treatment)* [1997] 2 FLR 426.
11 British Medical Association, The Law Society (2010) *Assessment of Mental Capacity*, 3rd edn, The Law Society, London, pp. 170–2.
12 General Medical Council (2008) *Consent: patients and doctors making decisions together*, GMC, London, paras 26–7.
13 Department of Health (2001) *Good Practice in Consent Implementation Guide: consent to examination or treatment*, DH, London, p.20, para 3; Welsh Assembly Government (2002) *Good Practice in Consent Implementation Guide: consent to examination or treatment*, WAG, Cardiff, p.17, para 3.
14 Royal College of Anaesthetists (2010) *For Patients: introduction*. Available at: www.rcoa.ac.uk (accessed 7 February 2011).
15 Association of Anaesthetists of Great Britain and Ireland (2010) *Pre-operative Assessment and Patient Preparation: the role of the anaesthetist*, AAGBI, London.
16 General Medical Council (2008) *Consent: patients and doctors making decisions together*, GMC, London, para 9.
17 Mason JK, Laurie GT. (2011) *Mason and McCall Smith's Law and Medical Ethics*, 8th edn, Oxford University Press, Oxford, pp.109–10, para 4.112.
18 *Sidaway v Board of Governors of the Bethlem Royal Hospital* [1985] AC 871; *Pearce v United Bristol Healthcare NHS Trust* (1999) 48 BMLR 118.
19 General Medical Council (2008) *Consent: patients and doctors making decisions together*, GMC, London, p.5.
20 *Sidaway v Board of Governors of the Bethlem Royal Hospital* [1985] AC 871.
21 *Sidaway v Board of Governors of the Bethlem Royal Hospital* [1985] AC 871.
22 *Bolam v Friern Hospital Management Committee* [1957] 2 All ER 118.
23 *Sidaway v Board of Governors of the Bethlem Royal Hospital* [1985] AC 871:888–9.
24 *Pearce v United Bristol Healthcare NHS Trust* [1998] EWCA Civ 865.
25 *Chester v Afshar* [2005] 1 AC 134.
26 *Chester v Afshar* [2005] 1 AC 134:144.
27 *Chester v Afshar* [2005] 1 AC 134:143.
28 General Medical Council (2008) *Consent: patients and doctors making decisions together*, GMC, London, p.34.

29 Department of Health (2009) *Reference guide to consent for examination or treatment*, 2nd edn, DH, London, para 18.

30 Mason JK, Laurie GT. (2011) *Mason and McCall Smith's Law and Medical Ethics*, 8th edn, Oxford University Press, Oxford, p.108, para 4.108.

31 *Birch v University College London Hospital NHS Foundation Trust* (2008) 104 BMLR 168.

32 Kennedy I, Grubb A. (2000) *Medical Law*, 3rd edn, Butterworths, London, p.702.

33 General Medical Council (2008) *Consent: patients and doctors making decisions together*, GMC, London, para 17.

34 General Medical Council (2008) *Consent: patients and doctors making decisions together*, GMC, London, para 16.

35 Department of Health (2009) *Reference Guide to Consent for Examination or Treatment*, 2nd edn, DH, London, p.13, para 20; Department of Health, Social Services and Public Safety (2003) *Reference Guide to Consent for Examination, Treatment or Care*, DHSSPS, Belfast, p.7, para 4.8.

36 General Medical Council (2008) *Consent: patients and doctors making decisions together*, GMC, London, para 14; British Medical Association (2009) *Consent tool kit*, 5th edn. BMA, London, pp.11–13, card 3.

37 General Medical Council (2008) *Consent: patients and doctors making decisions together*, GMC, London, para 15.

38 General Medical Council (2008) *Consent: patients and doctors making decisions together*, GMC, London, para 23.

39 Royal College of Surgeons of England (2008) *Good Surgical Practice*, RCSEng, London, para 4.1.

40 General Medical Council (2008) *Consent: patients and doctors making decisions together*, GMC, London, para 49.

41 See, for example, Human Fertilisation and Embryology Act 1990, Sch 3.

42 Department of Health (2001) *Reference Guide to Consent for Examination or Treatment*, DH, London; Department of Health (2001) *Good Practice in Consent Implementation Guide: consent to examination or treatment*, DH, London.

43 Department of Health (2009) *Reference Guide to Consent for Examination or Treatment*, 2nd edn, DH, London.

44 All consent guidance and consent form templates are available on the Department of Health website at www.dh.gov.uk (accessed 8 February 2011).

45 Consent publications are available from the health department in Wales at www.wales.gov.uk (accessed 9 February 2011), in Northern Ireland at www.dhsspsni.gov.uk (accessed 9 February 2011) and Scotland www.clinicalgovernance.scot.nhs.uk (accessed 9 February 2011).

46 General Medical Council (2008) *Consent: patients and doctors making decisions together*, GMC, London, para 40.

47 General Medical Council (2008) *Consent: patients and doctors making decisions together*, GMC, London, para 79.

48 GMC Professional Conduct Committee hearing, 27–30 May 2002.

49 *Re T (adult: refusal of treatment)* [1992] 4 All ER 649.

50 General Medical Council (2008) *Consent: patients and doctors making decisions together*, GMC, London, para 19.

51 Treatment must be under the direction of the approved clinician in charge of the treatment, which must be for the patient's mental disorder or the symptoms of it (Mental Health Act 1983, s 63), or in respect of certain treatments under the Mental Health Act 1983, s 62.

52 *Re T (adult: refusal of treatment)* [1992] 4 All ER 649.

53 *Vo v France* (2005) 40 EHRR 12.

54 *Re B (adult: refusal of medical treatment)* [2002] 2 All ER 449.

55 *X v Austria* (1980) 18 DR 154; *YF v Turkey* (2004) 39 ECHR 34; *Pretty v UK* (2346/02) (2002) 35 EHRR 1.

56 *Re B (adult: refusal of medical treatment)* [2002] 2 All ER 449:454.

57 *Re B (adult: refusal of medical treatment)* [2002] 2 All ER 449:465.

58 *Airedale NHS Trust v Bland* [1993] 1 All ER 821:866.

59 A copy of the letter can be found on the Royal College of Psychiatrists' website at www.rcpsych.ac.uk (accessed 9 February 2011).

60 Anon. (2009) Doctors 'forced' to allow suicide. *BBC News Online* (Oct 1). Available at: www.bbc.co.uk/news (accessed 9 February 2011).

61 Smith R, Laing A, Devlin K. (2009) Suicide woman allowed to die because doctors feared saving her would be assault. *Daily Telegraph* (Sep 30). Available at: www.telegraph.co.uk (accessed 9 February 2011).

62 Bingham J. (2009) Living wills law could be 'revisited' after Kerrie Wooltorton suicide case – Andy Burnham. *Daily Telegraph* (Oct 4). Available at: www.telegraph.co.uk (accessed 9 February 2011).

63   Anon. (2009) Doctors 'forced' to allow suicide. *BBC News Online* (Oct 1). Available at: www.bbc.co.uk/news (accessed 9 February 2011).

64   *Re C (adult: refusal of medical treatment)* [1994] 1 All ER 819; Mental Capacity Act 2005, s 2; Department for Constitutional Affairs (2007) *Mental Capacity Act 2005 Code of Practice*, The Stationery Office, London.

65   *St George's Healthcare NHS Trust v S, R v Collins and others, ex parte S* [1998] 3 All ER 673.

66   Department of Health (2009) *Better Blood Transfusion Toolkit*. Available at: www. transfusionguidelines.org.uk (accessed 9 February 2011).

67   Association of Personal Injury Lawyers (2001) Case notes, *APIL Newsletter* (Dec), p.27.

68   Further information is available from the central office of the Hospital Information Service for Jehovah's Witnesses by contacting his@uk.jw.org.

69   Watch Tower Bible and Tract Society of Pennsylvania (1995) *Family Care and Medical Management for Jehovah's Witnesses*, Watch Tower Bible and Tract Society of New York, New York.

70   *R (on the application of Burke) v General Medical Council* [2005] 2 FLR 1223.

71   NHS Blood and Transplant (2010) *Transplant Activity in the UK 2009–10*, NHSBT, Bristol, p.1.

72   NHS Blood and Transplant (2010) *Transplant Activity in the UK 2009–10*, NHSBT, Bristol, p.18.

73   Ingelfinger JR. (2005) Risks and benefits to the living donor. *N Engl J Med* **353**, 447–9.

74   NHS Blood and Transplant. *Frequently asked questions about kidney transplantation*. Available at: www.organdonation.nhs.uk (accessed 9 February 2011).

75   Spital A. (2004) Donor benefit is the key to justified living organ donation. *Camb Q Healthc Ethics* **13**, 105–9.

76   Cronin AJ. (2008) Allowing autonomous agents freedom. *J Med Ethics* **34**, 129–32.

77   Kennedy I, Grubb A. (2000) *Medical law*, 3rd edn, Butterworths, London, p.1758.

78   *The decision,* 'Whose kidney is it anyway?' Channel 4, 20 February 1996.

79   Human Organ Transplants Act 1989. Human Organ Transplants (Northern Ireland) Order 1989.

80   Human Tissue Authority (2009) *Code of Practice 2: Donation of solid organs for transplantation*, HTA, London, para 62.

81   Human Tissue Act 2004 (Persons who lack capacity to consent and transplants) Regulations 2006. SI 2006/1659.

82   NHS Blood and Transplant (2010) *Transplant Activity in the UK 2009–10*, NHSBT, Bristol, p.11.

83   Human Tissue Authority (2007) *Altruistic kidney donor meets stranger recipient in 'UK first'*. Press release, 14 December.

84   Human Tissue Authority (2009) *More altruistic living kidney donors coming forward to donate to someone they do not know*. Press release, 24 June.

85   Glannon W. (2008) Editorial – Underestimating the risk in living kidney donation. *J Med Ethics* **34**, 127–8.

86   Organ Procurement and Transplantation Network (2010) *Policies: Living Donation*, para 12.9.3. Available at: www.unos.org (accessed 9 February 2011).

87   Lavee J, Ashkenazi T, Gurman G, *et al.* (2010) A new law for allocation of donor organs in Israel. *Lancet* **375**, 1131–3.

88   National Collaborating Centre for Mental Health (2006) *Obsessive-compulsive disorder: core interventions in the treatment of obsessive-compulsive disorder and body dysmorphic disorder*, Royal College of Psychiatrists, British Psychological Society, London, p.25.

89   First M. (2004) Desire for amputation of a limb: paraphilia, psychosis, or a new type of identity disorder. *Psychol Med* **34**, 1–10.

90   See, for example, the documentary film: Gilbert M. *Whole*. 2003.

91   Bayne T, Levy N. (2005) Amputees by choice: body integrity identity disorder and the ethics of amputation. *J Appl Philosophy* **22**, 75–86, p.78.

92   This case was featured in a documentary on body dysmorphic disorder, *Horizon*, 'Complete Obsession', BBC2, 17 February 2000.

93   Ellison J. (2008) Cutting desire. *Newsweek* (May 28). Available at: www.newsweek.com (accessed 9 February 2011).

94   Kennedy I, Grubb A. (2000) *Medical law*, 3rd edn, Butterworths, London, p.771.

95   Skegg PDG. (1984) *Law, Ethics and Medicine*, Clarendon, Oxford, p.38.

96   *R v Brown* [1993] 2 All ER 75.

97   Law Commission (1995) *Consultation paper no 139: consent in the criminal law*. HMSO, London, p.46.

98   Bayne T, Levy N. (2005) Amputees by choice: body integrity identity disorder and the ethics of amputation. *J Appl Philosophy* **22**, 75–86, pp. 79–80.

99   Patrone D. (2009) Disfigured anatomies and imperfect analogies: body integrity identity disorder and the supposed right to self-demanded amputation of healthy body parts. *J Med Ethics* **35**, 541–545, p.543.

100   *R (on the application of Burke) v General Medical Council* [2005] 2 FLR 1223.

101 Gutridge K. (2010) Safer self-injury or assisted self-harm? *Theor Med Bioeth* **34**, 79–92; Gutridge K. (2010) Free to self-injure? In: Dickenson D, Huxtable R, Parker M. (eds.) *The Cambridge Medical Ethics Workbook*, 2nd edn, Cambridge University Press, Cambridge, pp.112–5.

102 Savulescu J. (2007) Autonomy, the good life, and controversial choices. In: Rhodes R, Francis LP, Silvers A. (eds.) *The Blackwell Guide to Medical Ethics*, Blackwell Publishing, London, pp. 17–37.

103 Bayne T, Levy N. (2005) Amputees by choice: body integrity identity disorder and the ethics of amputation. *J Appl Philosophy* **22**, 75–86, p.79.

104 *Horizon*, 'Complete Obsession', BBC 2, 2000 February 17.

105 First M. (2004) Desire for amputation of a limb: paraphilia, psychosis, or a new type of identity disorder. *Psychol Med* **34**, 1–10, p.9.

3: Treating adults who lack capacity

The questions covered in this chapter include the following.

- What is capacity?
- How should capacity be assessed?
- How can a person's 'best interests' be determined?
- Who may give consent to treatment on behalf of an adult who lacks the capacity to consent?
- Are advance decisions legally binding?
- When is compulsory treatment an option?

Consent and the alternatives

Except for the rare circumstances in which the law allows compulsory treatment for mental disorder, some forensic purposes and some investigations under public health legislation, consent from an adult is required before treatment or examination can take place. Where adults lack the capacity to make a necessary decision, it follows that the decision must be made by someone else on their behalf. In these circumstances, the nature of the doctor–patient partnership inevitably changes, with the emphasis shifting from a respect for individual decision making to a more welfare-oriented approach, with individual decisions being made on the basis of an assessment of the patient's needs and interests, although clearly involving the individual in the decision-making process as far as possible. A decision that an adult lacks capacity is a significant one, potentially involving the curtailment of significant rights and freedoms. Decision making in relation to adults lacking capacity has therefore long been an area of ethical and legal scrutiny. The period from 2000 through to 2010 also saw significant legal change in this area, with primary legislation appearing in both Scotland and in England and Wales. Separate legislation is also being developed in Northern Ireland.

Although the basic ethical issues remain consistent across the separate jurisdictions, there are nevertheless some variations in legal procedures. In order to avoid excessive repetition, this introduction begins with a discussion of the ethical issues common to all the jurisdictions. It also looks in some detail at the common law cases that have influenced both statute and professional practice and at issues directly related to assessing capacity. The chapter focuses principally on treatment, and although there is a small introductory piece on research involving incapacitated adults, further detail is provided in Chapter 14 on research and innovative treatment. Having established the background, the bulk of the chapter then focuses on the separate legal provisions in each of the various jurisdictions. In England and Wales the relevant legislation is the Mental Capacity Act 2005 (MCA); in Scotland, the Adults with Incapacity (Scotland) Act 2000. In Northern Ireland decisions are currently made under the common law. Further information on legal developments

Medical Ethics Today: The BMA's Handbook of Ethics and Law, Third Edition. Sophie Brannan, Eleanor Chrispin, Martin Davies, Veronica English, Rebecca Mussell, Julian Sheather and Ann Sommerville.
© 2012 BMA Medical Ethics Department. Published 2012 by Blackwell Publishing Ltd.

in Northern Ireland will be made available on the British Medical Association's (BMA) website.

The focus of this chapter is on the provision of treatment to adults who lack the capacity to consent. There will, of course, be occasions when these individuals will also have mental disorders that might make them eligible for treatment under mental health legislation. Many of the issues raised by mental health legislation are highly technical and are outside the scope of this chapter. There is some discussion, however, on the points of interface between the statutory provisions for mental health and mental capacity. It is anticipated that legislation being developed in Northern Ireland will bring together mental health and mental capacity provisions into a single piece of legislation.

Although each of the separate sections provides practical advice relevant to the specific jurisdictions, it is strongly recommended that doctors also acquaint themselves with the ethical issues raised in the preliminary discussion.

Proxy decision making and the role of those close to the patient

When patients lack the capacity to make decisions, others clearly need to make decisions on their behalf. Families and those close to the adult often feel that they are the natural decision makers, but the law is clear that they are only entitled to consent where they have been appointed as the patient's proxy decision maker. Legal provisions for patients to appoint proxy decision makers are available in England, Wales and Scotland, but currently there are no such provisions in Northern Ireland, although this may change. Unless appointed as legal proxies, relatives have no right to give consent to treatment, and responsibility will usually fall to the doctor in overall charge of the patient's care, who decides on the basis of the requirement to act and, in England, Wales and Northern Ireland, on the basis of an assessment of the patient's best interests. In Scotland, the legislation refers to the requirement that the intervention provide a 'benefit' to the patient but, in the BMA's view, in practice the two terms are generally likely to be interchangeable. Despite this, families and those close to adults who lack capacity have an essential role. The relevant sections in this chapter look at the scope and limits of that role. They describe the nature of decision-making capacity and provide advice on how it should be assessed. This chapter also looks at the importance of involving incapacitated adults to the fullest extent in decision making and at law and good practice in relation to proxy decision makers.

A decision about whether an adult lacks capacity is clearly a significant one. The presumption that all adults have the right to make their own decisions is a central feature of both law and ethical practice. Too hasty a decision that an adult lacks capacity can therefore lead to the violation of fundamental rights and freedoms. On the other hand, a failure to identify that an adult lacks appropriate decision-making capacity can mean that opportunities to provide necessary support and protection may be lost. The careful assessment of an individual's capacity is therefore central to the protection of their rights and interests and to the provision of good medical care.

Approaches to the care and treatment of adults who lack capacity have been changing. A number of factors have contributed to an increased sensitivity to the rights of adults who may either lack capacity to make specific decisions or who may be experiencing some cognitive decline. The process of developing statute in relation to adults lacking capacity has itself led to wide discussion and consultation and has given voice to patient and advocacy groups seeking to promote and protect the interests of incapacitated adults. A growing and increasingly articulate population of older people in the UK has also helped to overturn discriminatory stereotypes about the abilities of older people generally and has, once and for all, overturned the idea that decision-making ability necessarily declines with age. Recent years have also led to a recognition of the importance of respecting and promoting individual patient rights throughout the health and social care sectors and of respecting their wider human rights.[1] Combined, these changes have led to the recognition of the fundamental ethical obligation to place the patient at the centre of decision making, to enhance patients' decision-making abilities and to ensure that where decisions need to be made on behalf of adults, they reflect, as far as possible, their known wishes and values. A set of general ethical principles that relate to all treatment and welfare decisions involving incapacitated adults is given below.

Vulnerable adults: balancing freedom with protection

It is a fundamental principle in law and ethics that people with capacity have a right to make medical decisions that affect their own lives. Concerns are sometimes expressed, however, about adults who retain some decision-making capacity but whose health and circumstances make it more difficult for them to promote their own interests. Focus on these 'vulnerable adults' has been growing in recent years. These can include people with mental disorders or disabling physical conditions, people with drug and alcohol problems, displaced persons such as asylum seekers, and individuals in abusive relationships. It can also include frail older people with some cognitive or physical impairment. The pressures of some forms of institutional care can also heighten vulnerabilities. Health professionals frequently express concern about these capacitous vulnerable adults. While recognising that they have rights to make decisions about their life, it can nevertheless be challenging to health professionals to stand by when people remain in situations that may cause them harm, particularly where positive options are available, and where there are concerns that they may be subject to some coercion. There are no easy answers here. Competent decisions can only be overruled in exceptional circumstances and adults have the right to make choices in life that expose them to risk. In these situations, it is important that health professionals try, as far as possible, to maintain positive relationships with the individual and to continue to offer support. Options for treatment or support should ideally be discussed with the individual, and efforts should be made to ensure that such vulnerable adults are not 'lost' to health and social services.

Providing medical treatment in an emergency

In an emergency situation where consent cannot be obtained, doctors should provide treatment that they reasonably believe to be both medically necessary and in the patient's best interests, unless there is a valid and applicable advance decision refusing the necessary treatment. Where a decision can be put off until such a time as the individual is likely to regain capacity, or those close to the patient can be consulted, then it should be deferred.

If, in an emergency, a patient refuses treatment and there is doubt about his or her capacity to do so validly, doctors should take whatever steps are necessary to prevent deterioration of the patient's condition. Similarly, if a patient lacks capacity and a proxy refuses treatment that the doctor believes to be in the patient's best interests, emergency treatment should be provided. Once the patient has been stabilised, the normal procedures for making decisions about capacity and providing treatment should be followed.

When someone has attempted suicide and lacks the capacity to consent or refuse treatment, doctors will ordinarily be justified in attempting to save the individual's life. In these circumstances it will rarely be possible to be certain that the person had definitely intended to end his or her life, or that he or she had relevant capacity when the suicide attempt was made. In England and Wales, advance decisions refusing treatment have to be made in a specified format (see pages 114–115) and a hastily written suicide note should not be taken as a legally binding refusal. Even when the patient has attempted suicide and presents with an advance decision refusing treatment, there may be reason to doubt that the patient had capacity when it was made. When there is reasonable doubt about the validity of an advance decision, treatment should be provided in an emergency and then issues about capacity and the patient's intentions investigated subsequently. (For further information about emergency treatment, see Chapter 15.)

Advance decisions refusing treatment

Currently, advance decisions refusing medical treatment, sometimes referred to colloquially as advance directives or living wills, have been given statutory force only in England and Wales. In the UK's other jurisdictions, their lawfulness rests by and large by analogy with earlier English case law which made it clear that an unambiguous and informed advance decision refusing treatment is as valid as a competent contemporaneous refusal. Although neither Scotland nor Northern Ireland is under a legal obligation to follow English precedent, such cases are likely to be influential because they reflect the general principle of taking into account a person's known wishes. This is a principle given statutory expression in Scotland. Practical issues relating to advance decisions are discussed in each of the relevant sections in this chapter.

Advance decisions refusing medical treatment, particularly those refusing serious or life-sustaining treatment, have been the source of some controversy. Advance decisions are a means of enabling adults to exercise some control over decisions that may need to be made at a future time when they have lost the ability to make them. Doctors have expressed concerns in the past about a number of features of advance decisions. It can, for example, be extremely difficult to specify in advance the conditions that may arise or the kinds of treatment that will be offered. This can lead to difficulties in identifying the extent to which the decision is valid, and where there is doubt, doctors will ordinarily act to preserve life. For these reasons, when patients are considering drawing up a document to communicate advance decisions, it is a good idea to take medical advice in order to understand the likely course of any disorder and the treatments or interventions likely to be offered. It can also be difficult to anticipate in advance of serious illness how each individual will respond. Decisions made in full health and with full use of mental capacities may look different when in great pain or nearing the end of life. Advance decisions can have significant consequences and it is therefore important that anyone considering making them should be advised carefully to think through the likely implications.

The relationship with mental health legislation

There will be occasions when adults who lack capacity with respect to certain decisions fulfil the relevant criteria for treatment under both capacity and mental health law. Although treatment under either may be lawful, there are nonetheless significant distinctions between the regimes and in such circumstances careful consideration must be given as to which is the better approach. Although the following sections go into more detail with regard to the separate jurisdictions, the following general points should be taken into consideration.

- Where a patient retains capacity with respect to a decision for a mental disorder, capacity legislation cannot be used and, in the absence of consent, treatment can only be provided under mental health legislation.
- Where treatment is to be provided for a physical disorder, particularly where it is unlinked to a mental disorder, mental health legislation cannot be used.
- Where deprivation of liberty may be necessary, and the grounds for detention are met, consideration should be given to using mental health legislation in order to take advantage of its enhanced safeguards.

General principles

The following general principles should be taken into account when considering the medical treatment of a patient lacking capacity to consent. Patients are entitled to the following.

- *Liberty:* patients should be free from interventions that inhibit liberty or the ability to enjoy life unless the intervention is necessary to prevent a greater harm to the patient or to others. Treatment options should be the least restrictive possible while still being able to realise the goals of the treatment. Appropriate justification must be shown for the use of restraints and it is inappropriate for restrictive measures to be used as an alternative to adequate staffing levels.
- *Decision-making freedom:* patients' decision-making freedom should be promoted in a manner that is consistent with their needs and wishes. Where patients have fluctuating capacity, individual autonomy should be promoted to the greatest possible extent.
- *Dignity:* patients should be treated with respect and courtesy, and their social and cultural values should be respected.
- *Having their views taken into account:* patients' views should be taken into account even when they are considered in law to be incapable of making a decision.
- *Bodily integrity:* patients should be free from any medical interventions unless there are good therapeutic reasons for them.
- *Confidentiality:* incapacitated adults have the same right to confidentiality as other adults.
- *Having their health needs met:* patients' health needs should be met as fully as practicable, while recognising that the availability of resources may limit treatment options.
- *Being free from unfair discrimination:* treatment options should be considered on the basis of the patient's need and patients should not be treated differently solely because of the condition that gives rise to the incapacity.
- *Having the views of people close to them taken into account:* the views of those close to patients should be taken into account even when they are not entitled in law to make decisions on behalf of the patient.

In complex cases, for example where capacity may be in doubt, or the benefits and burdens of the treatment are finely balanced, it is advisable to discuss the matter widely with relevant individuals and, where necessary, to obtain a second opinion from another doctor. This can both assure the doctor proposing to treat the patient that the patient does lack capacity to decide and that the treatment is in the patient's best interests or for their benefit. The following steps are intended as a guide:

- consider whether there are alternative ways of treating the patient, particularly equally effective measures that may be less invasive, keep future options open and promote independence

- consider whether the proposals impact on the patient's human rights
- discuss the treatment within the healthcare team
- discuss the treatment with the patient insofar as this is possible
- consult relatives, carers and any proxy decision makers
- consider any anticipatory statement of the patient's views (valid and applicable advance decisions refusing treatment must be respected)
- consult other appropriate professionals involved with the patient's care in the hospital or community
- consider the need to obtain a second opinion from a doctor skilled in assessment of capacity or in the proposed treatment
- ensure that a record is made of the discussions.

Assessing an individual's decision-making capacity

There will be some circumstances, for example where an adult is unconscious, where an assessment of capacity is straightforward. In most other circumstances individuals will retain some level of capacity and will therefore be able to make some decisions. In accordance with both the law and good practice, every reasonable effort must be made to support individuals to make their own decisions. Although unconscious patients will clearly not retain any decision-making ability, in all other circumstances, adults are presumed to have capacity and it is important to avoid making blanket assumptions about an individual's decision-making ability. Similarly, earlier periods of incapacity should not be allowed to prejudice future assessments of capacity.

What is capacity?

Decision-making capacity refers to the everyday ability that individuals possess to make decisions or to take actions that influence their life. These range from simple decisions, such as when to get up and what to wear or to have for breakfast, to far-reaching decisions about serious medical treatment or complex financial investments. In a legal context it refers to a person's ability to do something that may have legal consequences, such as making a will, entering into a contract or agreeing to medical treatment. The starting point of any assessment of capacity must be the presumption that an adult has the capacity to make a specified decision unless there is evidence to the contrary.

More complex and far-reaching decisions are likely to require greater levels of decision-making ability, and the law recognises this by acknowledging that different decisions can require different tests of capacity. When assessing an individual's capacity, doctors must always consider the nature and implications of the decision that needs to be made as well as the patient's ability to make the decision. Ultimately, capacity is a legal concept and if there is doubt about a patient's capacity, the courts can be asked to decide, taking into account evidence from doctors as appropriate. Doctors may be involved in assessing capacity, not only for deciding about medical treatment, but they may also be asked to assess an individual's capacity to make other decisions, such as making a will. Different tests of capacity apply to different tasks. When doctors are asked to assess somebody's capacity they must therefore familiarise themselves with the relevant legal tests. The BMA publishes, jointly with the Law Society, advice on assessing capacity in a range of circumstances.[2] Two legal cases have been particularly influential in the development of the tests of capacity and although now codified, with some adjustments, they clearly illustrate the issues involved and are still useful for practitioners seeking to apply the statutory tests of capacity to decisions relating to medical treatment. In the first, a patient with a severe mental disorder was found to have the capacity to refuse treatment for a physical condition. In the second, a patient's severe needle phobia was found to invalidate her capacity to refuse a caesarean section.

Refusal of treatment for a physical condition by a mentally ill patient

C was a 68-year-old patient with paranoid schizophrenia. In 1993 he developed gangrene in a foot during his confinement in a secure hospital to which he had been transferred under mental health legislation while serving a 7-year term of imprisonment. He was removed to a general hospital, where the consultant surgeon diagnosed that there was an 85 per cent chance that he would die imminently if the leg was not amputated below the knee. C refused to consider amputation. He said that he would rather die with two feet than live with one.

C had grandiose and persecutory delusions, including that he had an international career in medicine during the course of which he had never lost a patient. He expressed complete confidence in his ability to survive aided by God, the good doctors and the good nurses, but acknowledged the possibility of death as a consequence of retaining his limb. He was content to follow medical advice and cooperate with treatment provided his rejection of amputation was respected. Conservative treatment was progressing well at the time of the hearing.

The High Court identified three necessary components of capacity to give consent to medical treatment. The patient must be able to:

- understand and retain the information relevant to the decision in question
- believe that information
- weigh that information in the balance to arrive at a choice.

The Court found that C's schizophrenia did impact on his general capacity, but what was relevant to the decision about amputation was that he had understood and retained the relevant treatment information, that in his own way he believed it and in the same fashion had arrived at a choice. The hospital was therefore not entitled to amputate his leg without his express written consent, nor could it do so in the future, even if his mental capacity deteriorated.[3]

In a second case, the Court of Appeal dismissed a 23-year-old woman's appeal against a decision to administer medical procedures required as part of a caesarean section.

Refusal of treatment due to phobia

MB was 40 weeks pregnant. The fetus was in the breech position. MB had a needle phobia and would not agree to a caesarean section because of the venepuncture involved. The Court of Appeal considered whether she had the capacity to decide about the procedure. Noting that adults are presumed to have capacity unless the contrary is proven, and that a woman with relevant capacity may for 'religious reasons, other reasons, for rational or irrational reasons, or for no reason at all, choose not to have medical intervention, even though the consequences may be the death or serious handicap of the child she bears, or her own death', the Court set out the relevant test of capacity.

A person lacks capacity if some impairment or disturbance of mental functioning renders the person unable to make a decision whether to consent to or refuse treatment. That inability to make a decision occurs when:

- the patient is unable to comprehend and retain the information that is material to the decision, especially as to the likely consequences of having or not having the treatment in question

- the patient is unable to use the information and weigh it in the balance as part of the process of arriving at a decision.

The Court found that MB's fear of needles dominated her thinking, and 'made her quite unable to consider anything else'.[4] She was found to lack the capacity to refuse treatment and it was therefore lawful for the doctors to administer anaesthetic in an emergency if it was in MB's best interests to do so. The Court also noted that it was obvious that MB was more likely to suffer significant long-term harm from death or injury to the baby than from receiving the anaesthetic against her wishes. It was likely, therefore, that should anaesthetic become necessary, it would be in her best interests to administer it.

Fluctuating capacity

One area that can raise particular difficulty relates to adults whose capacity may fluctuate. This could be, for example, where an individual has a bipolar disorder and may be in a temporary manic phase. Some treatments can also lead to periods of reduced capacity, and transient factors such as shock or grief can also have an impact on an individual's ability to make a specific decision. As with all such decisions, an assessment of capacity must be made on the basis of the decision in question at the time it needs to be made. Although if urgent treatment is required it may be necessary to make a decision during a period of incapacity, where a decision can be delayed until capacity improves then it should be. As emphasised throughout this chapter, unless it is an emergency and an immediate decision is required, all reasonable efforts should be made to enhance an individual's decision-making capacity.

Capacity to consent and to refuse

As discussed in Chapter 2, adults with capacity have the right to refuse medical treatment or diagnostic procedures for reasons which are 'rational, irrational or for no reason.'[5] An assessment of capacity is nonetheless commensurate with the seriousness of the decision and the more serious the decision, the greater the decision-making ability required. Generally, the measures that doctors propose are in the best medical interests of patients, and deciding not to follow medical advice can have serious implications. Therefore, although consent and refusal are opposite sides of the same coin, the courts have shown themselves more reluctant to accept weak evidence of capacity when refusal is at stake. This has sometimes meant, in practice, that patients are more likely to be regarded as lacking capacity when they refuse treatment than when they accept it.

Capacity being commensurate with the gravity of the decision

In a case involving a Jehovah's Witness who refused a blood transfusion, the Master of the Rolls said:

Doctors faced with a refusal of consent have to give very careful and detailed consideration to the patient's capacity to decide at the time when the decision was made. It may not be the simple case of the patient having no capacity because, for example, at that time he had hallucinations. It may be the more difficult case of a temporarily reduced capacity at the time when his decision was made. What matters is that the doctors should consider whether at that time he had a capacity which was commensurate with the gravity of the decision which he purported to make. The more serious the decision, the greater the capacity required. If the patient had the requisite capacity, they are bound by his decision. If not, they are free to treat him in what they believe to be his best interests.[6]

Unwise decisions

People are entitled to choose an option that is contradictory to that which most people would choose, but where their choice also appears to be a very reckless choice or to contradict their previously expressed attitudes, health professionals would be justified in questioning in greater detail their capacity to make a valid refusal, in order to eliminate the possibility that capacity may be impaired as a result of, for example, a depressive illness or a delusional state. A specialist psychiatric opinion may be required. Care should be taken, however, to ensure that there is not an excessive delay in obtaining an assessment, particularly where the patient may be requesting that treatment be discontinued. In these circumstances continued treatment in the face of a refusal could amount to an assault.[7]

Refusal rendered invalid by misinformation and undue influence

T was 20 years old and 34 weeks pregnant when she was injured in a road traffic accident. She had been brought up by her mother in accordance with the beliefs of the Jehovah's Witnesses, but did not become a member. On admission to hospital T twice refused a blood transfusion after having spent a period of time alone with her mother. A caesarean section was carried out, but the baby was stillborn. T's condition deteriorated and, had it not been for her advance refusal, the anaesthetist would have given her a blood transfusion. On the following day T's father and boyfriend decided to go to court to challenge the validity of the advance refusal. The challenge was upheld and the blood transfusion was given. The basis for this decision included, in the court's view, that T had been acting under the influence of her mother and the refusal did not represent a legitimate expression of T's free will. There were also serious doubts about her physical and mental state when refusing treatment and whether T had intended her refusal to apply to a situation that was life threatening. She had also been given misleading information about the availability and effectiveness of alternative treatments.

The Court of Appeal held that in such a circumstance doctors should accept that a refusal is valid only after considering whether capacity is diminished by illness, medication, false assumptions or misinformation, or whether the patient's will had been overborne by another's influence. In T's situation, it was held that the effect of her condition, together with misinformation and her mother's influence, rendered her refusal of consent invalid.[8]

Strictly speaking, undue influence refers less to capacity than the ability to exercise or to act upon that capacity. It is therefore more of an issue of voluntariness – the ability to provide valid consent is undermined rather than capacity itself.

Summary – assessment of individual's decision-making capacity

- Adults with capacity have the right to make health decisions on their own behalf even where those decisions do not appear to be in their objective best interests.
- When individuals lack the capacity to make specific decisions, others may need to make those decisions on their behalf.

- 'Next of kin' do not automatically have decision-making rights on behalf of incapacitated adults although they may need to be consulted as part of an evaluation of what is in the best interests of the adult.
- Decisions made on behalf of incapacitated adults must be made on the basis of an assessment of their best interests, or, in Scotland, their 'benefit'.
- The careful assessment of an individual's capacity is central to the protection of their rights and interests and to the provision of good medical care.
- Assessments of capacity must be decision specific.
- Valid and applicable advance decisions refusing treatment are legally binding.

Research and innovative treatment involving adults lacking the capacity to consent

Research, or the use of new or unproven interventions involving adults lacking capacity to consent to their participation, is an area of particular ethical sensitivity. Historical abuses of research in relation to vulnerable groups have led to the progressive development of stringent research governance frameworks in order to ensure that the interests of incapacitated subjects are protected. A balance is required, however, between the need to protect incapacitated adults and the requirement to ensure that research into both their care and the underlying conditions that give rise to incapacity is able to progress.

Although in seeking to achieve this balance there are some differences of approach in the separate UK jurisdictions, discussed in Chapter 14, there is nonetheless a great deal of common ground. A key source of ethical guidance for research governance in the UK is the World Medical Association's Declaration of Helsinki.[9]

Basic principles include the following.

- Adults lacking capacity to consent should not be included in research that is unlikely to benefit them personally, unless the research is necessary to promote the health of the population represented by the research subject.
- Incapacitated adults should only be enrolled in research where it is not possible to enrol adults with capacity.
- Research involving incapacitated adults must involve only minimal risks and burdens to the subjects.
- Where an adult is incapable of consenting to research, consent must be sought from a legally authorised representative.
- Any dissent or objection from an adult lacking the capacity to consent to participation in research should be respected, and the adult should either not be enrolled or withdrawn if they have already been enrolled.
- Research involving subjects who are physically or mentally incapable of giving consent may be undertaken only if the physical or mental condition that prevents giving informed consent is a necessary characteristic of the research population.

Providing treatment to adults lacking capacity – England and Wales

The provision of medical treatment to adults who lack the capacity to make those decisions is governed in England and Wales by the Mental Capacity Act 2005, which came into force in 2007. The Act provides a legal framework for decision making on behalf of people aged 16 or over who lack the capacity to make a specific decision themselves. (There are some exceptions in relation to the provision of medical treatment to children aged 16 and 17 years and these are dealt with separately below.) It also sets out the law for people who wish to make preparations for a time in the future when they may lack capacity to make certain decisions. The Act is based on two fundamental concepts drawn from the common law – lack of capacity and best interests. Before the powers of the Act can be used it must be established that an adult lacks capacity to make the decision in question and any subsequent decision made on his or her behalf must be based on an assessment of his or her best interests. The Act applies to a very wide range of decisions including welfare and financial decisions, but the focus in this section is on those relating to medical treatment.

Although the Act largely codifies and puts on a statutory footing the pre-existing common law position, it introduces some new provisions, including the following:

- the ability for individuals with the relevant capacity to nominate another person, an 'attorney', with legal authority to make health and welfare decisions at a time in the future when capacity is lost
- the power of the Court of Protection to appoint a deputy with legal authority to make specific decisions concerning the health and welfare of a person lacking capacity to make those decisions
- the development of safeguards to enable incapacitated adults to be enrolled in certain forms of research
- the development of safeguards which must be applied where an adult lacking capacity to consent requires care or treatment in circumstances that amount to a deprivation of liberty.

All doctors in England and Wales working with adults who lack, or who may lack, capacity need to be familiar with the Act's basic principles and its underlying provisions, and these are set out in some detail here. The Act is supported by a statutory Code of Practice which provides detailed guidance on how the Act should be used. Doctors making decisions on behalf of incapacitated adults have a legal duty to 'have regard' to the guidance given in the Code. Anyone requiring further information should refer both to the Code of Practice[10] and to the joint BMA/Law Society guidance, *Assessment of Mental Capacity*.[11]

The Mental Capacity Act 2005 – an outline

- The Act provides a comprehensive framework for decision making on behalf of adults aged 16 and over who lack the capacity to make specific decisions.
- Decision-making capacity refers to the everyday ability that individuals possess to make decisions or to take actions that influence their lives including decisions about medical treatment.
- Under the Act, a person lacks capacity if, at the time the decision needs to be made, he or she is unable either to make, or to communicate a decision as a result of an 'impairment of, or disturbance in the functioning of, the mind or brain'.[12]
- Where it is determined that individuals lack the capacity to make specified decisions, any such decisions made on their behalf must be made on the basis of an assessment of their 'best interests'.

The Act's basic principles

The Act sets out a number of basic principles that must govern decisions made and actions taken on behalf of incapacitated adults. Where confusion arises about how aspects of the Act should be interpreted it can be useful to refer back to these principles. Actions or decisions that clearly conflict with them are unlikely to be lawful, although there may be occasions when the principles are in tension with each other and some balancing may be necessary. Section 1 of the Act is given below. Brief descriptions of the principles follow. There is also further discussion of 'best interests' later in this section.

Mental Capacity Act 2005 – the principles

1. 'The following principles apply for the purposes of this Act.
2. A person must be assumed to have capacity unless it is established that he lacks capacity.
3. A person is not to be treated as unable to make a decision unless all practicable steps to help him to do so have been taken without success.
4. A person is not to be treated as unable to make a decision merely because he makes an unwise decision.
5. An act done or decision made, under this Act for or on behalf of a person who lacks capacity must be done, or made, in his best interests.
6. Before the act is done, or the decision is made, regard must be had to whether the purpose for which it is needed can be as effectively achieved in a way that is less restrictive of the person's rights and freedom of action.'[13]

A presumption of capacity

It is a fundamental principle of English law that adults have the right to make decisions on their own behalf and are assumed to have the capacity to do so unless it is proven otherwise. The responsibility for demonstrating that an adult lacks capacity rests with the person who challenges it.

Maximising decision-making capacity

Before it is decided that individuals lack capacity, everything practicable must be done to support them to make their own decisions. This refers principally to a variety of possible practical methods such as the use of advocates, language and communication support, and assessing capacity at the time most favourable for the individual. Consideration must also be given to the possibility that capacity may improve.

The freedom to make unwise decisions

This principle reflects the right, established at common law, that adults can make decisions which others consider unwise or irrational. The fact that an individual makes a rash, unwise or irrational decision is not itself proof of incapacity. Where such actions are out of character, or follow an accident or a period of illness, they may raise questions about capacity, but they are not in themselves determinative. What matters is the ability to make the decision, not the outcome.

Best interests

At the heart of the Act lies the principle that where it is determined that individuals lack capacity, any decision or action taken must be in their best interests. In practice, an assessment of best interests will depend upon the circumstances of each individual case.

The less restrictive alternative

Whenever people make decisions on behalf of adults who lack capacity, they must consider if it is possible to make a decision that is less restrictive of their fundamental rights or freedoms while still achieving the necessary goal and acting in the person's best interests.

Assessing capacity

When does a person lack capacity?

For the purposes of the Act, 'a person lacks capacity in relation to a matter if at the material time he is unable to make a decision for himself in relation to the matter because of impairment of, or a disturbance in the functioning of, the mind or brain'.[14] The Act uses a two-stage assessment of capacity.

- Is there an impairment of, or disturbance in the functioning of, the mind or brain? If so:
- is the impairment or disturbance sufficient that the person is unable to make that particular decision?

An assessment of capacity is task-specific: it focuses on the particular decision that needs to be made at the time it needs to be made. It does not matter if the incapacity is temporary, or the person retains the capacity to make other decisions, or if the person's capacity may fluctuate over time. The important point is whether the individual lacks capacity for the specified decision at the specific time the decision needs to be made. The inability to make the decision must, however, be a result of the impairment or disturbance already mentioned. The impairment or disturbance could be the result of a range of conditions including mental illness, learning disability, dementia, brain damage or intoxication. If the impairment is temporary and the decision can realistically be put off until such a time as the patient is likely to regain capacity, then it should be deferred.

Who should assess capacity?

The individual who wishes to make a decision on behalf of an incapacitated adult is responsible for assessing his or her capacity. Where consent to medical treatment is required, it is the responsibility of the health professional proposing the treatment to decide whether the patient has the capacity to consent. In hospital settings, treatment may involve multi-disciplinary teams, but ultimately the decision will rest with the professional responsible for the provision of treatment. The reasons why capacity is in doubt should be recorded in the medical record, as should details of the assessment process and its findings. More complex decisions may require more formal assessments and it may be helpful to seek the opinion of a colleague such as a psychiatrist or psychologist. Exceptionally, where disagreement persists, an application to the Court of Protection may be made.

How do you assess capacity?

Once it has been established that an individual is suffering from 'an impairment of, or a disturbance in the functioning of, the mind or brain' which may be affecting his or her decision-making capacity, attention must turn to identifying whether or not the impairment or disturbance is sufficient to affect his or her ability to make the specific decision. Under the Act, a person is regarded as being unable to make a decision if, at the time the decision needs to be made, he or she is unable:

- to understand the information relevant to the decision
- to retain the information relevant to the decision
- to use or weigh the information
- to communicate the decision (by any means).[15]

Where an individual fails one or more parts of this test, then they do not have the capacity to make the relevant decision and the entire test is failed.

In assessing capacity consideration should be given, where appropriate, to the views of those close to the individual. Family members and close friends may be able to provide valuable background information, although their views about what they might want for the individual must not be allowed to influence the assessment. Health professionals need to ensure that any assessment is not based on factors that are irrelevant to capacity. It must not, for example, be based simply on a person's age or appearance or any unfounded assumptions about their condition or behaviour. The focus has to be on the ability to make the decision in question at the time the decision needs to be made.

Enhancing capacity

Both ethically and legally, doctors are under an obligation to take all practical and appropriate steps to enable adults to make decisions on their own behalf. This is an area in which health professionals can make a significant difference to the protection of individual freedoms. In aiding an individual's decision-making capacity, the following questions may be helpful.

- Has all the information relevant to the decision been given to the patient, including any alternatives to the proposed treatment and the likely consequences of non-treatment?
- Has it been given in a form and in a way that is suitable to their understanding, for example by using simple language or visual aids or non-verbal forms of communication?
- Has consideration been given to involving someone to assist in communication, such as a relative, advocate or speech and language therapist?
- Are there certain times of day or particular locations that are more favourable for the individual?
- Can the decision, or information relating to the decision, be broken down into more manageable pieces?
- Have appropriate cultural, ethnic or religious factors been taken into account?

Uncertainties about capacity

Although the Act sets out a clear definition of lack of capacity, difficult judgements will still need to be made, particularly where there is fluctuating capacity, where a decision about capacity is disputed, or where some capacity is demonstrable but its extent is uncertain. In these circumstances, doctors should consider either a second opinion, or a referral to a colleague with more experience in assessing capacity or in treating the condition that may be causing the lack of capacity. It would be impractical, however, for professional experts routinely to be called upon in situations where assessments using the statutory test of capacity can be carried out by other decision makers. Responsibility rests with the person intending to make the decision on behalf of the person lacking capacity, not with the professional advising about capacity.

Ultimately, a decision about whether or not an adult has capacity is a legal one and, where there are disputes about an individual's capacity that cannot be resolved by using more informal methods, the Court of Protection can be asked for a judgment.[16]

What do you do when an individual refuses to be assessed?

Occasionally, individuals whose capacity is in doubt may refuse to be assessed. In most cases, a sensitive explanation of the potential consequences of such a refusal, such as the possibility that any decision they make will be challenged at a later date, will be sufficient for them to agree. However, if an individual refuses, in most cases no one can be required to undergo an assessment. Advice can always be sought from the Office of the Public Guardian.[17]

Summary – assessing capacity (England and Wales)

- Under the Mental Capacity Act 2005 people lack capacity if they are unable to make or communicate a decision because of an impairment of, or disturbance in the functioning of, the mind or brain.
- An assessment of capacity focuses on the specific decision that needs to be made at the time it needs to be made.
- The individual who wishes to make a decision on behalf of an incapacitated adult, or to carry out a proposed medical procedure, is responsible for assessing the patient's capacity to make the decision.
- Doctors are under an obligation to take all practical and appropriate steps to enable adults to make decisions on their own behalf.
- As a last resort, where uncertainties about an individual's capacity cannot be resolved informally, the Court of Protection can be asked for a judgment.

Best interests

The MCA makes it clear that, with a few exceptions discussed in more detail below, all decisions taken on behalf of someone who lacks capacity must be taken in his or her best interests. This is a statutory restatement of the former common law position and the Act has not therefore introduced changes to best practice. The Act does not define 'best interests' but provides a checklist of common factors that must always be taken into account when making a best interests judgement (see below). The Code of Practice does, however, make it clear that a best interests judgement is not exclusively an attempt to determine what the person would have wanted, although this must clearly be taken into account and regarded as a significant factor. It is instead as objective a test as possible of what would be in the person's actual best interests, taking into consideration all relevant factors. The Code of Practice and the checklist in the Act also make it clear that, in relation to medical treatment, a best interests test involves more than just an assessment of clinical interests, and extends to a consideration of the individual's wishes and values, where they can be identified.

'Best interests' checklist

When making a 'best interests' assessment, the following questions should be taken into account.

- Have you taken all reasonable steps to encourage the individual to participate in the decision?
- Have you considered whether the decision is discriminatory (i.e. whether it has been made solely on the basis of the person's age, appearance, condition or behaviour)?
- Have you tried to identify all the things that the person would take into account if they were making the decision for themselves?
- Have you taken into account the person's past and present wishes and feelings, expressed verbally or in writing, and any of the person's beliefs or values that might have a bearing on the decision?
- Have you considered whether the person might regain capacity in the future and, if so, whether the decision can be delayed until that time?
- Have you considered whether there are other options that might be less restrictive of the person's rights that are commensurate with the desired goal?
- In relation to life-sustaining treatment, are you clear that the decision is not motivated by a desire to bring about the person's death?
- Where appropriate, have you consulted with other people who may be able to provide information about the person's best interests, or any information about the individual's wishes, feelings, beliefs or values that might have an impact on the decision, including:
  - anyone previously named by the person to be consulted
  - anyone engaged in caring for the person
  - close relatives, friends or anyone who may have an interest in the person's welfare
  - any attorney appointed by the person
  - any deputy appointed by the Court of Protection?[18]

What should you take into account when assessing best interests?

Assessing the best interests of an individual lacking capacity can be a complex process. Although in an emergency situation, for example, the focus will be on meeting immediate clinical need, in other circumstances it will be important to develop a fuller picture of the individual's circumstances, needs, wishes and interests. In almost all circumstances, individuals are the best judge of their own interests, and even where an individual is assessed as lacking capacity, health professionals should, as far as possible, encourage them to participate in the decision-making process. On the same basis, any written statement of the patient's earlier wishes or feelings should be taken into account, even where they do not amount to a binding advance decision. It follows from this that consideration must be given as to whether the individual is likely to regain capacity. A decision should be delayed if it can reasonably be left until he or she regains the capacity to make it.

A crucial part of any best interests judgement will involve a discussion with those close to the individual, including family, friends or carers, where it is practical or appropriate to do so, bearing in mind that patients retain their rights of confidentiality. Unless it is an emergency, or it is genuinely impracticable to do so, any assessment of best interests should involve anyone nominated to act under a health and personal welfare Lasting Power of Attorney or any deputy appointed to make decisions by the Court of Protection. Although attorneys have rights of consent and refusal, any decision they make must still be in the incapacitated adult's best interests and an attorney cannot insist on treatment that, in the view of the treating health professional, is not clinically indicated.

Are there any exceptions to the best interests principle?

The legislation has provided for two circumstances where the best interests principle will not apply. The first is where someone has previously made an advance decision to refuse medical treatment while he or she had capacity. Where the advance decision is valid and applicable to the proposed treatment in the current circumstances, it should be respected, even if others think that the decision is not in the person's best interests. Advance decisions refusing medical treatment are discussed in more detail below. The second exception relates to the enrolment of incapacitated adults in certain forms of carefully controlled research. (This is discussed in more detail in Chapter 14.)

Challenges in assessing best interests

In 2010, the Court of Protection was asked to make a decision about the best interests of a patient with treatment-resistant schizophrenia. She was a chronic smoker and had developed either peripheral vascular disease or 'trench foot'. Diagnosis was complicated as she suffered from delusions and refused to let anyone look at her feet or discuss possible treatment. A number of her toes had fallen off, although she believed they would re-grow. The clinical team thought that the condition could lead to gangrene or septicaemia necessitating amputation, either electively or to save her life. The patient lacked capacity to make decisions about her healthcare and was likely to be highly resistant to any treatment. The Court of Protection was asked to make a decision about whether, should the need arise, it would be in her best interests to have an amputation, given that it was very likely she would have to be sedated and compulsorily treated. Medical experts differed as to what would be in her best interests. The Court held that, although ordinarily the strong presumption would be in favour of sustaining life, if the need for amputation to save the patient's life arose, it would be lawful to forgo it in favour of palliative care. In the judge's view, the provision of even life-sustaining treatment to a patient who did not understand the reasons for that treatment and whose resistance would mean that sedation and force might be required both for the procedure and any subsequent postoperative care, might not necessarily be in the patient's best interests.[19]

Summary – best interests (England and Wales)

- Decisions made on behalf of an incapacitated adult should be made on the basis of an assessment of his or her best interests, applying the checklist set out in the MCA.
- Best interests tests should be as objective as possible and should, where appropriate, extend beyond clinical factors.
- Advance decisions refusing treatment and certain forms of research are not subject to the best interests principle.

Acts in connection with care or treatment

The provision of treatment to adults without consent is potentially unlawful. The law has identified, however, that treatment can be provided to adults who lack capacity to consent where it is both necessary and in the patient's best interests. Section 5 of the Mental Capacity Act states that an action or intervention will be lawful (i.e. health professionals will have protection from liability) where the decision maker has a *reasonable belief* both that the individual lacks capacity, and that the action or decision is in his or her best interests. It applies to anyone making a decision on behalf of another, irrespective of whether they have a professional relationship with the incapacitated individual. In relation to medical treatment, it is applicable not only to an episode of treatment, but also to those necessary ancillary procedures such as conveying a person to hospital. All interventions under these powers must be in accordance with the principles of the MCA (see above). The Act also makes clear that anyone acting unreasonably, negligently or not in the person's best interests could forfeit the protection offered by the legislation.

How far do these powers extend?

There are limits to the defence provided by section 5 of the Act. A valid advance decision, and a valid decision by an attorney or a court-appointed deputy would take precedence. The Act also sets limits to the extent to which the freedom of movement of an incapacitated person can be restricted. An incapacitated person can only be restrained where there is a reasonable belief that it is necessary to prevent harm to the incapacitated person. Any restraint must be proportionate to the risk and of the minimum level necessary to protect the incapacitated person.

Although reasonable use of restraint may be lawful, the Act makes it clear that it will never be lawful to deprive a person of his or her liberty within the meaning of Article 5(1) of the European Convention on Human Rights, unless special safeguards are put in place.[20] The onus is on the person wishing to act to justify, as objectively as possible, his or her belief that the person being cared for is likely to be harmed unless some sort of physical intervention or other restraining action is taken. More detailed discussion of restraint, and of deprivation of liberty, is given below.

When is court approval required?

Before the Act came into force, the courts had decided that some decisions were so serious that each case should be taken to court so that a declaration of lawfulness could be made. The Act's Code of Practice[21] advises that the following cases should continue to go before the court:

- proposals to withdraw or withhold artificial nutrition and hydration from patients in a persistent vegetative state
- cases involving organ or bone marrow donation by a person lacking the capacity to consent
- proposals for non-therapeutic sterilisation
- cases where there is doubt or dispute about whether a particular treatment will be in a person's best interests
- cases involving ethical dilemmas in untested areas.

Practice Direction 9E issued under the Court of Protection Rules 2007 includes further examples of cases involving serious medical treatment which should be brought before the court.[22]

Summary – acts in connection with care and treatment

- An act or intervention will be lawful where the decision maker has a reasonable belief both that the individual has capacity and that the decision is in his or her best interests.

- It extends not only to the treatment itself but to any necessary ancillary procedures such as conveying a person to hospital.
- A valid advance decision or a decision by an attorney or court-appointed deputy would take precedence.
- An incapacitated person can only be restrained where there is a reasonable belief that it is necessary to prevent harm to the incapacitated person. Any restraint must be proportionate to the risk and of the minimum level necessary.

Care and treatment involving restraint or deprivation of liberty

There may be occasions when, in order to promote their interests, or to protect them from harm, health professionals need to consider using restraint when providing treatment to individuals lacking capacity. The Act defines restraint as the use, or the threat, of force in order to make someone do something they are resisting, or restricting a person's freedom of movement, whether they are resisting or not.[23] The Act permits the use of restraint only in order to prevent harm to a patient lacking capacity. Health professionals have a common law justification to use restraint where a patient who lacks capacity presents a risk of harm to others.

Restraint can take many forms, and health professionals need to be sensitive to the possibility that what may be seen as accepted practice actually involves a certain amount of restraint. Restraint can be overt, such as the use of bedrails that not only prevent a patient falling out of bed, but also prevent them leaving the bed at all. Restraint can also be covert and indirect, such as doors that are heavy and difficult to open. It can also extend to putting patients in low chairs from which they find it difficult to move. Restraint may be:

- physical – the individual is held by one or more persons or aids necessary for them to do what they want, for example spectacles or walking aids, are taken away
- mechanical – the use of equipment such as bedrails, tagging or mittens to stop patients removing nasogastric tubes or catheters
- chemical – involving medication such as sedation that does not have a direct therapeutic purpose
- psychological – for example telling patients that they are not allowed to do something, or not allowing visits or contact with family members, friends or carers.

When is restraint lawful?

Restrictive measures should only be used as a last resort and alternatives to restraint must always be considered first. Anybody proposing to use restraint must have objective reasons to justify that it is necessary. Any decision by a health professional to use restraint must be clearly documented, and the reasons, type and duration of restraint recorded in the medical record. They must also be able to show that the patient is likely to suffer harm unless proportionate restraint is used. A proportionate response will involve using the least intrusive form of restraint, and the minimum amount of restraint, to achieve the objective which must be in the best interests of the individual. Restraint should also only be used for the minimum amount of time necessary to achieve the desired goal. If these conditions are met, it is permissible to restrain a patient to provide necessary treatment. It also follows that in such circumstances there would be no liability for assault.

Deprivation of liberty

One of the more complex areas of the law involving adults lacking capacity relates to the distinction between restraint and care or treatment that amounts to a deprivation of liberty. Although the idea of depriving adults who lack capacity of their liberty may seem at odds with the underlying principles of the legislation, the issue nevertheless arises regularly in relation to adults who are accommodated in hospitals or care homes and are compliant but may be effectively deprived of their liberty without having the ability to consent to it. This issue was raised in relation to the *Bournewood* case whose name derived from the treating hospital (see below).[24]

The Bournewood case

HL was autistic and had profound learning disabilities. He lacked the capacity to consent to his admission to hospital and to his continuing stay. His contact with his carers was limited and he was both sedated and subject to continuing supervision. Those responsible for his care indicated that if he tried to leave they would prevent him by invoking mental health legislation. Commenting on the lawfulness of his treatment, the European Court of Human Rights found the following.

- HL had been deprived of his liberty contrary to Article 5(1) – the right to liberty – of the European Convention on Human Rights and Fundamental Freedoms (ECHR).
- The detention was arbitrary and not in accordance with a procedure prescribed by law.
- The lack of a procedure under which the lawfulness of his detention could be reviewed did not comply with Article 5(4) of the ECHR.[25]

Following the European Court ruling, a new statutory regime has been put in place for those incapacitated adults falling into what became known as the 'Bournewood gap'. This requires proper legal authorisation to be obtained before a person lacking capacity to consent can be given care or treatment in conditions which amount to a deprivation of his or her liberty. The regime, known as the Deprivation of Liberty Safeguards (DOLS), is complex and a very brief outline is given below. Healthcare professionals must, however, ensure they are familiar with the DOLS procedures, and are able to recognise when a deprivation of liberty may be occurring, in order to avoid acting unlawfully. Further details and guidance on implementing the DOLS procedures are available from the Deprivation of Liberty Safeguards Code of Practice.[26]

What is the difference between restraint and deprivation of liberty?

Drawing on the judgment in *HL v UK* (*Bournewood*), the Code of Practice holds that the difference between restraint and deprivation of liberty is a matter of degree and intensity, and will depend upon the circumstances of the particular case. The Code has identified the following factors that are likely to be relevant when assessing whether the circumstances of care might amount to a deprivation of liberty:

- restraint is used, including sedation, to admit a person to an institution where that person is resisting admission
- staff exercise complete and effective control over the care and movement of a person for a significant period
- staff exercise control over assessments, treatment, contacts and residence

- the individual will not be released into the care of others, or permitted to live elsewhere, unless the staff in the institution consider it appropriate
- a request by carers for a person to be discharged to their care is refused
- the person is unable to maintain social contacts because of restrictions placed on their access to other people
- the person is under continuous supervision and control.

How do you authorise a deprivation of liberty?

Under the Mental Capacity Act 2005, the deprivation of liberty of an adult lacking capacity to consent can be authorised in one of three ways:

- by the Court of Protection exercising its powers to make personal welfare decisions under the MCA 2005
- under the Deprivation of Liberty Safeguards as set out in the MCA 2005
- in order to give necessary life-sustaining treatment or to do any 'vital act' while a decision is sought from the court.[27]

Deprivation of liberty can still be authorised under mental health legislation, provided the conditions of that legislation are met. The High Court can also authorise such a deprivation under its inherent jurisdiction.

Deprivation of Liberty Safeguards

Under the DOLS, where it is necessary to deprive an individual of liberty, an application for authorisation must be made to an appropriate 'supervisory body', which in England will ordinarily be the commissioning body or local authority. In Wales it will be either the National Assembly for Wales or a Local Health Board. The application for a standard authorisation should be made in advance, when the supervisory body will set in motion a series of assessments which can take up to 21 days to complete. In urgent situations, when the person is already being deprived of his or her liberty, the care home or hospital can issue an urgent authorisation lasting 7 days. A standard authorisation must then be sought within the period of the urgent authorisation. Further information on the procedures for applying these safeguards is available from the Deprivation of Liberty Code of Practice.[28]

Summary – care and treatment involving restraint or deprivation of liberty

- Restrictive measures should only be used as a last resort and alternatives to restraint must always be considered first.
- Restraint may only be used where necessary to prevent harm to the person lacking capacity and in a way that is proportionate to the likelihood and seriousness of harm.
- Restraint should also only be used for the minimum amount of time necessary to achieve the desired goal.
- The difference between restraint and deprivation of liberty is a matter of degree and intensity and will depend upon the circumstances of the particular case.
- Any deprivation of liberty must be appropriately authorised.

Advance decisions refusing treatment

What is an advance decision?

Many people seek to have some influence over the course of future medical treatment at a time when they may lose the capacity to make decisions. These can take many forms, from statements of wishes and values, indications of preferences for certain forms of care or treatment, to explicit decisions or statements refusing individual treatments. Although all of these have an important part to play when health professionals are assessing treatment options for incapacitated adults, only specified refusals are potentially legally binding.

The MCA makes it clear that somebody who is aged 18 years or over and has the necessary mental capacity can refuse specified medical treatment for a time in the future when he or she may lose the capacity to make the decision. This is known as an advance decision. The Act's powers are restricted explicitly to advance decisions to refuse treatment and, although individuals can give written indication of the kinds of treatment they would like, advance requests for treatment are not binding on treating health professionals. A valid and applicable advance decision refusing treatment is as effective as a contemporaneous refusal.

Under the Act, an advance refusal of treatment is binding if:

- the person making the decision was 18 or older when it was made, and had the necessary mental capacity
- it specifies, in lay terms if necessary, the specific treatment to be refused and the particular circumstances in which the refusal is to apply
- the person making the decision has not changed his or her mind at a time when he or she had the capacity to do so
- the person making the decision has not appointed, after the decision was made, an attorney to make the specified decision
- the person making the decision has not done anything clearly inconsistent with the decision remaining a fixed decision.

Making an advance decision

Unless the decision relates to life-sustaining treatment, the Act does not impose any particular constraints or requirements on the form the refusal should take. The Act's Code of Practice nonetheless suggests that the following should be included:

- full details of the person making the advance decision including name, address and date of birth
- the name and address of the person's GP
- a statement that the document should be used at a point when the person lacks capacity
- a clear statement of the decision, the treatment to be refused and the circumstances in which the decision will apply
- the date the document was written and the date of any subsequent reviews
- the person's signature
- the signature of any witness.[29]

Advance decisions refusing life-sustaining treatment

The Act introduced new safeguards for advance decisions refusing life-sustaining treatment. Although ordinary advance decisions can be oral or in writing, an advance refusal will *only* apply to life-sustaining treatment where it is in writing, is signed and witnessed, and contains a statement that it is to apply even where life is at risk. Advance decisions cannot be used to refuse basic care, which includes warmth, shelter and hygiene measures to maintain body cleanliness. This also includes the offer of oral food and water, but not artificial nutrition and hydration.[30]

In an emergency or where there is doubt about the existence, validity or applicability of an advance decision, doctors can provide treatment that is immediately necessary to stabilise or to prevent a deterioration in the patient until the existence, and the validity and applicability, of the advance decision can be established. A doctor does not incur liability for carrying out or continuing treatment in the best interests of the patient unless, at the time, he or she is satisfied that a valid advance decision refusing it exists.

Do advance decisions apply to individuals subject to compulsory mental health powers?

Where a patient is subject to compulsory treatment under mental health legislation, an advance refusal relating to treatment provided for the mental disorder, for which compulsory powers have been invoked, will not be binding, although the treating professional should take such a refusal into account. This could include, for example, considering whether there are any other treatment options available that are less restrictive. An agreed advance treatment plan for mental health conditions can be helpful and would represent a kind of advance statement, although it would not be binding.

Summary – advance decisions refusing treatment

- Anyone aged 18 years or over with the necessary mental capacity can make an advance decision to refuse specified medical treatment for a time in the future when that treatment is proposed and he or she has lost the capacity to make the decision.
- An advance refusal will only apply to life-sustaining treatment where it is in writing, is signed and witnessed, and contains a statement that it is to apply even where life is at risk.
- In an emergency or where there is doubt about the existence or validity of an advance refusal of treatment, doctors can provide treatment that is immediately necessary to stabilise or to prevent a deterioration in the patient until the existence, and the validity and applicability, of the advance decision can be established.

Lasting powers of attorney

Prior to the MCA coming into force, some confusion existed among patients and health professionals about the ability of those close to incapacitated adults to make decisions on their behalf. Although legally it was clear that 'next of kin' had no lawful decision-making powers, this was not as widely understood as it might have been. One of the MCA's major innovations is the creation of a power of attorney enabling adults with the relevant capacity to nominate another individual – or individuals – to make health and welfare decisions on their behalf at a time in the future when they lose capacity. This is known as a Lasting Power of Attorney (LPA). It replaces the earlier Enduring Power of Attorney which related only to property and affairs. There are two types of LPA, one relating to property and financial affairs and one to health and personal welfare. The health and personal welfare

LPA covers personal, welfare and healthcare decisions, including decisions relating to medical treatment. Although an LPA in relation to property and affairs can be used by the attorney even when the donor still has capacity, an LPA dealing with health and personal welfare can only operate if the individual lacks capacity in relation to the issue in question.

Creating an LPA

The Act allows individuals aged 18 years or over who have capacity to appoint an attorney under a health and personal welfare LPA. In order for it to be valid a specific form must be used.[31] This must include the following:

- information about the nature and extent of the LPA
- a statement signed by the donors stating that they have read and understood the information and that they want the LPA to apply when they lose capacity
- the names of anyone (other than the attorney(s)) who should be told about an application to register the LPA
- a statement signed by the attorney(s) stating that they have read the information and understand the duties, in particular the duty to act in the donor's best interests
- a certificate completed by a third party, confirming that, in his or her opinion, the donor understands the nature and purpose of the LPA and, that no fraud or pressure has been used to force the donor to create the LPA. (Registered healthcare professionals can be certificate providers and, GPs in particular, may find they are asked by patients to fulfil this role.)

Registering a health and personal welfare LPA

Before a health and personal welfare LPA can be used, the adult must be assessed as lacking capacity to make the decision in question and the LPA must be registered with the Office of the Public Guardian (OPG). Until it is registered, the attorney will be unable lawfully to make decisions on the incapacitated adult's behalf. The OPG keeps a register of LPAs and, where there is doubt as to the existence of an LPA, a health professional can apply to search the register. A fee is, however, payable for this service.

The scope and extent of an LPA

The powers granted to an attorney will depend entirely on the wording of the LPA. If a health and personal welfare LPA has been registered, the attorney will have no authority to make decisions about the donor's finances or property. On the other hand, if a property and affairs LPA has been registered, the attorney will have no power to make any decisions about the care or medical treatment of the donor. The donor may also have included specific restrictions on the attorney's powers. It is therefore important that healthcare professionals carefully check the wording of the LPA. Even where a general health and welfare LPA has been created and no restrictions have been imposed by the donor, an attorney cannot:

- make treatment decisions if the donor has capacity
- consent to a specific treatment if the donor has made a valid and applicable advance decision to refuse that treatment after the creation of the LPA

- consent to or refuse life-sustaining treatment unless this is expressly authorised by the LPA
- consent to or refuse treatment for a mental disorder where a patient is detained and being treated under Part 4 of the Mental Health Act 1983
- demand specific treatment that health professionals consider not to be necessary or appropriate for the donor's particular condition.

Where attorneys are acting under a health and personal welfare LPA and are making decisions in relation to medical treatment, they must always act in the donor's best interests. Attorneys must also have regard to the guidance given in the Code of Practice.[32] If there is any doubt about an attorney's actions, and the matter cannot be resolved in any other way, an application can be made to the Court of Protection.

Enduring powers of attorney

Although it is no longer possible to make an enduring power of attorney (EPA), any that were created before 1 October 2007 and have been registered, at the time the donor has become or is becoming incapable of managing his or her affairs, will nonetheless remain legally effective. However, EPAs only cover decisions relating to property and financial affairs. Property and affairs LPAs will eventually replace the existing system of EPA, but this will inevitably take some years during which time the two systems will coexist.

Summary – lasting powers of attorney

- The Act allows individuals aged 18 years or over, who have capacity, to make a Lasting Power of Attorney appointing an attorney(s), to make decisions on their behalf at a time in the future when they lose capacity.
- Where attorneys are making health and welfare decisions, they must act in the donor's best interests.

Dispute resolution

It is always preferable to proceed with consensus in relation to medical treatment. In the overwhelming majority of cases, following discussion and an open exploration of available options, professionals providing treatment to incapacitated adults, and those close to them, agree on the appropriate course of care or treatment. However, there may be occasions where disagreements arise. These may relate to the following:

- whether an individual retains the capacity to make a decision
- whether a proposed decision or intervention is in an incapacitated person's best interests
- whether the decision or intervention is the most suitable of the available options.

It is clearly in everybody's interests that disagreements are resolved as soon as possible, and with consensus. Broadly speaking, disputes can be resolved either informally, through discussion and negotiation, or formally through local or national complaints processes. Some disputes will be so serious that they may have to be referred to the Court of Protection, discussed in more detail below.

Importance of good communication

The majority of disputes can either be avoided, or settled rapidly and equably, by using good communication and involving all relevant individuals. Good communication skills are a key aspect of medical practice, and as health professionals will recognise, involve both listening to concerns as well as setting out the available options in a way that can be easily understood by all parties to the dispute. The MCA's Code of Practice[33] suggests that, where health professionals are involved in a dispute with those close to an incapacitated person, it is a good idea to:

- set out the different options in a way that can be clearly understood
- invite a colleague to talk the matter over and offer a second opinion or seek independent expert advice
- consider enrolling the services of an advocate (see below)
- arrange a meeting or case conference to discuss the matter in detail
- listen to, acknowledge and address worries
- where the situation is not urgent, allow the family time to think it over.

Mediation

Where the methods outlined above do not successfully resolve the dispute, it may be a good idea to involve a mediator. Any dispute that is likely to be settled by negotiation is probably suitable for mediation. A mediator is an independent facilitator and it is not the mediator's role to make decisions or impose solutions. The mediator will seek to facilitate a decision that is acceptable to all parties in the dispute. Several national organisations provide trained and accredited mediators.[34] In the event that disputes cannot be resolved by these means, application can be made to the Court of Protection.

Summary – dispute resolution

- In the overwhelming majority of cases, treatment is provided on the basis of consensus.
- The majority of disputes can either be avoided, or settled rapidly and equably, by using good communication.
- Where consensus cannot be achieved, consideration should be given to enrolling a mediator.

Court of Protection and court-appointed deputies

The Court of Protection

The MCA established a new Court of Protection with extensive powers to oversee the proper functioning of the Act. It is also now a court of record, meaning that it is able to set precedent. The Court has the power to rule on cases where there is doubt or dispute as to whether a particular treatment is in the best interests of an incapacitated individual and to make a declaration as to whether an individual has or lacks capacity to make decisions. The Court also has the power to rule on the validity of LPAs as well as to determine their meaning or effect. Reflecting the position before the introduction of the Act, the approval of the Court will be required for some forms of serious medical treatment (see page 110). The Court of Protection has all the powers of the High Court and appeals can be made against its decisions, with permission, both to circuit judges and to the Court of Appeal.

Court-appointed deputies

The new Court of Protection has the power to appoint a deputy or deputies as substitute decision makers with authority to make decisions on behalf of a person lacking capacity, who has not previously appointed an attorney under an LPA to make relevant decisions. Deputies will generally be appointed to make decisions about property and financial affairs, replacing the previous role of court-appointed receivers. In certain cases, however, deputies can be appointed to make decisions on health and welfare matters. Welfare deputies are likely to be appointed where an ongoing series of decisions is needed to resolve an issue, rather than a single decision of the Court. The Court, however, is required where possible to make a single decision in preference to the appointment of a deputy,[35] so the appointment of welfare deputies is rare. In the majority of cases, the deputy is likely to be a family member or someone who knows the patient well. The Court may appoint a deputy who is independent of the family, if, for example, there is a history of serious family dispute or the individual's health and care needs are very complex.

As with attorneys appointed under an LPA, deputies have to make decisions in the individual's best interests and must allow individuals to make any decisions for which they have capacity. Deputies must also have regard to the guidance given in the Code of Practice. Deputies cannot refuse consent to life-sustaining treatment – such decisions must be referred to the Court.

Deputies should inform the health professional with whom they are dealing that the Court has appointed them as a deputy. The deputy will have been provided with an official order appointing them, setting out the scope of their decision-making powers. Health professionals should review the order to confirm the extent and scope of the authority given by the Court.

Summary – Court of Protection and court-appointed deputies

- The Court of Protection oversees the proper function of the MCA.
- The Court has the power to rule where disputes arises as to whether a particular treatment is in the best interests of an incapacitated adult.
- Court of Protection approval is required for certain particularly serious forms of treatment.
- The Court can appoint a deputy or deputies with authority to make decisions on behalf of a person lacking capacity.

Independent mental capacity advocates

The MCA introduced the first statutory advocacy service in England and Wales. The purpose of the service is to support and represent particularly vulnerable adults who lack capacity to make certain decisions where there are no family members or friends or any other person, other than paid carers, either available or who are willing or appropriate to be consulted. An independent mental capacity advocate (IMCA) is independent of the healthcare professional making the decision and represents the patient in discussions about whether the proposed decision is in the patient's best interests. Although IMCAs do not have decision-making powers, they can nonetheless raise questions or seek to challenge decisions that appear not to be in the patient's best interests.

When should an IMCA be instructed?

The MCA imposes a legal obligation to enrol the services of an IMCA in two defined circumstances. If an adult lacks capacity and has no-one whom it is appropriate to consult an IMCA must be appointed where:

- an NHS body is proposing to provide, withhold or stop 'serious medical treatment' (see below), or
- an NHS body or local authority is proposing to arrange accommodation (or a change in accommodation) in a hospital or care home, and the stay in hospital will be more than 28 days, or the stay in the care home more than 8 weeks.[36]

While it is not compulsory, IMCAs can also be instructed in a care review of arrangements for accommodation or safeguarding adult procedures involving a vulnerable individual who lacks capacity, whether or not family members or friends are involved. IMCAs may also be involved in some cases where the Deprivation of Liberty Safeguards are applied (see pages 112–113).

An IMCA cannot be instructed if an individual has previously named a person who should be consulted about decisions that affect them and that person is willing to assist, or they have appointed an attorney under an LPA or the Court of Protection has appointed a deputy to act on the patient's behalf. There is also no duty to instruct an IMCA where there is a need to make an urgent decision, for example to save a patient's life. If a patient requires treatment while a report is awaited from an IMCA, this can be provided in the patient's best interests. It is also not necessary to instruct an IMCA for patients detained under the Mental Health Act 1983.

Responsibility for instructing an IMCA lies with the NHS body or local authority providing the treatment or accommodation.

Serious medical treatment

Serious medical treatment is defined in regulations[37] as treatment which involves providing, withdrawing or withholding treatment where:

- in the case of a single treatment being proposed, there is a fine balance between its benefits to the patient and the burdens and risks it is likely to entail
- in the case where there is a choice of treatments, a decision as to which one to use is finely balanced, or
- what is proposed would be likely to involve serious consequences for the patient.

Examples of serious medical treatment might include chemotherapy and surgery for cancer, therapeutic sterilisation, major surgery, withholding or stopping artificial nutrition and hydration, and termination of pregnancy.

Scope of an IMCA's powers

In order to provide necessary support to the incapacitated individual, IMCAs have powers to:

- examine health or social care records which are relevant and necessary to deal with the issue
- consult in private with the person lacking capacity

- consult people who may be in a position to comment on the incapacitated individual's wishes, feelings and beliefs
- ascertain what alternative courses, actions and options may be available to the incapacitated individual
- obtain an alternative medical opinion.

An IMCA is required to write a report to the NHS body or local authority responsible for the individual's treatment or care. This must be taken into account before the decision is made.

Summary – independent mental capacity advocates

- Where an individual lacks capacity and has no-one whom it is appropriate to consult, an IMCA must be instructed in relation to decisions involving serious medical treatment or changes in accommodation.
- Responsibility for instructing an IMCA lies with the NHS body or local authority providing the treatment.
- IMCAs do not have decision-making powers. Their role is to represent patients in discussions about whether a decision is in their interest.

The relationship with mental health legislation

As discussed on pages 96–97, the relationship between capacity law and mental health legislation can be complex. Decisions as to the regime under which treatment should be provided can have significant consequences in terms of both patient freedoms and the kinds of safeguards that are available to monitor any necessary use of restraint. Although attitudes toward people with mental disorders are changing, the use of compulsory mental health powers can still be seen as stigmatising. The choice of regime is clearly therefore an important issue for health professionals to consider when providing treatment to incapacitated adults.

Which regime is appropriate?

Where an adult lacks decision-making capacity, good practice, as laid out in the Code of Practice to the MCA, indicates that consideration should first be given to using capacity legislation. By and large the MCA permits a more flexible and informal approach and is likely to be perceived as less coercive and stigmatising. Health professionals should, however, consider using the Mental Health Act 1983 (MHA) to provide care and treatment to an individual without capacity where:

- it is not possible to provide care or treatment without depriving the individual of his or her liberty
- the treatment cannot be given under the MCA, for example because of a valid advance decision
- restraint in a way that is not permitted by the MCA is required
- assessment or treatment cannot be undertaken safely and effectively other than on a compulsory basis
- the individual lacks capacity in respect of some parts of the treatment but has capacity in respect of other parts and refuses a key element

- there is another reason why the individual may not receive treatment and as a result the individual or someone else may suffer harm.[38]

Interface between capacity and mental health legislation

There may be occasions in the treatment of individuals lacking decision-making capacity where it might be appropriate to use aspects of both statutory provisions. This is particularly likely where an individual without capacity is being simultaneously treated for both mental and physical disorders. The following key points should be taken into consideration.

- Where an individual has made an advance decision relating to treatment that is to be provided under the compulsory powers of mental health legislation, it is not binding.
- A valid and applicable advance decision for treatment for conditions that are not covered by the compulsory powers of the MHA will be binding.
- Where an incapacitated adult is subject to compulsory powers, all other decisions relating to the general care and treatment of the individual will be covered by the MCA.[39]

There may be circumstances in which either legal framework may apply and the question as to which Act is appropriate will be for the judgement of the health professional. If the patient retains capacity, the MCA cannot be used. If the treatment is for a physical condition, then the MHA is irrelevant, even if the patient has a mental disorder. Where detention is deemed necessary, the MHA must be used provided the relevant grounds are met. Where the care or treatment amounts to a deprivation of liberty and the MHA cannot be used, for example where the person lacking capacity is receiving care or treatment in a care home, then the DOLS under the MCA should be used to authorise the deprivation of liberty (see pages 112–113).

Summary – the relationship with mental health legislation

- There may be occasions where an adult lacking capacity can be treated under both mental health and mental capacity legislation.
- An individual cannot be treated under mental capacity legislation where he or she retains capacity.
- Where detention is deemed necessary, mental health legislation should be used, provided the necessary grounds are met.

Providing treatment to adults lacking capacity – Scotland

In Scotland, there is a general presumption that adults aged 16 years or over have the relevant capacity to make decisions about medical treatment. Where adults lack the capacity to consent to a specified intervention, the lawfulness of their treatment is regulated by the Adults with Incapacity (Scotland) Act 2000. The Act relates to a very wide range of potential decisions, but this section outlines the main features of the Act as it relates to medical treatment. All doctors in Scotland working with adults who lack, or who may lack, capacity should be familiar with the Act's basic principles and its underlying provisions, and these are set out in some detail here. Medical treatment under the Act is supported by a specific statutory Code of Practice which provides detailed guidance on how the Act should be used.[40] It can be useful to read this section jointly with the general ethical principles given at the beginning of this chapter.

The Adults with Incapacity (Scotland) Act 2000 – an outline

- The Adults with Incapacity (Scotland) Act 2000 sets out the framework for regulating interventions in the affairs of adults – people aged 16 years and over – who have, or may have, impaired capacity.
- Any intervention in the affairs of an incapacitated adult must be intended to benefit the adult.
- In an emergency, doctors may provide medical treatment that is immediately necessary to save life or avoid significant deterioration in a patient's health unless there is a valid advance refusal of the treatment in question.
- Other than in an emergency, or where there is a proxy decision maker, where an adult lacks capacity to make healthcare decisions, a certificate of incapacity must be issued in order to provide care or treatment.
- A welfare attorney, someone authorised under an intervention order, or a welfare guardian with powers relating to the medical treatment in question can give consent to treatment on behalf of the incapacitated adult.

The Act's basic principles

The Act sets out a number of basic principles that must govern decisions made and actions taken on behalf of incapacitated adults. Where confusion arises about how aspects of the Act should be interpreted it can be useful to refer back to these principles. Actions or decisions that clearly conflict with them are unlikely to be lawful, although there may be occasions when the principles are in tension with each other and some balancing may be necessary.

Benefit

Any intervention in the affairs of an incapacitated adult, including any treatment or investigation, will only be lawful where the person proposing it is satisfied that it will benefit the adult and that the desired benefit cannot be reasonably achieved without the intervention.

Minimum necessary intervention

Any intervention must be the least restrictive of the adult's freedoms consistent with the purposes of the intervention.

Take account of the wishes of the adult

When making decisions on behalf of incapacitated adults, the past and present wishes of the adult must be taken into consideration in so far as they can be ascertained.

Consultation with relevant others

When making a decision on behalf of an incapacitated adult, the views of those close to the patient must be taken into account, bearing in mind the duty of confidentiality to the patient, and any previously expressed wishes about disclosure of information. In particular, the views of the following people should be sought:

- the nearest relative and primary carer
- any guardian or attorney with powers relating to the decision
- any person whom the sheriff has directed should be consulted, and
- anyone who has identified themselves as having an interest in the welfare of the adult or the decision in question.[41]

Encourage the adult to exercise residual capacity

Adults should be encouraged to participate as far as possible in any decisions made on their behalf.

Assessing capacity under the Adults with Incapacity (Scotland) Act 2000

The Act stresses the importance of basing an assessment of capacity on the specific decision that needs to be made. Unless the patient is unconscious, capacity must not be regarded as an all or nothing condition. Even people with low levels of capacity retain the ability to make some decisions, and usually the ability to participate in far more. The Act's Code of Practice emphasises that adults should not be seen as lacking capacity solely because they are suffering from a specific condition or disorder, including the following:

- having a psychotic illness
- having dementia, particularly in the early stages
- having communication difficulties
- having a brain injury or other physical disability
- disagreeing with the advice or treatment offered by health professionals.[42]

When does an adult lack capacity?

The Act states that an adult lacks capacity if he or she is incapable of:

- acting;
- making decisions;
- communicating decisions;
- understanding decisions; or
- retaining the memory of decisions

in relation to any particular matter, by reason of mental disorder or of inability to communicate because of physical disability or neurological impairment.[43]

The definition of 'mental disorder' in the Act refers to the definition in the Mental Health (Care and Treatment) (Scotland) Act 2003. Under that definition, a person is not mentally disordered by reason only of sexual orientation; sexual deviancy; transsexualism; transvestism; dependence on, or use of, alcohol or drugs; behaviour that causes, or is likely to cause, harassment, alarm or distress to another person; or acting as no prudent person would act. A person shall not be regarded as unable to communicate if difficulties can be overcome by human or mechanical aids.[44]

In some situations assessing an individual's capacity will be a relatively straightforward process. In others, such as where capacity may be fluctuating, or the patient clearly retains some cognitive ability but the decision in question is quite complex, it can be more difficult. Patients' abilities can fluctuate because of a range of factors, including their medical condition, medication, the time of day or their mood. Doctors have a general ethical duty to enhance capacity when it is possible to do so, and should seek to engage patients in decision making when they are best able to participate.

Mental capacity is a multi-faceted concept. The Act's Code of Practice states that, in relation to medical treatment, an assessment of mental capacity will ordinarily try to establish whether the adult:

- is capable of making and communicating the decision
- understands the nature of what is being asked and why
- has memory abilities that allow the retention of information
- is aware of any alternatives
- has knowledge of the risks and benefits involved
- is aware that such information is of personal relevance to them
- is aware of their right to, and how to, refuse, as well as the consequences of refusal
- has ever expressed their wishes relevant to the issue when greater capacity existed
- is expressing views consistent with their previously preferred moral, cultural, family and experiential background
- is not under undue influence from a relative, carer or other third party declaring an interest in the care and treatment of the adult.[45]

It is a statutory duty to take into account the views of the patient, and when assessing capacity, carers and relatives can have valuable information about the patient and about his or her past and present wishes and feelings. Account should also be taken of the views of anyone else with an interest in the welfare of the adult. This does not, however, require the practitioner to go to undue lengths to seek out such people. In addition, care needs to be taken to respect confidentiality and to ensure that it is the view of the patient that others are putting forward and not their own, particularly where they may have a vested interest in the outcome of the decision. Enquiries should also be made as to whether the adult has an independent advocate to assist in making decisions. In the absence of a family member or friend willing to assist the adult in decision making, consideration should be given to appointing a professional advocate to support the patient.

Summary – assessing capacity under the Adults with Incapacity (Scotland) Act 2000

- Assessments of capacity must focus on the specific decision that needs to be made at the time it needs to be made.
- Doctors must enhance capacity as far as reasonably possible.
- It is a statutory duty to take into account the views of the patient if they can be ascertained.
- Where an adult lacks capacity, carers and relatives can have valuable information about the patient and must be consulted in so far as it is reasonable and practicable to do so.
- Adults with capacity can nominate an adult to make decisions on their behalf at the time in the future when they lose capacity by means of a welfare power of attorney.

Where an adult lacks capacity

Certificate of incapacity and the general authority to treat

Except for emergencies – and treatment in some circumstances under mental health legislation – treatment can only be given to adults lacking the capacity to consent to that treatment once a certificate of incapacity has been issued. Such a certificate must be made out by the healthcare professional proposing the treatment, although the responsibility for providing the treatment can be delegated to a suitably qualified colleague. In considering whether to issue a certificate of incapacity, the health professional must apply the basic principles of the Act as outlined above. Once a certificate has been issued, treatment can be lawfully provided under what the Act describes as a 'general authority to treat'. Although the Act originally allowed only 'registered medical practitioners' to issue a certificate of incapacity, a 2005 amendment[46] extended the provisions to include dental practitioners, optometrists and registered nurses, provided they have successfully completed relevant training in the assessment of capacity as prescribed in the Adults with Incapacity (Requirements for Signing Medical Treatment Certificates) (Scotland) Regulations 2007. A certificate issued by a health professional other than a registered medical practitioner will only be valid in his or her area of practice. Dentists, for example, can only authorise dental treatment.

Even where the patient has a proxy with welfare powers (see page 130), a certificate of incapacity must still be issued before treatment can be provided, unless the treatment is required in an emergency. The general authority to treat may not be used where a proxy has been appointed, the practitioner is aware of the appointment and it would be reasonable and practicable for the practitioner who issued the certificate to obtain his or her consent. Persons authorised under intervention orders and guardians (see page 130) with relevant powers should make themselves known to the practitioner who is treating the adult where they believe the patient's capacity is failing, or has been lost, and this information should be clearly recorded in the adult's medical notes. It would, however, be good practice to check with close relatives or the adult's social worker, if relevant, to see whether such an appointment is known to them. The Public Guardian keeps a list of registered proxies appointed under the Act and where practicable to do so, a request can be made for a search of the registers for the contact details of any proxy.

A certificate of incapacity must be set out on a specified form and must include brief details of the proposed medical treatment and the nature of the patient's incapacity. The certificate must also specify the length of time the authority is to remain valid. This must be a period of time relevant to the nature of the treatment and the patient's condition. Ordinarily this will be a period of up to a year, although regulations introduced in 2007 permit, in some circumstances, the issuing of a certificate for up to 3 years.[47] Decisions about whether to issue such a certificate will obviously have to be made following an assessment of the patient's condition and prognosis, particularly where capacity may fluctuate and some degree of improvement may be likely. According to the Code of Practice, the issuing of a 3-year certificate would only be appropriate where the patient was suffering from at least one of the following disorders which resulted in an inability to make the decision in question:

- severe or profound learning disability, or
- severe dementia, or
- severe neurological disorder.[48]

Although a certificate makes treatment lawful, it is good practice to review the patient's capacity and to renew the certificate at appropriate intervals, particularly where there may have been a change in the patient's condition or where new treatment regimes are being considered. It is a good idea to record these assessments in the patient's records. Where the patient's condition or the treatment required have changed, doctors should consider revoking the current certificate and issuing a new one that covers the altered circumstances or the new treatment. Where the professional who first issues the certificate ceases to be primarily responsible for the patient's treatment, the new practitioner should review the patient's circumstances. If they have not changed since the original certificate was issued, continued treatment would remain lawful until such time as the patient's condition or treatment changes or the certificate expires.

Issuing a certificate of incapacity

Health professionals who are considering issuing a certificate of incapacity need to consider five main issues:

- the nature of the treatment that is being considered for the patient – a certificate should only be issued where the doctor intends to provide a course of treatment
- the adult must be assessed as lacking the capacity to consent to the treatment decision in question
- any proxy with welfare powers should be contacted, where it is reasonable and practicable to do so – even where the patient has a welfare proxy, a certificate of incapacity has to be issued
- where a welfare proxy has been appointed and the practitioner is aware of this, consent to treatment should be obtained from the proxy where it is reasonable and practicable to do so
- any treatment must be in keeping with the Act's basic principles.

What does the Act mean by 'treatment'?

Under the Act, 'medical treatment' includes any procedure or treatment designed to safeguard or promote physical or mental health and, unless in an emergency, any such intervention would need to be authorised by a certificate of incapacity. Generally speaking, treatment relates to some positive action. According to the Code of Practice, a decision not to provide treatment would not seem to require a certificate, but any non-treatment decision must be in keeping with the Act's basic principles.[49] The Act does not address the question of whether a certificate is required for medical examination prior to treatment. The Code of Practice states that physical examination could be considered to come under the Act's definition of treatment but that a general and non-invasive examination may not necessarily require a certificate.[50] Where more intrusive or invasive examinations are indicated, or where there may be a risk of unintended sequelae, careful consideration should be given to the issuing of a certificate. Where an adult may be reluctant to be examined, again the issuing of a certificate should be considered.

A treatment plan approach

Although the Act states that certificates of incapacity relate to specific treatments, in cases where longer term care may be required it would be unnecessarily burdensome and bureaucratic to issue a separate certificate for each intervention. For some adults, where all that is required is a single episode of treatment, a certificate containing a brief description of the proposed treatment is sufficient. Such a certificate also extends to authorising any necessary postoperative care. In other cases, adults may have complex and ongoing needs and in these circumstances it may be appropriate to complete the certificate with reference to a treatment plan. The contents of a treatment plan are not specified by the Act but examples are provided in the Code of Practice.[51] A treatment plan should normally refer to the kinds of intervention that it is known, or that it would be reasonable to anticipate, that the adult might require in the future in order to safeguard or promote his or her physical or mental health. Consideration should also be given to the likelihood that the adult may be able to consent to specific interventions.

Given the potential scope and authority of a treatment plan, it is important that it strikes an appropriate balance between breadth and specificity. A plan that is too broad will be at odds with the decision-specific focus of the Act's basic principles. If it is too narrow it may need such frequent updating that it interferes with the ability to provide necessary treatment to the adult as and when it is required.

All adults are entitled to basic care which includes the provision of food and fluids, mobility support, basic hygiene and pain control. The Act's Code of Practice recommends including in any treatment plan the heading 'Fundamental Health Care Procedures' which authorises these necessary interventions, including any preliminary investigation they might require.[52]

However, treatment plans cannot authorise treatments, such as serious surgery, where written consent would be required if the adult retained capacity. In these circumstances a separate certificate of capacity must be issued. During the lifetime of the certificate of incapacity, other health conditions may arise. Where they require a single, discrete intervention, a separate additional certificate of incapacity can be drawn up. If ongoing care is likely to be required then it would be preferable to develop a new treatment plan and, where the plan goes beyond the existing certificate, to authorise it with a new one. In cases of ongoing incapacity, the treatment plan should be reviewed, at a minimum, yearly. This review should involve all healthcare professionals providing relevant care and treatment, the patient – to the extent that this is possible – and any proxies.

Taking into consideration the views of the patient

When healthcare professionals issue a certificate of incapacity, they are under a legal obligation to take into consideration the views and wishes of the incapacitated patient. All reasonable efforts should be made to discuss the matter in question directly with the incapacitated adult in order to determine what his or her wishes might be. Many incapacitated adults have communication problems and consideration should be given to whether communication aids would be helpful. Where verbal communication is not possible, non-verbal clues, such as distress responses to certain interventions, would obviously need to be taken into account. Consideration should also be given to enrolling the help of communication experts such as language therapists.

A crucial part of considering the views and wishes of the patient will involve identifying any written statement of wishes, particularly where it is not possible to communicate with the patient directly. In addition to potentially binding advance decisions to refuse treatment, which are discussed in more detail below, written statements that may not be binding but that indicate underlying attitudes and values can be extremely helpful. The patient's medical records can also contain indications of underlying views or prior wishes.

Advance decisions

Unlike in England and Wales, there is no statutory basis in Scotland for advance decisions refusing treatment, but as indicated in the Act's Code of Practice, where the advance decision contains an explicit advance refusal of treatment, and that refusal is relevant to the patient's circumstances, they may be binding.[53] They may also be given particular weight if they were made orally or in writing to a practitioner, solicitor or other independent professional person. In the BMA's view, an advance decision refusing treatment is likely to be legally binding if the following conditions apply:

- the patient is an adult and had relevant capacity when the statement was made
- the patient has been offered, or has had access to, sufficient accurate information to make an informed decision
- the circumstances that have arisen are those that were envisaged by the patient
- the patient was not subjected to undue influence in making the decision.

Further considerations include the age of the statement, medical changes since the time it was made that might have an impact on the patient's views, and the patient's current wishes and feelings.

An advance statement cannot authorise in advance procedures that an individual could not authorise contemporaneously. They cannot, for example, authorise illegal interventions, such as euthanasia, or request treatment that is not clinically appropriate. Unless an advance decision makes it abundantly clear that it is intended to apply during pregnancy, it is unlikely to be valid if the patient is pregnant.

In addition to potentially binding advance refusals of treatment, a competently made advance statement, either made orally or in writing, can clearly give a strong indication of the patient's earlier wishes and feelings, and any such statement should be given careful consideration. Where such statements are not binding, they should be viewed in the overall context of the patient's health needs and current circumstances.

Considering the views of those close to the patient

The Act makes clear that any practitioner making out a certificate of incapacity is under an obligation to take into account the views of those close to the incapacitated adult, in so far as it is reasonable and practicable to do so.[54] While health professionals do not need to go to undue lengths to identify everyone with an interest in the welfare of the adult, good practice would ordinarily suggest that enquiries should be made of the adult's visitors and reasonable efforts should be made to contact known relatives and partners. The consent of any proxy with welfare powers (see below) should be sought unless the treatment is to be provided in an emergency. Although the views of any proxy will be influential, any decision made on behalf of the incapacitated adult must still be in keeping with the Act's underlying principles (see pages 123–124). Where disputes arise, there are procedures for resolving them which are outlined below.

Proxies

The term 'proxy' is used to mean a guardian, a welfare attorney or a person authorised under an intervention order, with power in relation to any medical treatment referred to in section 47 of the Act. Welfare guardians and persons authorised under an intervention order can be individuals, professionals or social workers. There are requirements under Part 5 of the Act to involve proxies in decision making about medical treatment and to involve guardians and welfare attorneys who have relevant powers in decisions about research. Part 5 also provides a dispute resolution process where proxies and practitioners do not agree about a treatment decision, or where the practitioner and proxy are in agreement but someone else, who has a relevant interest, disagrees. The proxy, the practitioner responsible for the treatment of the adult and the person with a relevant interest all have a right of appeal to the Court of Session. Where a proxy has been appointed, and the practitioner is aware of this, he or she should be asked to consent to proposed treatment where it is reasonable and practicable to do so.

Welfare attorneys

Individuals, while they have capacity, can grant one or more people they trust powers to act as their continuing attorney or attorneys. A welfare power of attorney only comes into effect in the event of the donor's loss of capacity. All powers of attorney must be registered with the Public Guardian (Scotland). Information about setting up a power of attorney is available on the Office of the Public Guardian (Scotland) (OPG) website.[55]

Intervention orders and welfare guardianship

Under Part 6 of the Adults with Incapacity (Scotland) Act 2000 it is possible to apply to the sheriff for an intervention order to deal with clearly defined financial, property or personal welfare matters in relation to an adult on a one-off basis. The court can also appoint a guardian with powers over property, financial affairs or personal welfare or a combination of these. A guardian with powers over personal welfare is referred to as a 'welfare guardian'. Persons authorised under an intervention order, and welfare guardians, may be given power by the sheriff to make decisions about medical treatment on behalf of the adult, subject to certain exceptions relating to mental health legislation.

Medical practitioners have formal responsibility for providing reports of incapacity in relation to applications for intervention orders or guardianship. At least two such reports are needed for each application. In a case where the cause of incapacity is mental disorder, one of these reports must be made by a medical practitioner approved for the purpose of section 22 of the Mental Health (Care and Treatment) (Scotland) Act 2003.

Summary – providing treatment to adults lacking capacity (Scotland)

- Unless an emergency, treatment can only be given to adults lacking the capacity to consent to that treatment once a certificate of incapacity has been issued.
- When healthcare professionals issue a certificate of incapacity, they are under a legal obligation to take into consideration, as far as possible, the views and wishes of the incapacitated patient.
- Explicit and applicable advance decisions refusing treatment made by adults with the relevant capacity are likely to be binding.
- Any practitioner making out a certificate of incapacity is under an obligation to take into account the views of those close to the incapacitated adult, in so far as it is reasonable and practicable to do so.
- Proxies can include welfare attorneys, welfare guardians and persons authorised by an intervention order. Where the practitioner is aware of the appointment, proxies should be asked to consent to the proposed treatment if it is reasonable and practicable for them to do so.

Withdrawing and withholding treatment

The Act's Code of Practice indicates that 'generally treatment will involve some positive intervention in the patient's condition' and that 'simple failure to do anything for a patient would not constitute treatment'.[56] In other words, the focus of the treatment and proxy decision-making provisions of the Act is on the authorisation of treatment, not decisions to withhold treatment. As a decision made on behalf of an incapacitated adult will nevertheless be covered by the legislation, any decision to withhold treatment must be made in accordance with the Act's basic principles (see pages 123-124). Where a decision to withhold or withdraw treatment that has a potential to prolong life is being considered, doctors should also consult the BMA's publication *Withholding and Withdrawing Life-Prolonging Treatment*.[57] The Code of Practice makes clear that the Act does not affect the existing criminal law whereby anybody who unlawfully causes or hastens another person's death would be guilty of a criminal offence.[58] Neither does the Act change the law in relation to euthanasia, which remains a criminal act under Scots law.

Exceptions to the general authority to treat

Providing treatment under the Mental Health (Care and Treatment) (Scotland) Act 2003

The provisions of the Adults with Incapacity (Scotland) Act allow treatment to be provided for mental disorder, so it may not always be necessary to detain mentally disordered patients formally under mental health legislation. Where an incapacitated adult resists treatment for a mental disorder, however, the use of formal mental health powers should be considered, particularly given the extra safeguards the legislation provides. Advice can always be sought from a psychiatrist or mental health officer. In difficult cases, the Mental Welfare Commission for Scotland may also be able to advise. Where an adult is subject to formal mental health powers any treatment for mental disorder must be given under those powers rather than under incapacity legislation. Treatment for physical conditions can only be provided to adults lacking the ability to consent or refuse under incapacity legislation.

Special safeguards

Certain treatments are also subject to special safeguards. Neurosurgery for mental disorder (NMD) and deep brain stimulation (DBS) for example, cannot be given under incapacity legislation unless relevant conditions under mental health legislation are also fulfilled. There are also safeguards for certain treatments for patients being treated for mental disorder under mental health legislation, including provision of nutrition to the patient by artificial means.[59] In addition, regulations have been made under the Adults with Incapacity (Scotland) Act 2000 which specify that certain irreversible or hazardous treatments require special safeguards, in addition to those laid down in the Act's basic principles.[60] These treatments cannot be provided under the general authority to treat or the proxy consent provisions of the Act. These regulations do not apply in an emergency where treatment is immediately necessary to preserve life or prevent serious deterioration in health.

The following treatments require approval by the Court of Session, although it is still necessary for a certificate of incapacity to be issued:

- sterilisation where there is no serious malformation or disease of the reproductive organs
- surgical implantation of hormones for the purpose of reducing sex drive.

The following require approval by an independent practitioner appointed by the Mental Welfare Commission but again a certificate of incapacity is still required:

- drug treatment for the purpose of reducing sex drive, other than surgical implantation of hormones
- electro-convulsive therapy for mental disorder
- abortion (in addition to meeting the provisions of the Abortion Act 1967)
- any medical treatment that is considered by the medical practitioner primarily responsible for that treatment to lead to sterilisation as an unavoidable result.

There is a supplementary Code of Practice in relation to these treatments.[61]

Use of force or detention

The Act prohibits the use of force or detention unless it is 'immediately necessary', and only for as long as is necessary. In addition to being difficult to achieve in practice, imposing treatment on incapacitated adults clearly has the potential to damage relationships with health professionals and to undermine trust in carers. It is important therefore that force or detention is used only as a last resort, and with continual support and explanation for the patient. As arbitrary detention is prohibited by Article 5 of the European Convention on Human Rights, doctors will need to consider the impact of the Human Rights Act 1998 on their decisions. It can be useful to refer to the advice and guidance that emerged subsequent to the *Bournewood* case in England (see page 112). In addition, the Mental Welfare Commission for Scotland has published guidance on best practice in relation to the use of force or detention.[62] Basic principles from that guidance are given below.

- People who are in hospital, in care homes or receiving care in the community retain their full human rights, unless these have been restricted by a legal process and then only to the extent allowed by the law.
- Residents should always be involved in any discussion of restraint, no matter how disabled they are.
- Self-determination and freedom of choice and movement should be paramount, unless there are compelling reasons why this should not be so.
- Each care home or hospital should have an explicit policy which determines the balance between residents' personal autonomy and staff's duty to care. The principal aim of any policy should be to avoid restraint wherever possible.
- Restraint should never be used to cover any deficiency of service, lack of professional skill or defects in the environment.[63]

The Code of Practice also recommends that where an adult lacks capacity and resists treatment for a physical disorder, consideration should be given to an application for welfare guardianship.[64] This would allow the sheriff to make an order that the adult complies with the decision of the guardian. Alternatively, in cases where the adult may recover capacity, it may be more appropriate to seek an intervention order to authorise the required treatment.

Covert medication

As discussed in Chapter 1 (pages 39–40), covert medication would be unethical and un-lawful in relation to an adult with capacity. In Scotland, the Act's Code of Practice indicates that there may be occasions when it is permissible in relation to incapacitated adults.[65] It may, for example, be appropriate to use covert medication where there would otherwise be a risk of significant harm to the incapacitated adult and all other reasonable options have been explored. Any decision to use covert medication must be fully documented in the patient's record and must involve full discussion within the multi-disciplinary team. Covert medication must not be used merely because it would be more convenient. More detailed guidance including a covert medication care pathway is available from the Mental Welfare Commission for Scotland.[66]

Summary – exceptions to the general authority to treat

The following treatments or interventions fall outside the general authority to treat.

- Treatment under the Mental Health (Care and Treatment) (Scotland) Act 2003.
- Certain treatments subject to special safeguards, such as neurosurgery for mental disorder.
- The use of force or detention.

Dispute resolution

Clearly, it is better for all parties if medical treatment can be provided to adults lacking capacity consensually. Where all parties agree, and a certificate of incapacity has been issued, treatment can proceed on the basis either of the proxy's consent or, in the absence of a proxy, under the general authority to treat. Although, ideally, disputes should be infrequent it may not, of course, be possible always to achieve consensus. Discussion and ongoing consultation can help doctors to understand the patient's priorities, and help proxies and others close to the patient to understand the reasoning behind the clinical decision. Where agreement cannot be reached, the Act puts in place a procedure for resolving disputes. There are two sides to this procedure. Where a proxy or someone who has an interest in the incapacitated adult's care requests a treatment that the health professional does not believe will benefit the patient, that person should request a second opinion or use the relevant NHS complaints procedure. Where the health professional proposes a treatment but the proxy or somebody else close to the patient disagrees, then the Act sets out a procedure for resolving the disagreement. In these circumstances the health professional must obtain a second opinion from a medical practitioner nominated by the Mental Welfare Commission. The nominated practitioner must consult the proxy or other interested adult. Where the nominated professional agrees with the treating professional, treatment can go ahead despite the disagreement of the proxy, unless an application has been made to the Court of Session. Where the nominated practitioner disagrees with the treating professional, he or she can apply to the Court of Session for a ruling as to whether treatment can go ahead.

Appeal to the Court of Session

Ideally, appeals to the Court should be rare and any doctor considering approaching the Court should take legal advice in advance. All decisions about medical treatment, either under the general authority to treat or where there is a proxy, are nevertheless open to appeal to the Court. Any person with an interest in the personal welfare of an adult with incapacity may challenge a decision by appealing to the sheriff and then, by leave of the sheriff, to the Court of Session. This could be a treating doctor, another member of the clinical team, a proxy decision maker or someone close to the patient. While an appeal is pending, doctors should only provide treatment that is required in an emergency or is necessary for preventing a serious deterioration in the patient's health. Although the courts can instruct that a patient should receive specified treatment they cannot force a doctor to provide treatment contrary to his or her professional judgement.

Summary – dispute resolution

- Although, ideally, treatment decisions should be consensual, the Act contains a procedure for dispute resolution.
- Proxies or individuals with an interest in the incapacitated adult should, in cases of dispute, seek a second opinion or use the relevant NHS complaints procedure.
- Where the proxy disagrees with the treatment proposed health professionals must obtain a second opinion from a medical practitioner nominated by the Mental Welfare Commission.
- Ultimately appeal can be made to the Court of Session.

Providing treatment to adults lacking capacity – Northern Ireland

Although legislation relating to the provision of medical treatment to adults lacking capacity exists in Scotland and in England and Wales, at the time of writing such legislation was still in the process of being developed in Northern Ireland. Until such time as legislation passes on to the statute book, treatment for incapacitated adults in Northern Ireland is regulated by common law. When legislation does appear, information will be available on the BMA's website. In this section, a brief outline of the existing common law position is given. This should be read alongside the introductory section to this chapter which highlights the ethical issues engaged in this area and gives some of the background to the common law provisions. The basic principles in both the Scottish and English legislation were drawn from the common law and health professionals in Northern Ireland should consider them as guides to good practice.

Presumption of capacity

Legally and ethically all adults are presumed to have the capacity to make decisions on their own behalf. The presence of a physical or mental disorder alone, or the fact that an individual's decisions may be unwise, are not of themselves evidence that decision-making capacity is lacking. Capacity is always a decision-specific issue: does the individual have the capacity to make the specific decision at the time the decision is required? The presumption that an individual has capacity can be overridden, but the burden of proving that capacity is lost falls upon the person, such as the doctor, who questions it.

Best interests and necessity

In Northern Ireland, under common law, where adults lack capacity, no one else has the power to consent to medical treatment on their behalf. Clearly it would be unconscionable if incapacitated adults were, as a consequence, unable to gain access to necessary medical treatment. The common law therefore makes use of the concepts of 'necessity' and 'best interests'. Once it has been established that an adult lacks capacity, treatment can be provided where it is both necessary to intervene, and any intervention is regarded as being in the adult's best interests. More detailed information about the scope of a best interests decision, and how to assess a patient's best interests is given on pages 107–108.

Treatment in emergencies

The common law doctrine of necessity emerged from the requirement to render lawful emergency treatment to adults who lacked capacity because, for example, they were unconscious following an accident or other misfortune. In an emergency, therefore, where consent cannot be obtained, doctors should provide treatment that is immediately necessary either to preserve life or to prevent a serious deterioration in the patient's condition, unless, exceptionally, there is a binding advance decision refusing treatment. (For more on advance decisions, see pages 137–139.) Treatment in an emergency need not be restricted to what is immediately necessary but can also include steps that are required in order for recovery to become an option. Where decisions can reasonably be put off until such time as the adult is likely to regain capacity, or to permit, where appropriate, an assessment of capacity and a discussion with those close to the patient, then they should be.

If, in an emergency, a patient refuses treatment and there is doubt about his or her capacity to do so, doctors should take whatever steps are necessary to prevent deterioration of the patient's condition and then consider matters of capacity and consent. When it is clear that a patient has the capacity to refuse treatment, or has a valid advance refusal that is applicable to the circumstances, doctors cannot provide treatment unless it is authorised under mental health legislation.

Common law test of capacity

The common law sets out a three-stage test of capacity which was developed in the case of *Re C*,[67] which is discussed in more detail on page 99. *Re C* was influential in the development of the statutory tests of capacity that appear in both the Scottish and the English legislation. According to the common law therefore, an individual has the capacity to make a decision if, at the time the decision needs to be made, he or she can:

- comprehend and retain the relevant information
- believe the information
- weigh the information, balancing risks and benefits, in order to arrive at a choice.

This three-stage test has been elaborated over time and it is now widely accepted that when doctors are involved in assessing a patient's ability to make specified decisions, they will need to identify whether he or she is able to:

- understand in simple language what the medical treatment is, its purpose and nature and why it is being proposed

- understand its principal risks, benefits and alternatives
- understand in broad terms what will be the consequences of not receiving the proposed treatment
- retain the information for long enough to make an effective decision
- weigh the information in the balance
- make a free choice (i.e. free from any pressure or coercion).

Assessing capacity

The assessment of adult patients' capacity to make a decision about their own medical treatment is a matter for professional judgement and is subject to legal requirements. It is the personal responsibility of any doctor proposing to treat a patient to judge whether the patient has the capacity to give valid consent. Indeed, doctors constantly assess whether patients have the capacity to make the decision with which they are faced.

Doctors involved with direct patient care, whatever their specialty, should ordinarily be able to take a psychiatric history and conduct a basic mental state examination in order to identify cognitive problems, irrespective of their cause. GPs are often well placed to judge capacity, especially if they have a close, long-term acquaintance with the person being assessed. Where the person's capacity is uncertain or unclear, however, or the treating doctor does not feel able to make an objective assessment, specialist advice should be sought.

In cases where patients have borderline or fluctuating capacity, it can be difficult to assess whether the individual can make valid decisions on very serious issues. Doctors should be aware that capacity can be influenced by many things, including the patient's medical condition, medication, pain, fatigue, time of day and mood. Mental disorder and impairment may affect capacity, although do not necessarily prevent patients from making a valid choice. A very wide spectrum of ability is found within the group of patients whose competence to decide is permanently or temporarily affected. Doctors should aim to minimise the effects of factors that affect capacity, and allow patients to make choices when they are best able to do so.

The BMA publishes detailed practical advice about assessing capacity.[68] In many cases there is, of course, no doubt about a person's capacity. When there is, however, a comprehensive psychological investigation may be needed and any elective, non-urgent treatment should be postponed until the issues of capacity are resolved. The psychological investigation would seek to determine whether the adult:

- is capable of making a choice
- understands the nature of what is being asked
- understands why a choice is needed
- has memory abilities that allow the retention of information
- is aware of any alternatives
- has knowledge of the risks and benefits involved
- is aware of the decision's personal relevance to him or herself
- is aware of his or her right to refuse, as well as the consequences of refusal
- is aware of how to refuse
- is capable of communicating his or her choice
- has ever expressed wishes relevant to the issue when greater capacity existed
- is expressing views consistent with previously held moral, cultural, family and experiential values.

Assessing capacity to give consent to medical treatment is somewhat different from other capacity assessments because the assessor may also be the person proposing the treatment. If the procedure proposed is risky or involves innovative techniques, or if there is a divergence of opinion as to its benefits for the patient, additional safeguards are likely to be needed. These may include seeking advice from health and legal professionals and may involve making an application to the courts.

Factors affecting capacity and how to enhance capacity

In many cases, particularly where there are doubts about capacity, a patient's ability to make a decision can be enhanced, and doctors have a general ethical duty to enhance it when it is possible to do so. A number of factors can contribute to the enhancement of capacity. Doctors should seek, for example, to engage patients in decision making when they are best able to participate. The venue should be as non-threatening and welcoming as possible. GPs in particular may find that the patient's own home is a good choice because anxiety about unfamiliar surroundings may be inhibiting. Capacity, and simply the ability to participate, can be enhanced with treatment or symptom management. Management of pain, for example, can mean a patient is more able to take part in decision making. Similarly, the effects of medication can affect capacity. Whenever possible, patients should be given the opportunity to express their views when any detrimental effects of medication are absent or at a minimum. The effects of some medications take a long time to diminish, and doctors should consider whether it would be appropriate to allow time for these long-term effects to dissipate before assessing capacity. Similarly, depression and anxiety can be difficult to recognise, but may also interfere with capacity. Where there is doubt about mental state, a psychiatric opinion is often needed. It may also help if decisions are broken down into a series of smaller choices. Vulnerability to coercive influences should be acknowledged and minimised. It is important that people are not judged to be incapable of making decisions just because they have communication difficulties. Communication support must be offered if appropriate. Speech and language therapy may be helpful. Written and other forms of recorded information can also be used to enhance communication.

Advance decisions refusing treatment

There is currently no legislation covering advance decisions refusing treatment in Northern Ireland. Although the situation in England and Wales is now covered by the Mental Capacity Act 2005, earlier common law cases had established that, in certain circumstances, advance decisions refusing treatment made by adults with the relevant capacity, and based on sufficient information, would have the same status as a contemporaneous refusal. Although cases heard in England are not binding in Northern Ireland, in the BMA's view it is likely that, until such time as primary legislation is passed in this area, the courts in Northern Ireland will take a similar approach. The following basic principles emerge from the common law cases.

An advance decision refusing treatment is likely to be legally binding if:

- the patient is an adult and had the relevant capacity when the decision was made, and
- the patient has been offered sufficient, accurate information to make an informed decision, and

- the circumstances that have arisen are those that were envisaged by the patient, and
- the patient was not subjected to undue influence in making the decision.

In addition, the following points should be taken into account when considering whether an advance decision refusing treatment is likely to be binding.

- Adults are presumed to have capacity to make decisions unless the contrary is shown. As with all decision making, the test of capacity to make an advance decision refusing treatment is functional and the understanding required depends on the gravity of the decision.
- In cases of genuine doubt about the validity of an advance decision refusing treatment, the presumption is in favour of providing life-saving treatment. When there is doubt, and time permits, a declaration should be sought from a court.
- Any persons, including health professionals and carers, who knowingly provide treatment in the face of a valid advance decision refusing treatment may be liable to legal action for battery or assault.
- Advance requests for future treatment are not legally binding, although they may be helpful in assessing a patient's likely wishes and preferences.
- Unless an advance decision refusing treatment makes it unambiguously clear that it is intended to apply during pregnancy it is unlikely to be valid if the patient is pregnant.

Scope and nature of advance decisions refusing treatment

Although any statement of a patient's future wishes should obviously be given serious consideration, there are limits to the ability to influence future care. People cannot authorise or refuse in advance procedures they could not authorise or refuse contemporaneously. They cannot, for example, insist upon unlawful procedures, such as euthanasia, nor can they insist upon futile or inappropriate treatment. Advance decisions refusing treatment cannot extend to treatment for mental disorders provided under the authority of mental health legislation. In the BMA's view, it would also be inappropriate for patients to refuse in advance the provision of all forms of 'basic care' such as hygiene and any intervention designed solely for the alleviation of pain or distress.

Format of advance decisions refusing treatment

The case law does not give any guidance as to the required form in which an advance decision refusing treatment needs to be made. Oral statements can certainly be binding, particularly where they are supported by appropriate evidence – a note should be made of any such statement in the patient's medical record for example. There are, nevertheless, clear advantages to recording any advance decision refusing treatment in writing. Although there are no current legal requirements, in the BMA's view the following information should be included as a minimum:

- name and address
- name and address of GP
- whether advice was sought from a health professional
- a clear statement of the nature and circumstances of the refusal, or the contact details of someone who should be consulted about the patient's views
- a signature and the date the document was written or subsequently reviewed.

It is recommended that advance decisions refusing treatment are reviewed on a regular basis and at least every 5 years. The decision should also be reviewed if there has been a material change in the individual's condition or in available treatment options. There is no requirement for advance decisions refusing treatment to be witnessed or to be accompanied by a certificate of capacity. If doctors are asked to witness an advance decision they should consider whether the patient possesses the relevant capacity to make the decision. Where patients are concerned that the validity of an advance decision refusing treatment may be called into question after they have lost capacity, they may ask a health professional to make a more formal assessment and to certify that the individual had capacity at the time.

Storage of advance decisions refusing treatment

Storage of an advance decision, and notification of its existence, is primarily the responsibility of the patient. A copy of any written advance decision should be given to the GP to keep with the patient's medical record and, where possible, the patient should draw it to the attention of hospital staff before any episode of care. Patients should also be encouraged to make their friends, relatives or advocates aware of the existence of any advance decision refusing treatment, its general content and whereabouts. The development of integrated electronic care records will also hopefully lead to opportunities to indicate the existence of general advance statements as well as specific advance decisions refusing treatment.

Summary – advance decisions refusing treatment (Northern Ireland)

- Valid and applicable advance decisions refusing treatment made by adults with relevant capacity are likely to be binding.
- In cases of genuine doubt about the validity of an advance decision refusing treatment, the presumption is in favour of providing life-saving treatment.
- People cannot authorise or refuse in advance procedures they could not authorise or refuse contemporaneously.

Treatments requiring special safeguards

For the majority of day-to-day healthcare decisions, the procedures and principles set out in the common law and outlined in this section are perfectly adequate. The aim is agreement about treatment between health professionals, people close to the patient and the incapacitated adult, in so far as he or she has been able to express a view. There are some treatments, however, that are generally regarded as being more serious or controversial and require either special safeguards or, in case of the most complex or difficult decisions, referral to court.

In the BMA's view, formal clinical review, or second opinions should be sought in the following cases:

- restricting the movements of incapacitated adults to prevent them from harm
- medical treatment that, as a side effect renders people infertile, for example a surgical intervention for a gynaecological cancer, although court approval would be required where the aim of the intervention is sterilisation

- testing existing samples for serious communicable diseases after a health professional has suffered occupational exposure to body fluids
- withdrawing or withholding artificial nutrition and hydration from a patient who is not imminently dying.

In addition, the following procedures currently require court approval, although it should be noted that the courts may add or remove procedures in the future:

- non-therapeutic sterilisation
- withdrawing artificial nutrition and hydration from a patient who is in a persistent vegetative state
- organ or tissue donation
- where there is a dispute about whether a particular treatment will be in a person's best interests (this may include cases that introduce new ethical dilemmas or involve untested or innovative treatments).

Control, restraint and deprivation of liberty

There will be times when incapacitated adults may act in ways that present a risk to themselves or others and there will be occasions on which some degree of control or restraint may need to be used. Following the European Court of Human Rights' judgment in the *'Bournewood'* case (see page 112) an important issue for health professionals is the requirement to distinguish between restraint and deprivation of liberty and this is discussed in more detail on pages 112–113.

Deprivation of Liberty Safeguards – Northern Ireland

In 2010 the Department of Health, Social Services and Public Safety issued interim guidance for practitioners in relation to incapacitated adults whose care and treatment might amount to a deprivation of liberty, based upon current practice and the Mental Health (Northern Ireland) Order 1986 and pending the introduction of new mental health and mental capacity legislation.[69] The guidance points out that until new legislation is introduced, depriving incapacitated adults of their liberty would be unlawful and points instead to the use of mental health powers, including the use of guardianship. Until such time as new safeguards are developed, practitioners 'will need to continue to provide care and treatment for incapacitated patients, and it is important that neither the safety of those patients or the quality of the care they receive is jeopardised during the interim period'.[70] Practitioners must therefore take care to ensure that incapacitated adults are protected against the risk of arbitrary deprivation of liberty. (Further information on deprivation of liberty can be found on pages 112–113.)

Proposals for legal reform – Northern Ireland

In 2007, the Bamford Review of Mental Health and Learning Disability concluded its work with the publication of a report on the need for legislative reform in Northern Ireland.[71] Although no final decisions had been made as to the content of the legislation, at the time of writing the following policy proposals were considered likely to be reflected in the draft Bill:

- a single piece of legislation encompassing both mental capacity and mental health provisions applying to individuals aged 16 years or over
- capacity-based mental health powers
- legislation based on key principles of autonomy, justice, benefit and 'least harm'
- a presumption of capacity coupled with a decision-specific understanding of incapacity
- a two-stage test of capacity:
  i. diagnostic – does the person have a disturbance or impairment of the functioning of the mind or brain?
  ii. does the impairment mean the individual is unable to make the decision in question?
- incapacitated adults deprived of their liberty will be given a right of access to an independent judicial tribunal
- provisions for adults to nominate a health and welfare attorney to make decisions at a time in the future when capacity is lost.

The development of a single piece of capacity-based legislation covering both mental health and mental capacity would be innovative. As a result, if mental incapacity is the doorway to the legislation, mentally disordered individuals regarded as having the capacity to make a decision regarding mental health treatment could not be compulsorily treated. Such an approach was rejected during the development of legislation for England and Wales on the grounds of managing the risk that mentally disordered individuals could present to themselves and others.

References

1   See, for example: United Nations (2006) *Convention on the Rights of Persons with Disabilities*, UN, Geneva. Ratified by the UK Government in June 2008. Available at: www.un.org (accessed 12 January 2011).
2   British Medical Association, Law Society (2010) *Assessment of Mental Capacity*, 3rd edn, Law Society, London.
3   *Re C (adult: refusal of medical treatment)* [1994] 1 All ER 819.
4   *Re MB (medical treatment)* [1997] 2 FLR 426.
5   *Sidaway v Board of Governors of the Bethlem Royal Hospital* [1985] AC 871.
6   *Re T (adult: refusal of medical treatment)* [1992] 4 All ER 649: 661h–662a.
7   *Re B (adult refusal of treatment)* [2002] 2 All ER 449.
8   *Re T (adult: refusal of medical treatment)* [1992] 4 All ER 649.
9   World Medical Association (1964) *Declaration of Helsinki* (as amended), WMA, Geneva.
10 Department for Constitutional Affairs (2007) *Mental Capacity Act 2005 Code of Practice*, The Stationery Office, London.
11 British Medical Association, Law Society (2010) *Assessment of Mental Capacity*, 3rd edn, Law Society, London.
12 Mental Capacity Act 2005, s 2(1).
13 Mental Capacity Act 2005, s 1.
14 Mental Capacity Act 2005, s 2(1).
15 Mental Capacity Act 2005, s3.
16 For further information about the Court of Protection, see: www.publicguardian.gov.uk (accessed 13 February 2011).
17 For further information on the Office of the Public Guardian, see: www.publicguardian.gov.uk (accessed 13 February 2011).
18 Mental Capacity Act 2005, s 4.
19 Uncited case. Personal communication. Denzil Lush, 24 June 2010.
20 Article 5 provides a right to security and liberty of person. Article 5(1) states that any deprivation of liberty must be 'in accordance with a procedure prescribed by law'.
21 Department for Constitutional Affairs (2007) *Mental Capacity Act 2005 Code of Practice*, The Stationery Office, London, p.143.
22 Her Majesty's Courts Service (2007) *Practice Direction 9E: Applications relating to serious medical treatment*, HMCS, London.
23 Mental Capacity Act 2005, s 6(1)–(3).

24 *HL* v *United Kingdom* (45508/99) [2004] 40 EHRR 761.

25 *HL v United Kingdom* (45508/99) [2004] 40 EHRR 761.

26 Ministry of Justice (2008) *Mental Capacity Act 2005 Deprivation of liberty safeguards Code of Practice to supplement the main Mental Capacity Act 2005 Code of Practice*, The Stationery Office, London.

27 Mental Capacity Act 2005, s 4B. A vital act is defined as 'any act which the person doing it reasonably believes to be necessary to prevent a serious deterioration in P's condition'.

28 Ministry of Justice (2008) *Mental Capacity Act 2005 Deprivation of liberty safeguards Code of Practice to supplement the main Mental Capacity Act 2005 Code of Practice*, The Stationery Office, London.

29 Department for Constitutional Affairs (2007) *Mental Capacity Act 2005 Code of Practice*, The Stationery Office, London, p.164.

30 Department for Constitutional Affairs (2007) *Mental Capacity Act 2005 Code of Practice*, The Stationery Office, London, p.167.

31 LPA forms are available from the Office of the Public Guardian. Available at: www.publicguardian.gov.uk (accessed 13 February 2011).

32 Department for Constitutional Affairs (2007) *Mental Capacity Act 2005 Code of Practice*, The Stationery Office, London, pp.114–35.

33 Department for Constitutional Affairs (2007) *Mental Capacity Act 2005 Code of Practice*, The Stationery Office, London, pp.258–9.

34 See, for example: The National Mediation Helpline. Available at: www.nationalmediationhelpline.com (accessed 13 February 2011). The Family Mediation Helpline. Available at: www.familymediationhelpline.co.uk (accessed 13 February 2011).

35 Mental Capacity Act 2005, s 16(4).

36 Department for Constitutional Affairs (2007) *Mental Capacity Act 2005 Code of Practice*, The Stationery Office, London, pp.178–9.

37 Mental Capacity Act 2005 (Independent Mental Capacity Advocates) (General) Regulations 2006. SI 2006/1832.

38 Department for Constitutional Affairs (2007) *Mental Capacity Act 2005 Code of Practice*, The Stationery Office, London, pp.225–6.

39 Department for Constitutional Affairs (2007) *Mental Capacity Act 2005 Code of Practice*, The Stationery Office, London, pp.225–6.

40 Scottish Executive (2010) *Adults with Incapacity (Scotland) Act 2000 Code of Practice (third edition) for practitioners authorised to carry out medical treatment or research under part 5 of the Act*. SG/2010/57. Available at: www.scotland.gov.uk (accessed 26 April 2011).

41 Scottish Executive (2010) *Adults with Incapacity (Scotland) Act 2000. Code of Practice (third edition) for practitioners authorised to carry out medical treatment or research under part 5 of the Act*. SG/2010/57. Available at: www.scotland.gov.uk (accessed 26 April 2011), para 1.6.6.

42 Scottish Executive (2010) *Adults with Incapacity (Scotland) Act 2000. Code of Practice (third edition) for practitioners authorised to carry out medical treatment or research under part 5 of the Act*. SG/2010/57. Available at: www.scotland.gov.uk (accessed 26 April 2011), para 1.9.

43 Scottish Executive (2010) *Adults with Incapacity (Scotland) Act 2000. Code of Practice (third edition) for practitioners authorised to carry out medical treatment or research under part 5 of the Act*. SG/2010/57. Available at: www.scotland.gov.uk (accessed 26 April 2011), para 1.20.

44 Scottish Executive (2010) *Adults with Incapacity (Scotland) Act 2000. Code of Practice (third edition) for practitioners authorised to carry out medical treatment or research under part 5 of the Act*. SG/2010/57. Available at: www.scotland.gov.uk (accessed 26 April 2011), para 1.20.

45 Scottish Executive (2010) *Adults with Incapacity (Scotland) Act 2000. Code of Practice (third edition) for practitioners authorised to carry out medical treatment or research under part 5 of the Act*. SG/2010/57. Available at: www.scotland.gov.uk (accessed 26 April 2011), para 1.22.

46 The Smoking, Health and Social Care (Scotland) Act 2005, s 35(2)(b).

47 Adults with Incapacity (Conditions and Circumstances Applicable to Three Year Medical Treatment Certificates) (Scotland) Regulations 2007.

48 Scottish Executive (2010) *Adults with Incapacity (Scotland) Act 2000. Code of Practice (third edition) for practitioners authorised to carry out medical treatment or research under part 5 of the Act*. SG/2010/57. Available at: www.scotland.gov.uk (accessed 26 April 2011), para 2.12.

49 Scottish Executive (2010) *Adults with Incapacity (Scotland) Act 2000. Code of Practice (third edition) for practitioners authorised to carry out medical treatment or research under part 5 of the Act*. SG/2010/57. Available at: www.scotland.gov.uk (accessed 26 April 2011), para 2.37.

50 Scottish Executive (2010) *Adults with Incapacity (Scotland) Act 2000. Code of Practice (third edition) for practitioners authorised to carry out medical treatment or research under part 5 of the Act*. SG/2010/57. Available at: www.scotland.gov.uk (accessed 26 April 2011), para 1.35.

51 Scottish Executive (2010) *Adults with Incapacity (Scotland) Act 2000. Code of Practice (third edition) for practitioners authorised to carry out medical treatment or research under part 5 of the Act*. SG/2010/57. Available at: www.scotland.gov.uk (accessed 26 April 2011), annexe 5.

52 Scottish Executive (2010) *Adults with Incapacity (Scotland) Act 2000. Code of Practice (third edition) for practitioners authorised to carry out medical treatment or research under part 5 of the Act*. SG/2010/57. Available at: www.scotland.gov.uk (accessed 26 April 2011), para 2.20.

53 Scottish Executive (2010) *Adults with Incapacity (Scotland) Act 2000. Code of Practice (third edition) for practitioners authorised to carry out medical treatment or research under part 5 of the Act*. SG/2010/57. Available at: www.scotland.gov.uk (accessed 26 April 2011), para 2.30.

54 Scottish Executive (2010) *Adults with Incapacity (Scotland) Act 2000. Code of Practice (third edition) for practitioners authorised to carry out medical treatment or research under part 5 of the Act*. SG/2010/57. Available at: www.scotland.gov.uk (accessed 26 April 2011), paras 1.6.6–1.6.7.

55 www.publicguardian-scotland.gov.uk (accessed 13 February 2011).

56 Scottish Executive (2010) *Adults with Incapacity (Scotland) Act 2000. Code of Practice (third edition) for practitioners authorised to carry out medical treatment or research under part 5 of the Act*. SG/2010/57. Available at: www.scotland.gov.uk (accessed 26 April 2011).

57 British Medical Association (2007) *Withholding and Withdrawing Life-Prolonging Medical Treatment: Guidance for decision-making*, 3rd edn, Blackwell, Oxford.

58 Scottish Executive (2010) *Adults with Incapacity (Scotland) Act 2000. Code of Practice (third edition) for practitioners authorised to carry out medical treatment or research under part 5 of the Act*. SG/2010/57. Available at: www.scotland.gov.uk (accessed 26 April 2011), para 2.65.

59 Mental Health (Care and Treatment) (Scotland) Act 2003, s 16.

60 The Adults with Incapacity (Specified Medical Treatments) (Scotland) Regulations 2002 SSI 2002/275.

61 Scottish Executive (2002) *Adults with Incapacity (Scotland) Act 2000. Supplement to Code of Practice for persons authorised to carry out medical treatment or research under part 5 of the Act*. SE/2002/111. Available at: www.sehd.scot.nhs.uk (accessed 19 October 2011).

62 Mental Welfare Commission for Scotland (2006) *Rights, Risks and Limits to Freedom: Principles and Good Practice Guidance for Practitioners Considering Restraint in Residential Settings*, MWCS, Edinburgh.

63 Mental Welfare Commission for Scotland (2006) *Rights, Risks and Limits to Freedom: Principles and Good Practice Guidance for Practitioners Considering Restraint in Residential Settings*, MWCS, Edinburgh, pp.6–7.

64 Scottish Executive (2010) *Adults with Incapacity (Scotland) Act 2000. Code of Practice (third edition) for practitioners authorised to carry out medical treatment or research under part 5 of the Act*. SG/2010/57. Available at: www.scotland.gov.uk (accessed 26 April 2011), para 2.59.

65 Scottish Executive (2010) *Adults with Incapacity (Scotland) Act 2000. Code of Practice (third edition) for practitioners authorised to carry out medical treatment or research under part 5 of the Act*. SG/2010/57. Available at: www.scotland.gov.uk (accessed 26 April 2011), para 2.60.

66 Mental Welfare Commission for Scotland. (2006) *Covert Medication: Legal and Practical Guidance*. MWCS, Edinburgh.

67 *Re C (adult: refusal of medical treatment)* [1994] 1 All ER 819.

68 British Medical Association, Law Society (2010) *Assessment of Mental Capacity*, 3rd edn, Law Society, London.

69 Department of Health, Social Services and Public Safety (2010) *Deprivation of Liberty Safeguards (DOLS) Interim Guidance*, DHSSPS, Belfast.

70 Department of Health, Social Services and Public Safety (2010) *Deprivation of Liberty Safeguards (DOLS) Interim Guidance*, DHSSPS, Belfast, para 20.

71 Bamford Review of Mental Health and Learning Disability (Northern Ireland) (2007) *A comprehensive legislative framework*. DHSSPS, Belfast.

4: Children and young people

The questions covered in this chapter include the following.

- Who can give consent for the medical treatment of children?
- When do young people become competent to make their own decisions?
- Are there differences between consent and refusal?
- When do the courts need to be involved in decisions?
- What are doctors' responsibilities with respect to child protection?

Combining respect for autonomy with best interests

During childhood and adolescence, most people attain the maturity that eventually allows them to take responsibility for their own lives. In this phase of development, children and young people sometimes seek to exercise their autonomy in a way that conflicts with other people's views of their best interests. Doctors, parents and others who care for young people can be torn between respecting the values of young people developing their autonomy and protecting those same individuals from the possibly adverse effects of their perceived inexperience. This raises questions of who is best able to judge what is in an individual's interests. In other sections of this book, while recognising that autonomy has some limits, and that many patients involve people close to them in decision making, we have strongly supported the view that judgements should be made by competent patients about their own situation. From an ethical viewpoint, therefore, a decision by a competent young person, which is based on an appreciation of the facts, demands respect. Both law and ethics stress that the views of children and young people must be heard. In some cases, however, their views alone do not determine what eventually happens.

Combining respect for autonomy with support for minors encourages children and young people to make all those decisions that they feel comfortable and able to make. This is the message of the Children Act 1989, Children (Scotland) Act 1995 and the Children (Northern Ireland) Order 1995, which stress that children's views should be heard in decisions that affect them. Children and young people sometimes refuse medical treatment because they lack the maturity and understanding to consider the long-term implications of their choices. Their anxieties may be focused on the short-term effects, such as fear of injections, in which case they may not be expressing a considered choice in favour of non-treatment. On the other hand, a child's refusal of treatment that is based on awareness of the long-term consequences, and is compatible with the child's view of his or her best interests beyond the short term, is likely to be a valid expression of choice. Adults who are responsible for providing care retain a duty to intervene if the child or young person appears to be exploited and/or abused, or if decision making seems seriously awry by the usual standards of what a reasonably prudent person in the patient's position would choose. In the former case, it may mean contacting social services. In the latter, as a starting point, it should mean further discussion with the child or young person

Medical Ethics Today: The BMA's Handbook of Ethics and Law, Third Edition. Sophie Brannan, Eleanor Chrispin, Martin Davies, Veronica English, Rebecca Mussell, Julian Sheather and Ann Sommerville.
© 2012 BMA Medical Ethics Department. Published 2012 by Blackwell Publishing Ltd.

and family. In cases of decision making for immature children, there must be a reasonable presumption that the parents have the child's best interests at heart. Such a presumption cannot be taken for granted, however, and, when there seem to be grounds for doubt, decisions should be evaluated carefully. There may be further difficulty where the parents themselves take different views.

Has human rights legislation changed things for children?

Over recent decades, society has paid increasing attention to the rights of groups of individuals who have been previously ignored. For example, societal attitudes towards the civil liberties of mentally disordered and elderly people have changed, with a consequent emphasis on the rights of individuals to exert self-determination and to receive assistance or services to maximise their liberty. The rights of children and young people have also been the focus of reappraisal. In 1989 the UN General Assembly adopted the Convention on the Rights of the Child, and this was ratified by the UK in 1992.[1] The Convention set internationally accepted minimum standards on issues such as freedom from discrimination on grounds of disability (Articles 2 and 5), privacy (Article 16) and the child's right to have his or her views accorded due weight in relation to the child's maturity (Article 12). The Human Rights Act 1998 gave further weight to legally enforceable rights, derived from the European Convention on Human Rights. The rights particularly relevant in the care of children include recognition of:

- the right to life (Article 2)
- the right not to be subjected to inhuman or degrading treatment (Article 3)
- the right to liberty and security (Article 5)
- the right to a fair hearing (Article 6)
- the right to respect for private and family life (Article 8)
- the right not to suffer discrimination in relation to any of the other basic rights (Article 14).

How the rights should be applied in practice is evolving and becoming clearer as case law develops. It is possible that young people will seek to use these rights to demand that their competent choices are respected. Parents have already used their right to respect for family life to be involved in important decisions concerning their children if they believe they have been being prevented from doing so.[2]

Discussion of children's rights is complex because much of the normal focus on patient rights is directed at issues of choice, autonomy and self-determination. Health professionals have come to associate the notion of patient rights with the legally binding power of adult patients with capacity to refuse or limit certain treatments. Logically, the closer a young person is to achieving similar competence, the more the moral weight should shift towards prioritising that person's right of self-determination. However, legal cases where competent young people have sought to exercise such a right have shown the great difficulty society has in dealing with the emerging autonomy of young people (see pages 157–159). Their rights to choose are often limited if their health would be seriously jeopardised as a result of their choices.

Rights are not only possessed by young people who are able to express their views; the human rights of babies and young children are equally important, although protecting them rather than promoting their (future) autonomy may be the principal consideration. It falls to the parents, healthcare team and others involved in caring for the child to ensure that his or her rights are not breached. Rights must be protected from the moment of birth, and decisions about treatment, or non-treatment, of neonates made on the same case-by-case basis as decisions about older children who cannot express a view.

Scope of this chapter

This chapter covers the examination and treatment of people in England, Wales and Northern Ireland who are aged under 18 years, and under 16 years in Scotland. It covers people who completely lack competency to make decisions (babies) right through to children and young people who are competent to make complex decisions for themselves. Because in healthcare contexts the decision-making process for babies and very young children is usually straightforward, with people who have parental responsibility (see pages 160–166) usually deciding for their children based on advice from the healthcare team, much of the focus of this chapter is on situations in which children and young people are able to express their own wishes. We also seek to answer questions such as how to assess children's best interests, what to do when agreement cannot be reached and how the decision-making rights of parents are limited. Some specific areas of healthcare are covered towards the end of this chapter or in other chapters – for example, issues relating to contraception are discussed in Chapter 7, genetic testing of children in Chapter 9 and withholding and withdrawing treatment in Chapter 10. The term 'children' is used for people who are probably not mature enough to make important decisions for themselves, and 'young people' for those who may be.

General principles

Basic principles have been established regarding the manner in which the treatment of children and young people should be approached. These reflect standards of good practice,[3] which are underpinned by domestic and international law.

The welfare of children and young people is the paramount consideration in decisions about their care. They should:

- be kept as fully informed as possible about their care and treatment
- be able to expect health professionals to act as their advocates
- have their views and wishes sought and taken into account as part of promoting their welfare in the widest sense
- be able to consent to treatment when they have sufficient 'understanding and intelligence'
- be encouraged to take decisions in collaboration with other family members, especially parents, if this is feasible.

Communication

The development of a trusting relationship and good communication between health professionals and their patients are fundamental aspects of good practice. A good relationship between a health team and a child patient should establish a lifelong pattern of mutual trust and candour. As soon as they are able to communicate and participate in the decisions that affect them, children should be encouraged to express their views, ask questions and discuss their health worries. Young patients themselves should be able to set the pace for discussion. Sensitivity is required to ensure that they are not overwhelmed with information but given the time they need to absorb it. Translators and interpreters, including those who provide sign language, should be provided where necessary.

Communicating with children and young people

The General Medical Council (GMC) lists the following factors that doctors should give particular consideration to when communicating with children and young people:

a. 'involve children and young people in discussions about their care
b. be honest and open with them and their parents, while respecting confidentiality
c. listen to and respect their views about their health, and respond to their concerns and preferences
d. explain things using language or other forms of communication they can understand
e. consider how you and they use non-verbal communication, and the surroundings in which you meet them
f. give them opportunities to ask questions, and answer these honestly and to the best of your ability
g. do all you can to make open and truthful discussion possible, taking into account that this can be helped or hindered by the involvement of parents or other people
h. give them the same time and respect that you would give to adult patients'.[4]

Some children may not want to have full information, or they may need time to adjust to one aspect of the situation before receiving more details. Each patient is an individual and is entitled to be given information in a manner that is accessible and appropriate according to his or her level of understanding. Parents may try to insist on secrecy in order to protect their children from painful facts.[5] This situation poses difficult dilemmas that need to be carefully worked through with the family in the light of the circumstances of the case. There is research suggesting that children prefer to receive information and not telling a child may be detrimental to a child's well-being.[6] On the whole, the British Medical Association (BMA) and General Medical Council (GMC) promote the sharing of information if the child seems willing to know it, even when parents request secrecy, unless disclosing the information would cause serious harm.[7] Questions should always be answered as frankly and as sensitively as possible; where there is uncertainty about the diagnosis, treatment or likely outcome, this should be acknowledged.

Involving children

When medical advice or treatment is sought by children and parents together, health professionals should remember their role as the patient's advocate and ensure that children and young people are not excluded from decision making. Including them should be seen as the norm. If children are excluded from decision making, there must be justification for that stance.

Children who are able and want to participate in decisions should be helped and encouraged to do so. They need information about their condition and options, and doctors should take steps to enhance their ability to make decisions by providing information in a way the child finds most accessible. They should also give the child options about having parents or other third parties present, and talk to the child at a time when he or she is relatively relaxed, comfortable and free from medication that may affect the ability to choose. Children should not simply be considered incompetent to decide if they are unwilling to participate in decisions or agree to treatment, and should be able to change their minds later if they so wish. In practical terms, although small children may not be asked to make major decisions such as whether to undergo surgery, they should be given a voice on all the lesser points, such as whether parents accompany them to the anaesthetic room. In this way, many of the child's views can be respected and it can be feasible to offer alternatives, even to young children.

Competence to make decisions

In addition to involving all children, it is important to recognise when a young person under 16 years is able to make a valid choice about a proposed medical intervention. The landmark *Gillick* case[8] clarified the standard for competency in England, Wales and Northern Ireland; in Scotland, it is set by the Age of Legal Capacity (Scotland) Act 1991.[9]

Competency to make decisions

Mrs Gillick took her local health authority to court because it refused to assure her that her five daughters, all aged under 16 years, would not be given contraceptive advice and treatment without her knowledge and consent. The case followed the publication of a Department of Health and Social Security circular advising that doctors consulted at a family planning clinic by a girl under 16 years would not be acting unlawfully if they prescribed contraceptives, provided that they acted in good faith and to protect the young woman from the harmful effects of sexual intercourse. In seeking a declaration that this advice was unlawful, Mrs Gillick argued that a young girl's consent was legally ineffective and inconsistent with parental rights. She said that it was therefore necessary to involve parents.

This argument was rejected by the House of Lords, where the majority opinion was that the relevant test was whether the girl had reached an age where she had sufficient understanding and intelligence to enable her to understand fully what was proposed. If she had, a doctor would not be acting unlawfully in giving advice and treatment.[10]

In order for the consent of any person to be valid it must be based on competence, information and voluntariness. This can be broken down into several fundamental points:

- the ability to understand that there is a choice and that choices have consequences
- the ability to weigh the information in the balance and arrive at a decision
- a willingness to make a choice (including the choice that someone else should make the decision)
- an understanding of the nature and purpose of the proposed procedure
- an understanding of the proposed procedure's risks and side effects
- an understanding of the alternatives to the proposed procedure, and the risks attached to them
- freedom from undue pressure.

Whether a child has the competence to make a specific decision is a legal concept, but medical or psychiatric tests can be involved in the assessment. There are various ways of testing whether children are competent; no magical definition or 'right' method exists, but the 'functional' approach has the greatest support, and is adopted in GMC guidance. This approach relates the individual ability of the patient to the particular decision to be made. The nature and complexity of the decision or task, and the person's ability to understand at the time the decision is made, the nature of the decision required and its implications, are all relevant. Thus, the graver the impact of the decision, the commensurately greater the competence needed to make it. In short, as with adults (see Chapter 3), children and young people are competent to give consent to medical treatment if they are able to understand the nature and purpose of the proposed treatment, and to retain the information and weigh it in the balance to arrive at a decision. Although some children clearly lack competence due to immaturity, doctors should not judge the ability of a particular child solely on the basis of his or her age.[11] Doctors should also be mindful that a young person's competency can fluctuate because of a range of factors, including their medical condition, medication, the time of day or their mood. Doctors have a general ethical duty to enhance competency when it is possible to do so, and should seek to engage children and young people in decision making when they are best able to participate.

The case of M highlights that the courts generally require a high level of competency for a young person to refuse life-saving treatment, although in a similar subsequent case a hospital trust accepted a young person's refusal and the case did not go to court (see page 158).

M's refusal of a heart transplant

M was a 15-year-old girl who refused to consent to a heart transplant operation in 1999 when her own heart was failing. Her mother gave legal consent on her behalf, but health professionals were unwilling to proceed without M's agreement. M said she did not want to die but neither did she wish to have the transplant because this would make her feel different from other people.

'I understand what a heart transplant means, procedure explained...checkups...tablets for the rest of your life. I feel depressed about that. I am only 15 and don't want to take tablets for the rest of my life...I don't want to die. It's hard to take it all in...If I had children...I would not let them die...I don't want to die, but I would rather die than have the transplant...I would feel different with someone else's heart, that's a good enough reason not to have a heart transplant, even if it saved my life.'[12]

The case was heard in the High Court, and after listening to her views, Mr Justice Johnson decided that M was not capable of making the decision herself and he authorised the operation to go ahead despite her reluctance. 'Events have overtaken her so swiftly that she has not been able to come to terms with her situation', he said.[13] Once that decision had been made on her behalf, M agreed to comply with treatment.

Growth of competence

Mental abilities, social understanding and emotional appreciation increase greatly during childhood development. Young people become more able to consider the long-term consequences of their own actions and of what happens to them. They also tend to think about such consequences more in terms of their own sense of responsibility and to have a better awareness of the effects of what they do on other people. Some generalisations can undoubtedly be made about the time at which children develop particular traits, but individuals differ and development is a continuous but uneven process.

Health professionals who work with seriously ill children often comment that those who have undergone suffering and discomfort develop the ability to understand the implications of choices in the light of past experiences at an earlier stage than other children. Children who have already undergone treatment have a greater imaginative perception of what is being proposed when treatment options are put forward. They are also influenced by the level of support, information and encouragement from key adults around them: parents, nurses and doctors. There is some obligation on clinical staff to create environments in which children are enabled to engage in decisions to the optimum level of their competence.

Children of the same age differ significantly in their ability and willingness to participate. Some believe that, since it is their life that is being affected, they should decide. Others want to share the process with parents, or want parents to decide for them. It is important not to approach young patients with preconceptions about ability based on experience of other children and young people of a similar age.[14]

Assessing competence

Assessment of competence to take a specific decision regarding healthcare or treatment needs to be based on how that particular decision is worked through, rather than on any standardised tests (although these may be useful in alerting professionals to the possibility that a child is unusually mentally advanced or delayed in comparison with others of the same age). Assessment should take account of the following factors.

Cognitive development

- The patient should demonstrate having a concept of himself or herself in relation to other people as shown by an ability to recognise, for example, his or her own needs and the needs of others. This might be shown by talking about relationships with parents, siblings, relatives and peers.
- The patient should recognise and understand that there is a choice to be made and show a willingness to make it.

Structured tests of cognitive development provide general information, although may not be task-specific.

Ability to balance risks and benefits of treatment

Some abilities develop as much by experience as by cognitive development. The assessment should consider whether the child or young person has:

- an understanding of what the illness means and that treatment is needed
- an appreciation of what the proposed treatment involves and what the intended outcomes will be
- an understanding of the implications of both treatment and non-treatment and the consequences (this implies that the individual has a sense of himself or herself over time.)

These abilities might be demonstrated through talking about the illness or condition and about hopes and fears for the future. Assessors should be looking to see whether patients ask questions that show they understand, and/or whether they show understanding in response to direct questions from others. Play or drawings are a way for some children to reveal their level of understanding.

The following factors should also be considered.

- Unwillingness to participate should not be interpreted as incompetence. A young patient who is competent to make his or her own decisions may nevertheless choose to allow parents to make decisions on his or her behalf. This demonstrates the ability to choose.
- Information must be retained for long enough to make an informed decision. This can be tested by asking questions about the information which has been given. A child may become irritated or bored by this, as might adults, but this is not evidence of incompetence.
- Some children are clearly unable to make decisions because of their immaturity or lack of ability to communicate their wishes. Extreme care is necessary, however, in making the assumption that the inability or unwillingness of a child to communicate with a doctor indicates incompetence.
- Doctors must be aware that their role as assessor of competency can radically change the doctor–patient relationship and that if it is not handled sensitively there is a danger that assessment could undermine the trust, confidence and mutual respect on which the doctor–patient relationship should be founded.

Confidentiality and involving parents

Young people are not always aware of their rights to seek medical advice and treatment without involving their parents, despite information provided in schools, on websites and in the media explaining that young people may approach their GP for advice about any health issues, including topics that teenagers are typically reticent about discussing with adults: contraception, smoking, alcohol and other drugs, for example. Ideally, treatment decisions involve people close to the patient. In the case of an immature child, the parents, or parents and child together, will decide (see pages 155–156 on unaccompanied children and young people). Unless there are convincing reasons to the contrary, because of an increased risk of harm for example, doctors should try to persuade the patient to allow parents to be informed of the consultation, but should not override the patient's refusal to do so. In the BMA's view, even when the doctor considers the unaccompanied young person is too immature to consent to the treatment requested, confidentiality should still generally be maintained concerning the consultation. The BMA considers that doctors' duty of confidentiality is not dependent upon the competency of the patient and, unless there are very convincing reasons to the contrary, for instance if abuse is suspected, the doctor should keep confidential a minor's request for treatment such as contraception, even if the doctor believes the minor to be insufficiently mature for the request to be fulfilled (see Chapter 7). Children and young people should be informed in advance of consultations about how their confidentiality will be respected and the exceptional circumstances in which it might be breached.

Further advice should be taken from, for example, professional bodies such as the GMC and BMA if there is any doubt. For more detailed advice on confidentiality and the situations in which it may be breached, see Chapter 5.

Best interests

A fundamental ethical obligation in the provision of treatment is that of focusing on the interests of the patient and providing benefit for that person. Adults with capacity are allowed to make decisions for themselves to consent or refuse, even if their views are very different from those of the rest of society. They can refuse treatment when they feel they have had enough or choose to take some risks with their own health (see Chapter 2). Children and young people have not generally been given the same options. Traditionally, other people – usually their parents – have chosen for them. Increasingly, however, it is being recognised that children and young people have a lot to contribute to decision making. Although children are usually best cared for in the family, and parents are generally the best decision makers for young children, it is acknowledged that the interests of children and those of the parents are not always synonymous. Doctors should be alert to situations in which parents' decisions appear to be contrary to their child's interests.

Regarding the definition of best interests, it is customary to assume that a person's interests are usually best served by measures that offer the hope of prolonging life or preventing damage to health. Health professionals are accustomed to measuring benefit primarily in terms of physical gains. Thus, when medical treatment carries low risk and offers substantial benefit to the patient, it is clearly perceived as being in the person's interests. This is the situation in many of the day-to-day decisions involving children, although not all choices are that simple. The side effects and other burdens of treatment may not be matched by a genuine prospect of significant and sustained improvement. Alternatively, the promise of physical improvement may necessarily involve compromises that the patient considers unacceptable, such as the administration of blood products to a Jehovah's Witness. In all cases, it is increasingly recognised that an assessment of best interests must involve far more complex matters than physical criteria alone. The following factors are relevant:

- the patient's own wishes and values (where these can be ascertained)
- the patient's ability to understand what is proposed and weigh up the alternatives
- the patient's potential to participate more in the decision, if provided with additional support or explanations
- the patient's physical and emotional needs
- relevant information about the patient's religious or cultural background
- clinical judgement about the effectiveness of the proposed treatment, particularly in relation to other options
- where there is more than one option, which option is least restrictive of the patient's future choices
- the likelihood and extent of any degree of improvement in the patient's condition if treatment is provided
- risks and side effects of the treatment
- the views of parents and others who are close to the patient about what is likely to benefit the patient
- the views of other healthcare professionals involved in providing care to the child or young person, and of any other professional who has an interest in their welfare.

Preventing harm

Harm is often seen as being an actual injury or impairment, but patients may also be wronged if their own values are ignored, regardless of whether they are physically or psychologically damaged by this. Neglect, including medical neglect, is a harm. Arguably, by imposing treatment contrary to the will of a competent young person, physical harm may be prevented, but the individual is nevertheless wronged. The degree to which this is acceptable is dependent upon the scale of the potential harm in comparison with that of the wrong.

Prevention of suicide and treatment for drug addiction, depression or anorexia nervosa exemplify circumstances in which denying the wishes of an apparently competent minor do not usually raise profound ethical dilemmas. Chemotherapy for leukaemia is an example of a treatment that carries particularly unpleasant side effects. Children who have previously undergone this therapy, and therefore understand what is involved, may be reluctant to accept further treatment. Nevertheless, the chances of treating the condition successfully may be such that some pressure on the child to agree would be justifiable, with the parents' consent, and in England, Wales and Northern Ireland the courts may overrule even a competent child's opinion if there are anticipated benefits in the individual case (see pages 157–158).

On the other hand, the imposition of treatments that are either likely to bring only minimal improvement or which involve distressing side effects and have only a small chance of success cannot be easily justified if refused by a minor who understands the implications. The treatment proposed may not involve a question of life and death, but gradations of foreseeable improvement. Children with chronic illnesses who have undergone many medical and surgical interventions may be able to weigh for themselves whether the anticipated improvement is worth another period in hospital and it may be appropriate to defer to their opinions. Parents may find it hard to accept this, and doctors need to treat such situations with great care and sensitivity to the needs of all family members.

Emergencies

When consent is not obtainable, for example in an emergency when the patient is unable to communicate his or her wishes and nobody with parental responsibility is available, it is legally and ethically appropriate for health professionals to proceed with treatment necessary to preserve the life, health or well-being of the patient. An emergency is best described as a situation in which the requirement for treatment is so pressing that there is not time to seek consent or refer the matter to court.

If such an emergency involves a treatment to which the child or family are known to object, for example the administration of blood to a Jehovah's Witness, viable alternatives, such as the use of non-blood products, should be explored if time allows. In extreme situations, however, health professionals are advised to accommodate the family's wishes as far as possible, but to take any essential steps to stabilise the child, even against the family's wishes. Legal advice should be sought as a matter of urgency. Although there is some suggestion from the Scottish courts that a competent young person's refusal of treatment may not be overridden (see page 159), in the absence of a clear ruling that this includes lifesaving treatment, the BMA advises that emergency life-saving treatment should be given and an application made to a court as a matter of urgency. Emergency care is discussed further in Chapter 15.

Consent and refusal by competent young people

Ideally, medical decisions are made in partnership between the patient, the family and the health team, with the parental role gradually fading as the child develops in maturity. Ordinarily, it is valid consent from somebody legally entitled to give it that affords doctors the legal authority to provide treatment. In the case of children and young people, consent can come from any one of a number of sources: a young patient competent to the make the decision, people with parental responsibility who have capacity (and in some circumstances other carers such as grandparents or childminders[15]) or the courts. In Scotland it appears that the legal rights of parents, carers and the courts to give consent may be extinguished when a young person is competent to decide for himself or herself (see page 159).[16]

When consent is required in writing, which is now generally accepted to be the case when treatment involves sedation or general anaesthesia, there are model consent forms produced by some of the health departments.[17]

Consent from competent young people

People aged over 16 years are presumed to be competent to give consent to medical treatment, unless the contrary is shown.[18] Young people under this age who have sufficient understanding and intelligence to comprehend fully what is proposed may also give consent to treatment, regardless of their age.[19] Young people should always be encouraged to involve their parents, but nevertheless treatment may proceed without their knowledge, or against their wishes, if the young person is competent to decide and cannot be persuaded to include them.

The BMA welcomes this recognition of young people's autonomy, seeing it as productive of better relationships between doctors and young patients. Trust in the doctor–patient relationship is a matter upon which the BMA lays great emphasis and such trust should be established as early as possible.

Unaccompanied minors

A common enquiry to the BMA concerns the duties of doctors in respect of children and young people who seek medical care without an adult. Doctors should not prohibit children and young people making appointments and seeing a doctor without an accompanying adult. The GMC states that 'you should make it clear that you are available to see children and young people on their own if that is what they want. You should avoid giving the impression (whether directly, through reception staff or in any other way) that they cannot access services without a parent.'[20] There will be circumstances where it will be advisable to see a child for some of the consultation time without an accompanying adult, for example to ensure there is no undue pressure.

Although there are circumstances in which it is reasonable for doctors to want a parent present – because, for example, the child has a serious condition and needs help in complying with a treatment regime – an absolutist rule prohibiting young patients attending alone is not good practice and could lead to a complaint against the doctor. Establishing a trusting relationship between the patient and doctor at this stage will do more to promote health than if doctors refuse to see young patients without involving parents. Both ethically and contractually, GPs, for example, are required to provide immediately necessary treatment and so they need to ascertain the kind of care patients are seeking. Although doctors are now less likely to try to ban unaccompanied minors, they may remain anxious about seeing young patients – especially in very sensitive or complex situations – without any input from an appropriate adult. The possible provision of family or parental support needs to be at least raised in the consultation even though patients may reject the notion for various reasons and their views should usually be respected.

Where children and young people are having tests, health professionals should arrange in advance, where possible, how competent children and young people will collect the results, and what should happen if they fail to collect them. If a prior arrangement has not been agreed and the results are not collected, doctors should examine all reasonable options, including writing to or telephoning the patient, with due regard to confidentiality. If the young person lives with his or her parents and may not want the parents to know of the health interaction, for example a teenager awaiting the results for a sexually transmitted infection, this should be borne in mind when examining the best way of contacting the patient.

Chaperones

A parent or carer often acts as a chaperone[21] for children or young people, but in the case of unaccompanied children or young people, they may be unaccompanied because they do not wish a parent or carer to be present. In these cases, consideration should be given to the GMC's guidance which states 'you should think carefully about the effect the presence of a chaperone can have. Their presence can deter young people from being frank and from asking for help.'[22]

If a doctor needs to perform an intimate examination, however, the GMC's general advice is that wherever possible, a chaperone should be offered. If either the doctor or the patient does not wish the examination to proceed without a chaperone present, or if either is uncomfortable with the choice of chaperone, the doctor may offer to delay the examination to a later date when a chaperone (or an alternative chaperone) will be available, if this is compatible with the patient's best interests. If the patient does not want a chaperone, the doctor should record that the offer was made and declined.

Child donors

In Scotland, children under 16 years (including those who are deemed to be competent) may not be living solid organ donors. In England, Wales and Northern Ireland, solid organ donation by living children is permitted but is expected to be extremely rare.[23] The removal of organs for transplantation is not covered by the human tissue legislation and the Human Tissue Authority (HTA) advises that it will only consider children as potential solid organ donors where prior court approval to the removal has been obtained.

The use of living children as solid organ donors is controversial and raises serious ethical issues.[24] The BMA originally opposed all use of children as living solid organ donors but reconsidered its view during 2005. The BMA now takes the view that those who are able to give valid consent, including competent children, should be able to be altruistic living donors of whole organs provided there are adequate safeguards in place to avoid the risk of coercion. Unlike young incompetent children, competent children are able to gain personal satisfaction from their altruistic act and also to appreciate and understand the consequences of not being able to donate. The BMA considers that many competent children and young people would want to donate a kidney to a sick sibling and that the arguments against permitting this are not sufficiently strong to justify prohibiting such an action.

While any relative may be subject to pressure and coercion – irrespective of age – we accept that younger people may be more susceptible. It is not clear, however, that this pressure is likely to be any less on a 16-year-old than on a 15-year-old. The BMA supports the safeguards that are in place to identify pressure on any living donor, regardless of their age (see Chapter 2, pages 82–83). The BMA does not support the use of young children who are unable to consent as living solid organ donors.

Refusal by competent young people

England, Wales and Northern Ireland

When the views of competent young people come into conflict with those of doctors and other people responsible for the minor, the law may intervene as a last resort. People under 18 years can and do regularly give consent to complex and risky procedures, but there is some legal distinction between a young person's consent and refusal, at least in England, Wales and Northern Ireland. When giving consent to proposed treatment, the patient is accepting the advice of a qualified professional. Deciding not to follow medical advice can have serious implications, in terms of both the immediate physical effects of non-treatment and the possible closing down of options for future treatment. The courts have shown themselves more reluctant to accept the refusal of a minor, even when he or she is found to be competent.

The message from legal cases is that a young person's decision about a very serious matter is valid only when it concurs with the views of the doctor who proposes it. In these cases, the courts have said that children and young people have a right to consent to what is proposed, but not to refuse if this would put their health in serious jeopardy. Consent has been described in terms of 'key holders' protecting the doctor from litigation. A doctor needs only one key holder (i.e. consent), and in England, Wales and Northern Ireland, when a patient is under 18 years it could come from a competent young patient, a person with parental responsibility or a court. Thus, consent from a person with parental responsibility may override a young person's refusal.

The power to override a competent refusal

W was 16 years old and living in a specialist adolescent residential unit under local authority care. Her physical condition due to anorexia nervosa deteriorated to the extent that the authority wished to transfer her to a specialist hospital for treatment. W refused, wanting instead to stay where she was and to cure herself when she decided it was right to do so. The local authority applied to court to be allowed to move W and for authorisation that she could be given medical treatment without her consent if necessary.

The judge in the Family Division of the High Court concluded that W was competent to make a decision to refuse treatment, but that the court could, in exercising its inherent jurisdiction, override a refusal of medical treatment by a competent young person if that was in her best interests. W appealed against the decision. Her condition deteriorated significantly, and the Court of Appeal made an emergency order enabling her to be taken to, and treated at, a specialist hospital notwithstanding her lack of consent. In delivering its judgment, the Court of Appeal held that the Family Division judge had been wrong to conclude that W was competent, because a desire not to be treated was symptomatic of anorexia nervosa. The Court also said that its inherent powers were theoretically limitless and that there was no doubt that it had power to override the refusal of a minor, whether over the age of 16 or under that age, but competent to make the decision.[25]

Thus, the law in England, Wales and Northern Ireland is clear that, in the last resort, medical treatment can be imposed upon competent minors who refuse it, if the overall intended effect is to benefit them. Doctors are often unhappy with such a view and the BMA hopes that all possibilities of a compromise solution would be explored first, including bringing in mediation or independent advocates to work out measures that the young person may feel able to accept, without having to compromise too far, lose face or resolve the case through the courts.

If the expected outcome of a proposed procedure is relatively insignificant for the patient, it is unlikely to be justifiable to override his or her wishes. When a competent young person refuses treatment, doctors should consider the impact of complying on his or her long-term chances of survival, recovery or improvement. For example, an informed refusal of a procedure with a purely cosmetic outcome, or repeated chemotherapy that has not led to significant improvement in the past, is highly influential. It is difficult to envisage a situation in which it is ethically acceptable to provide elective treatment when a competent, informed young person consistently refuses it. There has been no guidance from the courts on this matter because there has been no reported legal case dealing with refusal of elective or prophylactic intervention. This is likely to be because of the reluctance of doctors to impose non-essential treatment on unwilling competent patients.

On the other hand, when non-treatment threatens life, or postponement would lead to serious and permanent injury, the ethical arguments for providing treatment against a young person's wishes are stronger. Doctors must act within the law and balance the harm caused by violating a young person's autonomy against the harm caused by failing to treat. In cases of doubt, legal advice should be sought.

The case of *Re M* (see page 150) highlighted that the courts will sometimes override a young person's refusal of life-saving treatment. Despite this, it is not always the case that, even after seeking legal advice, the courts will be approached to override a young person's refusal. Legal advice was sought, for example, in the case of Hannah Jones, a 13-year-old girl who refused a heart transplant.[26] The case did not go to court, and so should not be seen as setting a legal precedent, but it did receive extensive media coverage in 2008.

Hannah Jones' refusal of a heart transplant

Hannah Jones was diagnosed with leukaemia at the age of 4 years and had been in and out of hospital for most of her childhood. As a result of treatment for leukaemia her heart was damaged and she was advised, in 2007, to undergo a heart transplant at the age of 12. Hannah refused to undergo a transplant.

As a consequence of her refusal, which her parents supported, Herefordshire Primary Care Trust (PCT) sought legal advice on whether to seek a decision from the High Court on whether a transplant would be in Hannah's best interests. The PCT decided not to pursue legal action after a member of the local child protection team held a private meeting with Hannah and advised the PCT that Hannah was competent to make a decision.

The PCT's chief executive subsequently wrote to Hannah's parents stating '[t]he PCT concluded that it was not appropriate to seek a court order to require you to permit Hannah to be admitted to hospital...Hannah appears to understand the serious nature of her condition. She demonstrated awareness that she could die. Treatment options were discussed and Hannah was able to express her clear views that she did not wish to go back on a pump or to go into hospital for cardiac treatment.'[27]

This case should not been seen as setting a precedent however. Had the PCT decided to pursue legal action and take the case to court, the outcome may have been very different. As it happened, a year later, following a change in her condition, Hannah consented to a heart transplant.

Scotland

This chapter only covers the examination and treatment of people under 16 years in Scotland. If a competent young person refuses treatment it is very likely that its administration would be unlawful, even if that treatment was necessary to save or prolong life. There has been just one reported legal case, in which the sheriff ruled that, once children of any age are judged to be competent they can consent to or refuse treatment. This follows the situation for competent adult patients (see Chapter 2). Despite there being grounds for maintaining some distinction between consent and refusal (see page 157) some commentators argue that the Scottish position is the more logical.[28] The Scottish courts have not, however, made a definitive ruling on this matter and any doctor faced with a refusal of treatment by a competent young person should seek legal advice.

Competent young person's refusal of treatment

In the only reported Scottish case to deal with refusal of treatment and the scope of the medical treatment provisions of the Age of Legal Capacity (Scotland) Act 1991, an application was made to Glasgow Sheriff Court in respect of a 15-year-old patient. The patient had symptoms of a psychotic illness. He would not consent to treatment and also refused to remain in hospital. The doctors believed that he was capable of understanding the nature and possible consequences of treatment and was therefore legally competent to make decisions on these matters. The doctors also believed that the right to consent carried with it the right to refuse, and that his refusal could not be overridden by his mother's consent. Treatment would therefore be lawful only if it fell within the scope of the Mental Health (Scotland) Act 1984, section 18 of which permitted detention on the approval of a sheriff. The doctors were reluctant to use the mental health legislation because of the stigma attached to a detention order.

The patient's mother was prepared to give consent to his treatment and detention in hospital. It was argued on her behalf that, since she was prepared to consent, the proposed order was unnecessary. The sheriff, however, took the view that the decision of a competent young person could not be overruled by a parent. He concluded that logic demanded that, when a young person was declared competent, the young person's decision took precedence over that of a parent. Furthermore, he considered that the Age of Legal Capacity (Scotland) Act covered refusal as well as consent to treatment.

In the circumstances, the sheriff granted the detention order with the observation that, despite the stigma, the patient's serious illness and its treatment were the paramount considerations.[29]

This judgment is taken by some to suggest that a competent young person's refusal may not be overridden by a parent or a court. In fact, the sheriff was able to avoid the issue of whether a court could override a competent refusal because there was an alternative way of dealing with the patient and treatment was given under mental health legislation. When doctors are faced with a competent young person's refusal of lifesaving treatment, legal advice is essential.

Advance decision making

In UK jurisdictions, where a young person's contemporaneous refusal of treatment may not be determinative, it follows that advance decisions refusing treatment (ADRTs) (see Chapter 3) made by young people cannot be legally binding on health professionals. This is supported by statute. For example, in England and Wales, although the majority of the Mental Capacity Act 2005 applies to 16- to 17-year-olds, they are specifically excluded in the legislation from making an ADRT to refuse medical treatment (for more detailed guidance on the Mental Capacity Act see Chapter 3).[30] Young people may wish to express their wishes in advance, however, so that these can be given proper consideration in decision making and assessment of their best interests.

Summary – consent and refusal by competent young people

- Young people are presumed to be competent from 16 years old, and deemed competent under 16 years if they have sufficient understanding and intelligence to enable them to understand fully what is proposed.
- Competent young people may give valid consent to medical treatment.
- Young people should be encouraged to involve their parents, but are entitled to confidentiality.
- Young people must be given the opportunity to have their views heard, even if their refusal of treatment is not determinative.
- Doctors should seek legal advice if a competent young person refuses essential medical treatment, although emergency treatment should not be delayed.

Consent and refusal by people with parental responsibility

Parental responsibility

Where a child lacks competence to make decisions, those with parental responsibility may make them on their behalf. Parental responsibility is a legal concept that consists of the rights, duties, powers, responsibilities and authority that most parents have in respect of their children. It includes the right to give consent to medical treatment, provided the treatment is in the interests of the child. Parental responsibility is afforded not only to parents, however, and not all parents have parental responsibility, despite arguably having equal moral rights to make decisions for their children where they have been equally involved in their care. It is possible that parents who do not have parental responsibility could use the Human Rights Act 1998 to claim a right to be involved in any important decisions about their child's life, including decisions about medical treatment.

Both of a child's parents have parental responsibility if they were married at the time of the child's conception or at some time thereafter. Neither parent loses parental responsibility if they divorce, and responsibility endures if the child is in care or custody. It is lost, however, if the child is adopted. If the parents have never married, the mother automatically has parental responsibility at birth and retains this, with the exception of adoption, unless it has exceptionally been removed by a court. Unmarried fathers registered on the child's birth certificate also have parental responsibility for children whose births were registered from 15 April 2002 in Northern Ireland, 1 December 2003 in England and Wales and 4 May 2006 in Scotland. For births registered prior to these dates unmarried fathers do not automatically have parental responsibility. A father may acquire it in various ways, including by entering into a parental responsibility agreement with the mother, or through a parental responsibility order made by a court. Where there is any reasonable doubt, enquiries should be made to ensure the father has parental responsibility before relying solely on his consent. Some same-sex couples will both hold parental responsibility for a child.[31] Where there is reasonable doubt about who is eligible to give consent on behalf of a child, further enquiries should be made.

A person other than a child's biological parents can acquire parental responsibility by being appointed as the child's guardian (an appointment that usually takes effect on the death of the parents) or by having a residence order made in his or her favour, in which case parental responsibility lasts for the duration of the order. A local authority acquires parental responsibility (shared with the parents) while a child is the subject of a care order. Detailed guidance on parental responsibility is available from the BMA website.[32]

Apart from people with parental responsibility, any person who has care of a child, for example a grandparent or childminder, may do 'what is reasonable in all the circumstances of the case for the purpose of safeguarding or promoting the child's welfare'.[33] In Scotland, the primacy of any known wishes of the parents in these situations has statutory force.[34] If a carer brings a child for treatment, steps should be taken to ascertain the parents' views, and if there is doubt about authority to proceed, doctors should seek legal advice.

In England, Wales and Northern Ireland, parental responsibilities may be exercised until a young person reaches 18 years. In Scotland, only the aspect of parental responsibility concerned with the parents giving 'guidance' to the young person endures until 18 years; the rest is lost when the young person reaches 16 years. Doctors who are treating people over 16 years in Scotland should refer to Chapter 2.

Consent from people with parental responsibility

People with parental responsibility are entitled to give consent on behalf of their children provided the decision is in the best interests of the child. Usually, parents are presumed to make the right decision about their young child's best interests, and most decision making is, rightly, left to children and parents with appropriate input from the clinical team. In cases of serious or chronic illness, parents may need time, respite facilities, possibly counselling, and certainly support from health professionals, but in most cases they are best placed to judge their young child's interests and decide about serious treatment.

There are limits on what parents are entitled to decide, however, and they cannot expect demands for inappropriate treatment for their children to be met.

Parents requesting treatment

C was a 16-month-old girl with spinal muscular atrophy, a progressive disease that causes severe emaciation and disability. She was dependent on intermittent positive pressure ventilation. Her doctors sought authority from the High Court to withdraw the ventilation, and not to reinstate it or resuscitate C if she developed further respiratory relapse. They maintained that further treatment would cause her increasing distress, could cause medical complications and could do little more than delay death without significant alleviation of suffering.

The judge described C's parents as highly responsible Orthodox Jews, who loved their daughter, but who were unable to 'bring themselves to face the inevitable future'. The parents' religious beliefs prevented them from standing aside and watching a person die when an intervention could prolong that life. The mother's affidavit, which the judge described as very moving, said that 'in such a case the person that stands by will subsequently be punished by God'.[35] The doctor's treatment plan of withholding resuscitation and ventilation and providing palliative care was endorsed by the judge to 'ease the suffering of this little girl to allow her life to end peacefully'.[36]

The courts do not always agree with medical advice, however, when decisions depend on the quality of life rather than on the ability of the treatment to achieve its physiological aim. In 2006 the High Court agreed with the parents of Baby MB against the unanimous view

of the medical team and rejected an application from the NHS Trust for the withdrawal
of ventilation.

> **Baby MB**
>
> MB was an 18-month-old with spinal muscular atrophy, type 1. The court heard that
> except for some movement of his eyes and possible slight, but barely perceptible,
> movement of his eyebrows, corners of his mouth, thumb, toes and feet, he could not
> move. He could not breathe unaided and required positive pressure ventilation via
> an invasive endotracheal tube and was fed through a gastrostomy tube. There was no
> hope of any improvement in his condition and his condition would inevitably deteriorate.
> The regular interventions required to keep MB alive caused him discomfort, distress
> and in some cases pain. Although unable to express this in any meaningful way,
> his heart rate would suddenly rise, his eyebrow would move slightly and sometimes
> he produced tears. The medical team, including 14 consultants, all agreed that to
> continue ventilation was contrary to MB's best interests.
>
> The parents argued that, despite his disability, MB was able to experience pleasure
> from his existence which outweighed the burdens and any discomfort or pain. They
> said he recognised them and his siblings and appeared to gain some pleasure from
> being with them and from watching certain DVDs or listening to music. In rejecting
> the NHS Trust's application to withdraw artificial ventilation, Mr Justice Holman said, 'I
> must proceed on the basis that M has age appropriate cognition, and does continue
> to have a relationship of value to him with his family, and does continue to gain other
> pleasures from touch, sight and sound.' He concluded: 'I do not consider that from
> one day to the next all the routine discomfort, distress and pain that the doctors
> describe . . . outweigh those benefits so that I can say that it is in his best interests
> that those benefits, and life itself, should immediately end. On the contrary, I positively
> consider that as his life does still have benefits, and is his life, it should be enabled
> to continue.'[37]

Willingness to continue with treatment may reflect the fact that a decision to stop
striving to maintain life is psychologically more difficult to make for children than adults
or that outcomes may be less predictable for children due to a small evidence base
from which to judge the likely outcome. The high profile case of Charlotte Wyatt serves
as a reminder of the difficulty of accurately assessing prognosis in seriously ill young
children and the importance of keeping treatment decisions constantly under review. The
developmental potential of children is also important and paediatricians will consider the
potential for progression from lacking competency to possessing competency as a factor
in decision making.

> **Charlotte Wyatt**
>
> Charlotte Wyatt was born in October 2003 at 26 weeks' gestation. By October 2004
> she had not left hospital. She had chronic respiratory and kidney problems coupled with
> profound brain damage that left her blind, deaf and incapable of voluntary movement
> or response. She demonstrably experienced pain but her doctors doubted that she was
> able to experience any pleasure. It was expected that during the winter of 2004 she
> would succumb to respiratory failure that would prove fatal and the unanimous view
> of her medical team was that, should this occur, it would not be in her best interests
> to provide artificial ventilation; Charlotte's parents disagreed. The High Court was told
> that a realistic likelihood of her surviving for 12 months was around 5 per cent. The
> judge concluded that further invasive and aggressive treatment would be intolerable
> to Charlotte and should not be provided.[38]
>
> In January 2005 Charlotte's condition had visibly improved. The medical team ac-
> knowledged that there had been some improvements but said this did not change
> her underlying condition. More investigations into Charlotte's condition and prognosis
> were planned and her parents asked that the earlier judgment be stayed while these

investigations took place. The judge refused.[39] A further application was made in March 2005 for the earlier judgment to be discharged. Charlotte had, unexpectedly, survived the winter and her condition had improved such that her oxygen requirement was 50 per cent compared to 100 per cent in October 2004, she was able to respond to loud noises and she was no longer under constant sedation. Nevertheless, the judge found that there had been no change in her underlying condition and again refused the application. Mr and Mrs Wyatt appealed against this decision but their appeal was dismissed.[40]

When the case was reviewed again in October 2005 further improvements had been made and Charlotte had been able to leave hospital and visit her home on a couple of occasions. The court rescinded the earlier declaration.[41] Between then and February 2006, however, her condition markedly deteriorated. She had developed an aggressive viral infection and the healthcare team felt it likely that within a few hours intubation and ventilation would be required to keep her alive, treatment they considered would cause her unnecessary pain and would not be in her best interests. The court agreed and issued a declaration that it would be lawful to withhold intubation and ventilation.[42] Again, against medical expectations, Charlotte's condition improved.

At the time of writing, the last posting on the www.savecharlotte.com website, in December 2007, stated that Charlotte's condition was continuing to improve.

Refusal by people with parental responsibility

Notwithstanding the importance of the parental role, if it appears that parents are following a course of action that is contrary to their child's interests, it may be necessary to seek a view from the courts, meanwhile providing only emergency treatment (see page 154) that is essential to preserve life or prevent serious deterioration. When asked to decide about treatment, the courts recognise their duty to protect children and have almost invariably said that serious treatment should be given against the wishes of parents where there is a good chance of it succeeding or providing significant benefit to the child. The courts are required, in their decision making, to have regard to the rights given force by the Human Rights Act and to have the child's welfare as the paramount consideration.[43]

Despite the courts' usual acceptance of the medical advice in these cases where there is a clear treatment route to follow, this is not always the case.

Parental refusal: the case of 'C'[44]

C had biliary atresia, a liver defect, and was not expected to live beyond $2^1/_2$ years without a liver transplant. He had undergone major invasive surgery when he was $3^1/_2$ weeks old which was unsuccessful and appeared to cause him severe pain and distress. Both of C's parents were health professionals experienced in caring for young sick children.

C's mother argued that she did not want to expose her son to further distress and believed that it would be best for him to be cared for by her abroad, where his father was working. C was referred to a hospital carrying out liver transplants, but when an organ became available, C and his mother were abroad and could not be contacted. When they returned to England, the mother continued to oppose the operation.

The local authority asked the court to exercise its inherent jurisdiction to order that a transplant would be in C's best interests, to give permission to perform the surgery and to order that C be returned to England for the surgery. The Court of Appeal disagreed, and held that it would not be in C's best interests for the court to override the parents, to give consent and require him to be returned to the jurisdiction for the operation.

C later had the transplant with his mother's consent.

In deciding the case, Lord Justice Waite stated that:

the greater the scope for genuine debate between one view and another [about the best interests of the child] the stronger will be the inclination of the court to be influenced by a reflection that in the last analysis the best interests of every child include an expectation that difficult decisions affecting the length and quality of its life will be taken for it by the parent to whom its care has been entrusted by nature.[45]

The clinical evidence was unchallenged: C was very likely to die before he was 3 years old without a transplant and his doctors were optimistic that a transplant would give C many years of life and normal growth and development. C's welfare had to be the determining factor in the court's decision, but the judges recognised that his welfare depended on his mother who would be expected to care for him, probably alone because the father was abroad, through surgery and for many years afterwards. The court was apparently influenced by the parents being health professionals and the practical difficulties of ensuring compliance, particularly since the family was abroad. The decision may have been very different in different social circumstances, and the court's decision is controversial. The courts may not follow this precedent in cases that do not involve these particular circumstances. Doctors should seek legal advice if they are concerned about the willingness of parents to provide essential care following invasive procedures.

Disagreements between people with parental responsibility

Generally, the law requires doctors to have consent from only one person in order lawfully to provide treatment. In practice, however, parents sometimes disagree and doctors are reluctant to override a parent's strongly held views, particularly when the benefits and burdens of the treatment are finely balanced and it is not clear what is best for the child. Disputes between parents can be difficult for everybody involved in the child's care. Health professionals need to be able to distinguish between the genuine concern of the dissenting parent and an objection that is based on grounds other than the child's welfare, such as a marital dispute. Discussion aimed at reaching consensus should be attempted. If this fails, a decision must be made by the clinician in charge whether to go ahead despite the disagreement. The onus is then on the parent who refuses treatment to take steps to stop it. If the dispute is over an irreversible, controversial, elective procedure, for example immunisation where it is known one parent disagrees, or male infant circumcision for religious purposes (see pages 170–171), doctors must not proceed without the authority of a court.[46]

A common enquiry to the BMA concerns parents who do not communicate with each other but both want to be involved in their child's healthcare. For example, GPs are frequently asked to tell the parent with whom the child is not resident when the other parent brings the child to the surgery. Such situations are dealt with in Chapter 6 (pages 258–259).

Summary – consent and refusal by people with parental responsibility

Agreement between everybody who is involved in decision making is the aim. People with parental responsibility:

- are entitled to give consent to medical treatment on behalf of their child
- may refuse medical treatment, when this is consistent with their child's best interests
- may not insist that doctors provide treatment contrary to their clinical judgement.

The courts

In England, Wales and Northern Ireland, the courts have the power to authorise treatment on behalf of a person aged under 18 years. This power endures even if the young person is competent to make decisions for himself or herself. Thus, the courts are an ultimate arbiter because authorisation from a court can override a child's refusal and parents' refusal of a particular treatment if there is evidence that it would provide significant benefit. The courts cannot, however, require doctors to treat contrary to their professional judgement.

In Scotland, the courts have the same powers to authorise treatment on behalf of people aged under 16 years when the child is not competent to give valid consent for himself or herself. It is unclear whether a Scottish court may override the decision of a child if the medical practitioner believes the child is competent, although it is thought that this is unlikely (see page 159). Again, the courts cannot compel doctors to treat contrary to their professional judgement.

Court involvement is necessary in only a minority of cases; most decisions are of the type doctors and families are entitled to make and usually agreement is reached by the child, the people with parental responsibility, and the healthcare team. Their goal is the same – to benefit the child – and in the vast majority of cases it is possible to agree on the best route to achieve this. If, however, agreement cannot be reached in a reasonable period of time, which will depend on the nature and likely course of the patient's condition, lawyers may advise that it is necessary to seek a court order without delay. Court orders can be obtained swiftly from a judge over the phone. The courts have also indicated that interventions of certain types, for example decisions about sterilisation, organ donation and, if the parents disagree, immunisation and religious circumcision, must be referred to court. Detailed advice about the situations in which the courts may become involved is given in the BMA's *Consent, rights and choices in health care for children and young people*.[47] Doctors must take legal advice if there may be a need to involve the courts. Where a court is involved, various bodies look after the interests of the child by working with families and advising the courts on what it considers to be in the child's best interests.[48]

Going to court can be distressing for those concerned and it is essential that ongoing support is provided for the child, the parents, other relatives and carers, and the healthcare team. There are great benefits, however, in a legal system that can give rulings very quickly when necessary. The law can provide a protective role for both patients and the healthcare team who treat them and where there is disagreement that cannot be resolved.

Health professionals should not be deterred from seeking a legal ruling because of the risk of appearing confrontational; legal review can be beneficial for all parties. The risk of appearing confrontational is reduced if doctors, when referring to a court, explain that there is an apparently unresolvable and serious disagreement about what would be in the child's best interests, so the fairest way of deciding is to ask an impartial court of law to adjudicate. It is also important to remember that doctors have been criticised in the past for failing to seek advice from the courts where there is disagreement about the best course of action (see the case of *Glass v United Kingdom* below). Where a judge is asked to make a declaration, it is important that all parties are kept informed of developments and are given information about how their views can be represented.

The case of *Glass v United Kingdom* highlights the need sometimes to involve the courts as soon as possible when there is a dispute. Where possible the court should be approached early where disagreement is foreseeable, rather than at the point the situation becomes an emergency. Other than in an emergency situation, treatment must not be provided for a child or young person who lacks competency without the consent of someone with parental responsibility or the court.

Glass v United Kingdom

In March 2004, the European Court of Human Rights (ECtHR) awarded Carol Glass and her son David compensation after doctors treated David contrary to his mother's wishes, without a court order.

Born in 1986, David Glass was severely mentally and physically disabled, requiring 24-hour care. In July 1998 after surgery to alleviate an upper respiratory tract obstruction, David became critically ill and was put on a ventilator. Doctors thought he was dying. His condition improved briefly and he returned home only to be readmitted a few days later when doctors discussed the option of morphine to alleviate his distress. His mother refused, believing it would compromise his chance of recovery. She also made clear that she wanted David resuscitated if his heart stopped. Relations between the family and the healthcare team had completely broken down, to the extent that some members of the family were later prosecuted for physically attacking hospital staff. Although the doctor managing David's care noted the possible need for a court order in such cases of total disagreement, no order was sought and the morphine was provided without consent.

The Glass family argued that, when the dispute arose, the hospital should have involved the courts to clarify whether, despite his mother's objections, the treatment proposed was in David's best interests and that the doctors were wrong in believing the urgency of the case made that unnecessary. Although dismissed by UK Courts, the ECtHR held that David's Article 8 right to privacy under the Human Rights Act, and in particular his right to physical integrity, had been breached. The Court said it was clear that there was a dispute over treatment before the situation reached crisis point and the UK courts should have been used to settle the dispute before an emergency situation arose.[49]

Summary – the courts

- When agreement cannot be reached about treatment, doctors should approach their lawyers for advice.
- The courts may become involved and make a decision about treatment.
- The courts cannot require doctors to provide treatment contrary to their professional judgement.
- Where disagreement is foreseeable, an early approach to the court is advisable.

Refusal of blood products by Jehovah's Witnesses

As explained in Chapter 2, Jehovah's Witnesses have a conscientiously held religious opposition to the use of blood products for themselves. Parents often hold the same view regarding blood products in the medical treatment of their children. It is essential that doctors make every effort to accommodate beliefs rather than resorting to the most obvious medical option when that is contrary to the patient's or parents' wish, or looking to the courts as a first resort. Nevertheless, when discussion, negotiation and consideration of other options fail to resolve the situation and a child's life is at risk, it is likely that the courts will be involved. Courts have indicated that the administration of blood transfusions to Jehovah's Witness children against the wishes of their parents should not be carried out without the approval of a court,[50] although in an emergency doctors are unlikely to be criticised for intervening if this is the only option to save a child or young person's life or to prevent serious deterioration in their health.

Clearly, whenever time allows, attempts should be made to negotiate with the family to try to find an acceptable solution. Invariably, family members are anxious to save the child's life if this can be done in a way that does not contravene their beliefs. Sometimes this may be possible by referral to a specialist centre where techniques such as bloodless surgery are practised (see Chapter 2, pages 78–79).

When faced with a refusal of blood products by or on behalf of a young patient, the following must be borne in mind.

- It is important that health professionals should ensure that the situation is truly life-threatening, or seriously deleterious to health, and that there are no other feasible alternatives to the use of blood.
- The child and the parents should be given an opportunity to put forward their views and have these considered.
- The local hospital liaison committee for Jehovah's Witnesses, which may be able to advise on possible alternatives, can be contacted as long as the family or the competent young person agrees.
- If health professionals involved in the case consider blood products to be the only solution they can offer to save the life of the child, the patient or the patient's family may request that treatment be transferred to another facility where bloodless treatment is practised; such wishes should be accommodated where possible.
- When there is no alternative, legal advice should be sought and it may be necessary for the matter to be considered by a court.

Whenever time allows, there should be careful discussion with the young person and the family to ensure that the situation is fully understood. It is advisable for health professionals to discuss the implications with the young person separately to ensure that the young person's decision has been reached without any pressure.

As with all refusals of treatment, if patients are competent, informed and sure of their decision to refuse blood, there are significant ethical arguments for respecting that decision. The imperative to comply with refusal by parents is necessarily weaker than when children themselves make informed decisions; treatment may be given with consent from a competent young person even if the parents refuse. Despite these ethical arguments, the following case highlights that even with a competent young person's refusal, and the young person's parents' refusal, a court may still authorise treatment.

Overriding a refusal of a blood transfusion

P was a 16-year-old Jehovah's Witness with an inherited condition called hypermobility syndrome, the symptoms of which include a tendency to bleed because of the fragility of the patient's blood vessels. The patient was admitted to hospital with what appeared to be a ruptured aorta and both the patient and his parents expressed their objection to any treatment using blood or blood products. The doctors acceded to these views because the operation that would be necessary to cure what was then a suspected ruptured aorta was dangerous and likely to be unsuccessful; a blood transfusion was therefore considered futile. The crisis passed but the problem was unresolved. The doctors envisaged that a similar crisis may occur in which the use of blood products could become necessary to save P's life. The hospital asked the court to authorise the use of blood products, despite P's objections, should this become necessary.

There was no suggestion in the judgment that P lacked competency to make the decision or that he was not fully aware of the consequences of his decision. Mr Justice Johnson said there were 'weighty and compelling reasons' not to make the order but, nonetheless, looking at P's best interests in the widest sense 'medical, religious, social, whatever they be', P's 'best interests' in those widest senses will be met if I make an order in the terms sought by the NHS Trust with the addition of . . . 'unless no other form of treatment is available'.[51]

Mr Justice Johnson was mindful of the court's responsibility to ensure so far as it can that children survive to adulthood. He referred to a statement by Nolan LJ in *Re W* that: 'In general terms the present state of the law is that an individual who has reached the age of 18 is free to do with his life what he wishes, but it is the duty of the court to ensure so far as it can that children survive to attain that age.'[52]

Interestingly, the judgment in *Re P* makes no reference to the Human Rights Act although it must be assumed that the court believed that the decision was compliant with that legislation. These cases are always controversial and, in similar cases, legal advice should be sought.

Providing treatment against a child or young person's wishes

Just because consent from a child's parents, or from a court, makes providing treatment lawful does not mean that it has to be given. Doctors must look at whether the harms associated with imposing treatment on a patient who refuses, whether competently or not, should play a part in the decision about proceeding. How critical the treatment is, whether alternative, less invasive treatments are available, and whether it is possible to allow time for further discussion with the patient, are all factors to be weighed. As much time as is practicable should be taken for discussion, and treatment delayed if that is possible without jeopardising its likely success.

Once a decision has been made that it is lawful and ethically acceptable to override a refusal of treatment, in principle there cannot be an absolute prohibition on the use of force to carry it out. However, 'merely because treatment is in a competent patient's best interests does not mean the use of force is'.[53] Doctors must look at the patient's overall interests, and how imposing treatment may impact on human rights. For example, the European Court of Human Rights has held that force feeding a patient may amount to degrading treatment,[54] although doctors must consider whether this is a proportionate interference with rights given the expected benefits. Promoting the child's welfare in the broadest sense is the overarching consideration.

Parents can have an important role in persuading their children to cooperate with treatment, although, if the family is dysfunctional, for example if the relationship is abusive, the views of parents may not influence the child or could unduly influence the child. If attempts to persuade a young person fail, but it is judged to be in his or her best interests to proceed, rarely the only option may be to use restraint or detention.

Using restraint

In addition to being difficult to achieve in practice, imposing treatment on young people when they refuse could damage the young person's current and future relationships with healthcare providers and undermine trust in the medical profession. It is important for young people to understand that restraint of any form in order to provide treatment is used only as a matter of last resort and not until other options for treatment have been explained, discussed with the team, and explored. The child and the family must be offered continual support and information throughout the period of treatment.

Members of the health team benefit from being given an opportunity to express their views and to participate in decision making, although ultimate responsibility rests with the clinician in charge of care. All staff require support, and must not be asked to be involved in restraining a child without proper training. This should include respect for the child or young person, not verbal intimidation or making inappropriate threats or comments.

If, after due process, spending as much time as is practicable, it is impossible to persuade a child to cooperate with essential treatment, the clinician in charge of the patient's care may decide that restraint is appropriate.[55] The following points are relevant to any action taken.

- Restraint should be used only when it is necessary to give essential treatment or to prevent a child from significantly injuring himself or herself or others and should be the minimum necessary to achieve that aim.
- The effect should be to provide an overall benefit to the child and in some cases the harms associated with the use of restraint may outweigh the benefits expected from treatment.
- Restraint is an act of care and control, not punishment.
- Unless life-prolonging or other crucial treatment is immediately necessary, legal advice should be sought when treatment involves restraint or detention to override the views of a competent young person, even if the law allows doctors to proceed on the basis of parental consent.
- All steps should be taken to anticipate the need for restraint and to prepare the child, his or her family, and staff.
- Wherever possible, the members of the healthcare team involved should have an established relationship with the child and should explain what is being done and why.
- Treatment plans should include safeguards to ensure that restraint is the minimum necessary, that it is for the minimum period necessary to achieve the clinical aim, and that both the child and the parents have been informed what will happen and why restraint is necessary.
- Restraint should usually be used only in the presence of other staff, who can act as assistants and witnesses.
- Any use of restraint should be recorded in the medical records. These issues are an appropriate subject for clinical audit and review by external agencies.

Detaining children

Detaining children for the purpose of providing medical treatment raises serious legal issues. Legal advice is essential before children are detained outwith the provisions of mental health legislation, and court approval will be necessary. A court asked to rule on such an issue is required to have regard to the young person's rights under the Human Rights Act 1998, and whether, in the circumstances, detention is compatible with these. For example, the right not to be subjected to inhuman or degrading treatment (Article 3), the right to liberty and security (Article 5) and the right to a fair hearing (Article 6).

Cultural practices

Male circumcision

Male circumcision in cases where there is a clear clinical need is not normally controversial. The circumcision of male babies and children, when there is no clinical indication, is a controversial area. Parents ask for their children to be circumcised for a range of reasons, including their religion, to incorporate a child into a community or so that sons are like their fathers. There is a spectrum of views within the BMA's membership about whether non-therapeutic male circumcision is a beneficial, neutral or harmful procedure or whether it is superfluous, and whether it should ever be carried out on a child who is not capable of deciding for himself. The medical harms or benefits have not been unequivocally proven except to the extent that there are clear risks of harm if the procedure is performed inexpertly. The BMA has no policy on whether male circumcision is acceptable or not. Indeed, it would be difficult to formulate a policy in the absence of unambiguously clear and consistent medical data on the implications of the intervention. Detailed advice is available in a BMA guidance note.[56]

General advice about assessment of best interests is given on pages 152–153. In relation to non-therapeutic male circumcision, the BMA identifies the following factors as being potentially relevant:

- where appropriate, the patient's own ascertainable wishes, feelings and values
- the patient's ability to understand what is proposed and weigh up the alternatives
- the patient's potential to participate in the decision, if provided with additional support or explanations
- the patient's physical and emotional needs
- the risk of harm or suffering for the patient
- the views of parents and family
- the implications for the family of performing, or not performing, the procedure
- relevant information about the patient's religious or cultural background
- the prioritising of options that maximise the patient's future opportunities and choices.

Circumcision – best interests

J was a 5-year-old boy who lived with his mother, a non-practising Christian. His father, a non-practising Muslim, wanted him to be circumcised. Asked to decide whether J should be circumcised, the Court of Appeal considered all the factors relevant to J's upbringing and concluded that J should not be circumcised because of three key facts.

- He was not, and was not likely to be, brought up in the Muslim religion.
- He was not likely to have such a degree of involvement with Muslims as to justify circumcising him for social reasons.
- As a result of these factors, the 'small but definite medical and psychological risks' of circumcision outweighed the benefits of the procedure.[57]

It is essential that doctors should perform male circumcision only where this is demonstrably in the best interests of the child. The responsibility to demonstrate that non-therapeutic circumcision is in a particular child's best interests falls to his parents. The BMA is generally very supportive of allowing parents to make choices on behalf of their children, and believes that neither society nor doctors should interfere unjustifiably in the relationship between parents and their children. It is clear from the list of factors that are relevant to a child's best interests, however, that parental preference alone is not sufficient justification for performing a surgical procedure on a child.

When there is agreement that non-therapeutic circumcision is in a child's best interests, consent may come from competent children or people with parental responsibility. The BMA and the GMC[58] have long recommended that consent for non-therapeutic circumcision should be sought from both parents. Although parents who have parental responsibility are usually allowed to take decisions for their children alone, non-therapeutic circumcision has been described by the courts as an important and irreversible decision that should not be taken against the wishes of a parent.[59] It follows that, when a child has two parents with parental responsibility, doctors considering circumcising the child must satisfy themselves, where possible, that both have given valid consent. If a child presents with only one parent, the doctor must make every effort to contact the other parent in order to seek consent. If parents disagree about having their child circumcised, the parent seeking circumcision could seek a court order authorising the procedure, which would make it lawful, although doctors are advised to consider carefully whether circumcising against the wishes of one parent would be in the child's best interests. When a child has only one parent, obviously that person can decide.

All children who are capable of expressing a view should be involved in decisions about their care and have their wishes taken into account. The BMA cannot envisage a situation in which it is ethically acceptable to circumcise a competent, informed young person who refuses the procedure. When children cannot decide for themselves, their parents usually choose for them. Although they usually coincide, this chapter explains that the interests of the child and those of the parents are not always synonymous. There are, therefore, limits on parents' rights to choose and parents are not entitled to demand medical procedures contrary to their child's best interests.

As with all medical procedures, doctors must act in accordance with good clinical practice, have the necessary skills to perform the procedure, ensure conditions are hygienic and provide adequate pain control and aftercare.[60]

Summary – male circumcision

- The welfare of child patients is paramount and doctors must act in the child's best interests.
- Children who are able to express views about circumcision should be involved in the decision-making process.
- Both parents must give consent for non-therapeutic circumcision, where possible.
- When people with parental responsibility for a child disagree about whether he should be circumcised, doctors should not circumcise the child without the leave of a court.
- As with all medical procedures, doctors must act in accordance with good clinical practice, have the necessary skills to perform the procedure, ensure conditions are hygienic and provide adequate pain control and aftercare.
- Doctors must make accurate, contemporaneous notes of discussions, consent, the procedure and its aftercare.

Female genital mutilation

Female genital mutilation is a collective term used for a range of practices involving the removal or alteration of parts of healthy female genitalia. It is carried out by communities in Africa, South-East Asia and the Middle East, and by immigrants from those areas, for reasons ranging from hygiene and control to enhancement of male sexual pleasure. It involves suffering and mutilation and can give rise to very serious health risks. Female genital mutilation is illegal in the UK – in England, Wales and Northern Ireland under the Female Genital Mutilation Act 2003 and in Scotland under the Prohibition of Female Genital Mutilation Act 2005. Both Acts also make it a criminal offence, in certain circumstances, to carry out female genital mutilation abroad, and to aid, abet, counsel or procure the carrying out of female genital mutilation abroad, including in countries where the practice is legal.

There is a pressing need to raise awareness about the health and legal issues, and about the services and sources of information that are available among communities that practise female genital mutilation. There are a small number of specialist clinics offering reversal procedures, and doctors should encourage women who have been mutilated to consider this option before they become pregnant. Doctors must also be alert to the possibility that girls may be at risk of genital mutilation.

If it becomes apparent that a girl is at risk of female genital mutilation, either in the UK or abroad, the GP or other doctor caring for her, for example the community paediatrician, must ensure that there is discussion with the family about the health and legal issues. This may also involve counsellors, supportive local community groups or other clinicians with experience of working with communities that have a tradition of female genital mutilation. Doctors must ensure that their approach is sensitive to the beliefs and culture of the family, while remembering that female genital mutilation is illegal in the UK and that participation by any person, including a doctor, is a criminal offence. The aim is to find effective mechanisms for ensuring the protection of the child in a way that promotes her overall welfare. Doctors are unlikely to be able to initiate all of this work as individuals and should consider seeking help from social services, counsellors and other health professionals. In initial enquiries to seek general help, advice and information, it is unlikely to be necessary to identify the child or family.

Female genital mutilation is considered as a form of child abuse in the UK; it is illegal, performed on a child who is unable to resist, medically unnecessary and harmful, extremely painful and poses severe health risks. Members of communities that practise female genital mutilation do so, however, with the best intentions for the future welfare of their child and do not intend it as an act of abuse. When parents cannot be persuaded that their daughter should not be subjected to female genital mutilation, doctors will have to find sensitive ways to explain that steps may be taken to prevent the child from being mutilated. It is usually appropriate for doctors to contact social services, on public interest grounds, when they believe a girl is at risk of female genital mutilation, for example when a mother becomes pregnant again in a family whose existing daughters have been mutilated in infancy.

Parents' rights to control information about their young children may be overridden when this is necessary to protect the child from serious harm, although whenever possible, their permission for disclosure of information to social services, or another appropriate agency, should be sought. In judging how to broach the issue with parents, doctors must bear in mind the likely attitude of the parents in such circumstances and the risk that the child may simply disappear by being concealed within the community or sent to relatives abroad. This can be extremely difficult and doctors must take great care to ensure that their reactions are supportive of the child's overall welfare wherever possible.

Guidance offering advice for doctors caring for women who have undergone female genital mutilation, and how to protect girls at risk of the procedure, is published by the BMA.[61] Multi-agency guidance is produced by the Foreign and Commonwealth Office.[62]

Summary – female genital mutilation

- Female genital mutilation is illegal in the UK.
- In certain circumstances, it is a criminal offence to carry out female genital mutilation abroad, and to aid, abet, counsel or procure the carrying out of female genital mutilation abroad, including in countries where the practice is legal.
- Doctors must be alert to the possibility that girls may be at risk of genital mutilation.
- If it becomes apparent that a girl is at risk of female genital mutilation doctors must ensure that there is discussion with the family about the health and legal issues.
- Doctors must ensure that their approach is sensitive to the beliefs and culture of the family, while remembering that female genital mutilation is illegal in the UK and that participation by any person, including a doctor, is a criminal offence.
- It is usually appropriate for doctors to contact social services when they believe a girl is at risk of female genital mutilation.

Conjoined twins

Infants born with severe disabilities have the right to expect care and treatment appropriate to their needs. Conjoined twins are one example of children about whom difficult decisions may need to be made. Although some twins remain conjoined and survive well into adulthood, others are separated. Sometimes the separation of twins means that one will inevitably die. Conjoined twins raise complex dilemmas, involving themes of autonomy and interdependent interests. Usually, decisions about how to manage the twins' medical needs are made by the parents and medical team together. In 2000, however, a case arose in which parents and medical staff were faced with an exceptionally difficult decision that required the court to intervene.

Conjoined twins

Jodie and Mary were conjoined twins. They were joined at the lower abdomen and each had her own brain, heart, lungs, other vital organs and limbs. Mary was considerably weaker than Jodie, and her brain was described as having only primitive function. Her heart and lungs were not sufficiently strong to sustain her life if she was separated from Jodie. Had she been born a singleton, she would have died shortly after birth.

Although surgery would be extremely complex, the twins' doctors were of the opinion that it would be possible to separate them, but that separation would kill the weaker twin, Mary, within minutes. If the operation did not take place, both were expected to die within 3–6 months because Jodie's heart would eventually fail. If they were separated, Jodie would still need extensive medical care and treatment, but was expected to have a good length and quality of life.

The parents, however, said that they could not consent to separation if this would result in Mary's death. The twins were equally precious to their parents, who felt that it was 'not God's will' for them or anyone to choose death for one. They could not agree to kill one even to save the other.

The High Court issued a declaration that separating the twins would be lawful. Although the parents appealed, the High Court's decision was upheld by the Court of Appeal and the twins were separated. Mary died shortly after being separated from Jodie.[63]

In the case of conjoined twins Jodie and Mary, the Court of Appeal concluded that the twins' interests were best served by giving the chance of life to the stronger twin, Jodie, even if that had to be at the cost of the life of the weaker twin, Mary. The least detrimental choice was to separate the twins. It then looked to whether it was possible to achieve this in a lawful way, because Mary was a human being and separating the twins involved a positive act of killing her. The Court said that the reality was that Mary was killing Jodie. That provided the legal justification for the doctors coming to Jodie's defence and removing the threat of fatal harm to her presented by Mary. In these very exceptional circumstances, 'necessity' to act made intervention by the doctors lawful.

It was a case that the Court found extremely difficult. Aside from being legally complex, one of the judges described it as 'difficult because of the scale of the tragedy for the parents and the twins, difficult for the seemingly irreconcilable conflicts of moral and ethical values'.[64]

The Court noted that, although there were those who believed most sincerely that it would be an immoral act to save Jodie if this would involve ending Mary's life prematurely, there were also those who believed, with equal sincerity, that it would be immoral not to save Jodie if there were a good prospect that she could live a happy, fulfilled life if the operation was performed. Subsequent commentators have argued that it was wrong to deprive parents of their usual decision-making authority in a case that was so finely balanced.[65]

The Court went to great lengths to make clear that the case did not set a precedent for intentional killing in order to preserve the life of another. One of the judges, Lord Justice Ward, in emphasising the uniqueness of the case, said:

> Lest it be thought that this decision could become authority for wider propositions, such as that a doctor, once he has determined that a patient cannot survive, can kill the patient, it is important to restate the unique circumstances for which this case is authority. They are that it must be impossible to preserve the life of X without bringing about the death of Y, that Y by his or her very continued existence will inevitably bring about the death of X within a short period of time, and that X is capable of living an independent life but Y is incapable under any circumstances, including all forms of medical intervention, of viable independent existence.[66]

The BMA generally believes that parents are the best decision makers for their young children, but it also acknowledges that there are occasions on which the law should intervene to determine what is in children's best interests. Any doctor caring for conjoined twins and considering their separation must consider:

- the likely clinical outcome for both twins, with and without intervention
- the legal and moral rights of both twins
- the twins' best interests
- the views of the parents.

Where these factors lead to the conclusion that separating the twins would be the best course of action, and it is unlikely, or impossible, that both twins could survive the separation, legal advice is essential.

Child protection

In child protection cases, a doctor's primary responsibility is to the well-being of the child or children concerned. Where a child is at risk of significant harm, the interests of the child override those of parents or carers. It is imperative that doctors are aware of their responsibilities in protecting children. Doctors working with children and young people should be able to identify abuse and neglect,[67] and know how to respond appropriately. The BMA has produced guidance on child protection which is available via the BMA website;[68] as has the Royal College of General Practitioners (RCGP)[69] and the Royal College of Paediatrics and Child Health (RCPCH).[70] At the time of writing the GMC was in the process of developing new guidance for doctors working in child protection.

Victoria Climbié

Eight-year-old Victoria Climbié died as a result of 'the worst case of child abuse and neglect' the paediatric consultant responsible for her care immediately before she died had ever seen.[71] This brief outline of her case focuses on Victoria's contact with professionals during her time in England.

Victoria was born in the Ivory Coast in 1991 and went to live with her aunt in England in April 1999. It was not uncommon for children born in the Ivory Coast to be entrusted to relatives living in Europe who could offer improved financial and educational opportunities for them.

Shortly after their arrival in England, Victoria and her aunt were seen by a number of social services staff. No efforts were made either by the aunt or social services to enrol Victoria in any educational or day care activity. Victoria was registered with a GP in June 1999. She was seen by the practice nurse, who did not physically examine her because she was reported not to have any current health problems or complaints. Shortly afterwards, a neighbour noticed what may have been early signs of physical harm including a scar on her cheek. A few days later the neighbour made the first of two anonymous telephone calls to social services reporting her concerns about the way Victoria's aunt treated her.

In July 1999, Victoria and her aunt joined the aunt's new boyfriend in a one-roomed flat where Victoria had no bed and spent the nights in the bathroom. The signs of physical abuse appeared to increase considerably soon after the move. Later that month, Victoria's childminder was worried and took her to hospital. The accident and emergency doctor who saw Victoria thought that there was a strong possibility that her injuries were non-accidental and referred her to a paediatric registrar. The registrar found a large number of injuries to Victoria's body and agreed that some may have been non-accidental. She was admitted overnight, and the police and social services were informed. She left the following day with her aunt.

Just over a week later, Victoria was admitted to a second hospital with a severe scald. She stayed on the paediatric ward for 13 nights, during which time a number of the clinical staff noticed signs of serious deliberate physical harm. When Victoria's aunt and her boyfriend visited, Victoria appeared frightened of them. Her discharge to the care of her aunt was agreed by a police constable and social worker who visited Victoria in hospital. After her discharge, Victoria's contact with the outside world during the remaining 7 months of her life was limited and sporadic. Professionals saw her on only four occasions during this period, twice when her social worker made a prearranged visit and twice when she was taken to the social services office. The social workers visited and noticed nothing untoward. That Victoria was not attending school was commented on but not pursued. The aunt's application for rehousing was turned down because Victoria was not considered to be 'at risk of serious harm'. She was, however, advised to move out when she told the social worker that her boyfriend was sexually harming Victoria. They were due to move in with a friend, but this did not materialise and by the end of the day they were back in the boyfriend's flat. The following day Victoria's aunt retracted the allegations to a different social worker, who advised that they must not return to the boyfriend's flat while the matter was being investigated. They continued to live there, however, until Victoria's death 4 months later. She had no further contact with professionals of any kind until she was admitted to hospital on the night before her death.

A post-mortem examination revealed death by hypothermia, which had arisen in the context of malnourishment, a damp environment and restricted movement. The pathologist found 128 separate injuries on Victoria's body showing that she had been beaten by sharp and blunt instruments. Marks on her wrists and ankles showed that her arms and legs had been tied together. The pathologist said that it was the worst case of deliberate harm to a child that he had ever seen.[72]

Lord Laming's report into the death of Victoria Climbié after extensive abuse by carers stated that protecting Victoria would have 'required nothing more than basic good practice being put into operation'.[73] The Inquiry identified gross system failures, with individuals and agencies neglecting to take responsibility to act to protect Victoria from the horrific abuse she suffered. The Inquiry sought to understand the failings that led to Victoria's death, and identify improvements at national and local level. There were failings in many areas of Victoria's care. In her contact with health professionals, it was clear from the evidence to the Inquiry that information was known about Victoria but not documented in health records, or was recorded but not shared. Investigations and examinations were deferred, and sometimes erroneously assumed to have been carried out by somebody else. Necessary action was identified but not acted upon. Of the Inquiry's 108 recommendations, 27 related specifically to healthcare. They focused on improving communication, ensuring communication flow, ensuring that concerns are acted upon, record keeping and attributing clear responsibility for child protection to a single hospital consultant. The Inquiry also recommended that no child about whom there are child protection concerns should be discharged from hospital without the permission of the consultant in charge or other suitable senior doctor. There must be a documented plan for the future care of the child and an identified GP.

The report's recommendations formed the basis of changes in national policy and were reflected in the England and Wales Children Act 2004. Despite the impetus for change following Lord Laming's report into the death of Victoria Climbié, Lord Laming was called upon to carry out a further review following the death of another child – Baby P.

Baby P

Baby P was 17 months old when he died on 3 August 2007. The mother of Baby P, her partner and the lodger living in the house were found guilty of causing or allowing his death.

During his life, Baby P had contact with health professionals numerous times as a result of non-accidental injuries, resulting in hospital admissions. He was on Haringey Council's child protection register and was the subject of a multi-agency child protection plan involving social services, health services and the police. His mother was arrested twice as a result of Baby P's injuries.

Despite this, his post-mortem examination revealed 22 injuries, including a broken back and ribs, a forceful knocking out of a tooth, and the removal of a toe and finger nail.[74]

In the sentencing remarks it was noted that 'health professionals who saw Peter shortly before he died seem at the least to have missed the import of the injuries to him'.[75]

The GMC subsequently suspended a GP who had seen Baby P 14 times before his death. A consultant paediatrician who had allegedly failed to fully examine Baby P when he was brought in for a developmental check relinquished her registration.

The second Lord Laming report, in response to the Baby P case, was published in March 2009.[76] Lord Laming's main criticism was that reforms proposed by the report into the death of Victoria Climbié had not been implemented in practice. Lord Laming was also very critical of the complicated paperwork and tick-box assessment carried out by social services. He identified a disproportionate focus on meeting targets rather than managing risks. Recommendations relevant to health include the following.

• Putting in place the systems and training so that staff in accident and emergency departments are able to tell if a child has recently presented at any accident and emergency department and if a child is the subject of a Child Protection Plan. If there is any cause for concern, staff must act accordingly, contacting other professionals, conducting further medical examinations of the child as appropriate and necessary, and ensuring no child is discharged while concerns for their safety or well being remain.

- All adult mental health and adult drug and alcohol services should have well-understood referral processes which prioritise the protection and well-being of children. These should include automatic referral where domestic violence or drug or alcohol abuse may put a child at risk of abuse or neglect.

- The Department of Health should promote the statutory duty of all GP providers to comply with child protection legislation and to ensure that all individual GPs have the necessary skills and training to carry out their duties. They should also take further steps to raise the profile and level of expertise for child protection within GP practices, for example by working with the Department for Children, Schools and Families to support joint training opportunities for GPs and children's social workers, and through the new practice accreditation scheme being developed by the Royal College of General Practitioners.

The Care Quality Commission also published a review of the Baby P case[77] focused on the health sectors involvement in the case. The review highlighted problems such as a lack of communication, shortage of staff, lack of training, absence of child protection supervision, lack of awareness of child protection procedures and inadequate governance.[78]

As a result of these cases there has been renewed emphasis on child protection training for health professionals as well as for social workers. Doctors need to be aware of the way the inquiries' recommendations are being implemented and ensure they are following best practice guidelines, including those from the health departments[79] and GMC.[80]

Doctors must try to work positively with families to enhance coping and parenting skills. In some cases, however, it is not possible to do this and also ensure the safety of children. A child or young person who comes to a doctor with a suspicious injury or other evidence of abuse or neglect should be the central focus of the doctor's concern, not the family, although the doctor must also bear in mind the safety of others who may be at risk, for example, the child's siblings. Some doctors say they feel a divided loyalty when they have as patients other members of the family, including the alleged abuser, but adults responsible for providing care have a duty to protect vulnerable people. Health professionals do not have statutory powers to intervene in family life, so, if intervention is necessary, the matter must be passed without delay to an agency that has the relevant statutory powers, namely social services, the National Society for the Prevention of Cruelty to Children (NSPCC), or the police. Informal advice from the local child protection team may be helpful. Advice about confidentiality and disclosure of information is given below and also in Chapter 5.

Confidentiality and disclosure of information about abuse or neglect

Everybody is entitled to confidentiality, but when abuse or neglect occurs, other imperatives are likely to take centre stage. As with all areas of caring for children and young people, the patient should be involved as much as possible in decisions, and this includes decisions about the disclosure of information. The child's right to confidentiality should be explained, but it must also be emphasised that where there are grounds for concern, there is a professional duty to take action to prevent serious harm to patients and others.

This means that doctors must consider what action best promotes the welfare of the abused child and protects others from the risk of harm. Doctors must be able to justify any decision about whether or not to refer a case to an outside agency and much depends on the evidence or reason for the suspicion that a child or young person is being neglected or abused. The same applies to the way in which doctors should respond to requests for information from outside agencies such as social services.

Decisions about disclosure in this area are complex and must be taken carefully and without delay. If a competent child cannot be persuaded to agree to voluntary disclosure, and there is an immediate need to disclose information to an outside agency, he or she should be told what action is to be taken unless to do so would expose the child or others to an increased risk of serious harm. When a child lacks the competence to make decisions about disclosure, doctors must protect that child's interests and encourage the child's cooperation. It is clearly in the public interest to identify and prevent abuse or neglect of children.

Cases in which the patient does have the competency to take decisions about disclosure, but refuses to permit disclosure so that the child can be protected and action can be taken against an abuser, are very difficult. Although it is essential to ensure child protection, it is also ethically important to respect the wishes of a competent patient. Disclosing against a competent patient's wishes may be unproductive. The patient may feel betrayed and lose trust in the doctor, and could refuse to cooperate with any investigation of alleged abuse. If it is possible without exposing them or others to danger, patients should be given time to come to a firm decision about disclosure. Counselling and support in the interim may help the patient to decide, and are essential throughout. Doctors must weigh the advantages and disadvantages of disclosure versus non-disclosure and make a decision based on the individual circumstances. Disclosure without consent will be justified in some cases and it follows that doctors should never make promises of secrecy.

Disclosure in order to prevent abuse may involve the identification of alleged abusers, and may include information that the doctor has learnt in his or her professional capacity as the abuser's doctor. The doctor's primary responsibility is to the child, as the more vulnerable party, and where the interests of the child and the suspected abuser conflict, the latter's interests should always give way to the child's. Doctors should, however, treat all parties sensitively and professionally, and try to respect both parties' rights, wishes and interests in so far as this is conducive to promoting the best interests of the child or children concerned.

If it is possible to involve parents and carers in the decision to disclose information concerning abuse or neglect, this may be helpful in encouraging all parties to work together towards what is in the best interests of the family. A goal of child protection is to promote good parenting and family relationships. The interests of family members are often interrelated and solutions ideally involve working with all concerned. The consent or refusal of family members regarding disclosure will not always be determinative in the decision whether to disclose, and where permission is not forthcoming disclosure may still be justified. Sometimes, however, this is not only inadvisable but could increase the risks to victims of abuse.

Refusal of medical or psychiatric examination under the Children Act

Children have a statutory right to refuse to submit to medical or psychiatric examination or other assessment that has been directed by the court for the purpose of an interim care, supervision, child protection or emergency protection order, provided that the child is 'of sufficient understanding to make an informed decision'.[81] This provision of the Children Act and its equivalents in other UK jurisdictions is often quoted out of context, resulting in the erroneous impression that the Act gives young people a general statutory right to refuse examination for care or treatment. On the contrary, the provisions apply only in the limited cases specified in law as described above. Even in these cases, however, the English High Court has dealt with competent young people refusing examination under the Children Act in the same way as other refusals by competent young people, by overriding their statutory right to refuse.[82] This approach is controversial, and doctors faced with a competent young person refusing examination in such circumstances should seek legal advice, particularly in Scotland, where there may be less scope for overriding a competent young person's wishes. Legal advice should be sought if a court order is required swiftly from a judge over the phone.

Best practice in child protection[83]

- In child protection cases, a doctor's primary responsibility is to the well-being of the child or children concerned. Where a child is at risk of serious harm, the interests of the child override those of parents or carers. Never delay taking emergency action.
- All doctors working with children, parents and other adults in contact with children should be able to recognise, and know how to act upon, signs that a child may be at risk of abuse or neglect, both in a home environment and in residential and other institutions.
- Any doctor seeing a child who raises concerns must ensure follow-on care. In particular, children must not be discharged from hospital without a full examination if there are concerns.
- Efforts should be made to include children and young people in decisions that closely affect them. The views and wishes of children should therefore be listened to and respected according to their competence and the level of their understanding. In some cases translation services suitable for young people may be needed.
- Wherever possible, the involvement and support of those who have parental responsibility for, or regular care of, a child should be encouraged, in so far as this is in keeping with promoting the best interests of the child or children concerned. Older children and young people may have their own views about parental involvement.
- When concerns about deliberate harm to children or young people have been raised, doctors must keep clear, accurate, comprehensive and contemporaneous notes. This must include a future care plan and identify the individual with lead responsibility.
- All doctors working with children, parents and other adults in contact with children must be familiar with relevant local child protection procedures, and must know how to deal promptly and professionally with any child protection concerns raised during their practice.
- All doctors working directly with children should ensure that safeguarding and promoting their welfare forms an integral part of all stages of the care they offer. Where doctors have patients who are parents or carers, they must also consider the potential impact of health conditions in those adults on the children in their care.
- Wherever a doctor sees a child who may be at risk, he or she must ensure that systems are in place to ensure follow-up care.
- As full a picture as possible of the circumstances of a child at risk must be drawn up.
- Where a child presents at hospital, enquiries must be made about any previous admissions.
- Where a child is admitted to hospital, a named consultant must be given overall responsibility for the child protection aspects of the case.
- Any child admitted to hospital about whom there are concerns about deliberate harm must receive a thorough examination within 24 hours unless it would compromise the child's care or well-being.

- Where a child at risk is to be discharged from hospital, a documented plan for the future care of the child must be drawn up.
- A child at risk should not be discharged from hospital without being registered at an identified GP.
- All professionals must be clear about their own responsibilities, and which professional has overall responsibility for the child protection aspects of a child's care.

References

1   United Nations High Commissioner for Human Rights. Convention on the rights of the child 1989.
2   *W v UK* (1987) 10 EHRR 29. *Dundee City Council v M* (2004) SLT 640.
3   Advice on good practice from the health departments includes: Department of Health (2001) *Seeking consent: working with children*, DH, London. Welsh Assembly Government (2002) *Reference guide for consent to examination or treatment*, WAG, Cardiff. Department of Health, Social Services and Public Safety (2003) *Good practice in consent: Consent for examination, treatment or care*, DHSSPS, Belfast, part 2. Scottish Executive Health Department (2006) *A Good Practice Guide on Consent for Health Professionals in NHSScotland*, SEHD, Edinburgh.
4   General Medical Council (2007) *0–18 years: guidance for all doctors*, GMC, London, para 14.
5   Young B, Dixon-Woods M, Windridge KC *et al.* (2003) Managing communication with young people who have a potentially life threatening chronic illness: qualitative study of patients and parents. *BMJ* **326**, 305–8.
6   Leveton M, American Academy of Paediatrics Committee on Bioethics (2008) Communicating with children and families: from everyday interactions to skill in conveying distressing information. *Pediatrics* **121**, e1441–60.
7   General Medical Council (2007) *0–18 years: guidance for all doctors*, GMC, London, para 20.
8   *Gillick v Wisbech and West Norfolk AHA* [1985] 3 All ER 402.
9   Age of Legal Capacity (Scotland) Act 1991, s 2(4).
10 *Gillick v Wisbech and West Norfolk AHA* [1985] 3 All ER 402.
11 For detailed advice about assessing competence see: British Medical Association (2001) *Consent, rights and choices in health care for children and young people*, BMJ Books, London.
12 *Re M (child: refusal of medical treatment)* [1999] 2 FLR 1097: 1100C-1100D.
13 *Re M (child: refusal of medical treatment)* [1999] 2 FLR 1097: 1100G.
14 For discussion of children's abilities and willingness to participate in decisions see: Alderson P. (1993) *Children's consent to surgery*, Open University Press, Buckingham.
15 Children Act 1989, s 3(5). Children (Northern Ireland) Order 1995, art 6(5). Children (Scotland) Act 1995, s 5(1).
16 *Houston (applicant)* (1996) 32 BMLR 93. Children (Scotland) Act 1995, s 15(5)(b).
17 Department of Health, Social Services and Public Safety (2003) *Good practice in consent. Consent for examination, treatment or care*, DHSSPS, Belfast. Welsh Assembly Government (2002) *Reference guide for consent to examination or treatment*, WAG, Cardiff. At the time of writing, there were no standard forms for use in Scotland. The Department of Health in England was reviewing its consent forms from 2001 as part of a larger consent review. Available at: www.dh.gov.uk (accessed 13 April 2011).
18 Family Law Reform Act 1969, s 8(1). Age of Majority Act (Northern Ireland) 1969, art 4(1). Age of Legal Capacity (Scotland) Act 1991, s 1(1)(b).
19 *Gillick v West Norfolk and Wisbech AHA* [1985] 3 All ER 402. *R (on the application of Axon) v Secretary of State for Health* [2006] 2 WLR 1130. Age of Legal Capacity (Scotland) Act 1991, s 2(4).
20 General Medical Council (2007) *0–18 years: guidance for all doctors*, GMC, London, para 15.
21 Clinical Governance Support Team (2005) *Guidance on the role and effective use of chaperones in primary and community care settings*: Model chaperone framework, CGST, Leicester.
22 General Medical Council (2007) *0–18 years: guidance for all doctors*, GMC, London, para 15.
23 Human Tissue Authority (2009) *Code of Practice 2: Donation of solid organs for transplantation*, HTA, London, para 47.
24 Ross LF, Thistlethwaite R, American Academy of Paediatrics Committee on Bioethics (2008) Minors as living solid-organ donors. *Pediatrics* **122**, 454–61.
25 *Re W (a minor) (medical treatment: court's jurisdiction)* [1992] 4 All ER 627.
26 Dyer C. (2008) Trust decides against action to force girl to undergo transplant. *BMJ* **337**, a2480 (see also correction *BMJ* **337**, a2659).
27 Sections of the letter were published in several newspapers. For example: Smith R. (2008) Brave schoolgirl Hannah Jones turns down life-saving heart transplant to die at home with her family. *The Mirror Online* (11 November). Available at: www.mirror.co.uk (accessed 31 May 2011).

28   Thomson JM. (2002) *Family law in Scotland*, 4th edn, E Butterworths/Law Society of Scotland, Edinburgh, pp. 189–90. Wilkinson AB, Norrie KM. (1999) *The law relating to parent and child in Scotland*, 2nd edn, Green, Edinburgh. Sutherland EE. (1999) *Child and family law*, Clark, Edinburgh, para 3.71.
29   *Houston (applicant)* (1996) 32 BMLR 93. Children (Scotland) Act 1995, s15(5)(b).
30   For more details see: Department for Constitutional Affairs (2007) *Mental Capacity Act 2005: Code of Practice*, The Stationery Office, London, Chapter 12.
31   Civil Partnership Act 2004.
32   British Medical Association (2008) *Parental responsibility: guidance from the British Medical Association*, BMA, London.
33   Children Act 1989, s 3(5).
34   Children (Scotland) Act 1995, s 5(1)(b).
35   *Re C (a minor) (medical treatment), sub nom Re C (a minor) (withdrawal of lifesaving treatment)* [1998] 1 FLR 384 at 389.
36   *Re C (a minor) (medical treatment), sub nom Re C (a minor) (withdrawal of lifesaving treatment)* [1998] 1 FLR 384 at 389.
37   *An NHS Trust v MB* [2006] 2 FLR 319, para 102.
38   *Portsmouth NHS Trust v Wyatt* [2005] 1 FLR 21.
39   *Portsmouth NHS Trust v Wyatt* [2005] EWHC 117.
40   *Portsmouth NHS Trust v Wyatt* [2005] 2 FLR 480.
41   *Portsmouth NHS Trust v Wyatt* [2005] 1 FLR 554.
42   *Portsmouth NHS Trust v Wyatt*, 21 October 2005 (unreported).
43   Children Act 1989, s 1(1). Children (Northern Ireland) Order 1995, art 3(1). Children (Scotland) Act 1995, s 16(1).
44   *Re T (a minor) (wardship: medical treatment)* [1997] 1 WLR 242; [1997] 1 All ER 906; [1997] 1 FLR 502, CA.
45   *Re T (a minor) (wardship: medical treatment)* [1997] 1 FLR 502 at 514.
46   *Re C (welfare of child: immunisation)* [2003] 2 FLR 1095 CA. *Re J (a minor) (prohibited steps order: circumcision), sub noms Re J (child's religious upbringing and circumcision); Re J (specific issue orders: Muslim upbringing and circumcision)* [2000] 1 FLR 571.
47   British Medical Association (2001) *Consent, rights and choices in health care for children and young people*, BMJ Books, London.
48   The Children and Family Court Advisory and Support Service (CAFCASS) (England), CAFCASS Cymru (Wales), the Official Solicitor of the Supreme Court for Northern Ireland, and the Scottish Executive Solicitors' Office.
49   *Glass v United Kingdom* (61827/00) [2004] ECHR 103 (9 March 2004).
50   *Re O (a minor) (medical treatment)* [1993] 2 FLR 149. *Re S (a minor) (medical treatment)* [1993] 1 FLR 377.
51   *P (Medical Treatment: Best interests)* [2004] 2 FLR 1117, para 12.
52   *Re W (a minor)(medical treatment: court's jurisdiction)* [1992] 4 All ER 627.
53   Grubb A. (1997) Commentary: court's inherent jurisdiction (child): detention and treatment. *Med Law Rev* **5**, 227–33, p.231.
54   *X v Germany* (1985) 7 EHRR 152.
55   Royal College of Nursing (2003) *Restraining, holding still and containing children and young people: guidance for nursing staff*, RCN, London.
56   British Medical Association (2006) *The law and ethics of male circumcision: guidance for doctors*, BMA, London.
57   *Re J (a minor) (prohibited steps order: circumcision) sub noms Re J (child's religious upbringing and circumcision), Re J (specific issue orders: Muslim upbringing and circumcision)* [2000] 1 FLR 571.
58   General Medical Council (2008) *Personal Beliefs and Medical Practice*, GMC, London, paras 12–16.
59   *Re J (a minor) (prohibited steps order: circumcision) sub noms Re J (child's religious upbringing and circumcision); Re J (specific issue orders: Muslim upbringing and circumcision)* [2000] 1 FLR 571.
60   The Scottish Government has produced a range of leaflets on religious male circumcision for NHS staff and parents. Available at: www.scotland.gov.uk (accessed 3 March 2011).
61   British Medical Association (2011) *Female genital mutilation: Caring for patients and child protection*, BMA, London.
62   Foreign and Commonwealth Office (2011) *Multi-Agency Practice Guidelines: Female Genital Mutilation*, FCO, London.
63   *Re A (children), sub nom Re A (conjoined twins: medical treatment), sub nom Re A (children) (conjoined twins: surgical separation)* [2000] 4 All ER 961.
64   *Re A (children), sub nom Re A (conjoined twins: medical treatment), sub nom Re A (children) (conjoined twins: surgical separation)* [2000] 4 All ER 961: 968j–969a.
65   Gillon R. (2001) Imposed separation of Siamese twins: moral hubris by the English courts? *J Med Ethics* **27**, 3–4.
66   *Re A (children), sub nom Re A (conjoined twins: medical treatment), sub nom Re A (children) (conjoined twins: surgical separation)* [2000] 4 All ER 961: 1019bc.

67   National Collaborating Centre for Women's and Children's Health (2009) *When to suspect child maltreatment*, RCOG Press, London.

68   British Medical Association (2009) *Child protection: a tool kit for doctors*, BMA, London.

69   Royal College of General Practitioners (2009) *Safeguarding children and young people: a toolkit for general practice*, RCGP, London.

70   Royal College of Paediatrics and Child Health (2010) *Safeguarding Children and Young People: Roles and Competences for Health Care Staff*, RCPCH, London.

71   The Victoria Climbié Inquiry (2003) *Report of an inquiry by Lord Laming*, The Stationery Office, London, para 1.5.

72   The Victoria Climbié Inquiry (2003) *Report of an inquiry by Lord Laming*, The Stationery Office, London.

73   The Victoria Climbié Inquiry (2003) *Report of an inquiry by Lord Laming*, The Stationery Office, London, para 1.16.

74   Kramer HHJ. (2009) *R v (B)(The boyfriend of Baby Peter's mother)(C)(Baby Peter's mother) and Jason Owen*. Sentencing remarks Central Criminal Court, May 22, para 2. Available at: www.judiciary.gov.uk (accessed 3 March 2011).

75   Kramer HHJ. (2009) *R v (B)(The boyfriend of Baby Peter's mother)(C)(Baby Peter's mother) and Jason Owen*. Sentencing remarks Central Criminal Court, May 22, para 28. Available at www.judiciary.gov.uk (accessed 3 March 2011).

76   The Lord Laming (2009) *The Protection of Children in England: A Progress Report*, The Stationery Office, London.

77   Care Quality Commission (2009) *Review of the involvement and action taken by health bodies in relation to the case of Baby P*, CQC, London.

78   Care Quality Commission (2009) *Review of the involvement and action taken by health bodies in relation to the case of Baby P*, CQC, London, p.25.

79   Department of Health, Home Office, Department for Education and Employment (2010) *Working together to safeguard children: a guide to inter-agency working to safeguard and promote the welfare of children*, The Stationery Office, London. Department of Health (2006) *What to do if you are worried a child is being abused*, DH, London. Welsh Assembly Government (2007) *Safeguarding Children: Working Together Under the Children Act 2004*, WAG, Cardiff. Scottish Executive Health Department (2003) *Protecting Children: a shared responsibility. Guidance for health professionals in Scotland*, SEHD, Edinburgh. Department of Health, Social Services and Public Safety (2003) *Co-operating to safeguard children*, DHSSPS, Belfast.

80   General Medical Council (2007) *0–18 years: guidance for all doctors*, GMC, London. At the time of writing the GMC was in the process of developing new additional standalone guidance for doctors working in child protection.

81   Children Act 1989, s 38(6). Children (Northern Ireland) Order 1995, art 57(6). Children (Scotland) Act 1995, s 90. The Scottish legislation gives competent young people the right to refuse to submit to medical or psychiatric examination or other assessment that has been directed by the court or a children's hearing for the purpose of supervision requirement, assessment, protection or place of safety order.

82   *South Glamorgan CC v B sub nom South Glamorgan CC v W and B* [1993] FLR 574.

83   The bullet points are taken from British Medical Association (2009) *Child protection: a tool kit for doctors*, BMA, London. For more detailed guidance see Chapter 5 of: Department of Health, Home Office, Department for Education and Employment (2010) *Working together to safeguard children: A guide to inter-agency working to safeguard and promote the welfare of children*, The Stationery Office, London.

5: Confidentiality

The questions covered in this chapter include the following.

- Is all health information confidential?
- What does the law say about confidentiality?
- Is consent always needed before information is disclosed?
- What form should consent take?
- When may confidentiality be breached 'in the public interest'?
- When can health information be disclosed for purposes other than the provision of care?
- Is information about deceased patients confidential?

Glossary of terms

This glossary defines the way the British Medical Association (BMA) has interpreted the key terms and phrases used throughout this chapter.

Consent	Agreement to an action based on knowledge of what that action involves and its likely consequences.[1]
Express consent	Consent that is expressed orally or in writing. Also known as explicit consent. An articulation of patient agreement for the disclosure of information, freely given in circumstances where the available options and the consequences have been made clear.[2] Express consent is generally preferable because it is unambiguous.
Implied consent	In the context of sharing health information, consent that can be inferred if the patient has been informed that information is to be disclosed, the purpose and extent of the disclosure, and that they have a right to object, but have not objected.[3] Patients are normally considered to have given implied consent for sharing information within the healthcare team or with others providing their care.
Personal information	Information about people that doctors learn in a professional capacity and from which individuals can be identified.[4] Such information is subject to a duty of confidentiality.
Identifiable information	Information from which a patient can be identified. Name, address and full postcode will identify a patient; combinations of information may also support identification, even if the name and address are not included.
Healthcare team	Comprises the people providing clinical services for a patient, and the administrative and other staff who support the provision of his or her care.[5]
Disclosure	The provision of access to information about a patient, regardless of the purpose.
Public interest disclosure	Exceptional circumstances that justify overriding the right of an individual to confidentiality in order to serve a broader social interest. Decisions about the public interest must take account of both the potential harm that disclosure may cause and the interests of

Medical Ethics Today: The BMA's Handbook of Ethics and Law, Third Edition. Sophie Brannan, Eleanor Chrispin, Martin Davies, Veronica English, Rebecca Mussell, Julian Sheather and Ann Sommerville.
© 2012 BMA Medical Ethics Department. Published 2012 by Blackwell Publishing Ltd.

	society in the continued provision of a confidential health service.[6]
Anonymised information	Information from which individuals cannot reasonably be identified. Requires the removal of name, address, full postcode, identification numbers or any other detail or combination of details that might support identification.
Pseudonymised information	Information from which individuals cannot be identified by the recipient, but which enables information about different patients to be distinguished or to link information about the same patients over time. A 'key' might be retained by the service that coded the information so that it can be reconnected with the patient.[7]

The duty of confidentiality

Confidentiality is a fundamental requirement for the preservation of trust between patients and health professionals, and is subject to legal and ethical safeguards. Patients should be able to expect that information about their health which they give in confidence will be kept confidential unless there is a compelling reason why it should not. Patient confidentiality is a legal obligation which is derived from case law and it is a requirement established within professionals' codes of conduct. There is also a strong public interest in maintaining confidentiality so that individuals will be encouraged to seek appropriate treatment and share information relevant to it.

It should be recognised at the outset that confidentiality remains an area where there is often a variety of opinion, not least because standards and working practices in the health service continue to change and evolve. The move away from a single doctor–patient relationship towards a multi-disciplinary care team relationship, of which the patient is a part, means that there is increased emphasis on providing more seamless, integrated care and promoting partnership working.[8] This requires the dissemination of data more widely and more routine information sharing amongst those providing care. Patients must have information about the way health information is shared between health professionals and others providing their care in order to provide a secure ethical and legal basis for this. With the shift in the delivery of health services and patients increasingly accessing care through a range of public and private healthcare services, maintaining a reasonable balance between protecting patient data and ensuring their appropriate use presents a challenge. This chapter reflects the principles laid out in the General Medical Council (GMC) guidance on confidentiality[9] by which doctors must abide.

The chapter answers many of the questions that doctors most commonly ask the BMA. The confidentiality issues for doctors with dual obligations, when colleagues are sick or failing and in relation to public health, are covered in detail in other chapters. Issues surrounding patients' access to their own records are covered in Chapter 6 and confidentiality and genetic information is covered in Chapter 9.

General principles

GMC guidance states that '[p]atients have a right to expect that information about them will be held in confidence by their doctors'.[10]

The following basic principles underpin the advice in this chapter.

- Information must be readily available to patients explaining how their data will be shared within the healthcare team, in order to provide clinical care, unless they object.
- Consent should usually be sought for the use or disclosure of identifiable personal health information outside the healthcare team.
- Information may be used more freely if it is effectively anonymised and therefore de-identified data should be used wherever possible for purposes not directly connected with supporting the care of the patient.
- Exceptionally, when identifiable data are needed and it is not possible to obtain consent, information may be disclosed, with strict safeguards, either with support under the Health Service (Control of Patient Information) Regulations 2002 in England and Wales, where approval has been obtained, or where the balance of public interests supports disclosure.
- Disclosures should be kept to the minimum necessary to achieve the purpose.
- Doctors must always be prepared to justify their decisions about the use of personal health information.
- Information about patients must be properly protected to prevent malicious, thoughtless or inadvertent breaches of confidentiality.
- All people who come into contact with personal health information in their work should have training in confidentiality and security issues.

What data are confidential?

All identifiable patient information that doctors have learnt in a professional capacity is subject to the duty of confidentiality. Once information is anonymised effectively, it is no longer confidential and may be used more freely.

An informal discussion?

A GP and a dentist were both found guilty of breaching confidentiality after discussing a mutual patient during a round of golf.

The GP told the dentist that the patient had had a termination of pregnancy 2 years earlier. The dentist repeated this to his wife, who told a friend, who then revealed to the patient that she knew about the termination.

Both the doctor and dentist were found guilty of serious professional misconduct and suspended from their professional registers for 6 months.[11]

Both legally and ethically, information that doctors learn about a patient in the course of their professional duties is confidential. Therefore, any information contained in health records should be regarded as confidential. This might include:

- any clinical information about an individual's diagnosis or treatment
- a picture, X-ray, photograph, video, audiotape or other images of the patient (see Chapter 6, pages 247–253)
- who the patient's doctor is and which clinics the patient attends and when
- any social information that a doctor may learn about a patient, for example, information about family life
- anything else that may be used to identify a patient directly or indirectly.

Any of the information above combined with the patient's name or address or full postcode or the patient's date of birth may identify them. Even when such obvious identifiers are missing, rare diseases, drug treatments or statistical analyses which have very small numbers within a small population, may allow individuals to be identified.

Doctors often enquire about which particular pieces of patient information are classified as confidential personal health information. Common questions include whether a list of patients who have attended a surgery can be given to the police, for example after a petty theft has taken place, or whether a patient's name and address are pieces of confidential information. In the BMA's view, all information collected in the context of healthcare, including a patient's NHS number, are confidential and doctors must take appropriate measures to ensure that the data are kept confidential.[12] Sometimes breaches of confidentiality occur inadvertently or as a result of poor practice, rather than deliberate disclosures.

Keeping it confidential

In 2009, the GMC found a GP guilty of deficient professional performance for breaching confidentiality after he dictated a letter for referral within the reception area of the practice in which a number of other patients were located. The dictation included details of the procedure requested and details of the patient's family medical history. The GMC imposed conditions on the GP's registration for 12 months.[13]

Contacting patients

A common enquiry to the BMA is whether GP practices can leave messages for patients on home telephones. Doctors are obliged to protect patient information from disclosure to non-authorised third parties. Ideally, prior discussion with the patient will have identified an appropriate method of communication with regard to sensitive test results but the BMA recognises that this may not always be the case. Doctors should be mindful that there is the possibility that a home telephone may be answered by someone other than the patient.

The BMA's general advice is that if the telephone is answered by an individual other than the patient the practice should simply say they will call back another time – unless the patient has explicitly agreed that someone else can take a message. Similarly, if the phone is answered and the practice reaches the voicemail facility then no message should be left as there is no guarantee that the message will remain confidential from third parties.

While there are clearly practical advantages to leaving telephone messages for patients, the fact that a patient has an appointment at his or her GP surgery is confidential information. Therefore, unless the practice can guarantee that the message will be received by the correct patient it would be regarded as a breach of confidentiality to leave a telephone message on a patient's answering machine (even if clinical information was omitted) which might be accessed by non-authorised third parties, such as family members. Doctors should be aware that the GMC's guidelines on confidentiality specify that 'you must make sure that any personal information about patients that you hold or control is effectively protected at all times against improper disclosure'.[14]

Generally, the BMA advises that if the test results or other information that need to be relayed are foreseeably sensitive, the doctor and patient should agree beforehand how they will be communicated. For example, patients can telephone in for the results and perhaps be given a password if the information is particularly sensitive. Such a system might be appropriate for a teenager going for a pregnancy or HIV test without their parents' knowledge. In such cases, merely the fact of a telephone call from the surgery could be very sensitive, even if no message was left.

Texting patients appointment reminders

There are practical advantages to texting patients to remind them of appointments via their mobile telephone, although patients should be asked first if they are happy to receive a text message before this method of communication is used. Receiving a text is likely to be unproblematic for most patients; however, it is advisable to check first as there may be some patients who do not wish to be contacted in this way. The BMA recommends that patients registering with a practice are given the chance on the registration form to indicate if they do not wish to be contacted via their mobile.

Sometimes, there may be particular circumstances when a GP is aware of a reason why it may not be appropriate to send a patient a text message reminder and in these cases another method of communication should be used.

Implied consent for disclosure of information as part of the direct provision of healthcare

In relation to health information, most patients understand and accept that information must be shared within the healthcare team in order to provide care.[15] This might include, for example, information being shared when a patient is referred to another healthcare professional or a referral letter being typed by a medical secretary. The view of the BMA and that of the GMC[16] is that implied consent is acceptable for uses or disclosures of information that directly contribute to the diagnosis, care or treatment of a patient, and to the quality assurance of that care within the healthcare team. This includes record keeping, transfer of information within a healthcare team and between healthcare professionals providing care, and local clinical audit (see below). It can also include appropriate information sharing between health and social care providers, as long as patients are aware when health and social care providers are working together on their case so that they would not be surprised to learn how their information has been shared. The BMA recognises, however, that there is no clear demarcation between healthcare and social care and it is not always evident when it might be considered appropriate to share information with social care providers on the basis of implied consent. Informed opinion differs as to where the exact boundaries lie in this context. It should be emphasised that express consent should be sought wherever it is practicable to do so in any circumstances where there is a risk of misunderstanding. Where there is uncertainty doctors are advised to seek advice from their professional or regulatory body. (Liaison between health and social care is discussed further on page 211.)

In order for implied consent to be valid the GMC states that information must be 'readily available to patients explaining that, unless they object, personal information about them will be shared within the healthcare team'.[17] Such information can be provided in leaflets, posters, on websites and face-to-face.[18] In reviewing the information provided to patients, consideration should be given to whether patients would be surprised to learn about how their personal data are being used and disclosed.[19]

Occasionally, however, the particular circumstances of the case mean that the general rules are not suitable. In a small community, for example, the doctor may be aware that the medical secretary is known personally to the patient and it would be helpful to confirm that the patient understands that all surgery staff are under a strict contractual duty of confidentiality which prohibits them from unauthorised disclosures.

Sometimes two competing interests come into conflict, such as an individual's informed refusal to allow disclosure and the need to provide effective treatment to that person. A patient's refusal to allow information sharing with other health professionals may compromise the patient's safety, but if this is an informed decision by an individual with capacity it should be respected. Individuals may knowingly compromise their own safety but not that of other people. Health professionals, although not abandoning the patient, may ethically curtail the range of procedures they offer if the outcome could foreseeably be unsafe or ineffective owing to lack of information. Patients must be informed if this is an implication of their choice, and must be offered further advice about their options.

Some health information is so sensitive that it is subject to additional legal restrictions on disclosure to other health professionals, for example, information capable of identifying an individual examined or treated for any sexually transmitted infection[20] or restrictions under the Gender Recognition Act 2004 (see pages 198–199).

Clinical audit

It is acceptable to rely on implied consent for clinical audit undertaken within the healthcare organisation providing care. GMC advice states that if an audit is to be undertaken 'by the team that provided care, or those working to support them, such as clinical audit staff, doctors may disclose identifiable information, provided they are satisfied that the patient:

- has ready access to information that explains that their personal information may be disclosed for local clinical audit, and that they have the right to object, and
- has not objected'.[21]

Sometimes, audit is undertaken across organisational boundaries, for example medication reviews of GP records by local pharmacists. Commercial agencies are also sometimes involved in audit. When a third party is to be brought in to carry out an audit, a member of the health team responsible for the patient's care should produce anonymous data for this purpose. When this is not practicable, or identifiable data is essential, explicit consent should be sought before identifiable information is disclosed, in line with GMC guidance.[22] When this is not feasible, in England and Wales it may be possible to seek approval for disclosure under section 251 of the NHS Act 2006 and its supporting regulations (see pages 209–211).

Pharmaceutical companies are also sometimes interested in sponsoring the audit of aspects such as prescribing habits in return for basic information resulting from the project. Doctors offered such services should consider whether there would be any conflict with the GMC's requirement that doctors must not accept any inducement or gift that may be seen to affect their judgement (see also Chapter 13, pages 554–556).[23] They should also enquire about the uses to which information is likely to be put and ensure that no identifiable data are made accessible. This requires monitoring not only that patient names and addresses are excluded, but also that other identifiers are omitted to ensure anonymity (see pages 193–194).

Uses of data unconnected with the direct provision of patient care generally require express consent (see pages 207–218), unless the data are anonymised or approval has been obtained under the Health Service (Control of Patient Information) Regulations 2002 which give effect to the powers under section 251 of the NHS Act 2006 (see pages 209–211).

The only alternative routes for sharing health information, in the absence of patient consent, are when the law compels disclosure (see pages 194–198) or when it is justifiable in the public interest (see pages 199–206).

Summary – implied consent for disclosure of information as part of the direct provision of healthcare

- Implied consent is acceptable for uses or disclosures of information that directly contribute to the diagnosis, care or treatment of a patient, and to the quality assurance of that care, unless the patient objects.
- Patients need information about the way health information is shared between health professionals and others providing care. This may include those providing social care.
- Patients need information about the way their data are shared within the healthcare organisation for clinical audit.
- Implied consent is acceptable when the patient is aware that appropriate information sharing is taking place between organisations working in partnership to provide his or her care.
- Competent refusals to allow information to be shared must be respected.
- Explicit consent is generally needed in order for information to be shared outside the healthcare team providing care, unless the data are anonymised prior to disclosure or support is obtained under the Health Service (Control of Patient Information) Regulations 2002.

The law

This section examines the main legal requirements that impact on confidentiality. In the context of sharing confidential health information, there is no overarching statute with regards to disclosure or otherwise in this area and a multitude of professional and regulatory codes exist.[24] For example, the legal responsibilities in respect of confidential information cannot be gleaned from common law and statute alone, and health professionals must look at the overall effect of the law, not each aspect in isolation. Doctors who are uncertain about the application of the law should seek legal advice.

Data protection and human rights legislation do not apply after death, although the Department of Health, the GMC and the BMA all agree that the ethical duty endures beyond death. (Disclosures in relation to deceased people are discussed on pages 221–223.)

The common law

In the UK, much of the law affecting confidentiality is not set out in legislation. It is common law that imposes a duty on health professionals to respect the confidences of patients. This duty arises where information is, by its nature, confidential (such as health information)[25] or where it is imparted in circumstances where an obligation of confidence is implied (such as the doctor–patient relationship). This duty also arises when there is a public interest that confidentiality should be protected, or when the confider may suffer from revelation of the information.

The effect of the common law is that information may be disclosed with consent or where the law requires or permits it. Legal judgments have also established that confidentiality may be breached, but only when there is a public interest that overrides the patient's right to confidentiality (and also the public interest in maintaining a confidential health service[26]). Decisions are made on a case-by-case basis, and health professionals must be able to justify their decisions.

Data Protection Act 1998

The Data Protection Act 1998 governs the processing of data that identify living individuals – personal data – in the UK.[27] It permits, rather than requires, disclosure of personal data in some circumstances. The Act is not limited to electronic data. It incorporates other areas of law such as confidentiality, by its blanket requirement that data processing is 'lawful'. The Information Commissioner's Officer (ICO) oversees and enforces the Data Protection Act and can prosecute those who commit offences under the legislation.

At the heart of the Act are eight data protection principles which state that data must be:

- fairly and lawfully processed
- processed for limited purposes and not in any manner incompatible with those purposes
- adequate, relevant and not excessive
- accurate
- not kept for longer than necessary
- processed in line with the data subject's rights
- secure
- not transferred to countries without adequate protection.[28]

The Act's requirement that all data processing must be 'fair and lawful' means that patients must be informed when and what information about them is being processed (the 'fair processing requirement'), and the processing itself must meet all the legal standards that apply, including the common law duty of confidentiality.

There are additional rules for when sensitive personal data are processed. Under section 2(e) of the Act sensitive personal data includes information about a person's 'physical or mental health or condition'. In such cases the processing must not only meet at least one of the conditions in Schedule 2, which is necessary for processing personal data, but also in Schedule 3 of the Act.[29] The conditions that are most commonly relied upon for the purposes of processing health information under the Act are the following.

Schedule 2:

- that there is consent from the data subject
- that processing is necessary for the administration of justice.

Schedule 3:

- that processing is necessary for the vital interests of the data subject or another person
- that processing is undertaken by a health professional for 'medical purposes', something that is very broadly defined in the Act as 'preventative medicine, medical diagnosis, medical research, the provision of care and treatment and the management of healthcare services'.[30]

The scope of the conditions is so wide that almost any disclosure from patient records for NHS purposes is likely to come within their remit. Even if these conditions are met, however, the requirement for processing to be fair and lawful, which includes compliance with the common law, still stands.

Patients are also entitled to have access to and a copy of their information, except where there are grounds for believing that access to that information would be likely to cause serious harm to the individual or a third party, or where it would identify someone who is not a health professional or entail disclosure of another individual's identifiable data (see Chapter 6, pages 255–260). They are also entitled to have information corrected when it is inaccurate (see Chapter 6, pages 235–238).

The Data Protection (Processing of Sensitive Personal Data) Order 2000 (SI 2000/417) adds a further condition to Schedule 3. This permits processing which is in the 'substantial public interest' where necessary for the discharge of certain public functions, such as protecting the public against malpractice, or other seriously improper conduct or incompetence. Therefore, disclosure to the GMC in relation to an allegation of professional misconduct would be permitted without the requirement to seek consent under the Data Protection Act 1998;[31] however, patients whose personal information is being disclosed should usually be informed of the disclosure as a matter of good practice even if their consent is not required. (Disclosure to regulatory bodies for the purposes of investigating complaints is discussed on pages 196–197.)

Increased sanctions for data breaches

In April 2010, the powers of the Information Commissioner were strengthened by the ability to fine organisations for serious data breaches under section 55 of the Data Protection Act 1998. Penalties of up to £500,000 can be imposed on organisations who seriously contravene data protection principles.[32] At the time of writing, custodial sanctions for those found guilty of knowingly or recklessly obtaining, disclosing, selling or procuring the disclosure of personal data were also under consideration.[33]

Human Rights Act 1998

A right to 'respect for private and family life', under Article 8 of the European Convention on Human Rights, is guaranteed by the Human Rights Act 1998. This right is not absolute, and may be derogated from where the law permits and where 'necessary in a democratic society in the interests of national security, public safety or the economic well-being of the country, for the prevention of disorder or crime, for the protection of health or morals, or for the protection of the rights and freedoms of others'.[34] The effect is similar to that of the common law duty of confidentiality: privacy is an important principle that must be respected, but confidentiality may be breached where other significant interests prevail.

NHS Act 2006

In England and Wales, section 251 of the NHS Act 2006 gives the Secretary of State for Health power to make regulations permitting the disclosure of identifiable information without consent, in certain circumstances, where it is needed to support essential NHS activity and medical research. Organisations can apply to the Ethics and Confidentiality Committee (ECC) of the National Information Governance Board (NIGB)[35] to seek support for disclosure under the Health Service (Control of Patient Information) Regulations 2002, which give effect to the powers under section 251. These provisions are discussed on pages 209–211.

The Health and Social Care Bill introduced into Parliament in January 2011 contained proposals to abolish the NIGB and transfer its statutory functions to the Care Quality Commission (CQC). The proposals included a provision requiring the CQC to appoint a National Information Governance Committee until March 2015. (Up-to-date information can be found on the BMA website.)

Computer Misuse Act 1990

In the UK, it is an offence under the Computer Misuse Act 1990 to gain unauthorised access to computer material. This includes using another person's ID and password without authority in order to use, alter or delete data.

GMC guidance

All doctors must maintain the standards of confidentiality laid down by the GMC, or risk complaint for professional misconduct. The GMC states that when disclosing information about a patient, doctors must:

- 'use anonymised or coded information if practicable and if it will serve the purpose
- be satisfied that the patient:
  - has ready access to information that explains that his or her personal information might be disclosed for the sake of their own care, or for local clinical audit, and that they can object, and
  - has not objected
- get the patient's express consent if identifiable information is to be disclosed for purposes other than their care or local clinical audit, unless the disclosure is required by law or can be justified in the public interest
- keep disclosures to the minimum necessary, and
- keep up to date with, and observe, all relevant legal requirements, including the common law and data protection legislation.'[36]

NHS Care Record Guarantee

The NHS Care Record Guarantee[37] summarises the legal and policy position for patients on how their information will be used and safeguarded by the NHS. It sets out 12 commitments of the NHS in England to the confidentiality and security of patient information. It stresses patients' rights regarding the way their health information is used. The 12 commitments of the guarantee cover:

- patients' access to their own records
- controls on access by others
- how access will be monitored and policed
- options patients have to further limit access
- access in an emergency
- what happens when patients cannot make decisions for themselves.

There also exists a wide range of other similar policies and standards in the four nations which provide guidance for healthcare professionals to ensure that patients are fully involved with decisions about the use of their information and that information provided by patients is kept confidential.[38]

Summary – the law and professional standards

- The sum of the ethical and legal rules about confidentiality is that health professionals are responsible to patients for the confidentiality and security of the health information they hold.
- There should be no disclosure of any confidential information gained in the course of professional work for any purpose other than for clinical care (or direct support of clinical care) of the patient to whom it relates. There are three broad exceptions to this standard:
  - where there is appropriate consent
  - where the law requires disclosure or
  - where there is an overriding public interest in disclosure.
- Patients must be informed of the purposes for which their data will be processed.
- Professional guidance and numerous organisational policies reinforce the importance of respecting patient confidentiality.

Anonymous information

A principle that underpins the BMA's views on confidentiality and access to information is that information may be used more freely if the information is not identifiable in any way. Although there should be safeguards to prevent inappropriate use or abuse of even anonymous information, in general the Association believes that it is not ethically necessary to seek consent for its use. It should be noted, however, that, although studies have shown qualified support amongst patients for the use of anonymised data for research purposes, concerns remain that data from which name, date of birth and address have been removed, could be made identifiable or will not be fully anonymised.[39] Indeed, some patients take the view that it is still their information even if anonymised and therefore still wish to exercise control over how it is used.[40]

Usually, data can be considered to be anonymous where clinical or administrative information is separated from details that may permit the individual to be identified such as name, NHS number, date of birth and postcode. Even where such obvious identifiers are missing, rare disease, drug treatments or statistical analyses that have very small numbers within a small population may allow individuals to be identified. A combination of items increases the chance of patient identification. For example, pieces of information such as date of birth, diagnosis or postcode may not alone identify an individual, but may do so in combination. Similarly, an NHS number may replace other identifiers, but the information cannot be said to be anonymous as NHS numbers are widely used as identifiers and many people are able to translate the number into a name and address. Indeed, it is arguable that detailed information that is about an individual cannot be anonymised, and true anonymisation can arise only with aggregation. Usually, however, data can be considered to be anonymous where clinical or administrative information is separated from details that may permit the individual to be identified. Doctors must take reasonable steps to anonymise data to this extent and, if necessary, take technical advice about anonymisation before releasing data. While it is not ethically necessary to seek consent for the use of anonymised data, general information about the use of such data should be available to patients. Anonymisation is a permanent process. (Reversible anonymisation, or pseudonymisation, is discussed below.)

The Court of Appeal, in a decision about the sale of prescribing data, has clarified that there is no legal duty of confidentiality when data are anonymous.[41]

Confidentiality and anonymous data: the Source Informatics case

Source Informatics was an American company that wanted to obtain information about doctors' prescribing habits in order to sell this on to pharmaceutical companies, so that those companies could market their products more effectively. The identity of the prescribing doctors, and the products they prescribed, was of interest to Source, but the identity of patients was not. Source proposed that pharmacists should collect anonymous data by computer and pass it to Source for a fee.

In 1997 the Department of Health issued guidance that said this would involve a breach of confidentiality. Although the judge at first instance upheld this position, his decision was overturned in the Court of Appeal, which held that confidentiality was not breached when patients' identities were protected. The Department of Health's guidance was therefore withdrawn.[42]

Pseudonymised data

Pseudonymisation[43] is sometimes referred to as reversible anonymisation or 'key coding' of data. True patient identifiers, such as name, address or NHS number, are substituted with a pseudonym that allows the data to be reconstructed as required. Where those who are using data have no means to reverse the process, and so no way to identify an individual from the data they have (or from the data they have and any they may acquire), the data may be treated as anonymised and there is no common law requirement to seek consent for their use. Processing should still meet at least one of the requirements in each of Schedules 2 and 3 of the Data Protection Act, however, since it is probable that pseudomymised data fall within the Act's definition of 'personal data'. This point has not been tested in court, although the Information Commissioner advises NHS bodies and clinicians to apply the Act in these circumstances.[44] For those who have access to both pseudonymised data and the means to reconstitute them, on the other hand, they should be treated as identifiable.

Pseudonymisation is a useful technique where the identity of individuals is not important for the day-to-day uses of the data, yet it is important to be able to distinguish between individuals or to link data to identity at a later stage. The use of pseudonymised data is common in research (see Chapter 14).

As there remains a small risk of re-identification of pseudonymised data, additional safeguards are required, such as contractual obligations to only link data with the permission of the original data controller and not to disclose the data to third parties.

Statutory and legal disclosures

In addition to the overarching legal framework of the common law, human rights and data protection legislation, doctors are required by law to disclose certain confidential information, regardless of patient consent. They must be aware of their obligations to disclose in these circumstances and ensure that they do not disclose more information than is necessary. Statutory disclosures should not normally involve transfer of the entire record. Patients generally cannot refuse but they should usually be made aware of the purpose of the disclosure (and if they can appeal) and that it is to a secure authority.

Examples of statutory obligations to disclose information

- Public health legislation contains a number of powers designed to control the spread of infectious diseases. In the UK, legislation requires health professionals to notify local authorities of the identity, sex and address of any person suspected of having a notifiable disease, including food poisoning.[45] In England and Wales this obligation also extends to notifying local authorities of patients who have an infection or are contaminated in a way which could present 'significant harm' to human health.[46]
  Further statutory exemptions for communicable diseases and other risks to public health are covered under the Health Service (Control of Patient Information) Regulations 2002[47] specifically permitting disclosure to the relevant authority (see Chapter 20, pages 847–848).
- The Abortion Regulations 1991 requires a doctor carrying out a termination of pregnancy to notify the appropriate Chief Medical Officer.[48]
- In the UK, the Reporting of Injuries, Diseases and Dangerous Occurrences Regulations 1995 requires deaths, major injuries and accidents resulting in more than 3 days off work, certain diseases and dangerous occurrences to be reported to the relevant authority.[49]
- From April 2010, as part of the requirements of registration with the Care Quality Commission (CQC),[50] English NHS trusts must report serious patient safety incidents, deaths or events that may indicate risks to ongoing compliance with registration requirements.[51] Reports are usually made via the National Patient Safety Agency (NPSA) which will forward relevant information to the CQC. The NPSA has developed a national framework for reporting serious incidents in the NHS.[52] (In 2010, it was proposed that the NPSA be abolished as part of the Government's plan to reduce the number of arm's-length bodies.[53]) (For further discussion on reporting adverse events see Chapter 21, pages 873–875.)

There are also a number of regulatory bodies with statutory powers to require access to patient's records (see pages 196–197).

In any situation where disclosure is made in the absence of the subject's consent, careful consideration must be given to the question of to whom it is proper to disclose the information. This varies with the circumstances of the case and the objective that is sought. Where there is a statutory requirement for disclosure, the recipient of the information is usually identified and in such cases the information released should be the minimum to fulfil the requirement. Doctors should seek legal advice if they believe that complying with a statutory obligation to disclose information would cause serious harm to the patient or another person.

Laws affecting all citizens

In addition to laws specifically requiring disclosure by health professionals, doctors may also be affected by the disclosure statutes that apply to all citizens. These are the following.

- Terrorism Act 2000 – all citizens, including health professionals, must inform police as soon as possible of any information that may help to prevent an act of terrorism, or help in apprehending or prosecuting a terrorist.
- Road Traffic Act 1988 – in certain circumstances, all citizens, including health professionals, must provide to the police, on request, any information that may identify a driver alleged to have committed a traffic offence. This does not require health professionals to volunteer information about drivers, but they must respond to requests from a police officer.

Disclosure to courts, tribunals and regulatory bodies

The courts, including the coroner's courts, some tribunals, regulatory bodies and those appointed to hold inquiries such as the GMC, have legal powers to require disclosure, without the patient's consent, of information that may be relevant to matters within their jurisdiction. Some examples are given below.

- In England and Wales, the NHS Counter Fraud and Security Management Service (CFSMS) has powers to compel disclosure of information and documentation from all NHS bodies and those contracting with the NHS, for use in their investigations to prevent, detect and prosecute fraud in the NHS.[54] There are serious consequences for not complying with requests for disclosure.
- GMC assessors are entitled to access confidential patient health records under section 35A of the Medical Act 1983.
- Under the Health and Social Care Act 2008, the CQC has powers of inspection, entry and to require documents and information (including medical records) from English NHS trusts.[55]

A number of the regulatory bodies have codes of practice governing how they will access and use personal information.[56] The GMC advises that doctors should, where practicable, inform patients about such disclosures even if their consent is not required (unless to do so would undermine the purpose).[57] Disclosures in relation to the investigation of complaints and into the fitness to practise of health professionals are discussed on pages 214–215.

Applications for court orders must be served on patients and, if they object to the disclosure of the information, they must be given an opportunity to make representations to the court. However, often applications are served on healthcare organisations when they should be served on patients. In these circumstances the patient should be informed of the application so they can make their representations to court if they object. Where a court order is served, health professionals are required to disclose information when they believe on reasonable grounds that information falls within that requested by the court, and should disclose only as much information as is requested. Failure to comply with a court order to release records may be an offence, but doctors should object to the judge or presiding officer if they believe that the records contain information that should not be disclosed, for example because it relates to third parties unconnected with the proceedings. Whenever possible, patients should be informed of disclosures required by a court.

In the case of *R (TB) v Stafford Combined Courts* the High Court affirmed the importance of medical confidentiality and the right of the patient to make representations before medical information is disclosed.[58]

The right to make representations before disclosure

TB, aged 14 years, was the main prosecution witness in the trial of a 34-year-old man for sexual offences. At the time of the offences, TB was receiving psychiatric treatment. The accused's solicitors issued a summons to the NHS Trust to produce TB's medical records. The initial hearing took place in November 2005 when the NHS was represented but not TB. The defence argued that the alleged abuse was merely a fantasy of TB. The judge said that the defendant's right to a fair trial outweighed TB's right to confidentiality and ordered disclosure of her psychiatric records. These showed she had a history of self-harm and suicide attempts. Following the Official Solicitor's intervention, TB was belatedly asked to attend court. Without time to arrange legal representation, TB reluctantly consented to disclosure. She subsequently applied for judicial review on the basis that her right to privacy under Article 8 of the European Convention on Human Rights had been infringed because she had not been represented and had not been able to make representations. In its judgment the High Court agreed with her that the existing rules, which did not oblige the court to give her notice of the summons against the NHS Trust, were inconsistent with Article 8. In future no such application should proceed unless the patient has been told and given the opportunity to make representations.[59]

In Scotland, the system of precognition means there may be limited disclosure of information, to both the Crown and defence, without express consent from the patient in a forthcoming trial.[60] This must be confined solely to the nature of the injuries, the patient's mental state or pre-existing conditions or health, documented by the examining doctor, and the likely mechanism by which they occurred.

Disclosure to solicitors

Health records that are required for legal proceedings are usually obtained via the Data Protection Act 1998 (see pages 190–191). Health professionals releasing information to lawyers acting for their patients should ensure that the lawyer has provided them with the patient's written consent to disclosure and, where there is any doubt, confirm that the patient understands the nature and extent of the information to be disclosed. In practice, most solicitors provide the patient's signed consent when making the request for confidential information. If a solicitor acting for someone else seeks information about a patient, his or her consent to the release of the information must be obtained. Should the patient refuse, the solicitor may apply for a court order requiring disclosure of the information. Joint BMA and Law Society consent forms for the disclosure of records in England and Wales and Scotland are available to help improve the process of seeking consent by ensuring that patients are well informed about these matters.[61]

Disclosure to the police, social services and partner organisations

Some statutes permit, rather than require, disclosure. Unless the legislation is explicit about not needing consent, however, consent is still a legal and ethical requirement. An example is the Crime and Disorder Act 1998, which permits disclosure to partner organisations, such as the police, local authority or probation service.[62] While doctors should not obstruct a police investigation, there is no legal obligation on them to disclose confidential information if requested to do so (unless a court order has been obtained). Similarly, the Children's Act 1989 permits disclosure to other organisations such as local authorities, social services and schools.[63] In such cases, health professionals may only disclose information when the patient has given consent or there is an overriding public interest (see pages 199–206). In the case of a crime, GMC guidance recognises that there may be an overriding public interest to disclose information to assist in the prevention, detection or prosecution of 'serious' crime, especially crimes against the person (see pages 203–204).[64] (Information sharing as it applies to children and young people is discussed further on pages 220–221 and in detail in Chapter 4. For confidentiality as it relates to the provision of contraception to people aged under 16 years see Chapter 7, pages 271–275 and to the Sexual Offences Act 2003 see Chapter 7, page 273.)

Many health organisations have what is called a section 29 form for requests for disclosure to the police. Such forms usually require an explanation of the purpose for the disclosure and clarification of the information that is needed, enabling health professionals to consider whether the disclosure is justified and how it might be minimised where disclosure is deemed appropriate.[65]

If health professionals have any doubts about whether the disclosure requested by police, lawyers or others is a statutory obligation, they should ask the person or body applying for the information to specify the nature of the authority under which it is sought and seek advice where there is uncertainty.

Summary – statutory and legal disclosures

- Where a statutory requirement exists, doctors are obliged to disclose the required information regardless of patient consent.
- Patients should generally be told about the disclosure unless to do so would undermine the purposes of the disclosure.
- A court can order disclosure of information.
- There is no general legal obligation to disclose information to the police, but in the case of a crime causing serious harm there may be circumstances where disclosure is required in the public interest.

Statutory restrictions on disclosure

Health professionals are required by law to restrict the disclosure of some specific types of highly sensitive information.

Examples of statutory restrictions on disclosure in the UK

- The Gender Recognition Act 2004 allows transsexual people who have taken decisive steps to live fully and permanently in their acquired gender to apply for legal recognition of that gender. The Act makes it an offence to disclose 'protected information' when that information is acquired in an official capacity. It defines 'protected information' as information about a person's application to the Gender Recognition Panel for gender recognition and a person's gender history after that person has changed gender under the Act.[66]
- The NHS (Venereal Disease) Regulations 1974 provide that any information capable of identifying an individual who is examined or treated for any sexually transmitted disease, including HIV, shall not be disclosed, other than to a medical practitioner in connection with the treatment of the individual or for the prevention of the spread of the disease. In England and Wales, this obligation extends to all employees of trusts or commissioning bodies under the NHS Trusts and PCTs (Sexually Transmitted Diseases) Directions 2000. Guidance from the GMC states that these regulations do not prevent other healthcare staff, for example the patient's GP, from disclosing information with appropriate consent. The GMC recognises that there are different interpretations of the Regulations and Directions. In particular, there have been concerns that a strict interpretation would prevent the disclosure of relevant information, except to other doctors or those working under their supervision, even with the patient's consent, or to known sexual contacts in the public interest. The view

of the GMC is that the Regulations and Directions do not preclude disclosure if it would otherwise be lawful at common law, for example with the patient's consent or in the public interest without consent.[67]

- The Human Fertilisation and Embryology Act 1990 protects the confidentiality of the information kept by clinics and the Human Fertilisation and Embryology Authority (HFEA). Information can only be viewed by people working in licensed centres; by staff or members of the HFEA (plus, in certain circumstances, the Registrar General or a court); the person to whom the information relates; and another licensed centre to enable that centre to carry out its licensed functions.[68] Information can also be disclosed with the consent of each person identifiable from the information, in medical emergencies and in connection with specific formal proceedings.[69] Disclosure of information that identifies the patient to another party without the patient's explicit consent is a criminal offence. The Human Fertilisation and Embryology Act 2008 amends the 1990 Act to permit information protected under the Act to be disclosed for research purposes. This was given effect through the Human Fertilisation and Embryology (Disclosure of information for research purposes) Regulations 2010.[70] At the time of writing it was unclear what functions would remain with the HFEA following the Government's proposals to reduce the number of arm's-length bodies (see Chapter 8, page 314).

Disclosures in the public interest

In the absence of patient consent, a legal obligation to disclose or anonymisation, any decision as to whether identifiable information is to be shared with third parties must be made on a case-by-case basis and must be justifiable in the 'public interest'. Justifications that would generally warrant disclosures in the public interest include disclosure that is essential to prevent or lessen a serious and imminent threat to public health, national security, the life of the individual or a third party or to prevent or detect serious crime. The GMC also advises that, in some circumstances, a disclosure without consent can be justified in the public interest to enable medical research (see pages 207–209).[71] In all cases, the facts must be subject to close scrutiny as to whether there is a genuine necessity for disclosure. Ultimately, the public interest in specific cases can only be determined by the courts. There have been few cases dealing with this and so it is difficult to state the legal position with any certainty. The case of *W v Egdell* (below) is an example where the public interest in disclosure trumped the public interest in protecting confidentiality.

Disclosure in the public interest

W suffered from paranoid schizophrenia and shot and killed five people and injured two others in 1974. At his trial, his plea of guilty to manslaughter on the grounds of diminished responsibility was accepted and he was detained indefinitely in a secure hospital.

In 1986, the responsible medical officer recommended to the Secretary of State that W be transferred to a regional secure unit, which could eventually lead to him returning to the community. The Secretary of State refused consent. W then applied to a mental health review tribunal. To support his application for a transfer to a regional secure unit he sought a report from an independent consultant psychiatrist, Dr Egdell.

Dr Egdell's report did not support W's application. It disclosed that W had a long-standing and continuing interest in homemade bombs and did not accept the view that W was no longer a danger to the public. W withdrew his application to the tribunal and refused to consent to Dr Egdell disclosing the report to the medical officer at the secure hospital.

Dr Egdell, however, was of the view that the report should be known to those treating W, and disclosed the report to the medical officer. Copies were subsequently sent to the Secretary of State and the Department of Health and Social Security. W challenged this decision. The Court of Appeal held that it was necessary to balance the public interest in maintaining confidentiality against the public interest in protecting others against possible violence. W lost his case because Dr Egdell's disclosure had been in the public interest and in accordance with the advice of the GMC.[72]

This case demonstrates that a doctor has a duty not only to the patient, but also to the public and that the concept of 'the public interest' can override the duty of confidence to the patient in some limited circumstances.

As stated in the NHS Code of Practice on confidentiality, healthcare professionals are permitted to disclose personal information where the public good that would be achieved by the disclosure outweighs both the obligation of confidentiality to the individual patient concerned, and the wider public interest in a confidential health service.[73] As a supplement to the Code of Practice, the Department of Health has also produced guidance on public interest disclosures to assist NHS staff in making decisions on whether a breach of patient confidentiality can be justified in the public interest.[74] The guidance provides useful public interest exemplar cases.[75]

In the BMA's view, confidentiality is too important a principle to be sacrificed for vague goals or indefinable harms, but it should generally give way where there is some 'serious' threat to people. The BMA has identified threats to living people as significant in a way in which threats to property or financial interests generally are not. In line with this reasoning, the risk of an assault, a traffic accident or an infectious disease may be seen as more compelling grounds for disclosure than risk relating to fraud or theft.

In reality, such neat divisions are not entirely satisfactory and, in many cases, harm is multi-faceted. Serious fraud or theft involving NHS resources, for example, may harm individuals awaiting treatment. Even comparatively minor prescription fraud may reveal a serious harm if prescriptions for controlled drugs are being forged.

In this comparatively narrow sphere there is no broad consensus of how harm to people should be evaluated or from whose perspective it should be judged. For the victim who suffers harm or loss, it may be perceived in very different terms than by a decision maker outside the situation who is trying to weigh it up. The BMA's advice is that, where feasible, health professionals should try to envisage the seriousness of the potential harm from the viewpoint of the person likely to suffer it.

Some serious crimes almost invariably justify disclosure of relevant information to the police. Examples include murder, manslaughter, rape and child abuse (see below). Serious harm, however, is a much wider concept than that of serious criminal activity and it encompasses omissions, such as neglect, as well as acts. It must also take account of psychological as well as physical damage. Child neglect or abuse is an example of treatment whose psychological sequelae may be considerably more profound than the physical harm suffered, and the psychological damage may be experienced not only by the actual victim, but also by siblings who know of it. When considering non-consensual disclosure, health professionals rightly take into account that the degree of psychological harm for victims may be influenced by the manner in which the disclosure is handled.

Advisory bodies, such as the BMA, cannot tell doctors whether or not to disclose information in a particular case, but can provide general guidance about the categories of cases in which decisions to disclose may be justifiable. Doctors should be aware that they risk criticism if they fail to take action to avoid serious harm. Guidance can also be sought from Caldicott Guardians (senior NHS staff who are appointed to protect the confidentiality of patient information), indemnifying or regulatory bodies where there is any doubt as to whether disclosure should take place in the public interest. It may also be helpful to discuss situations on an anonymous basis with colleagues.

Balancing benefits and harms

A decision to disclose is often not based on the interests of the person concerned but is made to protect other people or the public at large. The decision to disclose is based partly on a balancing of several moral imperatives, including the risk and likelihood of harm if no disclosure is made, and the need to maintain the trust of the patient and the harms that may result from breach of confidence. Health professionals can be in an invidious position in having to weigh speculative as well as known facts, and assess whether a perceived harm can be better averted by making a disclosure or by maintaining the trust of an individual while attempting to persuade him or her to disclose voluntarily.

In some cases, although a duty of confidentiality is owed, the need to protect other people may tip the balance. This may be the case, for example, when domestic violence occurs in a family where children are at risk. In many cases, however, clear and unambiguous information upon which to judge the potential threat is unavailable. Non-consensual disclosure is generally considered justifiable in cases where the threat appears serious, and disclosure is likely to limit or prevent it occurring.

Urgency of the need to disclose

In all cases, delay is inadvisable when the risks are imminent, serious and foreseeable. Health professionals who are unable to persuade an individual to disclose voluntarily information that could prevent serious harm to other people are likely to be justified in disclosing without consent. In some cases, it is inadvisable to ask for consent (see below).

Involving the individual

It is desirable for individuals to be strongly encouraged to take responsibility for disclosure themselves, while being made aware that a reluctance to do so may oblige the health professional to take action. Persuasion may require time, counselling and repeated consultations. Health professionals must therefore weigh up the potential immediacy of the risk in relation to the likelihood of eventually persuading the individual and consider whether the objective of preventing harm is achievable by other means.

In some cases, it is clearly inadvisable to alert the individual to the fact that health professionals are considering disclosure. Such cases arise, for example, when telling the patient would exacerbate the threat, possibly also resulting in violence against the health professional, or it may give time to destroy evidence that is necessary to secure the long-term protection of the other people at risk. Typical examples are those involving paedophile activities or production of child pornography.

Making a disclosure

Decisions to disclose information in the public interest should ideally be taken by health professionals, with the advice of the Caldicott Guardian, although there may be some circumstances where other health staff may need to disclose.[76] Whenever possible, the clinician with overall responsibility for care must be consulted when a disclosure is made. Where serious incidents are reported it may be useful for the whole team to discuss the case on an anonymous basis in order to learn from the experience. Advice can also be sought from professional, regulatory and indemnifying bodies.

Disclosure without consent should reveal the minimum of information required to deal with the risk and careful thought must be given to the question of to whom the information should be released. Doctors should seek assurances that the information will be used only for the purposes for which it was disclosed.

A doctor must be prepared to justify any decision regarding disclosure, and may be asked to do so before the GMC. The reasons for disclosing without consent should be documented in order to demonstrate that a clear and balanced approach has been taken. In line with advice from the GMC, doctors must also be prepared to justify a decision not to disclose, for example if they believe this would not be in the best interests of a neglected or abused patient (see page 205).[77]

Examples of disclosure in the public interest

This section considers some examples of situations where doctors might have to consider disclosure in the public interest. Health professionals have clear moral duties to individual patients and to colleagues which may come into conflict with wider obligations to avert serious and preventable harm to others. This section takes some examples of situations where disclosure could be in the public interest, and discusses what doctors should do if patients refuse to permit this. Dangers arising from the health or performance of colleagues, and decisions to disclose information, are discussed in Chapter 21. Specific issues that arise in public health are discussed in Chapter 20.

The BMA does not seek to lay down blanket rules in such situations and recognises that there may be scope for negotiation with patients which allows them to make the disclosure at their own pace, without exposing others to risk. It is hoped there will be few such cases that cannot be resolved in this way. Doctors must bear in mind that they may have to justify the decisions they take and seek advice where there is doubt.

Health

When a person has a medical condition that puts others at risk, for example a risk of infection or because of dangerous behaviour, doctors must discuss with the patient how to minimise the risk to others. Ultimately, however, the doctor may need to disclose without consent if, for example, a Heavy Goods Vehicle driver has narcolepsy – and the patient needs to be aware of this.

Informing sexual contacts of patients with a serious communicable disease

In the case of patients with a sexually transmitted serious communicable disease, doctors should discuss with the patient the need to inform sexual partners and the options for safer sex. Exceptionally, if patients refuse to modify their behaviour or inform others, doctors are advised by the GMC that they may breach confidentiality and inform a known sexual contact of a patient with a sexually transmitted serious communicable disease (see below). Reckless transmission of HIV can amount to a criminal offence.[78]

> **GMC guidance on informing sexual contacts of patients with a serious communicable disease**[79]
>
> 'You may disclose information to a known sexual contact of a patient with a sexually transmitted serious communicable disease if you have reason to think that they are at risk of infection and that the patient has not informed them and cannot be persuaded to do so. In such circumstances, you should tell the patient before you make the disclosure, if it is practicable and safe to do so. You must be prepared to justify a decision to disclose personal information without consent.'[80]
> Wherever possible, patients should always be told before this step is taken.

The same considerations apply to circumstances where the potential disclosure relates to a colleague who poses a threat to the health of his or her patients by reason of illness, incompetence or addiction (see Chapter 21).

Public safety

A common example of what can be categorised as public safety occurs in connection with the assessment of patients with, for example, diabetes, epilepsy, defective eyesight or serious cardiac conditions who have been advised by health professionals to discontinue driving, but who nevertheless continue. When an individual has insight into the problem, it is advisable for health professionals to attempt to persuade that person to either discontinue the risky behaviour or agree to disclosure being made to a responsible body as one step towards a change of behaviour. In some cases, the individual is unable or unwilling to follow the recommended course of action and health professionals have to weigh up the likelihood of serious harm and the need to breach confidentiality. The GMC advises that where a patient continues to drive when they may not be fit to do so, doctors should contact the Driver and Vehicle Licensing Agency (DVLA) and disclose any relevant medical information, in confidence, to the medical adviser.[81]

Issues of public safety may similarly arise in circumstances where an individual who legitimately possesses firearms is thought by health professionals to be a risk because of drug or alcohol addiction or a medical condition such as depression (see Chapter 16, page 666). The police should be informed if anybody is thought to be at risk.

Serious crime and national security

Disclosure necessary for the prevention, detection, investigation or punishment of a serious offence is widely regarded as justifiable and desirable. The definition of what constitutes a 'serious' crime is a matter of debate. In the BMA's view 'serious crimes' are those that may result in serious harm or loss of life for individuals. These offences can be regarded as very substantially more significant than crimes involving theft, minor fraud or damage to property. The NHS Code of Practice on confidentiality provides some guidance on the meaning of serious crime and risk of harm (see below).

> **NHS Code of Practice on confidentiality: examples of disclosure to protect the public**
>
> *Serious crime and national security*
>
> 'Murder, manslaughter, rape, treason, kidnapping, child abuse or other cases where individuals have suffered serious harm may all warrant breaching confidentiality. Serious harm to the security of the state or to public order and crimes that involve

substantial financial gain or loss will also generally fall within this category. In contrast, theft, fraud or damage to property where loss or damage is less substantial would generally not warrant a breach of confidence'.[82]

Risk of harm

'Disclosures to prevent serious harm or abuse also warrant a breach of confidence. The risk of child abuse or neglect, assault, a traffic accident or the spread of an infectious disease are perhaps the most common that staff may face. However, consideration of harm should also inform decisions about disclosure in relation to crime. Serious fraud or theft involving NHS resources would be likely to harm individuals waiting for treatment. A comparatively minor prescription fraud may actually be linked to serious harm if prescriptions for controlled drugs are being forged. It is also important to consider the impact of harm or neglect from the point of view of the victim(s) and to take account of psychological as well as physical danger. For example, the psychological impact of child abuse or neglect may harm siblings who know of it in addition to the child concerned.'[83]

When it is not possible to seek consent for disclosure of information about a crime, the following conditions should be satisfied before relevant information is disclosed.

- The crime must be sufficiently serious for the public interest to prevail, and
- the disclosure would be likely to assist in the prevention, detection or prosecution of the serious crime.[84]

Part of the balance in considering whether to disclose will also depend on the extent and the nature of the disclosure required – namely, if particularly sensitive information is required – as well as the relative seriousness of the crime. A common enquiry to the BMA is the situation in which many GPs find themselves, when the police are investigating a crime near the practice premises and want to know who attended the surgery in a given time period. The fact of attendance is, in itself, confidential and should not be disclosed unless disclosure can be justified according to the criteria set out above.

Similarly, doctors are often asked to speculate on the identity of the perpetrator of a minor crime, such as the theft of personal belongings from healthcare premises. It is unlikely that such crime would be considered to be of sufficient severity to warrant a breach of confidentiality. The police do not have an automatic right of access to information and doctors should seek an explanation of the purpose for the disclosure in order to enable them to consider whether the disclosure is justified.[85]

Reporting gunshot and knife wounds

Gunshot and knife wounds raise issues that warrant special consideration. As a direct response to a request from the Association of Chief Police Officers, GMC guidance advises that all gunshot and knife wounds, unless they are as a result of accidental injury or self-harm, must be reported to the police on an anonymised basis whenever a victim arrives at hospital.[86] When the police subsequently attend the hospital, identifying details, such as name and address, can only be disclosed with patient consent or in the absence of patient consent where it is in the public interest or required by law.[87]

Safety in the workplace

Disclosure is justifiable when failure to do so in regard to the health status of an employee could foreseeably result in a substantial risk to others. For example, an occupational health doctor has a responsibility to take action if he or she is aware that the health of an employee threatens the safety of others (see Chapter 16, pages 674–676). Similarly, GPs may need to take action if they become aware that a patient they consider to be a threat to vulnerable people begins working with young children, elderly people or other vulnerable groups. The vetting and barring scheme, which came into force in England, Wales and Northern Ireland in 2009, requires people who are engaged in 'regulated activity' and who work with vulnerable groups to be registered with the Independent Safeguarding Authority (ISA). Any person who is thought to pose a risk should be reported to the ISA. (For further discussion see Chapter 19, pages 794–795.)

Action may also be necessary if a colleague poses a threat to the health of his or her patients by reason of illness, incompetence, misconduct or addiction. This issue is addressed in Chapter 21.

Abuse and domestic violence

Knowing what to do when patients do not want confidential information to be disclosed, despite this being the best way to ensure that they do not suffer harm or abuse, is very difficult for doctors. Abuse of dependent older people may fall into this category, as may domestic violence (see Chapter 15, page 640). Safeguarding children where there are concerns or beliefs about child abuse is discussed in Chapter 4, pages 177–178.

Patients with capacity have the right to object to information they provide in confidence being disclosed to a third party in a form that identifies them, even if this is to someone who might provide essential healthcare. Victims of abuse may be concerned that disclosure of what has occurred may lead to further maltreatment. There are no easy solutions, but doctors must bear in mind such factors as whether other people in institutions, or in the family, are also at risk. High-risk cases of domestic abuse are discussed in local Multi-Agency Risk Assessment Conferences (MARACs). Health professionals can make referrals to MARACs using the Co-ordinated Action Against Domestic Violence (CAADA) Risk Identification Checklist which helps referring agencies determine the level of risk.[88] Disclosure of information to MARACs or to any other agencies should be made with the consent of the patient. The exceptions to this are where confidentiality can be overridden either by a court order (or other legal requirement) or in the public interest. Public interest justifications in such cases usually relate to disclosures to prevent significant harm to third parties or to prevent or prosecute a serious crime, as discussed on pages 199–201.

Patients may need time to come to a firm decision about disclosure after having the benefits carefully explained. Counselling and support in the interim may help the patient to decide. Ultimately, in circumstances where an adult with capacity is at risk of serious harm and refuses to agree to the sharing of information that would seem to be in their best interests, this must usually be respected.

It is particularly important in the context of domestic abuse that patients are involved in all stages of the decision-making process, and that they retain as much control as possible over disclosures of information. When treating a patient who has disclosed domestic abuse it is the responsibility of the healthcare professional to emphasise that, although information given to them by the patient is confidential, there are limits to this confidentiality. Where a healthcare professional decides, after considering all the available evidence and the wishes of a patient with capacity, to disclose this information to an appropriate third party in the public interest, they should ensure that the patient will not be put at increased risk following disclosure.

Patients lacking capacity

Knowledge or belief of abuse and neglect of a patient lacking capacity (including a child) is an exceptional circumstance that will usually justify a healthcare professional making a disclosure in the public interest to an appropriate person or agency. Where health professionals have concerns about a patient lacking capacity, who may be at risk of abuse or neglect, it is essential that these concerns are acted upon and information is given promptly to an appropriate person or statutory body, in order to prevent further harm. If the healthcare professional has reason to believe a patient lacking capacity is at risk, then protection must take precedence over confidentiality. Where there is any doubt as to whether disclosure is considered to be in the patient's best overall interests, it is recommended that the health professional discusses the matter, on an anonymised basis, with a senior colleague, the Caldicott Guardian, their professional body or defence organisation. Health professionals should ensure that their concerns and the actions they have taken or intend to take, including any discussion with the patient, colleagues or professionals in other agencies, are clearly recorded in the patient's medical records.

GMC advice: neglect or abuse of people who lack capacity

'If you believe that a patient may be a victim of neglect or physical, sexual or emotional abuse, and that they lack the capacity to consent to disclosure, you must give information promptly to an appropriate responsible person or authority, if you believe that the disclosure is in the patient's best interests or necessary to protect others from a risk of serious harm. If, for any reason, you believe that disclosure of information is not in the best interests of a neglected or abused patient, you should discuss the issues with an experienced colleague. If you decide not to disclose the information, you should document in the patient's record your discussion and the reasons for deciding not to disclose. You should be prepared to justify your decision.'[89]

For further discussion on confidentiality when the patient cannot give consent see pages 218–220, or where a child lacks capacity see pages 220–221.

Summary – disclosure in the public interest

When considering disclosing information to protect the public interest, doctors must:

- consider how the benefits of making the disclosure balance against the harms associated with breaching a patient's confidentiality
- assess the urgency of the need for disclosure
- consider whether the person could be persuaded to disclose voluntarily
- inform the person before making the disclosure and seek consent, unless to do so would enhance the risk of harm
- reveal identifiable information only if anonymised information will not suffice
- reveal only the minimum information necessary to achieve the objective
- seek assurances that the information will be used only for the purposes for which it was disclosed
- be able to justify the decision
- document the reasons for disclosure or a decision not to disclose.

Secondary uses of patient information

Disclosure for purposes associated with providing healthcare

Patient health information is collected primarily to provide care for individual patients. Patient data are also necessary for a variety of other functions related to the provision of healthcare and in order for the NHS to function effectively. This section focuses on secondary uses of patient information within the NHS (or for social care purposes). Secondary uses where identifiable information goes beyond healthcare provision in the NHS are covered on pages 216–218.

Unless there is specific legal provision to suggest otherwise, express consent is generally needed to use or disclose identifiable information for purposes associated with healthcare, other than those disclosures that support the direct provision of care to patients and are covered on pages 187–189. The GMC states that: '[a]s a general rule, you should seek a patient's express consent before disclosing identifiable information for purposes other than the provision of their care or local clinical audit.'[90] Such purposes include public health surveillance, financial audit and teaching. The GMC further states that doctors should 'be satisfied that the patient has sufficient information about the scope, purpose and likely consequences' of the disclosure.[91] Safeguards are always essential for disclosure of identifiable information but arguably the more distant the data from the direct provision of patient care, the more robust the safeguards should be as the more unlikely it is that patients will be aware of it, or the uses to which such data will be put. As highlighted in this section, it is good practice to use anonymised data for any secondary purpose where it is practicable to do so and to raise patient awareness about such usage.

Medical research

The use of healthcare data for medical research is an evolving area of practice in which a number of ethical dilemmas are brought into sharp focus. Lively debate over this particular secondary use of data has taken place against a backdrop of significant advancements in computer technology, changes in the way information flows within healthcare settings, competing commercial interests and political pressures.

The NHS Constitution for England stresses the commitment to research in the NHS: '[t]he NHS aspires to the highest standards of excellence and professionalism . . . through its commitment to innovation and to the promotion and conduct of research to improve the current and future health and care of the population.'[92] It also stresses a commitment to confidentiality: '[y]ou have the right to privacy and confidentiality and to expect the NHS to keep your information confidential and secure'.[93]

As well as participation in clinical trials, many research projects are carried out using patient data. As is emphasised throughout this chapter, patients should be able to expect that information about their health, which has been given in confidence, will be kept confidential unless there is a compelling reason why it should not. At the same time, this right to confidentiality must be balanced against the improvements and advancements in patient care that can be brought about through good quality research projects. Researchers have long expressed concern that inflexible rules about obtaining consent for the use of identifiable data impedes improvements to patient care.[94] They also wish to take advantage of the new and valuable opportunities that have been opened up by the development of electronic records systems.

Clearly, it is in the interests of society and future patients to conduct research for the advancement of healthcare but there is also a public interest in a confidential health service and there are concerns that a reduction in the requirement for consent could lead to a loss of public trust in health services. As is stressed throughout this book, honest and open exchange between doctors and patients is the ideal, and patients need to be able to trust doctors and the health service not to share information without sufficient justification. It has been argued that to lower the bar for the requirement for consent for the use of identifiable information would threaten the nature of the therapeutic relationship between doctors and patients.[95] Most patients want research to be carried out but wish to be asked if their own identifiable data are used.[96] Patients and the general public surveyed by the Department of Health in 2008 were clear that they expected their consent to be sought for the use of their identifiable data for the purpose of medical research.[97]

The consequence of these competing interests is that a balance must be struck between maintaining confidence in a secure health service while trying to achieve the benefits research can bring to patient care and health service developments in the future. In 2009, the GMC published guidance that set out the circumstances when disclosures of identifiable information can take place for research purposes in the public interest (see below). (For further discussion on records-based research, see Chapter 14, pages 604–606.)

Guidance from the GMC

Guidance from the GMC identifies medical research as a justifiable reason for a public interest disclosure without consent if:

- it is necessary to use identifiable information; or
- it is not practicable to anonymise the information and, in either case not practicable to seek consent.[98]

The GMC also sets out a number of factors which must be taken into account in any consideration as to whether the research justifies a breach of confidentiality in the public interest:

- the nature of the information must be considered
- the use that will be made of it
- how many people will have access to it
- the security arrangements to protect further disclosure
- the advice of an independent expert advisor such as a Caldicott Guardian, should be sought
- the potential for harm or distress to patients.[99]

Research governance

All research, both within and outside the NHS, must be subject to approval by an appropriately constituted research ethics committee (REC), which has responsibility for considering confidentiality issues. However, REC approval is not sufficient to justify a breach of confidentiality as these committees cannot authorise unconsented disclosure or determine if disclosure is justified in the public interest. When faced with requests for access to identifiable data from researchers, the BMA believes that health professionals must assess each case on its individual merits. It may be difficult to make a judgement as to when the public interest constitutes a legitimate reason for disclosure for research but generally the REC's scrutiny will have assessed the risks and benefits. If in doubt as to whether research is in the public interest doctors should seek further advice from the GMC or the National Information Governance Board (see below).[100]

Additionally, doctors may be aware of specific circumstances in relation to their population of patients, or to individuals, which may not have been brought to the attention of the approving committee. In such circumstances doctors can contact the committee chair and explain their concerns. In some exceptional circumstances doctors, as part of their role as advocates for patients, may elect not to disclose information where there are particular concerns, for example if a patient has suffered a recent bereavement or where individuals have asked for their information not to be used for research purposes.

Chapter 14 addresses the issue of research governance, together with discussion of the particular questions that arise when the subjects of research are incapacitated adults or children who are unable to give consent to disclosure.

Looking towards the future

As traditional patterns of healthcare provision continue to change, with a move away from a personalised healthcare service to care being provided by a more diverse healthcare team, and with fewer patients having the established individual relationship with their doctor that predominated in the twentieth century, the ethical debate about the use of data within the healthcare setting will continue. There has also been wide-ranging discussion within the BMA regarding the way data flow within the healthcare system and the principles that should underpin any new data management system, so that it is deemed trustworthy and secure by patients and healthcare professionals alike. One of the recommendations put forward by a number of commentators is a call for the public to be much more informed about how their information is used.[101] This may encourage a wider discussion about the benefits of using medical records for research alongside considerations of confidentiality and consent and in which circumstances access by researchers should be permitted.

Honest brokers and safe havens

As part of the debate around the use of health data for research, the concepts of 'honest brokers' and 'safe havens'[102] have been introduced. Honest brokers have been described as 'trusted custodians of data' with responsibility for ensuring access in accordance with relevant law and practice and the decisions and guidance of relevant information governance boards. The role would have the responsibility for ensuring that coding and anonymisation processes are correctly specified and implemented. They would also carry out permitted statistical linkage of data and carry out appropriate data quality checks.[103]

Safe havens have been described as a 'designated physical or electronic area that provides the most appropriate level of security for the use of the most sensitive and confidential information'.[104]

The concept of honest brokers and safe havens in order to process and manage the disclosure of identifiable data, including its anonymisation or coding, was approved by the GMC in 2009 guidance on confidentiality.[105]

The Health and Social Care Bill, introduced into Parliament in January 2011, contained proposals to give the NHS Information Centre power to act as an honest broker for health and social care data.

Disclosures under section 251 of the NHS Act 2006

In England and Wales, section 251 of the NHS Act 2006 (originally enacted under section 60 of the Health and Social Care Act 2001) gives the Secretary of State for Health power to make regulations that allow for the common law duty of confidentiality to be set aside in specific circumstances, where anonymised information is not sufficient and where patient consent is not practicable. These regulations are manifested in the

Health Service (Control of Patient Information) Regulations 2002 and can only be used to support 'medical purposes' that are in the interests of patients or the wider public. Section 251 and the accompanying regulations came about because it was recognised that there were essential NHS activities, and important medical research, that required the use of identifiable information, but because patient consent had not been obtained for the use of confidential information for these purposes, there was no secure basis in law for these uses. For example, the first regulations included section 251 approval for cancer registries and support for the Health Protection Agency to collect data relating to communicable disease surveillance. When approached about disclosures to disease registries, other than cancer registries, doctors should check whether section 251 approval has been given in each case before disclosing identifiable information. The Act was intended largely as a transitional measure while consent or anonymisation procedures were developed, but it is now acknowledged that section 251 powers, or other statutory support, will be necessary in the longer term for some activities (see also pages 191–192).

Responsibility for administering powers under section 251 lies with the NIGB. The NIGB has delegated these powers to the ECC which, until 2009, was the Patient Information Advisory Group (PIAG). When deciding whether confidential patient information can be used within the NHS, the ECC considers a number of factors. NIGB has produced guidance on the ECC approval process and the relevant legislative requirements. The main factors that are taken into consideration are listed below.

The Health and Social Care Bill introduced into Parliament in January 2011 contained proposals to abolish NIGB and transfer its statutory functions to the CQC. The proposals included a provision requiring the CQC to appoint a National Information Governance Committee until March 2015. (Up-to-date information can be found on the BMA website.)

ECC approval process

Public interest considerations

- The public good that might be served by the research
- The risks to individuals (from a breach of confidence).

Data protection considerations

- Fair processing – taking account of the conditions that apply to fair processing for medical purposes (including medical research), have patients been made sufficiently aware of what is proposed?
- Is the minimum information required to satisfy the purpose being used?
- What will happen to the data after the research ends?

Considerations in respect of what is reasonably practicable

- Are there other, less sensitive, sources of data that could be used to satisfy the purpose, for example the electoral roll?
- What are the reasons for not obtaining patient consent?
- What prevents the researchers selecting a cohort from pseudonymised information?[106]

In Northern Ireland, the Privacy Advisory Committee can advise on some of the same considerations, although it has no statutory powers and so cannot give lawful authority to disclosures of identifiable information without consent. Discussions are ongoing about the need to introduce a new legislative framework for information governance in that jurisdiction.

In Scotland, patient information is brought together and managed at a national level by the Information Services Division (ISD), which is part of the NHS National Services Scotland. A Privacy Advisory Committee provides advice to the Caldicott Guardian for the ISD on the use of personal health information for research.[107] This does not have statutory powers and so the disclosures of potentially identifiable data without consent that are agreed need to rely on the public interest justification.

Social care

When patients with capacity are receiving care from, or are being referred for care to, social services, relevant information can be shared on the basis of implied consent provided that patients are aware that health and social care providers are working together in order to provide their care (see pages 187–189).[108] The Care Record Guarantee promises that patients will be told if information is to be shared with other organisations providing care, such as social services.[109] It is always preferable to obtain explicit consent where it is possible to do so; however, as mentioned earlier in this chapter, there are numerous benefits to integrated care pathways that enable the smooth transfer of care from the health service to social care. This can have particular advantages for older people or for those with long-term conditions. Patients have the right to object to their information being shared, although they should be informed of the possible detrimental effect to their care should they object to disclosure.

Common Assessment Framework

The Common Assessment Framework (CAF) Demonstrator programme, piloted in 2010, includes support for the sharing of information across health and social care. The project provides a model for how to proceed with both health records and social care records continuing to be held by the respective organisations but with certain information made available through a shared record to professionals in multiple organisations with the consent of the individual.[110]

When patients lack the capacity to choose, relevant information may be shared with other people or agencies, such as social services, carers or near relatives of the individual when:

- it is necessary in the individual's best interests
- the disclosure is not contrary to the individual's express request or known wishes
- information is released on a 'need to know' basis.

Access to medical records by Independent Mental Capacity Advocates (IMCAs) is covered on pages 219–220.

If a patient has fluctuating capacity or is likely to lose capacity, early discussion of this nature are beneficial and can help to avoid disclosures that patients would object to. This is discussed on pages 218–220 and in Chapter 3, page 100.

Public health

Public health surveillance and research rely on vast quantities of data. Data come from many different sources and their appropriate handling by public health physicians is essential. Anonymised data should be used wherever possible.

In some cases, the law requires the reporting of infectious diseases (see page 195 and Chapter 20, pages 847–848). Doctors must comply with such statutory requirements and tell patients what information will be disclosed and why, and reassure them that information will be used in an identifiable form only where required by law.

Where there is no statutory requirement to disclose information, and it is not possible to anonymise data, consent should be sought. Patients are generally happy for their information to be disclosed when there are good grounds and satisfactory safeguards to protect the data. Exceptionally, when it is not possible to seek consent, and it is not possible to prepare aggregated data (for example, when dealing with rare diseases that do not become adequately anonymised on aggregation), doctors in England and Wales may look to the NHS Act 2006 and consider applying for section 251 approval for the disclosure (see above). The Health Protection Agency and Director of Public Health in England and Wales have statutory support through the Health Service (Control of Patient Information) Regulations 2002 to support communicable disease surveillance and monitoring and prevent the spread of other risks to public health such as environmental hazards. In the rest of the UK, there is no support in law for disclosures of identifiable information without consent that do not meet a 'public interest' justification for breach of confidentiality (see pages 199–202).

Doctors' responsibilities in relation to protecting the public's health is covered in detail in Chapter 20.

Teaching

Teaching is an essential process but, in the BMA's view, the public interest does not justify the use of identifiable material for teaching purposes without appropriate consent. Wherever possible, anonymous information should be used. Patient identifiable materials cannot be used without consent even in the context of teaching hospitals, although there are no restrictions on anonymous information being used in teaching. GMC advice states that: '[w]hen it is necessary to use identifiable information about a patient, or it is not practicable to anonymise information, you should seek the patient's consent before disclosing it'.[111] Images should be pixilated where possible and identifying details obscured. (The use of recordings is covered in more detail in Chapter 6, pages 247–252. More information about the use of medical information for teaching can be found in Chapter 18, pages 755–756.)

Junior doctors and medical students accessing records

Where junior doctors are not part of the team providing care, they cannot have access to identifiable patient information without the express consent of the patient. If junior doctors are part of the healthcare team providing or supporting a patient's care, GMC guidance permits access to patient identifiable information, unless the patient objects.[112]

If students need access to a patient's personal information, but are not involved in providing or supporting the patient's care, the GMC advises that anonymised information should be used whenever possible.[113] If this is not practicable, then express consent should be sought.

The issues that arise when potential medical students want to observe medical practice are covered in Chapter 18 (see pages 756–757). The key principle is that doctors should seek the patient's express consent to a student observing their care.[114]

Patients who lack capacity

In the absence of any indication about the preferences of a patient who lacks capacity, the GMC advises that personal information should not be published from which the patient can be identified but personal information may be disclosed to medical and other healthcare students and trainees to the extent necessary for their education and training.[115] If it is practicable to use information from patients who have capacity this must be done instead.[116]

An individual with parental responsibility for a young child can give consent for information to be used in teaching (although consent should be sought from the young person once he or she attains competency to give consent if identifiable materials continue to be used).

Financial audit and other healthcare management purposes

Health records are often used for a number of standard financial and administrative purposes outside the direct provision of care. These include disclosures of information for financial audit purposes by GPs to commissioning bodies, health and social services boards (HSSBs), local health boards (LHBs) or health boards for Post-Payment Verification (PPV) and the Quality and Outcomes Framework (QOF). These bodies may also require information for other purposes, such as the quality assurance of care. The BMA has produced guidance for GPs on confidentiality and disclosure of information to commissioning bodies in primary care settings.[117]

Anonymous data often satisfies standard financial purposes and should be used where possible. GMC guidance states that: '[i]f you are asked to disclose information about patients for financial or administrative purposes you should, if practicable, provide it in anonymised or coded form, if that will serve the purpose. If identifiable information is needed, you should, if practicable, seek the patient's express consent before disclosing it'.[118] Wherever possible, clinical information should be recorded separately from financial and administrative information.[119] It should be noted that no identifying information should be used for financial purposes in relation to sexually transmitted infections in line with the NHS Trusts and PCTs (Sexually Transmitted Diseases) Directions 2000 (see pages 198–199).

The GMC further advises that:

> You must draw attention to any system that prevents you from following this guidance, and recommend change. Until changes are made, you should make sure that information is readily available to patients explaining that their personal information may be disclosed for financial, administrative and similar purposes, and what they can do if they object.[120]

The Confidentiality and Disclosures of Information: General Medical Services (GMS), Personal Medical Services (PMS) and Alternative Provider Medical Services (APMS) Directions 2005 and associated codes of practice provide a limited statutory basis for commissioning bodies, HSSBs, LHBs or health boards to obtain access to information held by general practices that identifies individual patients, where the use of anonymised information is not feasible and express consent cannot be obtained.[121] Where express patient consent cannot be obtained or the data cannot be practicably anonymised, circumstances that would permit implied consent must be put in place (see below). Care should be taken to determine the minimum requirements and disclose only data that are relevant in these situations.

The codes of practice from the English, Scottish, Welsh and Northern Irish health departments emphasise that the circumstances in which commissioning bodies, HSSBs, LHBs or health boards may need to access patient identifiable information without consent should be rare. The circumstances in which patient identifiable information would reasonably be required by commissioning bodies, and could lawfully be disclosed by the GP practice, include the following:

- where the practice is unable to anonymise data that is needed to support the wider functioning of the NHS, including the management of healthcare services, such as the QOF annual review process – the practice should make a judgement in the context of each request for information as to whether anonymisation is practicable
- where the commissioning body is investigating and assuring the quality and provision of clinical care
- where it is needed in relation to the management of the contract or agreement – for example, where remedial action is being considered
- where the commissioning body considers there is a serious risk to patient health or safety
- investigation of suspected fraud or any other potential criminal activity.[122]

Doctors should take steps to ensure that patients are made aware that their information might be used for broader medical purposes related to health service management, how it will be used, to whom it will be disclosed and for what purpose. (For further information on implied consent for information sharing, see also pages 187–189). The Information Commissioner has provided advice on methods by which this 'fair processing information' can be given to patients. Methods include the following:

- posters plus a standard information leaflet
- information provided face-to-face in the course of a consultation
- information included with an appointment letter from a hospital or clinic
- information in a letter sent to a patient's home.[123]

The Information Commissioner has also stated that a poster in the surgery or waiting room, or a notice in the local paper, is unlikely to be sufficient to meet the fair processing requirements of the Data Protection Act 1998 as not all patients will see or be able to understand such information.[124] Practices should also ensure that patients are aware of their right to object to any disclosure and appropriate procedures for objection should be put in place. The NHS Code of Practice on confidentiality also emphasises the importance of making it clear to patients when identifiable information is recorded or health records are accessed and of checking that patients have seen the available information leaflets.[125]

Complaints

When patients initiate a complaint, it is unlikely to be practicable for an investigation to take place without access to relevant parts of the health record. The use of identifiable information is therefore necessary and appropriate. However, patients should be made aware of who will see information about them, and the safeguards that are in place to minimise any risks to confidentiality. It may be necessary to explain to a complainant that their complaint cannot be progressed if they refuse to authorise disclosure. Advice should be sought from regulatory or indemnifying bodies if a decision needs to be made about whether information can be disclosed in the public interest in order for a complaint to be investigated. Guidance on maintaining confidentiality in NHS complaints procedures is available from the health departments.[126]

If complaints are heard in a public forum, or a forum to which the media has access, this should be made clear. Some complaints systems, including that of the GMC, protect complainants' identities from the press. Although patients should not be discouraged from pursuing legitimate complaints, it is important that they understand, in advance, if there is any potential for media usage of health information and speculation about their condition.

Sometimes patients involve their MP or other elected representative in the complaints process. The Data Protection (Processing of Sensitive Personal Data) (Elected Representatives) Order 2002 provides a basis for the disclosure of sensitive information by organisations responding to elected representatives acting on behalf of their constituents and in connection with their functions as a representative.[127] The NHS Code of Practice on confidentiality advises that where an MP states, in writing, that he or she has a patient's consent for disclosure this may be accepted without further reference to the patient.[128] However, only information relevant to the complaint should be disclosed and the patient should be copied into the response. Guidance from the Information Commissioner makes it clear that there may be circumstances when a healthcare professional responding to an MP is justified in contacting the constituent to inform them of the intended disclosures, particularly where it is possible that disclosure could cause distress.[129]

Patients are also entitled to authorise relatives or carers to act on their behalf and health professionals who are asked to disclose information in these circumstances must be satisfied that the patient has given valid consent to the disclosure.

Investigations into healthcare professionals' fitness to practise

Information may be disclosed if it is required under the statutory powers of a regulatory body for any of the healthcare professions, where that body determines that this is necessary in the interests of justice and for the safety of other patients (see pages 196–197). Doctors should discuss this with patients whenever possible. If patient records are requested, but not required by law, or if a healthcare professional is referring concerns about another health professional to a regulatory body, then patients' express consent must be sought if practicable, unless it can be justified in the public interest.[130] If patients withhold consent, or it is not practicable to seek consent, the anonymised records should be used wherever possible. Occasionally, the statutory body may require their disclosure even if the patient objects (see pages 196–197). In these circumstances, the GMC advises that doctors should contact the appropriate regulatory body to help decide whether the disclosure can be justified in the public interest.[131]

Summary – secondary uses of patient information: disclosure for purposes associated with providing healthcare

- In addition to the direct provision of care and ensuring the quality of that care, personal health information is used for purposes associated with healthcare such as public health surveillance, research, financial audit, teaching and complaints.
- Wherever possible, personal health information used for secondary purposes should be anonymised.
- Express consent is generally needed for the use of identifiable information for purposes associated with providing healthcare; however, in relation to NHS financial and

management requirements some specific disclosures without express consent may be legitimate.

- The GMC advises that doctors can disclose identifiable information without consent for research purposes if it is in the public interest and:
  - o it is necessary to use identifiable information
  - o not practicable to anonymise the information, and
  - o not practicable to seek consent.
- Any decision as to whether identifiable information can be shared with third parties in the public interest must be made on a case-by-case basis.
- In England and Wales, it may be possible to rely on the provision of section 251 of the NHS Act 2006 for the use of information without consent for some essential NHS activities.

Uses of health information for purposes not associated with providing healthcare

This section covers uses of health information for purposes not associated with providing health care. Disclosure of information to prevent harm is covered separately on pages 199–202, with examples given on pages 202–206.

Spiritual care

Hospital chaplains or other faith representatives can provide vital support and care to people in hospital. In the case of a patient with capacity, information about affiliation and clinical information should not be passed on to spiritual advisers without the patient's consent.

When patients lack the capacity to give consent, for example because they are unconscious, those close to the patient should be consulted prior to disclosure of information to explore the patient's wishes, feelings and beliefs.[132] Spiritual care is also discussed in Chapter 1, page 26.

Disclosure to the media

When doctors are asked to disclose information to the media, the usual rules about confidentiality apply. Express consent must be obtained if patients will be identifiable from details disclosed. Doctors should be aware that patients can be identified from information other than names or addresses such as their condition or disease, their occupation, their age and the area where they live, and ensure they do not breach GMC guidance on confidentiality if the patient has not given consent. Any disclosure should be limited to the minimum necessary in the circumstances. Hospital doctors may want to take advice from their trust's solicitors and GPs from their defence bodies. When the patient lacks capacity, legal advice should be sought.

Responding to criticism in the press

Sometimes patients use the media as a vehicle to complain. The BMA does not believe that entering into an argument about the facts of a case in the media is an appropriate way for doctors to respond to allegations made by patients. In these situations, the GMC states that: '[a]lthough this can be frustrating or distressing it does not relieve you of your duty to respect your patient's confidentiality. Disclosures of patient information without consent can undermine the public's trust in the profession as well as your patient's trust in you. You must not put information you have learned in confidence about a patient in the public domain without that patient's express consent.'[133]

Where misleading information has been presented to the media, doctors who wish to respond should limit their comments to pointing out that the information is inaccurate or incomplete. Patients, and others pursuing complaints on their behalf, should be informed of any forthcoming statement.[134]

Whether it would be lawful to use images of patients for whom consent is not available is not clear. Often their faces or voices can be disguised. (The use of recordings is covered in Chapter 6, pages 247–253). Doctors approached by the media to involve incapacitated adults in such projects must take legal advice. It would rarely be in the individual's interest to be identified.

Employment, insurance and other affairs

When third parties such as insurers or employers ask for information, doctors must have written consent from the patient or a person properly authorised to act on the patient's behalf. This should be provided by the third party, as either the original consent form or a copy. The GMC states that doctors should:

- be satisfied the patient has had sufficient information about the scope, purpose and likely consequences of the examination or disclosure, and the fact that relevant information cannot be concealed
- obtain or have seen written consent to the disclosure from the patient or a person properly authorised to act on the patient's behalf
- offer to show the patient, or give them a copy of, any report you write about them for insurance purposes before it is sent, unless:
  - they have already indicated they do not wish to see it
  - disclosure would be likely to cause serious harm to the patient or anyone else
  - disclosure would be likely to reveal information about another person who does not consent.[135]

An electronic copy of the signed form is sufficient, provided that the third party can satisfy the doctor that there are robust mechanisms in place to ensure that the form has not been tampered with in any way. When disclosure of the full record is necessary, patients should understand that they are giving consent to the release of the full record and the reasons why full disclosure is required. For insurance purposes, for example, often only specific relevant information is required. The use of medical information in insurance is covered in Chapter 16, pages 654–661. The BMA has also agreed joint guidance with the Association of British Insurers (ABI) to set out best practice and provide practical advice on the use of medical information in insurance.[136] Patients also have the right to add comments or change their mind about consent. Information about consent and their rights should be given to patients by the third party.

In the case of requests for information from government departments, such as the Benefits Agency, the GMC advises doctors that they may 'accept an assurance from an officer of a government department or agency or a registered health professional acting on behalf of that patient' that the patient has consented to the disclosure.[137] For example, the BMA has an agreement with the DVLA that doctors can accept that patients have consented to the disclosure of their information on the basis of trust.[138] The DVLA accepts liability in the unlikely event that doctors release information without patient consent having been obtained. In other cases information should not be provided unless evidence is produced.

GPs are sometimes asked to provide information to a patient's family or solicitor when the family is seeking to exercise a Lasting Power of Attorney (LPA). This can take the form of a property and affairs LPA or a personal welfare LPA.[139] Situations when the patient's capacity is in doubt can be very difficult for doctors. Relatives may report aberrant behaviour but, if the patient refuses to cooperate with an assessment of his or her capacity, it can be unclear to health professionals whether they would be justified in providing medical information that would enable another person to act in the patient's interests. The BMA's advice in such cases is that health professionals must assess the information that is available from the patient's record and from third parties. As discussed in Chapter 3, capacity is presumed in adults unless it is proven otherwise. Health professionals should attempt to discuss with patients their needs and preferences and weigh up whether they appear to be making a valid decision regarding the assessment or the sharing of information resulting from it.[140] (For further discussion on patients who lack the capacity to consent, see below and Chapter 3.)

Summary – secondary uses of patient information: uses of health information for purposes not associated with providing care

- There are a range of purposes for which patient data can be used which go beyond the purposes of providing healthcare.
- Explicit or express consent is generally needed for disclosure of information for purposes not associated with the provision of healthcare.

Adults who lack capacity to consent

In the BMA's view, confidentiality is owed to all patients, regardless of their age, status or mental capacity. The fact that individuals are unable to give valid consent (be it due to immaturity, temporary or permanent lack of capacity, or an inability to communicate) neither implies that their information can be less closely guarded nor that it cannot be used or disclosed when doing so would be in their interests or satisfies some broader public interest test.

Patients with mental disorders or learning disabilities should not automatically be regarded as lacking the capacity to give or withhold their consent to disclosure of confidential information. Unless unconscious, most people can make valid decisions about some matters that affect them. An individual's mental capacity must be judged in relation to the particular decision being made.[141] Therefore, if a patient has the requisite capacity, disclosure of information to relatives or third parties requires patient consent. One of the most difficult dilemmas for health professionals occurs where the extent of the patient's mental capacity is in doubt. In such cases health professionals must assess the information that is available from the patient's health record and third parties. They should attempt to discuss with patients their needs and preferences as well as assess their ability to understand their condition and prognosis. If there is still doubt about a patient's capacity to give or withhold consent to disclosure, health professionals should seek a second opinion.

In an emergency when patients are unable to make decisions, information should be made available where this is necessary to provide treatment or to avert immediate and serious harm to any person. It is likely to be extremely rare, but if the patient has previously made explicit that disclosure is not permitted, and has acknowledged that this could entail some personal risk, information must not be released unless it is essential to prevent another person from suffering serious harm. Emergency care is discussed further in Chapter 15.

Sharing information with relatives, carers and friends

If a patient lacks capacity, health professionals may need to share information with relatives, friends or carers to enable them to assess the patient's best interests. In England and Wales, the Mental Capacity Act 2005 permits information sharing where it is in the incapacitated person's best interests.[142] Where a patient is seriously ill and lacks capacity, it would be unreasonable always to refuse to provide any information to those close to the patient on the basis that the patient has not given explicit consent. The GMC states that doctors may need to share personal information with a patient's relatives, friends or carers to enable them to assess the patient's best interests.[143] This does not, however, mean that all information should be routinely shared, and where the information is sensitive, a judgement will be needed about how much information the patient is likely to want to be shared and with whom. Where there is evidence that the patient did not want information to be shared, this usually must be respected. GMC advice regarding disclosures about patients who lack capacity is to:

• make the care of the patient your first concern
• respect the patient's dignity and privacy, and
• support and encourage the patient to be involved, as far as they want and are able, in decisions about disclosure of their personal information.[144]

Proxy decision makers

In England and Wales, under the Mental Capacity Act 2005, formal proxy decision makers in the form of welfare attorneys and court-appointed deputies can be appointed to make decisions relating to health and welfare on behalf of the incapacitated patient. Where a patient lacks capacity and has no relatives or friends to be consulted, the Mental Capacity Act requires an IMCA to be appointed and consulted about all decisions about 'serious medical treatment'. While it will therefore be necessary for attorneys, deputies or IMCAs to have access to some information, it does not mean that they will always need to have access to all the patient's records. Relevant information to deal with the issue in question should be disclosed.

In Scotland, the Adults with Incapacity (Scotland) Act 2000 allows people over the age of 16 years who have capacity to appoint a welfare attorney to make health and personal welfare decisions once capacity is lost. The Court of Session may also appoint a deputy to make these decisions. The same principles as those in England and Wales apply in that health professionals may only disclose health information when it is of benefit to the patient.

In Northern Ireland, there is no mental capacity legislation. Information should therefore only be disclosed in accordance with the common law and in the patient's best interests.

For further information on statutory provisions for proxy decision makers under the Mental Capacity Act 2005 in England and Wales see Chapter 3, pages 115–117 and pages 119–121, and for Scotland see Chapter 3, pages 129–130. (For disclosures where health professionals have concerns about a patient lacking capacity who may be at risk of abuse or neglect, see page 206. For discussion on the special rules which apply when an individual cannot consent to participation in research, see Chapter 14, pages 597–599.)

Summary – adults who lack capacity to consent

- Most people with some degree of mental capacity can make some decisions about matters that affect them.
- An individual's mental capacity must be judged in relation to the particular decision being made at the specific time it needs to be made.
- When patient's lack capacity, information may be disclosed when this is in the patient's best interests.
- In England, Wales and Scotland, a patient with capacity can appoint a welfare attorney; however, welfare attorneys should only have access to information when this is of benefit to the patient and which is relevant to the issue in question.

Children and young people

Children who lack competence

Occasionally, children seek medical treatment but are judged to lack the competence to give consent. An explicit request by a child that information should not be disclosed to parents or guardians, or indeed to any third party, must be respected save in the most exceptional circumstances, for example where it puts the child at risk of significant harm, in which case the disclosure may take place in the public interest without consent (see Chapter 4, pages 177–180). Where a health professional decides to disclose information to a third party against a child's wishes, the child should generally be told before the information is disclosed. The discussion with the child and the reasons for disclosure should also be documented in the child's record.

People with parental responsibility may give consent for the sharing of information about children who lack the competence to decide. These issues are discussed in detail in Chapter 4. (For discussion on information sharing in relation to young people and the provision of advice on contraception and sexual health, see Chapter 7, pages 271–275.)

Competent young people

There is no presumption of competence for people under 16 years in England, Wales and Northern Ireland and those under that age must demonstrate they have sufficient understanding of what is proposed. However, children who are aged 12 years or over are generally expected to have the competence to give or withhold their consent to the release of information.[145] However, it is important that an individual assessment of maturity and understanding is made. In Scotland, anyone aged 12 years or over is legally presumed to have such competence.[146] If the young person is competent to understand what is involved in the proposed treatment, the health professional should, unless there are convincing reasons to the contrary, respect the young person's wishes if they do not want parents or guardians to know. However, every reasonable effort must be made to persuade the young person to involve parents or guardians, particularly for important or life-changing decisions.

Scotland – confidentiality and children's services

In April 2011, the Joint Inspection of Children's Services and Inspections of Social Work Services (Scotland) Act 2006 and all associated regulations were repealed. All joint inspections requested by the Scottish Ministers of services for children and for adults are conducted under the provisions of the Public Services Reform (Scotland) Act 2010 which extended joint inspections of children's services to include 'such other services as the Scottish Ministers may specify in respect of which such persons or bodies have inspection functions'.[147] The Act gives broad rights of access for inspectors to access service records, including patient's medical records, primarily for audit purposes.

Summary – children and young people

- The duty of confidence to a child is the same as that for any other person.
- An explicit request that information should not be disclosed to parents or another third party should be respected unless there are overwhelming reasons why a disclosure is warranted.
- People with parental responsibility may give consent for the sharing of information about children who lack the competence to decide.

Deceased patients

The BMA, GMC[148] and Department of Health[149] have long agreed that the ethical obligation to respect a patient's confidentiality extends beyond death. In 2007, the Information Tribunal in England and Wales upheld the decision of the Information Commissioner, who found that most information in medical records, including those of the deceased, is likely to be confidential and exempt from disclosure under section 41 of the Freedom of Information Act 2000.

Bluck v The Information Commissioner and Epsom and St Helier University NHS Trust

Mrs Bluck sought the disclosure of the medical records of her adult daughter, who had died in hospital. The hospital had admitted some liability and reached a settlement with her next of kin (her husband and children), who opposed the disclosure of the medical records. Mrs Bluck sought further information on the circumstances of her daughter's death. The Information Tribunal upheld a decision of the Information Commissioner that confidentiality in medical records should continue after the death of the patient, in part to safeguard the doctor-patient relationship and that, in this case, the records should not be released.[150]

Following the decision in this case the Information Commissioner issued a guidance note in 2008 to help public bodies consider requests for information about deceased individuals under the Freedom of Information Act and confirmed the exemption under section 41.[151] The Freedom of Information (Scotland) Act 2002 contains an exemption to the disclosure of deceased patients' records.[152] The duty of confidence, however, needs to be balanced with other considerations, such as the interests of justice and of people close to the deceased person. Ideally, doctors should therefore counsel their patients about the possibility of disclosure after death and solicit views about disclosure where it is obvious that there may be some sensitivity. Such discussions should be noted in the records.

When considering requests for information from the records of a deceased patient, the GMC advises doctors to take a number of factors into account:

- whether the disclosure of information is likely to cause distress to, or be of benefit to, the patient's partner or family
- whether the disclosure will also disclose information about the patient's family or anyone else. (Generally third party information should not be disclosed but sometimes information relating to the patient will also be clinically relevant for family members.)
- whether the information is already public knowledge or can be anonymised or coded
- the purpose of the disclosure.[153]

Are relatives entitled to information from the deceased's medical record?

Family members have no legal right of access to the health records of the deceased patient (other than those contained in the Access to Health Records Act 1990 – see below); however, doctors have always had discretion to disclose information to a deceased person's relatives or others for appropriate purposes when there is a clear justification. A common example is when the family requests details of the terminal illness because of an anxiety that the patient might have been misdiagnosed or there might have been negligence. Disclosure in such cases is likely to be what the deceased wanted and may also be in the interests of justice. Refusal to disclose in the absence of some evidence that this was the deceased patient's known wish exacerbates suspicion and can result in unnecessary litigation. In other cases, the balance of benefit to be gained by disclosure to the family, for example of a hereditary or infectious condition, may outweigh the general obligation of confidentiality to the deceased. Information should not be disclosed if the patient gave it in the past with the specific understanding or expectation that it would be kept confidential. No information at all can be revealed if the patient requested non-disclosure except where there is a public interest justification.

The authorisation of a surviving relative or next of kin is not required for disclosure of confidential information, although the view of those who were close to the patient may help doctors decide if the disclosure is appropriate.

A family member or another third party may have a statutory right of access under the Access to Health Records Act 1990 or the Access to Health Records (Northern Ireland) Order 1993. Unless the patient requested confidentiality while alive, a 'personal representative and any person who may have a claim arising out of a patient's death' has a right of access to information directly relevant to the claim.[154] Disclosure may take place unless it may cause 'serious harm' to an individual, or if it related to a third party other than a healthcare professional. (This is discussed further in Chapter 6, pages 259–260.)

Other circumstances in which access to the records of a deceased patient might be granted

A coroner or procurator fiscal may need information in connection with an inquest or fatal accident inquiry (see Chapter 12, page 500). There are also a limited number of additional circumstances in which the GMC advises disclosure, including for National Confidential Inquiries.[155]

Summary – deceased patients

- The ethical duty of confidentiality continues after a patient's death.
- Family members do not have an automatic legal right of access to the deceased's medical information.
- Doctors have the discretion to disclose necessary and relevant information about deceased patients for appropriate purposes.

References

1   General Medical Council (2009) *Confidentiality*, GMC, London, p.31.
2   Department of Health (2003) *Confidentiality: NHS Code of Practice*, DH, London, p.5.
3   General Medical Council (2009) *Confidentiality*, GMC, London, p.31.
4   General Medical Council (2009) *Confidentiality*, GMC, London, p.30.
5   General Medical Council (2009) *Confidentiality*, GMC, London, p.31.
6   Department of Health (2003) *Confidentiality: NHS Code of Practice*, DH, London, p.6.
7   General Medical Council (2009) *Confidentiality*, GMC, London, p.30.
8   Department of Health (2009) *NHS 2010–2015: from good to great. Preventative, people-centred, productive*, DH, London, paras 2.77, 2.85, 3.5. This stresses the importance of liaison between the NHS and adult social care services.
9   General Medical Council (2009) *Confidentiality*, GMC, London.
10 General Medical Council (2006) *Good Medical Practice*, GMC, London, para 37.
11 Anon. (1997) GP struck off after golf club gossip. *Pulse* (Mar 8), p.12.
12 The EU Article 29 Data Protection Working Party indicates that any information in health records should be regarded as confidential. Article 29 Data Protection Working Party (2007) *Working Document on the processing of personal data relating to health in electronic health records (EHR) 00323/07/EN, WP 131*, European Commission, Belgium, p.7.
13 General Medical Council Fitness to Practise Panel, 29–30 November and 13–14 December 2008 and 18 January 2009.
14 General Medical Council (2009) *Confidentiality*, GMC, London, para 12.
15 General Medical Council (2009) *Confidentiality*, GMC, London, para 25.
16 General Medical Council (2009) *Confidentiality*, GMC, London, paras 25–32.
17 General Medical Council (2009) *Confidentiality*, GMC, London, para 25.
18 General Medical Council (2009) *Confidentiality*, GMC, London, para 26.
19 General Medical Council (2009) *Confidentiality*, GMC, London, para 26.
20 An exception to the notion of implied consent for sharing information amongst the healthcare team is when a patient visits a genitourinary medicine (GUM) clinic. Under the NHS (Venereal Disease) Regulations 1974 and NHS Trusts and PCTs (Sexually Transmitted Diseases) Directions 2000, information regarding attendance at GUM clinics and any subsequent test results should not be shared with healthcare professionals (including the patient's GP) beyond those treating the sexual health problems.
21 General Medical Council (2009) *Confidentiality*, GMC, London, para 30.
22 General Medical Council (2009) *Confidentiality*, GMC, London, para 32.
23 General Medical Council (2006) *Good Medical Practice*, GMC, London, para 74.
24 This is discussed in Thomas R, Walport M. (2008) *Data Sharing Review Report*. Available at: www.justice.gov.uk (accessed 19 May 2011).
25 A key aspect of the *Campbell v MGN [2004] UKHL 22* case was the finding of the House of Lords that an obligation of confidence existed because of the *nature* of the information relating to

Ms Campbell's treatment for drug addiction, rather than a duty of confidence owed because of the relationship between her and the *Mirror* newspaper.

26 Maintaining public trust in a confidential health service is in the public interest and strongly supported by the courts. See *Ashworth Security Hospital v MGN* [2002] UKHL 29.

27 Personal data is defined under the Data Protection Act 1998 as 'data which relate to a living individual who can be identified – (a) from those data, or (b) from those data and other information which is in the possession of, or likely to be in the possession of, the data controller – and includes any expression of opinion about the individual and any intentions of the data controller or any person in respect of the individual'. Data Protection Act 1998, s 1(1).

28 Data Protection Act 1998, Sch 1, Part 1.

29 The full lists can be found in the Data Protection Act 1998, Sch 2 and 3.

30 Data Protection Act 1998, Sch 3, para 8(2).

31 Medical Act 1983, s 35A (as amended). The limiting factors are that the processing must be in the substantial public interest, and that it must be necessary for the discharge of a particular public function.

32 Information Commissioner (2010) *Information Commissioner's guidance about the issue of monetary penalties prepared and issued under Section 55C(1) of the Data Protection Act 1998*, ICO, Wilmslow.

33 Ministry of Justice (2009) *The knowing or reckless misuse of personal data: Introducing custodial sentences. Consultation paper CP22/09*, MOJ, London.

34 European Convention for the Protection of Human Rights and Fundamental Freedoms 1950, art 8(2).

35 The Health and Social Care Act 2008 established the National Information Governance Board as an independent statutory body to advise the Secretary of State for Health in England and Wales about the use of patient information and the lawful basis for disclosure of patient identifiable information under the Health Service (Control of Patient Information) Regulations 2002. SI 2002/1438.

36 General Medical Council (2009) *Confidentiality*, GMC, London, para 9.

37 National Information Governance Board (2009) *NHS Care Record Guarantee*, NIGB, London.

38 These include: Department of Health (2010) *The Caldicott Guardian Manual*, DH, London; Department of Health (2003) *Confidentiality: NHS Code of Practice*, DH, London; Scottish Executive Health Department (2003) *NHS Code of Practice on Protecting Patient Confidentiality*, SEHD, Edinburgh; Northern Ireland Executive (2009) *Code of Practice on Protecting the Confidentiality of Service User Information*, DHSSPS, Belfast.

39 Department of Health (2008) *Summary of Responses to the Consultation on the Additional Uses of Patient Data*, DH, London.

40 Department of Health (2008) *Summary of Responses to the Consultation on the Additional Uses of Patient Data*, DH, London, p.25. Concerns over anonymisation were also expressed in: The Royal Academy of Engineering (2010) *Privacy and prejudice: Young people's view on the development and use of Electronic Patient Record*, RAEng, London, pp.28–9.

41 *R v Department of Health (Respondent), ex parte Source Informatics Ltd (Appellant) and (1) Association Of The British Pharmaceutical Industry (2) General Medical Council (3) Medical Research Council (4) National Pharmaceutical Association Ltd (Interveners)* [2000] 1 All ER 786.

42 *R v Department of Health (Respondent), ex parte Source Informatics Ltd (Appellant) and (1) Association Of The British Pharmaceutical Industry (2) General Medical Council (3) Medical Research Council (4) National Pharmaceutical Association Ltd (Interveners)* [2000] 1 All ER 786.

43 Department of Health (2003) *Confidentiality: NHS Code of Practice*, DH, London, p.5 defines pseudonymised information as 'like anonymised information in that in the possession of the holder it cannot reasonably be used by the holder to identify an individual. However it differs in that the original provider of the information may retain a means of identifying individuals. This will often be achieved by attaching codes or other unique references to information so that the data will only be identifiable to those who have access to the key or index. Pseudonymisation allows information about the same individual to be linked in a way that true anonymisation does not.'

44 Information Commissioner (2002) *Use and disclosure of health data. Guidance on the application of the Data Protection Act 1998*, ICO, Wilmslow, p.5.

45 In England and Wales this is covered under the Public Health (Control of Disease) Act 1984 (as amended) and the Public Health (Infectious Diseases) Regulations 1988. In Scotland, similar provisions are contained in the Public Health etc (Scotland) Act 2008 and in Northern Ireland in the Public Health Act (Northern Ireland) 1967 (as amended). See Chapter 20 for further details.

46 The Health Protection (Notification) Regulations 2010. SI 2010/659, regulations 2(b) and (c). Health Protection (Notification) (Wales) Regulations 2010. SI 2010/1546, regulations 2 (b) and (c).

47 The Health Service (Control of Patient Information) Regulations 2002. SI 2002/1438, s 1(a–d).

48 In England and Wales, doctors completing the notification form must provide a patient reference number, date of birth and postcode wherever possible as laid down in Department of Health (2009) *Guidance note for completing the abortion notification form HSA4*, DH, London. In Scotland, doctors must

give the name, address, postcode and date of birth as well as a patient reference number as in Abortion (Scotland) Regulations 1991. SI 1991/460, s.41.

49 The Reporting of Injuries, Diseases, and Dangerous Occurrences (Amendment) Regulations 1989. SI 1989/1457.

50 Registration with the Care Quality Commission by all NHS trusts is a requirement under the Health and Social Care Act 2008.

51 Care Quality Commission (2010) *Essential Standards of Quality and Safety: The Care Quality Registration Regulations*, CQC, London.

52 National Reporting and Learning Service (2010) *National Patient Safety Agency. National Framework for Reporting and Learning from Serious Incidents Requiring Investigation*, NPSA, London.

53 Department of Health (2010) *Liberating the NHS: report of the arms-length bodies review*, DH, London.

54 NHS Act 2006, Part 10, s 195-210. NHS Wales (Wales) Act 2006, s 143–58. Both the Department of Health (England) and the Welsh Assembly Government have published codes of practice for the use of these powers.

55 Health and Social Care Act 2008, s 62–4.

56 A number of the regulatory bodies who have statutory powers to require disclosure of information are listed in General Medical Council (2009) *Confidentiality*, GMC, London, pp.33–4.

57 General Medical Council (2009) *Confidentiality*, GMC, London, para 19.

58 *R (on the application of TB) v The Combined Court at Stafford* [2006] EWHC 1645 (Admin).

59 *R (on the application of TB) v The Combined Court at Stafford* [2006] EWHC 1645 (Admin).

60 General Medical Council (2009) *Confidentiality*, GMC, London, para 23. Precognition is the practice of taking a factual statement from witnesses before a trial.

61 British Medical Association, The Law Society (2003) *Consent form (Releasing health records under the Data Protection Act 1998) – for England and Wales*, BMA, London. British Medical Association, The Law Society of Scotland, Scottish Executive Health Department (2004) *Consent form for access to patient's records by solicitors (Releasing health records under the Data Protection Act 1998)*, BMA, London.

62 Crime and Disorder Act 1998, s 115.

63 Children Act 1989, s 47.

64 General Medical Council (2009) *Confidentiality*. GMC, London, para 54.

65 Section 29 of the Data Protection Act 1998 refers to disclosures in relation in crime.

66 Gender Recognition Act 2004, s 22.

67 General Medical Council (2009) *Confidentiality: Disclosing information about serious communicable diseases*, GMC, London, pp.20–1.

68 The list of disclosures which are permitted under the 1990 Act can be found in: Human Fertilisation and Embryology Authority (2009) *Code of Practice*, 8th edn, HFEA, London, box 30A.

69 Human Fertilisation and Embryology Authority (2009) *Code of Practice*, 8th edn, HFEA, London, box 30A.

70 Human Fertilisation and Embryology (Disclosure of information for research purposes) Regulations 2010. SI 2010/995. These powers are similar to the powers given under the Health Service (Control of Patient Information) Regulations 2002.

71 General Medical Council (2009) *Confidentiality*, GMC, London, para 36.

72 *W v Egdell and Ors* [1990] 1 All ER 835.

73 Department of Health (2003) *Confidentiality: NHS Code of Practice*, DH, London, p.34.

74 Department of Health (2010) *Confidentiality: NHS Code of Practice – Supplementary Guidance: Public Interest Disclosures*, DH, London.

75 Department of Health (2010) *Confidentiality: NHS Code of Practice – Supplementary Guidance: Public Interest Disclosures*, DH, London, pp.13–15.

76 For example, statutory obligations to report serious incidents as part the Care Quality Commission registration requirements.

77 General Medical Council (2009) *Confidentiality*, GMC, London, para 63.

78 This was confirmed by the English and Scottish courts in the early part of the twenty-first century. National Aids Trust (2006) *NAT Policy Update: Criminal Prosecution of HIV Transmission*, NAT, London.

79 General Medical Council (2009) *Confidentiality: Supplementary Guidance Disclosing information about serious communicable diseases*, GMC, London, p.20. The GMC defines the term 'serious communicable disease' as applying to any disease that can be transmitted from human to human and that can result in death or serious illness. It particularly applies to, but is not limited to, HIV, tuberculosis and hepatitis B and C.

80 General Medical Council (2009) *Confidentiality: supplementary guidance. Disclosing information about serious communicable diseases*, GMC, London, para 10.

81 General Medical Council (2009) *Confidentiality: supplementary guidance. Reporting concerns about patients to the DVLA or to the DVA*, GMC, London, para 7.

82 Department of Health (2003) *Confidentiality: NHS Code of Practice*, DH, London, p.35.

83   Department of Health (2003) *Confidentiality: NHS Code of Practice*, DH, London, p.35.
84   General Medical Council (2009) *Confidentiality*, GMC, London, para 54.
85   In 2008, NHS Scotland agreed an information sharing document with the Scottish police which provides some guidance in this area when read in conjunction with GMC guidance on public interest disclosures. Scottish Government (2008) *Information Sharing Between NHS Scotland and the Police*, Scottish Government, Edinburgh.
86   General Medical Council (2009) *Confidentiality: Supplementary guidance. Reporting gunshot and knife wounds*, GMC, London, paras 5–9.
87   General Medical Council (2009) *Confidentiality: Supplementary guidance. Reporting gunshot and knife wounds*, GMC, London, paras 12–15.
88   Co-ordinated Action Against Domestic Abuse (2009) *CAADA – DASH MARAC Risk Identification Checklist*, CAADA, Bristol.
89   General Medical Council (2009) *Confidentiality*, GMC, London, para 63.
90   General Medical Council (2009) *Confidentiality*, GMC, London, para 33.
91   General Medical Council (2009) *Confidentiality*, GMC, London, para 34(a).
92   Department of Health (2010) *The NHS Constitution for England*, DH, London, p.3.
93   Department of Health (2010) *The NHS Constitution for England*, DH, London, p.7.
94   Academy of Medical Sciences (2006) *Personal data for public good: using health information in medical research*, AMS, London. This report suggests that emphasis on the need to obtain explicit consent has impeded valuable research projects by introducing biases that made results difficult to interpret. See also: Academy of Medical Sciences (2011) *A new pathway for the regulation and governance of health research*, AMS, London. This report highlights the differences in research findings when restricted or incomplete data samples are accessed and the implications if research findings from such datasets are taken forward.
95   Case P. (2003) Confidence matters: the rise and fall of informational autonomy in medical law. *Med Law Rev* **11**(2), 208–36.
96   Medical Research Council (2006) *The Use of Personal Health Information in Medical Research: General Public Consultation Final Report*, MRC, London, p.55. This survey found that 79 per cent of respondents felt that they had the right to be consulted about any use of identifiable personal data for research purposes, even if it made the research impractical.
97   Department of Health (2008) *Summary of Responses to the Consultation on the Additional Uses of Patient Data*, DH, London, p.6. Fifty-three per cent of respondents from the general public thought that identifiable data should never be used for research purposes without consent.
98   General Medical Council (2009) *Confidentiality*, GMC, London, para 42.
99   General Medical Council (2009) *Confidentiality*, GMC, London, para 44.
100 National Information Governance Board (2011) *Identifying and contacting research participants*, NIGB, London.
101 Thomas R, Walport M. (2008) *Data Sharing Review Report*, para 8.13. Available at: www.justice.gov.uk (accessed 19 May 2011). Brown I, Brown L, Korff D. (2010) Using NHS patient data for research without consent. *Law, Innovation Technol* **2**(2), 219–58.
102 Thomas R, Walport M. (2008) *Data Sharing Review Report*, paras 8.78–8.79. Available at: www.justice.gov.uk (accessed 19 May 2011). This report discusses the concept of safe havens. It also recommends that the NHS should develop a system to allow approved researchers to work with healthcare providers to identify potential patients, who may then be approached to take part in clinical studies for which consent is needed – this has been termed the 'consent for consent' dilemma. See also: Academy of Medical Sciences (2011) *A new pathway for the regulation and governance of health research*, AMS, London p.59.
103 Care Record Development Board (2009) *Report of the Care Record Development Board Working Group on the Secondary Uses of Patient Information*, DH, London, para 5.1.2.
104 Care Record Development Board (2009) *Report of the Care Record Development Board Working Group on the Secondary Uses of Patient Information*, DH, London, para 5.1.3.
105 General Medical Council (2009) *Confidentiality*. GMC, London, para 49.
106 National Information Governance Board (2011) *Identifying and contacting patients for medical research*, NIGB, London.
107 Further information on the Privacy Advisory Committee is available on the NHS National Services Scotland website: www.nhsnss.org (accessed 1 February 2011).
108 General Medical Council (2009) *Confidentiality*, GMC, London, para 25.
109 National Information Governance Board (2011) *NHS Care Record Guarantee*, NIGB, London, para 5.
110 NHS Connecting For Health *Health and Social Care Integration programme*. Available at: www.connectingforhealth.nhs.uk (accessed 1 February 2011).
111 General Medical Council (2009) *Confidentiality: Supplementary guidance. Disclosing information for education and training purposes*, GMC, London, para 3.

112   General Medical Council (2009) *Confidentiality: Supplementary guidance. Disclosing information for education and training purposes*, GMC, London, para 9.

113   General Medical Council (2009) *Confidentiality: Supplementary guidance. Disclosing information for education and training purposes*, GMC, London, para 10.

114   General Medical Council (2009) *Confidentiality: Supplementary guidance. Disclosing information for education and training purposes*, GMC, London, para 12.

115   General Medical Council (2009) *Confidentiality: Supplementary guidance. Disclosing information for education and training purposes*, GMC, London, para 17.

116   General Medical Council (2009) *Confidentiality: Supplementary guidance. Disclosing information for education and training purposes*, GMC, London, para 13.

117   British Medical Association (2007) *Confidentiality and disclosure of information to PCTs in primary care settings*, BMA, London.

118   General Medical Council (2009) *Confidentiality: Supplementary guidance. Disclosing information for financial and administrative purposes*, GMC, London, para 3.

119   General Medical Council (2009) *Confidentiality: Supplementary guidance. Disclosing information for financial and administrative purposes*, GMC, London, para 2.

120   General Medical Council (2009) *Confidentiality: Supplementary guidance. Disclosing information for financial and administrative purposes*, GMC, London, para 4.

121   Department of Health (2005) *Confidentiality and Disclosure of Information: General Medical Services (GMS), Personal Medical Services (PMS) and Alternative Provider Medical Services (APMS) Directions 2005*, DH, London. Department of Health (2005) *Confidentiality and Disclosure of Information: General Medical Services (GMS), Personal Medical Services (PMS) and Alternative Provider Medical Services (APMS) Code of Practice*, DH, London. Scottish Executive Health Department (2005) *Confidentiality and Disclosure of Information: General Medical Services (GMS), Section 17c Agreements, and Health Board Primary Medical Services (HBPMS) Directions 2005*, SEHD, Edinburgh.

Scottish Executive Health Department (2005) *Confidentiality and Disclosure of Information: General Medical Services (GMS), Section 17c Agreements, and Health Board Primary Medical Services (HBPMS) Directions 2005 Code of Practice*, SEHD, Edinburgh. Welsh Assembly Government (2005) *Confidentiality and Disclosure of Information: General Medical Services and Alternative Provider Medical Services Directions 2006*, WAG, Cardiff. Welsh Assembly Government (2005) *Confidentiality and Disclosure of Information: General Medical Services and Alternative Provider Medical Services Directions 2006 Code of Practice*, WAG, Cardiff. Department of Health, Social Services and Public Safety (2006) *Confidentiality and Disclosure of Information: General Medical Services and Alternative Provider Medical Services Directions (Northern Ireland) 2006*, DHSSPS, Belfast. Department of Health, Social Services and Public Safety (2006) *Confidentiality and Disclosure of Information: General Medical Services (GMS) and Alternative Provider Medical Services (APMS) Code of Practice*, DHSSPS, Belfast.

122   Department of Health (2005) *Confidentiality and Disclosure of Information: General Medical Services (GMS), Personal Medical Services (PMS) and Alternative Provider Medical Services (APMS) Code of Practice*, DH, London, paras 30–2. Scottish Executive Health Department (2005) *Confidentiality and Disclosure of Information: General Medical Services (GMS), Section 17c Agreements, and Health Board Primary Medical Services (HBPMS) Code of Practice*, SEHD, Edinburgh, paras 29–31. Welsh Assembly Government (2005) *Confidentiality and Disclosure of Information: General Medical Services and Alternative Provider Medical Services Code of Practice*, WAG, Cardiff, paras 29–31. Department of Health, Social Services and Public Safety (2006) *Confidentiality and Disclosure of Information: General Medical Services (GMS) and Alternative Provider Medical Services (APMS) Code of Practice*, DHSSPS, Belfast, paras 30–2.

123   Information Commissioner (2002) *Use and disclosure of health data. Guidance on the application of the Data Protection Act 1998*, ICO, Wilmslow, p.8.

124   Information Commissioner (2002) *Use and disclosure of health data. Guidance on the application of the Data Protection Act 1998*, ICO, Wilmslow, p.8.

125   Department of Health (2003) *Confidentiality: NHS Code of Practice*, DH, London, p.21.

126   Department of Health (1998) *NHS complaints procedures: confidentiality,* HSC 1998/059, DH, London. Department of Health (2009) *Listening, responding, improving: a guide to better customer care. Advice sheet 2: Joint working on complaints*, DH, London. Scottish Executive Health Department (2005) *NHS Complaints Procedure Guidance: Including Statutory Directions*, SEHD, Edinburgh. Northern Ireland has not published guidance on the confidentiality aspects of complaints procedures.

127   The Data Protection Act (Processing of Sensitive Data) (Elected Representatives) Order 2002. SI 2002/2905.

128   Department of Health (2003) *Confidentiality: NHS Code of Practice*, DH, London, p.43.

129   Information Commissioner (2006) *Data Protection Technical Guidance Note Disclosures to Members of Parliament carrying out constituency casework*, ICO, Wilmslow.

130   General Medical Council (2009) *Confidentiality*, GMC, London, paras 18 and 20.

131   General Medical Council (2009) *Confidentiality*, GMC, London, para 20.

132 Department of Health (2009) *Religion or belief: a practical guide for the NHS*, DH, London.
133 General Medical Council (2009) *Confidentiality: supplementary guidance. Responding to criticism in the press*, GMC, London, para 3.
134 In *Ashworth Security Hospital v MGN* [2002] UKHL 29, the House of Lords ruled that the management of a high security mental hospital still had an independent interest in keeping health records confidential even when the data subject had put the information in the public domain.
135 General Medical Council (2009) *Confidentiality*, GMC, London, para 34.
136 British Medical Association, Association of British Insurers (2010) *Medical information and insurance*, BMA, London.
137 General Medical Council (2009) *Confidentiality*, GMC, London, para 34.
138 This is also confirmed by Department of Health (2010) *Standard General Medical Services Contract*, DH, London, clause 450. National Health Service (Primary Medical Services) (Miscellaneous Amendments) Regulations 2010. SI 2010/578, s 10(7)(3)(e).
139 The Mental Capacity Act 2005 replaced the Enduring Power of Attorney (EPA) with the LPA.
140 Further advice, including a chapter on the practical aspects of the assessment of capacity, is given in: British Medical Association, The Law Society (2010) *Assessment of mental capacity: guidance for doctors and lawyers*, 3rd edn, The Law Society, London.
141 Doctors should follow the guidance laid out in: Department for Constitutional Affairs (2007) *Mental Capacity Act 2005 Code of Practice*, The Stationery Office, London.
142 The Act provides a checklist of common factors that must be taken into account when making a best interests judgment. Mental Capacity Act 2005, s 4.
143 General Medical Council (2009) *Confidentiality*, GMC, London, para 62.
144 General Medical Council (2009) *Confidentiality*, GMC, London, para 59.
145 British Medical Association (2001) *Consent, Rights and Choices in Health Care for Children and Young People*, BMA, London, para 7.3.
146 General Medical Council (2007) *0–18 years: guidance for all doctors*, GMC, London, para 53.
147 Public Services Reform (Scotland) Act 2010, s 115(1)(b).
148 General Medical Council (2009) *Confidentiality*, GMC, London, para 70.
149 Department of Health (2003) *Confidentiality: NHS Code of Practice*, DH, London, p.13.
150 *Bluck v The Information Commissioner and Epsom and St Helier University NHS Trust* [2007] EA 2006/0090. See also: *Nicholas Lewis (Claimant) v Secretary of State for Health (Defendant) and Michael Redfern QC (Interested Party)* [2008] EWHC 2196 (QB).
151 Information Commissioner (2008) *Freedom of Information Act. Practical guidance: Information about the deceased*, ICO, Wilmslow.
152 Freedom of Information (Scotland) Act 2002, s 38.
153 General Medical Council (2009) *Confidentiality*, GMC, London, para 70.
154 Access to Health Records Act 1990, s 3(1)(f). Access to Health Records (Northern Ireland) Order 1993, s 5(e).
155 General Medical Council (2009) *Confidentiality*, GMC, London, para 71.

6: Health records

The questions covered in this chapter include the following.

- What should be put in health records?
- How much control do patients have over what does and does not go into health records?
- How long must records be kept?
- Are there special rules for photographs and videos?
- Are there any limits on patients' rights of access to their health records?
- How can patients access their electronic records?
- What measures are in place to protect electronically held data?

The importance of health information

The quality of health data and the clinical content of health records underpin the provision of high-quality and continuous patient care. Health records are accessed by a wide range of health professionals in various care settings and, clearly, the decisions they make about diagnosis and treatment must be based on accurate clinical information about the patient. Health records are, therefore, a key element of medical practice. The information stored within them is also crucial for the development of treatments and other health services in the future.

Many national health policy strategies since the start of the twenty-first century have stressed the importance of a greater focus on giving patients more information, greater choice and increased control over their healthcare. If services are to be developed in order to meet these ambitions, good quality health information is essential. Aligned to this, the implementation of electronic patient records systems in the NHS means that the structure and content of the health record is becoming ever more important. Increased priority is attached to standardising approaches to record keeping with a view to encouraging consistency, incorporating best practice and improving the quality of records so that they can be used to enable improvements in care and services for future patients. It should be highlighted at the outset that this is a rapidly evolving area of practice, which is subject to technological changes and advances, as systems develop in order to meet the requirements of clinical communication and information governance policies.

Many of the ethical issues that arise in relation to health records are to do with confidentiality and disclosure of information. These issues are dealt with in Chapter 5. This chapter focuses on the practical aspects to do with records and record keeping and does not address the principles concerning confidentiality which apply to all health records. This chapter includes practical information about a number of electronic and paper systems used for sharing, accessing, storing and transmitting records. These systems are continually revised in line with developments in new technology and models of sharing clinical information.

Medical Ethics Today: The BMA's Handbook of Ethics and Law, Third Edition. Sophie Brannan, Eleanor Chrispin, Martin Davies, Veronica English, Rebecca Mussell, Julian Sheather and Ann Sommerville.
© 2012 BMA Medical Ethics Department. Published 2012 by Blackwell Publishing Ltd.

The principles underlying the practical aspects of record keeping discussed throughout the chapter apply to all identifiable patient information, whether it is stored electronically or on paper.

Records and record keeping

Health records exist to provide a record of patients' contact with healthcare providers and are fundamental to good clinical practice. They act as an aide-memoire for healthcare professionals and facilitate communication with and about patients. Some specialties also make use of hand-held records, for example a multi-disciplinary hand-held record is often used for maternity patients and patients with diabetes.[1] The primary purpose of the health record is to support continuous patient care, but, as mentioned in the introduction, it is recognised that good quality health data are also essential to support and develop better patient care and improve communication and quality assurance of the care and services delivered. Health records contain information that is useful for clinical audit, financial planning, management, monitoring hospital performance, disease registers, research aimed at improving patient care in the future, and for coroners to undertake a thorough investigation of a death. Data quality and accuracy are essential in order for health records to be effective for such purposes. A continuous process of maintenance, or housekeeping, is necessary in order to maintain high quality.

Health records are also crucial in responding to complaints or claims (see pages 232 and 235–236). As is discussed further in Chapters 5 and 20, the medical record is increasingly used for a range of social purposes at the request of patients.

The information doctors put in health records falls into four broad categories:

- description from the patient or perhaps a relative or friend concerned about the patient's health
- observation by the health professional, including the outcome of examinations or tests
- an interpretation of these two sets of information, usually in the form of diagnosis or assessment of the problem
- documentation of the problem's management, including treatment, referral, prescription and outcome.

Health records may include notes made during consultations; prescribed medication; correspondence between health professionals, such as referral and discharge letters; results of tests and their interpretation; X-ray films; videotapes; audiotapes; photographs and tissue samples taken for diagnosis. They may also include reports written for third parties such as insurance companies.

General principles

The following principles apply to all types of records, whether they are held electronically or on paper.

- The primary purpose of health records is to support direct care to the patient.
- Good quality records are factual, accurate, contemporaneous and legible.
- Records must be stored and handled securely.

- Offering to share the content of records with patients and/or authorised proxies can help to strengthen the doctor–patient relationship, empower patients and improve accuracy.
- The use of data for secondary purposes including public health, audit, teaching, NHS administration and health research is core to the functioning of the health service.

Content of health records

In providing good clinical care, the General Medical Council (GMC) states that doctors must:

- keep clear, accurate, legible records, reporting the relevant clinical findings, the decisions made, the information given to patients and any drugs prescribed or other investigation or treatment
- make records at the same time as the events you are recording or as soon as possible afterwards.[2]

The key information that is recorded includes:

- presenting symptoms and reasons for seeking healthcare
- relevant clinical findings and diagnosis
- options for care and treatment discussed with the patient
- risks and benefits of care and treatment options, as explained to the patient
- decisions about care and treatment, including evidence of the patient's agreement
- action taken and outcomes.

In 2008, the Royal College of Physicians (RCP), supported by NHS Connecting for Health, published standards for the structure and content of medical records and communications when patients are admitted to hospital in the UK.[3] The standards, approved by the Academy of Medical Royal Colleges and published by the Department of Health, incorporate 12 generic record keeping standards which are applicable to any patient's medical record. Several of the standards, such as date and time of entry, will be automatically recorded in electronic records. Others, such as the frequency of record entries, are designed to be more flexible. The standards specify that a unique patient identifier (NHS number in England and Wales, Community Health Index in Scotland, Health and Care number in Northern Ireland) must be used on every page in the record and that information such as advance decisions to refuse treatment and cardio-pulmonary resuscitation (CPR) decisions must be clearly recorded. The RCP has also created a set of standardised headings and definitions for hospital admissions, handover and discharge communications. The content of all hospital patient records, electronic and paper, should be structured using these headings.[4] Standardised structure and content of medical records are essential not only for patient care but also for the financial management arrangements of the NHS. Sound financial management relies on the accurate reporting of clinical activity data as this information directly links to the payments trusts receive for work they carry out[5] and to payments received by GP practices under the Quality and Outcomes Framework (QOF) in England.

Some matters that are recorded in health records are speculation, or may later prove to be incorrect. Doctors should not be wary of recording reasonable speculations when these have a bearing on decisions about care or treatment. It is not uncommon for doctors to provide treatment based on an interim diagnosis that later investigations disprove.

It is important that the health records show a continuous record of all action taken and outcomes, and this type of information should remain on the records even if further investigation suggests a different approach. The records should, of course, indicate clearly such changes in approach, and put any previous diagnoses and management into context.

Personal views about the patient's behaviour or temperament should not be included in health records unless these have a potential bearing on treatment. Where behaviour or temperament is being recorded, the record should include a factual account. Recording the patient's actual words or phrases can be helpful. It should be remembered that patients have a right of access to their health record (see pages 255–258) and that other healthcare professionals may access the record; therefore, when adding comment or opinion doctors should consider how these might be viewed by the patient or another healthcare professional.

In line with GMC guidance, and the above-mentioned national record keeping standards, records should be made promptly. A contemporaneous record is more likely to be an accurate reflection of actual events, rather than an interpretation with the benefit of hindsight. Retrospective documentation may suggest that a course of action was based on dubious reasoning, or needs extensive justification. It is also important that records show clearly the reasoning behind treatment or management. Documenting the thought processes not only benefits health professionals using the records in the future, it explains matters to patients reading the records and may also protect the health professional in cases of litigation.

Altering medical records

If after the contemporaneous note has been made it becomes clear that more information should have been included, a fresh entry should be made, dated accordingly, with an explanation of why additional information is now considered necessary. In addition, a dated reference to the new note may properly be made to the original note so as to make clear that the content of the original note has subsequently been modified.

Even if additional, or non-contemporaneous, entries to a record are entirely accurate, the mere fact of altering it could jeopardise a legal case. (For removing information from health records, see also pages 235–236.) Medical defence bodies have warned that they have acted on behalf of doctors who are facing criminal charges in such cases for attempting to pervert the course of justice.[6] It is not unusual for a doctor to make a late entry in a medical record, for example when a GP sees a patient but does not immediately have access to the notes to make an entry. Doctors must, however, take care when amending medical notes to avoid potential accusations of evidence tampering. Medical notes are expected to be contemporaneous – if the events occurred previously the notes should clearly specify this. Any note must clearly show the date on which it is made – there must be no suggestion that the entry purports to have been made at an earlier time and date. While there may be an innocent explanation as to why a note was not made at the time stated, this can lead to the suggestion that notes have been tampered with.

Tampering with records

In 2010, the GMC found a GP guilty of acting dishonestly in amending the medical records of six patients. The GP also admitted altering the medical records of 32 patients. The doctor was suspended for 12 months.[7]

Should all interactions in relation to patients be recorded in medical records?

The primary purpose of the health record is to support patient care. Any information that is clinically relevant should be recorded. However, health records can also be a rich source of social information – for example, if a person is living in a house with children. They contain more than just 'health' information in order to create a holistic overview of a patient, and patients should generally be aware of this during their interactions with health professionals. In the view of the British Medical Association (BMA), for medico-legal purposes, every interaction in relation to a patient should be recorded in the patient's health record – for example, all correspondence from social services.

On occasions, the BMA has been asked whether unsubstantiated but serious allegations, for example child abuse, should be recorded in the GP records. Although in some instances it may be appropriate to record serious allegations where there is supporting evidence, doctors must exercise great care and caution in this area. Where an allegation is recorded, efforts should be made to establish the veracity of the allegation, for example seeking relevant follow-up information from social services as to whether the allegation was found to be substantiated, unfounded or malicious.

This is a difficult area and ultimately it is a matter of judgement for the individual GP to decide whether it is appropriate to record an allegation. Should the GP choose to record a particular piece of information, this should be done using the correct 'read code'. For example, while a patient is on the sex offenders register, the appropriate code should be present in the record. After the patient has been removed from the register, the record should reflect this change has occurred by removal of the code from display (although it will be retained in the audit trail) and replaced with a code to indicate that the patient has a criminal record.[8]

This process records the facts, keeps the record live and accurate and hides but does not lose past offences so as to avoid stigmatisation but still allows for protection.

Aggressive behaviour

Doctors sometimes ask whether they may record in a health record that the patient has been aggressive or threatening to staff. Patients should be aware, perhaps through the use of notices in waiting rooms, that such behaviour will not be tolerated and any incidents will be documented in their records. In England, the Personal Demographics Service (PDS) includes a classification for violent patients.[9] The PDS provides formal guidance with criteria to follow before the indicator can be marked.[10] Dealing with violent and aggressive patients is addressed in Chapter 1 (see pages 55–57). (For discussion of electronic records, see pages 239–243.)

Child protection case notes

A common enquiry from GPs is whether child protection case conference notes should be kept with the child's GP record. In the BMA's view it is likely that this information is both clinically relevant and necessary to promote the interests of the child. If the GP is to provide effective care to the child then it is vital that information relating to child protection concerns is included in the GP record. The same principle would apply to any siblings.

Adoption

What to record about the fact that a patient has been adopted raises a number of questions about record keeping. The fact of adoption may not, in itself, be medically relevant, but the fact that a child is not genetically related to his or her parents may be. Similarly, if the true parents are known to be carriers of a genetic condition, this may have implications for the child's future care. It is worth noting, however, that many children are not the genetic child of those whom they assume to be their father and assumptions about genetic ties may not always be true.

In the BMA's view, decisions about whether to include information on adoption must be taken on a case-by-case basis. Parents of adopted children are encouraged to be frank with them about the fact of adoption. It may be helpful to talk to parents about whether they are planning to tell the child about his or her adoption so that the risks of inadvertent disclosure are minimised should the child access his or her records later on in life. It could be harmful, and at least distressing, for individuals to discover inadvertently, and when unprepared, that their background is not as they had been led to believe.[11] (Telling children about donor insemination is discussed in Chapter 8, pages 329–330.)

Guidance from the Department of Health states that a new health record with a new NHS number should be created for an adopted child, unless the child is already aware of his or her adoption. Both GP and hospital records should be transferred to the new identity.[12]

Questions also arise as to how the fact of adoption is recorded in the child's record. With the use of electronic record systems, if the adoption is coded it is likely to be easier to find and identify for a health professional checking the record for any potentially harmful content before providing access at a later date. Free text entries may be hidden in years of consultation records and are much more likely to be missed. This should be borne in mind when making a record of the adoptive status of the child.

Facilitating access to records

Doctors should ensure that their manner of keeping records facilitates access by patients. Patients are entitled to see, and have copies of, their health records by submitting a subject access request under the Data Protection Act 1998 (see pages 255–258); however, developments in electronic systems across the UK now enable online access to health records for a number of patients (see pages 257–258 for enabling patient access to electronic records and also page 242 for online patient portals). Occasionally, information has to be withheld, for example, where it identifies a third party such as a family member or when it might cause serious harm to the patient or another person (see pages 256–257). Doctors should order or highlight records so that when patients seek access to their records, any information that should not be disclosed can be separated easily from the information to be disclosed.

Documenting patients' views about confidentiality

If patients express views about future disclosure to third parties, this should be documented clearly in the records. There are 'read codes' controls for uploading record content to the Summary Care Record (see pages 241–242), for example, and the Personal Demographic Service (see page 233) contains fields that relate to sharing of the detailed care record (see pages 239–241). Occasionally, it may appear to doctors that disclosure of information will become an issue at a time when the patient is unable to express a view, if he or she becomes incapacitated for example, or after his or her death. Doctors may want to counsel their patients about such future disclosures and record their wishes in the records.

Summary – content of health records

- Health records must be clear, accurate, factual, legible and contemporaneous.
- Health records must include relevant clinical findings, decisions made, information given to patients, drugs or treatment prescribed.
- Any subsequent additions or amendments to information and the reasons for these should be clearly indicated.
- Health records may also include patients' expectations and wishes, for example, advance decisions to refuse treatment.
- Health professionals' personal views about a patient's behaviour should not be included if they have no bearing on healthcare.
- Health records should be structured in line with national generic standards in order to ensure a common approach to record keeping across the NHS.
- Health records are also important for medico-legal purposes and care should be taken to ensure that entries are appropriately dated to avoid allegations of tampering.
- Health records must identify clearly information that the patient does not want revealed to third parties.

Omitting information from health records

Patients sometimes ask their doctor not to make a note of some clinical fact. Doctors have a duty to record medical information or episodes of care in the patient's record and could be open to criticism if relevant clinical information was omitted from the record and the patient suffered harm because of it. Explaining to the patient how confidentiality will be ensured can help to allay concerns about inadvertent disclosure. In some cases, with electronic records, another level of security can be offered such as limited access to named clinicians.

On some occasions patients take steps to avoid information being recorded in their GP record as they do not wish certain information to be disclosed. For example, a patient may choose to go outside his or her GP practice and attend a genitourinary medicine (GUM) clinic. Patients should be encouraged to allow their usual GP to be informed about care they are receiving elsewhere, and be reassured that all doctors are legally, professionally and contractually obliged to keep information about patients confidential. Ultimately, though, a patient's choice to object to a particular piece of health information being shared with the GP must be respected.

Removing information from health records

Closely linked to requests to omit information from records is when patients ask for information to be removed. Reasons for a request for removal may be very similar to requests for information to be omitted, although these can be more difficult to handle. The circumstances when it might be appropriate to permanently remove information from paper records are extremely rare and in the case of electronic records, an audit trail will always record where changes have been made. The Information Commissioner's Office (ICO), the National Information Governance Board for Health and Social Care (NIGB) in England and Wales, and the BMA all agree that information in health records should never be removed or changed without an explanation being recorded.[13] The general principles discussed below are relevant to both deletions from paper and electronic records. There are, however, some specific considerations which are applicable to electronic records and these are covered in a separate section below. NIGB has also produced detailed guidance for patients and healthcare professionals on requesting amendments to health and social care records.[14]

It is important that notes provide a contemporaneous record of consultations and information gained about patients. To remove relevant medical information may, for example, give the impression that the notes have been tampered with for an underhand reason, and may make later treatment and care decisions seem unsupported. Interventions generally reflect important aspects of the patient's contact with caregivers and an accurate record is essential. If it becomes obvious that interventions were inappropriate, this must be reflected clearly in the notes. The fact that a particular treatment was given may have long-term implications, however. It follows that doctors must take care to ensure that the records show all significant aspects of care, and clearly identify any decisions that were later found to have been inappropriate so that future carers do not misinterpret the patient's medical history.

It is obviously important that records do not contain inaccurate information or information that may mislead another health professional who uses them. Indeed, the Data Protection Act 1998 gives patients a right to have inaccurate records amended. Should records contain inaccurate information or information that may mislead another health professional who uses them, clear amendments or additions which highlight factual inaccuracies should be made, while allowing the original information to remain legible as an audit trail.

Patients sometimes request the removal of information that is 'social' or which they feel is not relevant to their health and so should not have been recorded. The BMA has no objection to the deletion of such information, provided that both parties agree, and it is done in a way that makes clear that the record has not been inappropriately changed. Doctors may consider that some social information is relevant, however, and could be used, for example if a GP was asked to comment on suitability for clinical assistance with reproduction. Decisions must be made on a case-by-case basis, taking into account the particular circumstances. If a decision to remove irrelevant information is taken, a deletion should be made clearly, with an explanation that the deletion is of irrelevant information.

If patients ask for relevant information to be removed from their records, doctors should explain why the information should be included and reassure the patient that, except where disclosure is in the public interest or a legal requirement, nobody outside of the care team can access the record without the patient's consent. Doctors should make it clear to patients that even though they will be assumed to have given implied consent for their information to be shared within the healthcare team, they have the option to object if they wish, although refusal could jeopardise their care. Doctors may also reassure patients that everybody who comes into contact with personal health information has legal and contractual obligations to keep it confidential. If the patient's primary concern is insurance or employment, doctors should point out that they could not be untruthful in a report.[15] Doctors should explain that they cannot omit relevant information of which they are aware from a report, because to do so would be dishonest and may risk sanction by the GMC.

Transsexualism

GPs sometimes ask what to do with the records of people who are transsexual. Such records should reflect the gender, names and titles by which these persons are commonly known. Once a gender recognition certificate has been obtained, new NHS numbers are available for these patients. In Scotland and Northern Ireland, NHS numbers are not changed until the patient has undergone surgery. Information about gender reassignment surgery should be kept in accordance with the usual rules about retaining medically relevant information. It would be inappropriate to remove all reference to a person's pre-surgery gender, for example. Further information on managing the medical records of transsexual patients is available from the Department of Health.[16] The Gender Recognition Act 2004 is discussed in Chapter 5, page 198.

Removing information from electronic records

The principles that apply to deletions to paper records should also apply to electronic records. An advantage of electronic records systems is that they automatically keep an audit trail about what has been changed in a record, when it was changed and who has changed it. Information can be removed from the record, but the audit trail will always keep the record complete in case of any further investigation into the care provided. Patients may not know that making changes to an electronic record leaves traces which cannot be completely deleted. Doctors may need to explain that it is necessary for a record to remain complete for legal reasons.

For multi-contributory records, with different healthcare professionals adding data to the same record, it is likely that there will be data controllers in common for the information held. Each organisation needs to ensure that all data protection requirements are being met. This does not necessarily mean that each organisation will be accountable for meeting all the requirements, but there needs to be a clearly documented agreement on how data controller responsibilities will be satisfied, including clarification for patients regarding with whom they should speak when they have concerns about the accuracy of their records. Further work is needed in order to provide clear guidance to organisations on their legal responsibilities in a multi-contributory record environment.

There are also some complexities concerning shared records and the removal of information where data is drawn from one record to construct another, for example the summary care record (SCR) is compiled initially with data which has been extracted from the GP practice record. In June 2009, the Information Commissioner agreed that an SCR can be completely deleted at the patient's request, without keeping an audit trail of its contents, unless the record has been used, or could have been used, during the course of treatment.[17] It should, however, be noted that this does not mean that the information in the other electronic records systems from which the SCR data was originally extracted should be deleted, and so the original records and audit trails remain complete.

Electronic records, including SCRs, are discussed in detail on pages 239–243.

Disputes over accuracy of records

The importance of good communication between doctor and patient and the value of shared decision making is stressed throughout this book. It is, of course, preferable for the content of the record to be agreed with the patient; however, the BMA recognises that agreement may not always be reached. Both patients and health professionals have a strong interest in the record being an accurate reflection of the process and outcome of diagnosis. When disputes occur and the health professional and patient cannot agree about the accuracy of an entry, both the Department of Health and NIGB advise that a note should be made in the record of when and how the patient's view conflicts with that of a health professional.[18] Ideally, any disputes should be resolved at a local and informal level. However, if this avenue is not successful at resolving the dispute, the patient has the right to go through the formal complaints process of the organisation they are dealing with or take the complaint directly to the ICO.[19] Defence bodies are also of the opinion that adding a note to the record which explains the dispute is the best way of dealing with this issue.[20]

If there is a dispute about the accuracy of information which was recorded by a previous GP, doctors should take reasonable steps to ascertain the veracity of the records. If this is not possible, a note explaining the patient's views should be appended to the records. Health professionals who use the records in the future will therefore be aware that the information may not be reliable. The NIGB guidance on requesting amendments to health records provides advice to patients about what to do if they disagree with what is in their record.[21]

Summary – removing information from health records

- When making decisions about care and treatment it is important to have a complete record.
- Circumstances where it might be appropriate to completely remove information from a paper record are extremely rare.
- Information should not be changed or removed without a clear explanation being recorded in a way that makes it clear why it has been altered.
- Electronic records keep an automatic audit trail which will always maintain a complete record.

Tagging records

In the past, doctors occasionally tagged patients' paper records to draw immediate attention to a piece of information, which may be clinical or social. Such systems often used coloured stickers so that everybody who saw the file knew that the patient was, for example, diabetic, allergic to certain medication or linked to an at-risk register. The BMA expressed concerns about such systems as they potentially compromise confidentiality because, as well as drawing the attention of health professionals to important information, they may incidentally alert all staff to clinical details or social facts such as child abuse. Tagging records in this way is acceptable only when it is the sole effective system and involves less risk of inadvertent disclosure than the available alternatives.

With the introduction of electronic records, there are a number of different systems that can record and display important coded or free text clinical information as soon as the record is opened by the appropriate health professional.

Where important social information needs to be displayed on the front page of a patient's electronic record (or tagged for paper records), patients should be told this and their consent sought. Where this applies to the records of young children, permission will usually come from their parents until the child is able to decide for himself or herself. Patients' wishes about the display of information as soon as their electronic record is opened should be respected unless there is an overriding public interest that warrants a breach of confidentiality, for example when there is a risk of future violence. Dealing with violent patients is discussed in Chapter 1, pages 55–57.

Electronic records

NHS organisations have long made use of a wide range of IT systems. Most GP practices, for example, use IT systems both for administrative and clinical purposes and all NHS hospitals have used basic Patient Administration Systems (PAS) for a number of years. Since the early part of the twenty-first century, there has been a significant expansion in electronic patient record technology in all parts of the UK. The general principles that apply to paper-based records, discussed at the start of this chapter, are common to any form of electronic health record. All health records are also subject to a duty of confidentiality (this is discussed in Chapter 5). A wide range of issues relevant to electronic patient records in general practice are discussed in the Department of Health, BMA and Royal College of General Practitioners' joint guidance document, *The good practice guidelines for GP electronic patient records.*[22]

Electronic record systems can bring obvious benefits to patient care. Storing and transferring patient information electronically has the potential to improve patient care and safety as well as allowing clinicians to communicate more quickly and accurately and to identify relevant information more easily. Electronic data can also be used for a range of purposes, other than direct care provision, such as healthcare audit and research (this is discussed in Chapter 5, pages 207–216). Electronic systems also maintain an audit trail indicating who has accessed patient information and for what purpose. This information can be viewed by GPs and Caldicott Guardians (senior NHS staff who are appointed to protect the confidentiality of patient information) and is available to patients on request. The Care Record Guarantee (CRG) for NHS Care Records in England describes how the NHS will protect confidential health information held both electronically and on paper.[23] Of course, technology can also make data potentially vulnerable to unauthorised or inappropriate access and the appropriate safeguards must be in place in order to protect electronic data – this is discussed on pages 243–245.

Shared detailed care records

One of the features of the implementation of electronic records systems is the concept of a shared electronic record for an individual patient that is accessible by the GP and health professionals working in local community and hospital care settings. This is often referred to as the 'shared detailed care record' and makes information available across organisational boundaries. The Data Protection Act 1998 requires that data are processed 'fairly and lawfully', so patients should be aware of the extent of the potential sharing of their health record. Information should be readily available explaining to patients how their health information will be shared. In reviewing the information provided to patients, consideration should be given to whether patients would be surprised to learn about how their personal data is being used and disclosed.[24] Patients also have the right to ask for information not to be made available across organisational boundaries other than for direct clinical communication.

In 2009, the BMA endorsed the guidance from the Royal College of General Practitioners which incorporates principles for shared electronic records.[25] The guidance provides a framework within which shared electronic patient records should operate and includes the following principles.

- Health organisations should be able to explain to patients who will have access to their records and must make information available to patients about such disclosures.
- Health professionals should respect the wishes of those patients who object to particular information being shared with others providing care through a shared record system (except where disclosure is a legal requirement or justified in the public interest).
- Clear rules are needed on who has responsibility for content within and between organisations.
- Each organisation should be responsible for its own organisational shared record; there should be a guardian (or team) within each organisation with clinical and information governance responsibilities for that organisation's shared records, in order to ensure best practice is followed.
- With more than one health professional having access to the record, there needs to be clear guidance about which health professional is responsible for taking the necessary action on the information contained within the record.[26]

In the UK, there are various programmes to deliver forms of shared electronic records for patients (see below).

Shared detailed care records in the UK

England

In England, a centralised approach dependent on nationally negotiated inflexible contracts with a limited number of suppliers has evolved into a more localised approach to delivering shared detailed electronic records. This approach focuses on interoperability between systems rather than wholesale system replacement. Various models for delivering shared electronic records are emerging. Some systems present data from existing organisation systems as a shared view, which can be tailored to suit local requirements. Others rely on holding data on a central server with the ability to set permission to allow inter-organisation record access and editing when a patient is being cared for by multiple organisations.

Information governance has been a fundamental part of these developments, to ensure that access to data is appropriate and not excessive in accordance with the Data Protection Act principles (see Chapter 5, page 190). The approach for national systems in England has been based on the use of a 'smartcard', which controls who has access and the level of access. The user's name, photograph and unique user identifier are held on the smartcard together with an associated personal identification number (PIN) in order to access clinical data contained in shared records.

'Role-based access' controls limit what parts of the record can be viewed according to job role, area of work and activity. For example, a doctor involved in providing treatment will need to see information about a patient's health, whereas a receptionist may only require contact and appointment details, not medical information. Systems should have audit trails, which show who has viewed and edited records and at what time. Records must conform with the interpretation of the case of *I v Finland*.[27] In this case the European Court of Human Rights ruled that Finland had not protected a nurse's right to privacy because the district health authority had installed a system which allowed staff who were not involved in her care to access her data. Any unnecessary disclosure of personal data is also likely to contravene the Data Protection Act 1998 (see Chapter 5, pages 190–191).

Scotland

In 2009, the ehealth programme in Scotland announced the development of a clinical portal (or electronic window) that will allow members of the healthcare team to view defined information about individual patients in a 'virtual' electronic patient record. The data are drawn from information held on different systems including the Emergency Care Summary (ECS), a summary record made available in out-of-hours settings, and Scottish Care Information (SCI) Store, a repository of information including test results and clinical communications. Access should only be available to authorised clinicians.

Wales

In Wales, the Welsh Clinical Portal, provided by Informing Healthcare, the IT programme in Wales, will provide a single point of access into various databases, in 'read-only' format via a webpage. It will enable access to key information held in systems and on databases across NHS Wales such as medication, referral and discharge information. Ordering tests and investigations will also be possible via the portal. Controls and audits for access to clinical information should be in place.

Northern Ireland

In Northern Ireland, an Electronic Care Record (ECR) enables clinicians to view a composite view of data held in different systems.

National summary records

While shared detailed care records aim to share relevant clinical information at a local level, summary care records are intended to provide a summary of key health information from GP practices which can potentially be accessed by healthcare professionals anywhere in the country working in out-of-hours or other unscheduled care settings. The BMA believes that patients must be offered a choice and sufficient information to make an informed decision about whether they want a summary care record and must be able to change their mind at any time.

National summary records in the UK

England

The Summary Care Record (SCR), which is being implemented in England, consists of a core record containing demographic information and details of medications, allergies and adverse reactions. Upload of this core information can proceed on the basis of implied consent following an appropriate public information programme, which includes patients being offered the choice to opt-out of having an SCR created. Access to the information held on the SCR is permissible only with the explicit consent of the patient unless it is an emergency situation where a patient is unable to state their preference. (Access to long-term incapacitated adult patients' records other than in an emergency is governed by the principle of best interests unless access is authorised by a person who has legal authority to make decisions on behalf of the incapacitated patient. A similar position exists in Scotland, Wales and Northern Ireland (see below) where 'consent to view' models have been implemented following public information programmes. Any future changes to the scope of the SCR will require further discussion but the focus should be on the information required to care for a patient in an emergency. As a principle, any additional information will be added only with the explicit consent of the patient.

A competent young person is entitled to have an SCR created, and an informed decision of this sort should be respected. Where the child lacks competence, and a parent wishes to dissent on behalf of the child then they should not generally be prevented from doing so unless it is felt to be in the child's best interests to have a SCR. There may specific circumstances where a clinician feels that the best interests of the child concerned may justify the creation of an SCR and he or she is not persuaded by the arguments made to support dissent.

Scotland

The Emergency Care Summary (ECS) service was implemented in Scotland in 2006. Medications and allergies are uploaded on an implied consent basis and, with explicit patient consent, a palliative care summary can be added.[28] The ECS is being expanded to include a Key Information Summary (KIS) to replace the Special Notes process between GP practices and out-of-hours services. Information on the KIS will be generic and it is proposed that it will include information such as main diagnoses, care and support information, such as home care or power of attorney, and key information such as views on resuscitation. Patients will decide what information they wish to be added and shared.

Wales

The Individual Health Record (IHR) in Wales comprises a standard data extraction from GP systems which includes medication, medical history, allergies, current problems, test results, GP encounters and vaccinations and immunisations. Certain information, which is deemed to be sensitive, is automatically excluded from the upload.

Northern Ireland

An Emergency Care Record (ECR), similar to the ECS in Scotland, is being implemented in Northern Ireland.

Online patient portals

Various online patient portals are being developed across the UK. These include 'Healthspace' in England,[29] 'My Health Online' in Wales and a patient portal in Scotland. Commercial companies are also developing patient portals. Functionality varies but can include the ability for patients to view elements of their health records online, book appointments, order repeat prescriptions and input information such as blood pressure readings. (Access to health records by patients is discussed on pages 255–260.)

Can patients opt out of having electronic health records?

Doctors have asked if patients can opt-out of having an electronic record and have their health information remain paper-based. The BMA is of the view that patients generally do not have a right to paper records. With many healthcare processes becoming electronic, for example ordering and receiving tests, imaging and prescribing, it is extremely difficult for GP practices and trusts to properly care for patients who wish to have paper records. Hybrid systems also run the risk that pertinent clinical information might be missed by a member of the healthcare team who is unaware that information is held elsewhere.

Enquiries regarding opting out of electronic records are often the result of anxieties about information sharing, rather than the presence of an electronic record per se. Sometimes patients can be reassured if they are informed about the inbuilt protections of the electronic health record, such as restriction of access to those who are providing care and an audit trail to show who has accessed the record.

The BMA recognises that there are elements of any health record that patients may feel particularly sensitive about and wish to restrict access to such information. Most electronic systems will allow data to be stored within the patient electronic record but in a hidden area with a flag in the record to indicate that the information is not generally available without the patient's permission. Where electronic systems do not offer extra layers of protection for the data, alternatives might be explored through discussion with a Caldicott Guardian.

Summary – electronic records

- Electronic records are subject to the duty of confidentiality common to paper-based records.
- Patients must be aware of how their data are shared and stored or have information readily available to them explaining the potential sharing of their health record.
- Patients can limit how much information is shared.
- Access to clinical information should be restricted to those providing clinical care to the patient.
- Patients must be informed about any upload of their clinical data to a national database and have the opportunity to opt out.

Security

All health professionals, and everybody employed by, or working under contract to, a healthcare establishment, have legal and contractual obligations of confidentiality. Maintaining patient confidentiality is a requirement of employment under the NHS and many independent sector contracts. Voluntary staff who are not employees should be asked to sign a confidentiality contract stating that they understand the obligation of confidentiality and will not breach it. In addition, doctors have particular obligations relating to the storage and use of health information, and may be held responsible for any breaches of confidentiality resulting from insecure handling. Doctors could face criminal charges as well as private actions by patients if they fail to provide adequate protection for health information.[30] The GMC states that doctors must:

- make sure that any personal information is effectively protected at all times against improper disclosure
- ensure that any staff they manage are trained and understand their responsibilities towards protecting personal information.[31]

Each organisation should have security, information governance and records management policies in place, which should be endorsed by its highest governance authority, for example the Board or all GP partners, and updated at regular intervals.[32] In England, NHS Connecting for Health has published an online *Information Governance Toolkit* which aims to bring together all the requirements, standards and best practice on handling personal information.[33] The tool kit provides a way for organisations to see whether information is handled correctly and protected from unauthorised access, loss, damage and destruction. All NHS organisations in England must complete the tool kit assessment which measures progress against a series of standards. The BMA, in conjunction with NHS Connecting for Health, has produced best practice guidelines in order to highlight responsibilities for both individuals and organisations in protecting electronic patient information.[34] In addition, the Department of Health has issued technical guidance on information security management of both electronic and paper-based health information.[35] As discussed in Chapter 5, the Information Commissioner has the power to fine organisations for serious data breaches under the Data Protection Act (see page 191). This is particularly relevant for healthcare organisations in view of the fact that they handle large quantities of highly sensitive data on a daily basis.

Protection is needed against both external threats, such as burglary, and internal threats such as inappropriate access by staff. Even the simplest security measures can be effective:

- lock doors, offices and filing cabinets
- avoid leaving paper or computer files open where they may be seen by others
- do not leave files unattended
- password protect computer systems and do not share passwords with other people
- change passwords at regular intervals to prevent anyone else using them
- always clear the screen of a previous patient's information before seeing another
- always log out of any computer system or application when finished.[36]

Staff in GP practices may know people who are patients of the practice. The BMA is aware of cases in which GP reception staff have inappropriately accessed the records of family members or acquaintances. Strict rules against unauthorised access should be part of staff contracts and there should be security measures in place to prevent inappropriate 'browsing' of records. In larger practices, having more than one member of staff on duty at all times can help. Electronic systems should make use of the ability to restrict individuals' access to a level that is suitable for their job (see pages 239–241). Electronic systems also maintain an audit trail indicating who has accessed patient information.

When records are stored remotely, for example on a centralised server, doctors must ensure that the remote facility has adequate safeguards to protect the information. This includes use of secure server connections and the appropriate encryption technology to ensure patient identifiable information is kept confidential. The Information Commissioner has said that, while he does not necessarily expect each GP practice, for example, to develop its own IT system capable of concealing the identities of patients from those who do not need to know them, he does expect those who are developing IT systems for use by GPs to build in such a capability and would certainly consider action against a GP (or any other data controller) who did not make use of the features available on a system for maximising the privacy of patients.[37] Sometimes there may also be a case for files on desktop computers to be encrypted if they contain sensitive data and are used in an area where they are at significant risk of being stolen or accessed improperly.

Sending patient information abroad

In 2010, concern was expressed in the media that the NHS was sending millions of confidential medical notes to India for transcribing.[38] The Data Protection Act 1998 is clear that personal data must not be transferred outside the European Economic Area (EEA) without adequate protections for the rights of data subjects equivalent to those provided by the Act. Data controllers have a duty to ensure that information exchanges at this level are compliant with the Act and that the appropriate protections are in place. Where doctors are aware that exchanges of patient information are taking place in this way, and have concerns about confidentiality, then they must raise these concerns by following the advice of the GMC on raising concerns about patient safety.[39]

GPs are also advised to take only necessary information with them when they leave the surgery to visit patients, because occasionally records have been stolen from doctors' cars. In many cases, the danger of possible loss or theft is outweighed by the improved quality of care that can be provided when the health records are available, but all reasonable precautions must be taken to ensure that identifiable information is not left unattended in risky situations and that appropriate levels of protection are deployed for electronic data being taken home on portable equipment, for example encryption techniques (see page 246).

For the record

The Information Commissioner has said that the NHS was amongst the worst offenders in 'unacceptable' rates of loss of data in the UK. The ICO criticised NHS trusts for data being stolen, lost in transit or mislaid by staff. The ICO also noted that 'far too much' personal data was being unnecessarily downloaded from secure servers onto unencrypted laptops, USB sticks and other portable media.[40] In one instance a trust lost three unencrypted USB sticks containing sensitive information about cancer patients[41] and in another a memory stick containing sensitive patient information, in addition to details about staff, was found in a supermarket car park.[42] It should, however, be noted that NHS organisations are actively encouraged to report data loss incidents and this may go some way towards explaining the high levels of data breaches which are brought to the attention of the ICO.

Health records should be stored in a secure way, with proper environmental control and adequate protection against fire and flood. Where records that are not in regular use are held only in electronic form, extra care may be needed to prevent corruption or deterioration of the data. Re-recording or migration of data may also need to be considered as equipment and software become obsolete.

Summary – security

- Doctors must ensure any personal information is effectively protected at all times.
- NHS organisations should have security policies in place to protect patient information.
- Both electronic and paper-based health information require safeguards against inappropriate access.
- The *Information Governance Toolkit* draws together the legal rules and guidance on how organisations should handle personal information.

Transmission

When transmitting patient details electronically, by fax, email, memory sticks or other portable devices, doctors are responsible for ensuring that identifiable information does not arrive in the wrong hands. The GMC states that doctors must follow policies and procedures designed to protect patients' privacy where they work and when using computer systems.[43] Whenever possible, clinical details must be separated from demographic data so that, should information fall into the wrong hands, it cannot readily be linked to an individual.[44] Obvious measures, such as using a unique identifying number rather than the patient's name and address, may be useful. In addition, it is BMA and Department of Health policy that all data transmitted in electronic format across the NHS must be encrypted.[45] Commissioning bodies, trusts and health boards should have policies in place to ensure the recommended encryption standards. NHS Connecting for Health has issued guidance on the use of encryption to protect identifiable and sensitive information when it is necessary to transfer data.[46] NHS Wales has the *National Encryption Framework* and *Encryption Code of Practice* which outlines the requirements to aid secure data transport[47] and a similar encryption policy exists in Scotland.[48] The only exception is the exchange of clinical information between NHSmail accounts because encryption technology is applied as part of the service (see below). Particular care should be taken with memory sticks to ensure that data are encrypted. NHS Connecting for Health has produced guidelines which detail the recommended encryption standards for when it is necessary to transfer data across removable media.[49]

The measures outlined above are necessary both to protect confidentiality and to ensure that doctors do not breach their obligation under the Data Protection Act 1998 to take adequate precautions to protect the confidential nature of information being transmitted. When information is being transmitted by fax, it is sensible to enquire whether the receiving machine is in a publicly accessible area, such as a waiting room, or in a private office. The BMA recommends that identifiable information should be faxed only when the receiving machine is known to be secure both during and out of working hours. Doctors should also make sure that, when data are being sent by email, messages will be received and dealt with, including if the intended recipient is absent, for example on holiday.

All members of staff should be aware of the procedures for the safe handling of confidential information.

NHSmail

NHSmail is an email service provided by the NHS for staff in England and Scotland. It is the only NHS email system accredited for the secure transfer of clinical data. This allows clinical information to be emailed to colleagues, who have NHSmail accounts, without the need for additional encryption as each email is encrypted during transition. The service uses technology to monitor for any potential security breaches. The BMA, in conjunction with Connecting for Health, has produced guidance on NHSmail.[50]

Transfer of GP records

The health records of a patient who leaves a GP practice are transferred to the patient's new GP via the commissioning body or primary care organisation. Many transfers of electronic records between GP practices in England are completed using the 'GP2GP' system, which enables an almost instantaneous transfer of a patient's electronic health record. If a patient leaves a computerised practice for a paper-based practice, a hard copy of his or her medical record at that date should be sent to the commissioning body or primary care organisation inside the manual record envelope, for onward transmission to the patient's new GP. It is essential that a complete and uncorrupted version of the record exists at all times, in the interests of both patients and doctors. The transfer of electronic patient records from one practice to another is discussed in detail in the Department of Health, BMA and Royal College of General Practitioners' joint guidance.[51]

Recordings

The increasing use of technologies such as video and picture messaging has made it considerably easier to record, copy and transmit images of patients. Doctors may be interested in using new technologies to aid rapid diagnosis and consultation and therefore improve patient care. Doctors need to bear in mind that when used for clinical purposes such images form part of the patient's medical record and the same standards of confidentiality, and the same requirements for consent to disclosure, apply (see Chapter 5).

A small number of exceptions to these requirements are covered in this section. The guidance here does not apply to CCTV recordings of public areas in hospitals and surgeries, which are the subject of separate guidance from the Information Commissioner.[52]

The general principles about record keeping covered in this chapter apply to all types of records. (This excludes pathology slides containing human tissue which are the subject of discussion in Chapter 12, although images of such slides are covered by this guidance.) The guidance in this section reflects the basic principles of the GMC guidance on making and using visual and audio recordings of patients.[53]

When making or using recordings the GMC states that doctors must:

- give patients the information they want, or need, about the purpose of the recording
- make recordings only where there is appropriate consent or other valid authority for doing so
- ensure that patients are under no pressure to give their consent for the recording to be made
- where practicable, stop the recording if the patient requests this, or if it is having an adverse effect on the consultation or treatment
- anonymise or code the recordings before using or disclosing them for a secondary purpose,[54] if this is practicable and will serve the purpose
- disclose or use recordings from which patients may be identifiable only with consent or other valid authority for doing so
- make appropriate secure arrangements for storing recordings
- be familiar with, and follow, the law and local guidance and procedures that apply where they work.[55]

The exceptional use of covert surveillance is discussed in Chapter 1 (pages 41–42).

Recordings made as part of a patient's care

The GMC identifies six categories of recordings for which consent to make the recordings is implicit in the consent given to the investigation or treatment, and does not need to be obtained separately:

- images of internal organs or structures
- images of pathology slides

- laparoscopic and endoscopic images
- recordings or organ functions
- ultrasound images
- X-rays.[56]

It is, however, clearly good practice to tell patients that images are being made as part of their care or treatment.

When these images are anonymous, the GMC advises that that they may be disclosed for use in research, teaching, training or other healthcare-related purposes, without consent, although doctors should, where practicable, explain that such recordings may be used in anonymised form for secondary purposes.[57] Of course, these images, when used in connection with a case history, could make a patient identifiable, and would therefore require permission. The making of other recordings and images that contribute to patient care, and which fall outside the list above, generally require express patient consent.[58] The GMC advises that, where practicable, doctors should explain any possible secondary uses of the recording in an anonymised form when seeking consent to make the recording. This discussion should be recorded in the patient's medical record.[59]

The images and recordings in the list above are, when presented alone, intrinsically anonymous. Other images or recordings may be anonymised by removing identifying details. Anonymisation must be effective;[60] simply putting a bar across a patient's eyes would not be sufficient, for example. The GMC advises that, when deciding whether a recording is anonymous, doctors should bear in mind that apparently insignificant details may still be capable of identifying the patient.[61] Extreme care should be taken about the anonymity of such recordings before using or publishing them without consent in journals or other learning materials.[62] The *British Medical Journal* publishes a patient consent form for use wherever a patient might be identifiable from a case report, illustration or paper published in the journal.[63]

The GMC draws a distinction between the use of these types of recordings for healthcare-related purposes such as teaching and research and the publication of images in media that are intended for a broad public audience and which are widely accessible to the public – such recordings are discussed below.

Adult patients who lack capacity

Where adults lack the capacity to consent to an identifiable recording for assessment and treatment purposes, agreement should be sought from someone with the lawful authority to consent on their behalf. Where no individual has legal authority to make the decision on a patient's behalf, it may be in the patient's best interests to discuss the making of the recording with family or friends close to the patient. Where there are no family members or friends available or willing to be involved in such a discussion or where treatment must be provided immediately, recordings may still be made where they form an integral part of an investigation or treatment in accordance with relevant legislation or common law (see Chapter 3).[64]

Where a recording has already been made as part of the patient's care, but may also be of value for a secondary purpose, the GMC advises that the recording should be anonymised wherever that is practicable and will serve the purpose.[65] (Recordings for use in widely accessible public media are distinct from other secondary purposes and are discussed on pages 250–251.) In relation to identifiable recordings used for secondary purposes the law in relation to adults lacking capacity is untested. In the BMA's view it is difficult to see how such a decision could be in the individual's best interests. Legal advice should be sought on a case-by-case basis for the use of identifiable recordings for reasons other than treatment and research. Involving incapacitated adults in research is dealt with separately below and in Chapter 14, pages 597–599.

Children or young people

Parents usually authorise recordings of their young children, while competent young people choose for themselves. The same advice for adults with capacity on use and disclosure of recordings made as part of care also applies to children and young people.

Recordings made for research, teaching, training and other healthcare-related purposes

Consent is required before making recordings for secondary purposes such as teaching, training, the assessment of healthcare professionals and research. It is good practice to get the patient's written consent but, if this is not practicable, the patient's oral consent should be obtained.[66] The GMC advises that before making the recording, doctors should explain:

- the purpose of the recording and how it will be used
- how long the recording will be kept and how it will be stored
- that patients may withhold consent, or withdraw consent during or immediately after the recording, and this will not affect the quality of care they receive or their relationship with those providing care.[67]

In some cases, although no recording has been planned, a recording of an unexpected development during the treatment process that would be valuable for teaching purposes may be made. Where the patient has capacity to consent their permission must be sought to make the recording.[68]

After a recording has been made, patients should be given the opportunity to see it and to withdraw consent for its future use. It is good practice to reaffirm consent for all continued use of identifiable recordings.

It is common for video recordings to be used as a teaching tool. Some bodies, including the BMA, have been concerned that doctors are not able to exercise adequate control over such visual teaching material, which could be copied illegally. It is difficult, if not impossible, to police provisions that all material must be withdrawn if the patient revokes consent to its use, although all efforts should be made to destroy or anonymise such material. One solution is that video recordings can be edited and anonymised by obscuring or pixelating identifying features. Although this is not universally possible, it is recommended that this procedure be followed wherever feasible. Patients' facial expressions, however, are important for some purposes, such as teaching that involves neurological and neuropsychological conditions. If anonymisation is not possible, consent from the patient is essential.

Except when patients have given specific consent to other arrangements, patient-identifiable recordings should remain part of the patient's confidential medical record, subject to the same safeguards as other data (see Chapter 5).

Adults who lack capacity

In England, Wales and Scotland it is lawful under the relevant mental capacity legislation to involve adults who lack capacity in research provided it is related to the condition with which they have been diagnosed; audio and visual recordings may form a part of such research. (This issue is covered in Chapter 14, pages 250–251.) Incapacitated patients should be given the opportunity to withdraw their consent for the use of the recording if they regain the capacity to make a decision.

In making audio or visual recordings for other secondary purposes the GMC states that doctors must be satisfied that:

- the recording is necessary, and benefits the patient or is in their best interests
- the purpose cannot be achieved in a way that is less restrictive of the patient's rights and choices.[69]

The law in this area is untested and doctors should seek legal advice on a case-by-case basis.

Children or young people

A person with parental responsibility may consent on behalf of a child or young person who lacks the competence to a planned or unplanned recording for secondary purposes. The GMC advises that the recording should stop if the child or young person objects verbally or through their actions, if they show distress in other ways about the recording or if the person with parental responsibility asks for the recording to stop.[70]

Minors must be able to withdraw consent upon attaining maturity. When the minor continues to be a patient, there should be opportunities to discuss permission as he or she becomes able to decide.

Documenting suspected cases of child abuse sometimes involves photographic records of children's bodies. Although usually parental consent should be sought, if alerting the parent would put the child at increased risk, photographs may be taken without consent. Particular care must be taken with such sensitive material. Practitioners must ensure that it is stored safely and disclosed only for the purposes intended.

Stillborn babies and neonates who are on the point of death are sometimes photographed at the request of the parents, but photographs should not be used for any other purposes, unless the parents indicate that this would be acceptable. Great sensitivity is required regarding this issue.

Recordings for use in widely accessible public media (television, radio, internet, print)

In general, the rules relevant to making recordings for secondary purposes also apply to recordings for use in widely accessible public media, for example to inform the general public. There are, however, some issues that are specific to recordings used in this context.

No identifying material may be published in textbooks or journals, or used for teaching without express patient consent (this should usually be in writing). For recordings or images that are not included in the list on pages 247–248, the GMC advises that patient consent is required to make a recording that will be used in widely accessible public media even if it is considered non-identifiable.

Sometimes, doctors may wish to publish a recording of a patient which was made as part of their care, although consent was not obtained at the time of recording. In these circumstances, patient consent must be obtained if the patient is, or may be, identifiable.[71] GMC guidance states that if the recording is anonymised, it is good practice to seek consent before publishing, bearing in mind the difficulties in ensuring that all the features of a recording that could identify the patient to any member of the public have been removed.[72]

Patients should understand that, once material is published and in the public domain, it is unlikely to be possible to withdraw it from circulation. Where a video recording has been made for a broadcast, doctors should check that patients understand that, once they have agreed to the recording being made for the broadcast, they may not be able to stop its subsequent use. The GMC states that if patients wish to restrict the use of material they should be advised to obtain agreement in writing from the programme maker and the owners of the recording before recording begins. That aside, the BMA takes the view that consent is not blanket permission but should be periodically renewed, giving the option to withdraw material from use or limit its future use. This is particularly important for children and young people. The GMC is clear that doctors must not participate in making or disclosing recordings of children or young people who lack competence, where it is believed that they may be harmed or distressed by making the recording or by its disclosure or use, even if a person with parental responsibility has given consent.[73]

Adults who lack capacity

As discussed above (and in Chapter 3), there are specific legal requirements for making recordings of adults who lack capacity, and using or disclosing such recordings. Legal advice should be sought in this area. The GMC states that in making audio or visual recordings for other secondary purposes, doctors must be satisfied that the recording is necessary and benefits the patient or is in their best interests, and that the purpose cannot be achieved in a way that is less restrictive of the patient's rights and choices.[74]

Children or young people

In the case of young children who are unable to decide for themselves, the consent of parents is needed and, as with all recordings used for secondary purposes, agreement for continued use should be re-confirmed at regular intervals. It may not be possible for material that has been published in the public domain to be completely withdrawn; however, where it might be possible to restrict distribution or withdraw the recording from circulation this should be done if a young person revokes consent on attaining maturity.

Telephone and other audio recordings

The monitoring and surveillance of telephone calls is subject to regulations by the Telecommunications Act 1984, which imposes a duty on those responsible for the call system to ensure that every reasonable effort is made to inform callers that their call might be recorded.

Calls to doctors' surgeries and to medical advice lines and similar services can obviously involve particularly sensitive information. In these circumstances it is important that callers are informed that their call may be recorded. Covert recordings of calls from individual patients should not be made.

In many areas, not only in health care, telephone calls are recorded for medico-legal purposes. Where telephone calls to a practice or out-of-hours service are recorded for these purposes, patients need to be told that conversations are being recorded and why. A failure to do so could mean that these recordings are unlawful. Information should also be available concerning how long recordings are kept and how patients can access them. As a general rule, the BMA encourages doctors to share information with patients whenever possible. If patients want to listen to recordings this should be facilitated, if possible via the doctor who usually provides their care. The recording forms part of the patient's medical record, and could be accessible under the access provisions of the Data Protection Act (see pages 255–260).

The BMA supports the use of tape-recording facilities for recording a discussion with a healthcare professional when a diagnosis or course of treatment is being discussed, when the aim is to assist patients to understand and recall facts. Doctors worry, however, if they feel that they are being recorded for future complaints or litigation, and may be less likely to want to express opinions freely. This issue is discussed further in Chapter 1 (pages 40–41).

Deceased patients

As discussed in Chapter 5 (pages 221–223), the duty of confidentiality continues after a patient has died. Where a recording was made when a patient was alive, doctors should follow a patient's known wishes after their death. This means that if a recording was made with the patient's consent for a specific purpose, it may be used after their death, provided there is no reason to believe that consent was withdrawn before the patient died.[75] However, if the recording will be in the public domain or the patient is identifiable, the GMC advises that consideration needs to be given to consulting the patient's family.[76] Legal advice should also be sought in these cases.

Storing and disposing of recordings

Recordings made as part of the patient's care form part of the medical record and must be treated in the same way as other medical records. The advice from the UK health departments on records retention, discussed on pages 253–255, should be followed.

For recordings made for secondary purposes, the GMC advises that doctors must be satisfied 'that there is agreement about the ownership, copyright, and intellectual property rights of the recording'.[77] Further advice can be sought from a Caldicott Guardian.

Summary – recordings

- Audio and visual recordings form part of health records.
- For the making of certain recordings which are part of patients' care or treatment, separate consent is not required.
- Consent should be sought to make recordings for secondary purposes.
- When consent is not available because the patient lacks capacity, recordings may be made for treatment purposes and consent sought from someone close to the patient or a proxy decision maker.

- Images from which it is impossible to identify the patient – generally, internal images and images of pathology slides – may be used for teaching, audit or research without consent, but such uses of identifiable images require consent.
- Extreme care should be taken about ensuring the anonymity of recordings before they are used or published in learning materials and media that is widely accessible to the public.
- Patients should understand that, once material is published and in the public domain, it is unlikely to be possible to withdraw it from circulation.

Ownership

For most purposes, establishing who owns the information or health record is not significant. What matters is who has control of records and information. The question of who owns health records is sometimes asked, however. In law, the concept of ownership of information is very underdeveloped. Many differentiate between the information, which belongs to the patient, the opinion, which the doctor brings to that raw information, and the documentation of this process. Private doctors, or occasionally their employers, are considered to own the records they make (for discussion of what happens to records when private practitioners retire or leave their employer, see page 255). NHS records are understood in law to be the property of the Secretary of State for Health. However, the Data Protection Act 1998 makes it a statutory requirement for data processing to meet common law standards for confidentiality (see Chapter 5, pages 190–191). The Act applies to all manual and computerised health records, and clearly prohibits inappropriate conditions being imposed by data 'owners'.

Retention of records

The primary purpose of making and maintaining health records is the provision of healthcare to the patient. Records serve many other useful purposes, however, and, with appropriate authorisation, may be useful for research, teaching, audit and litigation, virtually without limit of time, although there are legal rules governing the time limits within which actions for personal injuries or death may be brought.

The Department of Health for England, the Scottish Executive Health Department, National Assembly for Wales and the Department of Health, Social Services and Public Safety in Northern Ireland publish codes of practice which give detailed guidance about the retention of health records to help the NHS meet its legal obligations in the management of its records.[78] A basic summary of the main points for GP and hospital records is given in Tables 6.1–6.3. However, these tables only include extracts from the relevant schedules and doctors should refer directly to the schedules themselves for more detailed information specific to each of the devolved nations. The recommendations apply to NHS records irrespective of the form in which the records are held and the BMA advises private practitioners to follow the same rules (unless the records can be transferred to the patient's new doctor). As is highlighted throughout this chapter, record holders are under a legal and ethical obligation to maintain records safely and securely. The retention of human tissue of any form is covered in Chapter 12.

Although the guidance refers to minimum periods for which records must be retained, there may be occasions on which records need to be retained for longer. It is important to bear in mind that the fifth principle of the Data Protection Act 1998 prohibits the retention

Table 6.1 Recommended minimum lengths of retention of GP records (England, Wales and Northern Ireland)[101]

Type	Retention period
GP records	10 years after death or after the patient has permanently left the country unless the patient remains in the European Union. In the case of a child, if the illness or death could have potential relevance to adult conditions or have genetic implications for the family of the deceased, the advice of clinicians should be sought as to whether to retain the records for a longer period. Electronic patient records must not be destroyed, or deleted, for the foreseeable future.
Maternity records	25 years after the birth of the last child.
Records relating to persons receiving treatment for a mental disorder within the meaning of mental health legislation	20 years after the date of the last contact; or 10 years after the patient's death, if sooner.
Records relating to those serving in HM Armed Forces	Not to be destroyed.
Records relating to those serving a prison sentence	Not to be destroyed.

Table 6.2 Recommended minimum lengths of retention of hospital records (England, Wales and Northern Ireland)

Type	Retention period
Maternity records (including all obstetric and midwifery records, including those of episodes of maternity care that end in stillbirth or where the child later dies)	25 years after the birth of the last child.
Children and young people (all types of records relating to children and young people)	Until the patient's 25th birthday or 26th if the young person was 17 at conclusion of treatment, or 8 years after death.
Mentally disordered persons (within the meaning of any Mental Health Act)	20 years after the date of last contact between the patient/client/service user and any health/care professional employed by the mental health provider, or 8 years after the death of the patient/client/service user if sooner.
All other hospital records (other than non-specified secondary care records)	8 years after the conclusion of treatment or death.

Table 6.3 Summary of minimum retention periods for personal health records (Scotland)

Type	Retention period
Adult	6 years after last entry, or 3 years after the patient's death.
Records relating to children and young people (16 years on admission)	Until the patient's 25th birthday, or 26th if an entry was made when the young person was 17; or 3 years after death of the patient if sooner.
Mentally disordered person (within the meaning of any Mental Health Act)	20 years after date of last contact between the patient/client/service user and any health/care professional employed by the mental health provider, or 3 years after the death of the patient/client/service user if sooner and the patient died while in the care of the organisation.
Maternity records	25 years after the birth of the last child.
GP records	For the patient's lifetime and 3 years after the patient's death. Electronic Patient Records (GP only) must not be destroyed, or deleted, for the foreseeable future

of personal data for longer than necessary. Although the definition of 'necessary' will vary, where a decision is made to retain records for longer than the periods given below, it is important that this is supported by explicit reasons, which should ordinarily be recorded in the records. Doctors must be careful to ensure that, if it is known that records may be needed in litigation, they are not destroyed. Private practitioners are unlikely to be criticised if they retain records for the minimum period recommended by the NHS.

It should be noted that the guidance specifies that electronic records must not be destroyed for the foreseeable future.

Disposal

When doctors are responsible for destroying records, they must ensure that the method of destruction is effective and does not compromise confidentiality. A record of the destruction should be kept. Incineration, pulping and shredding are appropriate methods of destroying paper records. Doctors must similarly ensure that electronic data are deleted effectively, when appropriate. Again, this may involve incineration or other methods of physical destruction.

Private records

When private practitioners retire and there is a successor for their practice, the records should be passed to the new doctor. If there is no successor, records should be stored securely for the appropriate period (see page 254) or, with the patient's consent, passed to another doctor who is providing care. Patients should be informed of any changes in arrangements for their records – this is a requirement of the Data Protection Act.

Private doctors should make a will with instructions for how their records should be handled after their death. Ideally, the records should be transferred to another doctor to take responsibility for their safe-keeping. If there is no arrangement for succession to a private practice, the person administering the estate distributes the deceased's property. If no doctor can be found to take the records, one option is for the records to be given to the patients to take with them to their next doctor. Alternatively, and if there is no other reason to retain records, those falling outwith the recommended minimum retention periods for NHS records may be destroyed. Those administering a deceased doctor's estate should bear in mind that the patients to whom the records relate are entitled to expect that their confidentiality will be maintained. Patients may have a right to sue the holder of the records if information about them is wrongly disclosed. To minimise risks to confidentiality, therefore, ideally a registered health professional should sort through records to establish which ones may be destroyed. Those with custody of records should bear in mind that patients also retain their rights of access to their records (see below).

For information about occupational health records see Chapter 16, pages 673–679.

Access to health records

Access by patients

Doctors have long had the discretion to show patients the contents of records and the BMA encourages doctors to give patients informal access to their records.

Patients have a statutory right of access to information about themselves, as enshrined in the Data Protection Act 1998.[79] This covers all health records, including reports written to satisfy the requirements of mental health legislation and medical reports written by independent doctors who have no other professional relationship with the patient. The BMA and the Department of Health have both produced guidance on access to health records requests.[80]

The Access to Medical Reports Act 1988 and Access to Personal Files and Medical Reports (Northern Ireland) Order 1991 relate specifically to medical reports for insurance or employment purposes that are written by the patient's own doctor and give rights of access to them (see also Chapter 16, page 653). The GMC advises doctors to offer to show patients any reports they write about them for employment and insurance purposes.[81] The caveats to this advice are that the disclosure must not cause serious harm to the patient or anyone else and that the disclosure would not reveal information about another person. There are limited rights of access to information about deceased patients in the Access to Health Records Act 1990 and Access to Health Records (Northern Ireland) Order 1993 which are covered below and in Chapter 5, pages 221–223.

Patients, including young people, may apply for access to their own records, or may authorise a third party, such as their solicitor, to do so on their behalf (subject to the exemptions listed below). It is not necessary for patients to give reasons as to why they wish to access their records and copies must be provided if requested. The Data Protection Act 1998 also requires that copies are accompanied by an explanation of any terms that might be unintelligible to the patient or the person requesting access to the records. There is a schedule of fees that may be charged, which vary according to whether the records are held manually or on computer, and whether a copy is requested.[82]

Disproportionate effort

The circumstances in which it would not be possible to supply permanent copies of health records when such requests are made by patients are extremely rare. However, the Data Protection Act 1998 does not require that permanent copies be supplied if 'disproportionate effort' is involved in doing so. The Act does not define 'disproportionate effort' but health professionals are advised to consider the length of time it will take to provide the information, how difficult it might be to provide it, whether extra staff need to be employed to carry out the request and the size of the organisation in relation to these factors. Decisions as to what is disproportionate effort must be made on a case-by-case basis. For a request to involve disproportionate effort it is important that the effort, rather than the cost, be disproportionate regardless of whether the request for copies is for X-rays or any other types of health records.

Information that should not be disclosed

The Data Protection Act 1998 exempts certain categories of data from its subject access provisions. Information should not be disclosed if:

- it is likely to cause serious physical or mental harm to the patient or another person
- it relates to a third party who has not given consent to the disclosure (where that third party is not a health professional who has cared for the patient)[83]
- it is requested by a third party and the patient had asked that the information be kept confidential

- the records are subject to legal professional privilege or, in Scotland, to confidentiality as between client and professional legal adviser (this may arise in the case of an independent medical report written for the purpose of litigation)
- it is restricted by a court order
- it relates to the keeping or using of gametes or embryos or pertains to an individual being born as a result of *in vitro* fertilisation,[84] or
- in the case of children's records, disclosure is prohibited by law, for example, adoption and parental order records and records of the special educational needs of children in England, Wales, Scotland and Northern Ireland.[85]

Circumstances in which information may be withheld on the grounds of serious harm are extremely rare, and this exemption does not justify withholding comments in the records because patients may find them upsetting, although it may be helpful to discuss any potentially distressing entries with patients in advance of access and an offer to do so whenever patients wish to see their medical records would be considered to be good practice. Where there is any doubt as to whether disclosure would cause serious harm, the BMA recommends that the appropriate professional discusses the matter anonymously with an experienced colleague, the Caldicott Guardian or defence body. Withholding access solely because disclosure would be embarrassing for doctors, or may give rise to legal claims against them, is not acceptable.

Doctors should, of course, bear in mind that patients may read what they write. Records should not be amended because of a request for access. If amendments are made between the time that the request for access was received and the time at which the records were supplied, these must only be amendments that would have been made regardless of the request for access. (Removing information from records is covered on page 237.)

Copying letters to patients

The NHS Constitution for England includes a pledge that '[t]he NHS commits to share with you any letters sent between clinicians about your care'.[86] Copying letters to patients is not a contractual obligation for doctors, although the BMA believes it is good practice. It is also strongly recommended by the Department of Health.[87] The BMA has produced guidance on copying letters to patients which highlights a number of benefits this practice can bring. For example it:

- provides reassurance that clinical correspondence has taken place
- ensures that misunderstandings can be corrected or explained
- provides a valuable written point of reference for patients who are unable to remember complex important information.[88]

Enabling patients to access electronic health records

With increased use of electronic records, many patients can access their own records directly via internet connections controlled by passwords and PIN numbers. Different electronic systems have been developed to enable this process in the UK. The Royal College of General Practitioners has produced guidance for health professionals on patients reading their own electronic health records.[89] The guidance outlines the principles that should apply to such systems and covers the security and accessibility considerations that may arise. It applies to record access in both primary care and hospital settings. It is vital that electronic systems include robust technical controls and that appropriate measures (identity checks and PIN/password systems, for example) are taken to secure and control access to personal data in health records without providing access to confidential information about other people.

Access to the records of children and young people

All competent young people, whatever their age, may exercise a statutory right of access to their own health records.[90] Additionally, people with parental responsibility have a statutory right to apply for access to their child's health records, unless a court has imposed specific conditions to the contrary or providing access would conflict with the interests of the child. (Parental responsibility is discussed in Chapter 4, pages 160–161.[91]) This is an area where the tension between parents' rights and young people's developing maturity can come into conflict. It may be necessary to discuss parental access alone with young people if there is a suspicion that they are under pressure to agree.

If patients are minors (under 16 years in Scotland, under 18 years in the rest of the UK) but capable of giving consent, parents can apply to have access to their records only with the young person's consent. As discussed in Chapter 4, parents should ideally help young people to make medical decisions and should be aware of information about their child's care. In some cases, however, young people may wish to keep confidential from their parents some of the matters they have raised with their doctor. Contraceptive advice, examination for sexually transmitted infections, assistance in stopping smoking or drug abuse are examples of matters that young people may wish to conceal from their parents, although doctors should encourage them to involve the parents whenever possible.

In cases in which a child cannot understand the nature of the application, but parental access would be in his or her interests, the law allows such access. Parental access to a minor's medical record should not be allowed when it conflicts with the child's interests. Any information that the child previously gave in the expectation that it would not be revealed should not be released, although it must be noted that, exceptionally, doctors can breach the confidentiality of any patient if they consider that there are sufficiently serious grounds to justify it (see Chapter 5).

Parents may exercise this aspect of their parental responsibility separately from one another. If one parent applies for access, there is no requirement to inform the other, although if this would be in the child's best interests it may be appropriate in some cases. GPs in particular can find themselves in a difficult position when separated parents, independently of each other, want information about their child's healthcare. Some parents who do not live with their child ask the GP to contact them each time the child is brought to the surgery. There is no requirement on GPs to agree to such requests, which could become time-consuming if the child presents frequently. It is clearly better if parents are able to communicate with each other about their child's health, although doctors may agree to contact a parent under certain circumstances, for example if something serious arises. In any case, both parents may apply for access to the health records at reasonable intervals of time, provided that they have parental responsibility. Doctors are also usually prepared to discuss the child's health informally without requiring that the procedures in the legislation are followed. The aim is to ensure that both parents are involved in the child's healthcare without imposing a disproportionate burden on the doctor. Only if disclosure to either parent would be contrary to the child's interests, or contrary to a competent child's wishes, should information be withheld from those with parental responsibility.

A problem may arise if a young person who has been prescribed contraception refuses to allow her doctor to grant parental access to her medical record in order to conceal this fact, even though the doctor believes it would be in her best interests for her parents to be informed. The decision to prescribe in such cases turns on the competence and understanding of the patient, so it would follow that a patient capable of making up her mind about contraception should also be able to control access to her health record. More difficult perhaps is the case of a young person who requested contraception that the doctor declined to prescribe on grounds of a lack of comprehension of what was involved. Such decisions are subject to the doctor's clinical judgement in each case, but, unless there are very convincing reasons to the contrary, the doctor should keep this type of request confidential even if he or she believes the patient is insufficiently mature for the request to be granted. If, however, the doctor considers the child to be at risk of exploitation or abuse, the limits of confidentiality should be discussed and the young person told that information may exceptionally need to be disclosed. If the child cannot be persuaded to agree to voluntary disclosure, and there is an immediate need to disclose information to an outside agency, he or she should be told what action is to be taken, unless to do so would expose the child or others to increased risk of serious harm.[92] (Child protection issues are discussed in detail in Chapter 4, pages 174–180.)

Access to the records of incapacitated adults

As discussed in Chapter 5, information can be shared with people who are close to an incapacitated patient when this is in his or her interests. In some circumstances a third party may exercise rights of access to the patient's records. When the patient is incapable of managing his or her own affairs, a proxy decision maker or court-appointed deputy may seek access to the records under the Data Protection Act. Access should be restricted to the information necessary for the appointee to carry out his or her functions. Disclosure is acceptable insofar as it is commensurate with the best interests and previous wishes of the patient. Information given by patients at a time when they were competent and believed it would be kept confidential cannot be disclosed subsequently to other people. Confidentiality and issues relevant to sharing information with people close to incapacitated adults are discussed in Chapter 5, page 219 and Chapter 3.

Access to the records of deceased persons

As is discussed in Chapter 5, pages 221–222, most information in medical records is likely to be confidential and exempt from disclosure under section 41 of the Freedom of Information Act 2000 (FOIA).[93] The Freedom of Information (Scotland) Act 2002 contains an exemption to the disclosure of deceased patients' records.[94]

Statutory rights of access are set out in the Access to Health Records Act 1990 and Access to Health Records (Northern Ireland) Order 1993.[95] Access may be sought by any person who may have a claim arising from the death of a patient, and rights of access are limited to information directly relevant to that claim. For example, a personal representative or executor can access information that is necessary in relation to the management of the deceased's estate, as can an individual who was a dependent of the deceased and who has a claim relating to that dependency that has arisen from the death.

Information may be withheld if:

- it identifies a third party who has not given consent for disclosure, unless that person is a health professional who has cared for the patient

- in the opinion of the relevant health professional, it is likely to cause serious harm to somebody's physical or mental health, or
- the patient gave it in the past on the understanding that it would be kept confidential.

It follows that doctors should counsel their patients about the possibility of disclosure after death and solicit views about eventual disclosure where it is obvious in the circumstances that there may be some sensitivity. Such discussions should be documented in the records. In addition to the legal provisions, people who were close to a deceased patient often ask to see the records in order to learn more about the illness of their loved one. As discussed in the previous chapter, doctors have always had discretion to disclose information to deceased persons' relatives or others for appropriate purposes when there is a clear justification. Confidentiality and handling requests of this nature are covered in Chapter 5, page 222.

Summary – access to health records

- Patients and their representatives are entitled to have access to their records and to have copies of them.
- Patients may authorise a third party, such as a lawyer, to access records on their behalf.
- Parents with parental responsibility may have access to their child's records if this is in the child's best interests and, when the child is competent, if he or she gives consent.
- People appointed to manage the affairs of mentally incapacitated patients may have access to information necessary to fulfil their function.
- Information may be withheld if revealing it may cause serious physical or mental harm to the patient or, in certain circumstances, it relates to a third party who is not a health professional who has cared for the patient.
- Doctors should facilitate information access by patients, and be willing to show them the contents of their records.

Access to medical reports

The Access to Medical Reports Act 1988 and Access to Personal Files and Medical Reports (Northern Ireland) Order 1991 give patients rights in respect of reports written about them for employment or insurance purposes. They cover reports written by the applicant's GP or a specialist who has provided care. The extent to which occupational health physicians are subject to the legislation has long been a matter of debate. The degree of contact and nature of consultations with employees are likely to be relevant and the Faculty of Occupational Medicine advises that ultimately it is for occupational physicians to determine whether their activities amount to the provision of care defined by the legislation.[96] Reports written by an independent medical examiner are not covered. However, patients are entitled to access these reports under data protection legislation (see pages 255–258).

The administrative requirements of the legislation fall mainly upon the body that requests the report (the applicant). Applicants must inform patients of their rights, including the folowing:

- to withhold permission for the company to seek a medical report (that is, to refuse consent to the release of information)

- to have access to the medical report after completion by the doctor either before it is sent to the company or up to 6 months after it is sent
- if seeing the report before it is sent, to instruct the doctor not to send the report
- to request the amendment of inaccuracies in the report.

Patients must be informed when a report is sought and notified in writing of their rights. From the time that the doctor is notified that the patient wants to see the report, the patient has 21 days in which to do so and the doctor should not dispatch the report during this period. If the patient does not contact the doctor within that 21 days, the doctor may send the completed report to the applicant. If the patient sees the report and withdraws consent for it to be released, it must not be dispatched and the doctor should inform the applicant.

Patients are entitled to have any factual inaccuracies in the report corrected. If the doctor does not agree that there is an error, he or she must append a note to the report regarding the disputed information. Doctors must not comply with patients' requests to leave out relevant information from reports. If a patient refuses to give permission for certain relevant information to be included, the doctor should indicate to the applicant that he or she cannot write a report, taking care not to reveal any information the patient did not want revealed.[97] Alternatively, the report can be sent but the doctor must indicate that certain, medically relevant, information has been withheld at the request of the patient.

Looking towards the future

With the increase in electronic records, it is now much more feasible for patients to access their own health records directly. Record access by patients may become an integral part of the care process in the future, particularly in the context of shared decision making with health professionals.[98] There is increasing evidence that there are benefits for both patients and health professionals in direct patient record access. For example, a study undertaken in 2009 demonstrated that patients can find access to their record reassuring in terms of being fully informed about their care and it can reinforce confidence in GPs.[99] With the potential for patients to access their record through a wide variety of media in the future, such as viewing their records online or via mobile devices, health professionals will need to consider how they might adapt to this cultural change and new ways of working while, at the same time, ensuring that patient groups who may make less use of new technologies are not disadvantaged. Of course, record access by patients should be considered an additional way of supplying patients with the information they may require to manage their care, rather than a substitute for information communicated by health professionals in consultations. Further work is required in order to address some of the complexities associated with patient access, to ensure that shared record access is successful.[100]

There is also likely to be increased focus on the quality of health data as the requirement to capture information for a variety of purposes grows. Examples include quality metrics, performance monitoring, service commissioning and appraisal and revalidation. The continued improvement of the quality of data contained in health records is essential in order to improve patient care, directly, by ensuring clinicians are making decisions based on accurate information, particularly when it is from different care settings and mistakes may not be immediately apparent, and indirectly, when analysing data to improve the quality of clinical care. Continued investment in existing successful IT developments, data quality and supporting infrastructure will be necessary in order to ensure the benefits are available to patients and the health professionals who care for them.

References

1 In Scotland hand-held health records are available for gypsy and traveller communities. In England, a similar record is available for asylum seekers.

2 General Medical Council (2006) *Good Medical Practice*, GMC, London, paras 3 (f) and (g).

3 Department of Health (2008) *A Clinician's Guide to Record Standards – Part 2: Standards for the structure and content of medical records and communications when patients are admitted to hospital*, DH, London. Available at: www.rcplondon.ac.uk (accessed 8 February 2011).

4 The headings include admission, handover and discharge, and example templates can be downloaded and used to create paper proformas that can be customised for use by individual hospitals and trusts. Department of Health (2008) *A Clinician's Guide to Record Standards – Part 2: Standards for the structure and content of medical records and communications when patients are admitted to hospital*, DH, London. Available at: www.rcplondon.ac.uk (accessed 8 February 2011).

5 Audit Commission, Royal College of Physicians (2009) *Improving clinical records and clinical coding together*, Audit Commission, London. The financial management system of Payment by Results pays trusts for the work that they do.

6 Medical and Dental Defence Union of Scotland (2009) *Risk Alert: Altering medical notes* (4 June), MDDUS, Glasgow.

7 General Medical Council Fitness to Practise Panel, 22 March – 5 May 2010.

8 It should be noted that different computer systems handle the recording of a patient on a register in different ways so the ways to implement any change in the record will vary.

9 In England, the Personal Demographic Service is the national electronic database of NHS patient demographic details. In Scotland, the Community Health Index initiative provides patient demographic information. In Wales, the Welsh Demographic Service stores demographic information. In Northern Ireland, the Health and Care Number index is the central demographic system.

10 Connecting For Health, *Personal Demographics Service, Violent Patient Indicator*. Available at: www.connectingforhealth.nhs.uk (accessed 8 February 2011).

11 It should be noted that adoption records are exempt from subject access requests under the Data Protection Act 1998 (see pages 256–257).

12 Connecting For Health, *Adoptions*. Available at: www.connectingforhealth.nhs.uk (accessed 1 February 2011).

13 National Information Governance Board for Health and Social Care (2010) *Requesting amendments to health and social care records*, NIGB, London, p.8.

14 National Information Governance Board for Health and Social Care (2010) *Requesting amendments to health and social care records*, NIGB, London.

15 The BMA has agreed joint guidance with the Association of British Insurers (ABI) to set out best practice and practical advice on the use of medical information in insurance. British Medical Association, Association of British Insurers (2010) *Medical information and insurance*, BMA, London.

16 Department of Health (2008) *Guidance for GPs, other clinicians and health professionals on the care of gender variant people*, DH, London, p.19.

17 Bowcott O. (2010) NHS patients given right to delete electronic record. *The Guardian on-line* (May 26). Available at: www.guardian.co.uk (accessed 28 February 2011).

18 National Information Governance Board for Health and Social Care (2010) *Requesting amendments to health and social care records*, NIGB, London, p.11. Department of Health (2010) *Guidance for Access to Health Records Requests*, DH, London, p.13.

19 National Information Governance Board for Health and Social Care (2010) *Requesting amendments to health and social care records*, NIGB, London, p.12. Department of Health (2010) *Guidance for Access to Health Records Requests*, DH, London, p.13.

20 National Information Governance Board for Health and Social Care (2010) *Requesting amendments to health and social care records*, NIGB, London, p.16.

21 National Information Governance Board for Health and Social Care (2010) *Requesting amendments to health and social care records*, NIGB, London, pp.11–13.

22 Department of Health, British Medical Association, Royal College of General Practitioners (2011) *The good practice guidelines for GP electronic patient records* (version 4), DH, London.

23 National Information Governance Board (2011) *NHS Care Record Guarantee*, NIGB, London, p.13.

24 General Medical Council (2009) *Confidentiality*, GMC, London, para 26.

25 Royal College of General Practitioners, Connecting for Health (2009) *Informing shared clinical care: final report of the Shared Record Professional Guidance Project*, RCGP, London.

26 The BMA has produced specific guidance on this point: British Medical Association (2010) *Acting upon test results in an electronic world*, BMA, London.

27 *I v Finland* (20511/03) [2008] ECHR 623 (17 July 2008).

28 Further information can be found at: www.scotland.gov.uk.

29 Information on how to register is available at: www.healthspace.nhs.uk (accessed 28 February 2011).

30 Department of Health (2003) *Confidentiality: NHS Code of Practice*, DH, London, pp.16–19.

31 General Medical Council (2009) *Confidentiality*, GMC, London, paras 12 and 15.

32 Department of Health (2006) *Records management: NHS Code of Practice*, DH, London. This is a guide to the required standards of practice in the management of records and includes guidance on what should be included in each organisation's records management policy. The Department of Health, in conjunction with the BMA and Royal College of General Practitioners, has also produced guidance on managing electronic records, information governance issues and security for GP practices. See: Department of Health, British Medical Association, Royal College of General Practitioners (2011) *The good practice guidelines for GP electronic patient records* (version 4), DH, London.

33 Department of Health. *Information Governance Toolkit*. Available at: www.igt.connectingforhealth.nhs.uk (accessed 28 February 2011).

34 NHS Connecting for Health, British Medical Association (2008) *Joint Guidance on Protecting Electronic Patient Information*, BMA, London.

35 Department of Health (2007) *Information Security Management: NHS Code of Practice*, DH, London.

36 Department of Health (2003) *Confidentiality: NHS Code of Practice*, DH, London, pp.16–19. Connecting for Health, British Medical Association (2008) *Joint Guidance on Protecting Electronic Patient Information*, BMA, London.

37 Information Commissioner (2002) *Use and disclosure of health data: Guidance on the application of the Data Protection Act 1998*, ICO, Wilmslow, p.5.

38 Ungoed-Thomas J. (2010) NHS sends confidential patient records to India. *The Times* (April 4). Available at: www.timesonline.co.uk (accessed 28 February 2011).

39 General Medical Council (2006) *Good Medical Practice*, GMC, London, para 6.

40 Anon. (2010) 'Unacceptable' level of data loss. *BBC News Online* (November 11). Available at: www.bbc.co.uk/news (accessed 28 February 2011).

41 Information Commissioner (2009) *NHS staff to improve data handling after details of cancer patients go missing*. Press release, October 27.

42 Anon. (2010) Health records found in Asda car park. *BBC News Online*, (May 5). Available at: www.bbc.co.uk/news (accessed 28 February 2011).

43 General Medical Council (2009) *Confidentiality*, GMC, London, para 14.

44 General Medical Council (2009) *Confidentiality*, GMC, London, para 15.

45 British Medical Association (2002) *Consulting in the modern world*, BMA, London, p.6. NHS Connecting for Health (2009) *Guidelines on use of encryption to protect identifiable and sensitive information*, DH, London.

46 NHS Connecting for Health (2009) *Guidelines on use of encryption to protect identifiable and sensitive information*, DH, London.

47 NHS Wales, *National Encryption Framework*. Available at: www.wales.nhs.uk (accessed 28 February 2011).

48 NHS Scotland, *Encryption Policy*. Available at: www.srr.scot.nhs.uk (accessed 28 February 2011). NHS Scotland (2008) *eHealth Mobile Data Protection Standard*, NHS Scotland, Edinburgh.

49 Department of Health, *Information Governance Toolkit*, DH, London. Available at: www.igt.connectingforhealth.nhs.uk (accessed 28 February 2011).

50 British Medical Association, Connecting for Health. *NHSmail guidance*. Available at: www.connectingforhealth.nhs.uk (accessed 19 May 2011).

51 Department of Health, British Medical Association, Royal College of General Practitioners (2011) *The good practice guidelines for GP electronic patient records* (version 4), DH, London.

52 Information Commissioner's Office (2008) *CCTV Code of Practice*, ICO, Wilmslow.

53 General Medical Council (2011) *Making and using visual and audio recordings of patients*, GMC, London.

54 Secondary purposes are health-related uses that are not designed to benefit the patient directly, for example, teaching, assessment of healthcare professionals and students and research. General Medical Council (2011) *Making and using visual and audio recordings of patients*, GMC, London, para 5.

55 General Medical Council (2011) *Making and using visual and audio recordings of patients*, GMC, London, para 8.

56 General Medical Council (2011) *Making and using visual and audio recordings of patients*, GMC, London, para 10.

57 General Medical Council (2011) *Making and using visual and audio recordings of patients*, GMC, London, paras 11, 12 and 17.

58 General Medical Council (2011) *Making and using visual and audio recordings of patients*, GMC, London, para 13.

59 General Medical Council (2011) *Making and using visual and audio recordings of patients*, GMC, London, para 14.

60 Further advice on anonymising information is available from the Information Commissioner's Office. Information Commissioner's Office (2007) *Data Protection Technical Guidance: Determining what is personal data*, ICO, Wilmslow, section C.

61 General Medical Council (2011) *Making and using visual and audio recordings of patients*, GMC, London, para 17.

62 General Medical Council (2011) *Making and using visual and audio recordings of patients*, GMC, London, para 17.

63 BMJ editorial policies available at: www.bmj.com/bmj/authors/editorial-policies/ (accessed 28 February 2011).

64 General Medical Council (2011) *Making and using visual and audio recordings of patients*, GMC, London, paras 18–19.

65 General Medical Council (2011) *Making and using visual and audio recordings of patients*, GMC, London, para 20.

66 General Medical Council (2011) *Making and using visual and audio recordings of patients*, GMC, London, para 24.

67 General Medical Council (2011) *Making and using visual and audio recordings of patients*, GMC, London, para 25.

68 General Medical Council (2011) *Making and using visual and audio recordings of patients*, GMC, London, para 27.

69 General Medical Council (2011) *Making and using visual and audio recordings of patients*, GMC, London, para 31.

70 General Medical Council (2011) *Making and using visual and audio recordings of patients*, GMC, London, para 34.

71 General Medical Council (2011) *Making and using visual and audio recordings of patients*, GMC, London, para 38.

72 General Medical Council (2011) *Making and using visual and audio recordings of patients*, GMC, London, para 39.

73 General Medical Council (2011) *Making and using visual and audio recordings of patients*, GMC, London, para 44.

74 General Medical Council (2011) *Making and using visual and audio recordings of patients*, GMC, London, para 31.

75 General Medical Council (2011) *Making and using visual and audio recordings of patients*, GMC, London, para 47.

76 General Medical Council (2011) *Making and using visual and audio recordings of patients*, GMC, London, para 48.

77 General Medical Council (2011) *Making and using visual and audio recordings of patients*, GMC, London, para 57.

78 Department of Health (2006) *Records management: NHS Code of Practice*, DH, London. Scottish Government (2008) *Records Management: NHS code of practice (Scotland) Version 1.0*, Scottish Governemnt, Edinburgh. National Assembly for Wales (2000) *Welsh Health Circular 71: For The Record*, National Assembly for Wales, Cardiff. Department of Health, Social Services and Public Safety (2005) *Good Management, Good Records*, DHSSPS, Belfast. Department of Health, Social Services and Public Safety (2000) *Preservation, Retention and Destruction of GP Medical Records Circular HSS (PCC) 2000/1*, DHSSPS, Belfast. At the time of writing the DHSSPS was consulting on the *Good Management, Good Records* publication. The updated version will cover GP medical records as well as hospital records and will replace *Preservation, Retention and Destruction of GP Medical Records Circular HSS (PCC) 2000/1*.

79 Data Protection Act 1998, s 7 and 8.

80 British Medical Association (2008) *Access to health records: Guidance for health professionals in the United Kingdom*, BMA, London. Department of Health (2010) *Guidance for Access to Health Records Requests*, DH, London.

81 General Medical Council (2009) *Confidentiality*, GMC, London, para 34.

82 British Medical Association (2008) *Access to health records: Guidance for health professionals in the United Kingdom*, BMA, London.

83 Information Commissioner (2006) *Data Protection Technical guidance note: Dealing with subject access requests involving other people's information*, ICO, Wilmslow.

84 The Data Protection (Miscellaneous Subject Access Exemptions) Order 2000. SI 2000/419.

85 The Data Protection (Miscellaneous Subject Access Exemptions) Order 2000. SI 2000/419.

86 Department of Health (2010) *The NHS Constitution for England*, DH, London, p.7.

87 Department of Health (2003) *Copying letters to patients: Good practice guidelines*, DH, London.

88 British Medical Association (2009) *Defining best practice for copying letters to patients: Guidance for consultant doctors*, BMA, London.

89   Royal College of General Practitioners (2010) *Enabling Patients to Access Electronic Health Records: Guidance for Health Professionals*, RCGP, London.

90   General Medical Council (2007) *0-18 years: guidance for doctors*, GMC, London, paras 53–5.

91   British Medical Association (2008) *Parental Responsibility: Guidance from the British Medical Association*, BMA, London.

92   British Medical Association (2009) *Child protection: a tool kit for doctors*, BMA, London.

93   *Bluck v The Information Commissioner and Epsom and St Helier University NHS Trust* [2007] EA/2006/0090.

94   Freedom of Information (Scotland) Act 2002, s 38.

95   British Medial Association (2008) *Access to health records: Guidance for health professionals in the United Kingdom*, BMA, London. Department of Health (2010) *Guidance for Access to Health Records Requests*, DH, London.

96   Faculty of Occupational Medicine (2006) *Guidance on ethics for occupational physicians*, FOM, London, para 3.41.

97   British Medical Association (2009) *Access to medical reports*, BMA, London.

98   Royal College of General Practitioners (2010) *Enabling Patients to Access Electronic Health Records: Guidance for Health Professionals*, RCGP, London.

99   Fisher B, Bhavnani V. (2006) How patients use access to their full health records: a qualitative study of patients in general practice. *J R Soc Med* **102**(12), 539–44.

100   Royal College of General Practitioners (2010) *Enabling Patients to Access Electronic Health Records: Guidance for Health Professionals*, RCGP, London.

101   The tables quote the advice given in: Department of Health (2006) *Records management: NHS Code of Practice*, DH, London. Similar advice is provided in the schedules relevant to each of the devolved nations.

7: Contraception, abortion and birth

The questions covered in this chapter include the following.

- What factors should be considered when a person aged under 16 requests contraception?
- Can a woman with severe learning disabilities be sterilised?
- In what circumstances is abortion lawful?
- Should prenatal genetic testing be offered for adult onset disorders?
- Is it acceptable to continue to provide life support for a permanently unconscious pregnant woman in order to give her fetus the greatest chance of survival?
- Should women be able to choose to deliver by caesarean section?
- Can a woman refuse a caesarean section if that refusal would result in the death of a viable fetus?

The nature of reproductive ethics

The increasing ability of people to exercise control over fertility and reproduction has led to major changes in the way people live their lives. Women are now able to exercise choice over whether and when to have children to a greater extent than ever before. This chapter and Chapter 8 discuss the issues that arise throughout an individual's 'reproductive career'. They cover the decision of whether to have children (issues around contraception, sterilisation and abortion), dilemmas raised by pregnancy and birth, and the increased ability to help people to have children through assisted reproduction. The issues discussed concern not only individuals but, in some cases, their families and society at large. Although inevitably much of the discussion focuses on the rights and duties of women, as those who physically bear children, this is in no way intended to dismiss or undermine the important role of men in reproduction. Although emphasis is often placed on the provision of contraception to young women, boys and men also need advice about contraception and sexual health. Similarly, although decisions about the progress of a pregnancy ultimately rest with the woman carrying the fetus, fathers also have a role in decision making, particularly when they intend to take an active part in bringing up the child.

Reproduction differs from many other areas of medical practice because of its complexity and because tension can sometimes arise between the rights of women to make decisions about their own bodies and the moral duties owed to embryos and fetuses. It is this aspect of reproduction that is at the root of many of the ethical, legal, social and psychological questions that continue to be of concern to society. Control over one's body, abortion, reproduction and parenthood are matters about which most people hold strong views. For many, such views are based on moral, religious or cultural convictions. Given the existence of such diversity of opinion, it is clear that some of these questions

Medical Ethics Today: The BMA's Handbook of Ethics and Law, Third Edition. Sophie Brannan, Eleanor Chrispin, Martin Davies, Veronica English, Rebecca Mussell, Julian Sheather and Ann Sommerville.
© 2012 BMA Medical Ethics Department. Published 2012 by Blackwell Publishing Ltd.

can never be resolved to the satisfaction of all sections of society, but will be the subject of continuing ethical debate. Broad areas of moral consensus can, however, be sketched out after wide ranging consultation and public debate, and these form the basis of legislation, guidance and practice in this area.

General principles

When considering questions about contraception, abortion and birth, the following general principles should apply.

- The confidentiality of all patients, including those aged under 16, should be respected except in exceptional cases.
- Young people who are sufficiently mature to understand the nature and implications of the treatment requested are able to give valid consent, but parental involvement should be encouraged.
- No treatment may be provided to an adult who has capacity without valid consent.
- Adults are presumed to have capacity unless there is clear evidence to the contrary. (Being in labour does not, in itself, affect decision-making capacity.)
- Women should be encouraged to participate to the greatest possible extent in decisions about their pregnancy.
- A woman who plans to carry her fetus to term has special moral responsibilities towards the unborn child, but neither health professionals nor society can force her to fulfil those duties.
- Discussion about reproduction inevitably focuses primarily on women, but the role of men should not be undermined. Contraception and sexual health are the responsibility of both sexes.

Autonomy, rights and duties

The autonomy of pregnant women

It is an accepted principle of medical law and ethics that adults with capacity have the right to refuse any treatment or medical intervention, even if that refusal results in their avoidable death. The courts have held that this rule applies equally to a woman who is pregnant even if she is carrying a viable fetus capable of being born alive. The fetus, up to the moment of birth, does not have any separate legal interests capable of being taken into account by a court, and therefore the legal position is that the woman's right to refuse treatment overrides all other legal considerations.

> **Refusal of caesarean section**
>
> MB was 40 weeks pregnant and the fetus was in breech position. She signed a consent form for a caesarean section delivery, but refused to consent to a venepuncture because of her fear of needles. She subsequently gave and then withdrew her consent to the anaesthetic. The health authority sought and obtained a declaration that it would be lawful to perform a caesarean section, with the necessary anaesthetic, to deliver the fetus. MB appealed against this decision. The Appeal Court heard the case immediately and rejected it on the grounds that, because of her needle phobia, MB

temporarily lacked capacity and was unable to give a valid refusal. On the following day she agreed to the anaesthesia and a healthy male infant was delivered by caesarean section.

Despite rejecting MB's appeal, Lady Justice Butler-Sloss restated the legal position that a pregnant woman with capacity has an absolute right to refuse treatment, even if that refusal would result in the death or serious handicap of the child she is carrying. It was made clear that, in such cases, the courts do not have the jurisdiction to declare medical intervention lawful and the question of best interests does not arise. If a pregnant woman with capacity refuses medical intervention, the doctors may not lawfully do more than attempt to persuade her to accept the treatment. If that persuasion fails, there are no further steps that can be taken.[1]

Although refusals of treatment that would save an unborn child are uncommon, official statistics on maternal deaths do occasionally report cases in which women have died after not seeking or declining various treatments.[2] Such cases are deeply tragic for the individuals and families concerned and the health professionals who offer treatment, but they have been seen as a risk that society must allow in order to protect the integrity and autonomy of all patients with capacity. Some fear that usurping the decision-making rights of a pregnant woman with capacity demeans women in general and sets a precedent for invading the bodies of some patients in order to benefit others. The idea that a woman should be forced to undergo surgery for another's benefit has been widely rejected.

Does the fetus have any legal rights?

Although in the case of MB it was confirmed that the fetus does not have any legal rights capable of being taken into account in considering a woman's refusal of caesarean section, it is not the case that the embryo or fetus is totally without legal protection. There are, for example, restrictions in law on the use of human embryos for research (see Chapter 14, pages 616–620) and there are limits applied to the availability of abortion. Lady Justice Butler-Sloss referred to this inconsistency saying:

> Although it might seem illogical that a child capable of being born alive is protected by the criminal law from intentional destruction, and by the Abortion Act from termination otherwise than as permitted by the Act, but is not protected from the (irrational) decision of a competent mother not to allow medical intervention to avert the risk of death, this appears to be the present state of the law.[3]

The case of MB was considered before the Human Rights Act 1998 came into force in the UK and therefore did not specifically discuss rights under the European Convention of Human Rights. It has subsequently been suggested that the right of 'everyone' to have their life protected by law, under Article 2 of the convention, could extend to the embryo or fetus. The European Court of Human Rights has, however, rejected this suggestion – see the case of *Vo v France* below – arguing that this issue falls within the 'margin of appreciation' for interpretation by individual states.

Vo v France

Mrs Vo attended the Lyons General Hospital for an antenatal check up in her sixth month of pregnancy. On the same day, another women, also called Mrs Vo, was due to have a coil removed at the same hospital. There was a mix up in identity which resulted in an attempt by a doctor to remove a coil from the pregnant Mrs Vo. In doing so he pierced Mrs Vo's amniotic sac, causing a substantial loss of amniotic fluid and the subsequent failure of Mrs Vo's pregnancy.

Mrs Vo brought criminal proceedings against the doctor on the basis of unintentional homicide. The Lyons Court of Appeal found him guilty, but the judgment was subsequently overturned by the Court of Cessation on the basis that the offence of unintentional homicide could not be applied to the unborn.

The case was subsequently taken to the European Court of Human Rights. Mrs Vo argued that the 'term "everyone" ("toute personne") in Article 2 of the Convention was to be taken to mean human beings rather than individuals with the attributes of legal personality';[4] embryos and fetuses, therefore, should come under the scope of Article 2.

The European Court held that it was not possible to decide in the abstract whether an embryo or fetus is classed as a person under Article 2 of the Convention and concluded that:

> It follows that the issue of when the right to life begins comes within the margin of appreciation which the Court generally considers that States should enjoy in this sphere, notwithstanding an evolutive interpretation of the Convention... Having regard to the foregoing, the Court is convinced that it is neither desirable, nor even possible as matters stand, to answer in the abstract the question whether the unborn child is a person for the purposes of Article 2 of the Convention.[5]

Do we have duties towards embryos and fetuses?

The fact that there is a straightforward legal precedent for the situation in which a woman refuses treatment that could save the life of her fetus does not mean that the situation is unproblematic or straightforward from an ethical perspective. Most of those who accept that embryos and fetuses do not have rights nevertheless believe they are deserving of respect by virtue of their potential for development and for becoming the holder of rights after birth. As a society we do not regard human embryos and fetuses as having the same status as children or adults, but neither do we consider them to be merely cells or tissues. This 'special status' is reflected in the law, which gives them some protection. The extent of the duties owed to embryos and fetuses depends upon gestational age because the nearer they come to developing individual rights, after birth, the stronger their claim to protection. This approach of increasing duties owed according to age can be seen to underpin the legal limits for permissible interference. In the UK, human embryos, up to 14 days after fertilisation, may be used for carefully controlled and licensed research (see Chapter 14, pages 616–620); abortion is permitted in some circumstances up to 24 weeks' gestation and, in more restricted cases, up to term (see pages 283–284). The Human Fertilisation and Embryology Act 1990 (as amended) also enforces legal duties towards those who are not only unborn, but also not yet conceived – future or possible people – in its requirement to take account of the welfare of any future child before offering fertility treatment (see Chapter 8).

Although all members of society have certain duties and responsibilities, a pregnant woman who plans to carry a fetus to term can be seen to have particular moral obligations towards that unborn child. This means that she has a responsibility not to harm the unborn child deliberately and also to take positive steps to protect it. The general view of the British Medical Association (BMA) is that some duties are owed to the fetus even though its claims may not override the mother's claim to autonomy over her body. The fact that a woman is perceived to have moral responsibilities towards the fetus, however, does not mean that she can or should be forced, legally or ethically, to fulfil those duties.

Is there a right to reproduce?

A woman's right to refuse life-prolonging treatment is one of a number of 'rights' that are frequently appealed to in relation to reproduction. A distinction is often made between negative and positive rights or between a liberty and a right. Negative rights simply involve being free from interference and are based on the notion that the state should not interfere with essentially private decisions. In terms of reproduction, this confers the right not to be prevented from procreation, for example by non-consensual sterilisation. Positive rights, however, would include the right to demand appropriate healthcare. In terms of reproduction, this would include a positive obligation on the state and health professionals to support the individual's reproductive choices, including providing reproductive technology for every person who requires it. Claims to positive rights are often seen as problematic in that they suppose that there is a corresponding obligation on other people to supply what the right holder claims. In the UK, there is not a positive right to assistance to reproduce (see Chapter 8, pages 316–319).

Contraception

The continuing high number of unwanted or unintended pregnancies in the UK demonstrates a clear need for better access to, and uptake of, contraceptive information and services. Cooperation has been encouraged for many years between various agencies, including health and education services, the voluntary sector, and service users to try to improve family planning services. This includes recognition of the need for specific training to enable providers to assess, and explain to patients, the range of contraceptive methods available and to provide general advice about sexual health to accompany the provision of contraceptives. Most women who seek contraceptive advice and services do so from their GP practice, although many younger women tend to prefer the anonymity of specialist clinics. From April 2008 to March 2009 about one-fifth of women aged 16–49 who required family planning services in England went to community contraceptive clinics; most of the remainder went to their GPs.[6] In the exceptional circumstance where patients are registered with a GP practice that has opted out of providing contraceptive services, the GP practice's commissioning body should find an alternative provider of contraceptive services for patients.[7] It is important to maintain a diversity of provision of advice and services, including specialist sexual and reproductive health clinics in parallel with GP services, in order to offer patient choice.

Contraception and teenagers

Public policy

More than one-quarter of young people are sexually active before the age of 16 years in Britain.[8] Young people in particular need access to contraceptive advice because of the high teenage conception rates in Britain. Teenage pregnancy is often associated with low educational attainment, poverty, emotional difficulties and being a child of a teenage mother.[9]

An early report by the Social Exclusion Unit (whose functions have now transferred to the Social Exclusion Taskforce) found that one of the main reasons for the high number of teenage pregnancies (under 18) in England was a lack of accurate knowledge about contraception. Another important explanation was young people's low expectations about their future.[10] The young women studied did not see any prospect of obtaining a job and expected to end up on some form of state benefit. Many of those questioned also felt that society was giving mixed messages about young people and contraception. Although young people are bombarded by images of sexuality in the media, and sexual activity amongst young people is seen as the norm, there is still a reluctance to talk to young people about sex and contraception. One teenager told the Unit that it seems, sometimes, as if sex is compulsory but contraception is illegal.[11] Some suggest that the high teenage pregnancy rates are reflective of wider social problems and the breakdown of the family unit in modern day Britain,[12] despite teenage pregnancy rates being at their lowest in 20 years.[13]

Evidence shows that ignoring the issue does not lead to less sexual activity among young people, but to more unwanted pregnancies. In 2009, in England and Wales, approximately 38,300 under-18-year-olds became pregnant, and around 7,200 were under 16.[14] In 2008, in Scotland approximately 3,900 under-18-year-olds became pregnant, around 710 of whom were under 16.[15] In Northern Ireland 1,300 15- to 19-years-olds conceived and delivered live babies in 2009.[16] The teenage pregnancy rates for the UK's four nations are the highest in Europe.

In 1999, the UK Labour Government launched a cross-government teenage pregnancy strategy with a target of halving the under-18 conception rate in England by 2010. This target was not reached; by 2010, teenage pregnancy rates had fallen but only by 11 per cent, with a 23 per cent decrease in the under-18 birth rate.[17] In 2010, the Teenage Pregnancy Independent Advisory Group was abolished. At the time of writing it was not clear what the new Government's strategy would be in tackling teenage pregnancy, with some expressing concern that the widespread cuts in public spending, and the proposed mass re-organisation of the NHS, would have a detrimental effect on falling teenage pregnancy rates.[18]

The devolved nations have also identified teenage pregnancy as an issue, with the Scottish Government setting a national target to reduce the pregnancy rate of under-16-year-olds by 20 per cent by 2010, which was not achieved;[19] and Northern Ireland's Department of Health, Social Services and Public Safety (DHSSPS) has identified teenage pregnancy as an issue to be addressed under the Promoting Social Inclusion initiative.[20]

Research carried out by the Teenage Pregnancy Unit,[21] under the previous Labour Government, showed clearly that 'just say no' messages are not effective, but what can work is a campaign that does not lecture but tells young people to take control, be prepared, be responsible and not to feel pressurised into having sex before they are ready. Health professionals, particularly GPs, have an important role in reinforcing these messages because many young people are likely to turn to their family doctor if they have confidence that their requests for contraceptive advice or treatment are kept confidential.

Studies show that young people rank a confidential and friendly sexual health service most highly in their preferences for sexual health services[22] followed by an easily accessible service in terms of location and opening times. Teenagers express concern about confidentiality regarding:

- deliberate breaches of confidentiality, for example if an under 16-year-old revealed she was pregnant, teenagers thought the doctor would have to tell her parents
- informal, inadvertent breaches of confidentiality by staff, for example mentioning a teenager's recent visit to the surgery in the course of a conversation with a parent
- 'gossipy' receptionists
- confidential information being sent in the post and intercepted by parents.[23]

Every opportunity should be taken to offer reassurance to young people that the duty of confidentiality owed to them is the same as the duty to an adult.

Consent and confidentiality

Controversy about the issue of 'underage' contraception is a recurring phenomenon, particularly in relation to the provision of oral contraceptives and Long Acting Reversible Contraception (LARC) to those under the age of 16.

Provision of contraception to people aged under 16

In England, in July 2004, the Teenage Pregnancy Unit published guidance on providing advice and treatment relating to sexual health to people under 16.[24] The guidance clarifies that the Sexual Offences Act 2003 does not affect the duty of care and confidentiality of health professionals to young people under 16, including those under 13. The key points of the guidance are set out below.

- All young people under 16 have the right to confidential advice from health professionals about sexual health/sexually transmitted infections (STIs), contraception and relationships.
- Research with young people identifies anxiety about confidentiality as a major deterrent to asking for contraceptive advice.
- The duty of confidentiality is not, however, absolute. Where a health professional believes that there is a risk to the health, safety or welfare of a young person or others which is so serious as to outweigh the young person's right to privacy, they should follow locally agreed child protection protocols.
- A doctor or health professional is able to provide contraception, sexual and reproductive health advice and treatment, without parental knowledge or consent, to young people aged under 16, provided that:
  - ○ they understand the advice provided and its implications
  - ○ their physical or mental health would otherwise be likely to suffer and so provision of advice or treatment is in their best interest.
- However, even if a decision is taken not to provide treatment, the duty of confidentiality applies, unless there are exceptional circumstances as referred to above.

A judicial review of the guidance was granted to Mrs Sue Axon, the mother of two daughters who argued that her right to know, under Article 8 of the European Convention on Human Rights, about matters related to her children's health should override the duty of confidentiality. Mrs Axon lost her case.[25]

The BMA has clear policy, based on the Gillick judgment (see below),[26] that the patient's maturity and understanding of the nature of the consultation and of the treatment proposed should be the guiding factors. It is sometimes argued that very young patients may not understand either the concept of confidentiality or the implications of the treatment they request. They may have an erroneous impression of the purpose of contraceptives. An example would be that of a 9-year-old seeking contraceptives because she knows older friends have them. Kennedy[27] raises this hypothetical case, but such cases are likely to be exceptional. Minors who seek contraception are usually either sexually active or intending to be so. In such cases, when patients understand the treatment, their autonomy and confidentiality should be respected. The BMA emphasises the importance of the doctor trying to persuade the patient to agree to parental involvement but, if the patient refuses, there is a duty to maintain the confidentiality of the consultation.

Competency to make decisions

Mrs Gillick took her local health authority to court because it refused to assure her that her five daughters, all aged under 16, would not be given contraceptive advice and treatment without her knowledge and consent. The case followed the publication of a

Department of Health and Social Security circular advising that doctors consulted at a family planning clinic by a girl under 16 would not be acting unlawfully if they prescribed contraceptives, provided that they acted in good faith and to protect the young woman from the harmful effects of sexual intercourse. In seeking a declaration that this advice was unlawful, Mrs Gillick argued that a young girl's consent was legally ineffective and inconsistent with parental rights. She said that it was therefore necessary to involve parents.

This argument was rejected by the House of Lords, where the majority opinion was that the relevant test was whether the girl had reached an age where she had sufficient understanding and intelligence to enable her to understand fully what was proposed. If she had, a doctor would not be acting unlawfully in giving advice and treatment.[28]

Before providing contraception to young people, health professionals must:

- consider whether the patient understands the potential risks and benefits of the treatment
- consider whether the patient understands the advice given
- discuss with the patient the value of parental support (doctors must encourage young people to inform parents of the consultation and explore the reasons if the patient is unwilling to do so) – it is important for persons aged under 16 who are seeking contraceptive advice to be aware that, although the doctor is obliged to discuss the value of parental support, he or she will respect their confidentiality (see Chapter 5)
- take into account whether the patient is likely to have sexual intercourse without contraception
- assess whether the patient's physical or mental health or both are likely to suffer if the patient does not receive contraceptive advice or treatment
- consider whether the patient's best interests would require the provision of contraceptive advice or treatment or both without parental consent.[29]

Even if the doctor is unwilling to supply contraception on the grounds of the patient's immaturity, he or she still maintains a general duty of confidentiality unless there are exceptional reasons for disclosing information without consent. Such reasons could occur when, for example, the request for contraception arises in the context of sexual exploitation, incest or other sexual abuse. In such exceptional cases the doctor has a duty to protect the patient and this may eventually involve a breach of confidentiality, although with counselling and support the patient may feel able to agree to disclosure. Nevertheless, it is important that doctors avoid making completely unconditional promises about secrecy to individual young people, while at the same time making it clear that confidentiality as a general principle extends to all consultations.[30]

Obligatory reporting

In the summer of 2005, some Child Protection Committees issued guidance imposing a requirement to report all sexually active people under the age of 13 (and in some cases under the age of 16) to the police. A number of health bodies, including the BMA, challenged this guidance arguing that, while reporting to social services or the police should always be considered where the individual is very young, the obligation of health professionals is to act in the best interests of the patient and this requires flexibility. Revised guidance was subsequently issued which removed an obligation to report in all cases.

Changes to the law on sexual offences in Northern Ireland

The law on sexual offences in Northern Ireland changed in 2008. The Sexual Offences (Northern Ireland) Order 2008 came into effect on 2 February 2009 and provides a new legislative framework for sexual offences. It amends existing legislation and has important implications for all health professionals, including doctors, and particularly those who treat or advise children and young people.

Doctors in Northern Ireland have long been concerned about their ability to provide healthcare in the context of their duty under criminal legislation to report evidence of unlawful sexual activity between children. This aspect of the law placed doctors in a difficult situation whereby they themselves risked committing a criminal offence if they failed to report underage sexual activity involving their patients, even where there were no child protection concerns. The broader public health implications of the law, which had the potential to deter young people from seeking the advice of health professionals on sexual health matters for fear of being reported to the police, were also of concern to doctors.

This situation has now changed. The new law in Northern Ireland closely follows that in England and Wales and removes the duty to report information about certain offences. The Order ensures that health professionals, amongst others, are not liable to prosecution when they are acting to protect a child or young person, including those with a mental disorder. Doctors are not therefore under a duty to report sexual activity involving a child aged 13–15 years old where the other party is under 18. This exclusion does not apply to information about offences against children under 13 (as set out in Articles 12–15 of the Order), which must still be reported.

The new legislation also brings Northern Ireland into line with the rest of the UK on when young people are deemed to be able to consent to sexual activity. Specifically, the age of consent has been reduced from 17 to 16 years.

Provision of contraception to young people with learning difficulties

It is generally accepted that, if they wish to do so, young people with learning difficulties should be able to experience aspects of life from which they may have been protected in the past, including sexual relationships. It may be, however, that these are something that they explore at a later stage than many of their peers because most young people with significant learning difficulties have a highly supervised life. Clearly, there is no justification for providing contraception – particularly using invasive methods – if there is no evidence that the young person is interested in an intimate relationship and there is no identifiable risk of pregnancy. Doctors consulted in relation to a request for contraception for a young person with learning difficulties need to bear in mind the points made previously concerning contraception for any minor. Also, as with other patients, they need to ensure that any product supplied is the most appropriate for that patient's needs.[31] Some young women with a learning disability can be reliable pill takers, although they may require help from their carers. Implants or other long-term contraceptive methods, such as a hormonally loaded intrauterine system, are appropriate for some patients. It is lawful to provide contraception to a young person who is incapable of giving consent if a person with parental responsibility consents to the treatment, or if it is in the best interests of the patient. Obviously, however, lack of capacity to consent to the treatment would raise concerns about the individual's capacity to consent to sex, if that is the purpose of providing contraception. In cases of doubt or difficulty, doctors should seek legal advice.

Emergency hormonal contraception

The development of drugs that prevent the establishment of pregnancy after intercourse has provided another option for women when a regular contraceptive method has not been used or has failed. There were approximately 397,000 prescriptions dispensed for emergency contraception in 2009/10 in England; with approximately two-thirds prescribed by GPs and one-third at NHS community contraceptive clinics.[32] The main barriers to emergency contraception use is confusion about the timescale within which it must be taken and access, particularly outside normal opening hours. Although it is often referred to as the 'morning after pill' it can be taken up to 72 hours after intercourse, although it is most effective when taken within the first 24 hours. An emergency contraception licensed in May 2009 – ulipristal acetate - can be taken up to 5 days after intercourse. Fears that making access to emergency contraception easier would encourage promiscuity and discourage the use of more reliable contraception appear to be unfounded. Research evidence shows that women with ready access to emergency contraception use it neither irresponsibly nor as an alternative to other methods.[33]

Changes introduced throughout the UK in January 2001 enabled emergency contraception to be sold by pharmacists to women aged 16 or over, without a doctor's prescription.[34] The BMA strongly supported this change while recognising, along with the Royal Pharmaceutical Society of Great Britain, that pharmacists would need specific training in giving advice about contraception and sexual health, and would require facilities for private discussions in order to protect confidentiality.[35] Whether provided by doctors, nurses or by pharmacists, it should usually be accompanied by advice and counselling on sexual activity, future contraception and related matters such as sexually transmitted infections.[36]

The principles involved in the provision of contraception to people aged under 16 apply equally to emergency contraception. The BMA believes that a range of measures are needed to bring down the number of teenage pregnancies and that access to emergency contraception through pharmacies could have been extended to those under 16. There appears to be moves to extend provision to this age group – for example, in 2009 Abertawe Bro Morgannwg University Health Board, which covers Swansea and Bridgend in South Wales, accredited some pharmacies to dispense free emergency contraception to all age groups, including under-16-year-olds.[37] Pharmacists can provide emergency contraception to people aged under 16 if specified in patient group directions (see Chapter 13, page 560).

Emergency 'contraception' or early abortion?

There has, in the past, been some uncertainty about whether certain types of contraceptives that prevent implantation, such as emergency hormonal contraception and intrauterine devices, should be classed as abortifacients, which could be issued only under the terms of the Abortion Act 1967. This question was addressed in a parliamentary answer in May 1983, in which the Attorney General stated that the provision of postcoital contraception designed to prevent implantation does not constitute 'procuring a miscarriage'.[38] This view was tested and confirmed in the case of *R v HS Dhingra*[39] in 1991 and by a judicial review in 2002 (see below).

Judicial review on emergency contraception

The Society for the Protection of the Unborn Child applied for a judicial review of the decision of the Secretary of State for Health, made in 2000, to make emergency contraception available from pharmacists without a prescription. The claimant contended that the 'morning after pill' was not a contraceptive but an abortifacient because it procured a miscarriage within the meaning of the 1861 Offences Against the Persons Act. Its use, therefore, would be lawful only if prescribed by two doctors, as required by the Abortion Act 1967. The Secretary of State argued, however, that the meaning of 'miscarriage' was the loss of a fertilised egg that had become implanted in the endometrium of the uterus. Emergency contraception causes the loss of an egg before implantation, so there is no miscarriage and therefore no criminal offence.

The judge, in the High Court, held that the decision had to turn on the meaning of 'miscarriage' now and not its meaning in 1861. Today, miscarriage is taken to mean the termination of an established pregnancy and therefore the application was dismissed.[40]

Conscientious objection to the provision of contraceptive services

Although GPs are not obliged by their terms of service to provide contraceptive services, most do so. When a practice does not offer contraceptive advice it is important that patients are made aware of this fact and are advised of alternative practitioners or family planning services.

Although, legally, the use of contraceptives that are capable of preventing implantation does not constitute an abortion, the BMA recognises that some doctors, believing that life begins at fertilisation, may have an ethical objection to their use. Those who take this view may choose not to provide such services. In the BMA's view, however, doctors with a conscientious objection to providing contraceptive advice or treatment have an ethical duty to refer their patients promptly to another practitioner or family planning service. (For further details on the guidance of the General Medical Council (GMC) on conscientious objection, see page 289.)

Summary – contraception

- Health professionals have an important role in assisting people to avoid conception if they so wish, particularly among young people.
- The provision of contraception should be accompanied by advice and information about sexual health.
- Young people who are sufficiently mature to understand the implications are able to give valid consent to treatment, but parental involvement should be encouraged.
- Confidentiality of all patients, including those aged under 16, should be respected except in exceptional circumstances where there is serious concern about exploitation or abuse.
- Emergency hormonal contraception is an important step in the drive to reduce unwanted pregnancies and should be made available to those who need it.
- Health professionals with a conscientious objection to some or all forms of contraception are not obliged to provide them, but they have an ethical duty to refer their patients promptly to another practitioner.

Sterilisation

Male or female sterilisation is usually expected to produce permanent sterility (although this is not necessarily the outcome). Although some people have conscientious objections to sterilisation for contraceptive purposes, within society as a whole it appears to be viewed as an acceptable form of family planning, as long as individuals are adequately informed of the implications of the procedure and no pressure is exerted upon them. Reliance on sterilisation for contraceptive purposes is highest amongst older women.[41] Non-consensual sterilisation of those who are unable to give valid consent has, however, been the subject of intense debate.

Consent

As discussed in Chapter 2, the patient's agreement to treatment is valid only when adequate information about the procedure and its implications has been provided. This should include information about the likelihood of success and the possibility that the procedure could fail. The degree of patient understanding should be commensurate with the gravity of the treatment, in other words, where the procedure is irreversible, a high level of understanding is needed. Some men enquire about storing their semen prior to sterilisation in case their circumstances change in the future. Some clinics agree to semen storage; a limited number of treatment centres are also able to store oocytes prior to treatment likely to affect a woman's future fertility. Information about centres licensed to store gametes is available from the Human Fertilisation and Embryology Authority (see Chapter 8, page 314).

The same considerations about information and consent apply whether the intention is to sterilise the patient or, as with hysterectomy, permanent sterility is an inevitable side effect of a procedure undertaken for medical reasons. As part of the consent process, discussion should take place about the likelihood of the patient already being pregnant and how to proceed if that is found to be the case.

Inadequate consent for hysterectomy

In 2002, a consultant obstetrician and gynaecologist was found guilty of serious professional misconduct by the GMC for his management of a patient's total abdominal hysterectomy and bilateral salpingo-oophorectomy. The patient had been referred to the consultant by her GP because of symptoms of abdominal pain and vaginal discharge. Part of the case against the doctor was that he had failed to ensure that the patient understood the nature and purpose of the operation and that she had given her informed consent. The GMC's Professional Conduct Committee found that, during the course of the operation, the doctor had cause to suspect that the patient may have been pregnant but nonetheless continued with the operation, without her consent, thereby terminating the pregnancy. This action was held to be inappropriate because the doctor knew, or should have known, that the patient had not given her consent for termination of pregnancy and yet he made no effort to consult her about it, despite the fact that the operation would prevent her from ever having any children. The consultant was severely reprimanded.[42]

Any treatment affecting an individual's reproductive capacity also has potential implications for that person's partner or future partners. In the past, consent to treatments such as sterilisation was sought routinely from the patient's partner. This is now acknowledged to be inappropriate because it is for the individual patient to decide whether to be sterilised. Partners should be consulted only if the patient has given specific consent, although it is good practice to encourage patients to discuss such procedures with their partners.

Sterilisation of people with learning disabilities

Sterilisation as a contraceptive

Sterilisation is occasionally requested for young people with serious learning difficulties. Of course, every case requires assessment and balancing of the relevant factors, but sterilisation for contraceptive purposes should not normally be proposed for young people aged under 18 because of its irreversible nature. Even when there are exceptional circumstances in which there is agreement that sterilisation is the best option for a young person, court authorisation is essential.[43]

Individuals with learning disabilities have varying degrees of difficulty in making decisions that influence the course of their lives. Like all patients, they should be encouraged to make for themselves all those decisions whose implications they broadly understand and with which they feel comfortable. The rights of people with learning disabilities to enjoy sexual relationships in private has been an issue of historical debate, and sterilisation of those who lack the capacity to give valid consent has been controversial. Debate on this issue has focused primarily on proposals to sterilise women – where the consideration must include the risks of harm arising from the pregnancy as well as the difficulties of bringing up a child – but sterilisation of men with learning disabilities has also been proposed. Proposals to sterilise those who are not able to give consent present a number of difficulties. The harm against which it seeks to protect may not be sufficient to justify the intervention, or it may be proposed more for the benefit of carers than the individual. There are also concerns that it may more easily expose the patient to sexual abuse and misdirect attention towards preventing pregnancy rather than protecting vulnerable people from abuse. It has also been argued that non-consensual sterilisation can be seen as contravening a fundamental freedom to reproduce. Article 12 of the European Convention on Human Rights (the right to marry and found a family) is frequently referred to in this context.

As a matter of principle, contraceptive services for people with learning difficulties should not impede the exercise of autonomy more drastically than is essential to protect against an unwanted pregnancy. Advances in the development of contraceptive devices mean that, for many patients, other less drastic methods of contraception are available and these should always be considered before sterilisation – for example oral, injectable, subdermal implants or intrauterine contraception. In the past hysterectomies, or sterilisation, may have been carried out prematurely on young women who could have coped successfully with other forms of contraception and who might have been capable of making their own decisions about motherhood at a later stage. This point was implicit in a 1976 case where the judge refused to authorise the sterilisation of an 11-year-old girl, pointing to the frustration and resentment the patient would be likely to experience in later life, arising from her inability to have children.[44] To perform a sterilisation on a woman for non-therapeutic reasons and without her consent, the judge said, would be a violation of the individual's basic human rights to have the opportunity to reproduce. A similar point was made in the 1989 case of *Re F* (see below).

Sterilisation of a woman with severe mental disorder

F was 36 years old and suffered from a severe mental disorder. She was described in court as having the verbal capacity of a 2-year-old and the general mental capacity of a 4- or 5-year-old. F had been a hospital inpatient for more than 20 years and over that period had made great progress such that she was given increased freedom within the confines of the hospital. Her mental capacity was not, however, expected to improve. Over time, F had developed a sexual relationship with another patient. It was said that the psychiatric consequences for F of becoming pregnant would be 'catastrophic'. Consideration had been given to the option of preventing F from forming sexual relationships, but the view was taken that this could be achieved only by seriously restricting her already limited freedom. Less invasive methods of contraception had been considered, but none was suitable, so an application was made for a declaration that it would not be unlawful to sterilise F despite her being unable to give consent. All parties were agreed that sterilisation would be in F's best interests, but a number of legal and procedural issues needed to be resolved.

The House of Lords ruled that the common law allowed doctors to give medical or surgical treatment to an adult patient who is incapable of consenting when it is in the best interests of the patient to do so. Where the treatment proposed was sterilisation for non-therapeutic purposes, however, it was recommended that an application should be made to the court for a declaration that the operation was not unlawful and was in the patient's best interests.[45]

Sterilisation (unless for therapeutic reasons) is one of a small number of procedures that must not be carried out without applying for a court declaration. This is because of its intended irreversible nature, which deprives the individual of what is, according to one judge, 'widely and rightly regarded as one of the fundamental rights of a woman, the right to bear a child'.[46]

This 'right to reproduce' has also been raised, in the specific context of Article 12 of the European Convention on Human Rights, in a more recent case about male sterilisation.

Sterilisation of a man with Down syndrome

In *Re A*, an application for the sterilisation of a 28-year-old man with Down syndrome was rejected. A was cared for by his mother, who supervised him, but who was concerned that when, given her ill health, he moved into local authority care he may have a sexual relationship and be unable to understand the possible consequences. The judge at the High Court found that, although A was sexually aware and active, he did not understand the link between intercourse and pregnancy. Nevertheless, the judge refused the declaration on the basis that the effect on A would be minimal.

A's mother took her case to the Appeal Court but it was dismissed. Although decided shortly before the Human Rights Act 1998 came into force, in dismissing the appeal Lady Justice Butler-Sloss warned that the courts should be slow to take any step that could infringe the rights of those who are unable to speak for themselves. The case was decided on the basis that sterilisation would not be in A's best interests, taking account of medical, emotional and all other welfare issues. It was made clear in the judgment that the concept of best interests in such cases relates to the mentally incapacitated person, not to carers or other third parties.

It was noted that should the circumstances change however, for example if A's freedom was diminished because of a fear that he might form a sexual relationship, a reapplication for sterilisation could be made to the court.[47]

Hysterectomy for heavy menstrual bleeding

Concern is sometimes expressed that hysterectomy for heavy menstrual bleeding may be sought primarily for the benefit of carers rather than in the interests of the patient herself. Although attention is often drawn to the difficulty of separating out the 'interests' of individuals in the family context, the court will need to be convinced that sterilisation is the best option for the young woman.

Hysterectomy may, in the past, have seemed appropriate treatment for a young person who is approaching adulthood and who will never achieve the capacity to make a valid choice about treatment to manage heavy menstrual bleeding. In most cases, however, the objective of menstrual management can be achieved by lesser means than surgery. Given that evidence-based clinical guidelines examining these issues have been published by the National Institute for Health and Clinical Excellence (NICE),[48] it is hard to see how doctors could be satisfied that no less intrusive means of treatment is available. Oral or injectable contraception or a hormonally loaded intrauterine device may regularise and lighten menstrual bleeding. It must also be borne in mind that most women with a learning disability can manage their own menstruation with appropriate education and support. Some may need assistance from their carers. In many cases, referral to special learning disability services rather than to gynaecological services is most appropriate. In all cases where surgery is being considered, doctors must take legal advice and it is likely that a court ruling will be needed.[49]

Summary – sterilisation

- As with other irreversible procedures, those seeking sterilisation should be given sufficient information about the procedure and its implications in order to make an informed decision.
- Patients should be encouraged to discuss sterilisation with their partners, but the decision of whether to involve the partner rests with the patient.
- Sterilisation of those who are unable to consent, except where there are unambiguous therapeutic grounds, will require a court declaration.

Abortion

BMA policy

The BMA represents doctors who hold widely diverse moral views about abortion. In the 1970s and 1980s, the Association approved policy statements supporting the 1967 Abortion Act as 'a practical and humane piece of legislation'.[50] The BMA does not consider that abortion is unethical but, as with any act having profound moral implications, the justifications must be commensurate with the consequences. The BMA's advice to its members is to act within the boundaries of the law and of their own conscience. Patients are, however, entitled to receive objective medical advice and referral as appropriate to another practitioner, regardless of their doctor's personal views for or against abortion. Patients should be offered counselling and support before and after the procedure.

Background to the abortion debate

In order to understand the very contentious background to the abortion debate, it may be helpful to mention briefly the main strands of the argument. People generally give one of three common types of response to abortion: prochoice, anti-abortion and the middle ground that abortion is acceptable in some circumstances. The main arguments in support of each of these positions is set out below.

Arguments in support of abortion being made widely available

Those who support the wide availability of abortion consider the matter to be primarily one of a woman's right to choose and to exercise control over her own body.

These arguments tend not to consider the fetus to be a person, deserving of any rights or owed any duties. Those who judge actions by their consequences alone could argue that abortion is equivalent to a deliberate failure to conceive a child and, because contraception is widely available, abortion should be too. Others take a slightly different approach, believing that, even if the fetus has rights and entitlements, these are very limited and do not weigh significantly against the interests of people who have already been born, such as parents or existing children of the family. Most people believe it is right for couples to be able to plan their families and for women to have control over when they become pregnant. Although contraception is understood to be the appropriate means to avoid unwanted pregnancy, all methods have a failure rate. When contraception fails, or when couples fail to use it effectively, many people accept that abortion is preferable to forcing a woman to continue with an unwanted pregnancy.

Arguments against abortion

Some people consider that abortion is wrong in any circumstance because it fails to recognise the rights of the fetus or because it challenges the notion of the sanctity of all human life. They argue that permitting abortion diminishes the respect society feels for other vulnerable humans, possibly leading to their involuntary euthanasia. Those who consider that an embryo is a human being with full moral status from the moment of conception see abortion as intentional killing in the same sense as the murder of any other person. Those who take this view cannot accept that women should be allowed to obtain abortions, however difficult the lives of those women or their existing families are made as a result. Such views may be based on religious or moral convictions that each human life has unassailable intrinsic value, which is not diminished by any impairment or suffering that may be involved for the individual living that life. Many worry that the availability of abortion on grounds of fetal abnormality encourages prejudice towards any person with a handicap and insidiously creates the impression that the only valuable people are those who conform to some ill-defined stereotype of 'normality'.

More recently, some have shifted the arguments on to the pregnant woman and have argued that abortion is wrong because of the psychological and health consequences for a woman, although evidence in support of this is elusive and controversial.[51]

Some of those who oppose abortion in general nevertheless concede that it may be justifiable in very exceptional cases when termination is seen as the lesser moral offence. This could include cases such as where the pregnancy is the result of rape, or the consequence of the exploitation of a young girl or a woman lacking capacity. Risk to the mother's life may be another justifiable exception, but only when abortion is the only option. It would thus not be seen as justifiable to abort a fetus if the life of both fetus and mother could be saved by implementing any other solution.

Arguments used to support abortion in some circumstances

Many people argue that abortion may be justified in a greater number of circumstances than those conceded by opponents of abortion, but that it would be undesirable to allow 'abortion on demand'. To do so could incur undesirable effects, such as encouraging irresponsible attitudes to contraception. It could also lead to a devaluation of the lives of viable fetuses and trivialise the potential psychological effects of abortion on women and on health professionals. These types of argument are based on the premise that the embryo starts off without rights, although having a special status from conception in view of its potential for development, and that it acquires rights and status throughout its development. The notion of evolving fetal rights and practical factors, such as the increasing medical risks and possible distress to the pregnant woman, nurses, doctors or other children in the family, gives rise to the view that early abortion is more acceptable than late abortion.

Some people support this position on pragmatic grounds, believing that abortions will always be sought by women who are desperate and that it is better for society to provide abortion services that are safe and can be monitored and regulated, rather than to allow 'back street' practices.

The law on abortion in England, Scotland and Wales

In England, Scotland and Wales, a registered medical practitioner may lawfully terminate a pregnancy, in an NHS hospital or on premises approved for this purpose, if two registered medical practitioners are of the opinion, formed in good faith:

'(a) that the pregnancy has not exceeded its twenty-fourth week and that the continuance of the pregnancy would involve risk, greater than if the pregnancy were terminated, of injury to the physical or mental health of the pregnant woman or any existing children of her family; or
(b) that the termination is necessary to prevent grave permanent injury to the physical or mental health of the pregnant woman; or
(c) that the continuance of the pregnancy would involve risk to the life of the pregnant woman, greater than if the pregnancy were terminated; or
(d) that there is a substantial risk that if the child were born it would suffer from such physical or mental abnormalities as to be seriously handicapped.'[52]

(The above conditions are lettered, and ordered, as set out in the Act, which differs from the HSA1 form completed by doctors authorising, or referring a patient for, termination of pregnancy.)

In addition, when a doctor 'is of the opinion, formed in good faith, that the termination is immediately necessary to save the life or to prevent grave permanent injury to the physical or mental health of the pregnant woman'[53] the opinion of a second registered medical practitioner is not required. Nor, in these limited circumstances, are there restrictions on where the procedure may be carried out, and doctors have no legal right to conscientiously object to participation.

The Abortion Act was amended in 1990 to remove the pre-existing links with the Infant Life Preservation Act 1929, which had made it illegal to destroy the life of a child that is capable of being born alive, with an assumption that this would be so after 28 weeks' gestation. Thus, terminations carried out under (b)–(d) above may be performed at any gestational age.

Serious handicap

The question of what constitutes a 'serious handicap' under section 1(1)(d) of the Act is not addressed in the legislation. It is a matter of clinical judgement and accepted practice. Practical guidance for health professionals involved with terminations for fetal abnormality is available from the Royal College of Obstetricians and Gynaecologists which, amongst other things, offers guidance on counselling and support for women and their partners in this period of emotional shock and distress.[54] The types of factor that may be taken into account in assessing the seriousness of a handicap include the following:

- the probability of effective treatment, either *in utero* or after birth
- the child's probable potential for self-awareness and potential ability to communicate with others
- the suffering that would be experienced by the child when born or by the people caring for the child.

The question of how 'serious handicap' should be defined was raised in the courts in 2003. The Reverend Joanna Jepson sought a judicial review of the decision of the Chief Constable of West Mercia Constabulary not to pursue a prosecution of doctors who terminated a pregnancy at more than 24 weeks' gestation, where the fetus had been diagnosed with bilateral cleft lip and palate. The police authorities had undertaken an investigation of the case and were satisfied that 'the abortion was due to a bilateral cleft palate and was legally justified and procedurally correctly carried out'.[55] Reverend Jepson challenged this decision on the basis that bilateral cleft lip and palate was not a 'serious handicap' and therefore the abortion had been unlawful. After hearing the application Lord Justice Rose and Mr Justice Jackson held that the case raised serious issues of law and issues of public importance and so granted permission for a judicial review. The judicial review was stayed as subsequent to that decision the police re-investigated the case fully. The police sent a file to the Crown Prosecution Service (CPS) who announced in March 2005 that the doctors involved would not face prosecution. The Chief Crown Prosecutor for West Mercia CPS, Jim England, said that the doctors had decided in good faith that a substantial risk existed that the child would be seriously handicapped if born.[56]

Publication of national data on abortion

Following the Joanna Jepson case in 2004, the Department of Health altered the way it presented the annual abortion statistics for England and Wales due to concerns that individuals could be identified. As a result, the abortion data from 2003 only listed and provided data for specific groups of medical conditions for which the abortion was carried out if there were 10 or more cases in total.

The ProLife Alliance (PLA) sought to obtain the previous level of detail for the 2003 abortion data. When the Department of Health was not forthcoming with this, the PLA lodged a complaint to the Information Commissioner. The Information Commissioner,[57] and subsequently the Information Tribunal,[58] supported the PLA's application and ordered the Department of Health to disclose the disputed information.

The Department of Health subsequently appealed this decision but the appeal was lost.

Late gestation abortion

In October 2004, the Chief Medical Officer (CMO) was asked by the Secretary of State for Health to investigate allegations that women beyond the legal limit for abortion in Britain were being helped by the British Pregnancy Advisory Service (BPAS) to obtain abortions abroad. The CMO published a report[59] in September 2005 concluding that there was no evidence that BPAS had acted illegally, although its handling of calls from an undercover journalist was criticised. A number of recommendations were made for improving its procedures, including a call for the Department of Health to develop, with the relevant professional bodies and the Healthcare Commission, an agreed best practice protocol for dealing with late gestation abortion cases, to be adopted by the NHS and all independent sector providers.

Early medical abortion

In England, Wales and Scotland, the vast majority of abortions take place in the first trimester of pregnancy. In 2009, 91 per cent of abortions in England and Wales were carried out at 12 weeks or earlier,[60] and 94 per cent of abortions in Scotland were carried out at 13 weeks or earlier.[61] These percentages have remained constant over the last decade. Most people take the view that where a woman has made up her mind to seek an abortion and meets the legal criteria, it is better for the abortion to be carried out earlier in pregnancy rather than later, where this is an option. It is safer for women, with a lower risk of complications,[62] and is less traumatic for all concerned. For example, the risk of haemorrhage at the time of abortion is 0.88 in 1000 at less than 13 weeks' gestation, rising to 4 in 1000 beyond 20 weeks' gestation.[63]

Early abortion also opens up the opportunity, up to 9 weeks' gestation, for a woman to have a medical abortion rather than a surgical abortion. (Medical abortion is possible after this time but may take longer, involve more drugs and require more care.[64]) Medical abortion is considered to be less invasive and less expensive than surgical abortion.[65] A medical abortion typically involves taking mifepristone (formerly known as RU486) to block the hormones that help a pregnancy to continue, and then later on (usually 2 days later) the prostaglandin misoprostol, which makes the uterus expel the embryo/fetus, usually within 4–6 hours.

Mifepristone has been available since 1991 in England, Scotland and Wales for early medical abortions. A 1990 amendment to the Abortion Act specifies that the Secretary of State's power to approve premises for termination of pregnancy includes the power to approve premises for the administration of medicinal terminations. Without this amendment, the administration of mifepristone would have been lawful only if carried out on premises approved for surgical terminations. Those considering administering mifepristone should discuss with the woman the advantages and disadvantages of this technique compared with surgical abortion.

The additional ethical issue raised by the use of mifepristone is that it is said that it makes abortion too 'easy', the implication being that women may undertake the procedure too lightly.[66] Some have predicted that the availability of such early abortion may result in a diminished sense of moral responsibility to avoid unwanted pregnancy, leading couples to neglect to take contraceptive measures. Others, however, have argued that the decision to terminate an unplanned pregnancy is unlikely to be trivialised in this way and have criticised the attitude that appears to claim that abortion requires punitive aspects for the woman in order to be taken seriously.[67] The Royal College of Obstetricians and Gynaecologists emphasises the benefit of being able to offer a choice of methods.[68]

The Department of Health, in England, commissioned a project to assess the safety, effectiveness and acceptability of early medical abortions in non-traditional settings – for example, in primary care settings. These non-traditional settings fell under the 'class of places' provisions of the Abortion Act (section 1(3A)) which gives the Secretary of State for Health powers to approve other 'class of places' to perform medical abortions. The 2008 final report evaluating the project noted that there were 'no discernable differences between the pilot sites and their matched comparator sites in terms of safety, effectiveness or acceptability of non-traditional sites for the administration of early medical abortions'.[69]

Early medical abortion – home administration

There has long been disagreement between the Department of Health and the British Pregnancy Advisory Services (BPAS) about what constitutes 'any treatment for the termination of pregnancy' under the Abortion Act, specifically whether a woman taking the second set of drugs – misoprostol – in an early medical abortion is considered to be undergoing the 'treatment' and is therefore required to be present in premises permitted under the Act.

BPAS went to the High Court to challenge the Department of Health's view that the legislation requires women to take both sets of drugs in an approved place. BPAS argued that 'treatment' stops at the point of prescription and women should be able to go home, if they choose, to take the second set of drugs.

The High Court rejected BPAS's claim while going on to say that there was scope within the legislation for the Secretary of State to approve changes to where misoprotol could be taken.[70] The Secretary of State for Health was noted in the judgment as accepting that a number of countries permit home administration of misoprostol but did 'not wish to introduce a new practice simply because it is deemed safe elsewhere in the world without fully piloting, evaluating the system and developing the appropriate protocols and standards to ensure that it is safe and acceptable for women in Great Britain'.[71]

Following the case, BPAS was clear that it would continue to push for women to have the choice to take the second set of drugs at home, and given the Secretary of State's comment in the judgment, this may be a possibility. Details of any future changes in this area will be posted on the BMA website.

Selective reduction of multiple pregnancy

The increased use of fertility treatment has led to higher numbers of multiple pregnancies. Careful monitoring of ovulation induction and a reduction in the maximum number of embryos replaced in *in vitro* fertilisation treatment can help to reduce the number of multiple pregnancies, but despite concerted efforts to reduce the number (see Chapter 8, pages 314–316) this cannot be avoided in all cases. High order multiple pregnancies are known to be associated with higher rates of mortality and morbidity for mothers and their babies. The greater the number of fetuses the greater the likelihood of preterm delivery and adverse consequences for the health and development of each baby.[72] Risk may be reduced by 'selective reduction', or multi-fetal pregnancy reduction, which involves killing one or more of the fetuses *in utero* in order to give the others a greater chance of a healthy outcome. There is evidence that the perinatal and obstetric outcomes after reduction of four or more fetuses are improved but whether the same applies to triplets reduced to twins remains controversial.[73] There are some who also see the procedure as posing medical, ethical and psychosocial problems, not least because of the paucity of information about how women and their partners cope with the experience and its after effects. The limited research that has been published suggests that most mothers considered that they had made the right decision regarding multi-fetal pregnancy reduction but there are undoubtedly complex psychological factors in the short and long term.[74]

Until 1990, the legality of selective reduction of multiple pregnancy was unclear because the Abortion Act referred to the termination of a 'pregnancy' and, in selective reduction, the pregnancy itself is not terminated. This was clarified by section 37(5) of the Human Fertilisation and Embryology Act 1990, which amended the Abortion Act explicitly to include 'in the case of a woman carrying more than one fetus, her miscarriage of any fetus'. Thus, selective reduction of pregnancy would be lawful provided the circumstances matched the criteria for termination of pregnancy set out in the 1967 Act and the procedure was carried out in an NHS hospital or premises approved for terminations. The same ethical and legal considerations apply to termination of all or part of a multiple pregnancy as to the termination of a singleton pregnancy. Under the new section 5(2) of the Abortion Act, selective reduction of a multiple pregnancy may lawfully be performed if:

'(a) the ground for termination of the pregnancy specified in subsection (1)(d) of [section 1] applies in relation to any fetus and the thing is done for the purpose of procuring the miscarriage of that fetus; or

(b) any of the other grounds for termination of the pregnancy specified in that section applies.'

It has been suggested that a general risk of serious handicap to the fetuses, if the multiple pregnancy is not reduced, would not be covered by the Act and the risk must be to a specific fetus. However, where there is an increased risk to the mother, as a result of the multiple pregnancy, the selective reduction may be lawful under section 1(1)(a), (b) or (c) of the Act (see page 283).[75]

Like gender selection (see Chapter 8, page 345–347), selective reduction is a procedure that has arisen from medical necessity, but which could arguably be offered as a consumer choice to parents who are not prepared to accept a natural multiple pregnancy (see below).

Abortion of a healthy twin

In August 1996, it was reported in the media that a 28-year-old woman had aborted a healthy twin at 16 weeks' gestation on the grounds that she would be unable to cope with two babies.[76] The woman, Miss B, was reported to have one child already and to be in 'socially straitened circumstances'. She allegedly told her consultant that she would keep one baby but could not keep two, and if she could not have selective reduction, she would terminate the pregnancy. This case caused widespread disquiet, not only amongst those who were fundamentally opposed to abortion or those who objected in principle to selective reduction. Some believed that it was wrong to use selective reduction for 'social' reasons, while others thought that aborting any fetus at 16 weeks for purely social reasons was unacceptable.[77]

The BMA considers selective termination to be justifiable when the procedure is recommended for medical reasons (both physical and psychological). Women who have a multiple pregnancy should be carefully counselled when medical opinion is that continuation, without selective reduction, will result in the loss of all the fetuses, but they cannot be compelled or pressured to accept selective abortion. The Association does not, however, consider it acceptable to choose which fetuses to abort on anything other than medical grounds. When there are no medical indications for aborting a particular fetus, the choice should be a random one. The Association would not consider it acceptable, when making this decision, to accede to the parents' desire for a male or a female child. (For further discussion of sex selection, see Chapter 8, pages 345–347.)

Abortion on grounds of fetal sex

Fetal sex is not one of the criteria for abortion listed in the Abortion Act and therefore termination on this ground alone has been challenged as outwith the law. There may be circumstances, however, in which termination of pregnancy on grounds of fetal sex would be lawful. It has been suggested that if two doctors, acting in good faith, formed the opinion that the pregnant woman's health, or that of her existing children, would be put at greater risk than if she terminated the pregnancy, the abortion would arguably be lawful under section 1(1)(a) of the Abortion Act (see page 283).[78] The Association believes that it is normally unethical to terminate a pregnancy on the grounds of fetal sex alone, except in cases of severe sex-linked disorders. The pregnant woman's views about the effect of the sex of the fetus on her situation and on her existing children should nevertheless be carefully considered. In some circumstances doctors may come to the conclusion that the effects are so severe as to provide legal and ethical justification for a termination. They should be prepared to justify the decision if it were challenged.

Conscientious objection to abortion

The Abortion Act has a conscientious objection clause that permits doctors to refuse to participate in terminations, but which obliges them to provide necessary treatment in an emergency when the woman's life may be at risk. The BMA supports the right of doctors to have a conscientious objection to termination of pregnancy and believes that such doctors should not be marginalised. Some have complained of being harassed and discriminated against because of their conscientious objection to termination of pregnancy. There have also been reports of doctors who carry out abortions being subjected to harassment and abuse. The Association abhors all such behaviour and any BMA members who feel they are being pressured, abused or harassed because of their views about termination of pregnancy should contact the BMA for advice and support.

Legal scope

The scope of the conscientious objection clause in the 1967 Act was clarified by the House of Lords in 1988.[79] In that case, a doctor's secretary (Janaway) refused to type the referral letter for an abortion and claimed a conscientious objection under the Act. The House of Lords, in interpreting the word 'participate' in this context, said that the word should be given its ordinary and natural meaning; that is, in order to claim conscientious exemption under section 4 of the Act, the objector had to be required to actually take part in administering treatment in a hospital or approved centre. The same view emerged in a parliamentary answer in December 1991.[80] This made it clear that conscientious objection was intended to be applied only to participation in treatment, although hospital managers were asked to apply the principle, at their discretion, to those ancillary staff who were involved in the handling of fetuses and fetal tissue.

In the Janaway case the judge said that the signing of the certificate would not form part of the treatment for the termination of pregnancy. This would seem to support the view that GPs cannot claim exemption from giving advice or performing the preparatory steps to arranging an abortion, if the request meets the legal requirements. Such steps include referral to another doctor as appropriate.

The BMA believes that in the event of seeing patients seeking advice on abortion, doctors should tell them immediately of the existence of a conscientious objection and of their right to see another doctor, although the consultation may continue if the patient and doctor both agree. In the event of seeing a patient seeking such a procedure, the doctor must, in line with GMC guidance, tell them of their right to see another doctor and ensure that the patient has sufficient information to exercise their right; but if the patient cannot readily make their own arrangements to see another doctor, the doctor must ensure that arrangements are made, without delay, for another doctor to take over their care.

GPs with a conscientious objection, who are working in a group practice, may ask a partner to see patients seeking termination. Practices may wish to state in advance if GPs in their practice have a conscientious objection to abortion, for example in their practice leaflets.

General Medical Council – conscientious objection

The General Medical Council advises that:

> If carrying out a particular procedure or giving advice about it conflicts with your religious or moral beliefs, and this conflict might affect the treatment or advice you provide, you must explain this to the patient and tell them they have the right to see another doctor. You must be satisfied that the patient has sufficient information to enable them to exercise that right. If it is not practical for a patient to arrange to see another doctor, you must ensure that arrangements are made for another suitably qualified colleague to take over your role.[81]

The position of medical students was clarified in a personal communication with the Department of Health that has been passed to the BMA for information. This made clear that the conscientious objection clause may be used by students to opt out of witnessing abortions.

The BMA's advice is that those who have a conscientious objection should disclose that fact to supervisors, managers or GP partners (whichever is appropriate) at as early a stage as possible so that this fact can be taken into account when planning provisions for patient care. In addition, it is the BMA's view that all deaneries should implement appropriate policies for equality and diversity within their training schemes including:

- the responsibilities of employers to have protocols to deal with issues of conscientious objection without any individual being disadvantaged
- the responsibilities of trainees to inform the employer of any conscientious objection issues in advance of taking up a post.

Distinction between legal and moral duties

In some cases a distinction can be made between legal and ethical obligations. Although noting the legal view, the BMA considers that some things that fall outside the legal scope of the conscience clause, such as completion of the form for abortion, are arguably an integral part of the abortion procedure and thus fall morally within its scope. Other preliminary procedures, such as clerking in the patient, are incidental to the termination and are considered outwith the scope of the conscience clause, both legally and morally. Nevertheless, where such tasks are unavoidable, health professionals and other staff must pursue a non-judgemental approach to the women concerned.

Delays in referral

Much concern has been expressed about avoidable delays in referral. Unreasonable delay with the intention, or the result, of compromising the possibility of a termination being carried out is unethical and may possibly leave the practitioner open to litigation. Referral need not be a formal procedure. In some cases, it may simply consist of arranging for the patient to see a partner in the practice. In other cases, it involves arranging a specific appointment with a colleague. It is not sufficient simply to tell the patient to seek a view elsewhere because other doctors may not agree to see her without an appropriate referral. The Royal College of Obstetricians and Gynaecologists has issued guidance on recommended referral times.[82]

Questions about abortion in job applications

The BMA is frequently asked what enquiries may be made about a doctor's views on abortion in job advertisements and at interview. The Department of Health published guidance on this issue in 1994,[83] which states that, for training grade posts, no reference to abortion should be included in the job advertisement or the job description, and applicants should not be questioned about their attitude to termination of pregnancy prior to the appointment. For most career grade posts, no information should be included in the advertisement but, if certain conditions have been satisfied, reference may be included in job descriptions and some questions may be asked at interview. At interview, however, enquiries about duties that relate to termination of pregnancy should be confined to matters of professional intention and not extend to questions about the applicant's personal beliefs. The Department of Health has confirmed that this guidance is not intended to cover the advertising of career posts that have little content other than termination of pregnancy duties.[84] Trusts can therefore advertise explicitly when the duties of career posts are entirely for the termination of pregnancy. Similar guidance was published by the Scottish Executive in 2004.[85]

Calls for reform of the Abortion Act

In 2007, the House of Commons Science and Technology Committee (replaced by the Innovation, Universities, Science and Skills Committee from November 2007 to November 2009) conducted an inquiry into the scientific developments relating to the Abortion Act 1967.[86] The inquiry focused on the scientific and medical evidence relating to the 24 week time limit; the medical, scientific and social research relevant to the impact of suggested law reforms to first trimester abortion; and evidence of long-term or acute adverse health outcomes from abortion or from the restriction of access to abortion. The Committee concluded, amongst other things, that:

- at least in the first trimester, the requirement for two doctors' signatures should be removed
- the GMC should make clear that conscientious objectors should alert patients to the fact that they do not consult on abortions and that if the issue arises during a consultation that they have a duty to immediately refer the patient to another doctor for the consultation
- subject to training and professional standards, nurses (and midwives) could be permitted to carry out early medical and surgical abortions.

However, not all members of the Committee were happy with the final recommendations. A minority report was published by two of the 11 members of the Committee.[87]

The BMA supported many of the inquiry's findings. For example, at the BMA's annual meeting in June 2007 the BMA had agreed new policy that the Abortion Act should be amended so that first trimester abortion (abortions up to 13 weeks) is available on the same basis of informed consent as other treatment, and therefore without the need for two doctors' signatures and without the need to meet specified medical criteria (see page 283). The proposed amendment would help ensure that women seeking abortion are not exposed to delays, and consequently to later, more costly and higher risk procedures. It was also agreed that any changes in relation to first trimester abortion should not adversely impact upon the availability of later abortions.

Shortly after the inquiry, a rare opportunity arose for the Abortion Act to be amended during the passage of the Human Fertilisation and Embryology Act 2008 (HFE Act).

There was extensive debate regarding the 24 week time limit, which the BMA, along with the Royal College of Obstetricians (RCOG) and Royal College of Nursing (RCN), lobbied to retain.[88] Amendments to the HFE Bill to reduce the time limit were lost, and the Abortion Act was unchanged.

The law on abortion in Northern Ireland

The Abortion Act does not extend to Northern Ireland, where the law on abortion is different and is based on the Offences Against the Person Act 1861, which makes it an offence to procure a miscarriage unlawfully. The *Bourne* judgment of 1939,[89] in which a London gynaecologist was found not guilty of an offence under this Act for performing an abortion on a 14-year-old girl who was pregnant as a result of rape, was based on an interpretation of the word 'unlawfully' in this Act. The defence argued, and the judge accepted, that in the particular circumstances of the case, the operation was not unlawful because continuation of the pregnancy would severely affect the young woman's mental health. In reaching this decision, the judge turned to the wording of the Infant Life (Preservation) Act 1929, which gave protection from prosecution if the act was carried out in good faith for the purpose only of preserving the life of the mother. This formed the basis of the judgment and extended the grounds for a lawful abortion to include cases in which 'the probable consequence of the continuation of the pregnancy will be to make the woman a physical or mental wreck'.

It is known that abortions are carried out in Northern Ireland and abortion is lawful in some circumstances.[90] However, without specific legislation, doctors are left with the task of interpreting the word 'unlawfully' as discussed in the *Bourne* judgment.

Abortion in Northern Ireland

K became pregnant at the age of 13 while in the care of a children's home. By the time of the court hearing in October 1993, K was 14 years old and 14 weeks pregnant. K wanted an abortion and had threatened to kill herself and the baby. She had cut her wrists with broken glass, declined food and punched herself in the stomach. The judge declared that abortion would be lawful in Northern Ireland in these circumstances and that an abortion would be in K's best interests. Although it had been declared lawful in Northern Ireland, no doctor could be found to carry out the termination, not because of any moral qualms but because of the fear of litigation. K was taken to Liverpool, where the abortion was performed.[91]

In the subsequent case of *Re A* the judge clarified the circumstances in which abortion would be lawful, stating that:

> The doctor's act is lawful where the continuance of the pregnancy would adversely affect the mental or physical health of the mother. The adverse effect must, however, be a real and serious one and it will always be a question of fact and degree whether the perceived effect of non-termination is sufficiently grave to warrant terminating the unborn child.[92]

Although case law has provided some clarification of the law in Northern Ireland, these cases also indicate the continuing legal uncertainty concerning the precise circumstances in which abortion is lawful. The BMA recognises the difficulties caused by this lack of legal certainty and supports the extension of the 1967 Abortion Act to Northern Ireland.[93]

Guidance on the law in Northern Ireland

In 2001, the Family Planning Association (FPA) sought a judicial review of the situation regarding termination of pregnancy in Northern Ireland, arguing that the Health Minister had acted unlawfully in failing to issue advice and guidance to women and doctors on the availability and provision of services to terminate pregnancy. In July 2003, the court rejected the FPA's claim. The judge, however, invited the Department of Health, Social Security and Public Safety (DHSSPS) to consider issuing guidance even though it was not legally required to do so.[94] The case continued and in October 2004 the FPA successfully appealed against the High Court's ruling. Lord Justice Nicholson said that doctors were not adequately aware of the principles that govern the law in Northern Ireland and new guidelines could help them.

Guidelines were published by the DHSSPS in March 2009 but they were subsequently withdrawn following a judicial review brought by the Society for the Protection of Unborn Children (SPUC). The High Court in Belfast[95] rejected SPUC's criticisms that the guidance would lead to a situation where abortion was easier to obtain in Northern Ireland, and noted that the guidance outlined the law correctly and could not be considered to be a misdirection. The Court requested, however, its withdrawal as 'those aspects of the Guidance dealing with counselling and with conscientious objection . . . fail to give fully clear and accurate guidance.'[96]

Concern was expressed that the guidance did not give healthcare professionals clear advice on what to do when approached by a woman concerned about the continuation of pregnancy but who did not satisfy the legal criteria to have an abortion, or what a healthcare professional should do, or is entitled to do, when he or she takes the view that a proposed abortion would be unlawful.

The DHSSPS was reported to be 'disappointed' by the ruling and subsequently re-issued the guidance for consultation, taking into consideration the Court's findings.[97] Details of any future changes in this area will be posted on the BMA website.

Women from Northern Ireland frequently travel to England or Scotland for termination of pregnancy, despite the fact that they are not entitled to NHS funding. Adequate provision should be made for the aftercare of these patients.

Conscientious objection

Doctors in Northern Ireland should follow the GMC's guidelines on personal beliefs (see page 289). It should be noted, however, that as the Abortion Act does not apply to Northern Ireland, nor do the provisions permitting conscientious objection under the Act. Doctors do not have a legal right to conscientious objection when a termination of pregnancy is lawful.

Consent for abortion

Abortion and young people

As with other medical interventions, a person who has sufficient understanding of the issues, and is acting free from pressure, may give valid consent to the termination of pregnancy, regardless of age (see pages 273–274). Some competent young women requesting abortion insist that parents must not be informed. Patients may fear, for example, that their parents will disown them or threaten them if they find out. Awareness of the potential emotional and psychological sequelae of abortion, however, makes doctors anxious about the lack of family support mechanisms for such patients. Counselling may help the patient to identify supportive adults within or outside the immediate family. Ultimately, however, a patient's request for confidentiality should not be overridden except in very exceptional cases (see Chapter 5). The courts have confirmed that a parent's refusal to give consent for a termination cannot override the consent of a competent young person.[98]

The case of P and the limits of parents' power to refuse abortion

P was aged 15 and in local authority care after a conviction for theft when she gave birth to a baby boy. Soon after the baby's birth, she became pregnant again and, as with her first pregnancy, her parents refused to consent to an abortion. Part of their objection was on religious grounds because P's father was a Seventh Day Adventist. P herself wanted to terminate her second pregnancy. The local authority made P a Ward of Court and asked the High Court to authorise a termination. P's father opposed this, suggesting that P should give birth and take care of the second child while he and his wife raised the first. The judge, however, concluded that the second pregnancy endangered P's mental health, impeded her schooling and endangered the future of P's existing child. She had no doubt that continuance of the pregnancy involved greater risk for P and her existing child than the risks of the termination. P's welfare, as a Ward of Court, had to be the judge's paramount consideration and the Court also had to consider the welfare of P's existing son. The judge concluded that the parents' objections did not outweigh the risks to P's mental health if the pregnancy continued. Termination was ruled to be in P's best interests.[99]

If a young pregnant person is assessed as lacking competence, somebody with parental responsibility can legally give consent for her to have a termination of pregnancy, provided the legal requirements of abortion legislation are met (see pages 283–284 and 291–292). In all cases, the patient's views must be heard and considered. If an incompetent minor refuses to permit parental involvement, expert legal advice should be sought. This should clarify whether the parents should be informed against the girl's wishes. A termination cannot proceed without valid consent, except in an emergency. This may require an application to the courts. If doctors believe that the patient is insufficiently mature to consent validly to termination of pregnancy, this raises the question of whether she was also unable to consent to sexual intercourse.

The first duty of health professionals concerns the welfare of the patient, who may need to be referred for specialist counselling. For more information about consent for termination of pregnancy see the BMA's separate guidance.[100]

Abortion and incapacitated adults

In November 2003, the High Court considered the circumstances in which a declaration from the court should be sought where it is proposed to terminate the pregnancy of an incapacitated adult.[101] Mr Justice Coleridge confirmed that where the issues of capacity and best interests are clear and beyond doubt an application to the court is not necessary. The following circumstances would, however, ordinarily warrant an application to court:

- where there is a dispute as to capacity, or where there is a realistic prospect that the patient will regain capacity, following a response to treatment, within the period of her pregnancy or shortly thereafter
- where there is a lack of unanimity amongst the medical professionals as to the best interests of the patient
- where the procedures under section 1 of the Abortion Act 1967 have not been followed (i.e. where two medical practitioners have not provided a certificate)

- where the patient, members of her immediate family, or the fetus' father have opposed, or expressed views inconsistent with, a termination of the pregnancy
- where there are other exceptional circumstances (including where the pregnancy proposed for termination may be the patient's last chance to bear a child).

Any cases falling near the boundary line in relation to any one of these criteria should be referred to court.

Involvement of fathers

Although women should generally be encouraged to discuss their decision to terminate a pregnancy with the father, male partners have no legal rights to involvement in the decision, as confirmed by the *Paton* case below and others.

Male partner opposing abortion

Mr Paton applied for an injunction to prevent BPAS and his wife from causing or permitting an abortion to be carried out. He originally argued that his wife had no proper legal grounds for seeking the termination of pregnancy and that she was being spiteful, vindictive and utterly unreasonable in doing so. He later accepted that the provisions of the Abortion Act had been correctly complied with, but contended that he had the right to have a say in the destiny of the child he had conceived. The judge referred to the highly emotional nature of such cases but confirmed that his task was to apply the law free of emotion or predilection. He considered the terms of the Abortion Act and concluded that the husband had 'no legal right enforceable in law or in equity to stop his wife having this abortion or to stop the doctors from carrying out the abortion.'[102]

Mr Paton took his case to the European Court of Human Rights, claiming that his Article 8 right to respect for family life had been breached. The Commission found that the decision insofar as it interfered with the applicant's right to respect for his family life was justified under paragraph (2) of Article 8 as being necessary for the protection of the rights of another person.[103]

Summary – abortion

- In England, Scotland and Wales abortion is lawful in the circumstances set out in the Abortion Act 1967 (as amended). Abortion is also lawful in more limited circumstances in Northern Ireland.
- In England, Scotland and Wales, doctors with a conscientious objection to abortion are not obliged to participate, except in an emergency situation where the woman's life may be at risk. Patients should, however, be referred to another health professional without delay.
- A young person aged under 16, who has sufficient understanding and competence, may consent to termination of pregnancy, but parental involvement should be encouraged.
- Although women should generally be encouraged to discuss their decision to terminate a pregnancy with the father of the fetus, male partners do not have the legal right to decide.

Prenatal screening and diagnosis

Some form of screening or testing is offered routinely to every pregnant woman in the UK. It is often presented as a standard part of antenatal care but, in fact, it raises significant ethical dilemmas that need to be addressed. The main issues are summarised below.

Prenatal screening

Prenatal screening is frequently used as a means of identifying those at higher than average risk of having a child with a disability, who are then offered more specialised testing. Prenatal screening may be by family history, serum screening, molecular tests or ultrasound. Ultrasound scanning is currently offered routinely to all pregnant women in the UK. Although undertaken to monitor the development of the fetus, it is also able to detect both major and minor defects. Often it is offered as 'routine' and some women have reported difficulties in refusing it. Concerns have also been expressed that women may accept screening unquestioningly without giving due consideration to the implications of an unfavourable result. Health professionals have a general ethical and legal duty to ensure that patients are given sufficient information to understand what is proposed and are given the opportunity to give or withhold consent. The BMA believes that, when giving information to patients, health professionals should present the possibility of refusing all prenatal screening as a reasonable and acceptable option.

In March 2008, NICE published clinical guidelines on antenatal care, setting out the standards that should be met in England and Wales, including what should be offered in terms of screening for fetal abnormalities.[104]

Prenatal genetic testing

Prenatal testing is offered to those who are known to be at risk of carrying an affected child. This may be because of previous affected pregnancies, a family history of a particular disorder or because they have been identified, from screening, as being at higher than average risk of having an affected child. The majority of prenatal testing is carried out during pregnancy using either amniocentesis or chorionic villus sampling. (Embryos may also be tested for some conditions before implantation; this is discussed in Chapter 8, pages 337–342.) It has been suggested that those who are at high risk of passing on a severe genetic disability have a duty to future generations and to their partner either not to reproduce[105] or to seek appropriate testing and termination of an affected pregnancy. Harris, for example, argues that an individual's moral obligation to future generations is both positive and negative. Not only must we not deliberately act to cause harm to our offspring, but we also have an obligation to remove dangers that would cause harm.[106] Depending upon the notion of harm in this context, this could be interpreted as a moral obligation for women to avail themselves of prenatal diagnosis and, where the child would be affected, to terminate the pregnancy. The BMA does not support this position, believing that it would be unacceptable to prevent people from reproducing or to force women to have testing and terminate affected pregnancies. Neither is it reasonable to impose on those who have genetic disorders moral responsibilities over and above those that apply to the rest of the population. Information should be provided and women and couples should be supported in whatever decision they make. When the parents disagree with each other about whether to seek testing, or about whether to terminate an affected pregnancy, they should each be given the opportunity to discuss their views and wishes. In some cases it may also be appropriate to offer expert counselling. If agreement cannot be reached, the woman's view about the progress of her pregnancy should hold sway within the constraints imposed by the law.

Objectives of prenatal diagnosis

In the past, some health professionals restricted access to prenatal diagnosis to those individuals who planned to terminate an affected pregnancy,[107] but this approach is now widely regarded as paternalistic and unacceptable. The BMA believes that parents should be given as much information as necessary to enable them to make an informed decision about whether to opt for testing and, if so, how to respond to an unfavourable result.

The termination of an affected pregnancy is one possible outcome of prenatal diagnosis, but there are a number of reasons why parents may wish to know the health of their fetus. For many people, prenatal diagnosis brings reassurance, but for those who receive an unfavourable result there can be practical benefits in having advance warning. In some cases, for example, knowledge of a disorder prior to the birth allows arrangements to be made for delivery at a specialised unit with facilities and expertise available to provide for the immediate medical needs of the child. Advance knowledge of disability can also prevent misdiagnosis and lead to earlier treatment or management of the condition. With a very small number of conditions, such as congenital adrenal hyperplasia, there is also the option of *in utero* treatment. When treatment is not a possibility, parents may still find it helpful to know in advance, to give them and their family time to come to terms with the child's disability, to find out more information about the condition, to access support networks and to plan for the child's future. Even with fatal conditions, some people prefer to 'let nature take its course', allowing time for the parents and their family to come to terms with the inevitability of the child's death.

Social implications

Some people see prenatal diagnosis not as part of a duty of care to the potential child, but as a personal and societal drive to eliminate non-standard individuals and to what has been termed the 'tyranny of normality', leading to an ever-narrowing definition of normality and tolerance. This, in turn, leads to higher expectations among parents and makes them less able to accept disability when it happens. This can manifest itself in anger when a child is born with a disability and can result in the parents grieving for the loss of the normal, healthy baby that, they considered, was almost guaranteed. Although disability is a fact of life, it is suggested that people are less able to cope because, with the emphasis on prenatal diagnosis, 'normality' within a narrow range of variation is expected.

There are also concerns that, as prenatal diagnosis becomes more widespread, those who decide not to have testing when they are known to be at risk of a genetic disorder, or who decide to continue with an affected pregnancy, may come to be seen as irresponsible. When the child will be severely disabled and require long-term and expensive treatment it is possible that society will become increasingly unwilling to pay for the necessary care, seeing the parents as 'to blame' for the birth and therefore individually responsible for the cost of treatment. In the USA there have been reports of private insurance companies attempting, unsuccessfully, in the past to withhold reimbursement for the medical care of children whose disability was detected before birth.[108] Any such moves in this country must be vigorously opposed. The availability of resources for the care and treatment of a disabled child must not be contingent on whether the parents knew of the disability before the child was born.

Little research has been undertaken into the effect of prenatal diagnosis on public attitudes towards disability, either to confirm or refute these predictions. It is important that the potential for increased discrimination is recognised and that public attitudes towards disability are carefully monitored.

Setting boundaries

A frequent question in relation to prenatal diagnosis is where the boundaries should be set. Is it acceptable, for example, to terminate a pregnancy because the child, if born, will develop a serious disorder in middle age? Could, and should, the technology be used to meet parental desires for children with particular characteristics or looks? The BMA has considered these questions in some detail and has reached the following conclusions.

- The criteria for prenatal diagnosis should be sufficiently flexible to allow for consideration of individual cases, when the following factors should usually be taken into account:
  - the sensitivity and specificity of the test and the level of predictability obtained from the results
  - the pregnant woman's own perception of the situation and her existing family circumstances
  - the severity of the disorder
  - the age of onset of the condition
  - the options available, including the possibility of effective treatment, either *in utero* or after birth.
- The BMA has concerns about the routine use of prenatal diagnosis for adult onset disorders, but accepts that, in some circumstances, after careful counselling and consideration, such testing could be appropriate.
- Genetic information and technology should be used primarily to reduce suffering and impairment. Their use for trivial reasons or as a means of satisfying parental desires for certain physical or enhancing characteristics in healthy children is inappropriate.

Summary – prenatal screening and diagnosis

- When giving information to patients about prenatal diagnosis, health professionals should present the possibility of refusing all prenatal screening and testing as a reasonable and acceptable option.
- When the parents disagree with each other about whether to seek testing, or about whether to terminate an affected pregnancy, they should each be encouraged to discuss their views and wishes. If agreement cannot be reached, the woman's view should hold sway within the constraints imposed by the law.
- Parents should not be seen as 'to blame' for the birth of a disabled child, irrespective of whether they refused testing or knew of the disability before the child was born.
- Medical technology should be used to reduce suffering and impairment and its use for trivial reasons or for satisfying parental desires for certain physical or enhancing characteristics is inappropriate.

Pregnancy

Protecting the fetus from harm during pregnancy

There has been considerable debate, both in the UK and elsewhere, about ways of protecting a fetus from harm caused by its mother's actions during pregnancy by, for example, smoking, or the abuse of alcohol or drugs. In *Re F* (see below) the Appeal Court rejected an application to make a fetus a Ward of Court in order to protect it from harm from its mother, who suffered from severe mental illness, abused drugs and had a nomadic lifestyle. It was held in that case that the Court did not have the power to make an unborn child a Ward of Court and that any such action would necessarily involve controlling the mother.

Attempt to make a fetus a Ward of Court

F was 36 years old and since her early twenties had suffered from severe mental disturbance, accompanied by drug abuse, and she suffered from delusions and hallucinations. She lived a nomadic existence, travelling through a number of European countries. F had a son, G, who had been taken into the care of long-term foster parents and adoption proceedings had commenced; F's access to her son had been terminated after repeated unsuccessful attempts at rehabilitation. F became pregnant again and, shortly before the anticipated date of delivery, the local authority applied to make the fetus a Ward of Court in order to protect it from possible harm arising from its mother's actions. The application was dismissed on the grounds that the Court did not have the jurisdiction to make a fetus a Ward of Court.[109]
This decision was upheld by the Court of Appeal.

Although a child may sue a third party for damages caused by negligent acts in the antenatal period, in England, Wales and Northern Ireland a child cannot sue its mother for harm caused by her actions during pregnancy (with the exception of harm resulting from a road traffic accident).[110] This followed a Law Commission report published in 1974.[111] Influential in its decision were the arguments that: the relationship between a disabled child and its mother would inevitably be difficult and the situation would be exacerbated if she was liable to pay compensation for the child's disabilities; it was not clear where the mother would find the funds to pay any compensation to the child without causing hardship to the rest of the family; and such a course of action could easily become a weapon in cases of matrimonial conflict. Concern was also expressed about the problem of setting limits to the type of maternal conduct that would render the woman liable for any subsequent disability. Although women should be alerted to the likely risks to the fetus caused by their behaviour, and should be encouraged to refrain from risky activities for the duration of the pregnancy, there is no way of compelling them to do so. Some authorities have tried to modify pregnant women's behaviour with the use of incentives (for a discussion on incentives see Chapter 20, pages 832–833). In Scotland, this issue remains open because there is no law excluding a claim by the child against its mother in relation to prenatal injuries, although it has been suggested that a Scottish court would be unsympathetic to such claims, on policy grounds.[112]

Encouraging healthy behaviour

In May 2004, the *breathe* project was launched in Glasgow to test routinely the carbon monoxide levels of consenting pregnant women, solely for the purpose of identifying whether they smoke.[113] It was proposed that women identified as smokers would be offered a referral to a smoking cessation link midwife, whereby a smoking cessation 'action plan' would be devised, including telephone support and counselling.

Routine screening of pregnant women

In addition to prenatal screening and testing of the fetus (see pages 294–297), pregnant women are offered screening for disorders for which treatment or appropriate management during pregnancy and birth can prevent the disorder being passed to the baby. A good example of this is screening for HIV infection. Guidance from the Royal College of Obstetricians and Gynaecologists and health departments state that all maternity units should offer and recommend HIV testing as a routine part of antenatal care. All doctors and midwives should be competent to obtain consent for these tests and should request the tests according to local protocols.[114]

This is consistent with BMA policy dating back to 1991 that all pregnant women should be offered routine screening for HIV antibodies. If a woman tests positive, the risk of vertical transmission to her baby can be reduced from 25–30 per cent to less than 1 per cent by the avoidance of breastfeeding, the use of antiretroviral drugs and delivery by elective caesarean section.[115] Clearly, the greater the ability to intervene effectively to prevent harm, the greater the argument for offering screening.

Providing life support to a pregnant woman for the benefit of a fetus

Decisions to withhold or withdraw life prolonging treatment are difficult and controversial, but they are even more so when the patient is a pregnant woman and withdrawing treatment would result in the death of an otherwise healthy fetus. Thankfully, such situations are rare, but when they occur they raise difficult legal and ethical questions about the acceptability of continuing to provide life support for the benefit of the fetus. These questions have yet to be properly resolved. This section explores some of the legal and ethical factors that would need to be taken into account. When there is no benefit to the pregnant woman of providing treatment, it is likely that a court declaration would need to be sought.

As discussed in Chapter 3, when adults do not have the capacity to give consent to medical treatment, mental capacity legislation, which sets out a framework for decision making on behalf of adults who lack the capacity to make decisions for themselves, must be followed. When starting or continuing treatment is not in the patient's best interests, it may be withheld or withdrawn, even if this results in the patient's death. If the woman has a valid advance decision refusing treatment (ADRT) refusing all life-prolonging treatment in the circumstances that have arisen and which specifically states that the ADRT should apply while she is pregnant, the ADRT should be followed. If the ADRT does not state that it should apply when the woman is pregnant, and the life of the fetus could be saved by continuing to provide life support to the mother, legal advice should be sought and it may be necessary to seek a court declaration.

In the absence of any clear expression of the patient's previous wishes, the primary duty of the doctor is to provide necessary and appropriate treatment for the mother. So, when life support is likely to provide clinical benefit to the patient, this should be provided. This is true even if the treatment will jeopardise the health or life of the fetus, because the mother's interests prevail over those of her fetus in such cases.[116] When, however, an alternative treatment could be provided that does not jeopardise the fetus, this would be the preferred option. If the fact of pregnancy itself jeopardised the chances of survival for the woman, the legal grounds for terminating the pregnancy would be met.

A more difficult situation arises when clinical assessment reveals that there is no hope of survival for the woman and, although continuing to provide life support would increase the chance of a successful live birth, it will involve prolonging the dying process for the mother. The question then arises as to whether treatment may be provided for the benefit of the unborn child or whether saving the child could be seen to be in the woman's emotional or psychological best interests.

Providing life support for a pregnant woman

Ms Karen Battenbough was 24 years old and 4¹/₂ months pregnant when a car accident in 1995 left her in a coma with virtually no chance of survival. She could breathe unaided and was given artificial nutrition and hydration to prolong her life. On 3 May 1995 she delivered a daughter by caesarean section; according to her family this was a baby she desperately wanted. She never regained consciousness and died in December 1996.[117] This case did not go to court and it is unclear from the media reports whether, had she not been pregnant, her doctors would have judged the provision of life-prolonging treatment to be in her best interests. The fact that treatment was continued after the delivery, however, implies that her doctors considered that she was deriving benefit from it. Even if there had been no clinical benefit, it is likely that the woman's previously expressed views about her pregnancy would have been influential in assessing that her best interests would be met by providing treatment to give the child the best chance of survival.

The case described above would have been more complex if the woman had not known she was pregnant before the accident, she had not planned the pregnancy and she had never discussed her views about pregnancy. In that situation, it would be difficult to argue that it would be in the woman's best interests to continue life support in order to increase the chance of a healthy child. Then, the only grounds for continuing to provide the treatment would be for the benefit of the fetus, but, in considering cases of enforced caesarean section, the courts have made clear that they do not have the jurisdiction to take the interests of the fetus into account.[118] Similarly, in a review of the common law on consent, McLean highlighted that 'the best interests test requires evidence that the intended intervention is for the benefit of the individual concerned. Thus, no attention should be paid to possible benefits to third parties.'[119] Peart *et al.* point out that, using the reasoning in Bland (see Chapter 10, pages 444–445), 'it would be unlawful to keep a pregnant woman in such circumstances on life support solely for the benefit of her unborn child, because it would not be in her best interests. Life support should be withdrawn and she should be allowed to die, regardless of the effect that this has on her unborn child.'[120] They go on to say, however, that it seems improbable that a court would sanction the withdrawal of treatment, if continuing it was not contrary to the woman's interests (or if she was perceived to have no interests) and it would be possible to save the life of the unborn child. They take the view that:

> ... a pregnant woman in [persistent vegetative state (PVS) or similar irreversible condition] ... has no interest in being alive, nor does she have an interest in being dead. Prolonging her existence until after the birth of her child therefore does not conflict with her interests, because she no longer has interests in any meaningful sense. ... We would therefore conclude that decisions about treatment of a pregnant PVS patient should be made in the interests of her unborn child, because the patient's condition and prognosis have effectively deprived her of the sort of interests which normally underpin treatment decisions.[121]

Although, intuitively, it would appear appropriate to save the life of a child, when this is possible without causing harm to the mother, this is not straightforward either legally or morally. Legally, treatment may be provided to adults lacking capacity only if it is in their best interests, or benefit in Scotland (see Chapter 3). To provide treatment in other circumstances would constitute battery. Given that under the current law the best interests test cannot include the interests of any third party, including a fetus, treatment cannot lawfully be provided to a woman who lacks capacity for the benefit of her unborn child. Arguments about 'not being contrary to interests', which have been proposed in the academic literature, have not been tested in the courts. From an ethical perspective, unless it is assumed that all women have moral obligations to their unborn children that can be enforced, such action could be seen as assault on the woman's autonomy, bodily integrity and dignity. It has been argued, for example, that keeping a woman on a ventilator when there is no benefit to her, in order to permit the safe delivery of her child would, in the absence of any indication of her wishes, involve a violation of her autonomy, be an act of disrespect, and would amount to treating her as a 'human incubator' or 'fetal container'.[122]

Where the woman's own wishes about the outcome of the pregnancy are known these will be taken into account in determining her best interests. The UK courts have not considered, however, a case where treatment is not in the best interests of a pregnant woman (or where she is perceived to have no interests) and where her own wishes are not known. The question of whether the presumption should be in favour of providing life support or withholding it, in such circumstances, remains unresolved. Should such a case arise, legal advice should be sought and a declaration from the courts may be needed.

Summary – pregnancy

- Women should be alerted to any risks to their fetus arising from their behaviour during pregnancy, but they cannot be compelled to refrain from such activities.
- Even where there are concerns that a mother's actions are putting her fetus at risk, the fetus cannot be made a Ward of Court.
- It is unclear whether, legally, life support could continue to be provided to a pregnant woman solely for the benefit of the fetus. If such a situation arises, legal advice should be sought.

Childbirth

Over the last 20 years there has been a shift towards greater patient choice in where and how to give birth, articulated initially in the Department of Health's 1993 report *Changing childbirth*,[123] and more recently in 2007 in *Maternity matters*.[124] Some women have exercised this choice to opt for more medical intervention, by requesting elective caesarean section as their chosen mode of delivery. Others have sought to reduce medical intervention by requesting natural, water or home births, by refusing a medically indicated caesarean section or induction of a post-maturity pregnancy. A small number of women have sought to have no medical intervention, choosing unassisted childbirth or 'freebirth'.[125] Wherever and however a woman wishes to give birth, she must be given adequate, accurate information to enable her to make an informed choice. There should be clear agreement among the health professionals involved about who takes responsibility for different elements of the woman's care. In most cases, a midwife assumes sole responsibility for normal deliveries, calling upon a doctor for assistance only if complications arise.

Home births and the role of GPs

Approximately 2 per cent of women have home births in the UK but, according to a statement from the Royal College of Obstetricians and Gynaecologists and Royal College of Midwives, it is believed that 8–10 per cent of pregnant women would like a home birth.[126] When a woman is considering a home birth, with the support of her midwife, she should be given sufficient information to enable her to make an informed decision, based on both the actual and perceived risks and benefits of giving birth outside a medical environment. With home births, as in hospital, the lead role is usually taken by the midwife, with medical assistance called upon or hospital admission arranged only if complications arise. In an emergency situation, the patient is likely to be admitted to hospital but, if called, the GP would be required to attend and to give such assistance as is reasonable, judged by the standards of an ordinary GP. In some cases, the patient's GP attends during the labour, in order to give personal support to the woman or to provide additional backup to the midwife who is managing the birth. However, the majority of GPs do not have obstetric skills and they are not expected to provide specialist intervention as part of an enhanced service. GPs who are asked to support a woman's choice of a home birth should ensure that their patient is aware of what, if any, additional training in obstetrics they have received, and the role they will take in the delivery. It is important that a woman is aware of the limitations of the support her GP is able to provide.[127]

When, in a particular case, GPs have concerns about the safety of a home birth, this should be discussed with the patient, midwife and obstetrician. Every effort should be made to reach a mutually acceptable position through discussion, negotiation and the offer of seeking another expert opinion. When agreement cannot be reached, it is important that the patient does not feel abandoned by any of the healthcare providers. Nor should GPs be excluded from their patient's care, because they have a continuing duty of care to the woman. Even if GPs make clear their concerns about the choice of a home birth, they are still obliged to attend if called in an emergency situation. Although women cannot be obliged to attend hospital or a maternity unit for delivery, they do not have a legal right to demand medical assistance in support of their choice of a home birth.

Many women who have wanted to give birth at home when there were no medical contraindications have been unable to do so because of a shortage of midwives. As part of a concerted effort to improve maternity services, in May 2001 the previous Labour Government announced the recruitment of 2,000 more midwives by 2005. It also announced a National Service Framework for children and maternity services to ensure that:

- women will have access to a midwife dedicated to them when in established labour 100 per cent of the time
- all women will have access to care delivered by midwives they know and trust
- there is an end to the lottery in childbirth choices, so that women in all parts of the country, not just some, have greater choice, including that of a safe home birth.[128]

The shortage remains despite these efforts.

Requests for caesarean section

The number of women giving birth by caesarean section has increased dramatically; just under 25 per cent of women in England and Scotland now give birth in this way.[129] Part of the explanation for this increase is that women are delaying childbirth until later in life and it is known that older mothers are more likely to deliver by caesarean section. However, research has found that, despite this correlation, the higher number of caesarean deliveries is not explained by higher rates of complications, as could be expected.[130] Instead, as the authors of the study suggest, the results may support existing speculation that physician and maternal preference has had a significant role in the increase.

Others see the increase in caesarean sections as evidence of defensive medicine by obstetricians and 'a process in which women are finally given less information and less choice and in which obstetricians appropriate the central role of childbirth at the expense of women'.[131] It has been suggested that maternal preference is, in fact, strongly influenced by the views of medical practitioners, many of whom have vested interests in making 'the well worried'.[132] Later research disputes this, however, citing instead that safety is women's prime concern. The debate around women requesting caesarean sections may misunderstand women's priorities and decision making.[133]

Whatever the reasons behind the increase, doctors should ensure that information is provided objectively and is, wherever possible, evidence based, acknowledging uncertainty where it exists. All requests for elective caesarean section should be assessed individually, taking account of the most recent guidance available.

In April 2004, NICE published clinical guidelines on caesarean sections.[134] The guidelines state that maternal request is not, on its own, an indication for caesarean section and that the reasons for such requests should be explored, discussed and recorded. This discussion should include the overall benefits and risks of caesarean section compared with vaginal birth. The guidelines confirm that an individual clinician has the right to decline a request for caesarean section in the absence of an identifiable reason but recommends that, in such circumstances, the woman should be referred for a second opinion.

Why women choose caesarean section

The reasons why women choose to deliver by elective caesarean section, rather than by a vaginal birth, has been the subject of much debate. Some have speculated that 'health has become secondary to a sexually attractive body'[135] and that the fear of genital damage represents another aspect of society's popular obsession with body image. A genuine fear of vaginal delivery, as well as concerns about the long-term sequelae and fear of harm to the baby, were reported in interviews carried out by Weaver et al. with women who said that the issue of caesarean section arose during their pregnancy.[136] An expert advisory group that considered the increased rate of caesarean sections in Scotland reported a variety of reasons why women choose this option, including bad experiences at previous vaginal delivery, fear of intimate examinations and previous sexual abuse.[137]

Views are mixed about whether women should be given the right to choose a caesarean section when this is not required for medical reasons. In Scotland, an expert advisory group appeared to support giving women that option. Its report concluded that 'women's views and preferences should be acknowledged as a major factor in the joint decision between clinicians and women to deliver by caesarean section'.[138] The recommendations went on to say that, when a decision is made for a caesarean delivery, in the absence of obstetric indications, clinicians must ensure that the woman has the necessary information to reach a truly informed choice.

Those who oppose giving women this choice stress that caesarean section is a major operation, carrying risks for both mother and child, and that to expose women and their unborn babies to those risks when there is no medical need to do so would be wrong and contrary to the doctor's duty of care. Those who support giving women the choice of caesarean section argue that, provided they are properly informed of the risks, women themselves are the best judge of what is right for them. In a society that is increasingly intolerant of risk, where antenatal screening and care is positively encouraged, it has been argued that women should be given the option of a caesarean section if they find that more acceptable.

Central to this debate is the balance of risks between vaginal and caesarean delivery. Caesarean section has traditionally been seen as exposing both mother and baby to higher risk than vaginal delivery. It has been argued, however, that much of the data on mortality and morbidity rates after caesarean section are taken from emergency caesareans, where there are existing complications, and that the risks of vaginal delivery are frequently underestimated.[139] More research and clinical guidance is needed to provide objective, comparative data about risk in order to assist those facing such requests. Some argue that, until there is evidence that elective caesarean section is at least as safe as vaginal delivery, it should not be offered when there are no medical indications. Others take the view that, in the absence of clear and undisputed evidence, the woman's own assessment of the risks and benefits to her should provide the crucial deciding factor.[140] This is an area that needs to be explored further because the closer the balance of risks between the two modes of delivery, the stronger the argument for allowing women to choose. Inevitably, however, the resource implications of giving all women the option of elective caesarean section, at far greater cost than vaginal delivery, cannot be ignored.

When presented with a request for a caesarean section on grounds of maternal preference, rather than medical necessity, the doctor should ensure that the patient is provided with up-to-date information about the relative advantages and disadvantages. The woman should be encouraged to discuss any fears or concerns, and steps should be taken to address these before deciding on the most appropriate course of action. An obstetrician who is concerned about the risks of carrying out an elective caesarean in these circumstances would not be obliged to comply with the request. The courts have frequently stated that they would not force doctors to act contrary to their clinical judgement. The doctor should discuss the concerns with the patient and explain the reasons for not wishing to proceed. If the patient still wishes to have a caesarean section, she should be offered the option of transferring to the care of another doctor. Where elective caesarean section is not provided on the NHS, the patient should be informed of this and offered a referral for private treatment if that is her wish.

Refusal of caesarean section

Health professionals who provide care for women during their pregnancy and labour aim to promote the greatest benefit to both mother and fetus, with the least risk. In a small number of cases, problems arise because the pregnant woman and her doctors fundamentally disagree about the action believed to be in the best interest of the mother or fetus, or because medical advice conflicts with the woman's beliefs, religious or otherwise. Pregnancy and labour are particularly recognised as processes in which women's wishes should be supported and health professionals normally try to accommodate patients' wishes when this can be done without incurring grave risks.

Questions inevitably arise, however, about the validity of the patient's decision when it conflicts with her known desire to have a healthy baby or when she is subject to involuntary compulsion. Such is the case where a woman wishes to deliver a healthy child, but refuses a caesarean section or other medical intervention that is considered necessary to achieve that aim. The courts have made clear that whether treatment may be provided without consent in such cases depends upon whether the woman has capacity to make the decision. Assessing capacity in this situation is not always easy and in some cases specialist psychiatric examination may be required. Despite the pain and distress that can be associated with childbirth, being in labour is not incompatible with having capacity to make decisions. For women over the age of 16, there should be a presumption that they are capable of giving or withholding consent, and that their decisions will be respected. The fact that the healthcare team disagrees with the decision a woman has made does not mean that she lacks capacity to make the decision. There are, however, some cases in which a woman becomes temporarily incapacitated during labour, for example if her refusal of treatment is caused by a needle phobia as in the case of *Re MB* (see pages 268–269). In these situations, attempts should be made to alleviate the reasons for the incapacity, wherever possible, in order to obtain a valid decision.

If the woman has capacity, her refusal must be respected. The courts will not consider cases of refusal by adults with capacity because the law, on this point, is clear. If she lacks capacity, the doctor in charge of her care must act in the woman's best interests, taking account of any previously expressed wishes (see Chapter 3). If there is genuine doubt about the woman's capacity, an application may be made to the courts to decide if treatment may be provided lawfully.

Refusal of caesarean section

Ms S was 36 weeks pregnant and had not previously sought antenatal care. She was diagnosed with pre-eclampsia and was advised that she needed urgent attention, bed rest and admission to hospital for an induced delivery. Although she understood that without this treatment both her life and that of the fetus were in danger, she rejected the advice, wanting her baby to be born naturally. S was seen by an approved social worker and two doctors, and was admitted against her will for assessment under the Mental Health Act 1983. She was then transferred to St George's Hospital where she continued to refuse treatment. An application was made to court, and was granted, to dispense with the need for her consent and a caesarean section was carried out, delivering a baby girl. Shortly afterwards her detention under the Mental Health Act was terminated.

Ms S appealed against the original judgment. Upholding the appeal, the decision from the Appeal Court was:

... while pregnancy increases the personal responsibilities of a woman it does not diminish her entitlement to decide whether or not to undergo medical treatment. Although human, and protected by the law in a number of different ways ... an unborn child is not a separate person from its mother. Its need for medical assistance does not prevail over her rights. She is entitled not to be forced to submit to an invasion of her body against her will, whether her own life or that of her unborn child depends on it. Her right is not reduced or diminished merely because her decision to exercise it may appear morally repugnant.[141]

It was further held that the Mental Health Act could not be used to detain an individual against her will merely because her 'thinking process is unusual, even apparently bizarre and irrational, and contrary to the views of the overwhelming majority of the community at large'.[142]

The BMA considers that health professionals should encourage pregnant women to consider carefully the options available to them and the implications of a refusal to accept a caesarean section in such cases. Usually, once women realise that acceding to the medical intervention recommended is the best, or perhaps only, way of saving the life of the fetus, they agree to the treatment. In the minority of cases in which women continue to oppose a caesarean section, and they have capacity to make that decision, the refusal must be respected. Health professionals must tread a delicate line between advising women honestly of the implications of their decisions and unreasonably pressurising them to consent to the intervention. The refusal of treatment is discussed further in Chapter 2.

Pain relief

Sometimes questions are raised with the BMA about whether a 'birth plan' that refuses any pain relief would be binding if the woman subsequently changed her mind during labour. A birth plan is one form of ADRT and, as such, becomes active only when capacity is lost. Women in labour generally retain capacity to give consent and so their contemporaneous decisions should be respected. Some women make birth plans that include a stipulation that any request for drugs during childbirth should be ignored. Doctors who become aware of such plans should discuss them in advance with the women concerned and explain that any contemporaneous requests for drugs will be taken to override the birth plan. It should be made unambiguously clear that a birth plan refusing particular interventions becomes active only if the patient does not have capacity to make decisions. (General discussion about advance decisions can be found in Chapter 3.)

Summary – childbirth

- In home births, as in hospital, the lead role is usually taken by the midwife.
- A GP who is approached about a woman's choice of a home birth should ensure that the patient is aware of the limitations of the support the GP is able to provide.
- Even if a GP makes clear his or her concerns about the choice of a home birth, the GP is still obliged to attend if called in an emergency situation.
- An obstetrician with serious concerns about the risks of carrying out a caesarean section requested for maternal preference rather than medical necessity, would not be obliged to comply with such requests.
- A refusal of medical intervention by a woman with capacity must be respected even if both she and her fetus may die as a result. When there is genuine doubt about the patient's capacity, an application may be made to the courts.
- Women in labour generally retain capacity to give consent. A birth plan refusing any pain relief during pregnancy would be overridden by a contemporaneous request for drugs.

Reproductive ethics: a continuing dilemma

Reproduction is an area that covers a number of different strands, all of which raise complex legal and ethical questions. This chapter's focus on contraception, abortion and birth seeks to provide guidance on the type of practical questions raised with the BMA, while also discussing some of the more unusual and perhaps more theoretical scenarios. These are issues that will continue to challenge doctors and society. The next chapter focuses more specifically on the issues raised by assisted reproduction, including some of the major policy decisions that require debate within society.

References

1 *Re MB (medical treatment)* [1997] 2 FLR 426.
2 Centre for Maternal and Child Enquiries (2011) *Saving Mothers' Lives: reviewing maternal deaths to make motherhood safer 2006-2008. The Eighth Report on Confidential Enquiries into Maternal Deaths in the United Kingdom*, Wiley-Blackwell, London, pp.75, 124 and 159.
3 *Re MB (medical treatment)* [1997] 2 FLR 426: 441.
4 *Vo v France* (2005) 40 EHRR 12, para 47.
5 *Vo v France* (2005) 40 EHRR 12, paras 82 and 85.
6 NHS Information Centre (2009) *NHS contraceptive services, England: 2008–09*, NHS Information Centre, London.
7 National Health Service (General Medical Services Contracts) Regulations 2004. SI 2004/291, s3, schedule 2.
8 Wellings K, Nanachal K, Macdowall W. *et al.* (2001) Sexual behaviour in Britain: early heterosexual experience. *Lancet* **358**, 1843–50.
9 Brook (2009) *Factsheet 2. Teenage conceptions: Statistics and trends*, Brook, London.
10 Social Exclusion Unit (1999) *Teenage pregnancy*, The Stationery Office, London.
11 Social Exclusion Unit (1999) *Teenage pregnancy*, The Stationery Office, London, p.7.
12 Anon. (2005) Teenage pregnancy: Why are rates rising? *BBC News Online* (May 27). Available at: www.bbc.co.uk/news (accessed 2 March 2011).
13 Department for Children, Schools and Families (2009) *Government Response to the 5th Annual Report of the Teenage Pregnancy Independent Advisory Group*, DCSF, London, p.4.
14 Office for National Statistics (2011) *Conceptions in England and Wales 2009*, The Stationery Office, London.
15 Information Services Division (2009) *Sexual Health: teenage pregnancy – table 1 by age of mother at conception: 1994–2008*. Available at: www.isdscotland.org (accessed 3 March 2011).
16 Northern Ireland Statistics and Research Agency (2010) *The Registrar General's Quarterly Report, Number 355*, Northern Ireland Statistics and Research Agency, Belfast.
17 Teenage Pregnancy Independent Advisory Group (2009) *Annual Report 2008/09*, TPIAG, London.
18 Anon. (2010) Teenage pregnancy rate 'will rise' without action. *BBC News Online* (December 14). Available at: www.bbc.co.uk/news (accessed 1 March 2011).
19 Information Services Division (2009) *Sexual Health: teenage pregnancy – table 1 by age of mother at conception: 1994–2008*. Available at: www.isdscotland.org (accessed 3 March 2011).
20 Department of Health, Social Services and Public Safety (2002) *Teenage Pregnancy and Parenthood: Strategy and Action Plan 2002–2007*, DHSSPS, Belfast.
21 Teenage Pregnancy Unit (2000) *Teenage pregnancy national campaign. Findings of research conducted prior to campaign development*, Department of Health, London.
22 Reeves C, Whitaker R, Parsonage RK. *et al.* (2006) Sexual health services and education: young people's experiences and preferences. *Health Education J* **65**(4), 368–79.
23 Brook Advisory Centres (1999) *You think they won't tell anyone. Well you hope they won't*, Brook, London.
24 Teenage Pregnancy Unit (2004) *Best practice guidance for doctors and other health professionals on the provision of advice and treatment to young people under 16 on contraception, sexual and reproductive health*, DH, London.
25 *R (on the application of Axon) v Secretary of State for Health* [2006] 2 WLR 1130.
26 *Gillick v Wisbech and West Norfolk AHA* [1985] 3 All ER 402.
27 Kennedy I. (1988) *Treat me right*, Oxford University Press, Oxford, p.112.
28 *Gillick v Wisbech and West Norfolk AHA* [1985] 3 All ER 402.
29 Fraser guidelines as outlined by Lord Fraser in *Gillick v Wisbech and West Norfolk AHA* [1985] 3 All ER 402.
30 General Medical Council (2007) *0–18 years: guidance for all doctors*, GMC, London. British Medical Association (2010) *Children and young people tool kit*, BMA, London.
31 McCarthy M. (2010) Exercising choice and control: women with learning disabilities and contraception. *Br J Learning Disabilities* **38**(4), 293–302.
32 NHS Information Centre (2009) *NHS contraceptive services, England: 2008–09*, NHS Information Centre, London, p.9.
33 Marston C, Meltzer H, Majeed A. (2005) Impact on contraceptive practice of making emergency hormonal contraception available over the counter in Great Britain: repeated cross sectional surveys. *BMJ* **331**, 271. Glasier A, Baird D. (1998) The effects of self-administering emergency contraception. *N Engl J Med* **399**, 1–4.
34 Prescription Only Medicines (Human Use) Amendment (No. 3) Order 2000. SI 2000/3231.
35 The Royal Pharmaceutical Society of Great Britain (2004) *Practice guidance on the supply of emergency hormonal contraception as a pharmacy medicine*, RPSGB, London.
36 British Medical Association (2008) *Sexually transmitted infections*, BMA, London.

37 NHS Wales (2010) *Pharmacies offering free emergency contraception.* Available at: www.wales.nhs.uk (accessed 4 March 2011).

38 The Attorney General (1983) *House of Commons official report (Hansard),* May 10, col. 236.

39 *R v HS Dhingra* – Birmingham Crown Court Judgment 24 January 1991. *Daily Telegraph* (Jan 25).

40 *R (on the application of Smeaton) v Secretary of State for Health* [2002] 2 FLR 146.

41 Office for National Statistics (2009) *Contraception and Sexual Health, 2008/09,* ONS, London, p.11.

42 General Medical Council, Professional Conduct Committee hearing, 27–30 May 2002.

43 In England and Wales - *Re B (a minor) (wardship: sterilisation)* [1987] 2 All ER 206. Department for Constitutional Affairs (2007) *Mental Capacity Act 2005 Code of Practice,* The Stationery Office, London, paras 6.18, 8.18 and 8.2. The Office of the Official Solicitor (2006) *Practice note (official solicitor: declaratory proceedings: medical and welfare decisions for adults who lack capacity),* Office of the Official Solicitor, London. In Scotland, contraceptive sterilisation of people aged over 16 is regulated by the Adults with Incapacity (Scotland) Act (see Chapter 3) and Adults with Incapacity (Specified Medical Treatments) (Scotland) Regulations 2002. SSI 2002/275. At the time of writing mental health and capacity legislation was being developed in Northern Ireland. It is likely to include a provision on sterilisation.

44 *Re D (a minor)* [1976] 1 All ER 326.

45 *Re F (mental patient: sterilisation), sub nom F v West Berkshire Health Authority* [1989] 2 All ER. 545–66.

46 *Re F (mental patient: sterilisation), sub nom F v West Berkshire Health Authority* [1989] 2 All ER. 545–52.

47 *Re A (male sterilisation)* [2000] 1 FLR 549.

48 National Institute for Health and Clinical Excellence (2007) *Heavy menstrual bleeding,* NICE, London.

49 *Re S (sterilisation: patient's best interests), sub noms Re SL (adult patient: medical treatment), SL v SL* [2000] 1 FLR 465.

50 British Medical Association Annual Representatives Meeting, 1978.

51 Royal College of Psychiatrists (2008) *Position Statement on Women's Mental Health in Relation to Induced Abortion,* RcPsych, London.

52 Abortion Act 1967 (as amended), s1.

53 Abortion Act 1967 (as amended), s1(4).

54 Royal College of Obstetricians and Gynaecologists (2010) *Termination of pregnancy for fetal abnormality,* RCOG, London.

55 *Jepson v The Chief Constable of West Mercia* [2003] EWHC 3318.

56 Dyer C. (2005) Doctors who performed late abortion will not be prosecuted. *BMJ* **330,** 688.

57 Information Commissioner (2008) *Decision Notice FS50122432.* Available at: www.ico.gov.uk (accessed 4 March 2011).

58 The Information Tribunal (2009) *Information Tribunal Appeal Number EA/2008/0074, 15 October.* Available at: www.informationtribunal.gov.uk (accessed 3 March 2011).

59 Chief Medical Officer (2005) *An Investigation into the British Pregnancy Advisory Service (BPAS) Response to Requests for Late Abortions,* DH, London.

60 Department of Health (2010) *Abortion statistics. England and Wales, 2009. Statistical Bulletin 2010/11,* DH, London.

61 Information Services Division (2010) *Scottish Health Statistics,* ISD Scotland, Edinburgh.

62 Royal College of Obstetricians and Gynaecologists (2004) *The care of women requesting induced abortion,* RCOG Press, London, p.23. At the time of writing an updated version of this guidance was out for peer review. The final version was due to be published in autumn 2011.

63 Royal College of Obstetricians and Gynaecologists (2004) *The care of women requesting induced abortion,* RCOG Press, London, p.8.

64 Royal College of Obstetricians and Gynaecologists (2004) *Abortion care: what you need to know,* RCOG, London.

65 Armstrong N, Donaldson C. (2005) *The Economics of Sexual Health.* FPA, London.

66 Henshaw RC, Templeton AA. (1992) Mifepristone: separating fact from fiction. *Drugs* **44,** 531–6.

67 Henshaw RC, Templeton AA. (1992) Mifepristone: separating fact from fiction. *Drugs* **44,** 531–6.

68 Royal College of Obstetricians and Gynaecologists (2004) *The care of women requesting induced abortion,* RCOG Press, London.

69 Ingham R, Lee E. (2008) *Evaluation of Early Medical Abortion (EMA) Pilot Sites Final Report,* DH, London, p.8.

70 *BPAS v Secretary of State for Health* [2011] EWHC 235 (Admin), para 32.

71 *BPAS v Secretary of State for Health* [2011] EWHC 235 (Admin), para 12.

72 Royal College of Obstetricians and Gynaecologists (2011) *Multiple Pregnancy Following Assisted Reproduction,* RCOG, London.

73 Wimalasundera RC. (2006) Selective Reduction and Termination of Multiple Pregnancies. In: Kilby M, Baker K, Critchley H, Filed D. (eds.) *Multiple Pregnancies,* RCOG, London.

74 Garel M, Missonnier S, Blondel B. (2005) Psychological effects of multi-fetal pregnancy reduction. In: Blickstein I, Keith LG. (eds.) Multiple Pregnancy: epidemiology, gestation and perinatal outcome, 2nd edn, Taylor & Francis, Abingdon.

75 Lee RG, Morgan D. (2001) *Human fertilisation and embryology: Regulating the reproductive revolution.* Blackstone Press, London, pp.254–6.

76 Phillips C, Hadfield G. (1996) A mother wanted me to abort one of her healthy twins. It may sound unethical but it was either that or for both babies to die. *Sunday Express* (Aug 4), pp.12–13.

77 Habgood J. (1996) Moral implications of aborting a twin and of destroying human embryos [letter]. *The Times* (Aug 7), p.15.

78 Morgan D. (2001) *Issues in medical law and ethics,* Cavendish Publishing, London, pp.147–9.

79 *Janaway v Salford HA* [1988] 3 All ER 1079.

80 Bottomley V. (1991) *House of Commons official report (Hansard),* Dec 20, col. 355.

81 General Medical Council (2006) *Good Medical Practice,* GMC, London, para 8.

82 Royal College of Obstetricians and Gynaecologists (2004) *The care of women requesting induced abortion,* RCOG Press, London.

83 NHS Executive (1994) *Appointment of doctors to hospital posts: termination of pregnancy, HSG (94) 39,* DH, London.

84 Department of Health (2003) personal communication, Feb 19.

85 Scottish Executive Health Department (2004) *Advertisements and job descriptions of doctors to hospital posts: termination of pregnancy. NHS Circular: PCS(DD)2004/8,* SEHD, Edinburgh.

86 House of Commons Science and Technology Committee (2007) *Scientific Developments Relating to the Abortion Act 1967, Twelfth Report of Session 2006–07,* The Stationery Office, London.

87 House of Commons Science and Technology Committee (2007) *Formal minutes Monday 29 October 2007.* Available at: www.parliament.uk (accessed 7 March 2011).

88 In 2005 the BMA debated a motion calling for a reduction in the time limit for abortion at the BMA's Annual Representatives Meeting. The motion was rejected, leaving BMA policy as supportive of the current legislation in this matter. See briefing paper: British Medical Association (2005) *Abortion time limits,* BMA, London.

89 *R v Bourne* [1939] 1 KB 687.

90 Lee S. (1995) An A to K to Z of abortion law in Northern Ireland: abortion on remand. In: Furedi A. (ed). *The abortion law in Northern Ireland: human rights and reproductive choice.* Family Planning Association Northern Ireland, Belfast.

91 Grubb A. (1994) Abortion and children. Re K (a minor), Northern Health and Social Service Board v F and G (1993). *Med Law Rev* **2**, 371–4. Lee S. (1995) An A to K to Z of abortion law in Northern Ireland: abortion on remand. In: Furedi A (ed.) *The abortion law in Northern Ireland: human rights and reproductive choice,* Family Planning Association Northern Ireland, Belfast.

92 Grubb A. (1994) Treatment without consent (abortion): adult. Re A (Northern Health and Social Services Board v AMNH) (1994). *Med Law Rev* **2**, 374–5.

93 British Medical Association Annual Representatives Meeting, 1985.

94 Anon. (2003) Abortion clarity request denied. *BBC News Online* (Jul 7). Available at: www.bbc.co.uk/news (accessed 3 March 2011).

95 *Society for the Protection of Unborn Children v Department of Health, Social Services and Public Safety* [2009] NIQB 92.

96 *Society for the Protection of Unborn Children v Department of Health, Social Services and Public Safety* [2009] NIQB 92, para 48.

97 Anon. (2009) Anti-abortionists win court bid. *BBC News Online* (November 30). Available at: www.bbc.co.uk/news (accessed 3 March 2011).

98 *Re P (a minor)* [1986] 1 FLR 272. *Re B (wardship: abortion)* [1991] 2 FLR 426.

99 *Re P (a minor)* [1986] 1 FLR 272.

100 British Medical Association (2011) *The law and ethics of abortion: BMA views,* BMA, London.

101 *An NHS Trust and D (by her litigation friend The Official Solicitor)* [2003] EWHC 2793 (Fam).

102 *Paton v British Pregnancy Advisory Service Trustees* [1978] 2 All ER 987: 991.

103 *Paton v United Kingdom* (1981) 3 EHRR 408.

104 National Institute for Health and Clinical Excellence (2008) *Antenatal care: routine care for the healthy pregnant woman,* NICE, London.

105 Dickenson D. (1995) Carriers of genetic disorder and the right to have children. *Acta Genet Med Gemellol* **44**, 75–80.

106 Harris J. (1992) *Wonderwoman and superman,* Oxford University Press, Oxford, p.178.

107 Green JM. (1995) Obstetricians' views on prenatal diagnosis and termination of pregnancy: 1980 compared with 1993. *Br J Obstet Gynaecol* **102**, 228–32.

108 Wertz DC. (1992) Ethical and legal implications of the new genetics: issues for discussion. *Soc Sci Med* **35**, 495–505.

109 *Re F (in utero)* [1988] 2 All ER 193.

110 Congenital Disability (Civil Liability) Act 1976.

111 The Law Commission (1974) *Report on injuries to unborn children (Law Com No. 60),* HMSO, London, paras 54–64.

112 Mason JK, Laurie GT. (2011) *Mason & McCall Smith's Law and medical ethics*, 8th edn, Oxford University Press, Oxford, para 10.87.

113 Anon. (2004) Breath test move for mums-to-be. *BBC News Online* (May 6). Available at: www.bbc.co.uk/news (accessed 4 March 2011).

114 Royal College of Obstetricians and Gynaecologists (2010) *Management of HIV in pregnancy (Guideline No 39)*, RCOG, London. NHS Executive (1999) *Reducing mother to baby transmission of HIV (HSC 1999/183)*, DH, London. Scottish Executive Health Department (2002) *Offering HIV testing to women receiving antenatal care (NHS HDL (2002) 52)*, SEHD, Edinburgh. Department of Health, Social Services and Public Safety (2002) *Infection screening for pregnant women and reduction of mother to baby transmission (HSS (MD) 11/02)*, DHSSPS, Belfast.

115 Royal College of Obstetricians and Gynaecologists (2010) *Management of HIV in pregnancy (Guideline No 39)*, RCOG, London, p.3.

116 Peart NS, Campbell AV, Manara AR. *et al.* (2000) Maintaining a pregnancy following loss of capacity. *Med Law Rev* **8**, 275–99.

117 Anon. (1996) Mother who gave birth in coma dies. *Daily Telegraph* (December 5).

118 *Re MB (medical treatment)* [1997] 2 FLR 426.

119 McLean SAM. (1998) *Review of the common law provisions relating to the removal of gametes and of the consent provisions in the Human Fertilisation and Embryology Act 1990*, Department of Health, London, para 1.7.

120 Peart NS, Campbell AV, Manara AR. *et al.* (2000) Maintaining a pregnancy following loss of capacity. *Med Law Rev* **8**, 275–99, p.290.

121 Peart NS, Campbell AV, Manara AR. *et al.* (2000) Maintaining a pregnancy following loss of capacity. *Med Law Rev* **8**, 275–99, pp.292–3.

122 Jones DG. (2000) *Speaking for the dead*, Ashgate Dartmouth, Aldershot, pp.96–9. Purdy LM. (1990) Are pregnant women fetal containers? *Bioethics* **4**, 273–91.

123 Department of Health (1993) *Changing childbirth*, HMSO, London.

124 Department of Health (2007) *Maternity matters: choice, access and continuity of care in a safe service*, DH, London.

125 Royal College of Obstetricians and Gynaecologists (2007) *RCOG statement on unassisted childbirth or 'freebirth'*. Available at: www.rcog.org.uk (accessed 3 March 2011).

126 Royal College of Obstetricians and Gynaecologists, Royal College of Midwives (2007) *Joint statement no.2 April 2007. Home Births*, RCOG/RCM, London.

127 BMA General Practitioners Committee (2007) *National enhanced service: intrapartum care, 2 May 2003 (updated January 2007)*, BMA, London.

128 Department of Health (2001) *Milburn announces £100 million boost for maternity units; 2000 extra midwives by 2005*. Press release, May 2.

129 NHS Information Centre (2010) *NHS Maternity Statistics, England: 2009-2010*, NHS Information Centre, London. Information Services Division (2010) *Statistical Publication Notice 2010, Births in Scottish hospitals, financial year 2008/2009*. Available at: www.isdscotland.org (accessed 3 March 2011).

130 Bell JS, Campbell DM, Graham WJ. *et al.* (2001) Do obstetric complications explain high caesarean section rates among women over 30? A retrospective analysis. *BMJ* **322**, 894–5.

131 Castro A. (1999) Commentary: increase in caesarean sections may reflect medical control not women's choice. *BMJ* **319**, 1401–2.

132 Bewley S, Cockburn J. (2002) The unfacts of 'request' caesarean section. *Br J Obstet Gynaecol* **109**, 597–605.

133 Kingdon C, Neilson J, Singleton V. *et al.* (2009) Choice and birth method: mixed-method study of caesarean delivery for maternal request. *BJOG* **116**(7), 886–95.

134 National Collaborating Centre for Women's and Children's Health (2004) *Caesarean section*, RCOG, London. Available at: www.nice.org.uk (accessed 13 October 2011).

135 Bastian H. (1997) Health has become secondary to a sexually attractive body. *BMJ* **319**, 1402.

136 Statham H, Weaver J, Richards M. (2001) Why choose caesarean section? *Lancet* **357**, 635. Weaver J, Statham H, Richards M. (2001) High rates may be due to perceived potential for complications [letter]. *BMJ* **323**, 284.

137 Expert Advisory Group on Caesarean Section in Scotland (2001) *Report and recommendations to the chief medical officer of the Scottish Executive Health Department*, SEHD, Edinburgh.

138 Expert Advisory Group on Caesarean Section in Scotland (2001) *Report and recommendations to the chief medical officer of the Scottish Executive Health Department*, SEHD, Edinburgh, p.5.

139 Paterson-Brown S. (1998) Should doctors perform an elective caesarean section on request? Yes, as long as the woman is fully informed. *BMJ* **317**, 462.

140 Revill J. (2006) Why mothers should be offered caesareans. *The Observer* (Mar 5), p.14.

141 *St George's Healthcare NHS Trust v S, R v Collins and others, ex parte S* [1998] 3 All ER 673: 692.

142 *St George's Healthcare NHS Trust v S, R v Collins and others, ex parte S* [1998] 3 All ER 673: 693.

8: Assisted reproduction

The questions covered in this chapter include the following.

- What responsibility do those providing fertility treatment have towards the resulting children?
- Should there be limits on who can have access to fertility treatment?
- To what extent should parents be able to express preferences about the character-istics of their children?
- What is the role of health professionals in surrogacy arrangements?

New reproductive technologies, new dilemmas?

The inability to procreate is a common and distressing problem. Although statistics can be only an approximate guide, 1 in 10 couples is said to be infertile and 1 in 7 experience some difficulty in conceiving. Assisted reproduction gives some of these people the chance to have children when nature has failed them. Although initially viewed as an experimental procedure, *in vitro* fertilisation (IVF) is now a well-established, routine and an increasingly common method of treatment for those who experience infertility. Between 1992 and 2006, 122,043 babies were born following IVF treatment in the UK and IVF births now account for just over 1.5 per cent of all babies born in the UK each year.[1] Over the same period the success rate increased by 70 per cent for women up to 43 years of age. By 2008, the average live birth rate per treatment cycle started (all ages) had reached 24.1 per cent.[2]

Although developments in assisted reproduction represent one of the success stories of the late twentieth century, they nonetheless raise moral and social issues of profound importance. The creation and use of human embryos outside the body promotes complex debate about fundamental questions such as when life and 'personhood' begin and at what stage people (or hypothetical people) begin to matter morally. When donated gametes or surrogacy are used, our basic concepts of family relationships, personal identity and the definitions of 'mother' and 'father' are challenged. Reproductive technology enables women to have children long after their natural reproductive ability has ceased and to an extent frees women from the restrictions imposed by their biological clock, albeit that they may not be able to use their own gametes. Sadly, public expectations often still exceed what can be delivered, in terms of both the technical possibilities and the level of success achievable. Techniques that were originally developed to help people to overcome some pathology that meant they were unable to reproduce are increasingly being used to allow people greater choice in their reproductive decisions. For many, this continual pushing against the barriers is regarded as a very positive and exciting step, allowing women to take greater control over their bodies and reproduction, but others express fear and anxiety about where it may lead and about the need for society to set some moral barriers that it will not cross.

Medical Ethics Today: The BMA's Handbook of Ethics and Law, Third Edition. Sophie Brannan, Eleanor Chrispin, Martin Davies, Veronica English, Rebecca Mussell, Julian Sheather and Ann Sommerville.
© 2012 BMA Medical Ethics Department. Published 2012 by Blackwell Publishing Ltd.

General principles

When considering the types of dilemma that arise with assisted reproduction, the following general principles should be kept in mind.

- The human embryo has a 'special status' which means it should be afforded some respect but not absolute protection.
- Doctors who help to initiate a pregnancy have particular duties to address the welfare of any future child.
- All people are entitled to a fair and unprejudiced consideration of their request for treatment, so individual cases should be considered and blanket restrictions should not be applied to certain groups.
- The selection of embryos should not be used for trivial purposes or to meet the desire of individuals for particular physical characteristics in their offspring.

Regulation of assisted reproduction

Over recent decades there has been an almost constant barrage of news, information and debate about developments in assisted reproduction, resulting in the UK having one of the most comprehensive regulatory mechanisms in the world. The starting point for this period of public debate was the Warnock Committee, which reported in July 1984[3] and laid the foundations for the enactment of the Human Fertilisation and Embryology Act in 1990.

The Warnock Committee

A Committee of Inquiry was appointed in 1982 under the chairmanship of the philosopher Mary Warnock (now Baroness Warnock) to consider 'recent and potential developments in medicine and science related to human fertilisation and embryology; to consider what policies and safeguards should be applied, including consideration of the social, ethical and legal implications of these developments; and to make recommendations'.[4] The fact that the Warnock report is still referred to some 25 years on shows the way in which the report, and the wide ranging debate that stemmed from it, helped to shape public opinion on these matters. This is not to say that its recommendations were uncontroversial, but they represented the beginning of a long process of education and debate that helped to shape the current regulatory framework.

Regulated activities

The Human Fertilisation and Embryology Act 1990 put in place in the UK a statutory regulatory mechanism for assisted reproduction and embryo research, as recommended by the Warnock Committee. The Act established the Human Fertilisation and Embryology Authority (HFEA) and made it a criminal offence to undertake certain activities without a licence from the statutory body. The activities that were licensable were:

- the creation and use of human embryos in vitro for both treatment and research
- the storage of gametes and embryos
- the use of donated sperm, eggs or embryos.

From 2007, this list was extended, by Regulations[5] to implement the EU Tissues and Cells Directive,[6] to include the use of fresh sperm or eggs in treatment. The HFEA now regulates all processes for the 'donation, procurement, testing, preservation, storage and distribution' of gametes or embryos for treatment. This means that 'basic partner treatment services' such as GIFT (gamete intrafallopian transfer) and intrauterine insemination (IUI) using partner's sperm, surgical procedures to collect sperm and eggs for treatment and 'non-medical fertility services', such as those delivered by internet sperm providers, also require a licence from the HFEA. Hence, NHS and private obstetrics departments and GP practices that offer insemination services to their patients are required by law to be licensed.

Non-medical fertility services

In 2009 the scope of the HFEA's new powers was tested with a criminal prosecution against the directors of an online sperm donation business. The company, Fertility1st (formerly known as Spermdirect and First4Fertility), was providing fresh sperm from anonymous donors to women for self-insemination without a licence from the HFEA. The company held a database of donors which could be searched according to physical characteristics and then registered users could order a fresh sperm sample, which was collected from the donor by courier and delivered to the purchaser with a syringe for insemination.

The directors of the company, Nigel Woodforth and Ricky Gage, argued they did not require a licence because they were simply acting as indirect brokers, matching women to potential sperm donors, without any direct dealing with the sperm samples or insemination process. The key legal issue at stake was whether the service offered constituted 'procuring' gametes, defined in the Human Fertilisation and Embryology Act 1990 (as amended) as to 'make available'.

In September 2010, they were found guilty and were each given a suspended jail sentence, in addition to a £15,000 fine and being ordered to complete 200 hours of unpaid work. They were also banned from working in the fertility sector in the future.[7] This was the first criminal prosecution under the Act.

The legislation imposes several duties on those providing licensed treatments, such as an obligation to take account of the welfare of any child born or affected by the treatment, the duty to use gametes and embryos in accordance with the consent obtained and the requirement to offer counselling to people seeking certain licensed treatments (excluding GIFT or IUI with partner sperm). The Act also permits research to be undertaken using human embryos within certain limits (see Chapter 14, pages 616–620).

The Human Fertilisation and Embryology Act 2008

Following a long period of consultation and review, the Human Fertilisation and Embryology Act 2008 received Royal Assent in November 2008 and the bulk of its provisions came into force on 1 October 2009. Much of the 2008 Act amended, and was therefore incorporated into, the 1990 Act and the Surrogacy Arrangements Act 1985. The remainder of the 2008 Act made new provisions for parenthood in cases of assisted reproductive technology, and stands alone as a new piece of legislation. The review of the law provided the opportunity to update the legislation on assisted reproduction to take account of scientific and medical developments, and changes in societal attitudes, since 1990. It also allowed Parliament to endorse and formalise the approach taken by the HFEA on major issues that had arisen since the 1990 Act was passed, such as the use of preimplantation genetic diagnosis for tissue typing (see pages 342–345) and to address emerging issues such as the use of human admixed embryos for research (see Chapter 14, pages 619–620).

Role of the Human Fertilisation and Embryology Authority

It is unlawful for a clinic or establishment to provide regulated activities (see above) without a licence from the statutory regulatory body, the HFEA. The HFEA is legally required to issue a Code of Practice that gives detailed guidance to clinics about their responsibilities under the legislation and the requirements of the Authority.[8] Every clinic is inspected at least every 2 years by a team of inspectors from the HFEA to assess the protocols, facilities and staffing, and to ensure compliance with the Act and the Code of Practice. The HFEA is also required to maintain a confidential register of information containing details of every cycle of IVF and donor insemination (DI) carried out in the UK, and of all donors and all children born as a result of licensed treatment.

One of the responsibilities of the HFEA is to provide information to the public about the services available. It does this primarily through its website which has a section written specifically for potential patients, including advice on choosing a clinic, information about IVF and donor treatment and an online 'choose a fertility clinic' search function. It also publishes individual centres' success rates annually, with comparisons to the national average, and clinic inspection reports.

Future of the HFEA

At the time of writing, the future of the HFEA was uncertain. In July 2010, as part of a Government-wide initiative, the Department of Health published a review of its arm's-length bodies.[9] This included proposals to abolish the HFEA by 2015, with its functions being divided between the Care Quality Commission, a new research regulator and the Health and Social Care Information Centre. Up-to-date information can be found on the website of the British Medical Association (BMA).

Monitoring the outcome of fertility treatment

Another role of the HFEA is to monitor the outcome of fertility treatments, provide advice and information and, where possible, take steps to reduce avoidable risk to women seeking treatment and any child born. An unintended, and generally unwelcome, effect of the more frequent use of assisted reproduction has been a large increase in the number of multiple births, including in some cases high order multiple births, which have serious consequences for both the individual families and NHS services. In 1996, 28 per cent of IVF cycles resulted in multiple births. The rate had reduced to 23 per cent by 2006 but was still considered by many, including the BMA, to be too high.[10] Major efforts have been made to overcome this problem, most notably by reducing the number of embryos that may be replaced in a single cycle of IVF. This policy has always been unpopular among some clinics and was unsuccessfully challenged in the courts.[11] In 2004, the HFEA amended its Code of Practice to permit a maximum of two embryos to be transferred in women under 40, and a maximum of three in women aged 40 or over. This policy halved the number of triplet pregnancies but had no effect on twin births.

In 2005, the HFEA set up an expert group to review the available data and to consider whether the HFEA's policy on embryo transfer needed to be reviewed. The group produced a report in October 2006.[12] The report concluded that the risks of multiple pregnancies were unacceptably high and that maintaining the status quo was not an option; the HFEA must take steps to address this by issuing guidance to centres to increase the number of single embryo transfers. Although twins occur as a result of natural conception, and are often seen by patients as a positive outcome of fertility treatment, particularly in view of the lack of NHS funding for IVF treatment, the expert group was clear about the risks:

> [c]ompared with singletons, twins are four times more likely to die in pregnancy, seven times more likely to die shortly after birth, ten times more likely to be admitted to a neonatal special care unit, and have six times the risk of cerebral palsy. Maternal morbidity and mortality is also increased due to late miscarriage, high blood pressure, pre-eclampsia, and haemorrhage amongst others.[13]

One of the suggestions for change was that for selected patients the maximum number of embryos to be transferred should be reduced to one. When the BMA's Medical Ethics Committee (MEC) considered this issue it discussed both the evidence of risk and the importance of autonomy. It believed that there needed to be clear evidence of a serious risk of harm in order to justify overriding a woman's informed choice to replace more than one embryo at a time. On balance, the Committee concluded that, although steps needed to be taken to reduce the number of twin births, the risks associated with twins were not sufficiently high to justify using the Authority's regulatory power to impose this on clinics and patients. Rather, it was felt that some basic steps should be taken to facilitate change short of using regulatory force. This should include providing patients and practitioners with more detailed information about the risks, encouraging research into the long-term health outcomes for IVF twins and encouraging good practice in the use of selective embryo transfer in good prognosis patients. Some clinics, for example, have reported very high success rates with single blastocyst transfer in selected patients.[14] Similar results were found in a review of randomised trials comparing the clinical effectiveness of elective single and double cleavage stage embryos. This found that, once frozen single embryo transfer cycles were taken into account, the birth rates of the two groups were similar and the multiple birth rate in the single embryo groups were comparable with that observed in spontaneous pregnancies.[15] In 2008, the HFEA issued Directions[16] requiring all licensed clinics to develop a written multiple births minimisation strategy by 31 January 2009. This strategy was to set criteria for identifying women most at risk of a multiple pregnancy, and therefore suitable for elective single embryo transfer, and to set out how the centre planned to reduce its multiple birth rate to no more than 24 per cent of the centre's live birth rate initially. A review of practice during the first year can be found on the HFEA's website.[17] The HFEA set a series of targets aiming to reduce multiple births to 10 per cent within 3 years. For the year beginning April 2011 the target was set at 15 per cent.[18]

Another area that is closely monitored by the HFEA is research into any possible health risks to children born following fertility treatment or to women undergoing IVF or related procedures.[19] In 2002, the HFEA set up a joint working group with the Medical Research Council to assess the existing knowledge about health risks and to suggest areas for future research. One of the issues highlighted in the subsequent report[20] was the difficulty of undertaking research due to the very strict confidentiality rules in the 1990 Act. The HFEA has been required, since 1991, to maintain a register of information with details of every treatment cycle of IVF and donor conception undertaken in the UK. This register contains a wealth of data which have not been accessible to researchers. Due to the terms of the Act, neither could links be made with other databases, such as the cancer registry, which could help to answer important research questions. This issue was addressed in the Human Fertilisation and Embryology Act 2008 which allowed for Regulations to be made to allow the HFEA to give limited access to identifiable data from the register to bona fide researchers where it was not possible to obtain consent.[21] One of the first projects to be approved was a proposal to compare cancer rates of women who have taken fertility drugs with those that have not.[22] The HFEA also amended its standard consent forms, from October 2009, to allow those having IVF treatment to consent to identifiable information being provided to researchers. By August 2010, however, only 37 per cent of patients had consented to their information being used for research.[23]

What, if any duties, are owed to 'hypothetical' people?

In most circumstances doctors' duties are primarily focused on the patient before them, but in assisted reproduction there is another party to be considered, that is, the child to be born as a result of medical intervention. What, if any, ethical obligations are owed to the unborn child has been the subject of ongoing debate. The BMA's general view is that the fetus deserves respect but does not have absolute claims that can override those of an autonomous person, usually the woman – the mother-to-be (see Chapter 7, pages 268–270). In the case of any form of assisted reproduction, however, the 'person' to whom a duty is owed is not only unborn, but also not yet conceived. Furthermore, at the time of deciding whether to offer treatment, there is no way of telling whether an actual child will come into existence because this will depend on whether or not the treatment, if provided, is successful. There has been considerable debate about whether duties can be owed to a 'hypothetical person' and whether a child could be harmed by being brought into existence or whether existence itself could be considered a 'harm' in some cases. Another way of looking at this issue is whether those professionals who are assisting someone to have a child have any moral responsibilities towards any child who might be born as a result of the treatment. If a health professional had serious concerns about the circumstances a child would or might be born into, and had strong grounds to believe that any child would be at serious risk of abuse or neglect, should he or she provide treatment? Whereas many individuals experiencing pain, abuse, neglect or other substantial disadvantages are nevertheless glad to have been born, most people would consider it wrong for health professionals to assist in the generation of a pregnancy knowing that the future child would, or was very likely to, be harmed.

In the BMA's view, as well as in the view of the law (see pages 319–323), doctors who are asked to intervene to help to establish a pregnancy have particular duties to consider the welfare of any resultant children.

Access to treatment

Is there a right to assistance to reproduce?

As people are able to exercise more choice over their reproductive decisions and are less governed by biological constraints, so some have increasingly perceived control over reproduction as a 'right'. This tendency to focus on reproductive rights gained added impetus when the Human Rights Act 1998 came into force in 2000, with appeals not only to natural and moral rights but also to enforceable legal rights. It is not surprising, therefore, that one of the first cases to be considered as a challenge under the Human Rights Act was a claim relating to Article 12 of the European Convention on Human Rights (the right to marry and found a family). The case of Gavin Mellor, however, gave an early and clear statement that the Human Rights Act does not give all UK citizens a right to assistance to conceive.

The right to found a family

Gavin Mellor was serving a life sentence for murder when he met and married his wife. In 1997, he applied for permission to be allowed to inseminate his wife artificially, arguing that Article 12 of the European Convention gave him the right to found a family. The Secretary of State refused the request on the grounds that artificial insemination was not needed for medical reasons but was sought in order to circumvent the normal consequences of imprisonment. Furthermore, the Home Secretary argued that there were serious concerns about the stability of the relationship, which had not been tested under normal circumstances.

Mr Justice Forbes held that the Secretary of State's decision did not contravene Mr Mellor's Article 12 rights. It had been clearly established that the Article 12 right to found a family did not mean that a person must be given, at all times, the actual possibility of procreating his descendants. In reality, what Mr Mellor was seeking was to be granted the privilege or benefit of being afforded access to artificial insemination services because an inevitable consequence of his lawful detention in custody was that it was impossible for his wife to conceive a child by natural means. The Secretary of State was therefore entitled to formulate a policy for dealing with such requests by prisoners and to decide whether the privilege should be made available in a particular case. The application was dismissed. In upholding this decision, at the Court of Appeal, Lord Philips emphasised that it will not always be justifiable to prevent a prisoner from inseminating his wife. In this case, however, there were no exceptional circumstances, for example to demonstrate that a refusal would not merely delay the founding of a family but would prevent it altogether.[24]

The 'exceptional circumstances' referred to by Lord Philips in the Mellor case (see above) were present in a subsequent case which had a different outcome. Kirk and Lorraine Dickson had also been refused permission to use artificial insemination while Mr Dickson was serving a life sentence for murder. They applied to the European Court of Human Rights on the grounds that the Secretary of State's decision breached their Article 8 (right to private and family life) and/or Article 12 rights. The Court unanimously rejected the application but the couple was given permission to appeal to the Grand Chamber. In December 2007, the Grand Chamber held by 12 votes to five that there had been a violation of Article 8 of the Convention because insufficient account had been taken of the fact that, due to the woman's age (43 when the application was made in 2001) and the term of imprisonment, this represented their only chance to have their own child.[25] The Grand Chamber concluded that the existing policy did not strike a fair balance between the public and private rights involved and placed the 'exceptionality' burden too high.

It has been suggested that the lack of NHS provision of fertility treatment, and its sporadic provision around the country, leading to 'postcode rationing', was also an area that could be challenged under the Human Rights Act. Article 14 (which is not a freestanding right) gives a right not to be discriminated against in the enjoyment of a substantive right under the Convention. Thus, it has been argued that the inconsistent funding of fertility treatment by the NHS discriminates against people (on grounds of their place of residence and ability to pay) in their enjoyment of their Article 12 right (the right to found a family).[26] Given the clear statement from the Court in the Mellor case, however, that the right to found a family is not an absolute one, the success of any such claim may be in doubt.

The Human Rights Act has been used successfully by lesbian couples to challenge a refusal to provide NHS-funded IVF treatment on grounds of their sexual orientation. In one case a Scottish Health Board argued that treatment had been refused because the couple did not meet the definition of an 'infertile couple' (with infertility defined as failure to conceive after 2 years of unprotected intercourse) not because of their sexual orientation.[27] After an initial hearing before the Court of Session, however, the Health Board reversed its decision and agreed to offer treatment.[28] A similar case arose in England in 2009 where a Primary Care Trust (PCT) initially refused to provide funding for IVF treatment to a lesbian couple but reversed the decision after a threat of legal action.[29] In both of these cases it was also argued that the refusal to provide treatment, based on their sexual orientation, breached equality legislation. The Equality and Human Rights Commission uses the example of a couple being refused fertility treatment because they are lesbians as one example of direct discrimination on grounds of sexual orientation.[30] This applies equally to private providers of treatment as to the NHS.

NHS funding

For many years there has been debate about whether involuntary childlessness is a medical issue deserving of a publicly funded medical remedy. Although the Warnock Committee concluded that it was, others disagreed, arguing that those affected by infertility are not 'ill' and most infertile people lead normal, healthy lives. Although it is recognised that considerable psychological morbidity and depression stems from involuntary childlessness, it is often seen as a social rather than a medical problem and of lower priority than other forms of treatment. This argument is sometimes put forward to justify the limited amount of NHS funding for fertility treatment.

In 2004, the National Institute for Health and Clinical Excellence (NICE) published a fertility clinical guideline.[31] Among its recommendations was that the NHS should offer three cycles of stimulated IVF to couples in which the woman is aged between 23 and 39 years who have an identified cause of their fertility problems or unexplained infertility of at least 3 years. NICE guidelines apply to England, Wales and Northern Ireland. Although NICE clinical guidelines have never been binding on commissioning bodies in the way that technology appraisals have been (see pages 552–553), the previous Labour Government stated, on many occasions, its commitment to funding IVF treatment and encouraged full implementation of the NICE guidelines. This commitment was repeated in February 2011 by the new Public Health Minister.[32] Implementation of this guidance has, however, been inconsistent and the provision of IVF treatment within the NHS remains subject to significant variation around the country. In 2008, the Department of Health established an Expert Group on Commissioning NHS Infertility Provision to identify barriers to implementation of the NICE guidelines in England, and in June 2009 this group published a commissioning aid setting out best practice for commissioners.[33] The paper also reported on a Department of Health survey of PCT provision in England, carried out in 2008, which showed clear improvements in the availability of IVF treatment. It found that two PCTs were temporarily not funding IVF, 30 per cent were providing three cycles of IVF, 23 per cent two cycles, 25 per cent one full cycle (including subsequent frozen embryo replacements) and 22 per cent one fresh cycle (stimulated cycle only).[34]

At the time of writing NICE was in the process of revising its guidance but was not expecting to publish before 2012.[35]

TheExpert Advisory Group on Infertility Services in Scotland (EAGISS) published its first report in 2000. Some amendments were made to the recommendations following a review of infertility funding in 2007 by the Scottish Executive.[36] Following this review NHS-funded IVF treatment should be made available to anyone who meets *all* of the following criteria:

- individuals with infertility of diagnosed cause (of any duration), for which assisted conception represents effective treatment or individuals with unexplained infertility of at least 3 years' duration
- female partner is aged less than 40 years at the time of treatment
- individuals that have not previously undergone a sterilisation procedure
- individuals who have no child living with them in their home
- individuals who have had less than three previous embryo transfers, funded from any source.

For those who meet the criteria, up to three NHS-funded cycles should be provided, including a minimum of two transfers of fresh embryos. As with the rest of the UK, however, implementation of the guidance has been variable.

In both Wales and Northern Ireland, eligibility criteria for funding for IVF treatment are set centrally. At the time of writing, in Wales those fulfilling the access criteria are able to access two cycles of IVF,[37] whereas in Northern Ireland patients are only able to access one.[38]

Welfare of the child

Decisions about access to fertility treatment may also be made on social grounds. Clinics offering licensable treatments are required, by law, to take account of 'the welfare of any child who may be born as a result of the treatment . . . and of any other child who may be affected by the birth'.[39] Although some see this as discriminatory against infertile people, because society does not generally attempt to prevent 'unsuitable' people from conceiving naturally,[40] others consider that by intervening with treatment to help people to have children doctors become party to the creation of a child and therefore have special responsibilities to ensure that these children will not be significantly disadvantaged. As discussed above (see page 316), the BMA supports this latter view.

The question of eligibility for treatment is a difficult one that demands social judgements that go beyond the purely medical and require multi-disciplinary and non-clinical assessments. However, if it is known that a couple's existing children have been physically and psychologically abused and taken into care, and it is considered very likely that future children might also be abused, it would, in the BMA's view, be inappropriate to help that couple to have more children. The situation is rarely so straightforward. If an individual has a history of violence, but has not offended for many years or has a history of alcoholism or of mild psychiatric problems, for example, should treatment be refused? What about those who have an unusual lifestyle or whose existing children 'look unkempt'? There is clearly a risk that individual opinions and prejudices about appropriate and inappropriate lifestyles and family makeup could unfairly influence judgement. Although health professionals must take account of the welfare of the resulting child before offering fertility treatment, such assessments must be carried out fairly and avoid prejudice.

The threshold for concern

In most cases of people seeking assisted reproduction, there are no grounds for concern about the welfare of any resulting child. The BMA has always taken the view that the assessments that take place should seek to identify those few cases in which a future child is at foreseeable risk of serious harm, rather than trying to assess, in advance, the likely quality of parenting. In the past, guidance from the HFEA required all clinics to make routine enquiries to patients' GPs and the list of factors to take into account included many subjective social enquiries, such as the stability of the relationship and the commitment to having children.[41] Many GPs were, understandably, concerned about being asked to answer such questions which required them to speculate about issues that were outside their knowledge and area of expertise.

The HFEA undertook a major review of its guidance on welfare of the child in 2005 and issued new guidance, now incorporated into the eighth *Code of Practice*, which makes clear that in assessing patients, clinics are seeking to identify those where there is a risk of 'significant harm or neglect'.[42] The *Code of Practice* advises that the following factors should be considered:

'(a) past or current circumstances that may lead to any child [mentioned above] experiencing serious physical or psychological harm or neglect, for example:
  (i) previous convictions relating to harming children
  (ii) child protection measures taken regarding existing children, or
  (iii) violence or serious discord in the family environment
(b) past or current circumstances that are likely to lead to an inability to care throughout childhood for any child who may be born, or that are already seriously impairing the care of any existing child of the family, for example:
  (i) mental or physical conditions
  (ii) drug or alcohol abuse
  (iii) medical history, where the medical history indicates that any child who may be born is likely to suffer from a serious medical condition, or
  (iv) circumstances that the centre considers likely to cause serious harm to any child [mentioned above].'[43]

The need for 'supportive parenting'

The 1990 Act required that, as part of the welfare of the child assessment, clinics should take account of 'the need of [that] child for a father'.[44] Although the HFEA never interpreted this statement as preventing single women or lesbian couples from having treatment, concerns had been expressed for some time that this provision could be used to justify discriminating against such patients and was open to challenge under both the Human Rights Act and equality legislation. The previous Labour Government made clear, early in the consultation process, its intention to remove this provision from the legislation. Although many organisations, including the BMA, supported this move the decision proved controversial and, as a compromise, the Government tabled an amendment at Report Stage of the Human Fertilisation and Embryology Bill 2008 in the House of Lords to replace the 'need for a father' with the 'need for supportive parenting'. In its briefing to Parliamentarians, the BMA expressed continuing concern about this amendment, which appeared to move away from the more objective 'foreseeable risk of serious harm' approach and towards a more subjective assessment that would result in prospective parents being subjected to intrusive questioning about their lives.[45] The amendment was, nevertheless, successful and is incorporated into the legislation.

The HFEA has provided the following definition of supportive parenting which centres should consider as part of the welfare of the child assessment:

> Supportive parenting is a commitment to the health, well being and development of the child. It is presumed that all prospective parents will be supportive parents, in the absence of any reasonable cause of concern that any child who may be born, or any other child, may be at risk of significant harm or neglect. Where centres have concern as to whether this commitment exists, they may wish to take account of the wider family and social network within which the child will be raised.[46]

The presumption that those seeking treatment are 'supportive parents' unless there is reason to believe otherwise goes a long way to address the BMA's concerns.

Individual assessments

Although assisted reproduction was originally developed to help heterosexual couples experiencing infertility, it also allows people to have children outside biological constraints. By using donated gametes, women who are past their normal reproductive age can have children and single women and members of lesbian couples can reproduce without the need for a male partner. The increasing use of assisted reproduction in these types of cases reflects growing societal acceptance of a broad range of family relationships, including single parenthood, and some more formal recognition of homosexual relationships.[47]

The Human Fertilisation and Embryology Act does not exclude any category of patient from treatment but focuses on the clinic's assessment of the prospective patient's ability to meet the needs of a child. All individuals are entitled to a fair and unprejudiced assessment of their circumstances. The BMA has consistently rejected the idea of applying inflexible rules on access to fertility treatment, believing instead that each application should be considered on its merits. Although aspects such as age may be one of a number of relevant factors to take into account, assessments should be made on the individual circumstances in each case rather than according to blanket restrictions applied to certain categories of people. Applying blanket restrictions on access to treatment is also likely to be unlawful.

Postmenopausal women

The use of donor oocytes was originally used as a treatment to help those of normal reproductive age who had a premature menopause. However, reports have focused on a small number of cases of this treatment being provided for women in their mid to late fifties. There have also been a small number of reports of women having children in their sixties and, in one case, at the age of 70.[48] Although at least some of these women were British, none of the women were reported to have had treatment in the UK. The HFEA has resisted calls to set an upper age limit for treatment, arguing that clinics have a responsibility to consider every case on its individual merits. However, it is able to monitor the use of oocyte donation for older women, through its information register (see page 314), and could require clinics to justify the decision to proceed in individual cases. The BMA supports this approach believing that, although age may be one relevant factor to consider, it is the ability of the parents to provide a safe and supportive environment to a child throughout his or her childhood that is the most relevant factor. Between 2004 and 2009, 121 women over 50 years of age received treatment with donor eggs in the UK.[49]

Non-traditional families

A small proportion of people seeking treatment with donor sperm are single women who would like to start a family but who have not found a suitable partner with whom to have a child. These women are often called 'solo mothers' (as opposed to 'single mothers') in order to distinguish them from those women who are caring for children alone as a result of the breakdown of their relationship.

While there is good evidence that children raised by single mothers are more likely to be disadvantaged, this does not appear to be the case for the children of solo mothers.[50] Solo mothers have carefully considered their options and have chosen to have a child in this way. They have not suffered a relationship breakdown and tend to be in a better financial position than single mothers. They tend to have good networks of support and early research shows that their children compare well, emotionally and psychologically, with children born by donor insemination to two heterosexual parents.[51] Such studies have, however, only taken place while the children are very young and so it is too early to tell whether the absence of a father has any detrimental effect in adolescence.

Some of those seeking treatment with donor sperm are in lesbian relationships. A substantial amount of research has been carried out on the parenting skills of lesbian couples. Initially, research focused on women who had started a family in a heterosexual relationship but continued to raise their children in a lesbian relationship. More recently, research has concentrated on lesbian couples who have a child through donor insemination at a licensed fertility clinic.

Social research on children born to these families has reported similar findings to those children born to solo mothers. Their emotional and psychological development is comparable with children born of donor insemination to two heterosexual parents. In fact, the second female parent often has greater parent-child interaction than do the fathers in the heterosexual couples.[52]

Although lesbian couples were able to have treatment together at licensed clinics, until recently they were unable to both be registered as legal parents of any resulting child from birth. This changed in April 2009 when the parenthood provisions of the Human Fertilisation and Embryology Act 2008 came into force, allowing both women to be named as parents on the birth certificate – the woman who carried the child being recorded as the mother and the female partner registered as the second parent. In fact, the legislation goes further and permits anyone to be the second legal parent, provided the mother and second parent are not in a prohibited relationship and both adults consent.[53]

Enquiries to GPs

Clinics are no longer required to make routine enquiries to GPs (see page 320) but are advised to seek consent from their patients to contact other individuals or agencies (which could include the patients' GP) where:

'(a) information provided by the patient (and their partner if they have one) suggests a risk of significant harm or neglect to any child

(b) the patient (and their partner if they have one) has failed to provide any of the information requested

(c) the information the patient (and their partner if they have one) has provided is inconsistent, or

(d) there is evidence of deception.'[54]

In the past, some GPs expressed concern about responding to such enquiries, believing they were being asked to decide whether their patients should be given treatment. In fact, the responsibility for making these decisions rests very clearly with the clinic offering treatment. The GP's role is limited to providing factual information that may be important for the clinic to take into account in reaching its decision. If a clinic requests information that appears to be asking the doctor to speculate or to go beyond the information available to him or her, the question should not be answered and the reason for this should be passed on to the clinic.

As in other cases, GPs should ensure that they have their patient's written consent before providing information to a third party. The clinic requesting information should enclose a copy of the patient's signed consent with any request for information and, if this is not enclosed, the information should not be provided without checking with the patient directly or asking the clinic to forward a copy of the consent form. Some GPs are concerned about their continuing relationship with the patient if they disclose information that may harm the patient's chances of being accepted for treatment. Clearly, the doctor must not knowingly provide false information or withhold relevant information at the patient's request. When sensitive information is to be disclosed, it is important that this is discussed with the patient. If the patient subsequently withdraws consent to the release of the information, this fact should be relayed to the clinic concerned. A failure to give consent or the subsequent withdrawal of consent to the provision of information is likely to raise concern in the clinic. The HFEA's *Code of Practice* advises that failure to give consent for disclosure should 'not, in itself, be grounds for denying treatment but the centre should take this into account in deciding whether to provide treatment. The centre should discuss with the patient (and their partner if they have one) the reason for refusing to provide consent.'[55]

Review of difficult cases

Although in many cases the decision to provide treatment may be straightforward, there are others where the issues are complex or controversial and additional advice is needed. Despite having some initial reservations about the use of clinical ethics committees, since 2000 the HFEA has positively encouraged clinics to establish such committees and to seek their advice whenever necessary.[56] In its eighth code of practice, for example, the HFEA highlights some types of cases where the advice of a clinical ethics committee should normally be sought.[57] The BMA supports the use of clinical ethics committees and would encourage all clinics to have access to such independent scrutiny of difficult cases. The role of such committees is to provide a forum for debate and discussion about complex or controversial cases. Such committees will often provide advice but their role is not to take over responsibility for the decision; this responsibility remains with the clinic.

Summary – access to treatment

- Doctors who help people to conceive have legal and ethical duties to take account of the welfare of the child that may be born as a result of the treatment.
- Assessments should be carried out fairly and avoid prejudice. They should seek to identify those cases where there is a foreseeable risk of serious harm.
- Assessments should be made on the individual factors in each case rather than according to blanket restrictions applied to certain categories of people.

- GPs who are asked to provide information to a fertility clinic should do so only with their patients' consent. They should not speculate, but provide only factual information.

Consent to the storage and use of gametes and embryos

The Human Fertilisation and Embryology Act requires that consent for the storage or use of gametes or embryos must be in writing and that, before giving consent, the person must have been given information and the opportunity to receive counselling. (The exception to this rule is the use of gametes in basic partner treatment services such as IUI.) Consent to storage of gametes or embryos must specify the maximum period of storage (if less than the statutory limit which, from October 2009, is 10 years for both gametes and embryos) and what should be done with the gametes or embryos if the person who gave the consent dies or is unable, because of incapacity, to vary or withdraw the terms of the consent. Consent to the use of gametes or embryos must specify whether they may be used for treatment with a specified person, for the treatment of others or for use in licensed research. Individuals may withdraw or vary their consent at any time up to the point at which the gametes or embryos are used in treatment or research. If certain criteria are met individuals may apply for an extension of the statutory storage period, permitting storage for up to a maximum of 55 years.[58]

Storage and use of gametes without effective consent

The consent provisions of the legislation were tested in 1997 in the highly publicised case of Diane Blood (see below).

Posthumous use of gametes

In 1995 Mr Blood contracted meningitis and died. Prior to her husband's death, Mrs Blood asked the doctors to remove sperm samples from him; two samples were taken and stored. Mrs Blood's subsequent request to use the samples in treatment was denied on the grounds that her husband had not given written consent, or received information or the opportunity for counselling, as required by the Human Fertilisation and Embryology Act, and therefore the stored sample could not lawfully be used. In her evidence, Mrs Blood claimed that she and her husband had a genuine commitment to having a family together and that they had even discussed what should happen if he should die before conception occurred.

The HFEA's refusal to permit either the use of the sperm in the UK or its export to another European country for treatment was challenged by Mrs Blood. The Appeal Court held that the HFEA was correct that the sample could not lawfully be used in the UK. In considering its decision on export, however, the Court held that the HFEA had taken insufficient account of Mrs Blood's right, under European law, to seek treatment in another country. The matter was referred back to the HFEA, which subsequently withdrew its objection, leaving Mrs Blood free to seek treatment in another country. She has since had two children after treatment with the exported sample.[59]

This case led to considerable debate in the media, the medical profession and amongst the public. There was tremendous support and sympathy for Mrs Blood and many people argued vociferously for her right to fulfil her husband's previously expressed wish to have a child. Others, including the BMA, although understanding Mrs Blood's desire to have her late husband's child, were concerned about the broader implications of subjecting adults who lack capacity to medical procedures from which they would not benefit personally, but which were essentially for the benefit of a third party. It is interesting that both those who argued for and against her right to use the gametes used 'best interests' arguments to support their case. In a subsequent review of the law on consent,[60] it was clarified that, legally, the best interests test required evidence that the intended intervention was for the direct benefit of the individual concerned and that no attention could be paid to possible benefits for third parties. The review also confirmed that the taking, storage and use of sperm in this type of situation was unlawful under UK law.

It had been expected that, once the law had been clarified, there would be no further cases of this type appearing before the courts. In 2008, however, a similar case was heard in the High Court.[61] The case involved L, whose husband H died unexpectedly in hospital following an appendectomy. L made an emergency application to the Court for an order authorising the removal of sperm from her husband within 24 hours of his death and the subsequent storage of the sperm. The judge was, erroneously, informed that the legal position regarding storage of sperm after death without consent, had been changed by the Human Tissue Act 2004 (see Chapter 12, pages 522–524) and, on that basis, authorised the removal and storage of sperm. The High Court subsequently confirmed that it has no power to authorise storage where the deceased had not given the consent required by the HFE Act and that the storage of H's sperm was therefore unlawful. The Court also confirmed that the sperm could not be used for treatment in the UK. A preliminary view was expressed that the HFEA has the power to authorise storage of sperm pending its consideration of an application for export of the sperm, although the HFEA has said it disagrees with this view.[62] In this case, however, the HFEA agreed not to take regulatory action against the clinic storing the sperm while the HFEA considered L's application for a direction authorising the export of the sperm to another country for treatment. The BMA has been unable to determine the outcome in this case.[63]

The Human Fertilisation and Embryology Act 2008 modified the consent provisions of the 1990 Act in relation to storage but only in relation to people who are expected to regain capacity. The new provisions permit the storage of sperm, without consent, where gametes are removed from a child or adult lacking capacity who is expected to regain capacity but to be left infertile. If the individual dies the gametes must be destroyed; subsequent use of the gametes requires the individual's written consent. The removal of gametes from those who lack capacity is authorised under the common law on the basis that it would be in the patient's best interests to preserve the option of having children in the future. These amendments would not apply to the cases of L or Diane Blood, where the men were already dead or, were alive when gametes were taken, but were not expected to recover.

Since the Diane Blood case the law has also been amended to permit women who conceive after the death of their partners to have the deceased partner's name included on the birth certificate. The successful passage of the Human Fertilisation and Embryology (Deceased Fathers) Act 2003 followed a declaration from the High Court that section 28(6) of the Human Fertilisation and Embryology Act was incompatible with the Human Rights Act.[64] (The 2003 Act was repealed in 2008 and its provisions incorporated into the 1990 Act (as amended).) Although the provisions allow the father's name to be entered onto the birth certificate, he is not the child's legal father for other purposes such as inheritance.

Storage and use following withdrawal of consent

During 2002, another attempt was made to use the courts to overcome a lack of the valid consent required by the Human Fertilisation and Embryology Act.

Storage and use of embryos following withdrawal of consent

In October 2001, Natallie Evans was diagnosed with precancerous tumours in both ovaries and was informed that she would need to undergo surgery to have her ovaries removed. Before the surgery she and her fiancé, Howard Johnston, received information and counselling and decided to have IVF in order to store embryos for future use. They each consented to the creation, storage and use of embryos using their gametes. Six months later the couple split up and Mr Johnston wrote to the clinic to withdraw his consent and asking for the embryos to be destroyed. The clinic notified Ms Evans that, as it did not have the consent of both parties to continue to store the embryos, it must destroy them. She applied to the High Court for an injunction to prevent the destruction arguing that Mr Johnston should not be permitted to withdraw his consent. The injunction was granted and the embryos were to remain in storage until the case was settled. Natallie Evans asked the courts to rule that she could use the embryos, while Howard Johnston argued that they should be destroyed.

Ms Evans lost her case in the English courts[65] and at the European Court of Human Rights.[66] It was held that there was an interference with Ms Evans' right to private life (Article 8) but this was proportionate and necessary in order to protect the rights of Mr Johnston as permitted under Article 8(2). It was also held that Schedule 3 of the HFE Act does not give a 'male veto' but gives each party an equal right to respect for their private lives and so there was no breach of Article 14. At the European Court of Human Rights, however, the decision was not unanimous. Two of the five judges took the view that the Act should allow exceptions, such that the individual circumstances could be considered, where the application of a rigid rule could lead to irreparable harm or to the destruction of the essence of one party's rights. Ms Evans appealed to the Grand Chamber of the European Court of Human Rights, the final arbiter, but her case was lost.[67] The embryos were subsequently destroyed.

Although the 1990 Act was clear that there must be valid consent for storage and use of gametes and embryos, Natallie Evans argued that the consent requirements, which essentially gave one party a veto over the use of stored embryos, were inconsistent with Articles 8 and 12 of the Human Rights Act. She also used the analogy that if she had become pregnant naturally, and the embryos were in her body, then her partner would have no say at all over the future of the pregnancy. However, there are clear differences between an embryo that is implanted, and is therefore inextricably linked to the pregnant woman, and one that is in storage. In the former case any attempt to end the pregnancy would involve carrying out an invasive procedure on the pregnant woman, which she is entitled, both legally and ethically, to refuse. Where the embryo is not implanted, the BMA believes it is essential that both partners' views about whether they wish to be parents should be considered.

As with Diane Blood, however, there was tremendous support and sympathy for Natallie Evans and fierce public and professional debate about the case. While some commentators, including the BMA, argued that the law was correct to treat both parties equally, others argued that this approach failed to recognise Natallie Evans' greater moral rights over the fate of their frozen embryos. The reasons given for this assertion varied including the 'fact that parenthood is a more crucial matter to women',[68] and on the basis of how much each party has to lose by the decision.[69] Howard Johnston had given his consent to the creation and storage of embryos on the understanding that his consent could be withdrawn at any time up until the embryos were used in 'providing treatment services'. This was taken by the Court of Appeal and the European Court of Human Rights to mean the point at which an embryo is placed within a woman. Although the law was clear, there was considerable debate about the point at which it is reasonable to allow people to withdraw their consent. It was argued, for example, that it should be the creation of embryos, and not their use in treatment, that represents the 'point of no return'.[70] This would allow either party to use embryos once they have been created (although this raises the question of how the resulting conflict would, or should, be resolved if both parties wish to use a single embryo).

Although the 1990 Act was found to be clear and consistent with the Human Rights Act, the issues surrounding this case were highlighted by the Department of Health when it was reviewing the legislation. A central concern was the apparent anomaly that while the consent of both parties is required to store embryos, one gamete provider can insist on embryos being destroyed, by withdrawing consent to continued storage, irrespective of the views and wishes of the other. In one case embryos were destroyed before the other gamete provider had been informed that consent had been withdrawn. As a result of publicity surrounding this case, the HFEA wrote to clinics advising them that they must make every effort to inform the other party when notified of withdrawal of consent to storage and, wherever possible, this should be done before the embryos are destroyed.[71] Through the 2008 Act, however, a 'cooling off period' of 12 months was added to the 1990 Act to give both parties time to negotiate agreement about the fate of stored embryos.[72] This allows embryos to remain in storage, lawfully, for up to 12 months following withdrawal of consent. This would not have helped Natallie Evans, because her partner was adamant that he did not want the embryos used in treatment, but may be helpful in future cases.

Summary – consent to the storage and use of gametes and embryos

- Except for basic partner treatment services, consent for the storage or use of gametes or embryos must be in writing and, before giving consent, the person must have been given information and the opportunity to receive counselling.
- Individuals may withdraw or vary their consent at any time until the gametes or embryos are used in treatment or research.
- It is lawful to collect and store gametes from patients who lack capacity where they are expected to regain capacity but to be left infertile. Consent is required for their use. If the patient dies, the gametes must be destroyed.
- Where one party withdraws consent to the storage of embryos, the other party must be notified and storage may continue for up to 12 months to allow time for agreement to be reached about the fate of the embryos. Where agreement cannot be reached after that time, the embryos must be destroyed.

Use of donated gametes or embryos

For many people who are infertile, the use of donated sperm, oocytes or embryos may provide the opportunity to have a much wanted child. Whenever there is professional involvement in providing treatment involving donated gametes or embryos the treatment may be undertaken only in a clinic licensed by the HFEA. Before offering treatment with donated gametes or embryos clinics are required to provide information about the importance of informing any resulting child, at an early age, that they were conceived using donated gametes or embryos.[73] They must also give prospective parents information about suitable ways of telling children this information. This was included in the 2008 amendments to the 1990 Act because of a general belief, shared by the BMA, that it is in the child's best interests to know the circumstances of their conception. This belief was combined with concerns that still only a small number of parents tell their children about their donor conception. This not only introduces secrecy, with an element of risk that the information will be disclosed inadvertently when the child is unprepared and unsupported, but also reduces the number of people who are able to take advantage of the removal of anonymity (see pages 330–333) and make contact with the donor and with half siblings.

During the passage of the 2008 Act through Parliament there was discussion about whether it was appropriate to compel parents to tell their children about their donor conception, such as by including 'by donor' on the birth certificate. Despite supporting increased openness between parents and their donor-conceived children, the BMA opposed such moves, believing that encouragement and support was a better option. The evidence from adoption is that disclosure of a child's genetic origins is best handled by parents at their own speed, but with ongoing support and advice. Different children mature at different rates and can absorb, understand and contextualise complex information at different rates. Parents are best able to understand their child's level of development and to choose the right time to disclose the information. In the BMA's view, the amendments to the legislation have achieved the right balance of encouragement and support but only time will tell how effective this strategy is. One of the factors that may, in practice, work against encouraging parents to tell their offspring about their donation conception, however, is the removal of donor anonymity. The BMA believes there is a risk that some parents, who are concerned about their child making contact with the donor when they reach 18, may be less likely to tell their child they were donor conceived now that donor anonymity has been removed (see pages 330–333).

Psychological studies of people born after gamete donation

Although more research is being undertaken in this area there is still a limited amount of evidence about the psychological effect on people born after donor conception. Concerns have been expressed that parents may feel or behave less positively towards children where there is no genetic link and that this could affect the child's psychological well-being.[74] The research carried out to date does not support this view and, in fact, has found higher levels of warmth and interaction in these families than in naturally conceived control groups (see below). It has also been suggested that people are likely to suffer psychological harm from knowing of their donor conception but not being able to trace their genetic parents, although there is no definitive research that assesses the impact of this on individuals.

A European study of assisted reproduction families was set up in the mid-1990s to compare family relationships and the social and emotional development of children in families created as a result of IVF and DI compared with control groups of families with naturally conceived and adopted children. The first phase of the study was undertaken when the children were aged between 4 and 8 years old,[75] and the second phase took place when each child reached the age of 11–12 years.[76] Both studies found that all groups were similar for many aspects of the quality of parent–child relationships. In the later study, to the extent that differences were found, these reflected mainly more positive functioning among the assisted reproduction families. There were no differences between the groups of children on any of the measures of psychological adjustment and no differences were identified between the IVF and DI families for any of the variables relating to parenting or the psychological well-being of the children. It was noted in the article, however, that only 8.6 per cent of DI children had been told about their genetic origins and so the ability of this study to assess whether people are harmed by being unable to access information about donors is very limited. Research on this specific question is further hampered by the traditionally high dropout rate among donor families taking part in longitudinal studies.

In 2006, Golombok *et al.* studied 34 surrogacy families, 41 donor insemination families and 41 oocyte donation families compared with 67 natural conception families when the children were 3 years of age.[77] The study assessed the psychological well-being of the parents, mother–child relationship and the psychological well-being of the children. No differences were found in the psychological well-being of parents or children in the different family groups. The significant difference was in the mother–child relationship where, in line with previous studies, the warmth and interaction between mother and child was found to be higher in families that had used assisted reproduction with donated gametes. This study reinforces previous findings that the absence of a genetic link does not appear to impact negatively on parent–child relationships.

Some research has been undertaken involving adults who know they were born as a result of gamete donation. This found some evidence of mistrust within families, feelings of loss caused by the lack of knowledge about their genetic background, and frustration in being thwarted in the search for their biological fathers.[78] Many individuals reported feelings of anguish, resentment and anger as well as a loss of a sense of self and of identity.[79] In a number of cases, those interviewed had found out at a late stage and in an unplanned and sometimes confrontational way. For many of these it was not clear whether their feelings were caused by when and how they found out, or by being unable to obtain information about the donor, or by a combination of both. A 2009 study, for example, found that those who were told about their donor conception at a young age were more accepting and appeared to experience fewer problems. This study recruited 165 donor offspring via a website (Donor Sibling Registry) that allows individuals to search for their donors or donor siblings.[80] The participants were aged between 13 and 61, with 89 per cent currently living in the USA and 2 per cent living in the UK. The study looked at their feelings about learning of their donor conception based on when they were told the information – 30 per cent had found out before the age of 3 years and 19 per cent had found out after the age of 18. The most common feeling reported – irrespective of age of disclosure – was curiosity. Those told during adulthood were more likely to report feelings of being confused, shocked, upset, relieved, numb and angry than those told before they reached the age of 18. Those told during adolescence or adulthood were more likely to report feeling angry about being lied to and betrayed. This study appears to suggest that donor conceived offspring respond more positively when told at an early age. This is in line with advice on adoption which also suggests that children benefit from early disclosure about the circumstances of their birth.

Telling children about their donor conception

Despite an apparent change in social attitudes towards donor conception and towards the 'rights' of the child to know of their genetic origin over the last decade, this does not appear to be reflected in the practice of parents telling children about the circumstances of their conception. In the 2006 study by Golombok *et al.* mentioned above, only 7.3 per cent of oocyte donation parents and 4.9 per cent of donor insemination parents had begun to tell their child by the time of their third birthday and 46 per cent of donor insemination parents and 22 per cent of oocyte donation parents had made a definite decision not to inform the child.[81] Interestingly, when the same group had been interviewed when the children were aged 1, 56 per cent of oocyte donation parents and 46 per cent of donor insemination parents said they planned to tell the child about their donor conception. Very similar results were found in a 2007 study of 21 embryo donation families where the children were aged 2–5 years old. At the time of interview, 9 per cent had told their child how they had been conceived, 24 per cent reported that they were planning to tell, 43 per cent had decided they would never tell the child and 24 per cent were undecided.[82]

The main reasons given for not telling in these studies were:

- to protect the child
- to protect the non-genetic parent
- it was unnecessary.

The first of these reasons is at odds with the strong emphasis on informing young people about important information that affects them, including medical information. Although, generally, non-disclosure of distressing news to very young children by their parents is accepted, as they develop understanding and reach maturity, their own interests and needs take precedence.

Studies of parental attitudes to disclosure have found that those who have disclosed, or are planning to do so, give the following reasons:[83]

- to avoid accidental discovery
- a desire for openness
- the child's right to know his or her genetic origin.

It is perhaps too early to determine the effect of the removal of anonymity on the willingness of parents to tell their children. The BMA has been concerned that this may make parents less likely to inform their offspring, because of concerns about them making contact with the donor – although this assertion is not backed up with research evidence. In fact, one small study of infertility counsellors in the UK suggested that parents may be more likely to disclose the information following the removal of donor anonymity[84] (although, as the author points out, a stated intention to tell does not mean that the parents will necessarily do so). In Sweden, where children have had a right since 1985 to find out the identity of the donor, a study of 148 donor-conceived children aged 1–15 years, published in 2000, found that 89 per cent of parents had not informed their children about the DI, although 41 per cent expressed an intention to do so.[85] In a 2007 Swedish study, however, 61 per cent of parents had told their children about their donor conception (although this study was small involving just 19 families).[86] Interestingly, this study reported that the views of healthcare staff had strongly influenced parents' views and a majority of those who had been encouraged to tell their children about their donor conception had done so. It is hoped that the new requirement on clinics in the UK to provide information about the importance of telling children will be similarly influential and will result in reduced secrecy.

Anonymity of donors

Although the two concepts are often confused, there is a difference between secrecy and anonymity. While the BMA wishes to reduce secrecy, and encourage more parents to tell their children about their donor conception, the Association has concerns about the removal of donor anonymity. Gamete and embryo donation has traditionally been undertaken on an anonymous basis; parents and those conceived by donation were able to gain some information about the donor, but not identifying information. In 2004 this changed when Regulations were introduced[87] to remove donor anonymity for future donors; the BMA did not support this change. From 1 April 2005 all new donors have donated on the understanding that identifying information would be provided, on request, to anyone aged 18 or over who was conceived by the donation. The Regulations also provided for past donors to agree voluntarily to give up their anonymity by re-registering with the clinic at which they donated. With this exception people who donated prior to April 2005 will remain anonymous.

One of the major arguments against removing donor anonymity has been the fear that it would lead to a reduction in the number of donors available, so that some people in the future may be unable to obtain treatment. As a result, it is feared that some will make private arrangements that will potentially put women at risk, because of the absence of screening for HIV and other infectious diseases. There is also concern that more women will go overseas for treatment where anonymous donors can be used but where there may be less rigorous safeguards and regulation. There is evidence that this has happened in other countries with one Danish clinic reporting that Swedish couples made up 39 per cent of the total number of treatment cycles carried out between 1983 and 1992 and a Finnish clinic reporting that Swedish couples made up 50 per cent of its patients.[88]

Although the number of DI treatment cycles carried out in the UK has dropped significantly, from 26,095 in 1992 to 4,153 in 2006[89] (at least in part because developments such as intracytoplasmic sperm injection have opened up other treatment options for male infertility), there is still a large unmet demand for donors. It is estimated that around 500 new sperm donors per annum are required to meet demand but in 2008 only 396 new donors were registered with the HFEA.[90] Although there was a fairly dramatic drop in the number of donors in the late 1990s and the early part of this century, rates have improved with new registrations in 2008 the highest since 1996.[91] The HFEA has pointed out, however, that despite the number of registered donors increasing in recent years (from 251 in 2005 to 396 in 2008) the number of patients treated over the same period has fallen (from 825 to 621).[92] It is suggested that one explanation for this could be the increased use of known donors who donate to one family only.

Arguments for and against anonymity

The main arguments in support of donors being identifiable are summarised below.

- Individuals born as a result of treatment have a 'right' to know their genetic parents.
- The situation of people born subsequent to donor conception is different from those conceived naturally because information about the donor is available and is held by a public body (the HFEA).
- Generally, ethicists argue for openness and transparency and, unless there are good reasons for withholding information, it is usually considered appropriate to share information with those for whom it has personal relevance.
- It is generally considered to be in the interests of those who are adopted to have access to identifying information about their birth parents, an interest that since the mid 1970s has been enshrined in law. Although there are differences between adoption and donor conception, it is not self-evident that those differences justify dissimilar treatment in terms of access to identifying information about genetic parents.

- It is possible that a policy supporting donor anonymity could be found to breach Article 8 of the Human Rights Act (the right to respect for private and family life).

A 'right' to information about donors?

Ms Joanna Rose was born in Reading in 1972 and, when she was 7 years old, discovered that she was born as a result of donor insemination (DI). The circumstances of the discovery were distressing and she was sworn to secrecy; she felt grief, confusion and guilt. As an adult Ms Rose tried to find information about the donor. Although she discovered that all records of her conception had been destroyed, she decided to pursue her challenge of the Department of Health's policy on donor anonymity on behalf of other people in the same situation.

The second claimant was EM, who was born in 1996 as a result of DI. Her parents had always been open with her about the DI and were unhappy at not having the information needed to answer her questions about the donor.

Neither claimant was seeking the provision of identifiable information against the wishes of the donor. They were, however, seeking access to non-identifying information about donors and the establishment of a 'voluntary contact register' (to allow contact to be made if the donor was willing). They claimed that the Secretary of State's failure to take this action breached his duties under Articles 8 and 14 of the Human Rights Act. In assessing the scope of respect for private and family life the Court held that it required that 'everyone should be able to establish details of their identity as individual human beings. This includes their origins and the opportunity to understand them. It also embraces their physical and social identity and psychological integrity.'[93] In May 2002, Mr Justice Scott Baker held that Article 8 was engaged in this case but, because the Department of Health was already addressing the issue, a decision was not made about whether this right had been breached.

Those who are against the removal of anonymity, including the BMA, use the arguments summarised below.

- There is no 'right' to know one's parents. Many people who were conceived naturally are not the children of those they believe to be their parents and, if such a right existed, paternity tests should be available to everyone (irrespective of the views of the 'parents'). There is also a conflict between the offspring's 'right' to know and the parents' right to privacy. (The BMA accepts, however, that people born after donation have a strong interest in knowing the identity of the donor and that this can be very important for some individuals.)
- More donors are likely to come forward if they are guaranteed anonymity. Although donor numbers have begun to increase, after a significant fall widely believed to be a result of concerns about the removal of anonymity, they have not reached the levels achieved in the early 1990s and nor have they reached the number required to fulfil demand. This means that some people are unable to receive treatment or may resort to private arrangements or treatment overseas where there may be less protection.
- It is still the case that a large number of parents decide not to tell their children that they were born following donor conception (see pages 329–330). Although anybody can make enquiries to the HFEA about whether they were born subsequent to a donation, it is difficult to envisage people doing so unless they have some reason to doubt their genetic parentage. The impact of removing anonymity is therefore likely to be limited.
- There is no definitive research showing the impact of the availability of identifiable information on parents' decisions about whether to tell their children about their origins. It could make it easier for parents because they have more information available to give to their children, or it could make it more difficult, because the fact the children may want to trace the donors could be perceived as threatening to the parents. If the

latter is the case and more families opt not to tell their children they were born after donor conception, there is a risk that the search for more openness could, in fact, lead to more secrecy. It is currently not possible to determine whether removing anonymity would lead generally to more or less openness.

Payment of donors

The question of whether sperm and oocyte 'donors' should be paid, in money or in kind, has been a matter of considerable debate for over two decades and still remains a contentious issue. It has also been a difficult issue for the HFEA, which has changed its position on more than one occasion. Section 12(e) of the Human Fertilisation and Embryology Act 1990 stated that: 'no money or other benefit shall be given or received in respect of any supply of gametes or embryos unless authorised by directions'. In July 1991, the HFEA issued a direction allowing payment to donors of up to £15 plus reasonable expenses, or 'other benefits' (defined as treatment services and sterilisation) for each donation.[94] This maintained the status quo at that time although, in practice, sperm donors were given money to donate but egg donors were not. In its second annual report, in 1993, the HFEA stated that its intention was that payment should be phased out in the longer term.[95] Striving towards this aim, a conference was held in June 1995 and, in its 1996 annual report, the HFEA announced its decision that 'a donation should be a gift, freely and voluntarily given'.[96]

Wary of the risk of seeing a serious drop in the number of donors, the HFEA decided to take time to consider the best way to implement this broad policy decision. In February 1998, the HFEA issued a consultation document on how to implement the policy and to consider how payment could be withdrawn without adversely affecting the supply of donors.[97] In December 1998, while still stressing its commitment to altruistic donation, the HFEA reversed its policy and decided, for pragmatic reasons, to continue to allow payment, in both money and other benefits. A new direction was issued on 7 December 1998 allowing all clinics to offer payment of up to £15 per donation, the reimbursement of expenses (including loss of earnings and child minding expenses), and treatment services or sterilisation in return for donation.[98] The difficulty the HFEA encountered with implementing its policy demonstrates the tension that can arise between principle and pragmatism. Purely altruistic, voluntary donations are considered preferable, but many people are unwilling to accept the likely consequence of adopting such a policy which would be a reduction in the number of donors.

The HFEA changed its position again in October 2005, following a further consultation exercise, to state once more that gamete and embryo donors should be reimbursed for actual expenses incurred including compensation for loss of earnings (based on rates paid for jury service) but should not be paid for their donation. This time, the change took effect almost immediately with new directions issued in January 2006 prohibiting any payment for donors (other than legitimate expenses or 'treatment services', see pages 334–336) with effect from 1 April 2006.[99] In 2011, the HFEA undertook a further consultation exercise on gamete donation, including the question of compensating donors.[100] In considering any payments to donors, however, the HFEA must ensure that its decision falls within the terms of the EU Tissues and Cells Directive which requires member stares to 'endeavour to ensure voluntary and unpaid donation of tissues and cells'.[101] Under the Directive, donors may receive compensation but this is strictly limited to making good expenses and inconvenience directly related to the donation. In October 2011, the HFEA decided to permit compensation of £750 for egg donors and £35 per clinic visit for sperm donors.

Arguments for and against payment

The BMA has, over the years, contributed to the debate on the payment of donors and, in its consideration of the issue, has taken account of the following arguments.

In support of payment:

- Individuals should be free to do whatever they wish with their own gametes, including selling them, provided they have given informed consent and are not harming anyone else.
- Without payment it is impossible to ensure that the supply of donors is maintained and fewer people will be able to have a child using donor conception.
- Prohibiting payment could lead to people paying for sperm in private arrangements and thus bypassing the clinics and the screening and counselling they provide.
- Payment that induces individuals to donate does not necessarily constitute exploitation. Arguably, donors are exploited only if, under different financial circumstances or with full information, they would have refused to donate. Removing payment for donation will not improve their financial situation and may remove one of the few options open to them to make money.
- Payment can be seen as compensating donors for their inconvenience, rather than as payment for the gametes themselves, and also as a way of symbolically ending the donor's involvement and rights in relation to any child born.

Against payment:

- Paying donors for sperm and eggs can be seen as degrading for the individual.
- Payment for gamete donors can be seen as treating people as commodities and, arguably, undermining the moral obligation to show respect for persons.
- Some people are reluctant to see an act as morally acceptable if the motive is self-interest rather than altruism.
- People may begin to expect payment and this will change the nature of the act, leading to an overall reduction in altruism in society and a demand for payment for other acts currently based on altruism, such as blood donation.
- Paid donors may be more likely to lie about any illnesses or risk factors.
- Payment in money or in kind constitutes exploitation.
- Children born following donation may be distressed to learn that the donor was paid.

The BMA's MEC debated all of these issues on a number of occasions and, in February 2011, concluded that donors should have their expenses reimbursed including a reasonable payment in lieu of loss of earnings (sufficient to remove a disincentive but not sufficiently high to act as an inducement to donate). There was not, however, agreement on the Committee about whether donors should also be paid for their inconvenience and/or discomfort.

Egg sharing

Some women donate oocytes altruistically, while others may receive a benefit in kind, such as 'egg sharing' arrangements. Under such schemes, women who need IVF but cannot afford to pay for it are offered the option of receiving free or reduced price IVF treatment in return for donating some of the eggs collected for the treatment of others or, in a small number of centres, for research. For many people, payment in kind is no different, morally, from payment in money. If this is the case, most of the arguments set out above apply equally to egg sharing and monetary payment. Unlike sperm donation, however, egg donation is not without risks. The biggest risk is ovarian hyperstimulation syndrome developing as a result of the drugs given to stimulate the ovaries. Usually the symptoms are very mild, but in around 1 per cent of cases the complications can require hospital treatment, and in a very small number of patients this condition has been fatal. Many people find the procedure of egg collection painful, although there is no evidence of any long-term problems. The fact that egg donation includes risks has been used both to justify and to exclude payment and other inducement for egg donors. Some argue that women should not be given any incentive for taking a risk, whereas others argue that women should be given some benefit or payment in order to compensate for the increased risk and inconvenience. It has also been argued that egg sharing is, in fact, morally preferable to purely altruistic donation because, with egg sharing, the woman is not exposed to any additional risk for the sake of another person.[102]

The main concerns that have been expressed about egg sharing relate to consent and, in particular, the risk of coercion or exploitation. The monetary equivalent of a free IVF treatment cycle is likely to be many thousands of pounds and can therefore be seen as a major incentive to donate. Those seen as most at risk of exploitation are women who want a child but could not otherwise afford to pay for IVF and so agree to participate in an egg-sharing scheme as their only way of receiving treatment. Concerns have been expressed that in their desire to have a child, these women may not give adequate consideration to how they would feel if their treatment is unsuccessful but the recipient becomes pregnant, and that failing to address this issue could result in psychological harm in the longer term. With treatment cycles undertaken since 2005 these women also have the knowledge that any children conceived from the donated eggs could make contact in the future. The question is whether, if these women are fully informed of the procedures, risks and possible outcomes, they should be prevented from making this decision for themselves. Some would argue that they should be, because they are in a vulnerable position in relation to decisions about their fertility, and the offer of such a large incentive could result in them making a decision, contrary to their better judgement, that they would not have made had their circumstances been different. Others argue that adults with capacity should be free to make these decisions for themselves and that it is patronising to assume they are not capable of making such decisions. Such schemes help two women with different problems, one wanting IVF treatment using their own gametes, the other needing IVF using donated eggs; prohibiting such schemes could be seen as detrimental to both.

Following a consultation exercise which illustrated an almost equal divide between support for, and opposition to, this practice,[103] the HFEA reported in its 2000 annual report that it had been persuaded that, if properly regulated and monitored, egg sharing could, in some cases, be beneficial to participants.[104] The HFEA therefore decided to allow egg sharing subject to strict guidelines designed to protect all those involved in the arrangements. These guidelines set out the requirements around the provision of information and counselling, consent and confidentiality. All centres participating in such schemes are required to have a written policy that should include the centre's procedures for determining how the eggs will be shared between the provider and the recipient. The guidelines state that 'if too few eggs are collected for sharing, the woman should be given the option of using all the eggs for her own treatment, at the agreed discount'.[105] In its eighth code of practice, the HFEA extended the principles of 'egg sharing' to sperm donors so that clinics could offer reduced price treatment in return for donation of sperm.[106]

In 2003, it came to public attention that at least one clinic was practising a modification of the egg sharing scheme known as 'egg giving'. Under these arrangements a woman would agree to go through an IVF treatment cycle where all eggs retrieved were donated, followed by a second cycle – at reduced cost – where all eggs were used for her own treatment. The HFEA reviewed this practice and, because of the additional discomfort and risk women were exposed to, it decided that this was not acceptable. Clinics were informed of this and this practice was specifically prohibited in the 2006 Directions on payment for donors.[107]

When the BMA initially considered egg sharing, it expressed serious concerns about the validity of the consent, given the very strong incentive provided, and did not support the use of such schemes. This position was reviewed in 2007 both in relation to egg sharing for research and egg sharing for treatment. The MEC first considered egg sharing for research purposes and concluded that, because women were not being subjected to any additional risk, and that payment for participation in research was generally accepted (and the fact that payment was 'in kind' rather than in money did not alter the acceptability of this), the MEC did not object to this option. As a result of this decision, the MEC decided to review its position on egg sharing for treatment to ascertain whether there were sound moral reasons for taking a different approach to egg sharing where the eggs were to be used in treatment. There clearly are practical differences, because the donation could result in the birth of a child, and the committee specifically considered whether that reason alone justified taking a different ethical approach. In reviewing its decision the Committee took account of the factors outline below.

- The continuing lack of NHS funding for IVF treatment making it impossible for some women to obtain treatment except through egg-sharing arrangements.
- The severe shortage of egg donors and, with the loss of donor anonymity, the risk of increasing difficulty in recruiting donors except through egg-sharing arrangements.
- The increasing emphasis on patient autonomy and recognition that women who need IVF are not 'vulnerable' such that they need protection from making decisions they may possibly regret at a later stage. In other areas the BMA has taken the view that, as long as patients are provided with accurate information, they should be free to make their own decisions about where their interests lie – the BMA's view on egg sharing was, in many ways, an anomaly in this respect.
- The lack of evidence of harm arising from egg-sharing arrangements – which has now been happening for many years.
- Anecdotal evidence from patients that appears to show that some women perceive the fact that another woman has became pregnant as a positive outcome rather than a 'risk' of such arrangements.[108]

Taking account of all of these factors, the MEC took the view that the benefits (both to egg providers and recipients) outweigh the harms and so the BMA should withdraw its opposition to egg-sharing arrangements. The BMA does not consider this view to be inconsistent with its continued opposition to payment for blood, bone marrow and organ donation because the situation with egg sharing is sufficiently different from other forms of donation. This is because any risks the woman is taking are for her own benefit and not for the benefit of the recipient and her motivation is not commercial but in order to receive a health benefit for herself.

> ### Summary – use of donated gametes or embryos
>
> - For treatments provided since April 2005 identifiable information about donors may be provided to offspring, from the age of 18, on request.
> - Before providing treatment with donated gametes or embryos clinics are required to provide information to prospective parents about the importance of telling any resulting children about their donor conception, and to provide them with information about how to do this.
> - The arguments for and against anonymity of gamete donors are finely balanced, but the BMA did not support the removal of anonymity and continues to have concerns about the consequences of this decision.
> - Egg, sperm and embryo donors may be paid legitimate expenses, including compensation for loss of earnings, but must not be 'paid' for their donation. At the time of writing, however, the HFEA was in the process of reviewing this decision.
> - The BMA supports the reimbursement of donors' expenses and payment for loss of earnings. The MEC did not, however, reach agreement about payment for the inconvenience and/or discomfort of donation.
> - 'Egg sharing', whereby a woman receives free or reduced cost IVF treatment in return for donating some of her eggs, is permitted subject to strict guidelines. The same principles can also be applied to sperm donation.
> - The BMA believes, in the context of the shortage of donor gametes, that the benefits of egg and sperm sharing arrangements outweigh the harms and therefore does not object to this form of payment in kind.

Preimplantation genetic testing

Preimplantation genetic diagnosis

Preimplantation genetic diagnosis (PGD) is one form of prenatal testing and, as such, the ethical considerations discussed in Chapter 7 also apply to preimplantation diagnosis. PGD involves the creation of embryos *in vitro* and the removal of one or two cells for analysis prior to implantation. For those who know that they are at risk of passing on a serious genetic disorder, this procedure offers the opportunity of selecting and replacing only those embryos that are free of the disease. This allows a woman to begin her pregnancy knowing that the child is not affected by the disorder for which there is known risk. The number of conditions for which this type of testing is available is limited, and only a small number of centres have the necessary expertise to undertake the biopsy and testing procedures. Although it has been suggested that increasing numbers of people may wish to seek PGD for 'frivolous' reasons, the BMA considers this to be unlikely. The invasive nature of the technique combined with the relatively low success rates for IVF treatment and the costs of the procedure are likely to deter its widespread adoption. The nature of the UK's regulatory regime also prevents inappropriate use of such technologies. It is a criminal offence to carry out PGD without a licence from the HFEA.

PGD was developed in the UK in the late 1980s and was used to avoid passing on serious conditions that affected children such as adrenoleucodystrophy and X-linked mental retardation.[109] A general provision was made for the licensing of this activity in the 1990 Act. Schedule 2 of the Act allowed the HFEA to issue licences to authorise 'practices designed to secure that embryos are in a suitable condition to be placed in a woman or to determine whether embryos are suitable for that purpose'.[110] What was deemed 'suitable' was a matter for the HFEA which restricted PGD to testing for serious diseases. Its system of licensing required each clinic to apply individually for every condition it wished to test for. Originally, the HFEA licensed conditions that developed in infancy or childhood and where the disease was life-threatening or severely threatened the child's quality of life. Over time, however, the range of disorders the HFEA was asked to license expanded, including some adult-onset conditions – such as Huntington disease – and some where there was a very strong chance (around 90 per cent) but not a certainty that an individual with the gene mutation would develop the condition.

In 2005, the HFEA undertook a public consultation exercise in anticipation of being asked to license PGD for conditions where parents were at risk of passing on a genetic susceptibility to particular cancers, such as breast, ovarian and bowel cancer.[111] In these cases, the penetrance was lower – ranging around 30–80 per cent (so that only that proportion of those people who carry the affected gene would go on to develop the cancer). This meant that a number of the embryos that would be discarded as 'affected' would never have developed the condition. These conditions were also different in that people who develop these conditions do not do so until adulthood and there is also screening and, in some cases, treatment available. In its response to the consultation the BMA argued that there was no reason to restrict access to PGD where there was a health reason for selecting embryos and the individuals concerned – based on first-hand experience – felt sufficiently strongly to want to go through IVF and PGD. The BMA took the view that such cases should be permitted subject to discussion and negotiation between the individuals and their healthcare team. Following the consultation the HFEA also supported PGD being available for serious, lower-penetrance, later-onset genetic conditions such as inherited breast, bowel or ovarian cancer.

When the Human Fertilisation and Embryology Act was reviewed it decided that the legislation should be far more explicit about embryo testing and what was, and what was not, an acceptable use of the technology. Schedule 2 of the Act now includes a specific section on embryo testing, which allows a licence to authorise embryo testing for one of the following purposes:

'(a) establishing whether the embryo has a gene, chromosome or mitochondrion abnormality that may affect its capacity to result in a live birth,

(b) in a case where there is a particular risk that the embryo may have any gene, chromosome or mitochondrion abnormality, establishing whether it has that abnormality or any other gene, chromosome or mitochondrion abnormality,

(c) in a case where there is a particular risk that any resulting child will have or develop –
    (i)   a gender-related serious physical or mental disability
    (ii) a gender-related serious illness or
    (iii) any other gender-related serious medical condition, establishing the sex of the embryo,

(d) [tissue typing – see below]

(e) in a case where uncertainty has arisen as to whether the embryo is one of those whose creation was brought about by using the gametes of particular persons, establishing whether it is.'[112]

The Act specifies that the HFEA may only authorise testing in relation to an abnormality where there is 'a significant risk that a person with the abnormality will have or develop a serious physical or mental disability, a serious illness or any other serious medical condition'.[113] The legislation also now explicitly requires the HFEA to approve particular conditions for embryo testing, because the HFEA 'must be satisfied' that the test to be carried out meets the criteria in the Act.

The HFEA has set out, in its code of practice, the factors that should be taken into consideration by centres in determining whether a condition is 'serious' as follows:

'(a) the views of the people seeking treatment in relation to the condition to be avoided, including their previous reproductive experience
(b) the likely degree of suffering associated with the condition
(c) the availability of effective therapy, now and in the future
(d) the speed of degeneration in progressive disorders
(e) the extent of any intellectual impairment
(f) the social support available, and
(g) the family circumstances of the people seeking treatment.'[114]

A further provision of the amended legislation states that embryos that are known to have an abnormality, involving a significant risk of serious physical or mental disability, serious illness or serious medical condition, must not be preferred for implantation to ones that do not have the abnormality. This is intended to address the, possibly hypothetical, case of an individual or couple wishing to have testing to ensure that they have a child *with* a particular serious condition – the examples used in debate were individuals wishing to have a deaf child or a child with achondroplasia. The HFEA has interpreted this to apply only where there is at least one unaffected embryo that is suitable for transfer.[115] This allows for the situation where PGD is sought to avoid a particular condition – for example a predisposition to breast cancer – but only affected embryos are collected and the woman or couple wish to proceed with treatment. In most cases those in this situation are likely to opt to try again in another treatment cycle but, for some, this may not be possible (for example, if the embryos had been stored prior to treatment that had left the woman infertile). Clearly, the welfare of the child provisions are engaged in this situation and the HFEA requires clinics to take this into account in their decision making and also advises that such cases should normally have the approval of a clinical ethics committee.

Revealing additional information

As new techniques for undertaking PGD are developed, the possibility of discovering increasing amounts of genetic information has arisen. Currently, PGD requires the specific gene mutation to be identified – limiting the number of conditions that can be tested for and delaying the process of testing. New techniques, such as preimplantation haplotyping (PGH)[116] and karyomapping,[117] are being developed which do not look for the specific mutation but rather identify which sections of the embryo's chromosomes are inherited from which grandparent and therefore whether the embryo has inherited chunks of chromosome that contain a faulty gene. If successfully applied in practice, this will increase both the number of conditions tested for and also reduce the time within which the test can be carried out.

The use of techniques such as karyomapping and PGH does raise other issues. Using these methods of diagnosis to identify serious conditions will also lead to increasing amounts of genetic information becoming available, including information about other, less serious, conditions or susceptibilities. Although much of the media attention has focused on the fact that this would allow any of the almost 15,000 genetic conditions to be tested for, the fact that the HFEA must approve each condition will ensure that testing for only 'serious conditions' is permitted. However, this raises questions about how much of the additional information obtained should be given to prospective parents, who will not have received information about the condition or conditions detected and have not given consent to it being identified. It also raises questions about the extent to which this information should be used to select which embryo(s) to replace. In some cases the information may be inadvertently and unintentionally discovered but in others the clinic may make a positive choice to identify this information. The BMA believes that these developments raise important issues that require further debate. The BMA's general view, however, is that, in discussion with patients, clinics should aim to replace the best quality embryos and those most likely to lead to a successful pregnancy.

Exclusion testing and PGD with non-disclosure

Some patients, who are at 50 per cent risk of inheriting a condition such as Huntington disease, want to have PGD to avoid having an affected child without finding out if they themselves carry the gene mutation. There are two ways in which this can be achieved. The first is by exclusion testing whereby embryos are tested to see whether they have inherited chromosomal material from the 'at risk' partner's affected parent (who either has the condition already or is known to carry the mutation). If they have, the embryos are classified as high risk and are discarded (although statistically 50 per cent of them will not be affected). If they have not, then the embryos can be replaced and will be free of the disease. This does not reveal the genetic status of the patient to either the clinic or the patient or couple. Although this procedure involves discarding some embryos that will be healthy, this is also the case where PGD is used to determine the sex of embryos in order to avoid serious X-linked disorders, which is specifically permitted in the legislation and is generally accepted. Exclusion testing also exposes some people to unnecessary medical treatment because half of them will not carry the gene and therefore would not require PGD. It also raises the possibility of a couple remaining childless, because of the low success rate of PGD, when a naturally conceived child would not be affected by the condition because the 'at-risk' parent is, unknowingly, free of the mutation. In 2009, because of concerns about providing unnecessary treatment, the Dutch Government restricted PGD for conditions like Huntington disease to those individuals who agreed to find out their own genetic status prior to testing.[118] The BMA does not support such restrictions and believes it is for informed individuals themselves to decide whether to seek exclusion testing.

In some cases, however, it is not possible to conduct exclusion testing because, for example, both parents of the 'at risk' patient are dead and there are no DNA samples available from them or an informative member of the family to identify the chromosomal material from the embryo's affected grandparent. In such cases, a request may be made for direct testing of the embryo, with the replacement of only unaffected embryos, but without disclosing to the prospective parents whether any of the embryos tested were affected (because this would reveal that the 'at risk' patient had inherited the condition). Such 'non-disclosure testing' requires IVF to create embryos for PGD and in half of cases will reveal that some embryos carry the mutation, hence will be affected and, by inference, that the 'at risk' parent will be affected by the disease. There is an equal chance that the embryos will be found to be unaffected and, by inference, that the parent is unlikely to be a carrier and go on to develop the disease in the future.

There is a strong possibility that, as a result of the test, the staff at the clinic will become aware of the patient's genetic status which the patient does not know and does not want to know. This can lead to a number of practical and ethical problems.

- Knowing important information that the patient does not wish to know places a burden on clinic staff.
- There is a risk of inadvertent disclosure of the information.
- If all embryos are unaffected, and therefore it is unlikely that the 'at risk' patient carries the mutation, future treatment cycles could be considered ethically problematic because IVF and PGD may not be necessary from a clinical perspective, or meet the legal criteria for PGD. To inform the patient of this, however, would reveal genetic information the patient does not want to receive. Carrying out 'dummy testing' in future treatment cycles would involve deceit and taking money for procedures not undertaken.
- If all embryos are affected, and so there are none available for transfer, the patient could infer his or her genetic status, even if they are advised before testing that there may be other reasons why no embryos are available for transfer. To proceed with a 'dummy' embryo transfer, however, in order to disguise this fact would involve an unnecessary medical procedure and what might be considered an unacceptable level of deceit.

Some clinics may choose to send the embryos to another clinic for testing in these cases, to reduce the likelihood of the staff at the clinic finding out the genetic status of the patient. This is not always possible and some clinics refuse to provide PGD with non-disclosure on the grounds that it places an unacceptable burden on their staff. Some patients may be willing to proceed on the basis that the clinic will try not to reveal their genetic status but accepting that the information may become available. Given this risk of disclosure and the very serious implications of predictive testing (see Chapter 9, pages 383–385), the BMA believes that such testing should only be undertaken after specialist counselling. While recognising the difficulties, the MEC was concerned that if PGD with non-disclosure was not permitted, and exclusion testing were not possible, there may be pressure on those at risk to have predictive testing against their better judgement, as their only way of ensuring they could have an unaffected child.

This issue was considered by the HFEA in January 2010. As a result of its deliberations new guidance was included in the *Code of Practice* in April 2010 requiring that:

- PGD with non-disclosure is carried out only in exceptional circumstances and, wherever possible, exclusion testing should be used instead
- patients are given the opportunity to receive genetic counselling prior to giving consent
- protocols are developed, within clinics, to minimise the chance of inadvertent disclosure, such as by using a different embryology laboratory to carry out the testing, in order to limit the number of staff who know the patient's genetic status
- no dummy embryo transfers may be performed
- written informed consent is obtained from the patient, including a statement that they have been informed:
  - of the risk of inadvertent disclosure
  - that where all embryos are suitable for transfer this is not evidence of the patient's genetic status
  - that where no embryos are suitable for transfer this is not evidence of the patient's genetic status

- ○   that dummy embryo transfers are not necessary or permissible
- ○   that, as a result of the request, treatment may go ahead that is not medically necessary – where the patient does not have the condition – information must be provided about the potential costs and risks of medically unnecessary treatment.[119]

Preimplantation genetic screening

A modification of the PGD technique is preimplantation genetic screening (PGS) which involves similar testing. However, rather than being used for fertile couples who wish to avoid having a child with a serious genetic disorder, genetic testing of embryos is undertaken for childless couples to screen for numerical chromosomal abnormalities (aneuploidy) to determine which embryos are most likely to result in a successful pregnancy. The technique has been used for patients at high risk of failure with IVF, specifically patients:

- of advance maternal age (over 35 years of age)
- with recurrent implantation failure
- who have experienced recurrent miscarriages
- with male factor infertility.

The theory behind PGS is that chromosomally normal embryos have a higher chance of successful implantation and live birth and therefore selecting those embryos for replacement should improve success rates in these patients. The effectiveness of this technique has been hotly debated and the evidence in support of it is, at best, equivocal.[120] This has led to accusations that until properly controlled studies have shown that screening is beneficial 'the widespread use of this expensive technology . . . by in vitro fertilisation centres is arguably unethical'.[121] It can also be argued, however, that if patients are adequately informed of the lack of clear evidence in support of such procedures, they should be free to decide whether to proceed. The HFEA's Code of Practice requires clinics to inform patients 'of the unproven nature of the procedure, in particular that more robust clinical and laboratory trials are needed to assess whether or not PGS can significantly increase live birth rates for different specific indicators and [that] it is likely that the method of fluorescent in situ hybridisation (FISH) on embryos, using a limited number of chromosomes, is not effective at increasing live birth rates'.[122] Recent studies involving a new screening technique – comparative genomic hybridisation (CGH) – which is able to test all chromosomes, appear promising. In one study, 45 couples underwent CGH and the results were compared with 113 matched controls. A total of 269 blastocysts were successfully analysed and 51.3 per cent were diagnosed as aneuploid. Following the transfer of embryos found to be normal, the implantation rate in the CGH group was 72.2 per cent compared with 46.5 per cent of those having embryos transferred in the control group.[123]

Selecting embryos on the basis of tissue type compatibility

Another modification to the standard model of PGD is the use of embryo testing to select embryos on the basis of tissue type compatibility. In 2001, shortly after the HFEA had carried out a public consultation exercise on PGD, it received an application to use this technology in conjunction with human leucocyte antigen (HLA) typing, not only to avoid the birth of a child with a severe genetic disorder, but also to select for replacement those embryos that were most likely to produce a child who would be a good tissue match for a very sick sibling. It was proposed that stem cells would be taken from the umbilical cord blood and so the child himself or herself would not be a donor nor be subjected to any intrusive or painful procedures. In December 2001, the HFEA considered the issues raised as a matter of principle and gave its approval to the procedure subject to a number of conditions, including a requirement that individual requests must be considered by the HFEA on a case-by-case basis. Another criterion was that the PGD must be carried out to avoid a serious disorder in the future child and not simply for tissue typing.[124] The HFEA subsequently considered the original application and one further application, the first of which it approved but the second (for a non-inherited condition) it turned down on the grounds that it did not meet the criterion that the embryo itself must be at risk of the condition. The HFEA was criticised for both of these decisions including, for the first decision, by the House of Commons' Science and Technology Committee, which said 'the HFEA's decision to allow tissue typing in conjunction with preimplantation genetic diagnosis went beyond the scope of its own public consultation. It is vital that the public are taken along with decisions of such ethical importance'.[125]

PGD with tissue typing for the benefit of a very sick sibling

Three-year-old Zain Hashmi had beta thalassaemia. His parents wanted to use PGD to avoid the birth of another child with the same condition and also to select for replacement those embryos most likely to produce a child who would be a compatible donor. The intention was to use stem cells from the umbilical cord blood to produce bone marrow for the transplant, thus the child himself or herself would not be subjected to any invasive, painful or risky procedures. Approval was given by the HFEA for this case.[126] Unfortunately, the Hashmis' attempts at treatment resulted in miscarriage and so no child was born as a result.

Three-year-old Charlie Whitaker suffered from Diamond–Blackfan anaemia, a rare life-threatening blood disorder. Although some children with Diamond–Blackfan anaemia inherit this condition from carrier parents, most cases arise as a result of a sporadic mutation. In this case, the parents were found not to be carriers and so the future child was at no greater risk of developing the condition than any other child. The couple wished to use PGD solely to provide a compatible donor for Charlie. As with the Hashmi case, stem cells would be taken from the umbilical cord blood and so the child himself or herself would not be used as a donor. The HFEA turned down this application on the basis that the PGD was not being carried out to avoid a serious disorder in the future child and so it did not meet the criteria set out by the HFEA.[127] The Whitaker's went to Chicago for treatment which was successful and in 2003 Mrs Whitaker gave birth to a son who was a tissue match for Charlie. In July 2004, Charlie underwent a transplant of stem cells from the umbilical cord blood and in August 2005 tests showed that the treatment had been successful.[128]

The Pro-life Alliance sought a judicial review of the decision in the Hashmi case, arguing that the HFEA had exceeded its legal powers. Under the Human Fertilisation and Embryology Act, the HFEA can issue treatment licences only for the provision of 'treatment services', defined as 'assisting women to carry children'. The Pro-life Alliance argued that the purpose of tissue typing was not to assist a woman to carry a child and that it could not therefore be licensed. In upholding the challenge, Mr Justice Maurice Kay held that, because the reason for requesting tissue typing did not arise from an impaired ability to conceive or to carry a child through pregnancy to full term and birth, it could not be argued that it was 'necessary or desirable' for the purpose of assisting a woman to carry a child.[129] This decision was overturned by the Court of Appeal, which rejected this narrow interpretation. Lord Phillips said that 'when concern as to the characteristics of any child that she may bear may inhibit a woman from bearing a child, IVF treatment coupled with PGD that will eliminate that concern can properly be said to be ". . . for the purpose of assisting women to carry children".[130] He went on to say that decisions about what choices should be allowed raise difficult ethical questions, responsibility for which Parliament has placed in the hands of the HFEA.

The Appeal Court's decision in this case (subsequently upheld by the House of Lords[131]) was formally welcomed by the BMA at its Annual Representatives Meeting in July 2003. The BMA did not, however, agree with the distinction the HFEA made at the time between cases where a future child was at risk and where PGD was requested solely for tissue typing. While accepting that the former cases were easier to justify, the BMA did not believe there was any morally relevant difference between the two cases. Rather, the BMA supported, in principle, the use of PGD combined with tissue typing in all cases where this was the best option for treatment for a sibling whose condition was life-threatening or very serious. The HFEA subsequently removed this distinction from its approval criteria.[132]

These so-called 'saviour sibling' cases were given formal approval by Parliament in 2008 when revisions to the 1990 Act were debated. The new section on embryo testing in Schedule 2 of the Act (as amended) specifically permits testing in cases where:

> a person ('the sibling') who is the child of the persons whose gametes are used to bring about the creation of the embryo (or of either of those persons) suffers from a serious medical condition which could be treated by umbilical cord blood stem cells, bone marrow or other tissue [excluding a whole organ] of any resulting child, establishing whether the tissue of any resulting child would be compatible with that of the sibling.[133]

Welfare of the child

A key concern in this type of case was the possibility of psychological harm resulting to the child who would be selected and born to be a donor. Would the child resent being 'selected' and feel less wanted or less respected as an individual? Alternatively, would the child feel proud of being uniquely able to save the life of his or her sibling? If treatment with cord blood were unsuccessful, would the child feel obliged to donate bone marrow? What would be the effect on the child's relationship with the parents if, despite treatment, the sibling died? Would the child feel guilty for having been unable to save him or her? Even now, nearly a decade after these cases were first debated, we do not know the answer to these questions. Yet these speculative risks of harm have to be balanced against the real harm to the individual who would suffer or die without this treatment, and to that person's parents and siblings. If PGD with tissue typing was not permitted, parents might continue to have children naturally in the hope of obtaining a match; the harm to those children, particularly if they are unsuitable as donors, needs also to be considered. The requirement in the Human Fertilisation and Embryology Act to take account of the welfare of the child usually focuses on the child who may be born as a result of the treatment, but the requirement specifically extends to taking account of the welfare of 'any other child who may be affected by the birth'.[134] Under the terms of the Act, therefore, it is entirely reasonable and appropriate to consider the welfare of other children in the family who may be affected, in a positive or a negative way, by the birth of the new child.

It is sometimes argued that selection by tissue typing involves children being born merely as a means to someone else's end rather than for their own sake. In reality, however, parents have children for many reasons that are often more to do with their own wishes and desires than the interests of the future child. As Gillon points out in another context,[135] it is not unusual for individuals to use each other as a means to an end.

In helping each other, we do not become merely a tool for achieving objectives. Nevertheless, such concerns need to be taken seriously in the debate. For those who believe that the risks to the selected child are sufficiently serious to override all other considerations, neither of the cases described above would be acceptable. The BMA does not, however, believe that selection by tissue typing is necessarily incompatible with the welfare of the child.

Summary – preimplantation genetic testing

- It is a criminal offence for a clinic to carry out PGD without a licence from the HFEA.
- The BMA does not support the use of PGD to select physical characteristics but believes its use is acceptable where there is a health reason for selecting embryos and the individuals concerned – based on first-hand experience – feel sufficiently strongly to want to go through IVF and PGD.
- The BMA supports the use of exclusion testing where patients wish to avoid the birth of an affected child without finding out their own genetic status.
- The BMA supports the use of PGD with non-disclosure in exceptional circumstances and with safeguards. Patients seeking this should be advised of the risk of inadvertent disclosure and encouraged to seek genetic counselling prior to testing.
- Clinics offering preimplantation genetic screening for aneuploidy should inform patients that there is not clear evidence that this procedure increases success rates.
- The BMA supports, in principle, the use of PGD combined with tissue typing in all cases where this is the best option for treatment of a sibling whose condition is life threatening or sufficiently serious to justify the use of PGD.

Sex selection

One of the choices that developments in reproductive technology has made possible is that of selecting the sex of future children. The most accurate means of selection is using PGD and selecting for replacement only those embryos of the desired sex (this is known as 'secondary selection' as selection takes place after fertilisation). It is also possible, with increasing accuracy, to make the selection before fertilisation takes place (primary selection) by separating out the X- and Y-bearing sperm and using the preferred sample for insemination. Sex selection is a widely accepted practice for medical reasons, where it is used to avoid the birth of a child with a severe disorder that affects only one sex (such as Duchenne muscular dystrophy which affects only boys) and this is now specifically permitted in the legislation.[136] More controversial, however, is its use for social or cultural reasons, which the HFEA has consistently refused to license and is now prohibited in the 1990 Act.

Request for sex selection

In 2001, Alan and Louise Masterton appealed to the HFEA to make an exception to its prohibition on sex selection for social reasons to allow them to have a daughter. The Mastertons had four sons and their only daughter (born after 15 years of trying for a girl) died in a bonfire accident at her home in 1999 at the age of 3 years. Mrs Masterton had been sterilised after the birth of her daughter and therefore required IVF to have another child. Mr Masterton argued that there was a pressing medical need for the procedure because of the effect on the couple, confirmed by a psychologist and their GP, of their strong desire for a daughter.

The HFEA said it could consider an application only from one of its licensed clinics in order to make an exception to its general rule, but the Mastertons were unable to find a clinic with the relevant expertise that was willing to take the case to the HFEA. The couple considered challenging this decision, using the Human Rights Act and claiming that the HFEA's refusal to consider their case was a breach of their right to a fair hearing and to respect for private and family life, but did not pursue this. They subsequently went to Italy, where IVF treatment produced only one male embryo. The embryo was not replaced, but was donated to another couple.[137]

Consultation and debate

In both 1993 and 2002, the HFEA undertook public consultation exercises to seek views on whether people should be permitted to select the sex of their children in the absence of any medical imperative. In the later consultation, a distinction was made between 'family balancing' (where the family already had children of one sex) and other social reasons. Both consultations found strong public opposition to sex selection for social reasons. A MORI poll commissioned by the HFEA, as part of the 2002 consultation exercise, found that 69 per cent disagreed with a statement that prospective parents should have the right to choose the sex of their child, with only 14 per cent agreeing.[138] The survey found no significant difference in opinion between primary and secondary selection. Following the consultation exercise, the HFEA concluded that sex selection for non-medical reasons should be prohibited and that the current regulatory mechanism should be extended to include sex selection by sperm sorting techniques which, at the time, were unregulated.[139]

The issue was reviewed again in 2004 by the House of Commons Science and Technology Committee which questioned the evidence base for the HFEA's rejection of sex selection. It criticised the HFEA for taking a precautionary approach to the issue and argued that the onus should be on those who wished to restrict reproductive autonomy, by prohibiting sex selection, to produce evidence of harm in support of their case. On balance the Committee found 'no adequate justification for prohibiting the use of sex selection for family balancing.'[140] This, more liberal, approach did not hold sway, however, and following further debate during the legislative process, the 1990 Act was amended specifically to outlaw sex selection for non-medical reasons.[141] This includes both selection by PGD and sperm sorting which was brought within the regulatory framework as a result of implementing the EU Tissues and Cells Directive (see page 313).

Although sex selection has been debated on many occasions by the public, parliamentarians and within the BMA, the same key arguments are made and disputed. The key arguments of those who believe that sex selection should be permitted are set out below.

• Freedom of choice should be encouraged if there is no evidence of foreseeable harm from allowing people to choose. Concerns that boys would be favoured if selection was permitted in the UK (which could affect the balance of the sexes or reinforce gender stereotypes) is not borne out by the evidence and most people in the UK say they want a 'balanced' family. A survey of sex preference in the UK found that 68 per cent would ideally like an equal balance of girls and boys; a small percentage wanted only boys (3 per cent) or only girls (2 per cent) while, if they could only have one child, 19 per cent would prefer a boy and 17 per cent would prefer a girl.[142] Furthermore, any perceived problems of this nature could be avoided by allowing sex selection only for family balancing.

- People would be able to exercise greater control over the size of their family. Some people continue to have children until they have a child of the desired sex and there could even be a risk that those of the undesired sex may be abused or neglected.
- Primary and secondary sex selection is preferable to people seeking abortion based on the sex of the fetus. It is argued that this is practised, although reasons other than gender choice are given in justification (see Chapter 7, pages 287–288).
- Some have no objection in principle to people choosing the sex of their child but believe that PGD, which is an invasive procedure involving the creation and destruction of embryos, should only be used for serious conditions and not for allowing people to choose the characteristics of their offspring for social reasons. Such people would support the use of sperm sorting techniques but not PGD.

Those who oppose sex selection for social reasons use the arguments set out below.

- It is wrong to base the acceptance of a child on its particular characteristics. Children should be accepted and loved unconditionally. If a child of the 'wrong' sex is conceived through a failure of the technology, this could result in termination of pregnancy or parents may have difficulty accepting the child, which could result in psychological harm.
- This technology should not be used for 'trivial purposes' or to meet the desire of parents for particular characteristics in their children. Once a decision is made to allow people to choose one characteristic it will be more difficult to prevent other choices, resulting in 'designer children'.
- Although the balance of the sexes is unlikely to be upset in the UK as a whole, it is possible that it could be an issue within some communities. In research on attitudes to infertility among South Asian communities in the UK, for example, a strong 'social need' for a male child was reported to be widespread and the failure to produce a male child was regarded as a form of infertility in some families.[143]
- Allowing sex selection in the UK would send the wrong message to other countries where gender imbalance is potentially a serious problem. It would make it more difficult for the UK to criticise clearly unacceptable practices in other countries and, by conceding that sex is an important issue for choice, could be perceived as reinforcing unacceptable gender stereotypes and the oppression of members of the less-favoured sex.

The BMA's view on sex selection

Sex selection has been debated many times both by the BMA's MEC and its Representative Body. Although, as on other issues, the BMA represents doctors with a wide range of views, the BMA has had policy since 1993 opposing sex selection for social reasons. This policy was reaffirmed in 1994. BMA policy does not differentiate between sex selection for 'family balancing', in families with one or more children of the same sex, and personal preferences for children of only one sex or for the sex of a first born child.

Summary – sex selection

- It is unlawful to select the sex of a future child for non-medical reasons. This applies to both the use of PGD and sperm sorting techniques.
- The BMA is opposed to sex selection for social reasons.

Surrogacy

The number of people using surrogacy is small in comparison with those using other forms of assisted reproduction, but for some it offers the only practical way of addressing the consequences of involuntary childlessness. It raises profound questions and the separation of maternity from social motherhood raises complex moral and legal issues.

A distinction can be made between 'partial' surrogacy (also known as traditional or straight surrogacy) and 'full' surrogacy (also known as host or IVF surrogacy). In partial surrogacy, the surrogate mother provides an egg, which is fertilised with sperm from the intended father or a donor. In full surrogacy, the woman who carries the fetus makes no genetic contribution to an embryo that she receives to gestate. The eggs and sperm used to create the embryos are usually those of the intended parents, although in some cases donated gametes may be used.

The BMA's views on surrogacy have changed over time. From advice to doctors to have no involvement with surrogacy came a growing recognition that surrogacy is as much a social issue as a medical one. This recognition led to the BMA's acceptance, in 1990, of surrogacy as a treatment of last resort.[144] The BMA's 1996 report saw surrogacy as an acceptable option when 'it is impossible or highly undesirable for medical reasons for the intended mother to carry a child herself'.[145] The apparent growing public acceptance of surrogacy has led to a reduction in the amount of secrecy surrounding the practice and to a corresponding increase in the number of people requesting advice and support from the medical profession about surrogacy arrangements.

The regulatory framework

The law on surrogacy is set out in the Surrogacy Arrangements Act 1985 (as amended), the Human Fertilisation and Embryology Act 1990 (as amended) and the Human Fertilisation and Embryology Act 2008. The main points are summarised below.

- The law sets out comprehensive restrictions on commercial activity and advertising by surrogacy organisations. Legislation makes clear that surrogacy organisations may charge for certain activities but only if they do not make a profit. They may also advertise the services for which they may charge. They may charge for:
  - initiating negotiations with a view to the making of a surrogacy arrangement – enabling interested parties to meet each other to discuss a possible surrogacy arrangement
  - establishing and keeping lists of people willing to be surrogates or intended parents.

  It is not illegal for an organisation to negotiate a surrogacy arrangement, but it is illegal for them to charge for doing so and, therefore, also illegal to advertise their willingness to do so.

- The 2008 Act upholds a long established legal rule that the woman who carries the child will be the child's legal mother and her husband or partner (provided he consents) will be the child's legal father or second parent. To transfer parenthood, it is possible for the intended parents (but not a single person) to apply for a Parental Order provided the following criteria are met:
  - the gametes of either one or both of the couple must have been used

- the couple must be married, civil partners or living as partners in an enduring family relationship
- one or both must be domiciled in the UK, Channel Islands or the Isle of Man
- the couple must both be over 18 at the time the order is made
- the surrogate and her partner or husband (if she has one) must agree unconditionally to the making of the order
- no money, other than reasonable expenses, has been paid to the surrogate
- the child must be living with the intended parents at the time they apply for the parental order
- the intended parents must apply for the parental order within 6 months of the child being born (but the surrogate mother's consent may not be given within 6 weeks of the birth).

Those who do not meet these criteria can still apply to adopt the child.

- Surrogacy agreements are unenforceable in law. This means that, if the surrogate mother wishes to keep the child, and any money she has been paid, she is entitled to do so (although, in practice, the legal situation is not always so straightforward – see the case reported below). Equally, if the intended parents decide they do not want the child, the surrogate mother is responsible in law for its welfare, regardless of its genetic makeup. In practice, although extremely rare, a child rejected by its birth mother and the intended parents is likely to be placed for fostering or adoption.
- Advertising (including by the potential surrogate mother or intended parents) that indicates that a person is willing to be a surrogate mother, that someone is looking for a surrogate mother or that a person or organisation will help to initiate a surrogacy arrangement, is prohibited (with the exception of advertising by non-profit making organisations – see above).
- Any organisation or establishment offering IVF or DI services, including those carried out as part of a surrogacy arrangement, must be licensed by the HFEA.

The need to review the law

There has been growing recognition over the last decade that surrogacy law needs to be reviewed. In June 1997 the Government set up a review group, chaired by Professor Margaret Brazier, to review certain aspects of surrogacy arrangements; after wide-ranging consultation, the group reported in October 1998.[146] The report made the recommendations below.

- There should be a new Surrogacy Act to replace the Surrogacy Arrangements Act 1985 and the surrogacy provisions in the Human Fertilisation and Embryology Act. Under the new Act:
  - surrogacy arrangements would continue to be unenforceable
  - the existing prohibition on commercial agencies and advertising would remain
  - there would be statutory provisions defining and limiting lawful payments to surrogate mothers
  - non-profit making agencies would be required to register with the Department of Health and comply with a surrogacy code of practice issued by the Department of Health
  - unregistered agencies would be prohibited

○   the existing provision for parental orders would be amended to make it a requirement that the surrogacy code of practice and the restrictions on payments had been respected.

• Payments to surrogate mothers should cover only genuine expenses associated with the pregnancy. The nature and level of expenses should be agreed before there is any attempt to initiate a pregnancy and documentary evidence should be provided of the expenses incurred. The new Surrogacy Act should define expenses in broad terms of principle, but what constitutes 'reasonable expenses', and the evidence required, should be set out in directions.

• The Department of Health should consider establishing requirements for full record keeping and reporting of specified statistics.

The BMA supported these recommendations, which reflected very closely the Association's own views set out in its 1996 publication (see above) and in its evidence to the review team. This area of law is complex and frequently misunderstood. Those using surrogacy often rely on volunteer groups for advice, rather than seeking expert legal advice. The courts have commented in the past that relying on legal advice from groups of 'well-meaning amateurs' has led to individuals being given incorrect advice, leading to complex legal issues.[147] There are also areas where the law itself has caused difficulties and where the courts have taken a very pragmatic approach to enforcing the legislation. In one case, for example, although the law states that surrogacy arrangements are unenforceable in law, the courts used a residency order to remove a child from the surrogate mother and place it with the intended parents – effectively enforcing the contract (see below).

Enforcement of a surrogacy arrangement

In 2007 the Court of Appeal upheld a County Court judge's ruling that a child (N) who was born as a result of a surrogacy arrangement should be taken from the surrogate mother (P) and her husband, who had cared for him for 17 months, and placed with the intended parents (the Js). The intended parents applied for, and were awarded, a residency order. Despite the fact that surrogacy arrangements are unenforceable in law, the judge decided that, in this case, the surrogate mother should be forced to give up the child because the intended parents were 'most likely to deliver the best outcome for him over the course of his childhood and in the end be most beneficial.'[148]

The Court heard that P had engaged in deception and had never intended to honour the surrogacy agreement. The judge found that P 'had deliberately embarked on a path of deception, driven by Mrs P's compulsive desire to bear a child or further children, and that she had never had any other objective than to obtain insemination by surrogacy, with the single purpose of acquiring for herself, and her family, another child.'[149] He acknowledged that P and her husband had been good parents to N but considered that the Court had a straightforward decision to make about who would make the best parents for N. Based on expert medical opinion, and the fact of P's deception in agreeing to the arrangement with the intention of keeping the baby, the judge decided to award residency to the Js.

There have also been a number of cases in which the courts have retrospectively authorised payments to surrogate mothers in order that a Parental Order can be made transferring legal parentage to the intended parents. In some cases, applying the apparent letter of the law would have been contrary to the courts' overriding obligation to promote the best interests of the child and the granting of a Parental Order has been designed to achieve that primary objective, notwithstanding the provisions of an apparently applicable measure of surrogacy law. The options before the court have been particularly stark in some of the international surrogacy agreement cases, such as the case of *X v Y* (see below) where, if the Parental Order had been refused the twins born as a result of a commercial surrogacy arrangement would have had no legal parents and no right to citizenship of any country.

Surrogacy arrangement in the Ukraine

A British couple entered into a commercial surrogacy arrangement with a married woman in the Ukraine. The surrogate gave birth to twins which were handed over to the British couple as planned. Under UK law (which applies even where the arrangement is made in another country) the surrogate mother and her husband were the children's legal parents. Thus, having no British parents, the children were not entitled to citizenship of the UK. Under Ukrainian law, however, once the surrogate mother had handed over the twins, she and her husband had no obligations, rights or duties regarding the children and the children had no right to residence or citizenship in the Ukraine. Thus, the children were effectively left with no legal parents and no right to live in either the UK or the Ukraine – as the judge said they were left 'marooned stateless and parentless' in the Ukraine. The Home Office agreed to give special discretionary entry clearance allowing the British parents to bring the children home while their long-term future was decided by the courts.

The British parents applied for a Parental Order, transferring legal parentage to them. One of the difficulties, however, was that the surrogacy arrangement was made on a commercial basis with a total of €27,000 (£23,000) being paid to the surrogate mother. In this case the Court decided that the children's welfare required that they be regarded as lifelong members of the applicants' family and therefore decided to retrospectively authorise the payment and grant the parental order. The parental order was made on 5 November 2008.[150]

The judge stated, however, that this case should act as a precautionary tale to others considering entering into a surrogacy arrangement overseas. He also observed that this case has raised issues that highlight the wisdom of the Government reviewing the law on surrogacy.

As this case illustrates, entering into surrogacy arrangements in another country can be problematic. In some parts of the world, commercial surrogacy agencies are permitted and surrogacy arrangements are legally enforceable. UK women offering to be a surrogate mother in other jurisdictions must therefore be aware of their legal obligations, especially whether the contract can be legally enforced. Those considering entering into an arrangement with a surrogate in another country should seek specialist advice about their legal position and that of any children resulting from the arrangement. There are complicated legal questions about which jurisdiction should apply, who should be considered the legal parents of the resulting child and, when the intended parents are from the UK, whether the child is entitled to enter the UK, if born abroad, and become a UK citizen.[151]

In addition, these cases demonstrate the need to review the law. Although the previous Labour Government had the option of making fundamental changes to the law on surrogacy during its review of the Human Fertilisation and Embryology Act, it chose not to do so, making only minor changes in relation to non-commercial surrogacy agencies and updating the Parental Order Regulations.[152] A thorough review of the area is required to identify the problems and challenges that need to be addressed focussing on the practicalities and real-life cases rather than high level principles.

Society's ambivalence about surrogacy

The Government's apparent reluctance to get to grips with surrogacy perhaps reflects a general ambivalence within government and society about the practice of surrogacy.

In its 1987 White Paper, which preceded the 1990 Act, the Government stated explicitly that the 'legislation should not give any encouragement to the practice of surrogacy arranged privately or on a non-commercial basis'.[153] The very late introduction of parental orders in the 1990 Act, however, which made it easier for intended parents to transfer legal parentage from the surrogate mother, was widely regarded as formal, and perhaps overdue, acknowledgement of surrogacy as an acceptable treatment for infertility. Surrogacy's transition to mainstream practice, however, is far from complete and society and government's views about surrogacy remain ambivalent. In 1994, for example, guidance was issued to inform local authorities and health authorities about parental orders, which advised that: 'a local authority needs to make enquiries when it knows that a baby has been or is about to be born as a result of surrogacy so as to be satisfied that the baby is not, or will not be, at risk as a result of the arrangement'.[154] This guidance, which was in force until 2010, gave the clear message that the fact of a surrogacy arrangement is, in itself, sufficient justification to trigger enquiries by social services. So what is it about surrogacy that has led to this level of unease?

Undoubtedly, part of the problem for surrogacy, in its attempts to achieve legitimacy, stems from the rare but high-profile cases where the arrangement fails to work as planned – where there are public, and often legal, disputes about who should have the child. As a matter of public policy it has been decided that surrogacy arrangements should not be enforceable which means there is always the chance that a surrogate mother will change her mind and keep the child, or intended parents will decide not to take the child. This means that both parties are entirely dependent on the good will of the other parties involved and entering into a surrogacy arrangement, either as a surrogate mother or an intended parent, will always entail an element of risk.

Payment

Some of the concerns clearly arise from the commercial aspects of surrogacy. Although often presented as 'expenses', payments of £10–15,000 or more are said to be common, which is arguably more in line with women being paid a fee – effectively a wage – to carry a child for another person, which is controversial. It has been suggested, for example, that surrogacy 'seems to rank with prostitution' because it 'degrades an act which should surely be a reflection of love into a mere commercial transaction'.[155] Some people have also argued that surrogacy is equivalent to 'buying' a child and that there is no meaningful difference between paying for the inconvenience of pregnancy and paying for the baby itself. This contravenes the general belief in our society that children should not be viewed as commodities. Others argue that any payment reflects compensation for the risks and inconvenience of the altruistic act of carrying a child for 9 months and for giving birth.

Validity of consent

The offer of quite substantial sums of money also raises concerns about the validity of the consent obtained. It is, perhaps, not the offer of payment itself that could invalidate the consent but the balance between the size of the incentive offered and the risks involved. If the risks are high, but the incentives are also high, then individuals are more likely to be swayed towards an action they would otherwise not take. In order for consent to be valid, an individual needs to have sufficient information to make an informed decision. But with surrogacy, it is sometimes questioned whether a surrogate mother can ever be sufficiently informed about how she will feel about giving up the child she has carried for 9 months and given birth to, particularly if her own egg was used and the baby resembles her own children. This is a similar argument to that used by those who oppose egg sharing (see pages 334–336) where the counter-argument was made that informed adults who have capacity should be able to make their own decisions and do not need protecting by regulation that restricts their reproductive autonomy.

Exploitation

Closely bound up with the issue of payment is the question of exploitation. Although clear evidence is lacking, there is a perception that, apart from surrogacy involving family or friends, the vast majority of surrogate mothers are significantly poorer and less educated than intended parents. The idea of richer women paying a poorer woman to carry out this very intimate and personal service for them in itself raises concerns about exploitation and social justice. Research into surrogacy, however, and in particular the views of surrogate mothers, does not demonstrate that they feel exploited. In a 2003 study, for example, interviews were conducted with 34 women who had given birth to a surrogate child 1 year previously. The main findings are summarised below.

- Most (91 per cent) were motivated by wanting to help a childless couple and only one person said that payment was a motivating factor (although it has to be acknowledged that they may not have wanted to express that motivation in front of the interviewer).
- None of the women reported any doubts or difficulties with handing over the child.
- Relations with the intended parents were good both before and throughout the pregnancy.
- 35 per cent of women experienced some difficulties immediately after the handover but this reduced to 15 per cent after 3 months and to 6 per cent after 1 year. (Interestingly, the number of women still experiencing some difficulties after 1 year was significantly higher for those who were known surrogates – i.e. a friend or sister.[156])

An important question, in relation to claims of exploitation, is whether surrogate mothers who are motivated by the financial side of the arrangement have a genuine choice or whether they are forced by their financial circumstances, and lack of other options, to undertake a procedure that is risky – both physically and emotionally – against their better judgement. Denying people this option would not improve the financial pressures they are facing and would simply remove one option available to them.

Although exploitation is frequently linked with payment, it needs to be acknowledged that family and friends can feel exploited and can feel real pressure to agree to participate in a surrogacy arrangement.

Risk of psychological harm to all parties

Concerns have been raised about the risk of harm to all of the parties involved. There is a limited amount of research into the psychological consequences of surrogacy for surrogate mothers,[157] intended parents[158] and the children born.[159] What limited research there is, however, appears to be reassuring, suggesting that while problems can arise they are by no means inevitable.

Concepts of motherhood

Some of the concerns expressed about surrogacy are likely to be more fundamental, resting on the notion of a natural and intimate bond between mother and child that is challenged by surrogacy arrangements. In the past when women had less control over their fertility, it was not unusual for children to be given away for adoption or to be brought up by other family members. Now, people have fewer children and, arguably, invest more heavily in them. Surrogacy challenges the traditional view of motherhood and the notion of a natural bond between mother and baby: the idea that a woman can go through a pregnancy and give birth intending to give away the child undermines traditional notions of maternal instinct and appropriate maternal behaviour. For some people surrogacy seems to go against the natural order in a way that is troubling and difficult to comprehend.

The legacy of informal surrogacy

It is also possible that the low-tech nature of some forms of surrogacy (self-insemination), which one might expect would be in its favour, might actually go some way to explaining some of the negative perceptions of the practice. So does surrogacy need to move over more into the medical arena in order to achieve respectability? Although there may be some advantages to such a move, in terms of the reduced risk of infection and the availability of counselling, some people may be unwilling to go through the expense, delay and inconvenience of 'medicalising' the arrangement. It also risks the establishment of a two-tier system with a regulated system for those who choose to go through the 'approved' route of medical involvement and an unregulated, and increasingly hidden, system for those who choose to go it alone.

The doctor's duties in the surrogacy arrangement

Whatever societal messages are given about the acceptability or otherwise of surrogacy arrangements, it is, nevertheless, the case that nowadays there is far less secrecy about the practice and far more medical involvement. This means that doctors are increasingly being asked for advice about, or help with, surrogacy arrangements and need to be aware of their own duties and responsibilities. Doctors have different responsibilities depending on the level of their involvement with the surrogacy arrangement. Once a surrogate pregnancy has been established, the practitioner's ethical obligations to the surrogate mother and child are no different from those owed to any other pregnant woman, although additional emotional support may be required. The duty of the healthcare team is to provide the appropriate level of support and guidance, both during and after the pregnancy.

Practitioners approached for advice by people considering self-insemination should encourage those concerned to consider the issues and implications very carefully and should ensure that they are aware of how to obtain accurate information about the medical, psychological, emotional and legal issues involved with surrogacy. They should also actively encourage those considering surrogacy to seek counselling and testing for infectious diseases. The responsibilities are greatest for those who are providing licensed treatment services aimed at establishing a surrogate pregnancy through IVF or DI. In such cases, the healthcare team must take all reasonable steps to ensure that all relevant issues have been carefully considered. Where there is professional involvement in the treatment, it can be provided only in clinics licensed by the HFEA and in compliance with the HFEA's *Code of Practice*. This includes storing sperm and embryos for a 6-month quarantine period, as well as taking account of the range of factors associated with the welfare of the child (see pages 319–323) for both the intended parents and the surrogate mother and her partner because either couple could eventually be caring for the child.

Summary – surrogacy

- The BMA considers surrogacy to be an acceptable option of last resort in cases where it is impossible or highly undesirable for medical reasons for the intended mother to carry a child herself.
- The law on surrogacy needs to be reviewed.
- Doctors' responsibilities vary depending on the extent to which they are involved with initiating a pregnancy.
- Once a surrogate pregnancy has been established, the doctor's ethical obligations to the surrogate mother and the child are no different from those owed to any other pregnant woman, although more support may be required.
- Practitioners approached for advice by those planning self-insemination should encourage those concerned to consider the issues and implications carefully, ensure they know how to obtain accurate information and encourage them to seek counselling and testing for infectious diseases.
- Doctors providing IVF or DI as part of a surrogacy arrangement must have a licence from the HFEA and follow the HFEA's *Code of Practice*.

Seeking treatment in other countries

It has always been possible for people to travel to other countries to receive treatment that is either not available or is more expensive in their home country. As a result of the strict regulatory mechanism in the UK, reproduction is one area where this has been a particular issue. Common reasons for people seeking cross-border care include easier and quicker access to donor oocytes (often from paid and/or anonymous donors), access to PGD to determine the sex of a future child for social reasons and those wishing to use the services of a commercial surrogacy agency, either as intended parents or as a surrogate mother. In March 2010, the results of the first study to estimate the extent of this practice were published.[160] Data were collected from 46 centres in six European countries (Belgium, the Czech Republic, Denmark, Slovenia, Spain and Switzerland). For a period of 1 month the clinics collected information from all overseas patients including their country of origin and their reason for seeking treatment abroad. Over the month 1,230 forms were completed (53 relating to patients from the UK), leading to estimates that 24–30,000 cross-border treatment cycles may be carried out each year. The main reason given for seeking treatment abroad was to avoid legal restrictions at home (a large number of patients were Italians seeking treatment in Spain following very restrictive legislation passed in 2004). Of the UK patients, 34 per cent cited access problems as their main reason for travelling abroad. More than 60 per cent of the women from the UK were over 40 and the shortage of donor eggs in the UK prompted many women to travel to Spain and Slovakia where donors are paid for inconvienience and eggs are more readily available. Given the high number of patients travelling overseas, the HFEA has produced specific information to advise those considering this option of the risks and the type of questions to ask when choosing a clinic.[161]

It is not unlawful for patients from the UK to go abroad for procedures that are unavailable or prohibited here (although there may be legal consequences – see, for example, page 351). Nor is it unlawful for doctors to promote, facilitate or participate in such treatment. If individuals are aware of the possible legal complexities and, where appropriate, any additional risks of seeking treatment elsewhere, it is a matter for them alone to decide whether to seek procedures that are not permitted in the UK. When licensed clinics are involved in facilitating or providing the treatment, however, there are legitimate questions about whether doctors have a responsibility to abide not only by the letter of the law, but also by the spirit of the legislation.

Those who take the view that clinics should abide by the 'spirit and essence' of the law, and therefore not help their patients to get around legal restrictions in the UK, make the following arguments.

- The Human Fertilisation and Embryology Act and the HFEA were intended to provide a comprehensive legal and ethical framework within which clinics in the UK should operate. This framework takes account of the social and cultural values, of public opinion and of accepted ethical standards within our society.
- In a shared care scenario, where most of the treatment takes place in the UK with the patient going overseas just for the part of the treatment that is prohibited in the UK, the clinic is acting outside this agreed and established ethical framework and, although not breaking the law, is providing treatment that is unlawful in the UK through a UK clinic.
- Such practices can be seen as a deliberate attempt to exploit a 'legal loophole' which could undermine confidence in the regulatory mechanism and in those providing the service.
- Those who choose to work in the UK and within the regulatory system have some responsibility to ensure that all of their work falls within the scope of what is legally permitted in the UK. Finding ways around the legal restrictions – by undertaking part of the treatment in a different country – has been described as representing 'flagrant disrespect and disregard' for both the regulatory body and 'the socio-cultural and ethical values of their home country.'[162]
- UK clinics benefit from the kudos and respectability they gain by being licensed by the HFEA yet some are acting outside the established moral framework.

Those who take the opposite view argue along the lines summarised below.

- Such practices are not unlawful. The Act regulates activities that take place within the UK and cannot place any restrictions on activities that take place in other countries.
- Parliament had the option of making such practices unlawful by adding an offence of 'aiding and abetting' to the legislation for example (as with assisted suicide), or making it unlawful for someone to take steps in this country to facilitate an activity whether the actual procedures takes place in this country or overseas (as it has done with the sale of organs or female genital mutilation) but it chose not to do so. When the law was reviewed and updated in 2008 there were no attempts to address this issue through legislation. The Science and Technology Committee report on human reproductive technologies, published in 2005, touched upon 'reproductive tourism' generally and concluded that attempts to curtail this practice 'would not be justified by the seriousness of the offence'.[163] In its 2005 review of the Act the Government supported this finding, arguing that attempts to control 'reproductive tourism' would be 'extremely difficult and probably not justified'.[164] (Neither report, however, clearly differentiated between patients themselves going overseas for treatment and licensed clinics providing them with assistance to do so.)
- Provided they are not breaking the law, those who are providing the service should be guided by their own conscience and views about what is, and is not, acceptable and what represents the best option for their patients. If the patient and those working in

the clinic do not personally believe that paying egg donors for their inconvenience is unacceptable, and both consider that going overseas is a better option than waiting for a donor to become available in the UK, then why should clinics not assist? Arguably, it is better for the clinic to refer to an establishment they know will provide a high quality service, or to be directly involved in the treatment themselves, than to expect the patient to find a clinic in another country where it may be more difficult to assess the quality of the service provided.

- If it is acceptable for clinics to accept referrals, and shared-care arrangements, from other countries that are made specifically to avoid legal restrictions in those jurisdictions, such as referrals for abortion from Ireland, for gamete donation from Italy or PGD from Germany, then why should UK clinics not help their patients to do the same? The reason such approaches would probably not be considered morally objectionable is that the procedures or activities they are seeking are lawful in the UK and are within the ethical framework that operates in the UK. So, perhaps the acceptability of such arrangements depends on the nature of the procedure itself and just how acceptable or 'unacceptable' society considers it to be. The type of procedures people usually seek overseas – paid and anonymous donation or sex selection for social reasons – are ones of which it can be said that the arguments for and against are finely balanced with reasonable people and reasonable arguments on either side of the debate. Would or should society, and the regulatory body, take a more restrictive approach if the procedures being sought were risky and unproven – such as reproductive cloning or the use of artificial gametes in treatment?

The HFEA sought legal advice about what, if any, powers it had to regulate the activities of those UK-licensed clinics that refer patients to clinics overseas or participate in shared-care arrangements. The advice was clear that the HFEA has 'little or no' remit over these matters and is therefore unable to intervene. It has, however, made clear that clinics should provide information to patients considering this option, about the advantages and disadvantages of going down this route.[165]

A law for the twenty-first century?

Some of the current hot topics in the field of assisted reproduction – such as anonymity and payment of gamete donors – have been the subject of debate since the 1980s and continue to elicit strong and conflicting views. Other issues, such as some of the possibilities and implications of PGD are new, based on new technologies and greater understanding of the genetic components of disease. Inevitably, as new techniques and possibilities develop, new ethical dilemmas and controversies will emerge. The Human Fertilisation and Embryology Act 1990 was in force for nearly two decades before being substantially revised and updated. During the review of the Act in 2008, attempts were made to 'future proof' the legislation by looking ahead to future developments. Only time will tell how successful these attempts have been.

References

1 Human Fertilisation and Embryology Authority (2008) *Long term trends in fertility treatment – birth rate*s. Available at: www.hfea.gov.uk (accessed 16 February 2011).
2 Human Fertilisation and Embryology Authority (2010) *Fertility Facts and Figures 2008*. Available at: www.hfea.gov.uk (accessed 16 February 2011).

3   Committee of Inquiry into Human Fertilisation and Embryology (1984) *Report of the Committee of Inquiry into Human Fertilisation and Embryology (Cmnd 9314)*, HMSO, London.

4   Committee of Inquiry into Human Fertilisation and Embryology (1984) *Report of the Committee of Inquiry into Human Fertilisation and Embryology (Cmnd 9314)*, HMSO, London, p.4.

5   Human Fertilisation and Embryology (Quality and Standards) Regulations 2007. SI 2007/1522.

6   European Parliament Council of the European Union (2004) Directive 2004/23/EC of the European Parliament and of the Council of 31 March 2004 on setting standards of quality and safety for the donation, procurement, testing, processing, preservation, storage and distribution of human tissues and cells. *Official J European Union*, **L102**, 48–58.

7   Anon. (2010) Suspended jail term for illegal sperm website pair. *BBC News Online* (12 October). Available at: www.bbc.co.uk/news (accessed 16 February 2011).

8   Human Fertilisation and Embryology Authority (2009) *Code of Practice*, 8th edn, HFEA, London.

9   Department of Health (2010) *Liberating the NHS. Report of the arms-length bodies review*, London, DH.

10 Human Fertilisation and Embryology Authority (2008) *Long term trends in fertility treatment: embryo transfer and multiple births*. Available at: www.hfea.gov.uk (accessed 16 February 2011).

11 *R (on the application of ARGC and H) v HFEA* [2003] 1 FCR 266.

12 Braude P. (2006) *One child at a time: reducing multiple births after IVF*, HFEA, London.

13 Braude P. (2006) *One child at a time: reducing multiple births after IVF*, HFEA, London, p.3.

14 Khalaf Y, El-Toukhy T, Coomarasamy A. *et al*. (2008) Selective single blastocyst transfer reduces the multiple pregnancy rate and increases pregnancy rates: a pre- and postintervention study. *B J Obstet Gynaecol* **115**, 385–90.

15 McLernon DJ, Harrild K, Bergh C. *et al*. (2010) Clinical effectiveness of elective single versus double embryo transfer: meta-analysis of individual patient data from randomised trials. *BMJ* **341**, c6945.

16 Human Fertilisation and Embryology Authority (2008) *Directions given under the Human Fertilisation and Embryology Act 1990: Multiple Births Minimisation Strategy (Ref: D.2008/5)*, HFEA, London.

17 Human Fertilisation and Embryology Authority (2009) *Authority Paper No 527: Multiple Births: Moving Towards a Year 2 Target* (9 December), HFEA, London.

18 Human Fertilisation and Embryology Authority (2010) *Letter to UK fertility clinics: from Mr Nick Jones, Director of Compliance, HFEA* (10 November), HFEA, London.

19 Human Fertilisation and Embryology Authority (2009) *HFEA statement on the risk of birth defects associated with assisted reproductive technology*. Press Release, 24 March.

20 Medical Research Council (2004) *Assisted Reproduction: a safe, sound future*, MRC, London.

21 Human Fertilisation and Embryology (Disclosure of Information for Research Purposes) Regulations 2010. SI 2010/995.

22 Human Fertilisation and Embryology Authority (2010) *F-2010-00205 – IVF patients and subsequent cancers* (27 September). Available at: www.hfea.gov.uk (accessed 16 February 2011).

23 Human Fertilisation and Embryology Authority (2010) *F-2010-00175 – Women consenting to research with identifiers* (17 August). Available at: www.hfea.gov.uk (accessed 16 February 2011).

24 *R v Secretary of State for the Home Department, ex parte Mellor* [2001] 2 FLR 1158.

25 *Dickson v United Kingdom* (2008) 46 EHRR 41.

26 Havers P. (2002) The impact of the European Convention on Human Rights on medical law. *Med Leg J* **70**(2), 57–70.

27 McIlwraith G, McGivern M. (2009) Lesbian couple sue NHS for refusing them IVF. *Daily Record* (February 27). Available at: www.dailyrecord.co.uk (accessed 9 May 2011).

28 Anon. (2009) Lesbian couple win fertility bid. *BBC News Online* (27 February). Available at: www.bbc.co.uk/news (accessed 17 February 2011).

29 Templeton S. (2009) Lesbian couple win fight for IVF on the NHS. *The Sunday Times* (19 July). Available at: www.thesundaytimes.co.uk (accessed 9 May 2011).

30 Equality and Human Rights Commission. *Your rights: sexual orientation*. Available at: www.equalityhumanrights.com (accessed 17 February 2011).

31 National Institute for Health and Clinical Excellence (2004) *CG11 – Fertility: assessment and treatment for people with fertility problems*, NICE, London.

32 Beckford M. (2010) Anne Milton MP: Health bodies shouldn't cut IVF funding. *The Telegraph* (9 February). Available at: www.telegraph.co.uk (accessed 9 May 2011).

33 Expert Group on Commissioning NHS Infertility Provision (2009) *Regulated Fertility Services: a commissioning aid*, DH, London.

34 Expert Group on Commissioning NHS Infertility Provision (2009) *Regulated Fertility Services: a commissioning aid*, DH, London, p.5.

35 National Institute for Health and Clinical Excellence (2010) *Nice outlines review of fertility guideline*. Press release, 6 October.

36 Scottish Executive Health Department (2007) *Report of the review of infertility services in Scotland*, SEHD, Edinburgh.

37 National Infertility Awareness Campaign. *NIAC Key Messages: Wales.* Available at: www.infertilitynetworkuk.com (accessed 16 February 2011).

38 Infertility Network UK. *Current criteria for access to fertility treatment in Northern Ireland.* Available at: www.infertilitynetworkuk.com (accessed 16 February 2011).

39 Human Fertilisation and Embryology Act 1990 (as amended), s13(5).

40 Harris J (1998) *Clones, genes, and immortality*, Oxford University Press, Oxford, pp. 92–7.

41 Human Fertilisation and Embryology Authority (2003) *Code of Practice*, 6th edn, HFEA, London, paras 3.11–3.24.

42 Human Fertilisation and Embryology Authority (2009) *Code of Practice*, 8th edn, HFEA, London, para 8.3.

43 Human Fertilisation and Embryology Authority (2009) *Code of Practice*, 8th edn, HFEA, London, para 8.10.

44 Human Fertilisation and Embryology Act 1990, s13(5).

45 British Medical Association (2008) *Parliamentary Brief. Human Fertilisation and Embryology Bill. Report Stage, House of Lords, 21 January 2008*, BMA, London.

46 Human Fertilisation and Embryology Authority (2009) *Code of Practice*, 8th edn, HFEA, London, para 8.11.

47 Civil Partnership Act 2004.

48 Ramesh R. (2009) The world's oldest mother. *The Guardian* (6 March). Available at: www .guardian.co.uk (accessed 9 May 2011).

49 Information received on 14 April 2010 from the Human Fertilisation and Embryology Authority under a Freedom of Information request: 121 women aged 51 years of age and over received treatment with donor eggs between 1 April 2004 and 31 March 2009.

50 Murray C, Golombok S. (2005) Solo mothers and their donor insemination infants: follow-up at age 2 years. *Hum Reprod* **20**(6), 1655–60.

51 Murray C, Golombok S. (2005) Solo mothers and their donor insemination infants: follow-up at age 2 years. *Hum Reprod* **20**(6), 1655–60. Murray C, Golombok S. (2005) Going it alone: solo mothers and their infants conceived by donor insemination. *Am J Orthopsychiatry* **75**(2), 242–53.

52 Brewaeys A, Ponjaert I, van Hall E. *et al.* (1997) Donor insemination: child development and family functioning in lesbian mother families. *Hum Reprod* **12**(6), 1349–59.

53 Jackson E. (2010) *Medical Law: Text, cases and materials*, 2nd edn, Oxford University Press, Oxford, pp. 791–8.

54 Human Fertilisation and Embryology Authority (2009) *Code of Practice*, 8th edn, HFEA, London, para 8.13.

55 Human Fertilisation and Embryology Authority (2009) *Code of Practice*, 8th edn, HFEA, London, para 8.13.

56 Human Fertilisation and Embryology Authority (2000) *Ninth annual report and accounts 2000*, HFEA, London, p.28.

57 Human Fertilisation and Embryology Authority (2009) *Code of Practice*, 8th edn, HFEA, London, para 10.13.

58 Human Fertilisation and Embryology (Statutory Storage Period for Embryos and Gametes) Regulations 2009. SI 2009/1582.

59 *R v Human Fertilisation and Embryology Authority, ex parte Blood* [1997] 2 All ER 687.

60 McLean SAM. (1997) *Consent and the law: review of the current provisions in the Human Fertilisation and Embryology Act 1990 for the UK Health Ministers*, Department of Health, London.

61 *L v Human Fertilisation and Embryology Authority and the Secretary of State for Health* [2008] 2 FLR 1999.

62 Human Fertilisation and Embryology Authority (2008) *Note of the judgment – L v (1) HFEA and (2) Department of Health.* Available at: www.hfea.gov.uk (accessed 17 February 2011).

63 The BMA attempted to find out the outcome of the application for export under a Freedom of Information request to the Human Fertilisation and Embryology Authority (HFEA). On 20 April 2010 the HFEA replied stating that the application for export had been decided by the HFEA's Regulation Committee but the committee minutes contained personal information regarding the individual concerned and were therefore withheld under section 40 of the Freedom of Information Act.

64 Rozenberg J. (2003) Diane Blood wins fight over husband's name. *The Telegraph* (1 March). Available at: www.telegraph.co.uk (accessed 9 May 2011).

65 *Evans v Amicus Healthcare Ltd and Others* [2004] 1 FLR 67. *Evans v Amicus Healthcare Ltd and Others* [2004] 2 FLR 766.

66 *Evans v The United Kingdom* (6339/05) [2006] ECHR 200 (7 March 2006).

67 *Evans v The United Kingdom* (6339/05) [2007] ECHR 264 (10 April 2007).

68 Grayling AC. (2003) Embryo case. *Evening Standard* (2 October).

69 Harris J. (2006) Head to head: frozen embryos. *BBC News Online* (7 March). Available at: www .bbc.co.uk/news (accessed 18 February 2011).

70 Draper H. (2007) Gametes, consent and points of no return. *Human Fertility* **10**(2), 105–9.

71 Leather S. (2003) *Withdrawal of consent to storage CH(03)03*, HFEA, London.

72 Human Fertilisation and Embryology Act 1990 (as amended), Sch. 3, para 4A.

73 Human Fertilisation and Embryology Act 1990 (as amended), s13(6C).

74 Golombok S, Murray C, Jadva V. *et al*. (2006) Non-genetic and non-gestational parenthood: consequences for parent–child relationships and the psychological well-being of mothers, fathers and children at age 3. *Hum Reprod* **21**(7), 1918–24.

75 Golombok S, Brewaeys A, Cook R. *et al*. (1996) The European study of assisted reproduction families. *Hum Reprod* **11**(10), 2324–31.

76 Golombok S, Brewaeys A, Giavazzi MT. *et al*. (2002) The European study of assisted reproduction families: the transition to adolescence. *Hum Reprod* **17**(3), 830–40.

77 Golombok S, Murray C, Jadva V. *et al*. (2006) Non-genetic and non-gestational parenthood: consequences for parent-child relationships and the psychological well-being of mothers, fathers and children at age 3. *Hum Reprod* **21**(7), 1918–24.

78 Turner AJ, Coyle A. (2000) What does it mean to be a donor offspring? The identity experiences of adults conceived by donor insemination and the implications for counselling and therapy. *Hum Reprod* **15**(9), 2041–51.

79 McWhinnie A. (2001) Gamete donation and anonymity: should offspring from donated gametes continue to be denied knowledge of their origins and antecedents? *Hum Reprod* **16**(5), 807–17.

80 Jadva V, Freeman T, Kramer W. *et al*. (2009) The experiences of adolescents and adults conceived by sperm donation: comparisons by age of disclosure and family type. *Hum Reprod* **24**(8), 1909–19.

81 Golombok S, Murray C, Jadva V. *et al*. (2006) Non-genetic and non-gestational parenthood: consequences for parent–child relationships and the psychological well-being of mothers, fathers and children at age 3. *Hum Reprod* **21**(7), 1918–24.

82 MacCallum F, Golombok S. (2007) Embryo donation families: mothers' decisions regarding disclosure of donor conception. *Hum Reprod* **22**(11), 2888–95.

83 Lycett E, Daniels K, Curson R. *et al*. (2005) School-aged children of donor insemination: a study of parents' disclosure patterns. *Hum Reprod* **20**(3), 810–19. Lalos A, Gottlieb C, Lalos O. (2007) Legislated right for donor-insemination children to know their genetic origin: a study of parental thinking. *Hum Reprod* **22**(6), 1759–68.

84 Crawshaw M. (2008) Prospective parents' intentions regarding disclosure following the removal of donor anonymity. *Human Fertility* **11**(2), 95–100.

85 Gottlieb C, Lalos O, Lindblad F. (2000) Disclosure of donor insemination to the child: the impact of the Swedish legislation on couples' attitudes. *Hum Reprod* **15**(9), 2052–6.

86 Lalos A, Gottlieb C, Lalos O. (2007) Legislated right for donor-insemination children to know their genetic origin: a study of parental thinking. *Hum Reprod* **22**(6), 1759–68.

87 Human Fertilisation and Embryology (Disclosure of Donor Information) Regulations 2004. SI 2004/1511.

88 Daniels K, Ericsson HI, Burn IP. (1998) The views of semen donors regarding the Swedish Insemination Act 1984. *Medical Law International* **3**, 117–34.

89 Human Fertilisation and Embryology Authority (2007) *A long-term analysis of the Human Fertilisation and Embryology Authority register data 1991–2006*, table 5. Available at: www.hfea.gov.uk (accessed 18 February 2011).

90 Human Fertilisation and Embryology Authority *Facts and figures for researchers and the media – donor statistics*. Available at: www.hfea.gov.uk (accessed 18 February 2011).

91 Human Fertilisation and Embryology Authority *Facts and figures for researchers and the media – donor statistics*. Available at: www.hfea.gov.uk (accessed 18 February 2011).

92 Human Fertilisation and Embryology Authority (2011) *Donating sperm and eggs. Have your say – donation trends*. Available at: www.hfea.gov.uk (accessed 18 April 2011).

93 *Rose v Secretary of State for Health and Human Fertilisation and Embryology Authority* [2002] 2 FLR 962; 964–5.

94 Human Fertilisation and Embryology Authority (1991) *Directions given under the Human Fertilisation and Embryology Act 1990. Giving and receiving money or other benefits in respect of any supply of gametes or embryos (D.1991/2)*, HFEA, London.

95 Human Fertilisation and Embryology Authority (1993) *Second annual report 1993*, HFEA, London, p.29.

96 Human Fertilisation and Embryology Authority (1996) *Fifth annual report 1996*, HFEA, London, p.23.

97 Human Fertilisation and Embryology Authority (1998) *Implementation of withdrawal of payment to donors*, HFEA, London.

98 Human Fertilisation and Embryology Authority (1998) *Directions given under the Human Fertilisation and Embryology Act 1990. Giving and receiving money or other benefits in respect of any supply of gametes or embryos (D.1998/1)*, HFEA, London.

99   Human Fertilisation and Embryology Authority (2006) *Directions given under the Human Fertilisation and Embryology Act 1990. Giving and receiving money or other benefits in respect of any supply of gametes or embryos (D.2006/1)*, HFEA, London.

100 Human Fertilisation and Embryology Authority (2011) *Donating sperm and eggs. Have your say*. Available at: www.hfea.gov.uk (accessed 18 April 2011).

101 European Parliament Council of the European Union (2004) Directive 2004/23/EC of the European Parliament and of the Council of 31 March 2004 on setting standards of quality and safety for the donation, procurement, testing, processing, preservation, storage and distribution of human tissues and cells. *Official J European Union* **L102**, 48–58.

102 Simons EG, Ahuja KK. (2005) Egg sharing: an evidence based solution to donor egg shortages. *Obstet Gynaecol* **7**, 112–6.

103 Blyth E. (2002) Subsidized IVF: the development of 'egg sharing' in the United Kingdom. *Hum Reprod* **17**(12), 3254–9.

104 Human Fertilisation and Embryology Authority (2000) *Ninth annual report and accounts 2000*, HFEA, London, p.28.

105 Human Fertilisation and Embryology Authority (2009) *Code of Practice*, 8th edn, HFEA, London, para 12.20.

106 Human Fertilisation and Embryology Authority (2009) *Code of Practice*, 8th edn, HFEA, London, para 12.5.

107 Human Fertilisation and Embryology Authority (2006) *Directions given under the Human Fertilisation and Embryology Act 1990: Giving and receiving money or other benefits in respect of any supply of gametes or embryos (D.2006/1)*, HFEA, London.

108 Lewis-Jones C. (2006) *Results of an on-line survey performed in 2006 by Infertility Network UK of egg sharers and recipients*. Available at: www.infertilitynetworkuk.com (accessed 18 April 2011).

109 Braude P, Flinter F. (2007) Use and misuse of preimplantation genetic testing. *BMJ* **335**, 752–4.

110 Human Fertilisation and Embryology Act 1990, Sch 2, para 1(1)(d).

111 Human Fertilisation and Embryology Authority (2005) *Choices and Boundaries: should people be able to select embryos free from an inherited susceptibility to cancer?* HFEA, London.

112 Human Fertilisation and Embryology Act 1990 (as amended), Sch 2, para 1ZA(1).

113 Human Fertilisation and Embryology Act 1990 (as amended), Sch 2, para 1ZA(2).

114 Human Fertilisation and Embryology Authority (2009) *Code of Practice*, 8th edn, HFEA, London, para 10.6.

115 Human Fertilisation and Embryology Authority (2009) *Code of Practice*, 8th edn, HFEA, London, box 10C.

116 Renwick P, Trussler J, Lashwood A. *et al*. (2010) Preimplantation genetic haplotyping: 127 diagnostic cycles demonstrating a robust, efficient alternative to direct mutation testing on single cells. *RMB Online* **20**(4), 470–6.

117 Handyside A, Harton G, Mariani B. *et al*. (2010) Karyomapping: a universal method for genome wide analysis of genetic disease based on mapping crossovers between parental haplotypes. *J Med Genet* **47**, 651–8.

118 Asscher E, Koops B-J. (2010) The right not to know and preimplantation genetic diagnosis for Huntington's disease. *J Med Ethics* **36**, 30–3.

119 Human Fertilisation and Embryology Authority (2009) *Code of Practice*, 8th edn (updated April 2010), HFEA, London, para 10.7–10.9.

120 Human Fertilisation and Embryology Authority (2008) *The Scientific and Clinical Advances Group: Preimplantation genetic screening* (SCAG (02/08)01), 21 February. Available at: www.hfea.gov.uk (accessed 22 February 2011). Human Fertilisation and Embryology Authority (2009) *Code of Practice*, 8th edn, HFEA, London, section 9, para T89.

121 Braude P, Flinter F. (2007) Use and misuse of preimplantation genetic testing. *BMJ* **335**, 752–4, p.753.

122 Human Fertilisation and Embryology Authority (2009) *Code of Practice*, 8th edn, HFEA, London, section 9, para T89.

123 Schoolcraft W, Fragouli E, Stevens J. *et al*. (2010) Clinical application of comprehensive chromosomal screening at the blastocyst stage. *Fertil Steril* **94**(5), 1700–6.

124 Human Fertilisation and Embryology Authority (2002) *HFEA confirms that HLA tissue typing may only take place when PGD is required to avoid a serious genetic disorder*. Press Release, August 01.

125 House of Commons Science and Technology Committee (2002) *Developments in human genetics and embryology. Fourth report of session 2001–02*. (HC 791), The Stationery Office, London, para 25.

126 Dyer C. (2002) Watchdog approves embryo selection to treat 3 year old child. *BMJ* **324**, 503.

127 Human Fertilisation and Embryology Authority (2002) *HFEA confirms that HLA tissue typing may only take place when preimplantation genetic diagnosis is required to avoid a serious genetic disorder*. Press release, August 01.

128 Anon. (2005) Charlie Whitaker cured by 'saviour sibling'. *BioNews* (22 August). Available at: www.bionews.org.uk (accessed 18 April 2011).

129 *Quintavalle v Human Fertilisation and Embryology Authority* [2003] 2 All ER 105.

130 *Quintavalle v Human Fertilisation and Embryology Authority CA* [2003] 3 All ER 257: 270.

131 *Quintavalle (on behalf of Comment on Reproductive Ethics) v Human Fertilisation and Embryology Authority* [2005] 1 WLR 1061.

132 Human Fertilisation and Embryology Authority (2004) *HFEA agrees to extend policy on tissue typing*. Press release, July 21.

133 Human Fertilisation and Embryology Act 1990 (as amended), Sch 2, para 1ZA(1)(d).

134 Human Fertilisation and Embryology Act 1990, s13(5).

135 Gillon R. (1999) Human reproductive cloning: a look at the arguments against it and a rejection of most of them. *J R Soc Med* **92**, 3–12.

136 Human Fertilisation and Embryology Act 1990 (as amended), Sch 2, para 1ZA(1)(c).

137 Seenan G. (2001) 'Designer baby' parents give away male embryo. *The Guardian* (5 March). Available at: www.guardian.co.uk (accessed 9 May 2011).

138 Corrado M, Collao K (MORI) (2003) *Sex selection: public consultation. Research conducted for Human Fertilisation and Embryology Authority*, HFEA, London.

139 Human Fertilisation and Embryology Authority (2003) *Sex selection: options for regulation. A report on the HFEA's 2002–03 review of sex selection including a discussion of legislative and regulatory options*, HFEA, London.

140 House of Commons Science and Technology Committee (2005) *Human Reproductive Technologies and the Law. Fifth Report of Session 2004–05*, Vol. 1 (HC 7-1), The Stationery Office, London, para 142.

141 Human Fertilisation and Embryology Act 1990 (as amended), Sch 2, para 1ZB.

142 Dahl E, Hinsch K, Beutel M. *et al*. (2003) Preconception sex selection for non-medical reasons: a representative survey from the UK. *Hum Reprod* **18**(10), 2238–9.

143 Culley L. (2005) Memorandum from Dr Lorraine Culley, De Montford University. In: House of Commons Science and Technology Committee. *Human Reproductive Technologies and the Law. Fifth Report of Session 2004-05*, Vol. 2 (HC 7-II), The Stationery Office, London, Ev 351–5, p.Ev 352.

144 British Medical Association (1990) *Surrogacy: ethical considerations*, BMA, London.

145 British Medical Association (1996) *Changing conceptions of motherhood: the practice of surrogacy in Britain*, BMA, London, p.2.

146 Brazier M, Campbell A, Golombok S. (1998) *Surrogacy. Review for health ministers of current arrangements for payments and regulation. Report of the review team*, The Stationery Office, London.

147 *Re G (surrogacy: foreign domicile)* [2007] EWHC 2814 (Fam).

148 *Re N (a child)* [2007] EWCA Civ 1053: para 12.

149 *Re N (a child)* [2007] EWCA Civ 1053: para 4.

150 *Re X & Y (foreign surrogacy)* [2009] 1 FLR 733.

151 Gamble N. (2009) Crossing the line: the legal and ethical problems of foreign surrogacy. *RMB Online* **19**(2), 151–2. *Re X & Y (foreign surrogacy)* [2009] 1 FLR 733.

152 The Human Fertilisation and Embryology (Parental Orders) Regulations 2010. SI 2010/985.

153 Department of Health and Social Security (1987) *Human Fertilisation and Embryology: A Framework for Legislation (Cmnd) 259*, HMSO, London, para 73.

154 Department of Health (1994) *Local Authority Circular (LAC (94) 25). Human Fertilisation and Embryology Act 1990. Parental Orders (Human Fertilisation and Embryology) Regulations 1994: Powers and Duties of Local Authorities, Health Authorities and Guardians Ad Litem*, DH, London, para 3.

155 Deech R, Smajdor A. (2007) *From IVF to Immortality: controversy in the era of reproductive technology*, Oxford University Press, Oxford, p.160.

156 Jadva V, Murray C, Lycett E. *et al*. (2003) Surrogacy: the experiences of surrogate mothers. *Hum Reprod* **18**(10), 2196–204.

157 Jadva V, Murray C, Lycett E. *et al*. (2003) Surrogacy: the experiences of surrogate mothers. *Hum Reprod* **18**(10), 2196–204.

158 MacCallum F, Lycett E, Murray C. *et al*. (2003) Surrogacy: the experience of commissioning couples. *Hum Reprod* **18**(6), 1334–42.

159 Golombok S, Murray C, Jadva V. *et al*. (2006) Non-genetic and non-gestational parenthood: consequences for parent-child relationships and the psychological well-being of mothers, fathers and children at age 3. *Hum Reprod* **21**(7), 1918–24.

160 Shenfield F, de Mouzon J, Pennings G. *et al*.; ESHRE Taskforce on Cross Border Reproductive Care (2010) Cross border reproductive care in six European countries. *Hum Reprod* **25**(6), 1361–8.

161 Human Fertilisation and Embryology Authority. *Considering fertility treatment abroad: issues and risks*. Available at: www.hfea.gov.uk (accessed 1 March 2011).

162 Heng BC. (2006) 'Reproductive tourism': should locally registered fertility doctors be held accountable for channelling patients to foreign medical establishments? *Hum Reprod* **21**(3), 840–2, p.841.

163 House of Commons Science and Technology Committee (2005) *Human Reproductive Technologies and the Law. Fifth Report of Session 2004–05*, Vol. 1 (HC 7-1), The Stationery Office, London, p.166.

164 Department of Health (2005) *Review of the Human Fertilisation and Embryology Act: a public consultation*, DH, London, para 2.60.

165 Human Fertilisation and Embryology Authority (2010) *Chief Executive's Letter: Cross border reproductive care: clinics' and HFEA's responsibilities*, CE (10) 03, HFEA, London.

9: Genetics

The questions covered in this chapter include the following.

- Does genetics raise different ethical issues?
- To what extent can genetic information be shared with relatives for whom it has personal relevance?
- Should children be tested at the request of their parents?
- Should incidental findings be disclosed?
- What is the role of health professionals when patients request paternity testing?
- What safeguards should be in place for direct-to-consumer tests?

The impact of developments in genetics

The field of human genetics has been characterised by rapid and spectacular advances in knowledge. For some it represents the panacea that will revolutionise medicine, with gene chip technology, individualised treatment regimens and the ability not only to predict, but also to avoid or cure most diseases. For others, optimism about the inevitable health benefits is counter-balanced by fears about the potential for genetic knowledge to be abused, or is moderated by an appreciation of the limits to what is feasible. Media reports of developments in genetics – such as positive research findings in relation to gene therapy (see pages 405–406) or the potential of new areas of enquiry such as epigenetics (see pages 404–405) frequently lead to vastly unrealistic expectations of new treatments or understanding of the causes of disease or behaviour. A balance is needed between keeping the public informed of important developments, in order to increase public understanding and confidence, and ensuring that this does not promote misplaced optimism among those affected by genetic conditions or inappropriate and unnecessary concerns. Where concerns are raised, they need to be assessed and kept under review. Concerns have been voiced, for example, that genetics will give an unwelcome boost to our almost obsessive striving for perfection and that it signals a rejection of disability (to the detriment of those living with disability). There is also concern that with increasing genetic information becoming available, for example through whole genome sequencing (see page 404), and the potential uses of genetic information by employers (see page 398) and insurance companies (see pages 396–398), new areas of discrimination will develop.

Although there have been major advances in genetic technology, the practical impact on the population, and on most health professionals, has been small. The considerable advances in scientific knowledge have not yet been translated into new products, tests or treatments with the potential to 'revolutionise medicine' as originally predicted. There have been significant benefits for a relatively small number of people with inherited disorders but not for the majority of users of the NHS. This is because most work has focused on highly penetrant genes of large effect – Mendelian single gene disorders such as Huntington disease and cystic fibrosis and, increasingly, more common conditions such as cancer but where there is a Mendelian subset where genes have high penetrance. A House

Medical Ethics Today: The BMA's Handbook of Ethics and Law, Third Edition. Sophie Brannan, Eleanor Chrispin, Martin Davies, Veronica English, Rebecca Mussell, Julian Sheather and Ann Sommerville.
© 2012 BMA Medical Ethics Department. Published 2012 by Blackwell Publishing Ltd.

of Lords report on genomic medicine, published in 2009, however, highlighted a shift in emphasis towards greater focus on more common, genetically complex disorders where individuals are identified as having an increased risk of developing a condition but where environmental factors are also highly influential; conditions such as heart disease and diabetes.[1] The use of genetic tests to improve prescribing practice (pharmacogenetics – see Chapter 13, page 576–577) will also undoubtedly increase over time. These shifts have the potential to make genetics far more relevant for large numbers of the population and increasingly to involve non-specialist health professionals. Genetics is no longer just an issue for a limited number of experts; it is an issue for doctors from all specialties, particularly general practice, oncology and obstetrics. That is not to say that all health professionals are expected to provide specialist genetic advice and, in most cases, referral to a specialist genetics unit continues to be the most appropriate course of action. An understanding of the basic science of genetics, however, together with knowledge of the conflicts and dilemmas that can arise and where to go for help, forms part of the core knowledge base required for all doctors.

Although this chapter focuses on information obtained from genetic testing, it needs to be recognised that this is not the only way in which genetic information may be obtained. Many doctors – particularly GPs – are familiar with their patients' family histories and genetic information can also be inferred from conversations with patients (for example, if a woman says that her mother and her daughter have both tested positive for the same *BRCA1* mutation, then it is obvious, without the need for a test, that she too has the mutation – as long as she is correct in her understanding of the family situation). Genetic information may also be obtained from non-genetic tests.

General principles

When considering the types of difficulties or dilemmas that arise with genetic technology, the following general principles should be kept in mind.

- It should not automatically be assumed that different rules should always apply to genetics. There are some ways in which genetic information is different from other types of medical information, but the extent and inevitable implications of those differences are often overstated. Individual situations need to be assessed to decide whether additional safeguards or protection are needed.
- Genetics usually affects families, so individuals should be encouraged to consider the impact of their decisions on others who may be affected by them.
- The same basic principles of consent and confidentiality apply to genetics as to other areas of medical practice.
- Patients should be encouraged to share genetic information with others for whom it has personal relevance but, except in very exceptional circumstances, confidentiality should be respected.

Does genetics raise different ethical issues?

There has long been debate about whether genetic information is 'special' in some way and therefore requires different rules and more protection than other medical information.[2] Arguments to justify these differences, however, are frequently not articulated and, in fact, many of the ethical dilemmas that arise in the genetic sphere are similar to those that arise in other areas of medicine. They centre on the traditional duties of health professionals to act in the patient's interests and to avoid harm. Facets of those duties are embodied in the accepted obligations to respect patient confidentiality, to provide information in order to obtain valid consent, to evaluate the risks and benefits of treatment and to aim for justice and equity in decision making. In some ways, however, genetics is different, primarily because of its familial nature, which requires that these general principles are supplemented by other considerations such as the inevitable inter-dependence of interests and the duties owed to other family members. Although these considerations are not exclusive to genetics, they mean that these decisions can be more complex than those in other areas of medicine. This does not mean that specific provision should always be made for genetics but that there are some areas in which the standard response is inappropriate or inadequate.

When considering whether, and, if so, what, additional protection is needed for genetic information, the primary question that arises is whether this information is fundamentally different from all other medical information. One difficulty in answering this question is that 'genetic knowledge' is not a homogeneous concept – it is not all predictive, or relevant to families, or medically significant – and different kinds of information have different implications. Nevertheless, the Human Genetics Commission has suggested that the following factors could be seen to distinguish genetic from other forms of information:

- the almost uniquely identifying nature of some genetic information, including its capacity to confirm, deny, or reveal family relationships;
- the fact that genetic information could be obtained from a very small amount of material (such as skin, saliva, blood spot or hair), possibly secured without the consent of the person;
- the predictive power of some genetic information, especially the predictive power across generations of certain rare genetic diseases;
- the fact that genetic information may be used for purposes other than those for which it was originally collected;
- the interest which some genetic information has for others, including relatives who may be affected by it themselves, insurers, and employers;
- the importance that genetic information may have for establishing susceptibility both to rare inherited disease and the effectiveness of some treatments;
- ... the stability of DNA which can be recovered from stored specimens or even archaeological material after many years.'[3]

Some of these factors are also true of other types of information. For example, a broad range of medical information could be used for purposes other than those for which it was collected, and may be of interest to third parties such as insurance companies. Genetic information is also not unique in being predictive: HIV infection is predictive of AIDS. There are also unique elements that require specific attention, such as the potential that information about one person may reveal information about another, perhaps without that person's knowledge or consent. Also, unlike most other medical data, genetic information can have huge social importance and affect how we perceive ourselves by revealing definitive, and perhaps previously unknown, knowledge about our parentage. It can challenge traditional notions of confidentiality given that, in some senses, information does not 'belong' to just one person. These differences inevitably create tensions which are explored throughout this chapter. Nevertheless, these differences need to be kept in perspective and individual scenarios and uses need to be considered to determine whether and how the situation is 'different' and, if it is, whether it is sufficiently different to warrant special rules or treatment.

An ethical framework

As with the rest of this book, the aim of this chapter is not to provide ready-made answers to specific questions, but to provide a framework and some indicators about how to think about the types of dilemmas that arise in genetics, in order to reach balanced solutions. Where the British Medical Association (BMA) has taken a view on a particular issue, this is stated, but, as in other areas, the Association is conscious of the need for flexibility and to be responsive to exceptional circumstances. In most situations, case-by-case decision making is likely to be more useful than firm and inflexible rules.

In the BMA's view, any framework for decision making in the genetic sphere should take into account and attempt to integrate three themes.

1. *Rights and their limits:* showing respect for patients' decisions and rights is seen as central to good practice. Placing emphasis on rights alone, however, without any mention of corresponding responsibilities and concern for others, cannot provide complete or convincing solutions; nor does it reflect the reality of how most people make decisions. In genetics, one person's moral claim to privacy or to refuse to know information can conflict with another's claim to be forewarned of matters affecting his or her life. If one person has a right to information, this implies that another person may have some responsibility to provide that information.
2. *Concern for others:* genetics necessarily deals with the relatedness of people based on shared DNA. Although the BMA stresses that concern for others can only very rarely justify disregarding an individual's informed decision, we believe that patients should at least take into account the needs of others as well as their own. Doctors should therefore ensure that patients are aware of the implications that their decisions may have for other people and encourage them to take these factors into account in the decision-making process. This concept, of a shared interest in genetic information and research, has been referred to by the Human Genetics Commission as 'genetic solidarity and altruism'.[4]
3. *Interdependence of interests:* whereas a concern for others implies acting altruistically in circumstances where there is no direct benefit for the individual, the concept of interdependence recognises that in helping others, the individual may also accrue indirect benefits such as improved family relationships and emotional support. From a very practical perspective, with genetics there is frequently an interdependence of interests within families because people's ability to access genetic testing and counselling depends upon other family members being willing to share information about familial risk.

Genetic testing of those with a family history of genetic disease

A key aspect of developments in genetics – and a central issue for health professionals – is the increasing ability to identify and test for particular gene mutations associated with disease. There are various forms of testing, each with different outcomes and implications. The main distinctions are as follows.

*   *Diagnostic testing:* where the symptoms are already manifest.
*   *Carrier testing for recessive or X-linked conditions:* where individuals may be at risk of passing on a genetic disease to their children but will usually be unaffected themselves.

- *Predictive or presymptomatic testing:* which is able to predict future illness with varying degrees of accuracy.
- *Susceptibility testing:* which is able to identify those at increased genetic risk of developing a particular disorder.

In addition to general concerns around consent and confidentiality, which apply to all genetic testing, there are some specific issues that are particular to the type of testing carried out. These are discussed later in this chapter.

Consent for genetic testing

As with any other medical assessment, genetic tests should be carried out only with the valid consent of someone eligible to give it. (For general information on consent see Chapters 2 and 4.) This could be an adult with capacity or someone with parental responsibility for a young child, provided the test is in the child's best interests. It could also be a young person who is considered sufficiently mature to make the decision, although with most genetic testing the young person should be encouraged to involve his or her parents in the decision.

Information and counselling

Any consent must be given voluntarily and free from pressure, and whoever is giving consent must be provided with sufficient information to enable him or her to make an informed decision. Because of the nature of genetic testing, this should include information about the implications for other family members, the importance of sharing information with those for whom it has personal relevance and the implications of withholding information from family members. The Joint Committee on Medical Genetics has recommended that the following information should be discussed during the process of seeking consent for genetic testing:

- the fact that a 'family history of a condition or disease, or genetic test results, has a potential benefit to other family members
- the fact that communication of certain aspects of information to family members may therefore be recommended
- the means of contacting those at-risk family members where relevant
- the fact that a summary of relevant clinical and genetic information will usually be sent to other appropriate health professionals
- the likely timescales for availability of test results
- the possibility of unexpected or incidental findings from genetic testing and how these might be managed
- the predictive nature of certain genetic tests (for example, indicating risks many years in the future rather than current risks)
- the routine practice of long-term storage of samples for possible future analysis and the patient's preferences regarding further testing if it becomes available
- the routine practice of using stored samples from one family member as quality assurance for clinical testing in another family member.'[5]

In some cases definitive information can be obtained from genetic tests (for example, about whether an individual will or will not develop a particular condition), but more frequently the outcome is knowledge of an increased, but often unquantifiable, likelihood of developing the condition or probability of having an affected child. An important role of health professionals is to help people to understand 'risk', both as a concept and what it means for their lives. Those who specialise in genetics are well aware of the complexities of probability and the difficulties many people have in understanding risk[6] and they adopt particular strategies to achieve the best possible understanding.[7] Special care is needed to explain this information in a way that patients can understand.

When the implications of testing are profound, particularly with presymptomatic testing, counselling may also be required to ensure the individual has received sufficient information for the consent to be considered valid. Genetic counselling includes not only the provision of detailed information and discussion of the options for, and implications of, testing but also the offer of psychosocial support. The process involves an attempt by specially trained professionals to help the individual or family to:

1) comprehend the medical facts, including the diagnosis, the probable course of the disorder, and the available management;
2) appreciate the way heredity contributes to the disorder, and the risk of recurrence in specified relatives;
3) understand the options for dealing with the risk of recurrence;
4) choose the course of action which seems appropriate to them in view of their risk and their family goals and act in accordance with that decision; and
5) make the best possible psychological adjustment to the disorder in an affected family member and/or to the risk of recurrence of that disorder.[8]

A central principle in genetic counselling since the 1970s has been that it should be non-directive; its goal is not to achieve a particular outcome, such as reducing the number of babies born with disabilities or to increase the number of people who seek testing, but to help individuals or families to reach the outcome that is right for them. There has been considerable debate over many years, however, about the extent to which this is either feasible or desirable.[9] The practice of UK genetics centres is to emphasise the importance of informed individual choice, while also exploring with patients the needs of other people in the family for whom genetic information has direct and personal relevance. The BMA believes that all people, not only those with genetic conditions, have moral obligations to consider the effect of their decisions on others; inevitably, however, there is more focus on these obligations in the case of genetic information because of its familial nature. This does not mean that individuals should be forced to meet those obligations, but it does provide justification for some departure from the usual model of impartiality, with some form of encouragement or persuasion not only permitted but actively promoted. Despite their general support for the principle of non-directiveness, for example, most international guidelines on genetic counselling advise counsellors to 'persuade' those being counselled to disclose genetic information to other family members who may be affected.[10] This issue is discussed further on pages 374–376.

Testing adults who lack capacity

It may sometimes be desirable to carry out a genetic test on an adult who lacks capacity to give valid consent. When the test is for that individual's direct benefit (for example, by facilitating treatment) this may be undertaken in England, Wales and Scotland with the authorisation of an appointed proxy or, when there is no proxy, a doctor may provide a test that is in the patient's best interests (or, in Scotland, would provide a benefit). In Northern Ireland such testing may be undertaken under the common law principle of best interests. More information about decision making for patients who lack capacity to consent is provided in Chapter 3.

In some circumstances, genetic testing of an adult who lacks capacity may be suggested, not for the direct benefit of the individual him or herself, but for the benefit of other family members, by contributing to family linkage or mutation studies. Sometimes, when patients are aware of pending incapacity, they make specific provision for this, in the form of advance consent for the future testing of a sample for the benefit of other family members. When this has not occurred, however, it can cause considerable distress to the relatives that the assumption appears to be that the relative would not give consent if able to do so. If the individual has had capacity in the past, and has had a close relationship with other family members, there are good grounds for assuming that he or she would wish to help them in this way. It could be argued, therefore, that allowing an individual to help his or her family, in a way that most people would want to do, falls within the definition of 'best interests', providing there is no or minimal risk or distress. Although the BMA believes these arguments are persuasive from an ethical perspective, it is not entirely clear that taking a sample from an adult who lacks capacity for this purpose would be lawful. This will be determined by a legal interpretation of 'best interests' (in England, Wales and Northern Ireland) and 'benefit' (in Scotland), which has not, so far, been forthcoming. The BMA sought to have this specific scenario clarified in the Mental Capacity Act 2005, when the legislation was being debated, but was unsuccessful. The issue is addressed in the *Mental Capacity Act 2005 Code of Practice* which implies that genetic testing for the benefit of others may be in the best interests of the patient, saying:

> The Act allows actions that benefit other people, as long as they are in the best interests of the person who lacks capacity to make the decision. For example, having considered all the circumstances of the particular case, a decision might be made to take a blood sample from a person who lacks capacity to consent, to check for a genetic link to cancer within the family, because this might benefit someone else in the family. But it might still be in the best interests of the person who lacks capacity. 'Best interests' goes beyond the person's medical interests.
>
> For example, courts have previously ruled that possible wider benefits to a person who lacks capacity to consent, such as providing or gaining emotional support from close relationships are important factors in working out the person's own best interests. If it is likely that the person who lacks capacity would have considered these factors themselves, they can be seen as part of the person's best interests.[11]

Despite this apparently reassuring advice, health professionals wishing to test incapacitated adults for the benefit of others will need to be able to justify the decision by explaining why, in the particular case, testing would be in the best interests of the adult who lacks capacity. Where there is genuine doubt about whether this test is met, legal advice should be sought.

The code of practice issued under the Adults with Incapacity (Scotland) Act[12] makes no reference to this scenario but the lawfulness of taking and testing a sample for the benefit of others will depend on whether the test also benefits the incapacitated adult. Although it has not been tested, it is likely that the Scottish courts would follow the English position and construe 'benefit' widely. However, where there is genuine doubt about whether this test is met, legal advice should be sought.

In some cases it may be possible to use an existing sample to carry out a DNA test for the benefit of other family members. It is lawful to analyse the DNA of a person who lacks capacity with the consent of an authorised proxy or where the test would be in that person's best interests or, in Scotland, with the consent of someone authorised to give it (on the basis that the test would benefit the adult who lacks capacity).[13] Where testing is requested principally for the benefit of other family members, however, the same considerations would apply as discussed above and decisions need to be made and justified on the basis of the individual facts of the case. Legal advice should be sought in cases of doubt. When considering the ethical and legal acceptability of taking or testing a sample from an adult who lacks capacity for the benefit of others, the BMA believes the following factors should be taken into account:

- any previously expressed wishes
- whether the information can be obtained by other means such as testing another relative who has the capacity to consent
- the potential harm to the individual being tested, including the level of invasiveness or risk of the test and the implications for that person of the information being available
- the degree of harm or benefit to others
- whether there are grounds to believe that most adults with capacity would wish to help others in this way
- taking account of all relevant factors, whether testing would be in the best interests of, or provide a benefit to, the adult who lacks capacity.

Non-consensual testing

Throughout the UK it is a criminal offence[14] to have human tissue or cells, including hair, nails and gametes, with the intention of analysing its DNA without qualifying consent, subject to certain limited exceptions (see below).

Qualifying consent

In relation to DNA analysis, 'qualifying consent' means:[15]

- for living adults with capacity and competent young people – their own consent
- for children and young people who are unable or unwilling to make a decision – a person with parental responsibility
- for deceased adults who had capacity before they died – the individual's own consent given before death, or if no decision was made, the consent of someone in a qualifying relationship with the individual immediately before death (see Chapter 12, page 523)
- for deceased children who did not give consent before they died – a person with parental responsibility or, if there is nobody with parental responsibility, someone who was in a 'qualifying relationship' with the individual before death (see Chapter 12, page 523).

For DNA analysis there is no requirement to contact relatives in the order they are listed and the consent of any qualifying relative will suffice.

Exceptions to the offence of non-consensual DNA testing

It is not an offence to have tissue with the intention of analysing its DNA without qualifying consent where:[16]

- the purpose of the analysis is medical diagnosis or treatment of that person
- it is used for the purposes of the coroner or procurator fiscal
- it is in connection with the prevention or detection of a crime or for the prosecution of a crime
- it is in the interests of national security
- the test is carried out on the order of a court or tribunal
- the material is from a living person and is used for:
  ○ clinical audit
  ○ education or training relating to human health
  ○ performance assessment
  ○ public health monitoring
  ○ quality assurance;
- the material is an identifiable 'existing holding' (was held before 1 September 2006) and is used for:
  ○ clinical audit
  ○ determining the cause of death
  ○ education or training relating to human health
  ○ establishing after death the efficacy of any drug or treatment
  ○ obtaining scientific or medical information about a living or deceased person that may be relevant to any other person (including a future person)
  ○ performance assessment
  ○ public health monitoring
  ○ quality assurance
  ○ research in connection with disorders, or functioning, of the human body
  ○ transplantation;
- where the DNA comes from an adult who lacks capacity and the use is:
  ○ in that person's best interests
  ○ for the purpose of an authorised clinical trial or other approved research
  ○ in Scotland, with the consent of someone eligible to give it under the Adults with Incapacity (Scotland) Act;
- in the course of research where the material comes from a living person, the material is anonymised and the research project has been approved by a research ethics authority (see Chapter 14, pages 615–616)
- where the Human Tissue Authority (HTA)[17] (or, in Scotland, the Court of Session) has ruled that consent may be deemed to be in place, where:
  ○ the donor is believed to be alive and to have capacity but cannot be traced, or
  ○ the donor is believed to be alive and to have capacity but has not responded to repeated attempts to obtain consent.

In addition, the offence does not apply to material that is:

- from the body of a person who died at least 100 years before the Act came into force
- an anonymous existing holding (held before 1 September 2006)
- an embryo created outside the human body.

Summary – consent for genetic testing

- Genetic tests should be carried out only with the valid consent of someone eligible to give it.
- Young people who are competent to decide may give consent for genetic testing, but they should be encouraged to involve their parents.
- The information to be provided should include details of the implications of the result for other family members and individuals should be encouraged to share information with those for whom it has personal relevance.
- Testing may be provided if it is in the best interests of an adult who lacks capacity (or, in Scotland, if it would benefit the patient), for example because it would facilitate treatment.
- Testing of an adult who lacks capacity for the benefit of other family members would be lawful only if it is considered to be in the best interests of the individual himself or herself.
- With specified exceptions, it is a criminal offence to have tissue with the intention of analysing its DNA without qualifying consent.

Confidentiality within families

The general principles of confidentiality apply equally to genetic information as to other information about health. With the results of genetic testing, however, there is the added dimension that the testing of one individual frequently has relevance for other family members. This can lead to a conflict between health professionals' duties to maintain patient confidentiality and their duty to protect others from avoidable harm.[18] The standard model of confidentiality requires that information remains confidential unless the individual consents to disclosure or there is an overriding public interest in sharing information, usually taken to mean that there is a risk of serious harm if the information is not disclosed.[19] It has been suggested, however, that genetic test results should not be considered as personal information – and therefore should not be subject to the usual rules of confidentiality. Rather, the results should be viewed as familial information, such that information may be shared with other family members unless there is a good reason why it should not be divulged.[20] The BMA does not accept this view and believes that, as with other areas of healthcare, information about or provided by one patient should not be shared with others unless consent has been obtained or there is a legal requirement or an overriding public interest to justify disclosure.

Individuals should always be encouraged to consider the implications of their decisions for other people. Most patients are willing to allow information to be shared with those for whom it has personal relevance. In a survey of patients with familial colon cancer, 93.3 per cent of respondents thought it was their duty to tell all at-risk family members about their diagnosis and the implications for relatives.[21] Despite this apparent willingness to share information, this communication frequently does not happen or the information passed on may be incomplete or inaccurate, leaving health professionals in a difficult position and unsure of their obligations towards other family members.[22]

There are two main ways in which genetic information about one individual directly affects another. First, testing for a dominant disorder may reveal information about the genetic status of certain other people and, in some cases, it may reveal information that the other person does not know and does not want to know.

The impact of genetic testing on others

If a woman whose maternal grandfather has Huntington disease sought presymptomatic testing, a positive result would reveal that her mother also carried the gene mutation. The daughter's test has given her information about her mother's genetic status that her mother does not have and may not want to know. The added complication is that if people know about both the daughter and the grandfather, the mother's genetic status can be inferred. This raises the question of how best to manage the situation so that, if the mother is to learn about her genetic status, she does so in a controlled and supportive manner. This is complicated by the fact that if the healthcare team tell the mother about her daughter's test result, without the daughter's consent, they would be breaching confidentiality. This scenario raises not only issues of confidentiality, but also of consent because, essentially, the mother is receiving information about her health as though she herself had been tested without her consent. For this reason, it is important to encourage the patient to involve other family members and health professionals in discussions about the decision to seek testing and to try to reach agreement about how to proceed. If agreement cannot be reached, however, testing should not be withheld solely on the grounds that it would reveal information about another person.

Two studies in the 1990s, from the Netherlands and the UK, found that this sort of situation arises only rarely. They showed that this type of testing made up less than 10 per cent of all predictive testing. In most of these cases, the intervening parent was either dead or agreed to be tested, or the person seeking testing withdrew the request when agreement could not be reached. In both studies the number of cases where testing was carried out despite the intervening parent disagreeing, or being unaware of the test, was around 1 in 500 of the total predictive tests.[23] Similar issues can arise when one identical twin wishes to seek presymptomatic testing but the other does not. Although no more recent data are available, anecdotal evidence suggests these dilemmas are continuing to perplex genetics professionals in the UK.[24]

Another way in which genetic information can have personal relevance for others is when an individual discovers that other family members may be at risk of passing on a disorder to their children. The mother of a son with Duchenne muscular dystrophy, for example, who has tested positive for carrier status, would have information that would be important for any sisters or daughters who were planning to have children, because they too could be carriers.

Experience has shown that in the vast majority of cases, once they are informed of the potential impact on other family members, people are willing to share information with relatives for whom it has personal relevance.[25] However, if after counselling and persuasion, the individual refuses to share the information, this should be respected unless the criteria set out by the General Medical Council (GMC) for disclosure in the public interest are met.[26] Such situations are likely to be rare but may include a scenario in which an individual refuses consent to share information with a family member who is at risk of a severe genetic disorder where some action can be taken to reduce its impact if information is provided. In such circumstances there may be grounds for breaching confidentiality. Such decisions are not easy, but the type of factors that should be taken into account in deciding whether the risks are sufficiently serious to breach confidentiality are the following:

- the severity of the disorder
- the level of predictability of the information provided by testing

- what, if any, action the relatives could take to protect themselves or make informed reproductive decisions if they were told of the risk
- the level of harm or benefit of giving and withholding the information
- the reasons given for refusing to share the information, for example mistaken beliefs about the nature of inheritance
- whether it is possible to identify the relatives without the assistance of the patient
- whether it is possible to inform relatives without identifying the patient.

With genetic conditions, however, there is often a high level of uncertainty both in terms of the level of predictability and the severity of the condition; there may be harms to a relative that can be avoided but, in most cases, all that can be disclosed is a risk, not a certainty. This makes the task of balancing benefits and harms particularly difficult. As with other situations where a breach of confidentiality is being considered, views should be sought from other members of the healthcare team and, where it is decided that a breach of confidentiality is justified, this should be discussed in advance with the patient whenever possible. Before disclosing information, careful consideration should be given to whether it is possible to inform relatives of their risk without identifying the patient.

Although some individuals are aware of a problematic family history, there are likely to be some cases where family members are unaware of their at-risk status. Giving them this information allows them to make their own decisions about whether to seek testing but also denies them a so-called 'right not to know'. Withholding the information, however, involves the doctor, or family, making decisions about what is best for that individual without consulting him or her, which goes against traditional notions of autonomy. Husted takes the view that the disclosure of information about genetic risk to unsuspecting individuals is 'a clear cut case of strong medical paternalism' because the decision to know or not to know has been taken out of the hands of the individual for his or her own good.[27] He says that making people aware of the information may at first appear to be an enhancement of autonomy, because it is only by having such information that individuals can make informed choices, but it is in fact a denial of autonomy, because it prevents them from making decisions without the interference of genetic information.

The difficulty is that it is impossible to find out whether an individual wishes to know information without revealing that there is information available that he or she may want to know. Laurie argues that those who wish to disclose information to unsuspecting individuals should be able to justify that decision by demonstrating that the benefits of disclosure outweigh the benefits, for the individual, of remaining in ignorance. This judgement will depend on a number of factors, including the type of disease, the risks, the availability of a therapy or cure and any evidence of prior expressions indicating a desire not to receive information.[28] Careful consideration needs to be given to the likelihood of harm arising from both disclosure and non-disclosure, and a decision needs to be reached by weighing up the arguments in each case. Where individuals are approached this is usually achieved over a period of time with an initial approach, perhaps through non-medical sources, seeking to determine how much information the individual wants to know. It has been suggested that the potential psychosocial harm to family members can appear to health professionals as a rather abstract concept, compared to the more tangible health implications of non-disclosure, which may lead them to be more inclined to prioritise the sharing of information over the desire to protect relatives from information that could be perceived as harmful.[29] The authors acknowledge, however, that it is rare for health professionals to intervene directly and, more frequently, the emphasis is on finding ways of encouraging communication within families.

The BMA is sometimes asked whether health professionals are under a legal duty to disclose information about genetic risk to relatives who may be affected by it. There is no clear answer to this question because it is not an issue that has been specifically addressed by the courts in the UK. The extent of the duty of care of health professionals has been considered in other cases, however, and is likely to focus on the proximity between the party allegedly having the duty of care and the third party who would be harmed.[30] Legal commentators have argued that in some limited circumstances it is feasible that a doctor could be considered negligent for not disclosing relevant information, but only when that doctor has an existing duty of care to the relatives.[31] In reality, the type of circumstances in which such a duty may arise would be where the benefits clearly outweigh the harms of disclosure and so most doctors would consider themselves to be under a moral duty to disclose the information.

The BMA believes that, when consent has been obtained to share information, or when, exceptionally, it is considered that a breach of confidentiality is justified, information should usually be passed to family members about their own risk, to allow them to decide whether to seek testing. When information is to be shared, people are likely to prefer to learn it in a controlled and supportive environment. There has been considerable debate about the role of genetics professionals in this process; whether it is simply to encourage and persuade their patients to share information with the family, to help identify who should be given what information or to provide ongoing support throughout the communication process. Studies indicating poor understanding of the condition and risk amongst relatives informed by the patient[32] lend weight to the argument that genetic professionals should have a greater role in supporting and assisting individuals to inform their families or personally contacting at-risk relatives.[33]

Use of confidential information by clinics

The fact that genetics clinics often see many members of the same family raises the question of whether it is appropriate and acceptable to use information obtained about one patient for the benefit of another. Lucassen and Parker[34] use the scenario of a woman, Helen, who is aware of a family history of breast cancer who seeks testing. She does not know that another member of her family, Angela, has already had testing and a mutation in *BRCA1* has been identified. The question they raise is whether the genetics team can use the information obtained from Angela's results to test Helen, without revealing any information to her – essentially asking whether there is a difference between use and disclosure of information. The answer is not straightforward and, to date, has not been tested at law. Using the traditional understanding of confidentiality, it could be argued that provided no information about Angela is disclosed to Helen, confidentiality would not be breached. It is possible, however, that a court might take a broader view of confidentiality with either unauthorised disclosure or use of information without consent considered a technical breach of confidentiality. This is because both data protection law and human rights legislation focus on confidentiality as concerning the *control* of confidential information rather than merely its disclosure. This includes control over the uses to which the information is put.

Unless a case is tested in the courts it is not possible to give a definitive answer to this question. This leaves health professionals in a difficult position with a risk of complaint for breaching confidentiality if they use the information and a complaint of failing to warn patients of a known risk if they do not. On balance, the BMA believes that health professionals would be well advised to err on the side of maintaining confidentiality in these circumstances while recognising that the use of information may be acceptable in some circumstances. In practice, many people who do not want confidential information disclosed to others may, nonetheless, be willing for the information to be used for the benefit of other family members. Seeking consent for such use is the best option but, in order for this consent to be in place in case a family member subsequently presents for testing, such discussion would need to form a routine part of the consent process. As with disclosure, however, the right to protection is not absolute and confidentiality may be breached where there is an overriding public interest. Patients should therefore be advised that in some circumstances their refusal to allow information to be used may be overridden.

Summary – confidentiality within families

- Genetic information in one person may also reveal information about another family member.
- Individuals should be encouraged to share information with others for whom it has personal relevance. However, if they refuse, confidentiality should be breached only when there is a legal requirement or there is an overriding public interest.
- Although some people may prefer not to know that they are at risk of a serious genetic disorder, it is impossible to find out their wishes without revealing that there is information they may want to know.
- The possible harms of disclosure and non-disclosure need to be considered, but the BMA believes that where consent is given to sharing information, or there are exceptional grounds to breach confidentiality, information should be given to family members to allow them to decide whether to seek testing.
- When information is to be shared, it is preferable for people to learn it in a controlled and supportive environment.
- It is possible that the courts could judge the use, as well as disclosure, of confidential information without consent as a breach of confidentiality. Ideally, therefore, consent should be sought routinely for the use of information obtained from test results for the benefit of other family members.

Diagnostic testing

Genetic tests are frequently used, in the same way as other diagnostic tests, to confirm a diagnosis once symptoms have begun to appear. Consent should be sought in the usual way, but should include information about the implications for other family members. In some circumstances the tests themselves may not be genetic tests *per se*, but still reveal information about a genetic condition. In these cases there should be close liaison with the regional genetics unit, and support and advice should be obtained before carrying out the test. It would be inappropriate, for example, for a patient to be informed by a cardiologist about a diagnosis of cardiomyopathy, or a neurologist about a diagnosis of Huntington disease, without there being some prior discussion, with the patient if possible or his or her relatives, about the genetic nature of the condition and the consequent implications for other family members.

Carrier testing for recessive or X-linked disorders

When individuals are known to be at risk of carrying the gene for an autosomal recessive disorder, an X-linked disorder or a balanced chromosomal rearrangement they may seek carrier testing in order to inform future reproductive decisions. If it is found that future children would be at risk, the couple may decide to remain childless, opt for preimplantation or prenatal diagnosis, or accept the risk and proceed in the knowledge that the child may be affected by the disorder. When the patient is an adult with capacity or a competent minor, before consent is sought, information should be provided about the reliability of the test, the nature of the disorder and the implications of carrier status. Young people should be strongly encouraged to involve their parents in the decision to seek carrier testing. However, when they are sufficiently mature to give valid consent, they understand the implications of carrier status and there is no suggestion that the consent is given under pressure, there are strong arguments for respecting the young person's wishes and carrying out the test.

In some cases the suggestion for carrier testing may come from other family members, with the support of the appropriate health professionals. In this type of 'active programme' affected individuals are invited to inform their relatives of their potential risk of being a carrier and invite them to seek genetic testing. When carriers are identified through this mechanism, they are encouraged to inform their relatives of the risk and so the testing continues. This proactive strategy is called cascade testing.

Carrier testing of adults who lack capacity

Carrier testing of an adult who lacks capacity is unlikely to be of direct benefit to the individual but there may be circumstances in which it would be of benefit to other family members. Testing in such cases may be considered ethically acceptable, but it would need to be shown to be in the best interests of the incapacitated adult in order to meet the legal criteria for testing (see pages 370–372). Where there is doubt about this, legal advice should be sought.

Carrier testing of children

The most ethically problematic aspect of carrier testing is dealing with parental requests for testing of young children who are not able to give consent for themselves. Given that, for most conditions, the children themselves are not affected by or do not have any symptoms of the disorder, the only direct benefit of knowing their carrier status is to make plans for reproduction when they are older. It has been argued that testing in childhood restricts the child's future choices without any immediate benefit and that the child, and later the adult, would be denied the option of not knowing his or her genetic status. It has also been suggested that testing at the request of a child's parents and giving the parents the results denies the child, and later the adult, the confidentiality he or she would expect if tested as an adult. Despite these concerns, many parents strongly believe they have a right to know this information and requests for such testing are fairly common. A study on parents' attitudes to testing the siblings of patients with cystic fibrosis, for example, found that 90 per cent would like to know the carrier status of their unaffected children and 91 per cent believed they had a right to the information.[35]

Parental views about carrier testing contrast sharply with the reported views of European clinical geneticists, a large majority of whom said they were unwilling or very unwilling to undertake a carrier test on a 6-year-old child on parental request for a range of autosomal recessive and X-linked disorders (59–84 per cent, depending on the condition).[36] This majority view is in line with international guidance on genetic testing of children.

(It is interesting to note, however, that, for every condition studied, there were some geneticists – 9–27 per cent, depending on the condition – who would be willing to test contrary to the recommendations of most professional bodies.) Guidelines from the European Society of Human Genetics, for example, which were revised in 2009, state that testing for carrier status should be discouraged until minors have the maturity and competence to understand the nature of the decision and its implications. They go on to say that, in some cases, testing might be considered in families where other children in the family have been identified as being carriers or as having the disorder.[37] The British Society for Human Genetics also produced revised guidelines on genetic testing of children in 2010 which recommended a presumption in favour of delaying testing until the child was able to contribute to the decision, but concluded: 'in each case where parents request genetic testing of a child when this is of no direct or immediate medical benefit, an assessment should be made of the balance of harms and benefits of such testing taking into account that decisions ought to be made in the child's best interests.'[38]

Together with health professionals, parents are responsible for the healthcare of their children until they themselves are sufficiently mature to take over this task. It is generally accepted that parents can, and indeed should, have access to information that is necessary for them to fulfil this role. The BMA's general view is that parents are the natural decision makers for their children and their views about where their children's best interests lie should be determinative unless their choices are clearly harmful to the child. Because there is no evidence that carrier testing in childhood is harmful (see below), the question is whether carrier testing should be seen as materially different in nature to other information that parents would expect to be able to find out about their children, and other decisions that parents would expect to be able to make on their children's behalf, such that a different approach should be taken. Although the information is of no immediate benefit to the child, there is a clear benefit in knowing the information before having children. One difference is that the information is not already available but is being generated after a specific request from the parents. If information about carrier status were to be discovered inadvertently, for example while undertaking diagnostic testing or from neonatal screening, the BMA believes it would be inappropriate to withhold this from the parents unless disclosing it would clearly be contrary to the child's interests. (Where it is known that this information may be discovered, however, this possibility should be discussed with the parents before the test is undertaken.) Does this mean that parents should also be able to request carrier testing?

It was suggested above that one of the factors to be taken into account in considering genetics is the interdependence of interests. This is an important factor when considering the genetic testing of children because the interests of the child cannot be considered in total isolation from the interests of the parents and other family members. The parents' educational and caring role may be considered to put them in the best position to decide when to tell the child, as well as to help the child to understand the implications of the test. They may feel, for example, that it is in the best interests of the child to have early knowledge of their carrier status to give the child a period of time to adapt and to come to terms with the information, rather than being presented with this knowledge during adolescence, which is often a difficult and emotional time. They may also feel that their own anxiety, caused by the continuing uncertainty about the child's carrier status, may affect their relationship with the child. It is important, however, to distinguish between the parents' opinion about what is in the best interests of the child and the parents' own wishes; the courts have stated that the wishes of the parents are 'wholly irrelevant to consideration of the objective best interests of the child'.[39] Sometimes, the request may come as a result of unresolved grief in parents who have lost a brother, sister or child from a distressing disease and have a strong desire to know whether their children are carriers of the same condition.[40]

Carrier testing of children in Finland

A study was carried out in Finland to consider long-term psychological consequences, experience, satisfaction and recall of the test results of 25 healthy siblings of patients with aspartylglucosaminuria.[41] The age at testing ranged from 1 to 17 years (12 were 10 years or under and six were aged 15 or over at the time of testing). Of the 25 tested individuals, 21 reported that carrier testing had not had any influence on their lives, two reported that it had had a positive influence by ensuring the information was available for family planning, one reported both positive and negative influences, and no information was given about the remaining person. Overall, the emotional, social and physical well-being of the young people tested was at least as good as those in the control group. All of those tested were satisfied with the carrier testing and had no concerns about their parents having made the decision on their behalf. In terms of accuracy of recollection, 23 of the 25 (92 per cent) remembered and understood their test result correctly. The authors point out, however, that there was also no evidence that testing in childhood had any benefits over testing in adulthood. They concluded that, despite their findings, they did not recommend testing in childhood because the result is not needed prior to the time for reproductive decisions to be made.

When the BMA considered this issue in 1997 it came to a similar conclusion to that set out in the Clinical Genetics Society's 1994 guidelines:[42] that the evidence of harm was not sufficient to justify a prohibition on carrier testing of young children, but, because of the lack of clear benefit there were good arguments for delaying testing until the child was old enough to make an informed decision. The BMA called for some flexibility, however, to deal with the exceptional cases where agreement to delay testing was not reached and when testing would be appropriate in the circumstances. A review of the content of international guidance on carrier testing of children, undertaken by Borry *et al.*[43] in 2006, revealed a strong preference for delaying testing with only the BMA and the Genetic Interest Group (also UK based) calling for a more flexible approach. In 2007, the BMA hosted a conference on genetic testing of children jointly with the Clinical Genetics Society, the Genetic Interest Group, CESAGen (the ESRC Research Centre) and the Society for Genomics, Policy and Population Health. It became evident at this meeting that carrier testing of children was still an issue on which there were disparate views and also on which practice differed around the country. Following this conference, the Clinical Genetics Society decided to review its guidance and the BMA also reviewed its position.

In reviewing its position, the BMA's Medical Ethics Committee (MEC) focussed on a number of changes that had taken place since its original decision.

- It is now far more common for people to know they are carriers of an autosomal recessive or X-linked disorder (through preconception screening, for example, or as a by-product of newborn screening or, increasingly, from full genome sequencing).
- Parents will often know the carrier status of some of their children (perhaps by prenatal diagnosis or neonatal screening) but not others.
- There is far greater understanding – particularly among children and young adults – about genetics and so the risk of misunderstanding the implications of the test may be diminishing.
- More generally, there appears to have been a shift in perception about the role of parents as being the natural decision makers for their young children, with the view increasingly being taken (within society as well as by the BMA) that parents, rather than

doctors, are best placed to make decisions for children unless the decision is clearly harmful to the child.

The MEC also recognised that while there had been only a limited amount of research into the effects of childhood carrier testing, that which had been undertaken did not find any emotional or psychological harm from early testing. Nevertheless, the type of concerns that are raised by those opposed to childhood testing include the following.

- There is no benefit to testing and so no justification for doing so until the young person is sufficiently mature to be involved in the decision.
- It is known that some parents fail to pass on information about carrier status to their children in a timely fashion.
- Where parents are very keen to know their daughters' carrier status when they are very young there is concern they may put unreasonable pressure on their children and mould their expectations in a way that gives little room for personal choice (for example, carriers of Duchenne muscular dystrophy being brought up with the expectation that they will not have any boys).
- There is also a risk that those found to be carriers may reject and fail to act on the information they receive because of the way the information was provided. If they were personally involved in the decision to test there may be more chance that they would feel more 'ownership' of the information and integrate the result into their future decisions in a constructive and helpful way.

After careful consideration, the MEC concluded that the risk of harm was not sufficiently high to justify treating carrier testing of children differently from other medical decisions made by parents. The BMA believes that parents are the most appropriate decision makers for their children unless the decision they seek to make is clearly harmful to the child or others. Parents should be informed of the lack of immediate benefit of testing and the advantages of waiting until the young person can make a personal decision. The BMA believes that those seeking carrier testing for their children should be encouraged to wait until the child or young person is sufficiently mature to make a personal decision but if, after discussion, they feel testing now is important and in the best interests of their child – and there are no other factors that might indicate that testing would be harmful – testing should be permitted. The revised guidance of the British Society for Human Genetics recommends delaying testing until the child is sufficiently mature to participate in the decision but states that the benefits and harms need to be balanced in each individual case.

Summary – carrier testing for recessive or X-linked disorders

- Before consent is sought, adults with capacity and competent minors should be given information about the reliability of the test, the nature of the disorder and the implications of carrier status.
- Young people should be encouraged to involve their parents in a decision to seek carrier testing.
- In order to be lawful, carrier testing of an adult who lacks capacity for the benefit of other people would also need to be in the best interests of the incapacitated adult. Where there is doubt, legal advice should be sought before proceeding.

- Parents seeking carrier testing for their children should be encouraged to wait until the child or young person is sufficiently mature to make a personal decision.
- If, after discussion, parents feel that carrier testing now is important and in the best interests of their child – and there are no other factors that might indicate that testing would be harmful – the BMA believes that testing should be permitted.

Predictive or presymptomatic testing

The type of genetic testing that is most frequently debated, and which has the potential for the most problems, is testing that can predict, before any symptoms have appeared, whether an individual will or is highly likely to go on to develop a particular condition in the future.

For genetic mutations associated with dominantly inherited conditions with complete or near complete penetrance, such as Huntington disease, having the gene mutation means the individual will go on to develop the disease at some stage, unless he or she dies of another cause before the disease manifests itself. When it is possible to treat the condition for which the individual is at risk or when some intervention, such as screening for early evidence of the disease, can facilitate treatment, early diagnosis would clearly be beneficial and so predictive testing, with valid consent and counselling, is relatively unproblematic. More controversial is testing for those conditions for which there is no useful medical intervention. This means, in practice, that individuals know they will go on to develop a very serious, and perhaps life-threatening, disorder in the future but they do not know when. Despite having this knowledge, there is nothing they can do to prevent or cure the disease. Most people who are at risk of such conditions do not want to know what is in store for them and the take-up rate of presymptomatic testing for Huntington disease, for example, is only about 18 per cent of those who are at risk.[44]

For some people, however, living with uncertainty is one of the most difficult aspects of being part of an at-risk family and to know for certain that they will develop the disease is better than not knowing. Having access to information about future disability enables them to plan their careers, families and lives to take account of their potential limitations. There can also be practical benefits, such as making arrangements for suitable care and support to be available, or moving to a house that can accommodate a wheelchair for example. It is important to keep these benefits in perspective, however, because in some respects uncertainty about whether an individual will develop the disease is replaced with uncertainty about when the disease will manifest and how severe it will be. The implications of testing need to be explored fully by the patient before consent is sought, particularly as some people seek testing in the expectation of a favourable result. Genetic counselling forms an integral part of the service offered in regional genetics centres and forms a critical part of the process of presymptomatic testing.

Initial fears that for healthy people to learn they are destined to develop a serious and incurable genetic disorder would inevitably cause severe distress, stigmatisation and suicide have not materialised. A worldwide assessment of people who have had a predictive test for Huntington disease, published in 1999, found that the vast majority did not experience any subsequent catastrophic event (defined as: suicide, assisted suicide or psychiatric problems resulting in hospitalisation). However, 44 people out of 4,527 in the study (0.97 per cent) did experience such an event within 2 years of receiving the result (some – including all those who committed suicide – being symptomatic at the time of the event).[45] Although significantly higher than in the general population, the attempted suicide rate in this group, which included some people who had not yet developed the condition, was not out of proportion when compared with overall suicide rates for people with Huntington disease or other serious progressive diseases.[46] Other recent studies have found high levels of depression after testing (affecting 58 per cent of carriers and 24 per cent of non-carriers in one study[47]) and an overall frequency of clinical adverse events within 2 years of testing (including clinical depression and a marked increase in alcohol use) of 6.9 per cent.[48] Despite this increase in adverse events among some participants, a number of studies have found significant overall reductions in psychological distress and depression 5 years after testing amongst both carriers and non-carriers.[49] Interestingly, the likelihood of psychological distress appears to be more closely linked to factors other than the outcome of the test, such as psychological state and distress prior to testing.[50] This might be because the benefit of relief from uncertainty applies to both carriers and non-carriers.[51] A 2010 qualitative study found both positive and negative effects from presymptomatic testing for Huntington disease.[52] Of the 10 participants, four expressed regrets about having the test and two of those individuals felt 'severe remorse'. A common reason given for these regrets was that knowing their status was a far heavier load then they had expected and 'the hope is gone'.

These studies show that predictive genetic testing can be carried out without harmful effects in the context of a carefully designed clinical programme that includes genetic counselling as part of the process, but that care and long-term support are required to minimise the risks associated with such testing. Not surprisingly, research shows that people who receive an unfavourable result tend to be more distressed than those whose tests show they are not carriers of the gene mutation. There is also evidence of some negative reactions among confirmed non-carriers which could be due to an important change in personal identity on discovering after many years that they are not, in fact, at risk as they previously believed.[53]

Personal experiences of presymptomatic testing

Sue Wright was 14 years old when, after her father's diagnosis, she found out that she had a 50 per cent chance of developing Huntington disease. She described her experience as 'a yo-yo-type of existence',[54] sometimes convinced she had the gene and at other times feeling guilty about worrying. In practical terms, it added complications with relationships, insurance and applying for a nursing job in New Zealand.

In March 1993, the gene was cloned and the option of testing became a reality. After counselling she decided to have the test, which showed that she was carrying the gene. She was shocked and described her feelings as being similar to a form of bereavement. Nevertheless, she said that both she and her partner 'felt more at peace now we knew I had the gene. I'm sure fear can build up around something that might or might not happen and sometimes it's better to know the truth. In the months since this time neither of us has regretted the decision at all.'[55]

Charlotte Raven, however, recounts her experiences rather differently.[56] Having found out in 2006 that her father had Huntington disease she decided to have the test assuming that, although finding out would be traumatic, this would be offset by the satisfaction of being able to make informed decisions. Having tested positive, however, she says she wished she did not know and she describes spending a considerable amount of time contemplating how to commit suicide. In her personal account of her experience, and her subsequent investigation into the condition and those living with it, she expresses surprise that only one in four people with the condition actually commits suicide. After having the test, she reports finding herself wondering every time she misplaced something whether this was the beginning of the onset of the condition.

Raven describes both the best and worst thing about the illness as the fact that 'it leaves intact the sufferers' ability to love their family' and concludes that for her 'suicide is a fantasy. Loving my daughter, I am doomed to live.'[57]

Given the profound implications of predictive testing, it is essential that the individual gives the matter full and careful consideration and makes the decision that is appropriate for him or her. It is clear from experience that patients sometimes seek testing as a result of pressure from a spouse or other family member.[58] Although it is important for patients to consider the effect of their decision on other people, it is for each individual to decide and testing should proceed only if the patient has given valid, and therefore unpressured, consent. Partners may have a legitimate interest in knowing the genetic status of the patient, particularly if they are making decisions together about whether to have children. This does not, however, justify pressure being exerted on the individual to seek testing or to receive the result of the test, unless that is the patient's own wish. Despite having no authority to make the decision, it is important that the relatives and partners of those seeking testing also receive support. Some studies have shown significant levels of distress amongst the partners of those who received an unfavourable result from testing.[59]

The report issued by the Advisory Committee on Genetic Testing (whose role was subsequently taken over by the Human Genetics Commission – which itself, at the time of writing, is scheduled to be replaced with a Department of Health 'committee of experts') on testing for late onset disorders[60] offers the advice below on the information needed by those who are seeking testing.

- Information on the disorder being tested for should be full and accurate, and should be presented in a clear and simple manner that is readily understandable.
- Full information should be provided on the test, its consequences and limitations, and its scientific and clinical validity.
- Individuals should be fully informed of potential adverse consequences, such as for insurance, employment and effects on other family members.
- Although written details are important, complex information should be provided face-to-face by an appropriately trained and experienced person.
- Voluntary organisations involved with genetic disorders can also be a valuable source of information for those considering genetic testing.
- Individuals should be given adequate time to absorb the information provided before a decision is taken to be tested or a result is given.

Health professionals caring for patients who have received an unfavourable presymp-tomatic test should be wary of relying too heavily on the test result and should remain open minded to other explanations for reported symptoms. There have been cases in which other conditions have been missed because the doctor wrongly attributed the clinical signs to the underlying predictive genetic test result.

Adults who lack capacity

Presymptomatic testing of an adult who lacks capacity for a severe genetic disorder for which no treatment is available may only proceed where it would be in the best interests of the individual patient. This could be because it would allow carers to take practical steps to improve the care of the patient or to plan financially for the individual's future. In very limited circumstances, such testing may be of benefit to other family members. Testing incapacitated adults for the benefit of others is discussed on pages 370–372.

Young people

With presymptomatic testing where there is no medical benefit, there would need to be good evidence that the patient is competent and has a high level of understanding of the issues in order for a person aged under 16 to be able to consent to testing. Any health professional providing presymptomatic testing to a person under 16 years of age must be prepared to justify that decision on grounds of the individual's competence. The doctor would also have a responsibility to ensure that sufficient information had been given, that the patient had understood this information and that he or she had received extensive counselling and considered the implications of a positive test for him or herself and for other family members. The young person should also be strongly encouraged to involve his or her parents or another adult in this important decision and, ideally, to wait a few years before having the test. Before proceeding with testing, health professionals should satisfy themselves that an appropriate support mechanism is available for the young person. Young people over 16 years of age are presumed to be competent to consent to testing, but parental involvement should still be strongly encouraged and the difficulties that young people may have in imagining their lives 10–20 years away should be acknowledged.

Children

The majority of predictive genetic testing that has been carried out in young children is for conditions that usually manifest in early childhood or where some medical intervention can usefully be applied. The benefits that accrue from presymptomatic testing for childhood onset disorders include appropriate diagnosis and management as well as options for preventive action or treatment. Testing for Duchenne muscular dystrophy, for example, can allow parents to meet at an early stage with specialist health professionals in order to plan for the future health needs of the child. Arguments about undermining the child's right to make decisions for himself or herself in the future and problems of confidentiality, which arise in relation to testing for adult-onset disorders, do not arise when the condition usually becomes manifest in very young children. However, where parents request testing of a young child for a disorder that usually develops around the teens, these factors need to be taken into account. Some people take the view that it is harmful to the child to know from an early age that he or she will go on to develop a severe genetic condition, whereas others argue that young children are better able to cope with such information and will grow up in the knowledge of, and accepting, their impending disability. In fact, both the benefits and harms of testing in these circumstances are largely unproven and decisions need to be made on the basis of the facts of individual cases, making an assessment of the child's best interests, taking account of the following factors:

- the age and maturity of the child
- the length of time between the request and the estimated age of onset of symptoms
- the views of the child regarding testing, if sufficiently mature to make a judgement
- the type of disorder and the potential medical, psychological and practical benefits of knowing the child's genetic status prior to the onset of symptoms
- why, and by whom, testing is being sought
- the potential benefits or harms for the child.

Occasionally, requests are received from parents who wish to have their children tested presymptomatically for adult-onset disorders. In some cases, early treatment or regular surveillance could bring some medical benefit to the child and in these cases a careful balance needs to be reached between the amount of benefit and the potential for harm. When there is no treatment or useful medical intervention, there is general agreement, both within the UK and internationally, that testing should be delayed until the child is old enough to make an informed, personal decision.[61] In view of the potentially serious harms of testing in these circumstances, the BMA believes there are grounds for limiting parental decision making in these cases and therefore supports this position.

A major area of concern is that the burden for children of knowing that in adult life they will develop a severe, incurable genetic disorder may be too great and rob them of a carefree childhood. It is feared that learning such news in childhood or adolescence could have a very negative effect on individuals' self-esteem and ability to function properly in society. Parents sometimes seek predictive testing for their children because they believe that, for them, knowing for certain that the child has or has not inherited the gene mutation will enable them to provide more appropriate care for the child. For some parents this may indeed be a benefit, but this needs to be weighed against the risk of harm resulting to the child. There are concerns, for example, that those who find their children to be affected by a late-onset disorder may reflect this in the way they behave towards them. They may treat them as ill before the disorder becomes manifest, or fail to give them encouragement to do well at school or to train for a career. An unfavourable result may also harm the future life opportunities of the child through disadvantages in insurance and employment (see pages 396–398). Although these disadvantages apply equally to adults, who are in a position to make the decision for themselves about whether those risks are worth taking, for children, this irreversible decision would be taken on their behalf. Given that most adults decide that the disadvantages outweigh the advantages of testing for conditions like Huntington disease, and that there is a risk of significant harm to the child, there are good arguments for not complying with parental requests. Those asking for the test should be given a detailed explanation about why it will not be undertaken. The fact that a child is not tested does not mean that he or she should not be informed of the risk of carrying the gene mutation and the possibility of testing in the future. Discussion about their situation with a genetic counsellor can be encouraged.

Although there are good reasons to believe that harm could result from presymptomatic testing of children for serious, late-onset disorders, because such testing is not generally undertaken there is no evidence to prove this. Some research has been carried out on the psychological effects of predictive testing for familial adenomatous polyposis (FAP), for which there are medical benefits to early testing. This found that children did not show clinically significant distress over a period of 1 year after predictive testing.[62]

Predictive testing of children for FAP

One study compared the emotional state of children (aged 10–16 years) and adults (aged 17–67 years) after predictive genetic testing for familial adenomatous polyposis (FAP). It found that children receiving positive or negative results did not experience greater anxiety or depression than adults having the same tests. In fact, the only difference between children and adults was that, among those with positive results, the children were less anxious and a smaller proportion of them had anxiety scores in the clinical range. The study also found that the children, as a group, did not show clinically significant distress over a period of 1 year after predictive testing. This latter finding is consistent with the results of an earlier study conducted on 41 children aged between 6 and 16 years before and 3 months after predictive testing for FAP. This study, carried out in the USA, reported that anxiety and behavioural problems remained in the normal range for the 3 months after testing.[63]

A more recent study, however, found a lack of understanding about the test and a lack of involvement of young people in the decision to be tested and made a number of recommendations for how to improve practice.[64] Although these studies provide some objective evidence about the psychological effects of predictive testing of children, there are significant differences where the condition is incurable and it is appropriate in these latter cases to take a more cautious approach.

Summary – predictive or presymptomatic testing

- When there is no useful medical intervention or treatment, many people choose not to have predictive genetic testing. However, for some, certainty that they will develop the disease may be preferable to living with the uncertainty of their at-risk status.
- Given the profound implications of predictive testing for severe, life-threatening disorders, it is essential that the individual gives the matter full and careful consideration and makes the decision that is appropriate for him or her.
- Evidence of capacity and a high level of understanding would be required in order for a person aged under 16 to be able to consent to presymptomatic genetic testing.
- The majority of predictive genetic testing in young children is for conditions that usually manifest in early childhood or where some medical intervention can usefully be applied.
- When there is no medical benefit to predictive testing in childhood for adult onset disorders, and the potential for serious harm, removing the option for the child not to know his or her genetic status cannot be justified.

Susceptibility testing

It is also possible to test for genes that identify risk factors for particular diseases where having the gene mutation indicates an increased risk, but not certainty, of developing the disorder. The likelihood of developing the condition varies, from very high with hereditary breast cancer to much lower with conditions such as Alzheimer disease and heart disease.

A large number of common disorders are known sometimes to have a genetic component, including some forms of cancer, coronary heart disease and diabetes. With those forms of breast cancer that are caused by mutations in the *BRCA1* gene, testing has a high predictive value with estimates of up to an 85 per cent lifetime risk of developing the condition. Many more disorders, such as heart disease, have a lower genetic component and the level of risk is more dependent upon the interaction between genetic and environmental factors. Thus, genetic testing for these disorders can identify only an increased susceptibility to a particular disorder, with varying degrees of predictability. With some conditions that give a very high level of predictability, there can be clear advantages to testing. For example, some people who know from information provided by an affected family member that they are at increased risk of being carriers of a *BRCA1* mutation, consider having a prophylactic double mastectomy. A genetic test to determine whether the gene mutation has been inherited can inform this decision. If the gene is not present, the risk reduces significantly and the mastectomy can be avoided. When the risk of developing the condition tested for is much lower, however, the benefits are far less straightforward.

Many of the advantages of presymptomatic testing for conditions like Huntington disease (discussed above) focus on the benefit of relief from uncertainty and of being able to plan for the future in the knowledge of impending disability. When the test result indicates only an increased risk of developing the disorder, particularly when this is low, the strength of these arguments is reduced. There may be other advantages, however, to knowing about increased susceptibility. The role played by environmental factors in these common disorders, for example, makes it possible, in some people, to alter their lifestyle to reduce the risk. In some ways, this type of testing is an extension of existing practice, rather than something totally new. Doctors have for many years identified those who are at high risk of cancer or heart disease and tried to encourage them to make changes to their lifestyle to minimise that risk. It remains to be seen whether such advice, based on genetic testing, will be any more successful than previous attempts to encourage people to live healthier lives. There is some evidence to support the concern that many people associate genetic tests with conditions that are not preventable and not treatable, which is likely to make it more difficult to encourage behavioural changes.[65] This can lead not only to a reluctance to take action to reduce the risk, because it is seen as inevitable, but also to increased levels of anxiety. A review of the available research evidence carried out by Marteau and Lerman[66] in 2001 found that providing people with DNA-derived information about risks to their health did not increase motivation to change behaviour beyond that achieved with non-genetic information. There was also some indication that people may adopt a fatalistic approach and, for some, genetic information may reduce motivation to change their behaviour. This may change, however, as understanding within society of the role of genetic factors in health and disease increases, particularly if information is backed up by counselling and positive health messages.

If susceptibility testing is to be of any benefit in common diseases like heart disease, attention needs to be paid to methods of presenting information in such a way that it motivates and encourages people to make the necessary lifestyle changes. The future use and availability of testing that gives only a relatively low predictive value depends upon there being some clear benefits to its use.

Summary – susceptibility testing

- When the test result indicates only an increased risk of developing the disorder, the benefits – in terms of relief from uncertainty – are less clear-cut than with predictive testing.
- Attention needs to be given to finding methods of presenting information about predisposition to disease in such a way that it motivates and encourages people to make the necessary lifestyle changes.

Incidental findings

Sometimes, additional, unsought or unexpected information is obtained during genetic testing and this is likely to become more common as the use of microarrays and increasingly whole genome sequencing become part of everyday practice. The information detected could, for example, concern a condition other than the one being tested for, the discovery of carrier status or be about misattributed paternity.[67] If there is a reasonable chance of other information being inadvertently·discovered from a particular test, this should be discussed with the patient, or the parent of a young child, during the consent process in order to ascertain the individual's wishes about disclosure. The discussion should give examples of the type of information that could be discovered and the procedures that will be followed in that event.

When information is discovered unexpectedly, and this discussion has not taken place, the BMA believes there should be a general presumption that significant information will be shared because it would be wrong deliberately to withhold it on the assumption that it would not be in the individual's interests to know. However, there may be exceptions to this rule, such as where it is judged that revealing the information could cause severe psychological harm to the patient or would be contrary to the interests of a young child. When such information is to be given, this must be done sensitively and taking a cue from the individual about how much information he or she is ready and willing to accept at that particular time.

Population genetic screening

Population screening involves testing members of a particular population for a disorder or condition for which there is no family history or other prior evidence of its presence. The population to be screened may be chosen for a number of reasons. It may be those who, because of their circumstances, would find screening useful. This could include screening those who are planning to have children for carrier status for common autosomal recessive conditions, such as cystic fibrosis, to enable them to make informed reproductive decisions, or the well-established programme of screening the Ashkenazi Jewish population for Tay–Sachs carrier status. They may be chosen simply because of their age (for example, some genetic screening is routinely carried out on neonates), or the population may be the self-selecting group who choose to avail themselves of screening, possibly through one of the services that offers screening direct to consumers (see pages 393–396). It has also been suggested that, in the future, screening may be offered routinely to the whole population to assess the genetic risk of predisposition to certain conditions such as heart disease and types of cancer, with a view to prevention and early intervention.[68] For further information about population screening see Chapter 20 (pages 824–827).

Screening for carrier status for autosomal recessive disorders

The possibility of population screening for carrier status for a range of autosomal recessive disorders has been under consideration for some time. The introduction of screening for carrier status for cystic fibrosis, for example, has been discussed by the UK National Screening Committee (UK NSC) at various times over a number of years although, currently, it is not recommended.[69] As a result, availability and methods of screening vary between areas. Such programmes as exist are mainly based in antenatal units (although the UK NSC does not recommend that pregnant women are offered carrier screening for cystic fibrosis). Screening during pregnancy is not ideal because it precludes some of the reproductive options available, such as preimplantation genetic diagnosis (see Chapter 8, pages 337–339) or the use of donated gametes. The ideal situation is for information about carrier status to be available when people are planning a pregnancy.

At the request of the UK NSC, the Human Genetics Commission set up an expert working group to consider the potential ethical, legal and social implications of preconception screening for a range of conditions including cystic fibrosis. It concluded that 'there are no specific ethical, legal or social principles that would make preconception genetic testing within the framework of a population screening programme unacceptable'.[70] It therefore recommended that preconception screening should be made available to all those who might benefit from it.

Despite the clear advantages to preconception carrier screening, its uptake so far in the UK has been minimal. One difficulty is identifying the population who would be most likely to want to use the service – those who are planning a pregnancy. Some people discuss their plans with their family planning clinic or GP, but many more do not. Another alternative is to offer screening to all people of reproductive age, although where this has been offered the uptake has been low, which could indicate a lack of interest in such screening[71] or, in the absence of any family history, an unwillingness to believe that the screening is necessary or relevant. Some people who are planning pregnancy may opt to seek carrier screening independently by using one of the services offered direct to consumers (see pages 393–396). Another option would be to offer carrier screening in the final year of secondary school, when young people are sufficiently mature to give valid consent and can be offered testing in conjunction with a formal educational component. Established school-based programmes offering voluntary testing for carrier status for various conditions are in place in Hong Kong, Marseille, Israel, Australia and Canada.[72] An outcome evaluation of two decades of school-based screening in Montreal found the average uptake to be 67 per cent. The study also showed that all couples in Montreal using prenatal diagnosis for Tay–Sachs disease acquired their knowledge of their carrier status through the school-based programme.[73] Although there are benefits to carrier screening in schools, a number of safeguards would need to be put in place before this could be contemplated. These include difficulties around pressures on consent, confidentiality, the risk of stigmatisation and the need to provide appropriate support mechanisms.

Neonatal screening

Neonatal screening has, historically, been less controversial than other types, because its main aim has been to identify affected neonates in order to instigate treatment at the earliest opportunity. Since the 1970s, for example, virtually all newborn babies have been screened to ascertain whether they have inherited the genetic defect for phenylketonuria (PKU). The benefits to such screening are clear-cut because early diagnosis and a special diet can avoid most of the adverse effects of this disorder. Most parents are very happy to give consent when they appreciate the benefits of the test; when they refuse, there may be grounds for arguing that the refusal is not in the best interests of the child and therefore is not a decision the parents are able to make on their child's behalf. It is interesting, however, that the Supreme Court of Ireland upheld parents' right to refuse PKU testing, despite the very obvious benefits to children and the minimally invasive nature of the heel-prick test.[74] No such cases have been considered by courts in the UK.

Although the evidence is less clear-cut than with PKU, the UK NSC now recommends neonatal screening for cystic fibrosis as part of the heel-prick test. However, a complication with neonatal screening for cystic fibrosis (and other disorders such as sickle cell disease, which is offered to certain populations) is that, in addition to identifying affected babies, some carriers may also be detected. This has raised concerns given that most guidance recommends delaying carrier testing until the child is old enough to make a personal decision (see pages 379–382). It has also led to a situation where parents know the genetic status of some, but not all, of their children. When carrier status is likely to be revealed during the course of the diagnostic test, this should be explained to the parents in the process of seeking consent. Information that is available should not be deliberately withheld from the parents (unless they have expressed a wish not to be informed), particularly because knowledge of the child's carrier status may have implications for their own future reproductive decisions. When babies are found to be carriers, the parents should be given help and support to decide when and how to inform the child of the carrier status.

The range of conditions tested for by the heel-prick test varies between different parts of the UK (see below). In Wales, for example, boys are routinely tested for Duchenne muscular dystrophy. Although there is no available treatment, there may be advantages to having an early, confirmed diagnosis of this condition, such as the ability to meet specialist health professionals, to seek genetic counselling and to plan for the future, and also for the parents to be able to make informed decisions about future reproduction. Another advantage for some families is the avoidance of the typically prolonged period of uncertainty before a firm diagnosis is obtained. The potential advantages of early diagnosis need to be balanced against the disadvantage of knowing of impending disability, perhaps a few years before the onset of symptoms. The UK NSC does not currently recommend newborn screening for this condition.[75]

Newborn blood spot screening in the UK (the 'heel-prick test')[76]

England: phenylketonuria (PKU), congenital hypothyroidism (CHT), sickle cell disease (SCD), cystic fibrosis (CF) and medium-chain acyl-CoA dehydrogenase deficiency (MCADD).

Scotland: phenylketonuria (PKU), congenital hypothyroidism (CHT), cystic fibrosis (CF), sickle cell disease (SCD) and medium-chain acyl-CoA dehydrogenase deficiency (MCADD).

Wales: phenylketonuria (PKU), congenital hypothyroidism (CHT), cystic fibrosis (CF) and (boys only) Duchenne muscular dystrophy.

Northern Ireland: phenylketonuria (PKU), congenital hypothyroidism (CHT), cystic fibrosis (CF), medium-chain acyl-CoA dehydrogenase deficiency (MCADD) and sickle cell disease (SCD). Screening for homocystinuria and tyrosinaemia is also offered.

Screening for predisposition to common disorders

As more information becomes available about the genetic contribution to complex, common disorders, the possibility of screening the full population for predisposition to particular disorders becomes an option. It has been argued, for example, that society could, at some time in the future, embrace large-scale screening for susceptibility to common diseases such as cancer.[77] The purpose would be to identify those who are at increased genetic risk, so that they can take steps to reduce those environmental aspects of risk that are amenable to change such as diet and exercise, or possibly to take prophylactic medication to reduce the likelihood of the condition developing, or to facilitate early intervention.[78] Many of the issues that arise with such screening are similar to testing those at risk because of a family history (see pages 388–389), but on a much larger scale and with the added inherent problems of population screening (see Chapter 20, pages 824–827). The success of any such programme depends upon information being presented in such a way as to motivate people to change their lifestyle or take other steps to reduce the risk.

Unless this can be achieved, the disadvantages of full population screening are likely to outweigh the benefits for the foreseeable future. Over time, however, the population is likely to become better informed about genetics and may find it far less threatening and accept genetic predisposition as simply one among many risk factors for common disorders.

Summary – population genetic screening

- Population screening involves testing members of a particular population for a disorder or condition for which there is no family history or other prior evidence of its presence.
- Screening for carrier status for autosomal recessive disorders should ideally be offered to those planning to have children, but this population group is difficult to identify.
- Some forms of neonatal screening (such as for cystic fibrosis) also identify some carriers of the disorder. Parents should be informed of this as part of the consent process and should be told of the results if they wish to know them.
- In the future it may be possible to undertake population screening to detect an increased predisposition to common disorders. Attention needs to be given to providing information in such a way that it motivates and encourages people to make the necessary lifestyle changes.

Genetic tests supplied direct to consumers

Growing public interest and knowledge about genetics has led to a range of genetic tests being provided in shops, by mail or via the internet, without the need to discuss the test or the results with a medical practitioner or other suitably qualified health practitioner. Demand for such services has been lower than initially expected, however, and it is not clear whether this is an area that will continue to grow. Initially, such services were restricted to carrier testing for autosomal recessive disorders, but this expanded to, among other things, paternity testing and testing aimed at providing dietary and lifestyle advice. In 2007, some companies introduced 'whole genome testing', raising the possibility of presymptomatic testing for serious, untreatable conditions being provided direct to consumers with no requirement for pre- and post-test counselling and support. Given the very serious implications of such testing, for the individuals and their families, and the risk of severe distress and anxiety (see pages 383–385), this is a matter of concern.

Although it would be feasible to restrict the advertising or sale of genetic testing kits in the UK, it is not possible to prevent people from using services in other countries, such as those accessed via the internet. In an attempt to address this problem the Human Genetics Commission published, in 2010, a common framework of principles for direct-to-consumer genetic testing services (see below).[79] The framework aims to promote high standards and greater consistency in the provision of direct-to-consumer tests amongst commercial providers at an international level. It is intended to apply to situations where genetic tests are marketed and supplied directly to consumers rather than to, or via, qualified medical professionals. The House of Lords Science and Technology Committee has expressed its support for such a code, suggesting that it should include a requirement on companies to make public information about the standards they follow and the accreditation required of them nationally. The House of Lords also called upon the Department of Health to publish information on its website about accreditation and quality assurance schemes for companies offering such tests as well as scientific data about the robustness of the tests themselves.[80]

Common framework of principles for direct-to-consumer genetic testing services – key points[81]

- Claims about clinical validity of genetic tests should be supported by relevant evidence published in peer reviewed scientific literature.
- The test provider should provide easily understood, accurate, appropriate and adequate information to consumers.
- Where the test involves inherited disorders consumers should be given the opportunity to receive pre-and post-test counselling.
- Written consent should be obtained.
- The test provider should take reasonable steps to ensure the sample provided for testing was obtained from the person identified as the sample provider.
- Requests to recover DNA from secondary objects should raise suspicion about non-consensual testing and should be declined.
- Except in exceptional circumstances direct-to-consumer genetic tests should not be provided to adults unable to give consent.
- Genetic testing of children should normally be delayed until the child is able to give consent unless earlier testing is clinically indicated; in these circumstances testing should be organised by a health professional.
- Interpretation of genetic test results involving inherited disorders should be carried out under the responsibility of an appropriately qualified professional, with recognised training and qualifications, and regulated by an appropriate professional body, who is employed by or working on behalf of the test provider.
- The results of genetic tests and the significance that should be attributed to a particular genetic test result should be described to the consumer in a format that is easy to understand.
- The test provider should not release genetic test results to any third parties, including insurance companies, health professionals or solicitors, without the specific consent of the provider.

The Nuffield Council on Bioethics has also considered the ethical issues raised by direct-to-consumer genetic profiling as part of its 2010 report, *Medical profiling and online medicine: the ethics of 'personalised healthcare' in a consumer age*.[82]

The BMA does not believe that all genetic tests, simply by being DNA tests, require additional protection. Rather, it is the implications of the test result, the likelihood of the result being misinterpreted and the risk of harm arising to those seeking testing, or others, that should determine whether restrictions should be applied. Patients should be free to seek information about their own health without interference from the state but, at the same time, the state has a duty to protect its citizens from avoidable, and foreseeable, serious harm. There may be circumstances in which serious harm could result from an individual receiving a genetic test result without the necessary information and support to both understand and come to terms with it. For example, research evidence has shown that, in carefully controlled situations, presymptomatic testing for Huntington disease can be undertaken without harmful results (see pages 383–385), but there are good grounds for believing that predictive testing without any professional support could result in serious harm. In such cases, the duty of the state to protect its citizens from harm may override the individual's wish to seek testing without the provision of counselling and professional support.

A predictive test for Huntington disease is, of course, at one end of a spectrum of tests that could be available direct to consumers. The implications of other genetic tests are less problematic. For example, carrier testing for an autosomal recessive disorder in a couple who are planning a pregnancy and in whom there is no family history raises far fewer concerns, provided adequate and appropriate information is available. Carrier testing does not usually provide information about the individual's own health, or predict future disease, although an unfavourable result would have implications for other siblings or existing children, who may find out that they are also at risk of being a carrier of the disorder.

As our knowledge and understanding of the genetic contribution to complex common disorders increases, the market for direct-to-consumer testing may grow. An important question, in relation to the need for regulation, is whether a genetic test that identifies an increased susceptibility to heart disease, for example, is significantly different from any one of the non-genetic tests that could give the same information, such as tests for cholesterol levels or blood pressure. In the light of the research quoted on page 389, about people's understanding of genetic tests, there may be more of a risk of a genetic test being misunderstood and taken to imply that the individual will definitely develop heart disease, rather than that he or she is at increased risk. This could lead to considerable anxiety and also make behavioural changes appear futile. There are also considerable uncertainties, both about the validity and clinical utility of genome-based tests for susceptibility to common complex diseases, that need to be addressed. Those seeking such testing must be provided with accurate information enabling them to understand the limitations of the information provided and to understand what the result means, and what it does not mean. The identification of an increased genetic susceptibility in one individual could also have direct implications for other family members and, in this respect, it is also different from other forms of testing. Nevertheless, while the benefits may be questionable, the magnitude of potential harm is significantly less than for predictive testing for serious, untreatable disorders and the balance, in this case, is likely to rest firmly on individuals being able to seek testing in a way that best suits their personal needs.

The BMA believes that testing with the involvement and support of health professionals should continue to be the norm for most patients, and is preferable, particularly where the test has profound implications for the individual, but recognises that this is difficult to enforce, particularly where UK citizens access services from companies based overseas. Where testing is provided direct to consumers, the most important factor is that individuals seeking testing have access to objective, factual information about the risks, benefits and implications of the type of testing they are seeking. One problem is that the commercial companies providing the information prior to testing have a vested interest in the individuals going on to have the test and may not therefore give sufficient weight to the reasons why someone may decide not to be tested. The BMA has called for official Government websites to provide accurate information for those considering testing, including the benefits of prior discussion with a health professional and information about what standards they should expect to receive from companies providing direct-to-consumer testing.

If health professionals become aware of an individual's plan to seek testing in another country, they should ensure that the patient is aware of the importance of receiving detailed information, of having the opportunity to ask questions and of the availability of professional support. They should also be informed that, unless there is effective, local regulation, there can be no guarantees about the standards in the laboratories undertaking the test. The BMA believes that information provided to people seeking testing, in this country and overseas, should encourage individuals to discuss their wish for testing with their GP or other relevant health professional.

Since 2006, with some exceptions (see pages 372–373), it has been a criminal offence to have human tissue with the intention of analysing its DNA without the necessary consent. The BMA has concerns about some websites that offer direct-to-consumer genetic testing with samples taken from cigarette butts, nail clippings, underwear, licked envelopes, used tissues, etc. where there appears to be a high risk that the samples have been collected covertly and without the necessary consent. While it is preferable for testing only to be available where mouth swabs are provided, this is difficult to enforce. The BMA also believes there are good arguments for restricting direct-to-consumer testing, other than paternity testing (see below), to requests from adults with capacity. Although it is difficult to guarantee this where there is no personal contact between the company and the individual being tested, including this stipulation may act as a deterrent by requiring parents to deliberately provide false information in order for their request for testing of their child to be complied with.

Summary – genetic tests supplied direct to consumers

- The BMA does not believe that all genetic tests, simply by being DNA tests, require additional protection. Rather decisions should be based on the implications of the test, the likelihood of misunderstanding and the risk of serious harm to the person being tested or others.
- The BMA believes that testing with the involvement and support of health professionals should continue to be the norm for most patients, and is preferable, but recognises that this is difficult to enforce.
- Those seeking direct-to-consumer genetic testing should have access to objective, factual information about the implications of testing and should be encouraged to discuss their plan with a health professional.
- The BMA believes that, other than paternity testing, direct-to-consumer genetic testing should be restricted to requests by adults with capacity.

Controversial uses of genetic information

Genetic information may be used for a variety of purposes, both medical and social. It is the non-medical uses that have been most controversial and for some time there have been calls for additional protection to be afforded to genetic information (see pages 408–409). Some of the more controversial uses are briefly discussed below.

Genetics and insurance

Insurance companies have always requested medical information in order to assess premiums, but their use of the results of predictive genetic tests has been one of the most controversial and frequently debated aspects of developments in genetics. From the patient's perspective, the main problem is perceived to be that those who have an unfavourable genetic test may be refused insurance cover or may be charged such a high premium that, in effect, they are unable to purchase the insurance they want. It is feared that this could deter people from having genetic tests that would be in their broader interests and which could, in some cases, help to delay or prevent the onset of a disorder. However, insurance companies are concerned about pressure to change the existing basis of the relationship whereby both the insurer and the insured have access to the same information in making decisions. They are concerned that if clients have information that they do not reveal to the insurer, they could take out high value policies knowing that they have a high chance of making a claim (known as 'adverse selection'). Without that relevant information, the insurance company cannot set the premiums at higher rates and so the company, or other policyholders, lose out financially.

The short-term solution to this problem has been an agreed moratorium until November 2017 on the use of predictive genetic test results by insurance companies for life, critical illness and income protection policies up to certain levels (see Chapter 16, pages 658–659). For policies over the stated financial limits only tests that have been specifically approved may be used (this currently only applies to tests for Huntington disease). The task of approving tests and monitoring compliance with the moratorium originally fell to the Department of Health's Genetics and Insurance Committee but this was disbanded in 2009. The monitoring role was then taken over by a genetics and insurance committee of the Human Genetics Commission although in 2010 the Government announced plans to abolish the Human Genetics Commission, replacing it with an expert advisory committee of the Department of Health.[83] It is unclear whether this committee will take over responsibility for overseeing the use of genetic tests by insurance companies.

Although the agreement between the Government and the Association of British Insurers refers to a moratorium on the use of 'predictive genetic test results', it does not, in fact, apply to all such tests, but only to 'unfavourable' test results. The impact of the moratorium has been to restrict insurance companies' use of results that would be detrimental to the person buying the policy, while still allowing individuals to use favourable results that increase their likelihood of obtaining policies at the standard rates.[84] In some ways this is a logical distinction, because it would appear unreasonable for a company to load an insurance policy on the basis of a family history when it is clear that the individual has not inherited the gene mutation involved, and therefore is not at increased risk. On the other hand, it seems contrary to principles of natural justice to prevent insurance companies from using information when it would help them, but to allow them to use the same information when it would help the consumer.

Although the moratorium – originally agreed in 2001 – was widely welcomed and received considerable positive media attention, its benefit to those at risk of genetic disorders should not be overstated. Those who have undergone predictive genetic testing have done so because of a family history of the disease. Although under the terms of the moratorium they are not required to disclose the result of an unfavourable test, they are still required to disclose their family history. In some cases patients have been refused insurance cover on the basis of a family history of Huntington disease, putting them in no better position than if they had declared an unfavourable test result.[85] In this situation, those at risk have the option of forgoing insurance cover or taking the test in the hope that it will be favourable but knowing there is a 50 per cent chance they will discover they will go on to develop a severe, untreatable condition. This clearly puts pressure on those individuals to have testing, which is something the moratorium was originally designed to avoid. The moratorium also applies only to predictive tests, not to diagnostic tests carried out once symptoms have begun to appear.

Continually renewing the moratorium for short periods is not a reasonable option because people who are seeking testing while the moratorium is in force need to know whether they will be required to divulge their test results to insurance companies at any time in the future. One way around this problem would be for special provision to be made for those who have tests carried out while the moratorium is in force. In the BMA's view, however, the moratorium should be an interim position while consideration is given to the range of options available for the longer term. The discussion should look more broadly at the use of medical information by insurance companies, rather than focusing solely on genetic information. In the BMA's view the review should also consider whether there are logical objective reasons or sound political reasons for treating genetic information differently from other medical information in the context of insurance. The BMA has explored these issues in more detail elsewhere[86] and will continue to contribute to this debate. (Practical advice for doctors who are asked to complete medical reports for insurance companies can be found in Chapter 16, pages 654–661.)

Genetics and employment

The use of genetic information by employers has been the subject of less public debate and this reflects the fact that, when enquiries were made during 2001[87] and again in 2006,[88] very few employers were seeking access to such information. The 2006 survey, undertaken by the Human Genetics Commission did, however, receive anecdotal reports of one case of inappropriate use of genetic information by employers. In that case a police force had refused to employ a successful recruit on the basis of a family history of Huntington disease despite expert medical opinion stating that the condition was unlikely to manifest until after retirement age. The BMA supports the principle that pre-employment medical reports should focus on the individual's current ability safely to carry out the work in question and genetic information should only be used by employers for that purpose.

In June 2005 the Information Commissioner published an Employment Practice Code[89] giving clear guidance on the use of genetic information by employers (see below). The Code advises employers to inform the Human Genetics Commission of any proposals to use genetic testing for employment purposes which will enable the HGC to monitor their use. As discussed in Chapter 16 (pages 672–673), however, the main problem for GPs when asked to complete pre-employment reports is responding accurately to general health questions – such as whether the patient has been referred to a specialist – when a referral was made for genetic testing or was connected with an unfavourable genetic test result. Practical guidance for health professionals about responding to such requests is provided on pages 672–673.

Information Commissioner's Employment Practices Code[90]

- Do not use genetic testing in an effort to obtain information that is predictive of a worker's future general health.
- Do not insist that a worker discloses the results of a previous genetic test.
- Only use genetic testing to obtain information where it is clear that a worker with a particular, detectable genetic condition is likely to pose a serious safety risk to others or where it is known that a specific working environment or practice might pose specific risks to workers with particular genetic variations.
- If a genetic test is used to obtain information for employment purposes ensure that it is valid and is subject to assured levels of accuracy and reliability.

More information about genetic testing and employment, and about the monitoring work being undertaken by the Human Genetics Commission, can be found at: www.hgc.gov.uk.

Paternity testing

Another common use of genetic information is to establish family relationships, usually but not exclusively paternity. In the past this involved the taking of blood samples, so health professionals were invariably involved in the process, but developments in technology have led to tests being carried out on other material, such as a few hair follicles or a mouth swab, without medical involvement. As a result paternity testing is now offered as a direct-to-consumer service, using home testing kits or tests obtained via the internet and sent off for analysis. Although samples from the putative father and the child are always required, it is no longer necessary for the mother to provide a sample in order to obtain a meaningful result. These developments have raised the possibility of samples being tested without the knowledge and consent of all parties.

Legal issues

Where the taking of a sample involves an invasive procedure, such as taking a sample of blood, a mouth swab or removing a strand of hair, consent is required for the taking of the sample. In addition, since 2006, with limited exceptions (see pages 372–373) it has been a criminal offence throughout the UK to have material that has come from a human body and consists of, or includes, human cells, with the intention of analysing its DNA without consent.[91] This law is intended to prevent testing without consent and was passed following a small number of high profile cases where paternity tests were undertaken surreptitiously using dental floss retrieved from celebrities' rubbish bins. People with parental responsibility may give consent on behalf of children or young people, but when they are capable of understanding the issues, the young people's own views should be sought and taken into account in deciding whether testing would be in their best interests. Each case must be considered on its merits. If, after discussion, a mature minor decides to withhold consent to paternity testing it may not be in that person's best interests to proceed, regardless of the views of the adults involved. In Scotland, someone with parental responsibility can only give consent if the young person is not competent to decide. (For more information on children's consent see Chapter 4.)

When the putative father has parental responsibility for a child, and can therefore give consent on behalf of the child, paternity testing could lawfully be undertaken without the knowledge or consent of the mother. The BMA believes this could be very harmful to the child, as well as to the family unit as a whole, and would prefer to see a situation in which the consent of the mother and the putative father (and the child, if sufficiently mature) is required for paternity testing. In the absence of such a requirement, if doctors are consulted they should encourage those seeking testing to discuss their plans with the child's mother and the BMA would advise doctors not to become involved if that advice is rejected. Irrespective of the outcome, confidentiality must be respected and no information about the discussion should be passed to the mother or the child without the man's consent. The need for a sample to be provided by the putative father means that testing would not be lawful without his consent and cooperation.

When one of the adults does not consent to paternity testing, it is possible for a direction to be sought from the court.[92] When the court issues a direction for the test to be carried out on a blood sample, this does not authorise the taking of blood without consent but 'inferences' can be drawn from an adult's refusal to provide blood for testing. If the person with parental responsibility refuses to consent to the testing of a child under the age of 16, this may proceed in England, Wales and Northern Ireland with an order from the court, which allows blood to be taken from a person under the age of 16 'if the court considers that it would be in his best interests for the sample to be taken'.[93] The courts have taken the view that in the vast majority of cases the child's best interests are served by learning the truth.

Paternity testing

Mrs R gave birth to twins in 1997. At the time of conception Mrs R was having sexual relationships with both her husband (Mr R) and Mr B. Both Mr R and Mr B believed themselves to be the father of the twins. Mr R was unaware of his wife's relationship with Mr B and became the twins' primary carer. The relationship between Mrs R and Mr B ended acrimoniously in 1999 and Mr B applied to the court for contact and parental responsibility. The result was a consent order for DNA testing, with which Mrs R did not comply. At the subsequent hearing, Mr B applied for a ruling that testing could be undertaken on the children without Mrs R's consent on the grounds that it would be in their best interests.

Mr R submitted a statement to the court in which he asserted his inability to continue as the primary carer of the twins, should the court order a test that established Mr B's paternity and that, in that event, he would forsake them. In weighing 'the advantage of scientific truth against uncertainty' the judge said he must 'consider the interest that the community has in establishing such certitude on the one hand and on the other hand the possible, and I believe, ... probably disastrous disintegrative effects of a finding that Mr B in fact is the father'.[94] The judge also took account of the fact that he thought it unlikely that the matter would become the subject of local gossip and that it was therefore also unlikely that the children themselves would ever get to know about the uncertainty concerning their paternity. He therefore dismissed the application, arguing that the tests would not be in the children's best interests.

In allowing an appeal against this decision, Lady Justice Butler-Sloss held that the judge had given insufficient weight to the importance of certainty. She referred to the leading case from the 1970s, in which Lord Hodson said: 'the interests of justice in the abstract are best served by the ascertainment of the truth and there must be few cases where the interests of children can be shown to be best served by the suppression of the truth'.[95] The application was submitted for retrial in order that all of the facts could be carefully considered. The final outcome of this case has not been reported.

Where adults lack the capacity to consent, the test can only be performed if it is deemed to be in their best interests. In England and Wales (Mental Capacity Act 2005) and Scotland (Adults with Incapacity (Scotland) Act 2000), patients can appoint proxy decision makers to make health and welfare decisions on their behalf, should they lose the capacity to do so themselves (see Chapter 3). If the incapacitated adult has appointed a proxy decision maker, he or she must be consulted and can give valid consent for procedures that are in the patient's best interests. If there is serious dispute or doubt as to whether the procedure would be in the patient's best interests, legal advice should be sought.

In Northern Ireland, no person can give consent on behalf of another adult. However, under the Regulations issued under the Human Tissue Act 2004, consent to test an existing sample may be deemed to be in place where the test is in the best interests of the individual.[96]

Ethical obligations

Although, legally, paternity testing may be undertaken without further investigation when the necessary consents have been obtained, from an ethical perspective, the BMA considers that health professionals should agree to provide assistance with testing only when this is considered to be in the best interests of the child. In some cases, the certainty of knowing may be better for the child than a persistent unresolved suspicion. However, there are likely to be cases in which, because of the ease with which such testing can be obtained, the test is requested without those involved having considered the likely impact of the result on all concerned. It is important therefore for health professionals to discuss with the adults concerned why the test has been requested and the implications for family relationships of receiving the result. The information given must be clear and unambiguous, and should raise, for discussion, the possibility that the results may provide distressing information that those who are seeking the test do not want to hear, and which may have a profound effect, with possible lifetime implications, for those involved.

When a decision is made to proceed with testing, patients would be well advised to use an approved service provider, which gives assurances about standards. An up-to-date list of accredited paternity testing services in England and Wales can be obtained from the Ministry of Justice at: www.justice.gov.uk.

Forensic use of genetic information

In 1995, the Government set up the UK National DNA Database. This initially recorded, as numerical representations, the DNA profiles of individuals who had been charged with, informed they would be reported for, or convicted of a recordable offence. With the appropriate authorisation, samples could also be taken from those suspected of being involved in a recordable offence when it was believed that this would tend to confirm or disprove the individual's involvement by comparison with samples left at the crime scene. Police powers were extended in England and Wales by section 10 of the Criminal Justice Act 2003 so that DNA may be taken without consent from anyone arrested for a recordable offence, including those where there was no crime scene sample. The profiles are added to the DNA database and can be used for speculative searches against samples found at both past and future crime scenes. By 2009 the database contained around 5 million DNA profiles.[97]

When the database was first set up, the sample and profile had to be destroyed if someone was acquitted of a crime or if it was decided not to proceed with the case. This was amended, for England and Wales, by the Criminal Justice and Police Act 2001, to allow the profiles and samples to be retained even if the individuals were acquitted of the crimes for which they were taken or if the case was dropped. Those who volunteered samples for elimination purposes could be asked to sign a consent form for their profile to be added to the database. This consent could not subsequently be revoked and any stored profile could later be used for speculative searches against samples left at scenes of crime (including both serious and more minor offences). Similar changes were made for Northern Ireland.[98] In Scotland, samples and profiles could be retained for 3 years after acquittal if the person arrested had been suspected of certain sexual or violent offences. Thereafter samples had to be destroyed unless a Chief Constable applied to a Sheriff for a 2-year extension.[99]

The 2001 amendments in England and Wales, permitting samples to be retained after the suspect had been acquitted or the charges had been dropped, were challenged unsuccessfully in the English courts. In December 2008, however, the case was heard by the Grand Chamber of the European Court of Human Rights which held that the indefinite retention of samples in these circumstances was a violation of the Article 8 right to respect for private and family life. At the time of writing, proposals to amend the length of time for which DNA profiles may be retained were being debated in the Protection of Freedoms Bill. Up-to-date information can be found on the BMA's website.

Retention of DNA samples and the Human Rights Act

S was a 12-year old boy, with no previous convictions, who was arrested and charged with attempted robbery. During the investigation his fingerprints and DNA samples were taken. On 14 June 2001 he was acquitted of the charge. Despite requests from his solicitor that the DNA sample be destroyed, it was retained and the profile was added to the DNA database. S's solicitor argued that this breached Articles 8 (right to private and family life) and 14 (freedom from discrimination in the enjoyment of substantive rights) of the Human Rights Act.

Similar arguments were made by the solicitor acting for a 38-year-old man who was arrested and charged with harassment of his partner. The partner decided not to pursue the case and it was dropped, but the DNA sample was retained and the profile added to the database.

Both cases were dismissed by the High Court. The Appeal Court held that the interference with the Article 8 right to privacy was real but not significant, and that the level of interference was proportionate and justified.[100] It also held that there was a clear objective difference between individuals from whom samples had been taken and those from whom they had not been taken, which was wholly different from the categories mentioned in Article 14 and the case did not, therefore, fall within that Article. The House of Lords also rejected the appeal.[101]

In December 2008, both cases were heard jointly by the Grand Chamber of the European Court of Human Rights. The Grand Chamber noted that, despite the widespread use of DNA databases, the UK was the only member state to permit the systematic and indefinite retention of DNA profiles and samples of persons who had not been convicted of any offence. The Grand Chamber held that the retention of samples, DNA profiles and fingerprints represented an interference with the Article 8 right to privacy and family life and concluded that:

> [t]he blanket and indiscriminate nature of the powers of retention of the fingerprints, cellular samples and DNA profiles of persons suspected but not convicted of offences, as applied in the case of the present applicants, fails to strike a fair balance between the competing public and private interests and [that] the respondent State has overstepped any acceptable margin of appreciation in this regard. Accordingly, the retention at issue constitutes a disproportionate interference with the applicants' right to respect for private life and cannot be regarded as necessary in a democratic society.[102]

In addition to this judgment, the Government's policy has also been criticised in reports from the Nuffield Council on Bioethics[103] and, its own advisory committee, the Human Genetics Commission.[104] In 2007, an ethics group was established to monitor the operation and use of the DNA database which is reported to have considered and rejected the possibility of a population-wide database.[105]

The involvement of doctors

Questions about whose samples should be taken, which profiles and samples should be retained and for how long are matters for society as a whole rather than for doctors. However, some aspects of the use of DNA analysis for criminal justice purposes are directly relevant to doctors. The process of taking samples for DNA analysis uses mouth swabs that are taken by police officers. Forensic physicians may, however, be involved with assessing or providing treatment to the suspect or victim from whom a sample is being taken, or the person may be a patient in hospital at the time the sample is required. The treating doctor should object if any part of the process of taking the sample would be detrimental to the patient's care, but it is not the role of the doctor to assess whether the patient has the capacity to give consent.

When required for elimination purposes, consent is required for the taking of the sample and for its use for the current crime under investigation. The ethics group for the

National DNA database has advised there should be a presumption that samples taken for elimination purposes will not be included on the database – even with consent.[106] At the time of writing, such samples are retained and, once consent has been given, this can never be revoked. When consent is sought for the taking and use of these samples, a clear distinction should be made between consent to take the sample and consent for future retention.[107] It is possible that the individual – who may be the victim of, or a witness to, a crime – may be under the influence of drugs or alcohol or, because of his or her experience, may be very nervous or distressed. In such cases, although a sample may be needed quickly in order to expedite the investigation, there are good arguments for delaying seeking consent for the retention of the sample until the individual is able to make a more objective and informed decision. At the time of writing, Parliament was debating changes to the rules relating to the storage and retention of DNA samples.

In the future, it is possible that DNA analysis in relation to criminal justice could affect doctors more directly. Depending on how the samples are analysed, for example, it is possible that a crime scene sample could lead to the putative offender being identified as having a particular genetic condition or a predisposition to a certain medical condition.[108] The police might then seek information about people attending clinics for that condition, or ask GPs for information from patients' records about those patients in the area with a similar medical background. In responding to such requests, the BMA believes that the usual duty of confidentiality would apply and that information should only be released where there is an overriding public interest (see Chapter 5). In practice, this is likely to mean that the crime would need to be a serious one and the police would need to have a suspect already identified, rather than making speculative searches involving the medical records of all patients with the condition or similar medical history. Providing the police with a list of all patients with a particular disorder without their consent, where there are no other grounds to suspect their involvement in the crime, is unlikely to be justified. In each case careful consideration would need to be given to whether disclosure was both necessary and proportionate. As with other circumstances, however, the police could obtain a court order requiring the doctor to release the information.

Developments in the use of genetic analysis by the criminal justice system

In its report on the forensic use of bioinformation, the Nuffield Council on Bioethics highlights, and raises concerns about, the increasing use of 'familial searching' where the database is searched to identify relatives of offenders. Although guidelines have been drawn up detailing the circumstances in which such searches may be made, these are considered to be 'operationally sensitive' and are not therefore available for public scrutiny.[109]

Use of familial searching of the DNA database

In January 2010, Paul Hutchinson was jailed for 25 years for the rape and murder of 16-year-old Colette Aram in 1983.[110] Mr Hutchinson was charged after police searched the DNA database using DNA retrieved from a paper towel found at a pub near where the murder took place. Although Mr Hutchinson's details were not on the database, the DNA of his son was included after he had been detained for a traffic offence. The database indicated a partial match and this led police to identify the perpetrator. Hutchinson pleaded guilty to the offences shortly before the trial began.

At the current time, DNA profiles are used to compare with samples left at crime scenes but the use of DNA samples could become more sophisticated in the future. It has been suggested, for example, that it could be possible to generate a 'genetic photofit' of offenders by, for example, identifying their sex, race, skin, hair and eye colour.[111] Although the science is currently a long way from making this possible, there have been moves in this direction. The Nuffield Council on Bioethics has, however, expressed serious concerns about the use of genetic analysis to determine the most likely ethnic origin of the suspect which, it says, could reinforce racist views of propensity to criminality.[112]

Summary – controversial uses of genetic information

- The BMA believes there needs to be further informed debate about the use of genetic information by insurance companies. One of the issues that needs to be addressed is whether there are sound logical and objective reasons, or good political reasons, for treating genetic information differently from other medical information in the context of insurance.
- The BMA supports the principle that pre-employment medical reports should focus on the individual's current ability safely to carry out the work in question and believes that genetic information should be used by employers only for that purpose.
- It is important for health professionals who are asked to assist with paternity testing to ensure that the adults concerned have considered the implications of testing, including those for family relationships, of receiving the result. Health professionals should be involved only when they consider this to be in the best interests of the child.
- When health professionals are present when DNA samples are taken for forensic testing, they should object if any part of the process of taking the sample would be detrimental to the patient's care.

Other developments

Whole genome sequencing

Whole genome sequencing is likely to have a major impact on genetics in the future. This term refers to the ability to provide a complete DNA sequence of an individual in a single test. Although, at the time of writing, whole genome sequencing is limited to a relatively small number of private providers, the pressure to utilise the technology will increase, particularly once it becomes cheaper to undertake full genome sequencing than, for example, to sequence the *BRCA1* and *BRCA2* loci together. The increasing use of such technology will raise complex issues that need to be explored. Inevitably such tests will produce vast amounts of information which is of variable clinical utility and questions arise about who should have access to the information, how it should be stored and what responsibility, if any, rests with health professionals to contact those individuals in the future should any of the genome sequence variants identified subsequently be linked with a serious Mendelian disease.

Epigenetics

Claims about the therapeutic possibilities arising from the decoding of human DNA have to an extent been qualified by recent developments in the field of epigenetics. Although DNA is generally regarded as the 'instruction manual' for the development of complex organisms, it has now been established that the genes themselves do not actually contain all the information necessary for that development. Our genes require further biochemical data in order to determine which proteins to code. This information is found not in the DNA itself but in the epigenome, a regulatory network of chemical switches that govern the activation of the genes. The epigenome, it is clear, is just as important to the development of a healthy individual as the DNA itself. Although the first map of the human epigenome was published in 2009, the complex interactions between the DNA and the epigenome have qualified some earlier optimism about the potential therapeutic possibilities of the genome project. Additionally, while DNA is largely passed on unchanged from parents to children, the epigenome is sensitive to environmental factors such as diet, early parenting or toxins. Furthermore, it is looking increasingly likely that individual epigenetic changes in one individual can be heritable. Our environment, or our lifestyle choices, can have an impact on the health of our offspring, even up to several generations.

Behavioural genetics

Another interesting, and potentially extremely significant, area of genetics inquiry relates to the potential impact of heritable factors on human behaviour. It is broadly accepted now that human behaviour is influenced by a complex mixture of inherited and environmental factors.[113] Research in genetics is seeking to identify both individual genes, and clusters of genes, that can influence an extremely wide range of behavioural traits. Researchers are gathering evidence that suggests that all of the 'big five' personality traits – extraversion, agreeableness (aggression), conscientiousness, neuroticism and openness – have a significant genetic contribution.[114] Although research to date indicates that the relationship between genes and behaviour is very complex – it is not the case, for example, that a single gene governs a specific personality trait, rather complex interactions of individual genes, gene clusters and environmental factors influence the development and expression of traits – the relationship between genetics and behaviour gives rise to a number of ethical issues. In theory at least, it raises the possibility that certain favoured traits could be selected for, either via embryo selection or forms of genetic manipulation. The ability to identify individuals with preferred personality characteristics could potentially lead to educational and work-based streaming with resulting costs in social equity. It also invites questions about a potential genetic base for fundamental human characteristics such as freedom of choice and moral judgement that could have far-reaching significance for human self-understanding. Although these issues are philosophically intriguing, they nonetheless remain extremely speculative and their impact on clinical applications of genetics is currently insignificant.

Gene therapy

For many years there have been high hopes that gene therapy will provide a cure for many genetic diseases, cancers and infections, such as HIV. The basic principle of gene therapy is to correct defective genes. This could be done in the following ways:

- if a gene is missing, it could be added
- part of an abnormal gene could be changed to make it function correctly
- the abnormal gene could be removed and replaced with a normal one
- a normal gene could be inserted to supplement the abnormal gene, which would be left in the cell.

Of these options the one considered most likely to succeed is the insertion of a gene, either where the gene is missing or to augment an existing defective gene. This is far more complicated than it sounds and, so far, only limited success has been achieved. First, a method must be found for transporting the new gene and for ensuring that it reaches only those cells that need to be treated. Ideally, although even more difficult technically, it should be inserted into the stem cells so that, when new cells are generated, they already have the correct gene in place. If the gene is inserted into other cells, the effect lasts only as long as those cells survive and the treatment needs to be repeated at regular intervals. As with all experimental treatments, things could go wrong: the new gene could go into the wrong cell, it may not work appropriately, or it could disrupt the normal working of another gene, causing unexpected side effects. For this reason, careful research and monitoring is needed. For those with serious genetic disorders such as cystic fibrosis, however, gene therapy may offer the best hope of a cure. The potential benefits of gene therapy are not restricted to single gene disorders and much of the research undertaken has been aimed at developing new forms of treatment for cancer. This work has focused on trying to reverse the basic changes in cells that lead to them becoming cancerous, by finding ways of inducing the body's natural defences to kill the cancerous cells, or by inserting a gene that can convert a harmless chemical into one that destroys cancer cells but does not affect other cells in the body, thus removing the usual side effects of cancer treatment. Similar investigations are being undertaken into the possible use of gene therapy for treating infections such as HIV. In the UK, all clinical trials have been assessed, approved and monitored on a voluntary basis by the Gene Therapy Advisory Committee (GTAC). By the end of 2008, 170 applications had been considered by GTAC, of which 145 were approved and 25 were either declined or withdrawn and around 1800 patients had participated in UK gene therapy trials.[115] In 2008, GTAC's remit was extended to cover the ethical oversight of clinical trials involving therapies derived using stem cell lines. In 2010, however, the Government announced plans to abolish GTAC and transfer its functions to the National Research Ethics Service (NRES).[116]

Theoretically, it would be possible to perform gene therapy using either somatic cells or germ cells. Alteration of the genes in the somatic cells affects only the individual treated, whereas altered genes in the germ cells would be passed on to the next generation. The BMA believes that the issues raised by somatic cell gene therapy are essentially the same as those raised by the development of other new medical techniques. As with any new treatment, research results must show that the procedure is safe and efficacious before the shift is made from research to clinical practice, and those seeking treatment must give valid consent, having been informed of the inherent risks and uncertainties (this is discussed further in Chapter 14). Alteration of a defective gene in a germ cell or in an early embryo, however, would enable future generations to benefit from the treatment, but the safety of these procedures is not proven and cannot be proved in the short term. In view of these concerns about the effect on future generations, there is widespread agreement that germ cell gene therapy should not be undertaken.

Genetic manipulation of the early embryo for treatment is prohibited in the UK by the Human Fertilisation and Embryology Act 1990 (as amended), which states that: 'a [treatment] licence . . . cannot authorise altering the nuclear or mitochondrial DNA of any cell while it forms part of an embryo'[117] except where this is permitted by regulations to prevent the transmission of a serious mitochondrial disease. The Human Fertilisation and Embryology Act was amended during 2008 to remove a similar restriction on re- search licences. Research involving the genetic manipulation of the early embryo may now be undertaken subject to approval by the Human Fertilisation and Embryology Authority.

Cloning

Since the birth of Dolly the cloned sheep in February 1997,[118] the possibility of human cloning has been a frequent topic of debate both in scientific circles and in the popular press. In the early days, much of the discussion was sensationalist, predicting the imminent and inevitable use of the technique to create genetically identical individuals. Yet this development opened up new opportunities for important research into the use of stem cell technology which has huge potential to benefit mankind. (Stem cell research is discussed in Chapter 14, pages 617–619.) Early on, sensible debate about these possibilities was frequently hampered by confusion caused primarily by the terminology used: the phrase 'human cloning' was used both in its conventional sense, to refer to the deliberate creation of genetically identical individuals, but also as a generic phrase to refer to this broader range of research activities. The BMA, like many other organisations, was concerned that the negativity associated with our commonsense understanding of 'cloning' may have a detrimental effect on the development of important and worthwhile scientific research. For this reason, the BMA produced a discussion paper for the World Medical Association,[119] which called for an informed and rational debate about the range of activities that had been included under the broad heading of 'cloning'. It also called for the phrase 'human cloning' to be used only in its conventional sense.

Dolly, the cloned sheep

On 27 February 1997, a group of scientists from the Roslin Institute in Edinburgh announced in *Nature* the birth of Dolly the sheep.[120] Dolly was born after the transfer of the nucleus of a cell from the mammary gland of a 6-year-old Finn Dorset ewe into an unfertilised oocyte with its own nucleus removed. In total, the nuclei from 277 cells were transferred into 277 unfertilised eggs. The oocytes were then stimulated to begin cell division and the resulting embryos were replaced in the uteri of adult sheep for gestation. In total, 29 viable embryos were derived and transferred into surrogate Blackface ewes. This led to just one birth – Dolly – who was the first example of an adult vertebrate being cloned from another adult (the same technique had been used previously to clone cells from sheep embryos). Dolly subsequently gave birth to lambs conceived normally. She died in 2003.

The BMA is opposed to the deliberate creation of genetically identical individuals and welcomed the passage of the Human Reproductive Cloning Act 2001 (subsequently repealed and replaced by amendments to the Human Fertilisation and Embryology Act), which put its illegality throughout the UK beyond any doubt. The BMA also believes that the Government should take an active part in moves to negotiate an international ban on human reproductive cloning. Despite this, the BMA recognises that many of the arguments expressed in opposition to human cloning are based on popular misconceptions and instinct rather than clearly articulated robust and logical arguments. It may be the case that the very serious safety concerns about human cloning are never satisfactorily overcome, or that the level of benefit to be derived from using it are not sufficiently high to surmount the inherent risks associated with any new technique. If that is the case then, although interesting from an academic perspective, debate about the ethical acceptability of human cloning loses its urgency because the safety concerns alone are sufficient to justify a prohibition. If in the future, however, it became possible to say, with a reasonable degree of certainty, that human cloning was safe, it would be essential to explore in more detail the motives of those who wish to use this technique and to consider the benefits, harms and likely consequences of allowing it. If we ever reach that stage, detailed consideration will be required to ensure that continued opposition to cloning is based on careful analysis rather than relying on ill-defined notions of 'human dignity', and that decisions are made on the strength of the arguments rather than simply on the strength of public opinion.

Law and regulation

For many years it has been recognised that, in order to realise the huge potential benefits that genetic technology has to offer while protecting against the potential harms, a clear and coherent regulatory mechanism is required. Although there is no statutory body for genetics in the UK, a series of voluntary and advisory bodies have been established that each have a clearly defined remit. After a strategic review of the framework for overseeing developments in biotechnology and genetics carried out in 1999, the Human Genetics Commission was established to advise the Government on how new developments in genetics would impact on people and on healthcare. In 2010, the Government announced its plans to abolish the Human Genetics Commission, replacing it with an expert advisory committee of the Department of Health.

For a number of years there has also been ongoing debate about whether the UK should introduce a genetic discrimination law. The Human Genetics Commission has been a strong proponent of the need for legislation to protect against genetic discrimination.[121] It argues both that there is anecdotal evidence of discrimination occurring and also that the perceived risk of future discrimination acts as a deterrent to people having genetic tests that may bring medical benefit. The former Labour Government, however, rejected these arguments in its review of equality legislation and announced in October 2008 that it did not intend to introduce specific statutory protection against discrimination on grounds of genetic predisposition.[122] The House of Lords Science and Technology Committee also concluded that '[w]e do not believe that at present there should be specific legislation against genetic discrimination, either in the workplace or generally'.[123] It went on to recommend, however, that the Human Genetics Commission should continue to monitor the situation.

This issue is extremely complex both in terms of whether legislation is needed and, if it is, how the scope of the legislation would be determined. The PHG Foundation, for example, criticises the Human Genetics Commission for calling for comprehensive legal protection against discrimination on *any* genetic grounds which covers not only all types of DNA-based information, but also family history. It suggests that 'the only logical conclusion from the HGC's suggestions is that the proposed legislation should apply to any human trait with a genetic component – in other words to all human characteristics and all ways of measuring or detecting them'.[124] Lemke[125] has also highlighted a number of theoretical, normative and practical problems in the debate on genetic discrimination. He highlights the difficulty of defining 'genetic information' and what forms of discrimination should be included in any such legislation. He points out that putting the emphasis on the method of testing would unfairly protect those who have a DNA-based test for predisposition to heart disease but not those who have a non-genetic test such as measuring blood pressure. It would also protect those who have a genetic test but not those whose risk is known by family history (as is the case currently with the moratorium on insurance, see pages 396–398). Placing the emphasis on those who have a 'genetic' condition or predisposition is also problematic because, as suggested by the PHG Foundation, as our understanding of the genetic component of common diseases grows, so it will become increasingly difficult to distinguish between genetic and non-genetic conditions.

Lemke[126] also highlights the difficulty of determining what forms of 'discrimination' should be outlawed. He points out that in much of the academic literature 'genetic discrimination' is defined as the 'unjustified unequal treatment of people owing to their genetic characteristics'. People however, adopt very different views about what forms of unequal treatment are 'unjustified'. Some believe that any unequal treatment based on actual or suspected genetic differences are unacceptable, whereas others take the view that some forms of unequal treatment are justified and morally appropriate. In fact, some would argue that in a risk-based insurance scheme, it is unfair to allow individuals who know they are at increased risk to access insurance at standard rates.[127] The Human Genetics Commission acknowledges that any statutory prohibition of genetic discrimination would need to be a qualified prohibition but points out that careful consideration would need to be given to the way in which the prohibition was qualified. It recommends that '[a]s a minimum some requirement to demonstrate the reasonableness of an exception and its proportionality to some legitimate end would usefully shift the burden of justification to those who would treat individuals differently on genetic grounds'.[128] The Human Genetics Commission acknowledges, however, that the tests of reasonableness and proportionality are likely to be met where insurance companies wish to use the results of DNA tests to distinguish between individuals on genetic grounds, once the moratorium has ended. It therefore suggests that consideration should be given to other measures to avoid 'undesirable social consequences' such as the development of a class of people who cannot get access to insurance (although arguably this already exists given that people with existing conditions or disabilities are likely to find it difficult to access such services).

The BMA has previously argued that it is anomalous that those with existing illness or disability have greater protection against unfair discrimination than those who are asymptomatic but know they will develop a condition in the future.[129] The best way of addressing this anomaly, however, requires a more detailed and comprehensive review of the evidence and options than the BMA has been able to conduct. The conflicting views expressed by those who have undertaken such reviews – the Human Genetics Commission, the House of Lords and the Government, for example – demonstrate that this is not just a question of fact but one of opinion and balance. A formal review of the issue is needed, taking account of the experiences of countries, such as the USA, that have introduced legislation[130] and those, such as Australia,[131] that decided after detailed consideration against specific genetic discrimination legislation.

References

1   House of Lords Science and Technology Committee (2009) *Genomic Medicine: 2nd Report of Session 2008–09*, Vol. 1 (HL 107–1), The Stationery Office, London.
2   Human Genetics Commission (2002) *Inside information: balancing interests in the use of personal genetic data*, HGC, London, pp.28–33.
3   Human Genetics Commission (2002) *Inside information: balancing interests in the use of personal genetic data*, HGC, London, p.30.
4   Human Genetics Commission (2002) *Inside information: balancing interests in the use of personal genetic data*, HGC, London, pp.37–8.
5   Joint Committee on Medical Genetics of the Royal College of Physicians, Royal College of Pathologists and British Society for Human Genetics (2011) *Consent and Confidentiality in Clinical Genetic Practice: guidance on genetic testing and sharing genetic information*, RCP, London, p.12.
6   Michie S, Lester K, Pinto J. *et al.* (2005) Communicating risk information in genetic counseling: an observational study. *Health Educ Behav* **32**(5), 589–98.
7   Marteau TM. (1999) Communicating genetic risk information. *Br Med Bull* **55**, 414–28.
8   This definition was drawn up by the American Society of Human Genetics in 1974 and is discussed in: Fraser FC. (1974) Current issues in medical genetics: genetic counseling. *Am J Hum Genet* **26**, 636–59, p.637.

9   Clarke A. (1991) Is non-directive genetic counselling possible? *Lancet* **338**, 998–1001.
10   Rantanen E, Hietala M, Kristoffersson U. *et al.* (2008) What is ideal genetic counselling? A survey of current international guidelines. *Eur J Hum Genet* **16**, 445–52.
11   Department for Constitutional Affairs (2007) *Mental Capacity Act 2005 Code of Practice*, The Stationery Office, London, para 5.48.
12   Scottish Executive (2010) *Adults with Incapacity (Scotland) Act 2000 Code of Practice (third edition) for practitioners authorised to carry out medical treatment or research under part 5 of the Act*. SG/2010/57. Available at: www.scotland.gov.uk (accessed 24 October 2011).
13   The Human Tissue Act 2004 (Persons who Lack Capacity to Consent and Transplants) Regulations 2006. SI 2006/1659.
14   Human Tissue Act 2004, s 45.
15   Human Tissue Act 2004, Sch 4.
16   Human Tissue Act 2004, Sch 4.
17   Human Tissue Authority (2007) *Non-consensual DNA analysis*, HTA, London.
18   Lucassen A, Parker M. (2004) Confidentiality and serious harm in genetics: preserving the confidentiality of one patient and preventing harm to relatives. *Eur J Hum Genet* **12**, 93–7.
19   General Medical Council (2009) *Confidentiality*, GMC, London, para 36.
20   Parker M, Lucassen A. (2004) Genetic information: a joint account? *BMJ* **329**, 165–7.
21   Kohut K, Manno M, Gallinger S. *et al.* (2007) Should healthcare providers have a duty to warn family members of individuals with an HNPCC-causing mutation? A survey of patients from the Ontario Familial Colon Cancer Registry. *J Med Genet* **44**, 404–7.
22   Lucassen A, Parker M. (2010) Confidentiality and sharing genetic information with relatives. *Lancet* **375**, 1507–9.
23   Harper PS, Clarke AJ. (1997) *Genetics, society and clinical practice*. Bios Scientific, Oxford, pp.38–9.
24   Parker M. (co-founder of Genethics Club) Personal communication, October 2010.
25   Hallowell N. (1999) Doing the right thing: genetic risk and responsibility. *Sociol Health Illness* **21**(5), 597–621.
26   General Medical Council (2009) *Confidentiality*, GMC, London, paras 67–9.
27   Husted J. (1997) Autonomy and a right not to know. In: Chadwick R, Levitt M, Shickle D. (eds.) *The right to know and the right not to know*, Avebury, Aldershot, p.57.
28   Laurie G. (2002) *Genetic privacy: a challenge to medico-legal norms*, Cambridge University Press, Cambridge.
29   Gaff CL, Clarke AJ, Atkinson P. *et al.* (2007) Process and outcome in communication of genetic information within families: a systematic review. *Eur J Hum Genet* **15**, 999–1011.
30   *Palmer v Tees Health Authority & Anor* [1999] Lloyd's Rep Med 351.
31   Laurie GT. (1999) Obligations arising from genetic information: negligence and the protection of familial interests. *Child Fam Law Q* **11**, 109–24.
32   Sermijn E, Goelen G, Teugels E. *et al.* (2004) The impact of proband mediated information dissemination in families with a BRCA1/2 gene mutation. *J Med Genet* **41**, e23.
33   Forrest LE, Delatycki MB, Skene L. (2007) Communicating genetic information in families: a review of guidelines and position papers. *Eur J Hum Genet* **15**, 612–8.
34   Lucassen A, Parker M. (2010) Confidentiality and sharing genetic information with relatives. *Lancet* **375**, 1507–9.
35   Balfour-Lynn I, Madge S, Dinwiddie R. (1995) Testing carrier status in siblings of patients with cystic fibrosis. *Arch Dis Child* **72**, 167–8.
36   Borry P, Goffin T, Nys H. *et al.* (2007) Attitudes regarding carrier testing in incompetent children: a survey of European clinical geneticists. *Eur J Hum Genet* **15**, 1211–7.
37   Borry P, Evers-Kiebooms G, Cornel M. *et al.* (Public and Professional Policy Committee (PPPC) of the European Society of Human Genetics) (2009) Genetic testing in asymptomatic minors: background considerations towards ESHG recommendations. *Eur J Hum Genet* **17**, 711–9. Borry P, Evers-Kiebooms G, Cornel M. *et al.* (Public and Professional Policy Committee (PPPC) of the European Society of Human Genetics) (2009) Genetic testing in asymptomatic minors: recommendations of the European Society of Human Genetics. *Eur J Hum Genet* **17**, 720–1.
38   British Society for Human Genetics (2010) *Genetic Testing of Children: Report of a working party of the British Society for Human Genetics 2010*, BSHG, Birmingham, p.4.
39   *An NHS Trust v MB and Mr & Mrs B (parents)* [2006] EWHC 507 (Fam): 16.
40   Harper PS, Clarke AJ. (1997) *Genetics, society and clinical practice*, Bios Scientific, Oxford, p.22.
41   Järvinen O, Hietala M, Aalto AM. *et al.* (2000) A retrospective study of long-term psychosocial consequences and satisfaction after carrier testing in childhood in an autosomal recessive disease: aspartylglucosaminuria. *Clin Genet* **58**(6), 447–54.
42   Clarke A. (1994) The genetic testing of children. Working Party of the Clinical Genetics Society. *J Med Genet* **31**, 785–97.
43   Borry P, Fryns J, Schotsmans P. *et al.* (2006) Carrier testing in minors: a systematic review of guidelines and position papers. *Eur J Hum Genet* **14**, 133–8.

44 Harper PS, Lim C, Craufurd D, on behalf of the UK Huntington's Disease Prediction Consortium (2000) Ten years of presymptomatic testing for Huntington's disease: the experience of the UK Huntington's Disease Prediction Consortium. *J Med Genet* **37**, 567–71.

45 Almqvist EW, Bloch M, Brinkman R. *et al.* (1999) A worldwide assessment of the frequency of suicide, suicide attempts, or psychiatric hospitalization after predictive testing for Huntington disease. *Am J Hum Genet* **64**, 1293–304.

46 Bird TD. (1999) Invited Editorial: Outrageous fortune: the risk of suicide in genetic testing for Huntington disease. *Am J Hum Genet* **64**, 1289–92.

47 Gargiulo M, Lejeune S, Tanguy M. *et al.* (2008) Long-term outcome of presymptomatic testing in Huntington disease. *Eur J Hum Genet* **17**, 165–71.

48 Almqvist EW, Brinkman RR, Wiggins S. *et al.* and the Canadian Collaborative Study of Predictive Testing (2003) Psychological consequences and predictors of adverse events in the first 5 years after predictive testing for Huntington's disease. *Clin Genet* **64**(4), 300–9.

49 Decruyenaere M, Evers-Kiebooms G, Cloostermans T. *et al.* (2003) Psychological distress in the 5-year period after predictive testing for Huntington's disease. *Eur J Hum Genet* **11**, 30–8. Almqvist EW, Brinkman RR, Wiggins S. *et al.* and the Canadian Collaborative Study of Predictive Testing (2003) Psychological consequences and predictors of adverse events in the first 5 years after predictive testing for Huntington's disease. *Clin Genet* **64**(4), 300–9.

50 Meiser B, Dunn S. (2001) Psychological effect of genetic testing for Huntington's disease: an update of the literature. *West J Med* **174**(5), 336–40.

51 Broadstock M, Michie S, Marteau T. (2000) Psychological consequences of predictive genetic testing: a systematic review. *Eur J Hum Genet* **8**, 731–8.

52 Hagberg A, Bui TH, Winnberg E. (2010) More appreciation of life or regretting the test? Experiences of living as a mutation carrier of Huntington's disease. *J Genet Counsel* **20**(1), 70–9.

53 Gargiulo M, Lejeune S, Tanguy M. *et al.* (2008) Long-term outcome of presymptomatic testing in Huntington disease. *Eur J Hum Genet* **17**, 165–71.

54 Wright S. (1996) It's a yo-yo type of existence. In: Marteau T, Richards M. (eds.) *The troubled helix,* Cambridge University Press, Cambridge, p.5.

55 Wright S. (1996) It's a yo-yo type of existence. In: Marteau T, Richards M. (eds.) *The troubled helix,* Cambridge University Press, Cambridge, p.7.

56 Raven C. (2010) To be or not to be? *Guardian Weekend* (16 January), pp.29-40.

57 Raven C. (2010) To be or not to be? *Guardian Weekend* (16 January), p.38.

58 Harper PS, Clarke AJ. (1997) *Genetics, society and clinical practice.* Bios Scientific, Oxford, pp.31–48.

59 Meiser B, Dunn S. (2001) Pyschological effect of genetic testing for Huntington's disease: an update of the literature. *West J Med* **174**(5), 336–40.

60 Advisory Committee on Genetic Testing (1998) *Report on genetic testing for late onset disorders*, DH, London.

61 Borry P, Stultiens L, Nys H. *et al.* (2006) Presymptomatic and predictive genetic testing in minors: a systematic review of guidelines and position papers. *Clin Genet* **70**, 374–81.

62 Michie S, Bobrow M, Marteau TM. (2001) Predictive genetic testing in children and adults: a study of emotional impact. *J Med Genet* **38**, 519–26.

63 Michie S, Bobrow M, Marteau TM. (2001) Predictive genetic testing in children and adults: a study of emotional impact. *J Med Genet* **38**, 519–26.

64 Duncan RE, Gillam L, Savalescu J. *et al.* (2010) The challenge of developmentally appropriate care: predictive genetic testing in young people for familial adenomatous polyposis. *Fam Cancer* **9**, 27–35.

65 Marteau T, Croyle RT. (1998) The new genetics: psychological responses to genetic testing. *BMJ* **316**, 693–6.

66 Marteau TM, Lerman C. (2001) Genetic risk and behavioural change. *BMJ* **322**, 1056–9.

67 Lucassen A, Parker M. (2001) Revealing false paternity: some ethical considerations. *Lancet* **357**, 1033–5.

68 Khoury MJ, McCabe LL, McCabe ERB. (2003) Population screening in the age of genomic medicine. *N Engl J Med* **348**(1), 50–8.

69 UK National Screening Committee. *Policy database*. Available at: www.screening.nhs.uk (accessed 2 March 2011).

70 Human Genetics Commission (2011) *Increasing options, informing choice: a report on preconception genetic testing and screening*, HGC, London, p.1.

71 Bekker H, Modell M, Denniss G. *et al.* (1993) Uptake of cystic fibrosis testing in primary care: supply push or demand pull? *BMJ* **306**, 1584–6.

72 Gason AA, Delatycki MB, Metcalfe SA. *et al.* (2006) It's 'back to school' for genetic screening. *Eur J Hum Genet* **14**, 384–9.

73 Mitchell JJ, Capua A, Clow C. *et al.* (1996) Twenty-year outcome analysis of genetic screening programs for Tay Sachs and beta-thalassemia disease carriers in high schools. *Am J Hum Genet* **59**, 793–8.

74 Laurie G. (2002) Better to hesitate at the threshold of compulsion: PKU testing and the concept of family autonomy in Eire. *J Med Ethics* **28**, 136–7.

75 UK National Screening Committee *Policy database*. Available at: www.screening.nhs.uk (accessed 2 March 2011).

76 UK National Screening Committee *Newborn blood spot screening across the UK*. Available at: www.screening.nhs.uk (accessed 2 March 2011).

77 Khoury MJ, McCabe LL, McCabe ERB. (2003) Population screening in the age of genomic medicine. *New Engl J Med* **348**(1), 50–8.

78 Clarke AJ. (1995) Population screening for genetic susceptibility to disease. *BMJ* **311**, 3–8.

79 Human Genetics Commission (2010) *A common framework of principles for direct-to-consumer genetic testing services*, HGC, London.

80 House of Lords Science and Technology Committee (2009) *Genomic Medicine: 2nd Report of Session 2008–09*. Vol. 1 (HL 107-1), The Stationery Office, London.

81 Human Genetics Commission (2010) *A common framework of principles for direct-to-consumer genetic testing services*, HGC, London.

82 Nuffield Council on Bioethics (2010) *Medical profiling and online medicine: the ethics of 'personalised healthcare' in a consumer age*, NCB, London.

83 Prime Minister's Office (2010) Public Body Review Published. Press statement, 14 October.

84 Association of British Insurers (2008) *ABI Code of Practice for Genetic Tests: June 2008*, ABI, London.

85 Genetic Interest Group (2007) *Discrimination law review consultation: response from the Genetic Interest Group*. Available at: www.gig.org.uk (accessed 4 March 2011).

86 British Medical Association (1998) *Human Genetics: choice and responsibility*, Oxford University Press, Oxford, pp.153–69.

87 Human Genetics Commission (2002) *Inside information: Balancing interests in the use of personal genetic data*, HGC, London, p.138.

88 Kennedy H. (2006) Letter to Lord Sainsbury of Turville. *Genetic Testing and Employment* (5 June). Available at: www.hgc.gov.uk (accessed 3 March 2011).

89 Information Commissioner's Office (2005) *The Employment Practices Code*, ICO, Wilmslow, para 4.5.

90 Information Commissioner's Office (2005) *The Employment Practices Code*, ICO, Wilmslow, para 4.5.

91 Human Tissue Act 2004, s 45.

92 Family Law Reform Act 1969, s 20. Law Reform (Miscellaneous Provisions) (Scotland) Act 1990, s 70. Family Law Reform (Northern Ireland) Order 1977, art 8.

93 Child Support (Pensions and Social Security) Act 2000, s 82. Child Support, Pensions and Social Security Act (Northern Ireland) 2000, s 65(3).

94 *H and A (children) (paternity: blood tests)* [2002] 1 FLR 1145: 1146.

95 *S v McC*; *W v W* [1970] 3 All ER 107: 123.

96 The Human Tissue Act 2004 (Persons who Lack Capacity to Consent and Transplants) Regulations 2006. SI 2006/1659.

97 Human Genetics Commission (2009) *Nothing to hide, nothing to fear? Balancing individual rights and the public interest in the governance and use of the National DNA Database*, DH, London, p.4.

98 Nuffield Council on Bioethics (2007) *The forensic use of bioinformation: ethical issues*, NCB, London, p.11.

99 Nuffield Council on Bioethics (2007) *The forensic use of bioinformation: ethical issues*, NCB, London, p.11.

100 *R (on the application of S) v Chief Constable of South Yorkshire, R (on the application of Marper) v Chief Constable of South Yorkshire* [2003] 1 All ER 148.

101 *R (on the application of S) v Chief Constable of South Yorkshire* [2004] UKHL 39.

102 *S and Marper v The United Kingdom* (30562/04 and 30566/04) [2008] ECHR 1581 (4 December 2008): para 125.

103 Nuffield Council on Bioethics (2007) *The forensic use of bioinformation: ethical issues*, NCB, London.

104 Human Genetics Commission (2009) *Nothing to hide, nothing to fear? Balancing individual rights and the public interest in the governance and use of the National DNA Database*, DH, London.

105 Jackson E. (2010) *Medical Law: text, cases and materials*, 2nd edn, Oxford University Press, Oxford, p.410.

106 Jackson E. (2010) *Medical Law: text, cases and materials*, 2nd edn, Oxford University Press, Oxford, p.410.

107 Home Office (2003) *Police and Criminal Evidence Act 1984 Code D: code of practice for the identification of persons by police officers*, Home Office, London.

108 Human Genetics Commission (2009) *Nothing to hide, nothing to fear? Balancing individual rights and the public interest in the governance and use of the National DNA Database*, DH, London, pp.79–80.

109 Nuffield Council on Bioethics (2007) *The forensic use of bioinformation: ethical issues*, NCB, London, pp.78–80.

110 Fresco A. (2010) 'Crimewatch' killer jailed for life after 26 years. *Times Online* (26 January). Available at: www.timesonline.co.uk (accessed 4 March 2011).

111 Nuffield Council on Bioethics (2007) *The forensic use of bioinformation: ethical issues*, NCB, London, pp.20–1.

112 Nuffield Council on Bioethics (2007) *The forensic use of bioinformation: ethical issues*, NCB, London, pp.80–1.

113 Nuffield Council on Bioethics (2002) *Genetics and Human Behaviour: the ethical context*, NCB, London.

114 Bouchard TJ. (2004) Genetic influence on human psychological traits: a survey. *Curr Direct Psychol Sci* **13**(4), 148–51.

115 Gene Therapy Advisory Committee (2009) *Fifteenth Annual Report*, Health Departments of the United Kingdom, London, p.11. An up-to-date list of approved research can be found on the GTAC website (www.dh.gov.uk/ab/gtac).

116 Department of Health (2010) *Reform of Department of Health Public Bodies*. Press release, October 14.

117 Human Fertilisation and Embryology Act 1990 (as amended), Sch 2, para 1(4).

118 Wilmut I, Schnieke AE, McWhir J. *et al.* (1997) Viable offspring derived from fetal and adult mammalian cells. *Nature* **385**, 810–3.

119 British Medical Association (1999) *Human 'cloning': a discussion paper for the World Medical Association*, BMA, London.

120 Wilmut I, Schnieke AE, McWhir J. *et al.* (1997) Viable offspring derived from fetal and adult mammalian cells. *Nature* **385**, 810–3.

121 Kennedy H. (2007) *Human Genetics Commission response to the Discrimination Law Review consultation. A Framework for Fairness: Proposals for a Single Equality Bill for Great Britain*, HGC, London.

122 House of Lords Science and Technology Committee (2009) *Genomic Medicine: 2nd Report of Session 2008–09*, Vol. 1 (HL 107-1), The Stationery Office, London, para 6.35.

123 House of Lords Science and Technology Committee (2009) *Genomic Medicine: 2nd Report of Session 2008–09*, Vol. 1 (HL 107-1), The Stationery Office, London, para 6.40.

124 Stewart A. (2007) HGC advocates legal ban on 'genetic discrimination'. *PHG Foundation News* (September 28). Available at: www.phgfoundation.org (accessed 4 March 2011).

125 Lemke T. (2005) Beyond genetic discrimination: problems and perspectives of a contested notion. *Genom Soc Policy* **1**(3), 22–40.

126 Lemke T. (2005) Beyond genetic discrimination: problems and perspectives of a contested notion. *Genom Soc Policy* **1**(3), 22–40, p.24.

127 PHG Foundation (2007) *The PHG Foundation's Response to the Discrimination Law Review Consultation: A Framework for a Fairer Future: Proposals for a Single Equality Bill for Great Britain*, PHG Foundation, Cambridge.

128 Kennedy H. (2007) *Human Genetics Commission response to the Discrimination Law Review Consultation: A Framework for Fairness: Proposals for a Single Equality Bill for Great Britain*, HGC, London, p.6.

129 British Medical Association (1998) *Human genetics: choice and responsibility*, Oxford University Press, Oxford, pp.174–5.

130 Genetic Information Non-discrimination Act 2008.

131 Australian Law Reform Commission (2003) *ALRC 96 Essentially Yours: The protection of human genetic information in Australia*. ALRC, Sydney, paras 9.49–9.55.

10: Caring for patients at the end of life

The questions covered in this chapter include the following.

- How do the goals of care change when the patient's condition is recognised as terminal?
- How can patients be helped to maintain control over the end of their life?
- How should doctors respond to requests from relatives to keep information from the patient?
- What factors should be considered when deciding whether to withhold or withdraw life-prolonging treatment?
- Are there additional factors to consider for clinically assisted nutrition and hydration to be withdrawn?
- When should a doctor question a colleague's decisions?
- What steps should health professionals take to support patients in the last days of life?

Issues covered in this chapter

This chapter focuses primarily on the care of patients who are diagnosed as approaching the end of life but it also sets out the British Medical Association's (BMA's) guidance on decisions to withhold or withdraw life-prolonging treatment from people who are not dying, when non-treatment will predictably result in death. It includes discussion of do-not-attempt-resuscitation (DNAR) decisions. There is a significant body of guidance about end of life care, including from the General Medical Council (GMC)[1] and from expert palliative care groups. Some broad themes, however, are echoed in all of the existing guidance and this chapter seeks to summarise them. The GMC's guidance begins from several presumptions, emphasising that while there is no absolute obligation to prolong life, treatment must generally start from a presumption in favour of doing so, unless that is known to be against the patient's wishes. There is also a presumption that adults have the capacity to make decisions for themselves unless there is evidence to the contrary and that doctors will support patients with impaired capacity to maximise their decision-making abilities.

Defining 'end of life'

The GMC says that patients are:

approaching the end of life when they are likely to die within the next 12 months. This includes those patients whose death is expected within hours or days; those who have advanced, progressive incurable conditions; those with general frailty and co-existing conditions that mean they are expected to die within 12 months; those at risk of dying from a sudden acute crisis in an existing condition; and those with life-threatening

Medical Ethics Today: The BMA's Handbook of Ethics and Law, Third Edition. Sophie Brannan, Eleanor Chrispin, Martin Davies, Veronica English, Rebecca Mussell, Julian Sheather and Ann Sommerville.
© 2012 BMA Medical Ethics Department. Published 2012 by Blackwell Publishing Ltd.

acute conditions caused by sudden catastrophic events. The term 'approaching the end of life' can also apply to extremely premature neonates whose prospects for survival are known to be very poor, and patients who are diagnosed as being in a persistent vegetative state (PVS) for whom a decision to withdraw treatment and care may lead to their death.[2]

In previous generations, many people died suddenly, at any age, from infectious diseases. Dying patients were often cared for at home without the kind of symptom relief expected today, which was distressing for all concerned. Families often witnessed the death of a relative. Within society today, contact with the dying has significantly decreased. The majority of all deaths are of people over the age of 65. By 2030, it is anticipated that almost half (about 44 per cent) will be of people over 85.[3] People who die at an older age often have complex multiple morbidities and are likely to have had a protracted period of illness or frailty. They may suffer from dementia, in which case they are usually cared for by generalists rather than palliative care specialists. Most deaths occur in NHS hospitals and nursing homes. Due in part to demographic changes in the population, it is estimated that the overall number of deaths will rise significantly between 2012 and 2030.[4] These factors have implications for how end of life care is delivered but our traditional reluctance to talk about death means that for many people, perceptions of the dying process are based more on television dramas and fictional accounts rather than actual experience or accurate information. This can generate unrealistic expectations in the public about what can be achieved in terms of prolonging life and about the limited success rate of measures such as cardio-pulmonary resuscitation (CPR). When people have unrealistic expectations, they are often shocked by the unpredictable nature of a terminal illness. The first issue covered in this chapter is the importance of good communication so that patients and families have accurate information to make key decisions.

Other topics addressed here are patient choice and advance planning at the end of life. Currently, 'for most of us, our death will be in an acute hospital under circumstances which were not set up to ensure peace, privacy, dignity, and the gathering of a family in the way they would choose'.[5] Most people say that they would like to spend their final days in their own home and die in their own bed (which may be in a nursing home or residential care home). The End of Life Care Strategy throughout the UK is committed to making such choices a possibility, wherever feasible.[6] In practice, however, over half of all patients die in hospital[7] and if current trends continue, by 2030 less than 1 in 10 will die at home.[8] Across the UK, repeated reports and investigations have noted that the quality of end of life care has been very variable and the option of accessing specialist palliative care services has been subject to geographical and other variations. End of life services and the barriers to provision of high quality palliative care in a range of settings came under intense scrutiny across the UK in the years up to 2010 and led to efforts being made UK-wide to address the gaps and establish quality markers for end of life services. In 2008, the Department of Health published its *End of Life Care Strategy*.[9] The recommendations in it were echoed in similar plans which were developed in Scotland, Wales and Northern Ireland.[10]

The main thrust of all of this planning was that people nearing the end of life should have more choice about where they are cared for and die. High quality services must be spread equitably across the UK, with emphasis placed on timely, personalised and dignified care, reflecting the individuality of each patient. The national strategies for end of life care in the four nations recognise the need for early identification of patients who are approaching the last 12 months of life so that a detailed assessment of their needs can take place and a care plan can be developed jointly with them. It is also agreed that better coordination is needed, with the aim of providing continuous high quality services in all locations and ensuring good communication between GPs, out-of-hours services, district nurses, ambulance staff, hospitals and specialist palliative care services. Care plans designed specifically for the last days of life pay particular attention to keeping patients comfortable until death, as well as the importance of treating the body with respect after death and supporting the family. Although there is wide agreement about what is needed in terms of improving end of life care, financial constraints, fragmented out-of-hours services and, historically, the relatively low profile of end of life services in NHS and social care, all make change difficult.[11] In 2010, however, additional funds for end of life care were pledged by the authorities in England, Scotland and Wales.

This intense scrutiny of end of life services was part of a wider acknowledgement that the aim of medicine is not always to postpone death but rather to make the dying process as comfortable and dignified as possible, once its inevitability is recognised. A good death should be the norm and not the exception. In this chapter, we take account of how for everyone, there comes a stage when the aim of care shifts from trying to improve the patient's condition to keeping the person free from distressing symptoms. This shift is a recognition of the natural progression of care. The patient (where possible and appropriate), the treating team and those close to the patient need to acknowledge and accept this. If they do not have an opportunity to do so, patients and their relatives may miss the chance of preparing for, and achieving, a good death.

The impact of early palliative care intervention in the disease trajectory has been shown to provide better quality of life and mood scores, lower depression scores and even some prolonged survival.[12] One of the key challenges for doctors is to make the transition from using all the invasive processes of modern medicine to accepting that cure is not possible in this instance and allowing natural death to occur. Identifying when it is the right time for the team to reassess current interventions and individualise care to meet the best interests of the individual requires attention to the patient's wishes, sound clinical judgement and good communication. Tools such as the Liverpool Care Pathway for the Dying Patient (LCP)[13] have been developed as a framework to guide practice in the last hours or days of life. (The LCP is discussed later on pages 426–427.) They should be instigated when the patient is dying, reversible causes of deterioration have been excluded and death is expected within hours or days. This can be problematic as disease trajectories are often unpredictable, making it difficult for clinicians to identify when a patient is nearing the end of life. Diagnosing dying, talking about it and about decisions to withhold or withdraw treatment are covered later in this chapter.

In the UK, people have diverse cultural and religious beliefs which can make a significant difference to how they approach illness and death. It is increasingly recognised that individual holistic assessment leading to appropriately tailored support is essential for living well in the final stage of life. Spiritual and pastoral care can also be very important in the final stage of life and are discussed in this chapter.

General principles

The general principles regarding provision of care for patients at the end of life include the following.

- It is important to recognise when death is approaching and to help people to prepare for it.
- Compassion and sensitivity are particularly important but honest communication is also essential, while recognising that people's desire for information can vary at different stages of their illness.

- Effective communication within the health team is vital so that mixed messages are avoided.
- Patients must be afforded dignity and privacy: the usual rules of confidentiality apply.
- Patients should have opportunities to maintain control over as many aspects of their care as possible, including by advance planning if they wish.
- Health professionals should be sensitive to patients' cultural and religious backgrounds.
- Care provided to dying patients includes helping people close to them to come to terms with the situation and to cope with their bereavement.

Communication when patients are approaching death

For some death comes quickly and unexpectedly but for many patients there is a period of time when it is clear that death is approaching. This should be identified as early as possible (ideally, when death is likely to occur within 12 months) so that discussion and planning with the patient can take place, without urgency. It is a time for helping patients and families to come to terms with the situation. The crucial importance of effective communication at this stage is well recognised. Poor communication leaves people very anxious and frustrated. Within palliative care services, considerable attention has been given to developing good communication strategies to handle difficult situations openly, such as when patients ask for details about how their death will occur, and to the use of verbal and non-verbal skills to facilitate discussion.[14] Attention has also been drawn to the type of blocking tactics that the health team may unconsciously use to shift the focus of the conversation away from patients' fears or which encourage patients to be more positive and more reassured than the situation warrants. Such tactics are not deliberately intended to curtail discussion but have that effect. Health professionals can become accustomed to using them, without realising they are doing so, or use them to protect their own emotional stability in a very stressful area of patient care.[15] (See also the section on dilemmas about how much detail to provide on pages 422–423.)

Provision of information

In order to achieve a good death, individual patients need the right care to be available in the right place and at the right time. To make informed decisions, they need to know that they are nearing the end of life and what type of care will be available at each stage. This means that patients, families and health professionals need to be able to overcome the stigma associated with talking about death. Honesty must be combined with sensitivity and compassion and health professionals need very good communication skills. Euphemisms should be avoided but, if they are used, it should be clear what is meant. The emphasis on speaking frankly about the end of life is a relatively new development and may not be expected by all patients, especially those who have grown up in another age or culture. In Britain, in the 1950s, for example, the vast majority of doctors (90 per cent) thought that they should withhold the truth from cancer patients. By the late 1970s, however, frankness was being widely adopted as a general policy.[16] All the current end of life guidance for health professionals emphasises the importance of giving patients detailed information, if they wish to have it. A project examining patients' feelings as they near the end of life showed that many felt frustrated and isolated because of the unwillingness of family and carers to discuss the prospect of death with them.[17] Due to stereotyped notions of what patients want, health professionals may expect older patients to want less detail so they sometimes offer more information, are more supportive and more willing to share decision making with younger rather than older people.[18] Health professionals need to look closely at their own expectations and behaviour patterns so that older patients are not disadvantaged by being denied opportunities to discuss their wishes and anxieties.

Although patients should be kept informed so that they can be involved in decisions affecting them, individuals may want information in differing amounts of detail or at a different pace, according to their own circumstances. Discussion around treatment options should be an ongoing process, during which information may need to be repeated. Options may also need to be discussed at several stages for practical reasons as many patients do not have a predictable pattern of need at the end of life. When they make clear that they want little information, it cannot be forced upon them but, in order for their consent to (or refusal of) medical treatment to be valid, they need to know the core facts (see Chapter 2). Health professionals should sensitively explore with patients their particular wishes so that information can be offered at a pace that suits their needs.

Listening to the patient

End of life care focuses on the values of compassion, empathy, advocacy and honesty as well as good medical and communication skills. Doctors generally approach dying patients with a deepened sense of how crucial it is to talk and listen to the patient. All patients should be given opportunities to discuss their wishes about medical and personal aspects of their care. Facilitating such discussion shows respect for their autonomy and can increase the likelihood of the patient achieving a good death. Patients generally want to understand what can be expected and be able to prepare for it. (See also section on advance care planning on pages 428–431.) Where possible, they are likely to want to have a choice about whether to remain at home or in a hospice or hospital setting. For some patients, access to spiritual or emotional support is also very important. Patients should also have an opportunity to say who they would like to be with them in their final days or hours.

People diagnosed with a terminal illness express a range of strong emotions. Much pioneering work on this was done by Elizabeth Kubler-Ross in the 1970s. Having worked with dying patients, she analysed their anxieties, hopes and frustrations, and identified the stages that their reactions generally pass through when told that they are dying.[19] Initially, she said, they tend to experience a sense of denial and isolation; they may be able to consider the possibility of their own death for a while but then retreat from that realisation. This may be followed by anger, rage or resentment which is difficult for those around the patient to cope with, as the anger is often displaced onto them. The next stage may involve patients' attempts at bargaining for an extension of life. Kubler-Ross said that this situation can arise when they feel guilty about something; she also thought that the interdisciplinary approach, involving a spiritual adviser could be particularly helpful in such cases. Many patients then experience depression – which may focus on past loss, anxiety about other people or preparatory grief, preparing 'for the impending loss of all the love objects'.[20] This depression she describes as a necessary form of emotional preparation and mourning, during which patients need to be able to express their sorrow, and a tool to facilitate the final stage of acceptance. Modern palliative care skills help health professionals to respond appropriately to the full range of patients' emotions by recognising, acknowledging, understanding and accepting them with empathy.[21]

Understanding that feelings of intense anger, sadness and denial are natural can help patients and their relatives to manage the situation. Some fear that medical technology will prolong their dying while others fear that treatment may be withdrawn prematurely.

The health team needs to explain the clinically appropriate options. If patients request a futile treatment, they need an explanation of why it is inappropriate (see page 442). At the root of the patient's request may be a misunderstanding, a fear of being written off or a more general anxiety. In some cases, there may be good reasons for continuing even a clinically futile treatment for a limited period to give the patient time to adjust. What is 'reasonable' needs to be judged on an individual basis in terms of the patient's best interests, taking account of factors such as why the patient wants the treatment, its effects and the potential opportunity costs for other patients. Patients may, for example, prefer a course of treatment that does not give the best clinical outcome but is most compatible with their lifestyle and values. As long as it does not disadvantage other people, patients' preferences at the end of life should usually take precedence over their strictly medical interests. Some patients may choose treatment that will reduce their awareness whereas others may prefer to tolerate a degree of pain or discomfort in order to remain more alert.

GMC guidance

When patients have the capacity to make decisions for themselves:

'(a) The doctor and patient make an assessment of the patient's condition, taking into account the patient's medical history, views, experience and knowledge.

(b) The doctor uses specialist knowledge and experience and clinical judgment, and the patient's views and understanding of their condition, to identify which investigations or treatments are clinically appropriate and likely to result in overall benefit for the patient. The doctor explains the options to the patient, setting out the potential benefits, burdens and risks of each option. The doctor may recommend a particular option which they believe to be best for the patient, but they must not put pressure on the patient to accept their advice.

(c) The patient weighs up the potential benefits, burdens and risks of the various options as well as any non-clinical issues that are relevant to them. The patient decides whether to accept any of the options and, if so, which. They also have the right to accept or refuse an option for a reason that may seem irrational to the doctor or for no reason at all.

(d) If the patient asks for a treatment that the doctor considers would not be clinically appropriate for them, the doctor should discuss the issues with the patient and explore the reasons for their request. If after discussion, the doctor still considers that the treatment would not be clinically appropriate to the patient, they do not have to provide the treatment. They should explain their reasons to the patient and explain any other options that are available, including the option to seek a second opinion or access legal representation.'[22]

Communicating with patients who are in denial

Denial and collusion are separate but related phenomena. Denial is often temporary and describes a psychological defence mechanism, occurring when a patient or family is unable to accept the reality of what is happening. Kubler-Ross saw denial as a healthy way of dealing with painful situations. Denial, she said, is a 'buffer after unexpected shocking news which allows the patient to collect himself and, with time, mobilise other, less radical defences.'[23] 'The need for denial exists in every patient at times, at the very beginning of a serious illness more so than towards the end of life. Later on the need comes and goes, and the sensitive and perceptive listener will ... allow the patient his defences without making him aware of the contradictions'.[24] She also found that, once the initial shock had passed, many patients were able to discuss their illness and imminent death with health professionals and some other people while colluding in the pretence that they were getting well with relatives and friends who the patient thought would not cope with the truth.

Collusion is a complex response occurring in those who are well aware of the facts but wish to protect the patient or one another by not acknowledging or discussing them. One aspect of collusion occurs when relatives ask that information be withheld from the dying person. In some families, the expectation is that patients themselves are not told about the implications of their diagnosis. Relatives may particularly ask for information to be withheld, when the patient is a frail older person who they think cannot cope with the truth. This situation has been a focus of attention within palliative care services where strategies are being developed to explore the relatives' feelings with them, including the reasons why they do not want the truth revealed to the patient. Wilkinson points out how stressful it is for relatives to keep up the pretence, particularly if patients ask questions which indicate that they have, or want, an idea of their true situation.[25] Pointing out to the family that the multi-disciplinary team needs to assess the patient's feelings and worries, which often include answering patients' questions about symptoms and outcomes, can provide an opening to permit a truthful discussion, if patients themselves appear prepared to be informed. Ultimately, all patients who are willing to receive information are entitled to have it. Families can also become upset that information about degenerative illness, for example, is given before the onset of acute symptoms and deprives patients of a period of 'blissful ignorance' but information, sensitively given, at an early stage can allow the patient time to accomplish plans that would be impossible later. Most patients want to be systematically informed and trust is lost if they later discover that important facts were withheld.

With terminal illness, both denial and collusion can occur and even when health professionals sensitively try to assist the patient and the family to face up to the inevitability of death, they may encounter strong pressures to preserve an overly optimistic approach. Although they try to prepare patients to receive factual information about their illness, this can be a slow process if patients are unready. If in denial, individuals are unlikely to want to discuss care plans but the opportunity to do so must be kept open for them so that they know that they can talk about their wishes when they want. They need to know that they will be offered treatment that is appropriate but also that the healthcare team will respect their wishes in terms of knowing when to stop. (Contemporaneous and advance refusals of treatment are discussed in Chapter 3.)

Reinforcing hope and positive attitudes

Keeping a strongly positive attitude in the face of serious illness is generally seen as a good thing and something that health professionals should encourage. Being positive is not the same as being in denial or ignoring the gravity of the situation. Hope is an important coping strategy for patients with a serious condition. Retaining a hopeful attitude, in full knowledge of the facts, can help them adhere to difficult or painful treatment regimes and help them support the people close to them. Many people also believe that keeping a positive outlook can potentially influence survival. The growth of websites with uplifting quotations about surviving, and learning from, life-threatening conditions are one facet of the drive to sustain positive attitudes in patients and families. These and other measures to promote positive thinking can be helpful for some people but not necessarily for all patients. When so much emphasis is placed on responding positively, some patients who feel unable to do so can blame themselves when their condition deteriorates, even if this is a predictable development. They may need support to avoid feelings of self-blame or regret when this happens.

The complex interaction between hopefulness and acknowledgement of reality was studied in some patients with small cell lung cancer in a project that observed the communication process from the initial diagnosis to the patients' eventual deaths.[26] Typically, the patients expressed unjustified optimism after the first course of chemotherapy and their interpretation of their prognosis remained considerably more optimistic than that of their doctors. This seemed to lead to doctors almost colluding with the false optimism by ceasing to mention the predictable poor prognosis openly and focusing on treatment options and timing. It was not that doctors withheld information but rather that they stopped mentioning the long-term prognosis while patients gratefully accepted the opportunity to 'forget' the future and concentrate on the present. A false focus on possible recovery can help patients and their relatives to cope with the situation during treatment but it might also make it more difficult for them later to accept and prepare for death. Relatives involved in the cancer study were interviewed after the patients' death and many regretted this lack of opportunity to prepare. The research also identified ambiguities in the use of language and the way certain phrases were interpreted radically differently by the doctor and the patients. A statement such as 'this tumour can be treated', for example, was used by doctors to indicate that a possible treatment existed which might prolong the patient's life but some patients interpreted it as meaning that they could be cured. Although this particular study focused on cancer patients, similar miscommunication can occur with any patient at the end of life, irrespective of the diagnosis.

Is it problematic if doctors collude and permit a false air of optimism to persist? Health professionals generally accept patients' need for unjustified optimism as a common coping strategy. For patients faced with life-threatening disease, hope and the triumph of optimism over reality can make life bearable, in the short-term. This situation requires health professionals to tread a careful path. It is important to give patients as much accurate information as they need in order to be able to retain control over the situation and to make decisions appropriate for themselves about future care. At the same time, it is important not to impose unwanted information in a way that could have the effect of removing a short-term coping strategy for the patient. Kubler-Ross provided examples of the difficult balance needed to refrain from contradicting patients or breaking down their denial when they want to live and claim to be recovering, while encouraging them to continue to take the steps necessary to keep them alive. As the GMC's guidance (see above) makes clear, doctors must not put pressure on the patient to accept the advice provided and, similarly, patients should not be pressured to receive distressing information. The crucial factor is for health professionals to take their cue from the patient, recognising that individuals require varying degrees of time and support to assimilate what they are told. When a patient's viewpoint seems seriously out of step with reality, care is needed to assess whether he or she has misunderstood the information or is not ready to accept it and is adopting the strategy of false optimism. The role of the health team in such situations includes attempting to help these patients, and those who are close to them, to face the reality in a compassionate way and within a timescale that is appropriate for them, bearing in mind that there may be very limited time available.

Dilemmas about how much detail to provide

Dilemmas about how explicit to be with patients can arise when there is little in the way of effective treatment and they have to choose whether or not to have the limited interventions which are available for them. This can often result in a situation where the patient hears a different message to the one intended by health professionals. Unless it is spelled out to them that the focus of palliative treatment is to give as good a quality of life as possible through symptom management, patients may initially assume that any treatment is intended to improve their condition, not just manage their symptoms.

One of the areas of care where dilemmas sometimes arise is that of telling patients about the value or otherwise of chemotherapy for advanced cancer. For patients with metastatic colorectal, pancreatic or non-small cell lung cancer, life expectancy is generally short and they have to cope with the reality of that prognosis at the same time as deciding whether to accept palliative chemotherapy. The treatment has a high risk of unpleasant or life-threatening side effects and, for many, a low chance of extending survival. In 2008, the UK National Confidential Enquiry into Patient Outcome and Death found that chemotherapy had probably caused or hastened death in just over one-quarter of the very sick patients for whom it was prescribed and who died shortly after.[27] Yet, each year, thousands of UK patients with incurable cancers are offered it and many accept it, with some opting for chemotherapy that only potentially offers an extra week of survival and a high level of toxicity.[28] It was often unclear whether patients had made a properly informed choice and studies looked at the reasons why they opted for chemotherapy and also at the verbal triggers used by doctors and patients either to provoke or deflect detailed discussion about the side effects.[29] It was found that patients' expectations are partly shaped by the media and the internet but also they tend to interpret what doctors tell them more optimistically than the facts warrant. The fact that some form of active treatment is offered gives a sense of hope which supports some patients in the period of adjustment while they come to terms with the distress of their diagnosis. Some patients prioritise survival over quality of life whereas others would prefer to risk having a shorter lifespan but without constant hospital visits. If the oncologist points out the potential benefits of palliative chemotherapy in terms of symptom control and quality of life, but does not discuss survival rates, some patients opt for it erroneously assuming that it will prolong life. On the other hand, if the doctor mentions the side effects and likely lack of benefit in terms of survival more than an extra couple of months, patients may refuse chemotherapy, without assessing the benefit it might give in controlling distressing symptoms. Sometimes health professionals are deliberately vague in giving patients the option of chemotherapy because they themselves feel the need to offer some active treatment, even when it is unlikely to provide significant or long-term benefit. Generally, 'patients may be offered and accept palliative chemotherapy because of a reluctance to confront the issues that surround dying'[30] and that reluctance can be felt by both sides. In one study, breast cancer patients who were actually given detailed information about their prognosis and the effect of such treatment made quite different decisions from those who did not have such details.[31] Having details also helped some other patients who did not want chemotherapy to justify their decision to relatives who wanted them to fight the disease.[32]

The BMA's ethical guidance emphasises the importance of good accurate communication between health professionals and patients so that properly informed choices can be made. It is important that patients understand the potential benefits but also the limitations of the treatment offered. Rather than avoiding the unpalatable details, health professionals need to give as accurate a picture as possible, in a sensitive manner.

Sharing information with those close to a patient with capacity

Although doctors sometimes find it easier to talk to the relatives rather than directly to an adult patient, this is potentially a breach of confidentiality unless the patient requests it.

While adults retain mental capacity, the sharing of information with relatives and others should not take place without their agreement. Some patients may not wish those close to them to be aware of the prognosis. In such circumstances, although confidentiality should be maintained, the doctor usually counsels the patient about the desirability of preparing the family. Vital last opportunities for communication or reconciliation may otherwise be lost. Part of the general perception of a 'good death' involves patients and those close to them supporting each other. Occasionally, patients request that information is given to their relatives rather than to themselves. This may be accepted when it is the patient's determined wish or it may be unavoidable if the patient has impaired or fluctuating mental capacity but it limits the individual's scope for exercising informed choice. Doctors should continue to offer patients the opportunity to change their mind and receive information at a pace and in a manner that is acceptable to them.

Communication when adults lack capacity

When patients lack capacity, any appointed proxy needs to be involved in decision-making (see Chapter 3). Advance decisions about care are also discussed in Chapter 3.

GMC guidance about adults who lack capacity

When a patient lacks capacity, the doctor must:

'(a) be clear what decisions about treatment and care have to be made
(b) check the patient's medical record for any information suggesting that they have made a potentially binding advance decision or directive refusing treatment
(c) make enquiries as to whether someone else holds legal authority to decide which option would provide overall benefit for the patient (an attorney or other legal proxy). You should bear in mind that the powers held by a legal proxy may not cover all healthcare decisions, so you should check the scope of their decision-making authority
(d) take responsibility for deciding which treatment will provide overall benefit to the patient, when no legal proxy exists, and you are the doctor with responsibility for the patient's care. You must consult those close to the patient and members of the healthcare team to help you make your decisions.'[33]

Communication among care professionals

Although ultimately the responsibility for deciding what treatment to offer rests with the clinician in charge of the patient's care, specialist palliative care advice may be needed or a second opinion from another clinician. It is also important that account is taken of the views of other professionals involved in the patient's care. (For communication after the multi-disciplinary team assessment, see page 428.) End of life care is heavily based on the concept of 'one team' within which good coordination is essential. Good communication between different agencies is also vital to the general provision of properly integrated care. As patients approach the end of life, considerable emphasis is given to the importance of regular review of their condition by the multi-disciplinary team, as changes in care may be needed at this uncertain time. In the last days of life, formal multi-disciplinary review should be undertaken every 3 days.[34] At this stage, comprehensive and clear communication is pivotal and the views of all concerned should be heard and documented. Poor communication between care providers means that patients and relatives are likely to be given conflicting messages about important matters such as the amount of time that the patient is likely to survive.

Communicating with complementary therapists

Patients may seek out and gain support from complementary or alternative therapies[35] but some of these have a weak or no evidence base (see Chapter 19, pages 786–788). Some, such as aromatherapy or massage can be a comforting adjunct to standard care and are supplementary to NHS treatment, while others are perceived as an alternative to standard care, making claims to alleviate the patient's condition. Patients may want to investigate all options and have the right to do so privately where the NHS does not fund them, but dilemmas may arise if the patient wants to combine conventional NHS care and alternative therapies in a way that impacts adversely on their medical care or involves the sharing of information or the commissioning of tests and X-rays from the healthcare team. The degree to which health professionals feel able to liaise with alternative practitioners depends on the type of therapy, whether it is regulated by law and whether it supplements conventional methods of diagnosis and treatment or claims to provide an alternative to them.

Some disciplines, such as osteopathy and chiropractic, are professionally regulated and so health professionals can liaise with such practitioners with confidence that they are competent in the therapies they provide and are legally accountable for them. Others, such as herbal medicine and homeopathy are not regulated in the same way, but claim to provide diagnosis and treatment. Doctors may be worried if patients choose these and decline treatments for which there is evidence of benefit. In such cases, they need to talk to the patient about their concerns, while recognising that ultimately patients can choose whichever therapy they want. Among the therapies that are often used by patients to supplement conventional medicine but which do not claim to have any diagnostic purpose are aromatherapy, massage, stress therapy, reflexology and hypnotherapy. Practitioners of these therapies can provide supportive care without impeding conventional treatment. Some other alternative disciplines which do not impede conventional care are perceived as lacking any credible evidence base, such as crystal therapy and iridology. Among the complementary disciplines that claim to provide diagnoses and treatment are Ayurvedic medicine and traditional Chinese medicine. Patients may derive a sense of reassurance that they are trying all options if they embark on such alternative solutions. Dilemmas arise for the healthcare team if patients appear to be pursuing unproven therapies that are potentially harmful or which they cannot afford. It can also be problematic if unregulated practitioners request medical tests or results from the healthcare team. Generally, doctors would need to be convinced that such interventions are necessary in the patient's interests before providing them.

Summary – communication when patients are approaching death

- Effective communication between care providers is crucial in end of life care.
- To make informed decisions about future care, patients need to know that they are approaching the end of life. Honesty and frankness combined with sensitivity and compassion are needed when providing information.

- For many patients, loss of control is one of their main fears. Individuals should have opportunities to discuss this, their illness, prognosis and fears about death but should not be pushed to do so if they are unwilling.
- The cue should be taken from the patient about the amount of information to be provided and the timing of it. The aim should be to encourage patients to receive information at a pace that suits them.
- It is both important to prepare patients to receive information and to recognise when they are in denial as part of the psychological process of coming to terms with their illness.
- When patients have capacity, information should not be shared with relatives without their consent. If they lack capacity, the views of their proxy decision makers must be sought.
- When relatives do not want a patient who has capacity to be informed about the diagnosis, it should be made clear to them that the doctor's primary duty is to ascertain and respect the patient's own wishes.

Diagnosing the dying patient and preparing for death

Patients should be diagnosed as early as possible. In some cases, recognising that a patient has a limited life expectancy may occur 12 months or so in advance of death. One of the tools that has been developed to identify such patients, and provide care for them in their last year, is the Gold Standards Framework.[36] Originally developed in 2000 in England by the Department of Health End of Life Programme for use in a primary care setting, it was subsequently extended to other parts of the UK and to other care settings.[37] Its main aims are to identify patients who will need palliative or supportive care, assess their needs, preferences and issues important to them and plan around those needs and preferences. It seeks to develop locally based systems to improve the organisation of care for patients in the last year of life.

To ensure appropriate and good quality care, it is essential that clinicians are able to recognise when a patient is dying, particularly when the individual enters the last hours or days of life. The diagnosis of dying is often complex, irrespective of previous diagnosis or history. Uncertainty is frequently an integral part of the process and there are occasions when a patient who was thought to be dying lives longer than expected and vice versa.[38] In 2009, for example, an analysis of over 4,500 hospital deaths indicated that health professionals were sometimes unable to judge that patients were dying. This led to inadequate implementation of appropriate care and poor communication with patients, relatives and in health teams. Even when it was clearly recognised on admission that some patients could not survive long, discussion that should have taken place about treatment limitation did not occur.[39] When dying patients are correctly assessed, practical planning tools such as the LCP (see page 433) help to manage their current symptoms and anticipate others likely to occur. They help health professionals assess what medication may be needed to maintain symptom control and whether consideration should be given to withdrawing medication that is no longer achieving its therapeutic aim. These pathways require regular and frequent review of the patient's condition by the healthcare team so that drug doses can be tailored to match the individual patient's needs. The use of pathways in the final days of life appears more evident with adult rather than paediatric patients, for whom the range of life-limiting conditions is very broad.

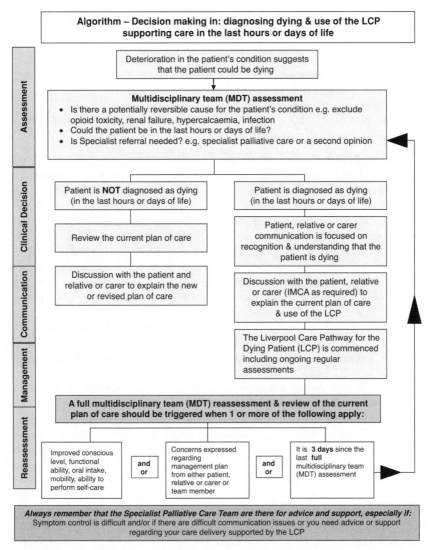

Figure 10.1 The Liverpool Care Pathway for the Dying Patient (LCP) algorithm. Reproduced by permission of The Royal Liverpool and Broadgreen University Hospitals NHS Trust and Marie Curie Cancer Care, operated under the MCPCIL, 2010.

It has been estimated that a small percentage (about 3 per cent) of adults diagnosed as dying and placed on the pathway will improve and need to be reassessed.[40] It is important that decisions are always made on an individual basis and that the judgement that the patient is dying does not automatically lead to withdrawal of treatment. The LCP includes an algorithm to support the clinical decision-making process in what is thought to be the last hours or days of life[41] (Figure 10.1). It is important that the diagnosis of dying is made by the multi-disciplinary team. As a minimum, the team involves a doctor and nurse but may also include other healthcare professionals or other staff, depending on the organisation providing care.

Communication after the multi-disciplinary team assessment

Assessment by the multi-disciplinary team needs to include the following:

- whether there is a potentially reversible cause for the patient's condition by, for example, excluding opioid toxicity, renal failure, hypercalcaemia, infection
- whether the patient could be in the last hours or days of life
- a decision about whether a second opinion or specialist referral, to a palliative care specialist for example, is needed.

If it is agreed that the patient is dying, this needs to be communicated sensitively. Good, comprehensive and clear communication is pivotal. All decisions leading to a change in care delivery should be explained to the patient (where possible and appropriate) and, unless the patient objects, to the family. (The LCP contains a model information sheet for relatives.) All relevant views should be noted and all subsequent decisions documented on the LCP. If after discussion, consensus about care is not reached, a second opinion may be needed. Initiating the LCP requires that healthcare professionals clearly articulate the date and time of starting it and this decision should be endorsed by the senior doctor ultimately responsible for the patient's care. Any changes at this stage should always be made in the best interests of the patient and bear in mind the needs of the relatives or carer. It is important, therefore, that these needs are reassessed regularly. The LCP recommends that ongoing assessments must occur at least every 4 hours and a full multi-disciplinary assessment should occur every 3 days but more often in response to significant changes in the patient's condition or in response to concerns expressed by relatives or other health professionals.

Most people die in hospital but this is not usually their preference. By means of the End of Life Care Strategy, health ministers have promised to give patients more choice about this throughout the UK. Some patients prefer to spend their last weeks in a hospice or specialist palliative care unit, either because they feel safer there or in order to relieve their family of the responsibility and burdens of care. The majority say that they want to remain at home for as long as possible and only be transferred to a specialist inpatient unit when death approaches. Although people's preferences about the place of death should be accommodated where possible, this is not always practical if relatives cannot provide home care or if the patient can only be kept pain and symptom free in a hospice or specialist unit. In some cases, it is not possible to put in place sufficient professional support at home. In Scotland, for example, many dying patients have received inpatient care far from their families when such hospital admissions could be avoided if more local support were available.[42] Across the UK, the most common reasons for admission to hospital or a hospice are breakdown of carer arrangements and problems controlling the patient's symptoms. There has been a trend of moving older people from care homes to hospital just before death.[43] Wherever possible, this should be avoided so that patients do not undergo unplanned transfers in the last days or hours of life. Community palliative care teams, combined with out-of-hours care and good interagency cooperation, should be able to provide care to patients in residential and nursing homes. The BMA has long campaigned, however, for the more equitable provision of such services as the level of provision remains inadequate for the increasing numbers of patients who could benefit from them.

Advance care planning

Making decisions in advance about future treatment is something that patients can choose to do at any stage of life, particularly if they have reason to fear a future loss of mental capacity. A valid competent advance decision refusing some or all medical treatment (a 'living will') is likely to be binding on health professionals (see Chapter 3, page 96). Advance care planning (ACP)[44] is different but builds on the same concept of patients making an advance statement of their wishes. For example, patients may express a clear wish for all active interventions, including CPR, in the event of a loss of mental capacity, or state a wish about where they want to be looked after. Care planning is a particularly important process for dying patients, their families and care providers. Unlike advance decisions, the process is not solely focused on what should happen if the patient loses the mental capacity to make decisions although care planning anticipates deterioration in the individual's condition, which may possibly involve impaired mental capacity.

Advance care planning

Advance care planning is defined as:

'a process of discussion between an individual and their care providers irrespective of discipline. If the individual wishes, their family and friends may be included. With the individual's agreement, discussion should be:

- documented
- regularly reviewed
- communicated to key people involved in his or her care.

Examples of what might be included are the individual's:

- concerns
- values or personal care goals
- understanding about his or her illness and prognosis and particular preferences for types of care or treatment that may be beneficial in the future.'[45]

ACP provides a framework within which terminally ill people can talk about their values, goals, their understanding of their prognosis and preferences for care. Many people want the chance to prepare themselves and their families but advance planning should not be forced on people who are in denial about their condition or are reluctant to discuss future treatment. An overemphasis on completing advance care plans can give the impression that this is something all patients must do whereas it should be a matter of individual choice. On the other hand, the amount of information and options that terminally ill patients want is often underestimated.

For many people, the loss of control over events at the end of their life is one of their main fears. Retaining control, particularly over pain relief and the management of other symptoms, is vital to them. Some aspects are not amenable to control but, for those matters that can be planned, patients should be offered the opportunity to say how they would like their care handled. Advance planning can offer patients a sense of reassurance. Details need to be truthfully and sensitively explained, so that patients do not have unrealistic expectations as sometimes there is a mismatch between the reality of patients' predicted short life-expectancy and their beliefs about it, creating 'a considerable gap between patients' hopes and what can usually be achieved'.[46] Patients' readiness to acknowledge their own condition and impending death is a key factor in any advance planning. They may also want to discuss what will happen to their body after death, including any wishes about organ donation.

What to discuss

The GMC advises that:

[p]atients whose death from their current condition is a foreseeable possibility are likely to want the opportunity to decide what arrangements should be made to manage the final stages of their illness. This could include having access to palliative care, and attending to any personal and other matters that they consider important towards the end of their life.

If a patient in your care has a condition that will impair their capacity as it progresses or is otherwise facing a situation in which loss or impairment of capacity is a foreseeable possibility, you should encourage them to think about what they might want for themselves should this happen, and to discuss their wishes and concerns with you and the health care team. Your discussions should cover:

(a) the patient's wishes, preferences or fears in relation to their future treatment and care
(b) the feelings, beliefs or values that may be influencing the patient's preferences and decisions
(c) the family members, others close to the patient or any legal proxies that the patient would like to be involved in decisions about their care
(d) interventions which may be considered or undertaken in an emergency such as cardio-pulmonary resuscitation, when it may be helpful to make decisions in advance
(e) the patient's preferred place of care (and how this may affect the treatment options available)
(f) the patient's need for religious, spiritual or other personal support.[47]

One of the aspects of care that may need to be discussed as part of advance care planning is the issue of nutrition as the patient approaches the end of life. Decisions may have to be made then about when and whether to introduce clinically assisted nutrition and hydration if there are problems maintaining oral feeding. In 2010, the Royal College of Physicians and British Society of Gastroenterology published detailed clinical and ethical advice about dealing with the uncertainties that can arise in relation to the transition from oral to clinically assisted feeding.[48]

GMC guidance on advance requests

'When planning ahead, some patients worry that they will be unreasonably denied certain treatments towards the end of their life, and so they may wish to make an advance request for those treatments. Some patients approaching the end of life want to retain as much control as possible over the treatments they receive and may want a treatment that has some prospects of prolonging their life, even if it has significant burdens and risks.

When responding to a request for future treatment, you should explore the reasons for the request and the degree of importance the patient attaches to the treatment. You should explain how decisions about the overall benefit of the treatment would be influenced by the patient's current wishes if they lose capacity. You should make clear that, although future decisions cannot be bound by their request for a particular treatment, their request will be given weight by those making the decision.

If a patient has lost capacity to decide, you must provide any treatment you assess to be of overall benefit to the patient. When assessing overall benefit, you should take into account the patient's previous request, what you know about their other wishes and preferences, and the goals of care at that stage (for example, whether the focus has changed to palliative care) and you should consult the patient's legal proxy or those close to the patient. The patient's previous request must be given weight and, when the benefits, burdens and risks are finely balanced, will usually be the deciding factor.'[49]

Another facet of advance planning may be discussion about the Preferred Priorities for Care (PPC).[50] This is a patient-held document to help health professionals understand and discuss patients' preferences. It records a family profile, carers' needs, the patient's preferences about care and the services available in the locality. It can aid communication and give individuals a way to discuss their preferences with family and friends. Not all patients want to engage in this and in some cases, a less structured discussion with the patient aimed at identifying his or her general wishes may be sufficient.

Palliative care

Palliative care is defined as 'an approach that improves the quality of life of patients and their families facing the problems associated with life-threatening illness, through the prevention and treatment of pain and other problems, physical, psychosocial and spiritual'.[51] When patients approach the end of life, palliative care brings together various forms of care to help them to live out their remaining days to the fullest extent and to prepare themselves for death. The principles underpinning it include the following:

- focus on quality of life, including good symptom control
- a whole person approach, taking account of the person's life experience and current situation
- care encompassing both the patient and the people close to the patient
- respect for patient autonomy and choice
- emphasis on open and sensitive communication with patients, informal carers and professional colleagues.[52]

Clinically, the focus is on keeping the person comfortable and free from distressing symptoms. Although opinions differ as to what a good death involves, most agree it is one in which pain and distress are well managed, the dying person and the relatives feel supported rather than abandoned, and a sense of closure is achieved.

In adults, palliative care has been particularly associated with cancer care at the end of life but is not restricted to either cancer or terminal care. It can provide supportive care for patients with other advanced progressive illnesses, such as cardiac, respiratory and neurological conditions. It focuses on maximising the patient's quality of life at all times within the parameters set by the disease, when cure or even effective disease control are not possible. Guidelines from the National Institute for Health and Clinical Excellence (NICE) emphasise the need for such support at all stages of a person's experience of life-threatening illness, stressing that palliative care involves the alleviation of pain and discomfort to improve a person's quality of life when a cure is not possible.[53] Palliative care may be provided in non-specialist settings or by specialist multi-disciplinary teams in specialist units such as hospices. Specialist palliative care professionals look after inpatients and work closely with primary care providers for patients at home or in residential or nursing homes. By their nature, palliative care services are holistic and put the patient at the centre. In line with NICE guidance, they also aim to provide 24-hour service, undertake a comprehensive needs assessment, give patients detailed information about their condition and provide good symptom control as well as psychological, social and spiritual support. Part of palliative care involves trying to enable patients to die in a place of their choosing and offer support to families through the illness and bereavement.

Quality markers

Quality markers aim to ensure that the same standards of care are offered across the UK and 10 of these are highlighted as having most potential to improve quality of care.[54] They centre on the need for good organisational planning, identifying early people who are approaching the end of life, consulting them about their wishes, having services continuously available day and night, ensuring that the workforce is trained in end of life care and monitoring and auditing the quality of that care. Ways of measuring whether patient choice works in practice include defined outcome measures, such as whether patients can be given a choice about place of death. Care standards are also measured through patient, carer and family feedback, such as by a patient or carer diary which can be more informative than questionnaires. Diaries of patients' experiences can be compared and analysed to inform service improvements and may be less of an imposition than asking people to complete repeated questionnaires.

The Liverpool Care Pathway for the Dying Patient (or equivalents)

When patients are recognised as dying, their treatment needs to be continually monitored and assessed. The best known tool to manage the care of dying adults is the Liverpool Care Pathway for the Dying Patient (LCP).[55] The LCP was developed in the late 1990s and has been continuously updated. Specialist palliative care services at the Royal Liverpool and Broad Green University Hospitals and the Marie Curie Hospice in Liverpool worked together to produce this integrated care pathway, based on the model of care in the hospice setting, with the aim of encouraging its use in other settings. In 2004, it was highlighted as an example of best practice by NICE.[56] LCP generic version 12 helps health professionals to focus on care in the last hours or days of a patient's life, ensuring that high quality care is tailored to individuals' needs when their death is expected. As with all other clinical guidelines, the LCP does not replace clinical judgement. Using it requires regular assessment, reflection, critical senior decision making and clinical skill. Changes in care at this complex, uncertain time need to be reviewed regularly by the multi-disciplinary team so that decisions are made in the best interests of patients with input from their family or carers. Good comprehensive clear communication is pivotal and all decisions leading to a change in care delivery should be communicated to the patient, where appropriate, and to the relative or carer. The views of all concerned must be listened to and documented.

If a goal on the LCP is not achieved, this should be coded as a variance. This is not a negative process but a response to the individual nature of the patient's condition and particular needs, as well as a reflection of the clinician's judgement and the needs of the relative or carer. The LCP does not preclude the use of clinically assisted nutrition or hydration or antibiotics; all such decisions should reflect an assessment of the patient's best interests. The responsibility for the use of the LCP generic document as part of a continuous quality improvement programme sits within the governance of an organisation and must be underpinned by an education and training programme. The main goals of the LCP are given below.

The Liverpool Care Pathway for the Dying Patient

Section 1 Initial Assessment Goals (joint assessment by doctor and nurse)

Goal 1.1 The patient is able to take a full and active part in communication

Goal 1.2 The relative or carer is able to take a full and active part in communication

Goal 1.3 The patient is aware that they are dying

Goal 1.4 The relative or carer is aware that the patient is dying

Goal 1.5 The clinical team have up-to-date contact information for the relative or carer as documented below

Goal 2 The relative or carer has had a full explanation of the facilities available to them and a facilities leaflet has been given

Goal 3.1 The patient is given the opportunity to discuss what is important to them at this time (e.g. their wishes, feelings, faith, beliefs, values)

Goal 3.2 The relative or carer is given the opportunity to discuss what is important to them at this time (e.g. their wishes, feelings, faith, beliefs, values)

Goal 4.1 The patient has medication prescribed on a prn basis for all of the following five symptoms which may develop in the last hours or days of life:
   o pain
   o agitation
   o respiratory tract secretions
   o nausea/vomiting
   o dyspnoea.

Goal 4.2 Equipment is available for the patient to support a continuous subcutaneous infusion (CSCI) of medication where required

Goal 5.1 *The patient's need for current interventions has been reviewed by the multi-disciplinary team*
   5a: routine blood tests
   5b: intravenous antibiotics
   5c: blood glucose monitoring
   5d: recording of routine vital signs
   5e: oxygen therapy

Goal 5.2 The patient has a 'do not attempt cardio-pulmonary resuscitation order' in place

Goal 5.3 *Implantable cardioverter defibrillator is deactivated*

Goal 6 The need for clinically assisted (artificial) nutrition is reviewed by the multi-disciplinary team

Goal 7 The need for clinically assisted (artificial) hydration is reviewed by the multi-disciplinary team

Goal 8 The patient's skin integrity is assessed

Goal 9.1 A full explanation of the current plan of care (LCP) is given to the patient

Goal 9.2 A full explanation of the current plan of care (LCP) is given to the relative or carer

Goal 9.3 The LCP Coping with dying leaflet or equivalent is given to the relative or carer

Goal 9.4 The patient's primary health care team/GP practice is notified that the patient is dying

This is reproduced with kind permission of the Marie Curie Palliative Care Institute Liverpool (MCPCIL) at Liverpool University.

Tools like the LCP are only as good as the team using them. The team need to reflect, challenge and critically discuss the patient's situation. It cannot be overemphasised that a robust learning and teaching programme must underpin the use of such tools. (See also pages 456–458 on training.)

Pain and symptom relief

When patients' condition is incurable, the goal of care shifts to maintaining their quality of life, by controlling pain and distressing symptoms. Recognition of the change in focus, by patients, relatives and staff, facilitates discussion about the management of death and bereavement. Some patients put the phase of struggling behind them and come to a degree of acceptance.

Use of opioids and sedatives: the principle of double effect

The principle of 'double effect' allows doctors to provide medical treatment that has both bad and good effects, as long as the intention is to provide an overall good effect. They can give sedatives and analgesics with the intention of, and in proportion to, the relief of suffering, even if as a consequence the patient's life risks being shortened. The moral distinction is between intending and foreseeing the harm. The intention of giving the drugs is to relieve pain and distress; the harmful, but unintended, effect is the risk of shortening life, which the doctor may foresee but not intend. Pain-relieving drugs, such as morphine, do not necessarily hasten death[57] but a common example of double effect is using morphine when it might do so. The administration of drugs which might hasten death is lawful and ethical when patients are terminally ill or dying, the drugs are in their best interests and the doctor's motive is the relief of suffering, not causing death. The actual treatment and dosage must be recognised as reasonable and proper within the profession.

Although the ethical and legal situation is clear, some doctors remain anxious about the degree of pain relief they can provide. They might be reluctant to increase a drug dosage to cope with patient's intractable pain or distress, in which case they need to take specialist advice. Some patients have been fearful that their mental distress or sense of panic, as well as physical symptoms, would not be adequately managed at the end of life. The case of Annie Lindsell highlighted the legal situation even though it did not proceed through the courts.

Annie Lindsell case and double effect

Annie Lindsell had motor neurone disease and sought a declaration from the court that it would not be unlawful for her GP to administer drugs for the relief of her mental distress when she became unable to swallow. Having seen others die of the disease, she was fearful of having to go through the final stages of choking and being unable to speak. Her GP had been warned by the Medical Protection Society that he might face a murder charge if he carried out her wishes to medicate her to relieve her distress. She asked the High Court to confirm that mental distress, as well as physical pain, could be treated with medication that could have the incidental effect of shortening her life. The GP said that he was not proposing to 'anaesthetise her to death' but he did believe 'in forthright and unhesitating relief of distress and pain, with no half measures'. Experts in palliative care gave advice that the regime proposed by the GP was in accord with best medical practice. Annie Lindsell withdrew her application after her doctor's plans for her care were supported by the medical experts; a declaration was therefore not required. This case merely restated the already existing legal position on double effect.[58]

Opioids are commonly used to treat pain and other symptoms of advancing disease. One of the feared side effects of strong or steadily increasing opioid use is respiratory depression. Experts argue, however, that when used appropriately, titrated against the patient's pain, the risk of respiratory depression is small and unlikely to have a significant effect on the patient's lifespan. When appropriately administered, 'there is evidence that sedation to alleviate distress in the last days of life does not shorten life'.[59] But even if life might be shortened as a result, the law and best practice allow such accepted measures to alleviate distressing symptoms that cannot be effectively managed by other means.

Fears that one's motives may be misinterpreted should not stand in the way of doctors providing good quality symptom control. If the intention is clearly to relieve pain and distress and the dosage provided is commensurate with that aim, the action is ethical and lawful. Once the patient's pain or distress has been relieved, if the dose is increased without further clinical indication, the doctor's motive in taking this step must be seriously questioned. When doctors are unable to relieve pain and are concerned about increasing the dose further, specialist advice should be sought from the local hospice or palliative care team.

Sedation at the end of life

Alleviating suffering is a very high priority in end of life care but intentionally reducing patients' awareness, even with their consent, is a serious matter requiring careful examination of doctors' motives and the availability of possible alternatives. Clearly, sedation can never be a substitute for personalised assessment and treatment of patients' physical symptoms and their psychological distress. Some people experience severe symptoms in the final days of life, either due to the terminal illness or to coexisting pathologies.[60] Specialist palliative care teams help patients with previously intractable pain, delirium, anxiety or dyspnoea to become comfortable and, in the majority of cases, symptom control can be achieved. In some cases, medication is given with the intention of relieving pain or agitation with the knowledge that one of the side effects is temporary sedation. Because the aim is to relieve patients' distress, often this does not mean reducing their consciousness to a level where all communication with them is impossible.[61] Various terms are used in the international literature to describe a deep level of sedation, including 'end of life sedation', 'total sedation', 'controlled sedation', 'sedation for intractable distress in the imminently dying'. Although there has been much debate on the subject, lack of common definitions has made it difficult to evaluate how much or how little, sedation is used and in what circumstances.[62]

Terminology

Refractory symptoms occur when 'all possible treatment has failed, or it is estimated that no methods are available for palliation within the time frame and the risk–benefit ratio that the patient can tolerate'.[63] This definition makes clear that the only intention in offering patients the option of sedation for refractory symptoms is to relieve intractable suffering at the very end of life. The team looking after the patient needs to have the expertise and experience to judge when symptoms are refractory, as opposed to those which are simply difficult to treat. Such symptoms include delirium, dyspnoea or severe pain.

Sedation may be offered which is mild (the patient is awake but with lowered consciousness), intermediate (the patient is asleep but can be woken to communicate) or deep (the patient is unconscious). In the UK, low dose sedation aimed at symptom control is an accepted part of terminal care. It is appropriate when necessary to use proportionately higher doses for those patients approaching death who are irreversibly confused, deeply agitated or in severe pain and whose symptoms cannot be relieved by any other means. Deep sedation is an option of last resort when patients experience severe symptoms that cannot effectively be relieved in the last days or hours of life.

Terminal sedation was a term used in north American studies in the 1990s but came to be seen as ambiguous as it could be conflated with the notion of sedation designed to terminate the patient's life.

Continuous deep sedation describes patients deeply sedated up until their death. Describing it as 'continuous' can give rise to anxiety as it might imply an ongoing situation when death is not expected imminently. In the Netherlands, there was some confusion in 2008 about whether such deep sedation had been given to some dying patients with the intention of hastening their death (see Chapter 11, page 466). In the UK, any measures aimed at intentionally hastening death, including by prolonged or deep sedation, would be unacceptable.

Palliative sedation is the term generally used in the UK. It is appropriate in exceptional cases where other measures are ineffective for patients who are very close to death. Many drugs used in palliative care have a sedative side effect and temporarily reduce patients' level of consciousness but 'palliative sedation' is defined as 'the use of specific sedative medications to relieve intolerable suffering from refractory symptoms by a reduction in patient consciousness, using appropriate drugs carefully titrated to the cessation of symptoms'.[64] It has been the focus of much debate both in the UK and internationally. The Association for Palliative Medicine has published guidance, emphasising that it is 'sedation while the patient dies and is not sedating the patient to death'.[65]

International debate

A group of palliative care experts systematically reviewed the literature on palliative sedation in 2007 and found significant differences both within and between countries as to how it was used.[66] They called for more research, the development of more internationally accepted standards and they agreed a number of recommendations. While it is the work of the health team to do all in its power to alleviate patients' symptoms and identify those which are refractory, the experience of suffering and distress are subjective. The expert group argued that only dying patients themselves can say whether their symptoms are so severe that sedation should be considered. So they defined intolerable suffering as that 'determined by a patient as a symptom or state that he or she does not wish to endure. If the patient cannot communicate, proxy judgement from family and/or caregivers is sought.'[67] Underlying this debate about palliative sedation, however, has been a persistent worry that it might lead to, or be seen as, a form of assisted dying which should never be the intention. In fact, the expert group found that retrospective studies strongly suggest that, when used appropriately, palliative sedation does not shorten life and 'presents no distinct ethical problem and should be regarded as acceptable medical practice'.[68] Problematically, however, the shortage of clear consensual guidelines has left some confusion. Where guidance exists, much attention focuses on the intention of the doctor initiating sedation. As a marker of the intention of the care team, the expert group said that the patient's drug record can sometimes provide useful evidence: 'repeated doses, titrated to ease an individual's distress, are the mark of proportionate sedation. Single large doses are the mark of ignorance or intentional harm.'[69]

As with any other good decision making, a partnership is needed which takes account of the clinical indications, the views of the patient and those of the multi-disciplinary team.

Good communication with patients and families is particularly crucial at this stage so that health professionals can assess how important it is for the patient to maintain a certain level of consciousness.

Case example of appropriate deep sedation

Randall and Downie provide a case example of appropriate deep sedation. A patient with capacity nearing death experiences intractable symptoms and requests sedation. He is distressed by dyspnoea (inability to breathe) due to a tumour obstructing the trachea but has refused a tracheostomy. Opiates and use of oxygen do not alleviate the problem and the patient will die due to loss of an adequate airway. There is a possibility that death may be hastened very slightly if sedation causes a decrease in respiratory drive but this is deemed unlikely by the clinical team. They recognise that death will occur soon with or without sedation and estimate that the intended benefit of alleviating the patient's distress outweighs the small risk of hastening death. The patient understands the risk and consents. The degree of sedation given has to be adequate and proportionate to the circumstances, avoiding an overdose but reducing the patient's awareness and consciousness enough to provide relief. 'It would be very difficult, if not impossible, to justify refusing to provide sedation adequate to relieve distress in this situation.'[70]

Whenever possible, patients nearing the end of life should be actively involved in decision making. In cases where palliative sedation may be appropriate, it should be discussed with the patient (or any appointed proxy decision maker for a person lacking capacity) making clear that the only aim is to alleviate refractory symptoms and not to hasten death.

The degree and timing of sedation must be proportionate to the situation and, other than in emergencies, the start dose should be low enough to permit patients to communicate with those around them. Refractoriness has a temporal component and the intermittent or temporary use of sedation reflects the fact that some patients' symptoms might respond to an alternative treatment or that their ability to tolerate the symptom might improve, following the stress reduction provided by temporary sedation.[71] Advice from palliative care specialists is recommended as the dosage must be carefully calculated to relieve distress but should still be the lowest possible to achieve a benefit. The patient's condition needs to be regularly reviewed.

Psychological or existential suffering

Some international debate has focussed on whether the refractory symptoms triggering palliative sedation include patients' psychological distress, panic and agitation, as well as refractory physical problems. There is a strong argument that while patients' psychological, spiritual or social needs might be a contributory factor to their distress, attempts can and should to be made to deal with these by other means than sedation. The expert group carrying out the international literature review in 2007 acknowledged that sedation as a response to psychological or existential distress in the dying patient would be very controversial and emphasised that other solutions should be sought. But they also noted the frequent interrelation of physical and psychological symptoms, as reflected in the concept of 'total' pain. The group called for a 'rigorous diagnostic approach, paying attention to the physical, psychological, social and emotional dimensions of the symptom' once all other possible solutions have been ruled out as ineffective or too risky or burdensome for the patient.[72] Multi-disciplinary management should be focused on all the patient's symptoms, physical and psychological, in the search for non-sedating alternatives that permit patients to complete any outstanding tasks at their life's end.

In 2009, the European Association for Palliative Care (EAPC) published a 10-point framework for the use of sedation in palliative care.[73] It acknowledged the risks of doctors providing sedation for the wrong reasons because, for example, they were 'fatigued and frustrated by the care of a complex symptomatic patient' or withholding it for the wrong reasons and persisting with ineffective alternatives due to anxieties that they might be perceived as hastening the patient's death.[74] It quoted data indicating that this is a misplaced fear, confirming palliative sedation does not necessarily hasten death. The EAPC emphasised that intermittent, mild sedation or 'conscious sedation' in which patients can respond to verbal stimuli should be the first option and deeper sedation only considered when the health team is sure that the patient's suffering is intense and definitely refractory, the patient's wish for it is explicit and death is anticipated within hours or days. Discussing whether 'severe non-physical symptoms, such as refractory depression, anxiety, demoralization or existential distress' should be considered as triggers for sedation, the EAPC noted that there was no consensus.[75] It said that if it were to be considered in such cases, special considerations would be needed.

European Association for Palliative Care – special considerations

Sedation for the management of refractory psychological symptoms and existential distress differs from other situations due to:

1. The difficulty of assessing whether the symptoms are truly refractory.
2. The severity of distress can be idiosyncratic. Psychological adaptation and coping are common.
3. Other standard treatment approaches have low intrinsic morbidity.
4. The presence of such symptoms does not necessarily indicate an advanced state of physiological deterioration.[76]

Sedation in such cases should only be considered for patients with advanced terminal illness. Repeated assessments would be needed by clinicians skilled in psychological care, who establish a relationship with the patient and family and try to address the symptoms by other accepted therapies for anxiety, depression and existential distress. Multi-disciplinary input is essential with representatives from psychiatry, chaplaincy, ethics and clinical care. If, in very rare situations, this strategy is considered proportionate and appropriate, it should only be initiated on a temporary respite basis for a pre-agreed time. Continuous sedation should only be considered after repeated trials of respite sedation, interwoven with intensive intermittent therapy.[77]

There appears to be no evidence that palliative sedation would be seen as appropriate in the UK for dying patients whose symptoms are predominantly psychological or existential. The expectation is that, as the EAPC suggests, other treatment approaches would be offered.

Intention of the doctor and patient

We have already emphasised that end of life care must be devoid of any intention deliberately to hasten the patient's death. Patients can refuse life-prolonging treatment or clinically assisted nutrition and hydration, and those decisions have the effect of hastening death, but they cannot receive assisted dying. (Clinically assisted nutrition and hydration is discussed on pages 444–446.) In 2000, it was suggested in the USA[78] that, in rare cases, terminally ill patients with intractable suffering might be able to request deep sedation while refusing to be artificially fed. It was argued that this could possibly provide a legal alternative for dying patients opposed to physician assisted suicide. Many, however, would perceive this as virtually indistinguishable from assisted dying, not least because sedation alone should be sufficient to eliminate suffering at the end of life. Combined with withdrawal of fluid and nutrition, it would be seen as only having the purpose of intentionally hastening death. Prolonged sedation in a patient not imminently dying also carried other risks for the patient who 'might suffer twilight periods of some awareness' or the possibility of 'awareness with distress and discomfort, but without adequate ability to signal distress'.[79]

When deep sedation is inappropriate

In 2007, Mrs Kelly Taylor who suffered from serious heart, lung and spinal conditions was expected to live less than a year. She had Eisenmenger and Klippel–Feil syndromes and needed to be fed artificially as eating was painful for her. She began a legal battle in February 2007 for a large dose of morphine to induce a coma-like state but her cardiologist, palliative care consultant and GP refused to comply with her request. As she had also made an advance refusal of nutrition and hydration if she were unconscious, the hospice providing care for her considered that her request was tantamount to euthanasia and in breach of the law. She argued that her request was lawful, because she was seeking pain relief, not death. Her lawyers also made the point that, to the extent that the law prevented her request being carried out, it required reinterpretation in the light of the Human Rights Act 1998. After a number of submissions on the law had been made by the parties, she withdrew her claims very shortly before the hearing in April 2007.[80]

Spiritual and pastoral care

One facet of 'whole person' care is offering the opportunity to receive spiritual or psychological support (see Chapter 1, page 26). For many patients, the spiritual dimension is immensely important, and particularly so at the end of life. This is not restricted to people who have a particular philosophy, world view or religious belief; many who have none of these things would like support to help them think about the values that have been important to them. A range of advisers may be helpful, including humanist counsellors, as well as hospital chaplains, rabbis, imams or other faith-based spiritual advisers. In a multi-faith, multi-cultural society such as the UK, it is important that professionals providing care and support to people nearing the end of life take account of individuals' varying spiritual needs. Ideally, these should be assessed before people reach the terminal or dying phase of illness. This gives them time to explore issues that may be troubling them before they reach the very end of life.[81]

The NICE guidelines[82] on palliative care identify the need to meet a person's spiritual needs as part of end of life support. When patients wish to talk to a hospital chaplain or other religious or spiritual adviser, every effort should be made to accommodate this but confidential information about patients should not be given to spiritual advisers by health professionals, without prior patient consent. Alternatively, the dying person may indicate a desire to discuss personal, moral or spiritual problems with health professionals. The GMC prohibits doctors from *initiating* discussion of their own religious or moral opinions with their patients, but they can respond if invited by patients to do so.[83]

When patients do have a particular spiritual or religious viewpoint, the Department of Health's guidance[84] places considerable emphasis on the rights of patients and health professionals to have that respected, as long as they do not seek to impose their views on others. It stresses that the NHS is committed to providing spiritual care for patients and there should be opportunities for consensual discussion, if patients initiate it, but proselytising must be avoided. (Doctors' personal beliefs are discussed in detail in Chapter 1, pages 32–33.)

Some people wish to observe specific traditions at the end of life or in the care of the body after death. The BMA emphasises the importance of identifying and respecting cultural and religious customs before and after death. One facet of a peaceful death may be the patient's knowledge that his or her beliefs concerning appropriate treatment of the body after death will be respected. There may need to be some discussion with the patient, if appropriate, or with those close to the patient, about how the body will be handled after death, while it remains on hospital or hospice premises, in order to conform with the individual's cultural or religious customs. Some patients may also wish to discuss whether their organs or tissue would be suitable for donation or research after their death. (Ethical issues regarding the management of deceased patients are discussed in Chapter 12.)

Summary – diagnosing the dying patient and preparing for death

- Care should be individually tailored and encompass physical, psychological, social and spiritual aspects of care. In so far as possible, individual preferences of place of death should be met.
- Honesty and truth telling are crucial facets of good communication at the end of life. Poor communication and lack of clear information are a source of distress for bereaved relatives.
- Good quality end of life care emphasises personalised and dignified care, focusing on the individuality of each patient.
- Patients' own views need to be heard and their wishes reflected in advance care planning. Patients with capacity should be involved in decision making about future treatment.
- Once it is recognised that the patient's condition is incurable, palliative care offers relief from pain and distressing symptoms. It also provides support for the patient's family.
- The Liverpool Care Pathway for the Dying Patient and equivalents provide a nationally accepted framework for care in the last hours or days of life.
- Loss of control over events is a fear for many patients. Giving them the opportunity to plan aspects of their care can have a positive psychological effect.
- Dying patients should have opportunities to discuss matters such as where they want to die.

Decisions to withhold or withdraw life-prolonging treatment

The BMA publishes detailed advice[85] on decisions to withhold or withdraw life-prolonging treatment. This is periodically updated to reflect best practice and changing case law. The GMC also includes guidance on this subject in its publication on end of life care.[86] Here we summarise the main factors to take into account when considering whether to withhold or withdraw life-prolonging medical treatment but clinicians making such decisions are also advised to refer to the specific BMA and GMC guidance. Prior to withdrawing or withholding such treatment, a senior clinician should talk to the patient, after reviewing the patient's notes, examining the patient and discussing options with the multi-disciplinary team. Where patients are mentally incapacitated, efforts should be made to ascertain their former views and any proxy decision makers should be consulted.

Sometimes, patients who have made an advance decision to refuse some forms of active treatment later want to reconsider that decision. It must be made clear that they can override their advance decision as long as they retain the mental capacity to do so but, in some situations, it may be ineffective to initiate active treatment at a later stage. This is something that patients should have considered carefully at the time they drew up their advance decision (see Chapter 3).

When patients with capacity approach the stage where the aim shifts from curative to supportive care, decisions about the benefits or otherwise of further active treatment need to be discussed with them. When patients lack capacity, the decision is made by an appointed proxy or the healthcare team on the basis of whether treatment would provide overall benefit (see Chapter 3). Any advance care plans that the patient has made need to be considered. It may be agreed that the focus of care should shift to the palliation of symptoms and preparing for death. It may also be agreed that, in the event of cardiac arrest, the patient will not be subjected to attempts at cardio-pulmonary resuscitation (see below). In some cases, decisions about continuation or withdrawal of clinically assisted nutrition and about instigation of hydration are needed. When treatment is unable to provide net benefit, there is no justification for continuing it. Most people do not want active treatment continued if it cannot help them or if it would merely prolong the dying process. If patients have either made an advance decision to refuse treatment, or if the treatment is unable to restore them to a level of health that they consider acceptable, it is inappropriate to continue it. Any decision to withhold or withdraw life-prolonging treatment, and the reasons for it, should be documented in the patient's notes. Doctors must be prepared to justify their decisions in every case.

Wishes of adults with capacity

The GMC highlights the benefits of patients being involved in advance care planning.[87] It can give them a sense of control and minimise misunderstandings which occur at times of emotional distress. Some may have planned whether or how they want continued treatment as they near the end of life. Those who retain capacity can change their advance plans if they wish. They should be involved in all decisions affecting their care and so the options should continue to be discussed with them. When informed of the implications, they have the right to decline medical treatment, without having to justify the decision. They can also refuse clinically assisted nutrition and hydration contemporaneously or in advance. Such refusals must be respected (see Chapter 3). Patients do not have the same right to refuse in advance basic care measures, such as normal oral feeding, intended to keep them comfortable. The refusal of a particular treatment does not imply a refusal of all treatment or all facets of care. The health team must continue to offer procedures that are intended to maintain patient comfort.

Requests for specific treatments are not generally binding on health professionals but they need to be taken seriously and, in the case of clinically assisted nutrition and hydration, there may be a duty to provide what the patient asks. In the case of *Burke v General Medical Council* (see below) the Court of Appeal stated that where a competent patient requests clinically assisted nutrition and hydration, or does so in advance of losing mental capacity, these must be provided.[88] The Court was careful to explain that this did not mean that patients had the right to demand *all* forms of treatment but rather that a fundamental aspect of the duty of care is to take reasonable steps to keep patients alive, where that is their known wish. The question of what is 'reasonable' needs to be considered in the context of each case.

Burke v GMC

Mr Burke was a 45-year-old man with a progressively degenerative condition (cerebellar ataxia with peripheral neuropathy). It was predictable that he would lose the ability to swallow, requiring clinically assisted nutrition and hydration but it was likely that he would retain mental capacity until close to death. Mr Burke was concerned that the GMC guidance, then available,[89] gave doctors the discretion to decide whether to provide or withdraw clinically assisted nutrition and hydration even if his death was not imminent. He challenged the guidance, claiming that it was incompatible with the Human Rights Act 1998.

In July 2004, Mr Justice Munby upheld the challenge, ruling that some parts of the GMC's guidance were not compatible with the Human Rights Act but his decision was overturned by the Court of Appeal. It said that there was no question of clinically assisted nutrition and hydration being withdrawn before the final stages of Mr Burke's disease because he had always made clear that he wanted it when he was no longer able to express his wishes. The Appeal Court held that 'autonomy and the right to self-determination do not entitle the patient to insist on receiving a particular medical treatment regardless of the nature of the treatment. In so far as a doctor has a legal obligation to provide treatment this cannot be founded simply upon the fact that the patient demands it.'[90] Explaining the relationship between a doctor's duty of care and a patient's request for treatment, the judge said that where artificial (clinically assisted) nutrition and hydration is necessary to keep the patient alive, the duty of care normally requires doctors to supply it, if that is the patient's known wish. Deliberately interrupting life-prolonging treatment, with the intention of ending the patient's life, despite the patient's express wish to be kept alive, would leave doctors potentially facing a murder charge.

If patients request treatment that is not clinically indicated, doctors are not obliged to provide it. The Appeal Court endorsed the principles put forward by the GMC that:

- the doctor decides what treatment options would provide overall clinical benefit for the patient
- the options are offered to the patient, with an explanation of the benefits, risks and side effects
- patients decide which, if any, of the treatment options they wish to accept
- if one option is accepted, the doctor will provide it
- if the patient refuses all the options and requests an alternative which was not offered, the doctor will discuss that treatment but is not obliged to offer it if he or she does not believe it to be clinically indicated, although a second opinion should be offered.[91]

Decisions on behalf of adults who lack capacity

Some adults who lack mental capacity have made advance care plans. If they have not done so, treatment decisions must be made in their 'best interests' in line with the Mental Capacity Act 2005 (England and Wales) and the common law (Northern Ireland). In Scotland, decisions are made on the basis of what would 'benefit' the incapacitated person in line with the Adults with Incapacity (Scotland) Act 2000. The respective codes of practice for these two pieces of legislation provide detailed guidance.[92] The GMC's end of life guidance[93] also talks in terms of 'overall benefit'. The concepts of best interests and benefit are clearly similar.

When patients lack mental capacity, their relatives are normally consulted about how treatment should proceed and an indication is sought about what the individual is likely to have wanted. Although they often have helpful insight, relatives do not necessarily determine what happens unless they have been formally appointed to make decisions on the patient's behalf. Such nominated proxies, any court appointed deputies or independent mental capacity advocates (IMCAs) should be consulted. (For the role of legally appointed proxy decision makers, see Chapter 3.)

As part of the assessment of what would be in the best interests or would benefit incapacitated patients, when specifically considering withdrawing or withholding life-sustaining treatment, consideration should include:

• the person's known wishes, including any written statements made when the person had capacity
• clinical judgement about the effectiveness or otherwise of the proposed treatment
• the likelihood of the person experiencing severe unmanageable pain or suffering
• the level of awareness individuals have of their existence and surroundings
• the likelihood and extent of any degree of improvement if treatment is provided
• whether the invasiveness, risks and side effects of the treatment are justified in the circumstances
• the views of any appointed healthcare proxy or welfare attorney (see Chapter 3)
• the views of people close to the person, especially close relatives, partners and carers, about what the individual is likely to see as beneficial.

Relatives and people close to an incapacitated person should be kept informed. The LCP (see pages 432–434) recommends explaining to them the plan of care when treatment is to be withdrawn. They need to understand that treatment is only withdrawn if it cannot benefit the patient or if the patient has refused it. The aim is to ensure that treatment is not continued when it is no longer in the patient's best interests. The courts have confirmed that, in such circumstances, the health team is not in breach of its duty to protect life under the Human Rights Act.[94]

Discussion within the healthcare team

Although ultimately the responsibility for treatment decisions rests with the clinician in charge of the patient's care, it is important that account is taken of the views of the multi-disciplinary team to reduce subjectivity or bias in situations of uncertainty. Nurses who have spent time with the patient may have particular insight into that person's wishes. Depending upon the treatment under consideration, a dietitian, speech therapist, psychologist or physiotherapist may also need to be involved.

Withdrawing or withholding conventional treatment

When patients are admitted after an injury or stroke, there may be initial uncertainty about the diagnosis, the effectiveness of treatment and the long-term prognosis. Initial focus is on stabilising the patient, so that a detailed assessment can take place. If it becomes evident that the patient cannot recover and is nearing the end of life, treatment is generally stopped and the focus is on palliative care. Decisions to withhold or withdraw treatment must be based on the best available clinical evidence and relevant guidelines. It is important that all decisions are made on an individual assessment of the patient, rather than in a blanket fashion.

Nutrition and hydration

When patients are nearing the end of life

Oral nutrition and hydration – by any method of putting food or liquid into a person's mouth – is usually part of essential nursing care which should be *offered* to all patients, including those who lack mental capacity, unless the burdens outweigh the benefits. For some patients, the pleasure of receiving oral fluids, for example, may be offset by the risks of developing frightening shortness of breath, by aspiration of the liquid. Moistening the patient's mouth for comfort is also an essential aspect of care to offer. Patients can refuse these things but, if they are willing, they should be supported to take food and liquids by mouth as long as it is safe to do so. If they cannot cope with oral feeding or it does not meet their nutritional needs, consideration is given to clinically assisted nutrition by nasogastric tube, percutaneous endoscopic gastrostomy or total parenteral nutrition. Decisions must be made on the basis of the individual's circumstances and many patients never need clinically assisted nutrition. Also although nutrition and hydration are often classed together, they should be assessed separately in relation to the individual's needs. For some patients, subcutaneous or intravenous fluids may avoid dehydration or decrease the risk of pressure sores so they may be continued after clinically assisted nutrition is deemed too invasive. The importance of regular clinical review cannot be overemphasised. Multi-disciplinary review should also take place on a regular basis. The LCP (see pages 432–434), for example, recommends daily assessment of the need for clinically assisted nutrition and hydration in the final days.

When patients are not nearing the end of life

This chapter focuses on the care of patients who are approaching the end of life but clinically assisted nutrition and hydration may also be withdrawn from patients who are not dying. In such cases, additional safeguards are required. The law relating to this decision was established by the case of Tony Bland (see below), in which it was held that it would not be unlawful to withdraw clinically assisted nutrition and hydration, even though the patient was not dying and this would lead to his death. It was subsequently confirmed that when withdrawing or withholding clinically assisted nutrition and hydration is in a patient's best interests, there is no breach of the patient's rights under Article 2 of the European Convention on Human Rights (the right to life). When people are not near death, safeguards must be in place to ensure that appropriate consideration is given to their individual circumstances and interests.

Withdrawal of artificial nutrition and hydration

Tony Bland was 17 years old when he was involved in the Hillsborough football stadium disaster in April 1989. His lungs were crushed and punctured and the supply of oxygen to his brain was interrupted. He suffered catastrophic and irreversible damage to the higher centres of the brain, leaving him in a persistent vegetative state (PVS). Bland could breathe unaided but he had no cognitive function. He was unable to see, hear, taste, smell, speak or communicate in any way or feel pain. Being unable to swallow, Tony Bland was fed artificially by a nasogastric tube. In 1992, an application was submitted to the court for a declaration that it would be lawful to withdraw all life-sustaining treatment, including artificial (clinically assisted) nutrition and hydration. The application had the support of Bland's family, the consultant in charge of his care and two independent doctors. In approving the application the House of Lords was satisfied that there was no therapeutic, medical or other benefit to Tony Bland in continuing to maintain his nutrition and hydration by artificial means. It was also held that the provision of artificial feeding by means of a nasogastric tube was 'medical treatment'.[95]

If a mentally incapacitated patient is not dying, has not made a prior refusal of clinically assisted feeding and could survive for a considerable time if so fed, non-provision of nutrition and hydration can be controversial. Some people regard clinically assisted feeding as essential care which should be provided unless the person is actually dying. Judgments in legal cases in England and Scotland,[96] however, have classified clinically assisted nutrition and hydration as medical treatments which – like any other medical intervention – may be withheld or can be withdrawn in some circumstances. Adults with mental capacity can refuse such interventions. If they lack capacity, clinically assisted nutrition and hydration are provided when in their best interests. It is established in common law that decisions not to insert a feeding tube, or not to reinsert it if it becomes dislodged, are medical decisions which are taken after assessment of the individual circumstances of the case. The GMC's guidance requires that a second clinical opinion is sought before clinically assisted nutrition or hydration is withheld or withdrawn from a person who is not imminently dying. This opinion should be sought from a senior clinician (medical or nursing) who has experience of the person's condition and who is not directly involved in the individual's care.[97] This is to ensure that, in this most sensitive area, the person's interests have been thoroughly assessed.

Patients in a low awareness or vegetative state

The vegetative state is a complex neurological condition for which clinical methods of diagnosis are limited. Retrospective clinical audits indicate that up to 40 per cent of patients thought to be in a vegetative state may have been misdiagnosed.[98] Diagnosis is based primarily on clinical history and detailed observation which may require repeated examinations to identify any evidence of awareness, comprehension of language or sustained, reproducible or voluntary responses to various stimuli. A patient's sensory impairments or other acquired conditions can mask such evidence. Brain imaging tools, such as positron emission tomography, functional magnetic resonance imaging and electroencephalography have been used to try and assess residual brain function. It is generally thought that while neuroimaging cannot confirm a diagnosis of vegetative state, it can be used to rule out a diagnosis of vegetative state and may provide information about the patient's prognosis. 'Limited data on prognosis show that quantitative measures of brain activity – in particular, activations beyond primary sensory cortices – are positively correlated with recovery from the vegetative state.'[99]

The complexities associated with diagnosis mean that great care and repeated examination is needed prior to a recommendation being made about treatment withdrawal from a patient who appears to be in a vegetative state. If such a patient is assessed as being in a persistent vegetative state (PVS), or in a state of very low awareness closely resembling PVS, and not imminently dying, any proposal to withdraw clinically assisted nutrition and hydration requires legal review in England, Wales and Northern Ireland. In Scotland, the withdrawal of clinically assisted feeding from a person in PVS does not require a court declaration in the same way but the Lord Advocate stated in 1996 that when such authority has been granted, the doctor would not face prosecution.[100] This left open the possibility of prosecution should the doctor not seek authority from the Court of Session.

In view of the sensitivity of such decisions, the English courts decided that a declaration should be sought in each case where it was proposed to withdraw clinically assisted nutrition and hydration from a patient in PVS. They initially only mentioned PVS patients, however, rather than patients with other serious conditions in which a decision to withhold or withdraw clinically assisted nutrition and hydration could also arise. In other serious cases where such a decision is needed, such as those who have suffered a serious stroke or have severe dementia, the decision has been based on whether providing the treatment would be in the best interests of the patient. This situation could change and up-to-date information can be found on the BMA's website. Legal advice should be sought if there is disagreement within the healthcare team or between the treating team and the family or if there is doubt about the patient's capacity, prognosis or best interests.

GMC advice on patients in a persistent vegetative state

'If you are considering withdrawing nutrition or hydration from a patient in PVS or a condition closely resembling PVS the courts in England, Wales and Northern Ireland currently require that you approach them for a ruling. The courts in Scotland have not specified such a requirement, but you should seek legal advice on whether a court ruling may be necessary in an individual case.'[101]

The BMA also recommends that trusts should have standard policies and guidelines on treatment withdrawal from patients in low awareness or vegetative states to ensure that proper procedures are followed.

Disagreements about treatment withdrawal

In most cases, agreement on what is in the patient's interests is reached after discussion between the healthcare team, the individual, or individual's family or the proxy decision maker. When disagreement arises, steps should be taken to address the issue without delay. Discussion, provision of more information and of a second clinical opinion can resolve some difficulties. If these fail, legal advice should be sought. Many disagreements can be resolved without the need for a full court hearing. Sometimes lawyers are able to give advice about how to proceed or a judge may make the decision in a medical emergency. It is important to remember that the law can provide a protective role for both patients and the healthcare team and whenever disagreement cannot be quickly resolved, legal advice should be sought. Legal review can be beneficial for all parties and doctors should not be deterred from seeking a legal ruling because of the risk of appearing confrontational.

Summary – decisions to withhold or withdraw life-prolonging treatment

- Difficult decisions to withhold or withdraw life-prolonging treatment arise if treatment can no longer provide sustained benefit to the patient.
- Reasons for not providing life-prolonging treatment must be clearly communicated to individuals who have capacity, or those close to people who lack capacity.
- Efforts should be made to communicate with people who appear to lack capacity.
- Advance care planning may indicate whether treatment should be withheld or withdrawn.

- Treatment cannot be provided if patients have made a valid refusal of it but basic care must be provided and patients with capacity can change their mind about refusing treatment.
- Decisions for incapacitated patients are made on the basis of their best interests or what would benefit them. Proxy decision makers need to be involved in the discussion.
- Oral nutrition and hydration should be maintained as long as the patient is willing and able to tolerate this but cannot be forced on patients who resist or refuse.
- The need for clinically assisted nutrition and hydration needs to be considered on an individual basis.
- As the need and desire for nutrition naturally decreases near the end of life, many patients do not need to have clinically assisted nutrition and hydration.
- Legal advice should be sought if disagreements arise about treatment withdrawal.

Cardio-pulmonary resuscitation

Cardio-pulmonary resuscitation (CPR) attempts to restore breathing and spontaneous circulation in patients who have had cardiac and/or respiratory arrest. It can be very invasive, including chest compression, electric shock, injection of drugs and ventilation, although electric shock alone can sometimes restore cardiac function. Patients and their families are often unaware of what is involved or that survival rates after cardio-respiratory arrest and CPR are low. They may also be unaware that attempting resuscitation carries risks, such as rib or sternal fractures, hepatic or splenic rupture, or that patients may be left with brain damage. It cannot prolong the life of people who are imminently dying from an injury or disease process and it might make their death painful or undignified. Patients for whom it is likely to be an option (or their relatives if patients themselves lack mental capacity) should know what is involved. People who have cared for relatives who underwent attempted CPR are far more aware of these risks and often less willing to accept them for themselves.

If and when to discuss CPR decisions with patients

An advance decision that may need discussion as part of care planning is that of whether to attempt resuscitation or record a 'do not attempt CPR' (DNACPR) decision. The term 'resuscitation' can be confusing and agreement not to attempt CPR should not be interpreted as an indication that other measures for that patient should be abandoned. If no DNACPR decision has been made, health professionals are sometimes unclear about when, and in what situations, they should talk to patients, especially older people, about CPR. Raising the subject can be distressing for patients and some may not want to discuss it, in which case it should not be forced upon them but they should be aware that there is information available when they want it. Others may want to talk about it as a way of gaining a better overall picture of what is likely to happen to them. The public often perceive CPR as being significantly more successful than it is in practice and this means that they often have unrealistic expectations about its benefits and consequently they also can be more disappointed by the clinical team's judgement that it would be unsuitable in specific cases.

Regarding when discussion should occur, much depends on the circumstances and the individual patient's wishes. A possible time for clinicians to consider and document the patient's CPR status could be at the initial assessment stage. If patients or their relatives have questions about CPR, or want an opinion about whether it would be likely to work for them, they should be answered truthfully and the reasons discussed. If the patient's condition makes a cardiac arrest likely, discussion should take place with a view to formulating a management plan with them. In some cases, earlier general discussions or advance care planning with patients will have already established such a care and treatment plan, including mention of palliative care and CPR. Healthcare professionals can help people, who are willing to do so, to plan for their future care in a sensitive and realistic manner, and this can include making it clear whether or not attempted CPR is likely to be needed and successful.

The GMC[102] advises that, when possible, doctors should give patients opportunities to discuss whether CPR should be attempted if there is a likelihood of cardiac or respiratory arrest which might be successfully reversed by CPR. Patients who want to discuss it need accurate information about the risks and burdens and should be told if the healthcare team believes that the burdens would outweigh the benefits.

GMC guidance on CPR

'As with other treatments, decisions about whether CPR should be attempted must be based on the circumstances and wishes of the individual patient. This may involve discussions with the patient or with those close to them, or both, as well as members of the healthcare team. You must approach discussions sensitively and bear in mind that some patients, or those close to them, may have concerns that decisions not to attempt CPR might be influenced by poorly informed or unfounded assumptions about the impact of disability or advanced age on the patient's quality of life.'[103]

'If a patient is at foreseeable risk of cardiac or respiratory arrest and you judge that CPR should not be attempted, because it will not be successful in restarting the patient's heart and breathing and restoring circulation, you must carefully consider whether it is necessary or appropriate to tell the patient that a DNACPR decision has been made. You should not make assumptions about a patient's wishes, but should explore in a sensitive way how willing they might be to know about a DNACPR decision. While some patients may want to be told, others may find discussion about interventions that would not be clinically appropriate burdensome and of little or no value. You should not withhold information simply because conveying it is difficult or uncomfortable for you or the healthcare team.'[104]

'Some patients may wish to receive CPR when there is only a small chance of success, in spite of distressing clinical and other outcomes. If it is your considered judgement that CPR would not be clinically appropriate for the patient, you should make sure that they have accurate information about the nature of possible CPR interventions. You should explore the reasons for their request and try to reach agreement; for example, limited CPR interventions could be agreed in some cases. Where the benefits, burdens and risks are finely balanced, the patient's request will usually be the deciding factor. If, after discussion, you still consider that CPR would not be clinically appropriate, you are not obliged to agree to attempt it in the circumstances envisaged. You should explain your reasons and any other options that may be available to the patient, including seeking a second opinion.'[105]

If patients have lost mental capacity, proxy decision makers should be consulted in the same way as mentioned above in relation to withdrawing and withholding treatment. If, after looking at the person's medical history, the healthcare team concludes that CPR would be very unlikely to be successful in restarting the heart and maintaining respiration, it should not be offered. The patient's family and proxy decision makers should be informed. An extreme example would be a patient in the final stages of a terminal illness, for whom death is approaching. CPR is unlikely to prolong life and could significantly increase the individual's suffering.

Patients in nursing homes and care homes

Nursing homes and care homes are sometimes unsure whether and how they should document patients' resuscitation status. All establishments that face decisions about attempting CPR, including care homes and ambulance services, should have a clear policy about it. These policies must be readily available to and understood by staff.[106] They should also be available to residents who want to discuss them. Residents can also talk to their GP about their wishes if they have firm views about refusing resuscitation. Ideally, the patient's wishes should be formally noted by both the doctor and the management of the residential facility. Otherwise, ambulance crews called out in the event of a patient's cardiac arrest may have to follow their own protocols to provide CPR. If a formal DNACPR order or advance decision to refuse treatment has been made, it should be readily available to any attending ambulance crew.

When patients are dying

It is not necessary to raise the issue if the patient has already stipulated that CPR should not be attempted or has reached the terminal stage of life. Dying patients should not be subjected to CPR as this would be futile and inappropriate. Occasionally, individuals or their relatives request that CPR be attempted in situations in which the healthcare team consider it futile and clinically inappropriate. Where the clinical view is that CPR would not restart the heart and breathing, this needs to be explained in a sensitive way, as set out in the GMC's advice quoted above. Health professionals should not agree to provide treatment that is clinically inappropriate but such discussions with patients are obviously very difficult and should be led by an experienced clinician, where possible. If the patient does not accept the decision and requests a second opinion, this should be arranged whenever possible. Similarly, if those close to the patient do not accept a DNACPR decision in these circumstances, despite careful explanation for its basis, a second opinion should be offered.

When patients are not dying

Attempting resuscitation is the default position if no DNACPR order has been made and the patient is not in the terminal stage of his or her illness. Sometimes, patients refuse CPR in advance because they believe that their underlying condition makes it unlikely to restore them to a reasonable quality of life. In some cases, however, patients with whom a DNACPR decision has been agreed, may experience cardiac or respiratory arrest from an easily reversible cause such as choking, induction of anaesthesia or a severe allergic reaction. In those kinds of cases where the condition can be successfully reversed, resuscitation is appropriate, unless the patient has previously specifically refused it with that kind of situation in mind. In the absence of other instructions or agreement, health professionals normally attempt CPR and other measures to sustain life. That may not always be the right decision or what the patient wanted which is why it is important to talk in advance to patients who may need CPR. It raises very sensitive and potentially distressing issues and so can be very difficult to discuss but doctors need to do so if cardiac arrest is likely to occur and CPR could be successful but it is unclear how the person feels about the risks involved. In advance discussion of cases where CPR is likely to restart the patient's heart for a sustained period, the benefits and risks should be discussed with individuals who have capacity and with those close to patients who lack capacity. Any such decisions, and the reasons for them, should be recorded in the medical notes.

When to attempt CPR

Attempting CPR is inappropriate for some patients, such as those for whom death from their underlying condition is imminent. For other patients, where there is no DNACPR order in place, no proper assessment has been made and the person's wishes are unknown, the presumption is that all reasonable efforts are made to revive the individual. Sometimes when CPR is started in such an emergency situation, clinical information soon emerges indicating that it is very unlikely to succeed and it would be inappropriate to continue.

CPR should not be attempted on people who have refused it unless there is evidence that they had a change of heart. Assumptions should not be made about people's wishes if the issue has never been discussed with them. It is sometimes erroneously assumed that patients who have multiple co-morbidities and a relatively poor prognosis should not be considered for CPR. It is important that decisions are made on a case-by-case basis. Blanket decisions against CPR solely on the basis of age or disability, rather than the individual's actual condition, are discriminatory and unacceptable.

Summary – cardio-pulmonary resuscitation

- CPR decisions should be made on the basis of an individual assessment.
- Provision of information is part of good quality care and patients' questions must be answered honestly.
- Attempting CPR is not appropriate when death, from the patient's underlying condition, is imminent.
- Where no decision has been made in advance there should be an initial presumption in favour of CPR but, if it is clear that CPR would not maintain the heart and breathing, it should not be attempted.
- Where the expected benefit of attempted CPR could be outweighed by the burdens, the person's own views are important.
- If the individual lacks capacity, an appointed proxy decision maker or those close to that person should be involved in discussions.
- If a person with capacity refuses CPR, or a person lacking capacity has a valid and applicable advance decision refusing CPR, this should be respected.
- A DNACPR decision does not necessarily override clinical judgement if the cause of the patient's respiratory or cardiac arrest does not match the circumstances envisaged and would be reversible.
- DNACPR decisions apply only to CPR and not to any other aspects of treatment.

Caring for children and young people

Caring for children and young people who are approaching the end of life differs from providing care for adults. Such patients may have complex, long-term conditions, during which they have long experience of inpatient and respite care. The use of care pathways in the final days of a child's care is not widespread, because the range of life-limiting conditions in paediatric care is very broad. Treatment needs to be holistic, flexible and family focused, so that parents are able – wherever possible – to stay with their children in treatment facilities. The needs of siblings have to be considered as the impact of a seriously ill child in the family is likely to have major implications for them. Families should have opportunities to provide feedback in a structured way about the services they receive.

Like adults, children should also have choices about where they spend their last days and where they die.

Communication with the young patient

Children and young people are individuals and can have differing needs and wishes in terms of information. Talking to seriously ill children presents particular difficulties from both an emotional and a practical perspective. Communication needs to be appropriate to their age, life experience and level of understanding. With younger children, this may involve toys, books or drawing pictures. In the past, a very protective attitude was adopted. Children and young people were not told about the implications of their illness or about treatment options. More recently, there is more recognition of the rights of young people to be involved. It has been accepted that they often want to participate in making decisions that affect them very closely. A child or young person who has already undergone a lot of treatment may have relatively mature opinions, based on experience, about the prospect of more. Young patients need to be given information in a manner they can understand and, with sensitive support, have the opportunity to talk about their fears and anxieties. This generally means involving somebody who is specifically trained in communicating with young patients. Families may request secrecy in order to spare the sick child from having to cope with distressing information but secrecy and poor communication can exacerbate anxiety. The child or young person's willingness or need to talk is a paramount consideration and health professionals need to take their cue from patients in deciding how much information they are ready and able to accept. With young children, communication is a three-way process involving the child, the parents and the healthcare team. The GMC has published specific guidance about communicating with children and making decisions with them.[107]

Talking to dying children and young people

A senior ward sister described her approach to discussions with children before surgery as follows:

I usually say to the child, 'what do you want to be told?' Sometimes the teenagers say, 'everything', but then you can see them edge away as if what I am saying is too much for them. I don't leave it at that. I say, 'What is it upsetting you?' I make sure that before the day of surgery they have an opportunity to voice their fears and uncertainties. These girls can be very protective of their mothers. They don't want to upset them by showing how worried they really are, and they put on a brave face when others are around. Sometimes it is important that they know more than they have asked for. I try to edge them forwards to accept a little more information each time we have a chat. I watch carefully to see how successful this is being – and I ration it out, particularly if they seem very anxious, only telling them one main thing at a time.[108]

Communication with parents

Parents and the child's siblings need special support during the child's illness and they should be given information honestly and sensitively. As with other situations of dealing with dying patients, excellent communication skills at all stages are required to ensure that the information is presented with compassion. Particularly difficult decisions arise for parents when withdrawing or withholding treatment requires discussion.

GMC advice on meeting parents' concerns

'You should be sensitive to the concerns and anxieties that parents may have when decisions have to be made about withdrawing or not starting potentially life-prolonging treatment. For example, parents may feel responsible for any adverse outcomes and want reassurance that all appropriate treatment for their child is being offered. You must listen to their concerns, consider carefully their views about changes in their child's condition and make sure they have access to information and support if they need or want it. You should try to make sure that they receive consistent, clear messages about their child's care or condition from different members of the healthcare team.'[109]

In a study of parents' experiences of treatment withdrawal from infants, communication problems – in terms of both what was said and the way the information was given – were by far the most common cause of dissatisfaction.[110]

Parents also need support after the child's death. Although the death of a loved one is always difficult, losing a child is particularly traumatic and parents may need specialist counselling in preparing them for what lies ahead and subsequently to help them to cope with their loss. In addition to the usual manifestations of grief experienced by most bereaved people, parents often feel intense guilt and anger at the unnaturalness of the death of a child. Although referral for specialist bereavement counselling may be appropriate, it is also essential that members of the healthcare team are able to provide clear and concise information in a sensitive and appropriate manner.

When there is disagreement

If parents and doctors do not agree about withdrawing or withholding treatment, the GMC[111] suggests involving an independent advocate, involving a senior colleague, seeking a second opinion or holding a case conference or ethics consultation. It also suggests the use of local mediation services but, if all else fails, legal advice should be sought. It says that approaching the court should be viewed as a constructive way of exploring the issues and providing reassurance that the child's interests have been properly considered. Ultimately, the court decides whether the provision of life-prolonging treatment would benefit or be in the best interests of the patient. It must make the child's welfare its paramount consideration. In exceptional cases, courts have been willing to authorise the withholding or withdrawing of life-prolonging treatment, against the parents' wishes, where it was considered that continued treatment would be contrary to the child's best interests. In 1997, for example, the High Court endorsed a doctor's decision to withhold artificial ventilation and refrain from resuscitating a 16-month-old girl with a desperately serious disease.[112] (This case is discussed in Chapter 4, page 161.)

Sometimes parents strongly disagree with each other and a court opinion may be needed. Although immensely stressful, going through the court process and hearing all the evidence presented in a formal way can help them come to a joint decision, as in the case of *RB*.

Baby RB

RB was born in October 2008. He was seriously ill, could not breathe on his own and was admitted to a special care baby unit where he spent the rest of his life on a ventilator. RB was diagnosed as having congenital myasthenic syndrome (CMS), an inherited muscular disorder. It proved impossible to identify the defective gene in RB's case and although he was trialled on each of the three known drugs for the condition, he showed no response. In the 13 months following his birth, RB was unable to control his muscles or limbs apart from making small movements of his lower arms and hands. Nor could he open his eyes. The medical evidence was that he probably felt the same pain and discomfort as any other child would. Expert opinion was that RB would be totally dependent upon artificial ventilation and feeding for life. Both his parents dedicated a lot of time to RB, both agreed that it would not be in his best interests to spend the rest of his life as an inpatient on a paediatric intensive care unit, but they disagreed about his long-term care. His father wanted RB to have a tracheostomy so that he could be connected to a portable ventilator and leave hospital but this would have also initiated a range of further operations to try and keep him alive. His mother and the treating clinicians supported the administration of a large dose of sedative and the removal of his ventilation tube which would result in his death. The case went to court in November 2009. The judge commended both parents and the treating medical team for having done everything that they possibly could to make RB's life bearable and viable. In the course of the week during which all the evidence was presented, the judge, Mr Justice McFarlane, and RB's father gradually reached the same conclusion, which was to support the decision of the mother and the treating team. The fact that three expert witnesses set out in a detailed manner the potential benefits and burdens for RB was, the judge said, compelling. He and RB's father came to agree that the only tenable outcome was the withdrawal of the intensive and invasive treatment that RB had depended upon from birth.[113]

Palliative care for children and young people

Palliative care for children and young people with life-limiting conditions is defined as 'an active and total approach to care, embracing physical, emotional, social and spiritual elements. It focuses on enhancement of quality of life for the child and support for the family and includes the management of distressing symptoms, provision of respite and care through death and bereavement.'[114] It centres on 'the need to maintain quality of life, not just in the dying stages, but also in the weeks, months and years before death and is characterised by concern for symptom relief, promotion of general well-being and psychological and social comfort for the child and family'.[115] Such care involves an active approach to the management of the child's symptoms and the provision of psychological, emotional and social support which ideally begins long before the dying stage. It requires the provision of flexible respite care and support for the family and siblings, throughout the illness, death and bereavement.

Children and young people often have complex, long-term conditions that require more specialist care and higher levels of home and community support than adults. Care also needs to take account of the child's or young person's emotional and cognitive development. Educational needs and the provision of play therapies may have to be planned. The continuing physical, emotional and cognitive development of children also influences all aspects of their care. The transition between active treatment and palliative care is often less clear for children than for adults, particularly when children have genetic disorders with different clinical manifestations to those encountered in other life-threatening conditions. Many professional and voluntary agencies are involved in different aspects of the care of a seriously ill child and the family. These services need to be properly coordinated.

In 2007, around 20,000 children and young people were estimated to need such care in England and recent estimates for the rest of the UK are hard to find.[116] In fact, an expert review 'found a poor information base with no nationally agreed figures on prevalence and little evidence of good needs assessments at either regional or local level'.[117] An enormous overlap was identified between children with disabilities and complex health needs and those requiring palliative care. Due to advances in medical care, many of these children are living longer and requiring more palliative care services. Fortunately, some conditions that were previously life-limiting are no longer inevitably fatal in childhood and this has profound implications for the services they require. The life expectancy of children with Duchenne muscular dystrophy, for example, has increased substantially so that the majority of children with the condition may be expected to reach adulthood.[118]

As many of these patients now have longer life expectancy, there are increasing numbers of adolescents with palliative care needs who may experience problems making the transition from child to adult services. Often, neither is entirely suitable for them. Successful transition to adult services must allow for the fact that adolescents undergo changes far broader than just their clinical needs and specialised resources have been developed to help manage this process.[119]

Withdrawing treatment from children and young people

General factors to be taken into consideration prior to any withdrawal or withholding of treatment are discussed above (see pages 440–441). They include ascertaining, where possible, the views of the patient and those of the parents. Where their wishes can be known, the child's own preferences about treatment should be taken into account even though they may not ultimately be determinative. Competent children and young people should be supported and given information in an accessible way. The GMC advises that doctors should not withhold information about diagnosis and prognosis unless the patient requests that or if the doctor considers that giving it might cause the patient serious harm.[120] Health professionals should work constructively with the child or young person to arrive at a consensus on the treatment options. Even children who are not mature enough to make decisions for themselves may have opinions about their care and these should be listened to so that the child's concerns can be addressed. (Children's consent and refusal are discussed in Chapter 4.)

Parents or people with parental responsibility for a baby or young child can give or withhold consent to treatment, on the child's behalf. Their decisions are usually determinative, unless they conflict seriously with the medical team's interpretation of the child's best interests. Parents' powers to withhold consent for a child's treatment are likely to be curtailed when the treatment refused is likely to provide a clear benefit to the child, when the statistical chances of recovery are good, or when the burdens and side effects of the treatment are insufficient to justify not giving it.

The Royal College of Paediatrics and Child Health has drawn up a framework for the withholding and withdrawing of life-sustaining treatment from children and young people.[121] This covers five broad situations:

- the 'brain dead' older child, where the criteria of brainstem death have been met and therefore further treatment is futile
- the 'permanent vegetative state' where the child cannot react or relate to the outside world and treatment withdrawal may be appropriate
- the 'no chance' situation where the child has such a severe condition that life-sustaining treatment would only delay death without significantly alleviating the child's suffering

- the 'no purpose' situation in which the child might be able to survive with treatment, 'but the degree of physical or mental impairment will be so great that it is unreasonable to expect them to bear it'
- the 'unbearable' situation in which the child and/or family conclude that no further treatment can be borne in the face of the child's progressive and irreversible illness.

The College advises that if cases fall outside these five categories, or if uncertainty or disagreement exist about the extent of likely future impairment, the child's life should be 'safeguarded in the best way possible'[122] until the issues are resolved. This may involve resuscitation in emergency situations. It emphasises that rigid rules should be avoided, even for conditions that appear hopeless, and decisions should never be rushed but must always be made by the team with all the available evidence.

The aim of the guidance is not to be prescriptive but to help professionals, patients and families to make very difficult decisions and to find common ground when differences of opinion arise. When agreement is not reached, it suggests various measures, such as obtaining an external expert clinical opinion or seeking legal advice from the Children and Family Court Advisory and Support Service (CAFCASS) or involving a clinical ethics committee.

Summary – caring for children and young people

- Children and young people need access to information in a manner appropriate to their age, experience and maturity.
- Parents should be involved in discussion and decision making. Care should be family-focused and flexible.
- Children and young people need opportunities to talk about their anxieties.
- Children and young people should have psychological and social support.
- Attention needs to be given to siblings during the child's illness and after the child's death.

After the patient's death

It is important for healthcare professionals to recognise that end of life care does not stop at the point of death. Verification and certification of death should be completed in a timely manner and, where necessary, referral made to the coroner or procurator fiscal (see Chapter 12).

Last offices

The UK consists of culturally diverse communities with some differing concepts of 'family' as well as different traditions and rituals concerning the deceased. The care that is given to the body of the deceased is referred to as last offices. It includes ensuring that the religious or cultural wishes of the deceased person are honoured and that the dignity and privacy of the body is maintained. Although these last offices involve comparatively simple procedures, they often have emotional significance for the bereaved family.

Bereavement support for those close to the patient

Arrangements may need to be made to provide support, including emotional and practical bereavement support, to the family. Good communication and team care should ideally have been initiated at an early stage and this may help to ease the pain of bereavement. Although expected deaths do not represent a shock to the staff who have been caring for the patient, the death of a loved one, however expected, is often a shock for friends and family. Much preparatory work falls to the nursing staff or to GPs. After the patient has died, it is usual and comforting to see death as a release for the patient, but a sense of guilt and fear of criticism often prevent people from also admitting beforehand that the death of the patient may represent a relief for them. The family should be encouraged to discuss any concerns and, if appropriate, should be offered counselling.

For parents, the death of a child is the most devastating experience they can have. The Royal College of Paediatrics and Child Health cautions health professionals against medicalising the family's grief or intervening inappropriately but says that information about support services and voluntary agencies should be available.[123] Hospitals should have appropriate policies in place so that staff are aware of the needs of different cultures at this time and so that the family can be given information, if relevant, about asking for a post-mortem examination or donating tissue or organs.

Support for the healthcare team

Caring for dying and bereaved people can also take a toll on health professionals at all levels. Forming necessarily impermanent, although rewarding, relationships with patients can be draining and being constantly exposed to suffering, helplessness, uncertainty, anger and loss can be hard for healthcare staff. Psychological support should be available for staff who may need help to cope with the psychological impact of their role. Employing bodies and colleagues of those caring for dying patients need to be sensitive to the possibility of 'burnout'. Staff at all levels should have access to counselling and support both within and outside the healthcare team.

Summary – after the patient's death

* Providing support for those close to the patient to help them to come to terms with their bereavement is an essential part of caring for dying people.
* Caring for dying and bereaved people can also take its toll on health professionals at all levels. All staff should have access to counselling and support both within and outside the healthcare team.

Training

Training for non-specialists

One of the challenges in improving end of life care for patients is that of achieving a high level of professional involvement. In particular, for some doctors, death may still be seen as a failure. Encouraging all health professionals to see the provision of high quality end of life care as a fulfilling role requires changes in such attitudes. Many non-specialist health professionals are already committed to that view and to using tools such as the Gold Standards Framework for end of life care (see page 426). Research of patients' views in Scotland, for example, indicated that patients and family carers increasingly had the confidence to allow the patient to die at home, when assured that their GP and local practice staff were committed to providing support for that.[124]

As part of the end of life care strategies across the UK, there has been renewed emphasis on training, including in communication skills at undergraduate and post-qualification level for any professional caring for seriously ill patients. Nevertheless, 'hundreds of thousands of NHS and social care staff deal with people at the end of their lives but many have had little or no training in this area.'[125] At the BMA's annual meeting in 2010, a resolution was passed urging the Association to campaign for better training in palliative medicine for all GPs and hospital doctors involved in managing dying patients. Increasing emphasis is also placed on health professionals in a variety of settings acquiring greater skills in pain and symptom management.

In the community, general palliative care services are provided by primary care teams, often supported by palliative care outreach services. For them, the high levels of specialist expertise acquired by colleagues, including palliative care clinical nurse specialists, can be very valuable. In most parts of the UK, GP practices have been particularly encouraged to work towards improving the care of patients who are approaching the end of life care. The Gold Standards Framework (see page 426) encourages GPs to identify such patients early and prospectively review their care provision with them.

End of life care should also be recognised as a core generic skill for hospital staff but, as yet, few have received specific preparation for it. In 2009, it was noted that 'repeated reports have demonstrated high levels of dissatisfaction and complaints regarding care of the dying in acute hospital settings'.[126] The solution must be training tailored to the healthcare professional's needs. The King's Fund suggested a variety of means for providing this, including by e-learning, apprentice-style learning and training by specialist palliative care providers.[127] In Wales, a role was identified for telecare systems, both in the discussion of treatment and care and also for the training and development of staff.[128] In Wales, the gap in continuity has been plugged by specialist palliative care teams developing integrated clinical records.[129]

Special attention also needs to be given to children's palliative care as a subspecialty of paediatrics. The Royal College of Paediatrics and Child Health recommended that all clinical and nursing staff should also have access to continuing education in communication, ethics and withdrawing and withholding treatment.[130] Child bereavement organisations and family support groups could also be involved in educational clinical ethics meetings.

Specialist palliative care services are delivered by multi-disciplinary teams, which include palliative medicine consultants, palliative care nurse specialists, social workers, counsellors and other staff who are able to provide both the psychological and social support needed. Specialist palliative care teams can either provide advice to those who are responsible for care, or take the lead in a patient's care – whether in the community, hospital or hospice – depending on that individual's needs. They have an important role in the education and training of the wide range of generalist staff who care for patients at the end of life.

The development of general palliative care services within hospitals, primary care and nursing homes has illustrated that the integration of palliative care principles into existing services is a viable and appropriate response which should be encouraged. In addition to their technical medical expertise and skills in pain and symptom control, all health professionals who care for dying patients need specific training in aspects of end of life care. They need to be able to recognise when individual patients and relatives (including the parents of a sick child) need counselling, more or less detail, or simply a breathing space prior to receiving more information. Training in terminal care assists professionals to deal with patients' psychological pain and distress as well as their physical symptoms. Senior clinicians who have developed the appropriate skills, such as consultants in palliative medicine, are invaluable role models.

Summary – training

- Regardless of how well intentioned doctors may be, their relationships with their terminally ill patients and their families can be severely and irrevocably damaged by inadequate communication skills.
- It is imperative that all doctors receive training in symptom control and communication skills as well as in recognising patients' needs for comfort, counselling and for more or less information.

References

1 General Medical Council (2010) *Treatment and care towards the end of life: Good practice in decision-making*, GMC, London.
2 General Medical Council (2010) *Treatment and care towards the end of life: Good practice in decision-making*, GMC, London, pp.86–7.
3 Addicott R, Ashton R. (eds.) (2010) *Delivering Better Care at the End of Life: the next steps*, King's Fund, London, p.2.
4 Gomes B, Higginson I. (2008) Where people die (1974–2030): past trends, future projections and implications for care. *Palliat Med* **22**, 33–41.
5 National Confidential Enquiry into Patient Outcomes and Death (2009) *Caring to the End? A review of the care of patients who died in hospital within four days of admission*, NCEPOD, London, p.3.
6 This is articulated in England in: Department of Health (2008) *End of Life Care Strategy: Promoting high quality care for all adults at the end of life*, The Stationery Office, London. In Northern Ireland, in: Department of Health, Social Services and Public Safety (2010) *Living Matters, Dying Matters. A Palliative and End of Life Care Strategy for Adults in Northern Ireland*, DHSSPSNI, Belfast. In Scotland in: Scottish Government (2008) *Living and Dying Well: a national action plan for end of life care*, Scottish Government, Edinburgh. In Wales in: Palliative Care Planning Group Wales (2008) *Report to the Minister for Health and Social Services*. Available at: www.wales.gov.uk (accessed 10 May 2011).
7 Richards M. (2010) The End of Life Care Strategy: 16 months on in the King's Fund. In: Addicott R, Ashton R (eds.) *Delivering Better Care at the End of Life: the next steps*, King's Fund, London, p.30.
8 Addicott R, Ashton R. (eds.) (2010) *Delivering Better Care at the End of Life: the next steps*, King's Fund, London, p.2.
9 Department of Health (2008) *End of Life Care Strategy: Promoting high quality care for all adults at the end of life*, DH, London.
10 Scottish Government (2008) *Living and Dying Well: a national action plan for end of life care*, Scottish Government, Edinburgh. In Northern Ireland, see: Department of Health, Social Services and Public Safety (2010) *Living Matters, Dying Matters. A Palliative and End of Life Care Strategy for Adults in Northern Ireland*, DHSSPSNI, Belfast. The All Wales Palliative Care Planning Group, set up with the remit of establishing the elements of a core palliative care service for adults and children, reported its recommendations to the Welsh Assembly in June 2008, see: Palliative Care Planning Group Wales (2008) *Report to the Minister for Health and Social Services*. Available at: www.wales.gov.uk (accessed 10 May 2011).
11 Richards M. (2010) The End of Life Care Strategy: 16 months on in the King's Fund. In: Addicott R, Ashton R. (eds.) *Delivering Better Care at the End of Life*, King's Fund, London, pp.30–3.
12 Temel JS, Greer JA, Muzikansky A. *et al.* (2010) Early Palliative Care for patients with metastatic non-small-cell lung cancer. *N Engl J Med* **363**, 733–42.
13 Ellershaw J, Murphy D. (2011) What is the Liverpool Care Pathway for the Dying Patient (LCP)? In: Ellershaw J, Wilkinson S (eds.) *Care of the Dying: a pathway to excellence*, 2nd edn, Oxford University Press, Oxford, pp.15–31.
14 Wilkinson S. (2011) Communication in care of the dying. In: Ellershaw J, Wilkinson S (eds.) *Care of the Dying: a pathway to excellence*, 2nd edn, Oxford University Press, Oxford, pp.88–9.

15 Wilkinson S. (2011) Communication in care of the dying. In: Ellershaw J, Wilkinson S (eds.) *Care of the Dying: a pathway to excellence*, 2nd edn, Oxford University Press, Oxford, p.89.

16 Buckman R. (1994) *How to break bad news a guide for health care professionals*, Papermac, London.

17 Schels W, Moorhead J. (2008) *Life before death*, Wellcome Collection Exhibition, April 2008. Reported in *The Guardian* 1 April 2008.

18 Adelman RD, Greene MG, Charon R. (1991) Issues in the physician-elderly patient interaction. *Aging and Society* **2**, 127–48.

19 Kubler-Ross E. (1970) *On death and dying*, Tavistock Publications, London.

20 Kubler-Ross E. (1970) *On death and dying*, Tavistock Publications, London, p.76.

21 Wilkinson S. (2011) Communication in care of the dying. In: Ellershaw J, Wilkinson S (eds.) *Care of the Dying: a pathway to excellence*, 2nd edn, Oxford University Press, Oxford, pp.100–1.

22 General Medical Council (2010) *Treatment and care towards the end of life: Good practice in decision-making*, GMC, London, para 14.

23 Kubler-Ross E. (1970) *On death and dying*, Tavistock Publications, London, p.35.

24 Kubler-Ross E. (1970) *On death and dying*, Tavistock Publications, London, p.37.

25 Wilkinson S. (2011) Communication in care of the dying. In: Ellershaw J, Wilkinson S (eds.) *Care of the Dying: a pathway to excellence*, 2nd edn, Oxford University Press, Oxford, pp.100–2.

26 The AM, Hak T, Koeter G. *et al.* (2000) Collusion in doctor-patient communication about imminent death: an ethnographic study. *BMJ* **321**, 1376–81.

27 Mayor S. (2008) UK audit shows need for greater caution with chemotherapy in very sick patients. *BMJ* **337**, 1130.

28 Munday DF, Maher EJ. (2008) Informed consent and palliative chemotherapy. *BMJ* **337**, 471.

29 Audrey S, Abel J, Blazeby JM. *et al.* (2008) What oncologists tell patients about survival benefits of palliative chemotherapy and implications for informed consent: qualitative study. *BMJ* **337**, 1752.

30 Munday DF, Maher EJ. (2008) Informed consent and palliative chemotherapy. *BMJ* **337**, 471.

31 Peele PB, Siminoff LA, Xu Y. *et al.* (2005) Decreased use of adjuvant breast cancer therapy in a randomized controlled trial of a decision aid with individualized risk information. *Med Decis Making* **25**, 301–7.

32 Audrey S, Abel J, Blazeby JM. *et al.* (2008) What oncologists tell patients about survival benefits of palliative chemotherapy and implications for informed consent: qualitative study. *BMJ* **337**, 492–6, p.494.

33 General Medical Council (2010) *Treatment and care towards the end of life: Good practice in decision-making*, GMC, London, para 15.

34 The Marie Curie Palliative Care Institute Liverpool (2009) *The Liverpool Care Pathway for the Dying Patient (LCP) Core Documentation*, MCPCIL, Liverpool.

35 Harris P, Finlay IG, Cook A. *et al.* (2003) Complementary and alternative medicine use by patients with cancer in Wales: a cross sectional survey. *Complementary Therapies in Medicine* **11**, 249–53.

36 See the National Gold Standards Framework (GSF) Centre overview for the history and growth of the GSF. Available at: www.goldstandardsframework.org.uk (accessed 10 May 2011).

37 Scottish Partnership for Palliative Care (2007) *Palliative and end of life care in Scotland: the case for a cohesive approach, Report and recommendations submitted to the Scottish Executive*, Scottish Partnership for Palliative Care, Edinburgh, p.18.

38 The Marie Curie Palliative Care Institute Liverpool (2009) *The Liverpool Care Pathway for the Dying Patient (LCP) Core Documentation*, MCPCIL, Liverpool.

39 National Confidential Enquiry into Patient Outcomes and Death (2009) *Caring to the End? A review of the care of patients who died in hospital within four days of admission*, NCEPOD, London, p.5.

40 Edmonds P, Burman R, Prentice W. (2009) End of life care in the acute hospital setting. *BMJ* **339**, 1269–70.

41 The Marie Curie Palliative Care Institute Liverpool (2009) *The Liverpool Care Pathway for the Dying Patient (LCP) Core Documentation*, MCPCIL, Liverpool.

42 Scottish Partnership for Palliative Care (2007) *Palliative and end of life care in Scotland: the case for a cohesive approach, Report and recommendations submitted to the Scottish Executive*, Scottish Partnership for Palliative Care, Edinburgh.

43 Help the Aged (2005) *Dying in Older Age: reflections from an older person's perspective*, Help the Aged, London.

44 NHS End of Life Care Programme (2008) *Advance Care Planning: A Guide for Health and Social Care Staff*, Department of Health. Available at: www.endoflifecareforadults.nhs.uk (accessed 10 May 2011).

45 NHS End of Life Care Programme (2008) *Advance Care Planning: A Guide for Health and Social Care Staff*, Department of Health. Available at: www.endoflifecareforadults.nhs.uk (accessed 10 May 2011).

46 Audrey S, Abel J, Blazeby JM. *et al.* (2008) What oncologists tell patients about survival benefits of palliative chemotherapy and implications for informed consent: qualitative study. *BMJ* **337**, 1752.

47 General Medical Council (2010) *Treatment and care towards the end of life: Good practice in decision-making*, GMC, London, paras 52–3.

48 Royal College of Physicians, British Society of Gastroenterology (2010) *Oral feeding difficulties and dilemmas*, RCP, London.

49 General Medical Council (2010) *Treatment and care towards the end of life: Good practice in decision-making*, GMC, London, paras 63–5.

50 NHS End of Life Care Programme (2007) *Preferred Priorities for Care*, Department of Health. Available at: www.endoflifecareforadults.nhs.uk (accessed 10 May 2011).

51 World Health Organization (2004) *WHO Definition of Palliative Care*. Available at: www.who.int (accessed 17 January 2011).

52 Addington-Hall J. (1998) *Reaching out: specialist palliative care for adults with non-malignant diseases*. Occasional paper 14. National Council for Hospice and Specialist Palliative Care Services and Scottish Partnership Agency for Palliative and Cancer Care, London.

53 National Institute for Clinical Excellence (2004) *Improving supportive and palliative care services for adults with cancer*, NICE, London.

54 Department of Health (2008) *End of Life Care Strategy: Promoting high quality care for all adults at the end of life*, DH, London.

55 The Marie Curie Palliative Care Institute Liverpool (2009) *The Liverpool Care Pathway for the Dying Patient (LCP) Core Documentation*, MCPCIL, Liverpool.

56 National Institute for Clinical Excellence (2004) *Improving supportive and palliative care services for adults with cancer*, NICE, London.

57 Sykes N, Thorne A. (2003) The use of opiods and sedatives at the end of life. *Lancet Oncology* **4**, 312–8.

58 Dyer C. (1997) Court confirms right to palliative treatment for mental distress. *BMJ* **315**, 1177.

59 Randall F, Downie RS. (2010) *End of Life Choices: consensus and controversy*, Oxford University Press, Oxford, p.104.

60 Randall F, Downie RS. (2010) *End of Life Choices: consensus and controversy*. Oxford University Press, Oxford, p.85.

61 De Graeff A, Dean M. (2007) Palliative sedation therapy in the last weeks of life: a literature review and recommendations for standards. *J Palliat Med* **10**(1), 67–85, p.79.

62 Randall F, Downie RS. (2010) *End of Life Choices: consensus and controversy*, Oxford University Press, Oxford, p.101.

63 De Graeff A, Dean M. (2007) Palliative sedation therapy in the last weeks of life: a literature review and recommendations for standards. *J Palliat Med* **10**(1), 67–85, p.69.

64 De Graeff A, Dean M. (2007) Palliative sedation therapy in the last weeks of life: a literature review and recommendations for standards. *J Palliat Med* **10**(1), 67–85, p.67.

65 Association for Palliative Medicine of Great Britain and Ireland (2009) *APM position on the use of sedation at the end of life*. Available at: www.apmonline.org (accessed 30 March 2011).

66 De Graeff A, Dean M. (2007) Palliative sedation therapy in the last weeks of life: a literature review and recommendations for standards. *J Palliat Med* **10**(1), 67–85.

67 De Graeff A, Dean M. (2007) Palliative sedation therapy in the last weeks of life: a literature review and recommendations for standards. *J Palliat Med* **10**(1), 67–85, p.68.

68 De Graeff A, Dean M. (2007) Palliative sedation therapy in the last weeks of life: a literature review and recommendations for standards. *J Palliat Med* **10**(1), 67–85, p.79.

69 De Graeff A, Dean M. (2007) Palliative sedation therapy in the last weeks of life: a literature review and recommendations for standards. *J Palliat Med* **10**(1), 67–85, p.70.

70 Randall F, Downie RS. (2010) *End of Life Choices: consensus and controversy*, Oxford University Press, Oxford, p.103.

71 De Graeff A, Dean M. (2007) Palliative sedation therapy in the last weeks of life: a literature review and recommendations for standards. *J Palliat Med* **10**(1), 67–85, p.70.

72 De Graeff A, Dean M. (2007) Palliative sedation therapy in the last weeks of life: a literature review and recommendations for standards. *J Palliat Med* **10**(1), 67–85, p.70.

73 Cherny NI, Radbruch L. (2009) European Association for Palliative Care recommended framework for the use of sedation in palliative care. *Palliat Med* **23**(7), 581–93.

74 Cherny NI, Radbruch L. (2009) European Association for Palliative Care recommended framework for the use of sedation in palliative care. *Palliat Med* **23**(7), 581–93, p.582.

75 Cherny NI, Radbruch L. (2009) European Association for Palliative Care recommended framework for the use of sedation in palliative care. *Palliat Med* **23**(7), 581–93, p.584.

76 Cherny NI, Radbruch L. (2009) European Association for Palliative Care recommended framework for the use of sedation in palliative care. *Palliat Med* **23**(7), 581–93, p.588.

77 Cherny NI, Radbruch L. (2009) European Association for Palliative Care recommended framework for the use of sedation in palliative care. *Palliat Med* **23**(7), 581–93, p.584.

78 Quill TE, Byock IR. (2000) Responding to terminal suffering: the role of terminal sedation and voluntary refusal of foods and fluids. *Ann Intern Med* **132**, 408–14.

79 Randall F, Downie RS. (2010) *End of Life Choices: consensus and controversy*, Oxford University Press, Oxford, p.108.

80 Laurence J. (2007) Woman goes to court in historic euthanasia case. *The Independent* (13 February). Available at: www.independent.co.uk (accessed 19 April 2011).

81 Speck P. (2011) Spiritual/religious issues in care of the dying. In: Ellershaw J, Wilkinson S. (eds.) *Care of the dying: A pathway to excellence*, Oxford University Press, Oxford, pp.107–26.

82 National Institute for Clinical Excellence (2004) *Improving supportive and palliative care services for adults with cancer*, NICE, London.

83 General Medical Council (2008) *Personal beliefs and medical practice*, GMC, London.

84 Department of Health (2009) *Religion or belief: a practical guide for the NHS*, DH, London.

85 British Medical Association (2007) *Withholding and Withdrawing Life-Prolonging Medical Treatment*, 3rd edn, Blackwell, Oxford.

86 General Medical Council (2010) *Treatment and care towards the end of life: Good practice in decision making*, GMC, London.

87 General Medical Council (2010) *Treatment and care towards the end of life: Good practice in decision making*, GMC, London, p.31.

88 *R (on the application of Burke) v General Medical Council* [2005] 2 FLR 1223.

89 General Medical Council (2002) *Withholding and withdrawing life-prolonging treatments*, GMC, London.

90 *R (on the application of Burke) v General Medical Council* [2005] 2 FLR 1223: 31.

91 *R (on the application of Burke) v General Medical Council* [2005] 2 FLR 1223: 50.

92 Department for Constitutional Affairs (2007) *Mental Capacity Act 2005 Code of Practice*, The Stationery Office, London. Scottish Executive (2010) *Adults with Incapacity (Scotland) Act 2000. Code of Practice, (third edition) for practitioners authorised to carry out medical treatment or research under part 5 of the Act*. SG/2010/57. Available at: www.scotland.gov.uk (accessed 26 April 2011).

93 General Medical Council (2010) *Treatment and care towards the end of life: Good practice in decision-making*, GMC, London.

94 *NHS Trust A v M; NHS Trust B v H* [2001] 1 All ER 801.

95 *Airedale NHS Trust v Bland* [1993] 1 All ER 821: 869.

96 See, for example: *Frenchay Healthcare NHS Trust v S* [1994] 1 WLR 601. *Re D (medical treatment)* [1998] 1 FLR 411. *Law Hospital NHS Trust v Lord Advocate* (1996) SLT 848.

97 General Medical Council (2010) *Treatment and care towards the end of life: Good practice in decision making*, GMC, London, para 121.

98 Monti MM, Laureys S, Owen AM. (2010) The vegetative state. *BMJ* **341**, c3765.

99 Monti MM, Laureys S, Owen AM. (2010) The vegetative state. *BMJ* **341**, c3765.

100 *Law Hospital NHS Trust v Lord Advocate* (1996) SLT 848.

101 General Medical Council (2010) *Treatment and care towards the end of life: good practice in decision making*, GMC, London, para 126. See also: Court of Protection Practice Direction 9E – Applications relating to serious medical treatment.

102 General Medical Council (2010) *Treatment and care towards the end of life: good practice in decision making*, GMC, London, para 137.

103 General Medical Council (2010) *Treatment and care towards the end of life: good practice in decision making*, GMC, London, para 132.

104 General Medical Council (2010) *Treatment and care towards the end of life: good practice in decision making*, GMC, London, para 134.

105 General Medical Council (2010) *Treatment and care towards the end of life: good practice in decision making*, GMC, London, para 139.

106 NHS Executive (2000) *Resuscitation policy, HSC 2000/028*, DH, London. Scottish Executive Health Department (2000) *Resuscitation policy, HDL (2000) 22*, SEHD, Edinburgh.

107 General Medical Council (2007) *0–18 years: guidance for all doctors*, GMC, London. It also has a section on children's care in: General Medical Council (2010) *Treatment and care towards the end of life: good practice in decision making*, GMC, London.

108 Alderson P. (1993) *Children's consent to surgery*, Open University Press, Buckingham.

109 General Medical Council (2010) *Treatment and care towards the end of life: good practice in decision making*, GMC, London, para 107.

110 McHaffie HE. (2001) *Crucial decisions at the beginning of life. Parents' experiences of treatment withdrawal from infants*, Radcliffe Medical Press, Oxford.

111 General Medical Council (2010) *Treatment and care towards the end of life: good practice in decision making*, GMC, London, para 108.

112 *Re C (a minor) (medical treatment) sub nom Re C (a minor) (withdrawal of lifesaving treatment)* [1998] 1 FLR 384.

113 *In the matter of RB (A Child)* [2009] EWHC 3269 (Fam).

114 Royal College of Paediatrics and Child Health, Association of Children with Life-threatening or Terminal Conditions and their Families (1997) *A guide to the development of children's palliative care services*, RCPCH, London and ACLTCF, Bristol, p.7.

115 Craft A, Killen S. (2007) *Palliative care services for children and young people in England: an independent review for the Secretary of State for Health*, DH, London, p.15.

116 Craft A, Killen S. (2007) *Palliative care services for children and young people in England: an independent review for the Secretary of State for Health*, DH, London, p.21.

117 Craft A, Killen S. (2007) *Palliative care services for children and young people in England: an independent review for the Secretary of State for Health*, DH, London, p.4.

118 Craft A, Killen S. (2007) *Palliative care services for children and young people in England: an independent review for the Secretary of State for Health*, DH, London, pp.22–3.

119 Craft A, Killen S. (2007) *Palliative care services for children and young people in England: an independent review for the Secretary of State for Health*, DH, London, pp.22–3.

120 General Medical Council (2010) *Treatment and care towards the end of life: good practice in decision making*, GMC, London, para 102–3.

121 Royal College of Paediatrics and Child Health (2004) *Withholding or Withdrawing Life Sustaining Treatment in Children: a framework for practice*, 2nd edn, RCPCH, London.

122 Royal College of Paediatrics and Child Health (2004) *Withholding or Withdrawing Life Sustaining Treatment in Children: a framework for practice*, 2nd edn, RCPCH, London, p.11.

123 Royal College of Paediatrics and Child Health (2004) *Withholding or Withdrawing Life Sustaining Treatment in Children: a framework for practice*, 2nd edn, RCPCH, London, p.36.

124 Scottish Partnership for Palliative Care (2007) *Palliative and end of life care in Scotland: the case for a cohesive approach*, Scottish Partnership for Palliative Care, Edinburgh, p.21.

125 Richards M. (2010) The End of Life Care Strategy: 16 months on. In: Addicott R, Ashton R. (eds.) *Delivering better care at the end of life: the next steps*, King's Fund, London, p.33.

126 Ellershaw J. (2010) Driving improvements in hospital. In: Addicott R, Ashton R. (eds.) *Delivering better care at the end of life: the next steps*, King's Fund, London, p.23.

127 Addicott R, Ashton R (eds.) (2010) *Delivering Better Care at the End of Life*, King's Fund, London, p.43.

128 Palliative Care Planning Group Wales (2008) *Report to the Minister for Health and Social Services*. Available at: www.wales.gov.uk (accessed 10 May 2011), p.13.

129 Palliative Care Strategy Implementation Board (2010) *Report to the Minister 2009–10*, Welsh Assembly Government, Cardiff.

130 Royal College of Paediatrics and Child Health (2004) *Withholding or Withdrawing Life Sustaining Treatment in Children: a framework for practice*, 2nd edn, RCPCH, London, p.38.

11: Euthanasia and physician assisted suicide

The questions covered in this chapter include the following:

- What is the law on different forms of assisted dying?
- What are the main ethical arguments about it?
- What is the BMA position on assisted dying?
- Can doctors give factual information about medication that might be used in a suicide?
- How should doctors respond to patients who ask for advice about going abroad for assisted dying?

The previous chapter discussed medical decision making as patients near the end of life. This chapter addresses different but related matters concerning the law, the ethical arguments and the policy of the British Medical Association (BMA) on euthanasia and assisted suicide. Doctors have a duty to try to provide patients with as peaceful and dignified a death as possible but the BMA considers it contrary to the doctor's role to hasten death deliberately or assist in a suicide, even at the patient's request. Current law prohibiting assisted dying is clear but debate within the profession and society about legalising it continues. This chapter looks at concepts of harm and benefit, autonomy and its limits. Consideration is given to the question of whether stepping beyond one legal boundary would lead inevitably to further steps (the 'slippery slope' argument) and whether permitting a previously forbidden action trivialises it or ultimately leads to it becoming routine.

All forms of assisted dying (defined below) are illegal in the UK but they remain a focus for heated discussion. The reasons are not hard to find. Commentators write eloquently about how people in western societies find it difficult 'to understand and pacify death'.[1] This trend is 'exacerbated by a widespread fear that modern medical death can strip a person of choice and dignity'.[2] Developing more opportunities for patient choice and control is seen by some people as an answer to such fears. Those who support the pre-eminence of patient choice may claim a right to use medical skills to bring about death prematurely, in hopes of avoiding pain or indignity. Many doctors find this approach counter-intuitive. The more closely they are involved with caring for dying people, the more likely doctors are to believe that there are other better options to minimise the risks of pain and indignity. (For doctors' views, see pages 467–469.)

Adults with capacity can refuse life-prolonging treatment, even when their decision will result in death (see Chapter 2, pages 75–77) and people who attempt suicide can also refuse resuscitation, if they have capacity (see Chapter 15, pages 630–633). However, they cannot receive active help to end their lives. Within a society where personal autonomy carries considerable weight, responses to the concept of assisted dying are often polarised. It highlights the tensions between respecting the autonomy of people who want to end their lives and ensuring that vulnerable people are not pressured to do the same.

Medical Ethics Today: The BMA's Handbook of Ethics and Law, Third Edition. Sophie Brannan, Eleanor Chrispin, Martin Davies, Veronica English, Rebecca Mussell, Julian Sheather and Ann Sommerville.
© 2012 BMA Medical Ethics Department. Published 2012 by Blackwell Publishing Ltd.

Assisted dying raises profound questions about society's values and the purpose of medicine. It stirs deeply held moral beliefs about the value of life and the qualities that make it valuable, the scope and limits of individual autonomy, and the balancing of benefit for one patient with the possibility of disadvantaging others.

General principles

The previous chapter established principles for good quality end of life care. In terms of requests for assisted dying, the BMA supports the following principles.

- Doctors should act within the law to help patients to achieve a good death.
- Patients should be able to control the dying process as much as possible and doctors need to listen to patients' views.
- Patient autonomy is an important principle but does not override other principles. A balance is essential.
- Individuals' personal choices should not be allowed to harm others.
- Intentionally causing premature death is prohibited and, in the BMA's view, does not fit with the ethos of medicine.
- Withdrawing or withholding treatment differs fundamentally from intentionally ending life.

In terms of other general principles, the BMA emphasises the importance of providing high quality care to all patients, without unfair discrimination. As it is not unlawful to commit suicide, the argument is sometimes made by advocates of assisted dying that it is discriminatory not to provide assistance for people who wish to kill themselves but are physically unable to do so. This was part of the argument made by Diane Pretty who took her case to the European Court of Human Rights (see pages 470–471). She had motor neurone disease which left her unable to end her own life when she wished. Her arguments were not accepted, however, and this is an area in which notions about perceived discrimination can be risky to patient groups who already experience some unfair discrimination in society. If it were accepted, for example, that people who lack the physical capacity to kill themselves should be assisted to die, it might be argued that it would be discriminatory not to extend that 'benefit' to people who lack the mental capacity to do the same thing. (See also the discussion of the 'slippery slope' on pages 479–483.)

Terms and definitions

Discussion about end of life care and assisted dying is often beset by definitional problems. In some opinion polls and surveys, for example, lawful withdrawal or withholding of treatment is conflated with euthanasia, as is palliative sedation at the end of life (see Chapter 10, pages 435–439). Patients' informed refusal of treatment, resuscitation or artificial feeding is sometimes seen as suicide. Many key concepts, such as that of 'intractable symptoms' in the dying patient remain undefined, giving rise to confusion. It remains difficult to find terminology that is clear and acceptable to everyone, for even some of the most fundamental concepts. Some find terms like 'assisted dying' over-euphemistic, for example, but 'killing' is also offensive to many. The BMA's understanding of the key terms is set out below.

Assisted dying is an overarching term to describe measures intentionally designed to terminate a person's life. It is normally applied to patients who voluntarily seek to end their lives and who have a terminal or degenerative condition. It includes euthanasia and physician assisted suicide but does not cover non-treatment decisions.

Euthanasia literally means a gentle or easy death. It is sometimes called 'mercy killing'. It describes deliberate steps by someone – usually a health professional – to end a patient's life. Legally, in the UK it is murder or manslaughter. Some ethicists say that the term should be reserved for the 'compassion-motivated, deliberate, rapid and painless termination of the life of someone afflicted with an incurable and progressive disease'.[3] In the 1990s, the House of Lords Select Committee on Medical Ethics adopted a similar definition, emphasising the intention behind the act, defining it as 'a deliberate intervention undertaken with the express intention of ending a life to relieve suffering'.[4] It is often proposed that – if legalised in the UK – it should only be available for patients with a terminal illness but elsewhere its use may be wider and involve patients whose suffering is unrelated to terminal illness (see pages 479–483). The term 'euthanasia' is sometimes qualified by the adjectives 'voluntary', 'non-voluntary' or 'involuntary'. Many advocates of euthanasia limit their support to the 'voluntary' category, where death is brought about at the patient's request. 'Non-voluntary euthanasia' describes the premature end of the life of a patient who does not have the mental capacity to request or consent to it. 'Involuntary' describes the euthanasia of a person who is capable of expressing a view but either refuses it or is not asked. All categories are prohibited in the UK. In the past, the qualifiers 'active' and 'passive' were also used. A positive intervention such as lethal injection, would be described as 'active euthanasia' and an omission to provide treatment was sometimes termed 'passive euthanasia'. There has long been agreement that these terms are misleading and should be avoided as they appear to equate completely ethical non-treatment with killing.

Assisted suicide and physician assisted suicide: it is not illegal for people to kill themselves nor to attempt suicide but helping or encouraging someone to do so is an offence in England, Wales and Northern Ireland. In Scotland, the law is less clear (see page 470). In England, Wales and Northern Ireland, an offence is committed if someone 'does an act capable of encouraging or assisting the suicide or attempted suicide of another person' if 'the act was intended to encourage or assist suicide or an attempt at suicide.'[5] The offence carries a penalty of up to 14 years' imprisonment and the offence can be committed regardless of whether the suicide or attempted suicide actually occurs. Assisting a suicide does not necessarily involve doctors but, when the subject is discussed, it is often envisaged that medical participation would be part of the process by, for example, determining the patient's prognosis, certifying the individual's mental capacity and providing a prescription for lethal drugs. Some jurisdictions that have formally legalised it, such as Oregon, give doctors such a role. Some people argue that the process of assisted suicide – where legal – should not involve doctors at all. (See pages 478–479 on the doctor–patient relationship.) Assisted suicide differs from euthanasia in that the patient is required to undertake the final act. It has been said that putting fatal drugs into a patient's hand may be morally preferable, because more likely to be voluntary, but less certain than euthanasia, which involves putting fatal drugs into a patient's arm.[6] The person who 'assists' provides the means or encouragement for the individual to end his or her own life. In some jurisdictions, a doctor might provide equipment, advice or drugs but need not, or may not be allowed to be, present at the death. The line between assisted suicide and euthanasia can be blurred when the patient is physically unable to begin, or to complete the steps to end life. For example, a person might be unable to swallow a lethal concoction or might vomit after taking it. Further assistance may be required which may then turn the situation into one of euthanasia.

Continuous deep sedation: as discussed in Chapter 10, 'palliative' or deep sedation may be offered to patients who are very close to death and experience distressing symptoms which cannot be effectively controlled by other measures. Continuous sedation when patients are not expected to die imminently has been perceived as 'slow euthanasia'.[7] Whether it would be ethical and lawful to use deep sedation depends on the doctor's intention and the context, including whether all feasible alternatives have been exhausted and the patient's symptoms are clearly refractory. (This is discussed in detail in Chapter 10, pages 435–439.) A reason for particular concern about the use of deep sedation in the Netherlands was that an increase in its use appeared to accompany a decline in euthanasia up to 2005. Continuous deep sedation can be used in the Netherlands for patients whose life expectancy is 2 weeks or less. A Dutch study[8] in 2008 reported that 1,200 fewer patients died as a result of euthanasia but 1,800 more died following deep sedation in 2005 than in 2001. This gave rise to speculation that continuous deep sedation, with few bureaucratic requirements, might have been seen by doctors as an alternative to euthanasia. Some of the sedated patients had previously requested euthanasia but failed to meet the legal criteria. The cause of this trend was never fully understood and 'meaningful interpretation of these findings is impeded not only by the legality and acceptance of euthanasia in the Netherlands, but more so by a persistent deficit of clearly defined taxonomy...the term "continuous deep sedation" is not precise enough to discern the reasoning and motives of clinicians needed to support relevant ethical analyses.'[9] A report of the Dutch Review Committee subsequently found that sedation was used less than originally thought.[10] Nevertheless, some concerns about the use of continuous deep sedation remain. Euthanasia and continuous deep sedation address different clinical problems[11] and if undertaken with the intention of hastening death, continuous or deep sedation would be unacceptable.

Withholding or withdrawing life-prolonging treatment is fundamentally different from assisted dying. Doctors must withhold or withdraw treatment when a patient with capacity refuses it or when a patient who lacks capacity has made a valid advance decision to refuse it. Nor can doctors give treatment that is futile in that it cannot achieve its aim or cannot provide a 'benefit' to the patient (see Chapter 10, pages 440–447). It may be predictable that the patient will die as a result but ending the person's life is not the doctor's intention. The overriding objective is to ensure that treatment that is not in the best interests of the patient is not given. In the past, it was sometimes argued that withholding life-prolonging treatment was similar to taking active steps to end life. Now, few believe that doctors must strive to prolong life at all costs, with no regard to the benefits or burdens to the patient.

Double effect: in 2009, a survey of UK doctors' views indicated that they 'may take decisions which they expect to contribute to the ending of life since they may take the view that an action is acceptable where the primary aim is to relieve the suffering of a person close to death'.[12] This reflects the principle of 'double effect' which allows doctors to provide medical treatment that has both bad and good effects, as long as the primary intention is to provide an overall good effect. While drugs such as morphine do not necessarily contribute to the hastening of death,[13] a commonly quoted example of double effect is the use of such pain relief which may risk shortening a patient's life. In order for the administration of drugs that might hasten death to be lawful:

- the patient must be terminally ill or dying
- the intervention must be in that person's best interests
- it must be a treatment accepted as reasonable and proper within the medical profession
- the motivation must be to relieve the patient's suffering.

If doctors were to continue to increase the dosage of such medication once the patient's symptoms were under control, the principle of double effect would not be engaged and the action may be seen as euthanasia.

Intention and motivation of doctors are crucial considerations in this debate. A person who deliberately acts to shorten another's life and fully intends that person's death satisfies the criminal law requirement of intention and commits a serious offence. Knowingly providing advice to help people kill themselves, or attempt to do so, may be an offence but whether it results in prosecution depends on the actual circumstances of the case. Guidelines issued in 2010 by the Director of Public Prosecutions (see pages 473–474) make clear that motive (combined with the prohibited action) plays a part in whether or not prosecution is seen as being in the public interest. Encouraging a vulnerable person to commit suicide for one's own personal gain would clearly be in a different moral category to acting solely out of compassion, although both are illegal. Our general guidance throughout this book is that doctors should be open and honest with their patients but caution is required if the doctor is asked for advice or information that will assist patients to kill themselves or kill someone else.

On the other hand, if the doctor's intention is to cease a futile medical treatment, it is legally and ethically acceptable to withdraw it, even if death is foreseeable as a result (see Chapter 10, pages 440–447). Even in cases where the intention is illegally to bring about a premature death, the individual's motive can have a mitigating or exacerbating effect. For example, the Criminal Justice Act 2003 recognises among other potentially mitigating factors in terms of the prison sentence given, a 'belief by [the] offender that the murder was an act of mercy'.[14]

Slippery slope is the metaphor often invoked in debates about assisted dying to describe situations in which one action might possibly be seen as permissible but would lead to undesirable consequences. Once an accepted boundary is breached, the argument goes, there will be no way of preventing a slide down the slippery slope to the breaching of other standards. There has been much debate about the usefulness or otherwise of the metaphor. Its utility depends on factors such as whether we believe society would be able to make limited changes while retaining crucial boundaries, whether it is possible to measure and limit the changes made, and the degree to which a wholesale change in standards is seen as undesirable. It might have been argued in the past, for example, that extending the franchise to all adult males rather than restricting it to the wealthy was a slippery slope leading to servants and women being able to vote. Before embarking on any major change, it is clearly important for society to assess the potential ramifications, including 'whether there really is a slippery slope, and how slippery in reality it is and whether clear points of arrest in the slide exist'.[15] In relation to euthanasia, it is often argued that a move towards acceptance of voluntary euthanasia would lead to the practice being extended to people who had not chosen it. As the first jurisdiction to openly accept assisted dying, the Netherlands is sometimes portrayed as an example of the slippery slope (see pages 480–482).

Public and professional views on assisted dying

Surveys of doctors' views

A blurring of terms has sometimes made it difficult to assess doctors' views in detail although broad trends opposing assisted dying appear to emerge consistently. In 2005, the House of Lords debated the Assisted Dying for the Terminally Ill Bill (also known as the

'Joffe' Bill). The detailed discussion and evidence taking generated much public and professional reflection. Among other matters, the Lords' Select Committee on the Bill noted the varying quality and scope of opinion polls involving doctors and agreed that 'most research is superficial in coverage and only a few attempts have been made to understand the basis of the opinions of doctors'.[16] While this view may limit people's confidence in the opinion polls, they cannot be dismissed entirely. The Lords' Committee also recognised that doctors appeared to be significantly less in favour of any legal change than the lay public and 'the closer the experience of end-of-life patients, the less sure professionals are about the prospect of a change in the law in favour of euthanasia'.[17] The same view was later echoed by a wide survey in 2009.[18] Despite differences in questions producing variability in results, repeated investigations show that doctors' organisations and most UK doctors appear to be opposed to the legalisation of euthanasia and physician assisted suicide. Their views tend to differ markedly from those expressed by the general population. Opposition to assisted dying is particularly strong among palliative care specialists and geriatricians; that is to say, in the specialities in which doctors have more contact with dying people.[19] Patients dying from cancer in hospices and palliative care units have been seen as particularly likely to make requests for an assisted death but some 'changed their minds in response to care provided, a pattern which is consistent with the view that care in such settings aims to address the fears that lie behind such requests'.[20]

Despite the difficulties in obtaining reliable data about illegal practices, other information obtained through anonymised surveys of doctors indicates that there is unlikely to be a significant level of clandestine assisted dying in the UK. The available evidence appears to indicate that the law is rarely broken and instances of physician assisted suicide or euthanasia are very low.[21] This was also the conclusion of the House of Lords Select Committee on Medical Ethics in 2005.[22]

Public views

The report of the Select Committee on the Assisted Dying for the Terminally Ill Bill[23] also contained a review of public opinion polls, concluding that such surveys generally produce 'one-dimensional' findings. It cautioned Parliament about how to weigh such information. Periodic surveys of social attitudes were seen by the Committee as unsuitable for complex questions about euthanasia, where public understanding of the implications of legislation could not be assumed. Despite the fact that it perceived such surveys as being of limited value, the report acknowledged that there was a significant level of sympathy in society for the concept of assisting sick people who want to end their lives.

Much emphasis is still put on public opinion polls despite the reservations about them expressed by the House of Lords. Since at least the mid-1990s, such polls show that a majority of the public think that patients with an incurable, painful disease should have the right to ask a doctor to end their life. Although such findings can partly depend on the wording of questions and the options offered, the evidence of public support for assisted dying appears consistent. Among doctors, and especially those working with the terminally ill, there has been concern that advocates of assisted dying often lack information about the alternatives or that they 'do not recognise adequately the clinical realities of managing serious illness and disability'.[24] At its annual meeting in 2010, the BMA called for better information to be available to the public about what can be achieved by good palliative care. Not all patients may want it but they should at least know the choices available. The BMA also called for better training in palliative medicine for all doctors involved with the care of dying patients so that high quality management could be better ensured.

Individual tragic cases continue to be influential in affecting public opinion. In December 2008, for example, following a controversial TV broadcast of the assisted suicide of a patient called Craig Ewert, a survey found that most people asked thought that relatives who take terminally ill people abroad for assisted suicide should not be prosecuted.[25]

BMA policy

The BMA first debated this issue in 1950 when it rejected the idea of euthanasia. Policy reinforcing that view was established in 1969, when the annual representatives meeting declared that doctors' fundamental objectives must be the relief of suffering and preservation of life. While such early policy statements categorically rejected euthanasia, later ones continued to do so but also acknowledged the existence of a wide spectrum of views within the membership. They also ceased to see preservation of life at all costs as the objective. Attention gradually turned from euthanasia carried out by doctors to assisted suicide where patients carried out the final act themselves. At the BMA annual representatives meeting in 2005, there was heated debate about this and a vote on three options: (a) to reaffirm the BMA's traditional opposition to all forms of assisted dying; (b) to withdraw opposition to assisted dying, recognising the law is primarily a matter for society and for Parliament but to press for robust safeguards if legal change occurred; (c) to support a system that allowed terminally ill patients with capacity to receive assisted dying within robust safeguards. The meeting voted by a narrow margin in favour of option (b). As had been made clear, 'assisted dying' in this context included both voluntary euthanasia and physician assisted suicide. Therefore the BMA became briefly neutral on both of these issues.

In the following year the BMA again discussed its policy on assisted dying and reversed the neutral policy of the previous year. It established the current policy which focuses on improvements in palliative care to allow patients to die with dignity and opposes all forms of assisted dying. Accordingly, since 2006, the BMA has lobbied against any proposals for legal change on assisted suicide or euthanasia.

The law

England and Wales

Taking another person's life may be murder or manslaughter, which are serious criminal offences. Acting in self-defence is an exception to the law but no exception is made for killing people at their request. So euthanasia is covered by the law on homicide.

Encouraging or assisting a person to commit suicide is covered in England and Wales by the Suicide Act 1961, as amended by the Coroners and Justice Act 2009, which makes assisting suicide an offence, punishable by up to 14 years' imprisonment. Section 2(1) of the Suicide Act made it an offence to aid, abet, counsel or procure the suicide or attempted suicide of another person (the substantive offence) but did not cover someone unsuccessfully trying to persuade a person to commit suicide. So, in the past, it had to be read in combination with section 1 of the Criminal Attempts Act 1981 which made it an offence *to attempt* the same things (the attempted offence). In 2009, Parliament amended the Suicide Act in the Coroners and Justice Act which covers England, Wales and Northern Ireland. The amended legislation replaced the substantive and attempt offences in the two Acts with a single offence expressed in terms of 'encouraging or assisting' the suicide or attempted suicide of another person.

At the same time, there was considerable debate about what constituted 'assisting' a suicide. In the 1980s, the High Court had considered whether advice published by the Voluntary Euthanasia Society breached the law.[26] It identified three criteria for an offence: that the accused knew that the individual was considering suicide, agreed to it and encouraged the suicide attempt. Concern later grew about whether the law was adequate to deal with encouragement or information sharing about suicide over the internet. The Coroners and Justice Act 2009 addressed this, making clear that a person providing information services about how to kill oneself potentially commits an offence even if it is not read by anyone known to the author.[27] In many cases, the intention to provoke suicide is enough but whether or not a prosecution is brought depends on the evidence and whether it would be in the public interest to prosecute.

Northern Ireland

Euthanasia is also illegal and a similar law to the Suicide Act applies in Northern Ireland. Assisting suicide has been a criminal offence there since the Criminal Justice (Northern Ireland) Act 1966. This also set a penalty of up to 14 years' imprisonment and was amended to match the law in England and Wales by section 60 of the Coroners and Justice Act 2009.

Scotland

In Scotland, homicide law covers euthanasia but there is some uncertainty about assisted suicide, as there is no specific law to match England's Suicide Act. In theory, someone who assists another person to kill him or herself could be prosecuted under homicide law.

Attempts to change the law

There have been various attempts to change the law, both via the courts and through Parliament. The Pretty case in 2001 was a key example.

Diane Pretty case

Diane Pretty sought to persuade the domestic and European courts of her entitlement to assisted dying by reference to the Human Rights Act 1998 and the European Convention on Human Rights. She had motor neurone disease, a progressive and degenerative illness, and knew that she was likely to die from respiratory failure. She feared her death would be frightening and distressing but she was unable to take her own life. Her husband was willing to help her commit suicide which would risk him being prosecuted under the Suicide Act 1961. Mrs Pretty tried, but failed, to obtain an undertaking from the Director of Public Prosecutions (DPP) that her husband would not be prosecuted and so she sought judicial review of the DPP's decision. In the House of Lords, Lord Steyn said that to succeed in her argument, Mrs Pretty would have had to persuade the House that the European Convention on Human Rights compelled member states to legalise assisted suicide.[28] The Lords found that there had been no *prima facie* violations of her rights.

Mrs Pretty took her case to the European Court of Human Rights. She claimed that the right to life (Article 2 of the European Convention on Human Rights) gave the right to choose whether or not to live, that failure to guarantee this right breached her right to be free from inhuman or degrading treatment (Article 3) and that the state was interfering with her private life (contrary to Article 8).

> The European Court was not persuaded that Article 2 conferred a right to die and said that it would be a distortion of language to interpret it so. Article 3 was primarily seen as imposing a duty on states to refrain from inflicting harm or suffering – a negative duty not a positive obligation to act. 'The suffering which flows from naturally occurring illness may be covered by Article 3, where it is exacerbated by treatment … for which the authorities can be held responsible' but in this case, the Government had not imposed treatment on her.[29]
>
> Under Article 8, people have the right to conduct their life in a manner of their own choosing. The Court recognised that in the face of growing technological sophistication in medicine, some patients would choose not to have their lives prolonged by it but that in Mrs Pretty's case, she was 'prevented by law from exercising her choice to avoid what she considers will be an undignified and distressing end to her life'.[30] The European Court was not prepared to exclude the possibility that this interfered with her right to respect for her private life. Nevertheless, the European Court concluded that the UK's blanket ban on assisted suicide was not disproportionate. Her claim was rejected in April 2002 and she died 12 days later.

Despite public interest in the possibility of doctors intervening to end life, there seems little indication that lawmakers welcome that debate. Attempts at legal change through the English and Scottish Parliaments have, so far, failed to progress and anxieties associated with the possibility of undermining the law of homicide are often part of the reasoning. This has been a continuous line of argument since at least the mid-1990s when an earlier House of Lords Select Committee on Medical Ethics agreed that, although it had heard moving evidence about deaths that were not peaceful nor uplifting, the arguments were insufficient to weaken society's prohibition of intentional killing. It saw the prohibition as the cornerstone of law and of social relationships.[31]

England and Wales

Among failed attempts in England to change the law on assisted dying was the Assisted Dying for the Terminally Ill Bill. It sought to allow adults with capacity who are suffering as a result of a terminal illness to receive medical assistance to die following a considered and persistent request from the individual suffering, and to make provision for a person suffering from a terminal illness to receive pain relief medication. The final report of the Select Committee on the Bill was published in April 2005.[32] It summarised the current law, the principles underlying the Bill, legislation in other countries and suggested amendments for a future Bill. Other points made included the following.

- Given the caveat about surveys, evidence exists for growing public sympathy for physician assisted suicide (PAS) for those who request it.
- Patient autonomy has limits but agreement is lacking on where the limits should be drawn.
- If autonomy is the key, there are arguments for not restricting assisted suicide to terminally ill people, especially given problems defining terminal illness.
- Attitudes of disabled people to the Bill appeared mixed. A few indicated support while others feared that it would make it harder for the disabled to access high quality care or that prejudice might pressure them to end their lives.
- Doctors tend to see the legalisation of euthanasia as less straightforward than the public. Although some support it, the majority appear opposed to any legal change. Those who would accept change would apparently be more likely to accept a move towards PAS than towards euthanasia.

- Covert euthanasia may exist but hard evidence is lacking and current structures make it unlikely that it occurs on the scale that some surveys suggest.
- If future legislation permits PAS, doctors need not necessarily be involved because assessing patients and prescribing could be sourced outside clinical services.
- Private medical practices specialising in PAS in future should be discouraged.
- If they are involved, doctors with a conscientious objection should not be obliged to refer patients on. It is the patient's responsibility to find a doctor without an objection.
- Palliative care is of high quality but inadequately resourced and unevenly spread in the UK and some doctors already fear prosecution if they provide adequate pain relief.
- Some patients – especially with degenerative diseases – suffer intractable distress despite palliative medicine.

In 2010, a Commission on Assisted Dying was hosted by the think tank Demos to promote debate on this issue. Its remit was to 'independently investigate whether there are circumstances in which it should be possible for people to be assisted to die, and whether the legal status quo is adequate, or whether any changes in the law are required'.[33] In the Commission's view, there was a need to address the topic at that time because 'the legal and ethical status of assisted dying in our society continues to be an unresolved public policy issue'.[34] It published a briefing on the legal, ethical and practical considerations for assisted dying legislation and invited responses. The BMA made clear its opposition to legal change.

Scotland

In 2004, Liberal Democrat MSP, Jeremy Purvis publicised a Bill to legalise 'mercy killing', based on the Oregon physician assisted suicide legislation (see pages 484–485). At the consultation stage, the Bill seemed to have public support (56 per cent of respondents in favour and 33 per cent opposed) but it failed to get the required number of supporting signatures from MSPs to be introduced into the Scottish Parliament. In 2009, Margo MacDonald MSP consulted on her proposed End of Life Choices Bill relating to the assistance that can be given to someone who wishes to die. She proposed that doctors should not be guilty of an illegal act if they fulfil certain conditions in helping patients to die. Over 400 responses were submitted to the consultation and, in its reply, the BMA stated its policy opposing physician assisted suicide and euthanasia. In December 2010, the End of Life Assistance (Scotland) Bill was rejected after the Stage 1 debate. The vote was 85 against, 16 for, with 2 abstentions.

What currently counts as 'assisting suicide'?

Doctors are aware that assisted dying is illegal but it may sometimes seem unclear where the exact boundaries lie. Handing somebody a cup containing a lethal cocktail of drugs is clearly assisting suicide but doctors may also need to ask questions in more apparently innocuous situations, for example, if patients request multiple repeat prescriptions for potentially lethal drugs. Clearly, some may need a large supply of their medication because they will be travelling away from home but, in cases where the doctor suspects an intention to self-harm, a request for a potentially fatal amount needs prior discussion with the patient.

Some criteria were established in the 1980s, when the courts[35] examined *A guide to self-deliverance* published by the Voluntary Euthanasia Society (VES, now called Dignity in Dying). The VES said that the fear of death often conflated two separate anxieties: fear of the state of non-existence and fear of the process of dying. Its booklet aimed to overcome the second of these. The court found that the booklet provided information which might deter some would-be suicides but could assist others to kill themselves so circumstances might arise in which supplying it would amount to an offence. Without proof of the necessary intent, however, it could not be said in advance of any particular case that supplying the booklet would necessarily be an offence.

Prior to 2009, relatives of terminally ill people had long been unclear whether accompanying a patient to Switzerland for assisted dying would result in prosecution. One of the early highly publicised cases occurred in 2002, when Reginald Crew died in Switzerland after using barbiturates supplied by the right to die organisation Dignitas. He had motor neurone disease and was accompanied by his wife and a television crew. Merseyside police investigated his death and concluded that there was insufficient evidence of an offence to pursue a prosecution under section 2(1) of the Suicide Act 1961.[36] By 2009, well over a hundred more British people were known to have died in Dignitas clinics. Some relatives who had accompanied patients were questioned by police on their return to the UK but charges were not brought, as the Director of Public Prosecutions (DPP) considered that, in the cases he examined, it would not be in the public interest. This did not remove the risks for subsequent accompanying relatives, as was highlighted by the case of Debbie Purdy.

Debbie Purdy case

Debbie Purdy had been diagnosed with multiple sclerosis in 1995 and she wanted reassurance from the courts that if her husband travelled with her to Switzerland, he would not be charged with having assisted her suicide. She argued that the DPP had illegally failed to provide guidance on whether travelling abroad with a patient in these circumstances breached UK law. In the court of first instance, the judge concluded that the existing guidelines were adequate and that relatives could not be given any guarantees that they would be safe from prosecution. This view was later reiterated by the Appeal Court which said that only Parliament could amend the law.

In July 2009, during the Lords Committee Stage of the Coroners and Justice Bill, Lord Falconer tabled an amendment, which was defeated, seeking to grant legal immunity to relatives who accompany patients to a country where assisted suicide is legal. In July, Debbie Purdy's case also reached the Law Lords who ruled that the DPP must produce clear, offence-specific guidelines on the circumstances in which a prosecution would be brought against those who help friends or relatives travel abroad for assisted suicide. The Law Lords reiterated that any change to the criminal law against aiding and abetting suicide remained a political matter for Parliament. They held that the right to respect for a private life, and the associated right to autonomy, was potentially infringed by the absence of a transparent policy covering those who need help to travel abroad for assisted dying. They agreed that Ms Purdy's right to respect for her private life included the right to clarity regarding the exercise of the DPP's discretion as to whether or not to prosecute.[37]

In February 2010, the DPP[38] produced a policy applicable to all acts of assisted suicide in England and Wales and the Northern Ireland DPP did the same. This set out the factors to be taken into account by prosecutors deciding whether to bring a case against a suspect accused of assisting a suicide. Prior to issuing the final policy, the DPP warned health professionals that they need to be particularly cautious and not take the new guidance lightly. He said that doctors needed to be very, very careful as there are 'a number of factors . . . that would indicate that they are more likely to be prosecuted than, say, family members'.[39]

Policy for prosecutors in respect of cases of encouraging or assisting suicide[40]

- Euthanasia remains murder or manslaughter. If someone causes the death of a person who has tried to commit suicide but fails and is only unconscious, causing their death believing it to be the express wish of the unconscious person is murder or manslaughter.
- Encouraging or assisting suicide remains a criminal offence with a penalty of up to 14 years' imprisonment.
- Whether or not a prosecution is brought depends on the evidence and the public interest.

Evidential stage

- Prosecutors first need to consider if there is evidence for successful prosecution. Any case that does not pass the evidential stage cannot proceed.
- The prosecution must prove the suspect carried out an act capable of encouraging or assisting a suicide or attempted suicide and the act was intended to assist a suicide or an attempted suicide.
- A person who arranges for someone else to do such an act is also liable.
- An offence may be committed even if the suicide attempt does not actually occur or could not occur – for example, if the suspect supplies harmless drugs believing them to be lethal.
- The suspect need not know or ever be able to identify the person who commits or attempts suicide.
- Websites that promote suicide may commit an offence if that is the intention behind them.
- Explaining the law on assisted suicide is not an offence.

Public interest stage

Each case is assessed on its merits. A number of factors have to be taken into consideration but it is not a matter of adding up the factors for or against prosecution: one factor may weigh more than many others in the decision. The factors set out by the DPP are not an exhaustive list.

Prosecution is more likely in the public interest when:

- the victim was under 18 or lacked mental capacity or had not reached a settled decision to commit suicide or did not initiate the idea of suicide
- the victim was physically able to commit suicide unaided
- the suspect would gain or benefit from the death or tried to influence or pressure the victim to die or had a history of violence or abuse against the victim
- the suspect was unknown to the victim and provided specific information via a website or publication, or if the suspect encouraged more than one victim or was paid by the victim or by people close to the victim to give encouragement or assistance
- the suspect was acting as a healthcare professional or person in authority, such as a prison officer and the victim was in his or her care
- the suspect was aware that the victim intended to commit suicide in a public place where members of the public might be present
- the suspect was acting as manager or employee of an organisation or group that specifically provides an environment in which people can commit suicide.

Prosecution is less likely in the public interest when:

- the victim had a clear settled wish or initiated the idea of suicide, had a terminal illness or disability or degenerative condition
- the victim needed help and was unable to act alone, or if the victim had attempted suicide before
- the suspect was motivated by compassion, had sought to dissuade the victim or if the suspect's actions were of only minor encouragement or assistance
- the suspect only helped reluctantly and reported the matter to the police and assisted them in their enquiries.

Case of Dr Wilson

In August 2010, the Crown Prosecution Service (CPS) announced that it would not bring prosecutions against three people arrested in relation to the suicide, in June 2009, of Caroline Loder, who had a neurological disorder. Dr Libby Wilson, a retired GP and co-founder of pro-euthanasia group Friends at the End (Fate), was the first person in the UK to be arrested after the new policy on assisted suicide was published early in 2010. Along with two men, Dr Wilson was questioned on suspicion of aiding, abetting, counselling or procuring a suicide. The patient, who had never met Dr Wilson, telephoned her twice and, having made a previous botched suicide attempt, asked for information from Dr Wilson about how to kill herself successfully on her next attempt. The CPS said there was insufficient evidence to prosecute one of the men, and it was deemed not to be 'in the public interest' to proceed against the other or against Dr Wilson, whose assistance was judged to have been minimal. Dr Wilson complained about the length of time it had taken the CPS to reach a decision and the fact that much still depended on how the word 'assist' was interpreted. She claimed that the patient had been determined to commit suicide and she had merely provided information, to which she thought the patient had a right.[41]

When doctors know or suspect that a patient or a patient's family intends to carry out assisted dying, they should investigate whether counselling or practical support could improve the patient's quality of life. The benefits of respite care and good palliative care should also be discussed if the patient is willing to consider those options. Doctors should avoid actions that might be interpreted as encouraging an attempt at suicide or assisted dying. This means not giving specific advice on what constitutes a fatal dose or on anti-emetics in relation to a possible planned overdose, not suggesting the option of suicide abroad nor writing medical reports specifically to facilitate assisted dying abroad, nor on any other aspects of planning a suicide. In many cases, however, doctors are unaware of the patient's intention. All patients have a statutory right to copies of their medical records (see Chapter 6, pages 255–258) and, even if they plan to travel abroad for assisted suicide, they need not give an explanation of what they intend to do with the information.

If a patient is depressed or suffering from a mental disturbance, therapy and counselling should be recommended. Patients who are terminally ill or feel that their quality of life is irretrievably low present a dilemma. Doctors should listen to patients who ask for assistance to commit suicide, and give them control of their decision making as far as possible.

Prescribing or supplying drugs with the intention of enabling patients to shorten their lives could lead to prosecution and, despite the example of the case of Dr Wilson, so could the provision of advice or literature on the subject. During debate on the Coroners and Justice Bill (as it then was) in 2009, Parliament also made explicit that an offence occurs when individuals disseminate information via media, such as the internet, which would be likely to encourage other people to end their lives. Putting people in touch with someone who will help them to end their life is also likely to be an offence. Doctors have to be honest with patients and explain that they will not act illegally but will do all they can to provide the care and support they need at the end of their lives.

Summary – the law

- UK law currently forbids assisted dying but some uncertainty can exist as to what actually constitutes 'assistance'.
- Prosecutors look at cases on an individual basis, bearing in mind a set of predefined factors.

- Doctors should make patients approaching the end of life aware of the potential benefits of well managed palliative care.
- Doctors who suspect that a patient or that person's relatives intend to carry out assisted dying need to try to discourage that attempt. They should explore whether additional support could be provided to improve the patient's quality of life.

Moral, legal and pragmatic arguments

The key principle underpinning the BMA's views on assisted dying is that it is unacceptable for individuals' choices to impinge pejoratively on others. Many doctors also believe it to be quite contrary to the ethos of medicine. Cases arise in which some people consider that assisted dying would be right for a patient but there is a risk that removing the traditional ban on intentional killing would have detrimental effects on perceptions of medical practice and the doctor–patient relationship. The strong consensus within the BMA is in favour of not changing the law but it is acknowledged that BMA members hold a spectrum of opinions on this issue.

Arguments for and against assisted dying

Ending a human life is a profound and disturbing concept. The large and scholarly literature on assisted dying reflects the attempts to marshal the arguments on either side and draw firm boundaries. Set out below is a brief summary and then a more detailed discussion of the key aspects that the BMA has debated.

Arguments in support of assisted dying

- Arguments for assisted dying are rights based, consequentialist and deontological. In terms of rights and consequences, assisted dying would allow some patients to achieve their aim of controlling their death and avoiding a situation which they fear will involve suffering or indignity. The main argument in favour of assisted dying focuses on this concept of patients' rights to choose.
- In terms of deontology, doctors have duties to respect patient choice and minimise suffering. They have special duties to their patients and cannot abandon patients who have unbearable pain.
- Human rights also provide a similar focus on individual entitlements.
- Quality of life is often portrayed as being more important than the patient's length of life and issues around sanctity of life.
- Opinion polls appear to show that the public support assisted dying being available in some cases.
- Both sides of the argument raise questions about the kind of society we want and whether respect for choices and compassion for suffering should overrule other considerations.

Arguments opposing assisted dying

- Arguments against assisted dying are also consequentialist and deontological. The consequentialist argument is that permitting assisted dying for some would put large numbers of other people at risk of harm.

- The deontological argument is that this would be contrary to the ethics of clinical practice. The purpose of medicine is perceived as being to improve patients' quality of life and the opposite of trying to foreshorten it.
- The issue of sanctity of life is sometimes raised as a cogent reason against assisted dying (although many opponents of assisted dying do not subscribe to the notion that life must be preserved at all costs, regardless of its quality).
- It would weaken society's prohibition on killing and undermine the safeguards against non-voluntary euthanasia. Society would embark on a 'slippery slope' with undesirable consequences.
- Effective and high quality palliative care can effectively alleviate distressing symptoms associated with the dying process and allay patients' fears.
- Only a minority of people want to end their lives. The rules for the majority should not be changed to accommodate a small group.
- Both sides of the argument raise questions about the kind of society we want and whether concern for the vulnerable and respect for life should count for more than individual autonomy.

Autonomy, human rights and the impact on others

Supporters on both sides of the debate about assisted dying have framed their arguments in terms of rights, not least due to the 'powerful political impact of rights-based arguments'.[42] Some of the strongest arguments for assisted dying are based on autonomy, empowerment, self-determination and the individual's human rights. People increasingly expect to exercise control over crucial aspects of their life and over matters that affect them, as long as they do not harm others. The counter-argument is that personal autonomy has limits even though, as the House of Lords noted, we do not all agree where those limits lie.[43] The crucial question is whether, in practice, allowing some people to choose death would be likely to harm others. If we are unsure but suspect that it might do so, then society needs to be cautious. The rights of one person or one group cannot be permitted to undermine disproportionately the rights of others.

Human rights arguments follow a similar pattern to the autonomy argument. Rights-based arguments in support of assisted dying turn on concepts such as the right to liberty, privacy, equality (if the patient needs help and cannot commit suicide as able-bodied people could do) and freedom of conscience.[44] Rights-based arguments against it feature the right to life and also the right to equality. This latter argument focuses on the impact legalisation might have on already marginalised or vulnerable groups. The limitations of trying to argue a human rights case in favour of assisted dying was illustrated by the case of Diane Pretty (see pages 470–471).

By limiting personal autonomy, society hopes to avoid a greater harm but opinion varies as to how serious the risks of that harm are. It is sometimes argued that a change in legislation would change society's attitudes. Old or disabled people might be seen as burdensome and put under pressure to end their lives. Legal safeguards designed to ensure the voluntary nature of assisted dying could fail to detect self-imposed pressure or subtle emotional coercion from relatives. Of patients who made use of Oregon's Death with Dignity Act 1994 during its first 5 years, 44 per cent cited their fear of being a burden to their family, friends and carers as part of their reasoning for wanting to end their life.[45] Some people might not see this as problematic as many of the choices we make in life are predicated upon doing the best we can for our children and friends. Nevertheless, issues of life and death are arguably in a different category from most other decisions and it would be an undesirable outcome if allowing assisted dying generated a perception that some lives are worth less.

If some people in the population came to be seen as less valuable, individuals might fear that a premature death would be selected for them. In the debates before the brief legalisation of euthanasia and PAS in Australia's Northern Territory, there was evidence of disquiet from the indigenous Aboriginal population. The Australian Select Committee on Euthanasia reported that some Aborigines were afraid to attend health clinics and hospitals for fear of doctors having 'the power to kill'.[46] In the early years of euthanasia being tolerated in the Netherlands, it was also alleged that some older people feared their lives would be ended without their consent.[47] This is more likely to be a suspicion among patient groups who already feel marginalised within the system of healthcare provision.

The doctor–patient relationship

As with many other aspects of the arguments around assisted dying, the need to preserve the integrity, and mutual trust, of the doctor–patient relationship is quoted by both sides of the debate. The BMA's position is that the special relationship between doctors and their patients risks being undermined, and trust lost, if doctors are permitted to end patients' lives. Although society relies on the integrity of the medical profession, Callahan argues that giving any group the power deliberately to take life is based on a dangerous illusion. The result, he says, will be the greater medicalisation of human experience. He predicts that allowing doctors to provide assisted dying will not solve 'the problem of an intolerable death, it simply treats the symptoms, while reinforcing and driving us more deeply into, an ideology of control'.[48]

However, others have argued that providing assisted dying could be a natural extension of the medical profession's role as relievers of suffering, especially when the doctor and patient have had a long relationship. It has been argued that doctors owe special duties to terminally ill patients and that 'the love and care one harbours for a particular dying person may impel one to intervene and hasten death. Care for another may make it morally impossible to simply step aside and watch a protracted illness run a painful course.'[49] For a minority of patients, pain relief technology cannot keep them comfortable other than by rendering them unconscious. If they consider such life meaningless without any prospect of recovery, they may prefer not to be kept alive. In 1991, Quill described[50] how he had helped one of his patients to end her life with barbiturates. She suffered from acute myelomonocytic leukaemia and believed that the treatment which offered a chance of survival would involve intolerable suffering. Quill provided the fatal drugs and argued that accompanying – and if necessary – assisting such patients to their death was a facet of his duty. He wrote about the need to offer partnership and non-abandonment to the dying in 'a bond of personal commitment and connection which supplements the more professional requirements of the doctor–patient relationship'.[51]

It is sometimes argued that the doctor's duty of compassion should permit assisted dying for people who fear they may suffer. This was part of the rationale in the Netherlands where it was argued that doctors faced a conflict of duties: the duty to obey the law and the obligation to alleviate unbearable and hopeless suffering. Crucial to the legal acceptance of assisted dying in the Netherlands was the argument that some patients found their suffering unbearable but, for the doctor, there was no reasonable alternative to relieve that suffering other than by ending the patient's life. The duty to the patient and the absence of an alternative triggered the defence of 'necessity' for doctors who provided assisted dying.[52] The Dutch law turned more on the concept of doctors' duties rather than patients' rights. (See also below on 'slippery slope' arguments.) The BMA, however, sees doctors' duties in a different light, as part of a continuing obligation to try to help patients achieve their own goals within a widely accepted moral framework that protects the weak as well as articulate autonomous patients.

Patients have various motives for considering ending their lives. Anxiety about possible future suffering is not the only motive. Of those who sought a lethal prescription in the first 5 years of Oregon's Death with Dignity Act, fear of inadequate pain control was a factor for only 22 per cent.[53] More relevant issues for some patients was the fear of being a burden on family or friends, losing their autonomy, having less ability to participate in activities that make life enjoyable and losing control of bodily functions. Skilled and compassionate palliative care, with good communication and patient involvement, can help with these issues. There will always be people, however, for whom palliative care does not meet their needs and wishes, for example those who believe that they have a right to choose when to die. Requests for euthanasia and PAS are therefore unlikely to be eliminated entirely.

Because doctors may legally withdraw life-sustaining treatment in certain circumstances (see Chapter 10, pages 440–447), some question why they should not go further. The BMA argues that this is not fundamentally about whether there is a difference between commission and omission – killing and letting die – but it is rather about the intention behind the doctor's actions. When treatment is withheld or withdrawn, the intention is not to kill but to refrain from providing an intervention that cannot benefit the patient. If doctors are authorised to kill deliberately or to help to kill, however carefully circumscribed the situation, they acquire an additional role that the BMA believes is alien to the traditional view of doctor–patient trust.

Some people argue that it would be possible to change the law to allow assisted dying but still protect the integrity and trust of the doctor–patient relationship. This was suggested to the House of Lords Select Committee on the Assisted Dying for the Terminally Ill Bill when it was proposed that, if legal change occurred, its implementation should be placed outside the healthcare service.[54] Some go further and say that a means of achieving this could be by excluding doctors completely from the process so that a non-medical official, such a judge or law-enforcement agent, would decide whether the criteria were met and a poison, rather than a medicinal drug, would provide the means of death. Adherents of this viewpoint argue that the purpose of medicine is to cure and palliate and so it is a perversion to use medicinal drugs for the deliberate ending of life, when effective poisons exist. Similarly, the doctor's role is one of improving health and welfare and so it is a distortion of the ethos underlying medical training to use it for contrary purposes. The counter-argument is that part of the doctor's role is to relieve suffering and if the only means to achieve that goal is by effectively hastening the person's death, doing so might be seen as acting in the interests of his or her overall welfare.

'Slippery slope' arguments

In this area of ethical debate, 'slippery slope' arguments are commonly invoked denoting an inevitable slide to an undesirable situation. Adherents of this line of reasoning argue that if assisted dying is accepted as a reasonable choice for people with capacity, it would be extended to the weak and vulnerable; the justification of death as a 'benefit' underpinning claims for a *right* to voluntary euthanasia would be applied to people such as the disabled, those with coexisting depression and patients with dementia. A common counter-argument is that relaxing the prohibition on assisted dying would mean that it could be regulated and include safeguards to protect the vulnerable. While it is illegal, it is said that we cannot judge accurately whether assisted dying already occurs in an unregulated manner. The removal of previously accepted barriers may reflect a positive recognition of changing moral views.

One way of attempting to assess whether assisted dying occurs secretly and whether vulnerable groups are particularly prone to be selected for it is by anonymous surveys. Seale's research on the attitudes of UK doctors is of interest here. In 2009, he canvassed the views of 8,857 doctors in different specialties, receiving 3,733 anonymous responses. Seale found that decisions that doctors took in the expectation, or with the intention, of ending a patient's life were not taken more often amongst the elderly, those dying in care homes or amongst patients with dementia. Palliative care specialists were particularly unlikely to report decisions intended to end life and, on the contrary, they found that some patients who asked for assisted dying changed their minds in response to the care provided. He concluded that there was no evidence of a clandestine slippery slope phenomenon in the UK, nor evidence to support claims that doctors were ignoring their patients' wishes but rather that they 'are sometimes willing to take actions that they think will hasten the end of life, but do so with a degree of caution and consultation that is particularly characteristic of UK medical practice'.[55]

The Netherlands due care criteria and Groningen Protocol

Some see the Dutch practice of assisted dying as an example of a slippery slope, in that the requirements of due care first applied to adults with capacity (who were not necessarily terminally ill) later encompassed other cases. The justification for permitting assisted dying in the Netherlands was the fact that in some cases the doctor's duty to preserve life came into conflict with the duty to prevent suffering. Doctors were seen to have an obligation to alleviate 'unbearable and hopeless suffering' but in some cases, it was only possible to do this by ending the patient's life. Doctors' defence in such cases was one of 'necessity'. Guidelines for euthanasia were first published by the Royal Dutch Medical Association in 1984, when the Dutch Supreme Court ruled that euthanasia (termination of life on request) and PAS were lawful in certain circumstances. This view was given statutory force by the Termination of Life on Request and Assisted Suicide (Review Procedures) Act 2001 which set out certain criteria. Before providing euthanasia or assisted suicide, doctors must:

- be satisfied that the patient has made a voluntary and carefully considered request
- be satisfied that the patient's suffering is unbearable, and that there is no prospect of improvement
- have informed the patient about his or her situation and his or her prospects
- have come to the conclusion, together with the patient, that there is no reasonable alternative in the light of the patient's situation
- have consulted at least one other, independent physician, who must have seen the patient and given a written opinion.[56]

Breaches of these rules were reported in the early years but were mainly procedural. They included, for example, allegations of failure to consult another practitioner before carrying out euthanasia.

Dr Chabot: assisted suicide in a case of psychological suffering

In the mid-1990s, the Dutch courts found that unbearable and hopeless psychological suffering, even in the absence of physical illness, was legitimate grounds for a doctor to assist suicide. Dr Chabot helped a 50-year-old woman to commit suicide. The woman's two sons had died: one from cancer, and the other had committed suicide. She had been abused by her alcohol-dependent husband. Dr Chabot, a psychiatrist, came to know his patient well over several months and concluded that she was not suffering from a diagnosable psychiatric disorder. He recommended antidepressants and psychotherapy but her wish was to commit suicide in a painless way. Dr Chabot thought that her condition fell within the Royal Dutch Medical Association's due care criteria, and provided her with a lethal drink, which she took in her own home. He reported the death to the coroner, and was charged under Article 294 of the Dutch Penal Code with assisting a suicide. His case went to the Supreme Court in 1994. The court ruled that psychological suffering could fulfil the necessary criteria for a lawful assisted suicide, because what mattered was whether the suffering was unbearable and hopeless, not its origin. Dr Chabot, however, had failed to obtain the opinion of an independent medical expert, as required by the due care criteria, and accordingly was found guilty of an offence. The Supreme Court declined to impose a penalty but Dr Chabot was reprimanded by a Medical Disciplinary Tribunal.[57]

Other breaches of the reporting criteria involved certifying the cause of death as natural but some cases of non-voluntary euthanasia were also reported.[58] In these too, the defence of 'necessity' was invoked as just as some patients with capacity experienced unbearable and hopeless suffering, so doctors treating incapacitated people might also be faced with the same conflict of duties between saving life and relieving suffering. As Lewis points out, 'a regime resulting from necessity as the mechanism of legal change does not necessarily require a competent request in cases where a patient is incompetent' but endures unbearable and hopeless suffering.[59]

Prins and Kadijk cases

Following discussion in the 1980s and 1990s in the Netherlands about the euthanasia of disabled babies, the lives of two severely disabled neonates were terminated in the mid-1990s. The doctors involved were prosecuted for murder. In response, they called upon the defence of necessity which applies equally to patients with and without capacity when the doctor is faced with the conflict between trying to preserve life and relieve the patient's unbearable and hopeless suffering. Continued medical treatment had been judged futile for both children and the doctors considered that they fulfilled the criteria of unbearable and hopeless suffering. Baby Kadijk, for example, had a chromosomal condition with other complications and, despite being given pain relief and sedation, she appeared to be in continued pain. Both sets of parents had requested that their child's life be ended. Both doctors had followed the procedural requirements by consulting colleagues and reporting the deaths as unnatural and both were acquitted.[60]

The Groningen University Hospital department of paediatrics developed a protocol for such cases, including in it the requirements derived from the Prins and Kadijk cases. This outlined criteria to be taken into account when ending the life of neonates and was known as the 'Groningen protocol'.

The 'Groningen protocol'

Criteria to be taken into account when ending the life of neonates:

- the suffering must be so severe that the newborn has no prospects of a future
- there is no possibility of a cure or alleviation with medication or surgery
- the parents must always give their consent
- a second opinion must be provided by an independent doctor who has not been involved with the child's treatment, and
- the deliberate ending of life must be meticulously carried out.

The protocol was adopted by the Dutch Paediatrics Association for national use in 2005. Opponents saw it as proof of the existence of a slippery slope, whereas supporters argued that it represented a reasonable response to the child's suffering and merely brought into the open practices that were already occurring clandestinely. Lewis points out that it is logical, given the reliance that had always been placed on the defence of 'necessity' which 'could be available if an incompetent person, whether child or adult, is experiencing unbearable and hopeless suffering, most likely following a decision that the continuation of life-sustaining treatment is medically futile'.[61] She goes on to argue that 'in order to show that legalisation causes a slippery slope from voluntary to non-voluntary euthanasia, one must show that (1) there has been an increase in the rate of non-voluntary euthanasia following the legalisation of voluntary euthanasia and (2) that the increase was caused by the legalisation of voluntary euthanasia'.[62] This cannot be proved as, although euthanasia rates have been monitored since legalisation, no data are available about the rate of non-voluntary euthanasia prior to that and nor is there evidence to link non-voluntary euthanasia rates and the law being passed to permit voluntary euthanasia. Furthermore, although the Dutch figures for assisted dying have varied, the overall numbers appear to have declined rather than increased since the legislation (from 3,527 in 1995 to 2,636 in 2009)[63] and the rate of non-voluntary euthanasia has also fallen from 0.8 per cent of all deaths in 1995 to 0.4 per cent in 2005.[64]

Despite the reasoning about 'necessity' when duties come into conflict, many people who support the concept of assisted dying would like to see it restricted to patients who both have capacity and are terminally ill. In Switzerland, assisting suicide is not an offence as long as the motive of the person doing the assisting is not a selfish one but failing to report all unnatural deaths is a breach of the regulations. The evidence so far indicates that unnatural deaths are properly reported but that the criteria for providing assistance vary.[65] Legally, the helper must have no direct interest in the death. In 2007, a Swiss psychiatrist was found guilty of manslaughter after helping three mentally ill patients to commit suicide.[66] His actions were considered illegal, despite the fact that the Swiss law is relatively relaxed on this matter, because he had acted out of self-interest. In this case, his motive was judged to be to spread his beliefs as he had been a former member of Exit (a right to die society) and had subsequently set up his own association. The option of obtaining a quick end to one's life with few restrictions has increasingly attracted patients from other countries, including some who are not terminally ill. The case of British patient, Daniel James illustrates this.

Daniel James case

Daniel James, was a 23-year-old rugby player, who had played for England under-16s, who was left paralysed from the the chest down after his spine was damaged while training with Nuneaton Rugby Club in March 2007. Despite surgery, he only regained the limited use of his fingers and said that his body had become a prison to him. He also told his parents that he lived in fear and loathing of his daily life. He was not terminally ill but could not adjust to his changed life and made three unsuccessful suicide attempts. He felt that other than starving himself to death, his only option was to travel to Switzerland, which he did with his parents. He was helped to die there in September 2008. His case was controversial, both because of the lack of a terminal medical condition and some people thought that, given time, he could have come to terms with his condition, as some other injured athletes had done. He was one of the youngest Britons to have travelled to Switzerland for an assisted suicide.[67]

Following the assisted suicide of a healthy German woman in Switzerland in 2005, the Swiss National Advisory Commission on Medical Ethics called for greater state supervision of right to die organisations and highlighted a number of unresolved questions including the implications for health professionals of death tourism. The patient in question had produced a false medical report, indicating that she had terminal liver cirrhosis but a routine autopsy showed this was untrue.[68] The Commission also noted a deep-seated ambivalence for health professionals leading to conflicting goals and made a series of recommendations about assisted suicide in hospitals and care homes. It pointed to some unresolved issues such as whether people with mental disorders or competent minors should be eligible for assisted dying, recommending that the mentally ill should be generally ineligible. The Commission supported the liberal approach of Article 115 of the Swiss Penal Code which permits assisted suicide as long as the assistance is not prompted by self-seeking motives. In 2009, the Swiss Justice Minister announced that parliament would consider tightening the rules on assisted dying by, for example, requiring patients to present two medical opinions that their condition is incurable and death is expected within a few months and that they are of sound mind.[69] (For more recent information, see the BMA website.)

Availability of alternatives to assisted dying

In 2000, when the BMA held a consensus conference on assisted dying, one of the strong recommendations arising from it was a call for continuing improvements in palliative care. Doctors who attended the meeting held a range of personal views and came from a variety of specialties but unanimously agreed that doctors have a duty to provide maximum support and quality care, particularly for patients nearing the end of life. Part of the BMA's current argument opposing assisted dying is that by focusing on that as a solution to people's natural anxieties about dying, society is having the wrong debate. Other aspects of end of life care which might provide some reassurance should be given more prominence. People fear many aspects of the dying process, including the possibility of not being listened to, being left in unrelieved pain, neglected, alone, or the opposite – that medical technology will take over and prolong or delay death. Callahan has drawn attention to how death dominated by technological medicine has become 'marked by undue fear and uncertainty, by the presence of medical powers not quite within our mastery, by a course of decline that may leave us isolated and degraded'.[70] He calls this the fear of 'wild' death – 'wild because it is alien from and outside of, the cycle of life, because modern technology makes its course uncertain, and because it seems removed from a full, fitting presence of the community'.[71] He contrasts this with the 'tame' death described by French historian, Aries, who wrote about how death needs to be faced and accepted as part of the natural order. Aries pictured a tolerable and familiar form of death, in which people felt supported by social solidarity and which they felt able to face without crippling fear.

This does not mean that society has to reject the advances and palliation available at the end of life through modern medicine but rather have more awareness of what can be provided by way of support. In Chapter 10, for example, we discussed measures such as the Liverpool Care Pathway which focuses very much on reducing non-essential medication at the end of life and concentrating instead on comfort measures, psychological and insight issues, spiritual support and good communication. Part of that process involves helping people find some sense of meaning and solidarity as they near death.

Callahan argues that many people fear that their death will be drawn out and become 'a violent death by technological attenuation'. He sees society's interest in euthanasia as an understandable and predictable response to this anxiety. Assisted dying appears to promise a controlled and peaceful death but Callahan says this is a mistaken view. 'Euthanasia will simply introduce another form of violence, that of consenting-adult killing. . .Euthanasia makes an obsession with control, already a source of medical damage, become still more a source of social damage.' He sees it as 'deforming' the end of life and deforming society. He concedes, however, that assisted dying might provide one kind of peaceful death for some people but, even so, 'the peaceful death of individuals ought not to be bought at the risk of significant societal harm. Nor should it be bought at the price of feeding an already excessive preoccupation with control, which generates its own pathologies.'[72]

The BMA takes the view that the widespread availability of high quality palliative care services would be likely to diminish the demand for assisted dying. Patients and their families need to know about such options, both in hospice-type settings and also as part of outreach care to people who want to die at home. The BMA has repeatedly expressed concern that good quality palliative care is currently not always available and that some groups continue to have poor access to it. In its debate on the Assisted Dying Bill, the House of Lords Select Committee also insisted that greater attention needed to be paid to the provision of palliative care or else some people would continue to see premature death as the only solution.[73]

Altering the rules to accommodate a minority – experience from Oregon

Another common argument in the debate about assisted dying is whether society should alter its traditional opposition to certain actions – which will affect everyone – at the behest of a relatively small group. On the other hand, the fact that a law only applies to a few citizens is not necessarily grounds for not having that law. In Oregon, for example, a majority of the population voted for the law to allow assisted dying even though experience so far is that only a minority of citizens make use of it.

Oregon's Death with Dignity Act (DWDA) came into force in 1997. It permits doctors to prescribe lethal drugs for competent patients over the age of 18. The action to end life, if it is taken, is carried out by the patient. Evidence suggests that the numbers who want assistance in dying continue to be small and that, year on year, more people obtain the prescription than use it. Many who obtain a prescription die of their underlying illness. Between 1998 and 2002, 198 lethal prescriptions were written but only 38 Oregonians died after using them, an average of less than 9 in 10,000 deaths per year.[74] By the end of 2008, when the law had been in force for over a decade, 401 patients had died under its terms.[75] In 2008, 88 lethal prescriptions were written and 54 patients died from using them; 22 people died of their underlying disease without using the drugs and 12 remained alive at the year's end. In 2009, 95 lethal prescriptions were written and that number went up to 96 in 2010.[76] Of the 96 patients who obtained prescriptions in 2010, 59 died from using the drugs, as did another six people who had obtained prescriptions in previous years, making a total of 65 known DWDA deaths in 2010 and a total of 525 since the law came into force. Two patients who took the drugs in 2010 regurgitated them and died later from their disease. Another 20 obtained prescriptions which they did not use but died of their underlying illness. Most patients who died under the Act were aged over 65 (median age 72), well educated, had healthcare insurance, suffered from cancer and were enrolled in hospice care at the time of death.

The fact that each year, more Oregon residents obtain lethal prescriptions than use them may indicate that some patients mainly want reassurance that they have another option rather than being trapped in a prolonged or distressing dying process. The main reasons for them wanting to end their lives were concerns about loss of autonomy, decreasing ability to participate in activities that made life enjoyable and loss of dignity. In the BMA's view, reassurance about some of these factors could be provided by less drastic means, such as better resourced palliative care, home support and well-integrated social and medical services.

Even though in Oregon few use the legislation, in other jurisdictions there might still be a risk of harm to the other people in society if there is significant existing inequity in how patients are treated. Marginalised groups, including the mentally disabled, are at greater risk of isolation, lack of support and self-harm. A New York State Task Force[77] articulated concerns that have been echoed more widely that:

> No matter how carefully any guidelines are framed, assisted suicide and euthanasia will be practised through the prism of social inequality that characterises the delivery of services in all segments of our society, including health care. The practices will pose the greatest risks to those who are poor, elderly, members of a minority group or without access to good health care.[78]

Although the data from Oregon do not appear to bear out such fears so far[79] and the UK healthcare situation is different to that of the USA, similar fears about marginalisation of the weakest members of society also motivated the conclusion of the House of Lords Select Committee on the Assisted Dying for the Terminally Ill Bill. Although it had been profoundly moved by the people and arguments in favour of euthanasia, ultimately it did not believe the arguments to be sufficient reason to weaken society's prohibition of intentional killing. The Committee acknowledged that 'there are individual cases in which euthanasia may be seen by some to be appropriate. But individual cases cannot reasonably establish the foundation of a policy which would have such serious and widespread repercussions.'[80]

Summary – moral, legal and pragmatic arguments

- Legalising assisted dying could have a profound and, in the BMA's view, detrimental effect on the doctor–patient relationship.
- The individual's right to choose is important but is limited if it would cause harm to others. It would be unacceptable to put vulnerable people in the position of feeling they had to consider precipitating the end of their lives.
- Not all slopes are slippery and not all change involves a downward slope. Choosing to remove some barriers need not necessarily result in others being abandoned but major changes in society may entail risks that need to be considered carefully.

- High quality palliative care services should be widely available for those who want it and the public should be better informed about such services.
- Despite the wide range of views among its membership, there is consensus within the BMA that the law should not be changed to permit assisted dying.

References

1 Callahan D. (1993) *The Troubled Dream of Life*, Simon & Schuster, New York, p.23.
2 Callahan D. (1993) *The Troubled Dream of Life*, Simon & Schuster, New York, p.23.
3 Boyd KM, Higgs R, Pinching AJ. (eds.) (1997) *The New Dictionary of Medical Ethics*, BMJ Books, London, p.90.
4 House of Lords (1994) *Report of the Select Committee on Medical Ethics*, The Stationery Office, London.
5 Coroners and Justice Act 2009, s 59. This amended the Suicide Act 1961 in England and Wales. The Coroners and Justice Act 2009, s 60 did the same for Northern Ireland.
6 Boyd KM, Higgs R, Pinching AJ. (eds.) (1997) *The New Dictionary of Medical Ethics*, BMJ Books, London, p.16.
7 Billings JA, Block SD. (1996) Slow euthanasia. *J. Palliat Care* **12**(4), 21–30.
8 Rietjens JA, van Delden JJ, Onwuteaka-Philipsen B. *et al*. (2008) Continuous deep sedation for patients nearing death in the Netherlands: descriptive study. *BMJ* **336**, 810–3.
9 Murray SA, Boyd K, Bycock I. (2008) Continuous deep sedation in patients nearing death. BMJ **336**, 781–2, p.781.
10 Regional euthanasia review committees (2009) *2008 Annual Report*. Available at: www .euthanasiecommissie.nl (accessed 12 May 2011).
11 Rietjens JA, van Delden JJ, van der Heide A. *et al*. (2006) Terminal sedation and euthanasia: a comparison of clinical practices. *Arch Intern Med* **166**, 749–53.
12 Seale C. (2009) Hastening death in end-of-life care: a survey of doctors. *Soc Sci Med* **69**(11), 1659–66.
13 Sykes N, Thorne A. (2003) The use of opiods and sedatives at the end of life. *Lancet Oncol* **4**, 312–8.
14 Criminal Justice Act 2003, s 269, Sch 21, para 11(f).
15 Boyd KM, Higgs R, Pinching AJ. (eds.) (1997) *The New Dictionary of Medical Ethics*, BMJ Books, London, p.239.
16 House of Lords Select Committee on the Assisted Dying for the Terminally Ill Bill (2005) *Assisted Dying for the Terminally Ill Bill [HL]* Vol I: Report, HL Paper 86-1, The Stationery Office, London, p.80 and Annex 7.
17 House of Lords Select Committee on the Assisted Dying for the Terminally Ill Bill (2005) *Assisted Dying for the Terminally Ill Bill [HL]* Vol I: Report, HL Paper 86-1, The Stationery Office, London, p.78 and Annex 7.
18 Seale C. (2009) Legalisation of euthanasia or physician-assisted suicide: survey of doctors' attitudes. *Palliat Med* **3**, 205–12.
19 Seale C. (2009) Legalisation of euthanasia or physician-assisted suicide: survey of doctors' attitudes. *Palliat Med* **3**, 205–12.
20 Seale C. (2009) Hastening death in end-of-life care: a survey of doctors. *Soc Sci Med* **69**(11), 1659–66.
21 Seale C. (2006) National survey of end-of-life decisions made by UK medical practitioners. *Palliat Med* **20**, 1–8. Seale C. (2009) End-of-life decisions in the UK involving medical practitioners. *Palliat Med* **23**, 1–7.
22 House of Lords Select Committee on the Assisted Dying for the Terminally Ill Bill (2005) *Assisted Dying for the Terminally Ill Bill [HL]* Vol I: Report, HL Paper 86-1, The Stationery Office, London.
23 House of Lords Select Committee on the Assisted Dying for the Terminally Ill Bill (2005) *Assisted Dying for the Terminally Ill Bill [HL]* Vol I: Report, HL Paper 86-1, The Stationery Office, London.
24 Royal College of Physicians (2010) Press release, 12 October.
25 Smith D, Templeton SK. (2008) Public in strong backing for right to assisted suicide. *Times Online* (December 14) Available at: www.timesonline.co.uk (accessed 18 May 2011).
26 *Attorney General v Able and others* [1984] 1 All ER 277.
27 Coroners and Justice Act 2009, s 61.
28 *R (on the application of Pretty) v Director of Public Prosecutions* (2001) UKHL 61.
29 *Pretty v UK* (2346/02) (2002) 35 EHRR 1.
30 *Pretty v UK* (2346/02) (2002) 35 EHRR 1, as quoted in: Jackson E. (2010) *Medical Law: text, cases and materials,* 2nd edn, Oxford University Press, Oxford, p.865.
31 House of Lords (1994) *Report of the Select Committee on Medical Ethics*, The Stationery Office, London.
32 House of Lords Select Committee on the Assisted Dying for the Terminally Ill Bill (2005) *Assisted Dying for the Terminally Ill Bill [HL]* Vol I: Report, HL Paper 86-1, The Stationery Office, London.

33 Bazalgette L, Bradley W. (2010) *The Commission on Assisted Dying: Key Research Themes*, Demos, London, p.6.

34 Bazalgette L, Bradley W. (2010) *The Commission on Assisted Dying: Key Research Themes*, Demos, London, p.6.

35 *Attorney General v Able and others* [1984] 1 All ER 277.

36 The Solicitor-General (2003) *House of Commons official report* (Hansard), Apr 10: col 346W.

37 Hirsch A. (2009) Debbie Purdy wins 'significant legal victory' on assisted suicide. *The Guardian* (July 30). Available at: www.guardian.co.uk (accessed 20 May 2011).

38 Director of Public Prosecutions (2010) *Policy for Prosecutors in respect of Cases of Encouraging or Assisting Suicide*, Crown Prosecution Service, London.

39 BMJ Podcast (2009) Dignified dying and physical barriers. Interview with Keir Starmer (September 25). Available at: podcasts.bmj.com (accessed 1 June 2009).

40 Director of Public Prosecutions (2010) *Policy for Prosecutors in respect of Cases of Encouraging or Assisting Suicide*, Crown Prosecution Service, London.

41 Mcardle H. (2010) Threat of charges dropped against suicide GP. *The Herald* (August 17). Available at: www.heraldscotland.com (accessed 24 May 2011).

42 Lewis P. (2007) *Assisted Dying and Legal Change*, Oxford University Press, Oxford, p.15.

43 House of Lords Select Committee on the Assisted Dying for the Terminally Ill Bill (2005) *Assisted Dying for the Terminally Ill Bill [HL]* Vol I: Report, HL Paper 86-1, The Stationery Office, London.

44 Lewis P. (2006) Assisted Dying and Legal Change, Oxford University Press, Oxford, ch 2.

45 Department of Human Services (2003) *Fifth annual report on Oregon's Death with Dignity Act*, DHS, Oregon, p.20

46 Legislative Assembly of the Northern Territory Select Committee on Euthanasia (1995) *Report of the Inquiry by the Select Committee on Euthanasia*. Vol. 2 *Transcripts of Oral Evidence* (Public Hearings, Thursday 6 April 1995, Opened: 14:10), Legislative Assembly of the Northern Territory, Darwin, section 2, para 3.

47 Segers JH. (1988) Elderly persons on the subject of euthanasia. *Issues Law Med* **3**, 429–37.

48 Callahan D. (1993) *The Troubled Dream of Life*, Simon & Schuster, New York, p.92.

49 Jecker NS. (1991) Giving death a hand: when the dying and the doctor stand in a special relationship. *J Am Geriatr Soc* **39**(8), 831–5.

50 Quill TE. (1991) Death and dignity: a case of individualized decision making. *N Engl J Med* **324**(10), 691–4, p.692.

51 Quill TE. (1996) *A midwife through the dying process*, Johns Hopkins University Press, Baltimore, p.64.

52 Lewis P. (2006) *Assisted Dying and Legal Change*, Oxford University Press, Oxford, ch 4.

53 Department of Human Services (2003) *Fifth annual report on Oregan's Death with Dignity Act*, DHS, Oregon, p.20.

54 House of Lords Select Committee on the Assisted Dying for the Terminally Ill Bill (2005) *Assisted Dying for the Terminally Ill Bill [HL]* Vol I: Report, HL Paper 86-1, The Stationery Office, London.

55 Seale C. (2009) Hastening death in end-of-life care: a survey of doctors. *Soc Sci Med* **69**(11), 1659–66.

56 Termination of Life on Request and Assisted Suicide (Review Procedures) Act 2001.

57 Sheldon T. (1994) The doctor who prescribed suicide: was the Dutch psychiatrist Dr Boudewijn Chabot right to help a sane, healthy woman to take her own life? *The Independent* (30 June). Available at: www.independent.co.uk (accessed 18 May 2011).

58 Keown J. (1995) Euthanasia in the Netherlands: sliding down the slippery slope? In: Keown J. (ed.) *Euthanasia examined: ethical, clinical and legal perspectives*, Cambridge University Press, Cambridge.

59 Lewis P. (2007) *Assisted Dying and Legal Change*, Oxford University Press, Oxford, p.167.

60 Lewis P. (2007) *Assisted Dying and Legal Change*, Oxford University Press, Oxford, ch 6.

61 Lewis P. (2007) *Assisted Dying and Legal Change*, Oxford University Press, Oxford, pp.133–4.

62 Lewis P. (2007) *Assisted Dying and Legal Change*, Oxford University Press, Oxford, p.171.

63 See: annual reports of the Regional Dutch Euthanasia Review Committees. Available at www.euthanasie.nl and in English at: www.laatstewilpil.org.

64 Van der Heide A, Rurup M, Hassen-de Wolf J. *et al.* (2007) End of life practices in the Netherlands under the Euthanasia Act. *N Engl J Med* **356**(19), 1957–65.

65 Fischer S, Huber CA, Mahrer Imhof R. *et al.* (2008) Suicide assisted by two Swiss right-to-die organisations. *J Med Ethics* **34**, 810–4.

66 Anon. (2007) Doctor sentenced over assisted suicides. swissinfo (July 6). Available at: www.swissinfo.ch (accessed 31 May 2011).

67 Booth R. (2008) 'He wasn't prepared for a second class life': why injured rugby star went to Switzerland to die. *The Guardian* (October 18). Available at: www.guardian.co.uk (accessed 18 October 2010).

68 Leidig M. (2005) Dignitas is investigated for helping healthy woman to die. *BMJ* **331**, 1160.

69 Boyes R. (2009) Swiss plan crackdown on suicide tourism that could spell the end for Dignitas clinic. *The Times* (29 October).

70 Callahan D. (1993) *The Troubled Dream of Life*, Simon & Schuster, New York, p.26.

71   Callahan D. (1993) *The Troubled Dream of Life*, Simon & Schuster, New York, p.26.

72   Callahan D. (1993) *The Troubled Dream of Life*, Simon & Schuster, New York, p.118.

73   House of Lords Select Committee on the Assisted Dying for the Terminally Ill Bill (2005) *Assisted Dying for the Terminally Ill Bill [HL]* Vol I: Report, HL Paper 86-1, The Stationery Office, London.

74   Department of Human Services (2003) *Fifth annual report on Oregon's Death with Dignity Act*, DHS, Oregon, p.20.

75   Department of Human Services (2009) *2008 Summary of Oregon's Death with Dignity Act*, Oregon Health Authority, Portland, p.2. Available at: public.health.oregon.gov (accessed 18 May 2011).

76   Oregon Public Health Division (2011) *Report on Oregon's Death with Dignity Act 2010*. Available at: www.oregon.gov (accessed 7 March 2011).

77   Lewis P. (2007) *Assisted Dying and Legal Change*, Oxford University Press, Oxford, p.38.

78   Report of New York State Task Force on Life and Law, *When death is sought: assisted suicide and euthanasia in the medical context*, quoted by: Lewis P. (2006) *Assisted Dying and Legal Change*, Oxford University Press, Oxford, p.38.

79   Battin MP, Van der Heide A, Ganzini L. *et al*. (2007) Legal physician assisted suicide in Oregon and the Netherlands: evidence concerning the impact on patients in 'vulnerable' groups. *J Med Ethics* **33**(10), 591–7.

80   House of Lords Select Committee on the Assisted Dying for the Terminally Ill Bill (2005) *Assisted Dying for the Terminally Ill Bill [HL]* Vol I: Report, HL Paper 86-1, The Stationery Office, London, p.48.

12: Responsibilities after a patient's death

The questions covered in this chapter include the following.

- What obligations do health professionals have towards their deceased patients?
- Is consent required for all interventions in relation to the deceased?
- Do relatives have a right to deceased patients' medical records or tissue samples?
- Should benefit for the living take precedence over protecting the dead as a general principle?
- Can relatives control what happens to a deceased person, including organ donation?
- Can cadavers be tested for infectious diseases to protect pathology staff?
- Who can confirm and certify death?

Scope of this chapter

Doctors have obligations to their deceased patients and their relatives. They also have general duties to promote public health and the public interest. Often it is difficult to reconcile all of these responsibilities.

In this chapter, we look at ethical and legal issues that arise after a patient has died, drawing attention to publications containing standards, guidance or other information that practitioners should be aware of. This chapter highlights the importance of the patient's own views about matters such as the future retention of diagnostic materials or tissue donation being discussed during the person's lifetime. After the person's death, people close to them must be consulted about proposed interventions under the human tissue legislation. More widely, considerable effort needs to be put into informing everyone in society about the immense benefits that can accrue from donation for transplantation, research and education.

Many of the issues covered here including post-mortem examinations, transplantation and use of tissue from deceased patients have been affected, in England, Wales and Northern Ireland by the Human Tissue Act 2004 and in Scotland by the Human Tissue (Scotland) Act 2006. The reformed legislation was intended to provide clarity about the requirement for consent which had been unclear in the past. The 2004 Act also established the Human Tissue Authority (HTA) as the regulatory body charged with ensuring best practice and issuing licences for certain activities (see pages 522–524).

There has also been significant legislative reform in the area of death certification which is manifested in the Coroners and Justice Act 2009. The Act has reformed the law in relation to the death certification process and modernised the coronial system in England and Wales, with the aim of establishing a more transparent and unified system for bereaved families and the wider public in the wake of the Shipman Inquiry[1] (see page 496). The implications of the legislative reforms in this area for doctors and bereaved families are the subject of discussion in this chapter along with aspects of the management of deceased patients.

Medical Ethics Today: The BMA's Handbook of Ethics and Law, Third Edition. Sophie Brannan, Eleanor Chrispin, Martin Davies, Veronica English, Rebecca Mussell, Julian Sheather and Ann Sommerville.
© 2012 BMA Medical Ethics Department. Published 2012 by Blackwell Publishing Ltd.

This chapter does not explore comparative religious or cultural attitudes to death, although health professionals need to be aware of such factors in the communities they serve. Issues around end of life care are the subject of discussion in Chapter 10.

General principles

The general ethical principles applicable to this sphere of practice include the following:

- the duty to show respect for people, living and dead
- the need to have clear and effective communication with people who were close to the deceased person
- the obligation to offer relatives as much information as they need about what will happen to the body after death
- the duty to balance this openness with the duty of confidentiality owed to the dead patient
- the need to demonstrate cultural awareness and sensitivity in relation to the management of the body
- the duty to bear in mind the public good and to promote ethical ways of maximising knowledge.

Terminology

Consent and authorisation in relation to interventions after death

A theme of this chapter is the importance society and the law attaches to obtaining consent for interventions after death. It can be argued that 'consent' is simply a misplaced notion when talking about dead persons because the reasons for valuing consent are to promote individual autonomy in a way that is inapplicable to deceased people. Partners and relatives may give their agreement or authorisation to procedures involving the dead person, but this proxy procedure is not 'consent' as we normally understand it (people agreeing to things being done to themselves). Nevertheless, the general language of consent is well understood by most people and is used in the legislation covering England, Wales and Northern Ireland and so it is likely to continue to be used in this context. It is also worth pointing out that the type of consent that is sufficient to count as 'appropriate consent' under human tissue legislation, even when it involves the dead person 'consenting' while still alive, is different to the type of consent required for treatment. For example, individuals can sign up to the donor register online without any opportunity for information giving or a capacity assessment. This is very different to what is commonly understood by 'informed' consent, which is the subject of discussion in Chapter 2.

The report by the Independent Review Group on Retention of Organs at Post Mortem in 2001 argued that it is more appropriate to talk of relatives' 'authorisation' rather than their 'consent'.[2] The semantics of consent and authorisation remain problematic to the extent that the Human Tissue (Scotland) Act 2006 uses the term authorisation while the Human Tissue Act 2004, applicable to England Wales and Northern Ireland, uses the term consent. Many people see advantages in continuing to use the term consent (even if not strictly correct) because it is a term well understood by both health professionals and the public. Consent is the central focus of the human tissue legislation (see pages 522–526).

Under the Human Tissue Act 2004, appropriate consent can come from three different sources – the deceased individual, their nominee or someone in a 'qualifying relationship', (see pages 523–524). For those practising in England, Wales or Northern Ireland, the HTA gives general advice about the law, process and practice of seeking consent to the removal, storage and use of human material after death in its consent code of practice.[3] It also stresses the importance of providing full and clear information in order to allow the person from whom consent is being sought to make an informed decision.[4] The general rules about who may give consent are covered on pages 523–526 and the basic requirements for different activities are summarised below. Human material that is imported for use in England, Wales and Northern Ireland (including material imported from Scotland) falls outside the scope of the Act but it is considered good practice to ensure that consent is in place. The HTA gives guidance in its code of practice on the import and export of human tissue.[5]

In Scotland, guidance about the implications of the Human Tissue (Scotland) Act for practice can be found in guidance from the Scottish Executive Health Department.[6] The general rules about who may give authorisation are covered on pages 524–526 and the basic requirements for different activities are summarised below. The 2006 Act does not include an exemption for imported material and so the consent rules in the Act also apply to bodies imported to Scotland.

Next of kin

This is a term in common usage but without definition in law. 'Families' or 'relatives' are often used as a shorthand way of indicating that people emotionally close to the deceased person need to be involved in decisions. For many adults without close family ties, however, cohabiting partners, carers or friends may be more in tune than blood relatives with the individual's values and intentions. Some adults may have formally nominated a person to make decisions after their death. Where they have not done so, human tissue legislation ranks persons in a 'qualifying relationship' ('nearest relative' in Scotland) and consent should be obtained from the person ranked the highest (see pages 523–526).[7] The codes of practice for England, Wales and Northern Ireland make clear that although lawful, careful consideration should be given before proceeding on the basis of one person's consent where it is evident that there are differences of opinion; decisions should be made on a case-by-case basis with inclusive discussion where possible.[8]

Society's and individuals' attitudes to deceased people

Respect for the wishes of the dead

Society expects that the advance wishes of people now deceased should carry some weight unless there are strong reasons to the contrary. Such reasons can include the public interest in conducting a post-mortem examination to ensure that the cause of death is identified and unlawful killing is revealed. Harris makes the point that 'the public interest serves principally the interests of existing and future individuals' rather than the past wishes of the deceased person.[9] He draws an analogy to how, in some areas, society feels entitled to overrule the prior wishes of dead people by, for example, demanding the payment of death duties, which are usually very much against those prior wishes. Nevertheless, in some other areas, the question of whose wishes should dominate is left vague. In the view of the British Medical Association (BMA), in the absence of an overriding societal need, or if the anticipated risks and benefits of an intervention are finely balanced, the wishes of the deceased person should be respected. Assessing risks and benefits can be complex. If the deceased individual carried an organ donor card, the removal of organs for transplantation could clearly benefit other people as well as respect that individual's former intent. On the other hand, if relatives know that the individual carried a donor card but still adamantly oppose donation, proceeding will cause them distress. If they cannot be persuaded to accept the wishes of the deceased person, their opposition may generate a difficult confrontational situation or, if publicised, might result in a backlash leading other people to refuse to donate. Doctors need to give careful consideration to these issues if the family is adamantly opposed to the wishes of their deceased relative. This is discussed further on pages 496–497.

Human tissue legislation is based on the premise that the individual's prior wishes should take precedence over the views of relatives and relatives do not have a legal right to override the wishes of the deceased. Interestingly, the Scottish legislation gives clear priority to transplantation, so that an individual's wish to donate his or her body for transplantation will override a wish to donate for anatomical examination. The justification for this was that where there was the possibility of saving lives this should be given precedence.

Treatment of the dead body

Individuals cope with loss in different ways. In her study of parents' response to the death of young children, McHaffie describes how 'death and involvement mean different things to different people' by reference to the deep anger felt by one father on seeing a nurse cuddling his dead baby.[10] In multi-cultural, multi-faith settings, diverse views exist about the importance of the dead body and how it should be treated. Families are often intensely protective of deceased relatives, perceiving them still as loved individuals. Feelings about the moral presence of the dead fade only as time passes. Nevertheless, many decisions, such as the donation of organs for transplantation, have to be made quickly when families are likely to feel least ready to consider them. Knowledge of the deceased individual's own wishes and intentions are therefore vitally important.

Dignified, respectful and culturally appropriate treatment of dead people is essential. Society is shocked by any perceived lack of respect for the dignity of human bodies. There was public outcry, for example, when the media reported that some corpses had had to be placed on the floors of hospital mortuaries or chapels of rest because the mortuary was too small. Such treatment was perceived as unacceptable.[11] As Jones points out, 'respect for the cadaver is respect for the relatives' grief'.[12]

Religion, tradition and moral intuition all lead us to show respect to dead people in order to honour the individuals they once were and in the hope that our own remains will be treated likewise. For those who are bereaved, the last acts of care and remembrance can be of vital importance in coming to terms with their loss. Parents continue to have very strong feelings of responsibility for a deceased child and therefore can experience guilt as well as distress if bereavement is compounded by what may appear to be unjustified interference with the corpse. Other relatives too may feel that they have failed in their protective duty if arrangements after death seem to be wrong. Death after invasive treatment often evokes the response from relatives that the deceased person 'has been through enough' and should not be exposed to further interventions such as a post-mortem examination. Although people who donate their bodies for scientific purposes sometimes describe the corpse as organic waste or an empty container, they may still worry about whether they will be treated respectfully.[13] Brazier points out that:

> [d]eath, especially sudden or untimely death, leaves the funeral of a relative or friend as the last service those who loved him or her can render to them. The reality of death, or loss, takes time to come to terms with. The dead infant, the wife succumbing to breast cancer at 35, the elderly father dying suddenly of a heart attack do not change their nature for their mother, husband or daughter. They remain Susannah, Lucy and Dad. How each bereaved mother, husband or daughter grieves will differ dramatically . . . The image of the newly dead person remains fixed in the mind of most bereaved families. Mutilation of the body becomes a mutilation of that image. Reason may tell the family that a dead child could not suffer when organs were removed. Grief coupled with imagination may overpower reason. Families grieve differently just as they live their lives differently. Respect for family life requires respect for such differences.[14]

Maintaining the integrity of the body is an important issue for some people and, even within specific religious faiths, individuals' views may differ. Disfigurement of cadavers arouses particular anxiety. Distress about the notion of their child's body being cut is a prevailing reason for parents to refuse an autopsy, for example, and reassurance about lack of disfigurement of the body is a potent factor in their agreement to it.[15]

Views about public dissection

Historically, society reserved procedures such as anatomical dissection for educational purposes for people about whom there was little societal concern: condemned criminals for whom it was part of a punishment extending beyond death, inmates of institutions or destitute persons.[16] For the public, the notion of dissection has long involved a mixture of repulsion and fascination. Such societal ambivalence was manifest when, in 2002, an autopsy was broadcast on television, provoking calls for the anatomist to be prosecuted.[17] Many people objected to the manner in which this took place, perceiving it as a misuse of the human body for entertainment. Others saw it as an educational experience, a reminder of our mortality and an attempt to demystify death for a public increasingly unfamiliar with the sight of dead people. In the early part of the twenty-first century, Professor Gunther von Hagens' travelling exhibition of preserved human bodies displayed in flamboyant and unconventional poses, *Body Worlds*, has proved popular as a tourist attraction at numerous worldwide locations, including England, where licences were granted by the HTA to hold the exhibition. (For further discussion on the use of bodies for public display, see pages 516–517.) The exhibition has aroused controversy with the public, with some taking the view that it is an opportunity to learn more about the human body while others have found the unconventional display of human bodies deeply offensive and insensitive. In 2005, it was reported that Edinburgh City Council had blocked the application for a *Body Worlds* show in 2003 on the grounds that some people could find it offensive.[18] In 2009, a French court ordered the closure of the *Our Bodies* exhibition on the grounds that it commercialised the body and lacked respect for the dead.[19] Since 2006, when the Human Tissue Act 2004 came into force, any activity classed as 'public display' requires a licence from the HTA (see pages 516–517).

Although, in purely practical terms, dead people cannot be physically harmed, profound societal abhorrence is generated by failure to respect human remains and any failure to consider the effect on relatives. Furthermore, even though dead people are not attributed rights, the use of improperly obtained cadavers or human material is generally recognised as a violation of accepted standards as well as being contrary to the law.

Attitudes of health professionals

Health professionals are expected to be both sensitive and stoic. Accustomed to dealing with death, they are also expected to remain compassionate, caring and open in their dealings with families for whom death may come as a shocking event. Traditionally, early medical training has sought to inculcate a dispassionate detachment and scientific interest in the cadaver, which make it hard to see it as the remains of a real person (see Chapter 18, pages 759–760). Nevertheless, dissecting human bodies or analysing human bones and tissue cannot occur in an ethical or cultural vacuum but must reflect society's moral intuitions. Jones reminds doctors that what is done to a dead body has relevance for human feelings about that person when alive: 'the cadaver and the person cannot be totally separated'.[20] Even molecular work should be viewed with ethical and human considerations in mind. As Jones notes, cadavers, body parts and tissues always come from particular individuals and 'they can never be completely dehumanised'.[21]

In the past, scientific work around post-mortem examinations and retention of tissue raised few ethical issues for health professionals but after 2000 it emerged as the focus of ethical debate which resulted in a demand for a review of the UK law (see below). The requirements for appropriate consent under the Human Tissue Act 2004, and authorisation under the Human Tissue (Scotland) Act 2006, stem from the notion of maintaining the dignity of the cadaver and ensuring relatives are brought into the decision-making process. It is obviously important for health professionals to be aware of cultural expectations towards dissection, and post-mortem examinations, and be sensitive to certain ways in which cadavers can and cannot be treated amongst diverse cultures. There can sometimes be tension and conflict between the needs of medical research and efforts to protect the dignity and respect for human tissue. As described by Jones, 'account needs to be taken of the dual importance of scientific and clinical research on the one hand, and informed consent and allied ethical considerations on the other'.[22]

Summary – society's and individuals' attitudes to deceased people

- Careful consideration needs to be given to potential benefits and harms in circumstances where the wishes of the deceased person are opposed to those of their relatives.
- Human bodies must be treated with dignity and respect.
- Health professionals must be aware of societal expectations and cultural sensitivities towards dissection and post-mortem examinations.

The impetus for law reform

The period of consultation and wide-ranging public debate which culminated in the enactment of the Human Tissue Act 2004 and the Human Tissue (Scotland) Act 2006 were hugely shaped by the high-profile events between 1999 and 2004 when UK post-mortem procedures were placed under a spotlight. The findings of public inquiries[23] into organ retention practices throughout the UK challenged public confidence and created a legacy of distress and anger. This section reflects on the events that focussed public attention on this area at the time.

Organ retention scandal

In 1999, it emerged that Alder Hey hospital had, for many years, been retaining organs and body parts following post-mortem examinations without the knowledge or agreement of the parents or family.[24] Many families were shocked and distressed to realise that by allowing a post-mortem examination on their child they were also deemed to have agreed to the long-term retention of organs and tissues. In January 2001, the then Secretary of State for Health, Mr Alan Milburn MP, reported to the House of Commons that one pathologist – Professor van Velzen – had ordered 'the unethical and illegal stripping of every organ from every child who had had a post-mortem' examination without the consent, or even the knowledge, of the parents.[25]

After the scandal at Alder Hey hospital it emerged that other hospitals had also been retaining organs and body parts without consent. A survey found that over 54,000 organs, body parts and stillborn children or fetuses had been retained in England since 1970 and were still held by pathology services.[26] There were similar findings in other parts of the UK.[27] Many of these organs had never been used for education or research and were simply left untouched on shelves.

The Human Tissue Act 1961 did not require explicit consent for organ retention for medical education or research. It only required practitioners to make 'such reasonable enquiry as may be practicable' to establish whether family members objected. The scope for interpretation that this provided often meant that in practice, many parents or relatives could not object to organ retention because they were never asked. Pathologists did not want to upset relatives by going into details and thought they were protecting them. In fact, this represented a clear breakdown between professional views and public expectations. The shift towards the concept of personal autonomy and rights of the individual which had occurred in other areas of medical practice was less apparent in this sphere.

One of the major criticisms arising from the subsequent inquiries[28] was the lack of clear information provided to bereaved parents. Even when they were consulted about organ retention, the literature was not explicit, referring to 'tissue' or 'samples of human material' when the intention was to retain whole organs such as hearts, brains and kidneys.[29] Similar issues arose in the 2010 Redfern Report.[30]

This inquiry was ordered in 2007 when it emerged that tissue and organs had been removed from deceased nuclear workers without consent at Sellafield in Cumbria between 1962 and 1992.

These events set the tone for wide-ranging proposals for reform of the law and pathology practice which, following consultation,[31] led to the introduction of the Human Tissue Act 2004 and the Human Tissue (Scotland) Act 2006. The bulk of the provisions of both Acts came into force in 2006. The legislation places a significant emphasis on consent and the views of the individual. The legislative and regulatory framework, and legal requirements for consent, are examined on pages 522–526.

Completely separate to the reform of the law on the use and retention of human material, significant flaws in the systems of death certification, coronial investigation and the issuing of cremation certificates were highlighted by the case of Dr Harold Shipman, whose murders of his patients remained undetected for decades (see below). The subsequent inquiry called for the introduction of more robust safeguards intended to detect such patterns of abuse and triggered legal review of all these areas. The events surrounding the Shipman case have shaped the changes to death and cremation certification and extensive reform of the coroner service. The legislative framework for implementing the reform of the process of death certification in England and Wales is included in Sections 19–21 of the Coroners and Justice Act 2009. Implementation of the reforms will broadly mirror that for introducing reforms to the coroner service and is expected to commence in April 2013.

Harold Shipman case

In January 2000, a Manchester GP, Dr Harold Shipman, was sentenced to life imprisonment for the murder of 15 patients. In July 2002, the first independent report following the inquiry into the case found that he had begun killing patients in 1975 and had murdered at least 215. It concluded that the true number of his victims could be far greater, but in some cases the evidence was inadequate to form an accurate view retrospectively. The inquiry sought to learn why Shipman had escaped detection for so long. Many of the deaths occurred suddenly, without prior life-threatening illness, and so should have been reported to the coroner. By carrying out death certification himself and persuading relatives that no post-mortem examination was needed, Shipman managed to avoid the involvement of coroners in all but a few cases. The inquiry found that a major weakness of the system had been the lack of exchange of information between those involved in the various stages of death certification, registration of the death and preparation for cremation. This meant that no person had an overview of the circumstances of the death. Relatives were neither able to find out what had been written nor asked to give their own views about the death. The death certification review was initiated and the inquiry also examined the system of cremation certificates.[32]

The Shipman Inquiry, chaired by Dame Janet Smith, went on to produce five further reports; the sixth and final report being published in January 2005.[33] In February 2006, the BMA and other organisations submitted evidence to the Reform of the Coroners System and Death Certification in England and Wales Inquiry which was then followed by draft legislation.[34] Following consultation the Bill was subsequently amalgamated into a larger piece of legislation which included several other fundamental changes to the judicial system. The Coroners and Justice Bill reached parliament in January 2009, was enacted in November 2009 and is expected to come into force in April 2013.

The Act will bring a number of key changes to the death certification and coroner systems including:

- the creation of a single system for secondary certification of deaths (covering both burials and cremation) that are not referred to the coroner
- the introduction of the 'medical examiner' role which centrally oversees the certification process of all deaths in both community and hospital settings.

The death certification and coroner provisions of the Act aim to unify the certification processes for cremation and burial while at the same time ensuring that all death certificates are subject to independent medical scrutiny. These provisions are intended to enable the identification and deterrence of criminal activity and poor practice in the wake of the recommendations of the Shipman Inquiry. (The legislation is discussed in greater detail on page 526.)

Duties and responsibilities after death

Respect for people: what duties do doctors have to dead persons?

Respect for persons is a fundamental part of medical ethics, but it is not obvious how it applies to dead people. Harris points out that, although differences of opinion exist about how to define a 'person' or when a person begins or ceases to exist, two aspects of respect for persons are widely accepted: respect for autonomy and concern for welfare.[35] In most respects, neither of these can be usefully applied to dead people. Autonomy 'as the ability and the freedom to make the choices that shape our lives, is quite crucial in giving to each life its own special and peculiar value'.[36] Concern for welfare provides the conditions under which autonomy can flourish. Personal consent is normally an important facet of autonomy, and it has been argued that such concepts are applied in any meaningful way only to those who are living. However, advance consent or refusal by a deceased person about posthumous interventions is now given greater prominence than was previously the case and is more closely aligned to other paradigm cases of consent in medical contexts. For example, the HTA code of practice on consent covering England, Wales and Northern Ireland confirms that where an adult has, while alive, given valid consent for any particular donation or the removal, storage or use of their body or tissue to take place following their death, then that consent is sufficient for the activity to be lawful.[37] This cannot be vetoed by those close to the deceased person although the HTA makes clear that healthcare professionals should consider the impact of going ahead with a procedure in light of strong and sustained opposition from the family, despite the legal basis for doing so.[38]

Doctors believe that they have a strong moral duty to respect the wishes of their deceased patients. Those who have had a relationship of care with a patient often express the sense that the moral duties owed to that relationship extend beyond the patient's death. Part of this almost retrospective duty of care may involve obligations to determine whether patients had received the best treatment, whether their diagnosis and treatment regimen were correct or whether avoidable errors that should be acknowledged were made. Doctors audit all of these things to improve practice for future patients and to promote the public interest, and give informed explanations to relatives, but they often also have a sense of 'owing' it to the deceased person. This sense of unfinished business may be a strong motive in asking for a hospital post-mortem examination, without which, in some cases, the presumed cause of death will be wrong or incomplete. Although it may not fall within the usual understanding of 'respect for persons', health professionals do feel a duty to respect the person's known wishes and the relationship that formerly existed. Ethical duties, such as that of confidentiality, also continue even though the patient is dead. From an ethical perspective, doctors are encouraged to assess what the deceased person would have wanted concerning disclosure. Even though it can be argued that dead people have no interests, public and professional expectations are that deceased patients' cultural and religious values should be respected, for example in the handling of the body and its disposal. Relatives also have a strong interest in ensuring that dead persons are handled appropriately and health professionals have an obligation to avoid harming them.[39] Obligations of confidentiality towards the deceased are discussed in the next section and in Chapter 5.

Do doctors have responsibilities to patients' families?

It is clear that doctors do have responsibilities to the families of deceased people. Among other obvious duties to offer support and information, the medical profession as a whole has an obligation to raise awareness about the benefits to be gained from procedures such as post-mortem examinations. Clearly, it can be difficult to convey this to bereaved families, but doctors need to discuss with them the reasons why a post-mortem examination is recommended, the information that may be revealed and how this information will be handled. Health professionals often continue to have contact with the family after a patient's death, especially in the primary care setting or as part of bereavement support or counselling. We discuss further below how the confidentiality owed to the deceased person can be balanced with the needs for information of a surviving partner or relative.

The difficulties of trying to argue that dead people are harmed by having their wishes or their confidentiality overturned by their relatives are obvious. On a practical level, individuals can neither be harmed nor helped once they are dead, although arguably some intangible harm may be done to their reputation and symbolic benefit may be derived from the implementation of their known wishes. The most immediate harms and benefits, however, are experienced by people who are close to the deceased and who have the satisfaction or distress of knowing that the dead person's values continue or fail to have an influence. Other people too may be distressed to become aware that their own wishes may not be respected after their death and indeed can be comforted by the knowledge that their wishes will be respected.

The importance of a more involved role for the family of the deceased in the bureaucratic procedures following death has long been stressed. The Cremation Regulations 2008 gave families in England and Wales the option to view cremation forms prior to cremation being authorised so they can raise any concerns about the death.[40] It is anticipated that this provision will be incorporated into regulations under the Coroners and Justice Act 2009 when it comes into force in 2013. (Up-to-date information is available on the BMA website.) The role of the medical examiner will facilitate increased communication between the coroner's office and bereaved relatives when the cause of death requires further investigation by the coroner. (For further details on cremation forms see page 504 and for further discussion on the role of the medical examiner see page 505.)

Summary – duties and responsibilities after death

- In assessments of harm and benefit, attention needs to be given to the potential distress to people who are emotionally close to the deceased person.
- In most circumstances the known wishes of the deceased person take precedence over the views of relatives.

Confidentiality after death

The moral basis of the duty of confidentiality is primarily to protect patients' privacy and respect their wishes. A common argument is that individual patients will lose faith in doctors if their confidentiality is not protected. When they are no longer alive, patients cannot be harmed in the same way, although the trust of the public at large may be diminished if confidentiality is routinely breached. The General Medical Council (GMC) emphasises that the duty of confidentiality is not extinguished by the patient's death,[41] but the extent to which it must be protected depends upon the circumstances. Factors to be taken into account include the following:

- the deceased person's former wishes
- the nature of the information
- whether disclosure is likely to cause distress to, or be of benefit to, the patient's family
- whether it is already public knowledge
- the use to which the information will be put
- whether the objective could be attained by anonymised data.

Therefore, the general principles, outlined in Chapter 5, should be observed. Disclosure should be kept to the minimum unless the patient indicated to the contrary.

Benefit and harm

As health professionals see themselves as owing a continuing duty to dead patients, doctors often have to make judgements about what the person might have wanted in a particular situation. The fact that the law says little about the confidentiality of deceased people does not mean that information or photographic records of dead individuals can be used in an unlimited way, nor does it mean that information cannot be disclosed for an appropriate purpose. Doctors have always had discretion to disclose information to a deceased person's relatives or others when there is a clear justification. In many cases, it is obvious that the deceased person would have wanted a partner or relative to have specific information. A common example is when the family requests details of the terminal illness because of an anxiety that the patient might have been erroneously diagnosed or there might have been negligence, or from a feeling of guilt that warning signs were missed within the family. Disclosure in such cases is likely to be what the deceased person would have wanted and may also be in the interests of justice. Refusal to disclose in the absence of some evidence that this was the deceased patient's known wish exacerbates suspicion and can result in pointless litigation. The statutory right of access to relevant parts of deceased patients' records by people with a claim arising from the death is discussed in Chapter 6, pages 259–260. In other cases, the balance of benefit to be gained by disclosure to the family, for example of a hereditary or infectious condition, may outweigh the obligation of confidentiality to the deceased. Relatives of the deceased frequently make the assumption that they have more or less automatic access to aspects of the deceased person's health information. In these circumstances, the former instructions and wishes of the deceased person need to be taken properly into account.

Traditionally, the BMA and the GMC have long upheld the general concept of a duty of confidentiality that extends beyond the patient's death, unless there is an overriding reason for disclosure. Periodically this view has been challenged. In the aftermath of events, such as the Shipman case (see page 496), there have been calls for relatives to have more routine access to information about the deceased patient's health and, potentially, a reduction in the notion that dead people are owed confidentiality. Unless there is a statutory requirement to disclose information about a deceased person, however, the ethics advice remains that individuals should be able to indicate in their lifetime if they do not wish relatives to have access to certain parts of their record. Relatives and heirs may have insurance or other legal claims arising from the death which mean that they have statutory rights of access to relevant parts of the deceased person's medical history (see Chapter 6, pages 259–260). In 2007, the Information Commissioner found that most information in medical records is likely to be confidential – this is discussed in Chapter 5, pages 221–223.

Despite the fact that there is no automatic right of access to the deceased person's health information, there is now a recognition that procedures relevant to coroner investigations and post-mortem examination should be more inclusive of, and sensitive to, the needs of bereaved families. This is reflected in the Charter for Bereaved People, brought in under the Coroners and Justice Act 2009, which states that the coroner's office will enable bereaved people to be 'informed and consulted' during the coroner investigation process.[42] As mentioned on page 504, cremation regulations which came into force in January 2009 allow the bereaved the option to view cremation forms before cremation takes place.[43] The Ministry of Justice has issued guidance to doctors which says that they need to bear in mind that some information requested on the forms may have been provided in confidence by the deceased person. Doctors completing the forms have the option of submitting that information on a separate piece of paper to the medical referee. This indicates to doctors that they should maintain a duty of confidentiality to the deceased and some information can be separated from the form which the family can see.

Thorough investigation of deaths can provide an early warning system of many hazards in the community. Patterns of preventable deaths may be identified in hospitals, on the roads, in the workplace or in the home. Identifying such patterns over time and geographical areas, while having regard to issues of confidentiality, requires sophisticated information handling. Forensic pathology services accumulate information and experience that has importance in terms of public health and safety. It has been argued that forensic pathology systems have an ethical responsibility to contribute to the prevention of deaths and injuries by identifying such patterns. Some have argued that this responsibility is of even greater significance to society than the judicial role of forensic pathology.[44]

Disclosing information to a coroner or procurator fiscal

Doctors must provide relevant information about a patient if this is requested by a coroner or procurator fiscal. The GMC states:

> [y]ou must assist the coroner or procurator fiscal in an inquest or inquiry into a patient's death by responding to their enquiries and by offering all relevant information. You are entitled to remain silent only when your evidence may lead to criminal proceedings being taken against you.[45]

There is also a statutory duty for organisations to respond to a request from a coroner under Rule 43 of the Coroners Rules. This rule deals with the prevention of further deaths and also requires coroners to report circumstances in which further deaths could occur if action is not taken to prevent them.[46]

Information on death certificates

Death certification is an important source of data not only for families, but also for society (although without the availability of data from post-mortem examinations, the reliability of death certificates cannot entirely be known). Since 1995, the BMA has been calling for an abbreviated version of the death certificate to be made available to relatives who need it purely for administrative purposes related to the death, such as closing bank accounts, thereby avoiding unnecessary distress or embarrassment to the families by disclosing the actual cause of death. The Coroners and Justice Act 2009 has, for the first time, enabled regulations to be made for the introduction of short death certificates which will omit the cause of death. At the time of writing no regulations had been prepared. (Up-to-date information on this can be found on the BMA's website.) The short death certificate can be provided in addition to the Medical Certificate of Cause of Death (MCCD) to enable families to inform most organisations of a death without having to reveal the cause of death.

Although the introduction of short death certificates will improve the situation in circumstances when the cause of death is particularly sensitive to the family, there may still be the potential problem of limiting disclosure when, for example, patients had not wished relatives to be informed of sensitive information relating to their illness. The GMC's 2009 confidentiality guidance points out that doctors must complete death certificates honestly and fully.[47]

In September 2008, the Office for National Statistics Death Certification Advisory Group revised its guidance for doctors completing MCCDs in England and Wales. It said that this was needed as doctors were unsure, following the Shipman case, how to describe the causes of death. It advises doctors to avoid stating causes such as 'old age', 'natural causes' or 'organ failure' without giving further explanation of the cause of death.[48]

Although the duty of confidentiality continues beyond the patient's death, such ethical obligations are overridden where there is a statutory duty to disclose. This can be problematic because death certificates are public documents, and surviving partners or family members may fear the consequences if full details are disclosed, for example where HIV infection or AIDS is the cause of death; nevertheless this must be stated on the death certificate, whatever the views of the patient and/or family.

Summary – confidentiality after death

- Ethically, the obligation of confidentiality extends beyond the patient's death.
- The duty of confidentiality needs to be balanced with other considerations, such as the interests of justice and of people close to the deceased person.
- All relevant information should be provided to a coroner or procurator fiscal in an inquest or inquiry into a patient's death.
- Despite the duty of confidentiality, death certificates giving the cause of death must be completed honestly and fully.

Certifying and confirming death

Who should certify and confirm death?

Confusion has often arisen about the distinction between confirmation of death and its certification. Any health professional can confirm that death has occurred, but a certification of death can be completed only by a doctor who attended the patient during that person's last illness. This doctor provides an opinion of the cause of death and certifies the cause of death, not the fact.

The law does not require a doctor:

- to confirm death has occurred or that 'life is extinct'
- to view the body of the deceased person
- to report the fact that death has occurred.

The law does require the doctor who attended the patient during the last illness to issue a certificate detailing the cause of death.

Although only a registered medical practitioner can legally certify death, nurses and other health professionals can confirm that death has occurred. It is common for nurses to confirm death in cases where the death is expected and there is an explicit policy or protocol specifying the nurse's role in this context.[49] Clearly, any professional who is expected to carry out this task must have appropriate training and assessment to ensure that it is carried out competently. Even though it is not a legal requirement for a doctor to confirm death, hospital rules may require that a doctor do so before a deceased patient is moved from the ward.

The law requires a doctor to notify the cause of death of any patient whom he or she has attended during that patient's last illness to the Registrar of Births and Deaths. Sometimes the police or ambulance services ask GPs to attend the body of a person who is said to be dead. The BMA advises that in these circumstances, and especially in the case of an on-call doctor, GPs should decline to attend and advise that the services of a forensic physician should be obtained by the caller. If a patient is declared to be dead by a relative, a member of staff in a nursing home, ambulance personnel or police, GPs would be acting correctly by prioritising the needs of their living patients. Where there are grounds for believing that the death was violent, unnatural or unexpected and of unknown cause, coroners and procurator fiscals must investigate if the body is lying within their district, even though the death may have occurred elsewhere. All suicides and any deaths in prison must also be investigated. All such deaths may be the subject of a post-mortem examination at the coroner's or procurator fiscal's direction. Generally, the death cannot be registered until the coroner's investigations are finished. The BMA's General Practitioner's Committee has produced detailed guidance on confirmation and certification of death.[50]

The method for confirming death can give rise to anxiety for relatives, particularly when patients are on life support and their heart is being kept beating artificially. In these cases it is not possible to use the usual tests – of cessation of the heart and breathing – and so death is confirmed by brainstem tests. These tests confirm that the brainstem has died and that recovery is impossible. Guidance from the Academy of Medical Royal Colleges specifies the safeguards that should be in place for diagnosing death in this way, including that the death should be confirmed by at least two doctors who have been registered for over 5 years, one of whom is a consultant.[51]

Which deaths should be referred to a coroner or procurator fiscal?

The current legal provisions governing the process for selecting deaths that should be reported to coroners in England, Wales and Northern Ireland are unsatisfactory and not clearly defined.[52] There is a common law duty to report a death to the coroner in circumstances where an inquest might be required. It applies to all citizens. Deaths should be reported to the local coroner in the following situations:

- the death was violent or unnatural
- the death was in prison or state custody
- the death was sudden or unexpected.[53]

Deaths should also be referred to the coroner if the person was detained or liable to be detained under the Mental Health Act 1983 (as amended) (this list is not exhaustive).[54] Many reports are also made by doctors because they do not fill the requirements of attendance for certifying death.[55] There is also a statutory duty for the registrar to report the decision to the coroner in certain situations, for example, if the death took place during surgery or if the death was caused by an industrial disease.[56]

As part of the Coroners and Justice Act 2009, medical practitioners in England and Wales have a statutory duty to report deaths to a coroner where the death meets one or more criteria set out in regulations.[57] It is anticipated that this duty will come into force in April 2013. At the time of writing no regulations had been prepared. (Up-to-date information on this can be found on the BMA website.)

In Scotland, such reports are made to the procurator fiscal, who fulfils a similar role in determining the precise cause of death and may order a post-mortem examination.[58] The following deaths must be reported to the procurator fiscal:

- sudden deaths
- deaths related to neglect or a complaint about medical treatment received by a health board or NHS trust
- certain categories of deaths of children
- certain deaths related to public health
- deaths associated with medical and dental care.[59]

These categories are not exhaustive.

Death certification process in England and Wales

At the time of writing it is anticipated that the death certification provisions in the Coroners and Justice Act 2009 will come into force in April 2013. A registered medical practitioner who attended the deceased prior to death ('the attending practitioner') is required to prepare a MCCD stating the cause of death to the best of his or her knowledge and belief. In order to complete the MCCD, the doctor must have attended the patient within 14 days leading up to the death, or seen the body after death and be sufficiently familiar with the patient to be sure of the cause of death. Commissioning bodies, local health boards and healthcare providers (both in the NHS and the private sector) will also be encouraged to provide the attending practitioner with information on circumstances leading to the death which may assist the attending practitioner in establishing the cause of death or deciding to make a referral to a senior coroner. Doctors who are not sure what to write as the cause of death on the MCCD can seek further guidance from the medical examiner (see below). It is hoped that this will reduce the number of deaths being unnecessarily referred to the coroner.[60]

The entire framework was reformed, from preparation of the MCCD by the doctor who attended the deceased to the return of the certificate to the medical examiner after the death has been registered. The aim was to create a more simple process, ensuring transparency and clarity for bereaved families by distinguishing who is involved and their specific roles and responsibilities. While the new legislation provides for a more rigorous scrutiny process, it is expected that this will not cause significant delays to funerals. The registrar can issue a deferral of registration to allow burial or cremation prior to registration where it is necessary to do so.

Independent scrutiny of the Medical Certificate of Cause of Death by a medical examiner

One of the key features of the death certification sections of the Coroners and Justice Act 2009 is the requirement that MCCDs are subject to independent scrutiny. After completion of the MCCD, the legislation requires that it should be passed to a medical examiner attached to the clinical governance team of a commissioning body (or local health board (LHB) in Wales). If the medical practitioner is unable to complete an MCCD, or if the death is violent or suspicious, the death must be reported to the coroner. The medical examiner will scrutinise the MCCD and investigate as necessary. This stage needs to be completed as speedily as possible to allow cremation or burial to take place promptly. It will include, for example, discussing the circumstances of the death with the doctor signing the MCCD and other clinicians involved in the deceased's care and, where necessary, with the family of the deceased. If the medical examiner is satisfied that all is in order, he or she will issue an authorisation to the family of the deceased to enable the death to be registered and burial or cremation to proceed (this will remove the existing responsibility for authorising burial from registrars and abolish the present cremation form system). A copy of the medical examiner's authorisation will be given to the funeral director to allow him or her to finish preparing the body for burial or cremation. If not satisfied, the medical examiner will have a duty to refer the case to a senior coroner for further investigation and to inform the family that he or she has done so. In this situation, the medical examiner should provide a recommendation on whether or not a post-mortem examination is likely to provide relevant information beyond that which is available from other sources (although the final decision to order a post-mortem examination will continue to remain with the coroner).[61] At the time of writing regulations are awaited which will provide further details about the preparation, scrutiny and confirmation of MCCDs, about the way the confirmed MCCD is notified and given to a registrar, and about how the death is referred to a coroner. (Up-to-date information is available on the BMA website.)

Cremation certificates

As part of the changes to the death certification process, which are expected to come into force in April 2013, the medical checks that are currently required before a cremation takes place will be replaced by two new forms which need to be completed alongside the MCCD. The first requires administrative information for the medical examiner and can be completed by clerical staff at a hospital or GP practice; the second documents more detailed information required for scrutiny by a medical examiner or coroner and must be completed by a doctor who attended the deceased during his or her last illness or, if that is not possible, by another doctor who has access to the notes and can discuss the death with a medical examiner and/or coroner. The medical examiner will incorporate the activities currently undertaken by the medical referee at the crematorium. As discussed above, the medical examiner, once satisfied, will confirm the cause of death and authorise cremation or burial and allow the death to be registered. The Cremation Regulations 2008 also gave families the option to view and discuss the cause of death prior to disposal of the body being authorised so they can raise any concerns about the death.[62] It is anticipated that this provision will be incorporated into regulations under the Coroners and Justice Act 2009. (Up-to-date information is available on the BMA website.)

Removal of medical devices before cremation

Cardiac pacemakers and other battery-operated devices may explode if cremated and must be removed. Fixion expandable nails will also explode unless vented or removed prior to cremation. The presence of most radioactive implants precludes cremation. It is the responsibility of the doctor certifying death to state whether or not such devices or implants are present. It may not be possible for a cremation to proceed if it is not possible to obtain such information, for example from the medical records, external examination or discussion with relatives.

Stillbirths

The certification and registration of stillbirths will change when the death certification provisions in the Coroners and Justice Act 2009 come into force in April 2013. Registration of stillbirths will be brought into line with that for other deaths and allow medical investigation to be carried out in appropriate cases by the medical examiner who will carry out the certification role currently undertaken by referees. (Up-to-date information is available on the BMA website.)

Role of the medical examiner

Medical examiners must be GMC registered medical practitioners with at least 5 years' experience who have been practising as such within the previous 5 years and who have received special training in the role. They will be appointed by commissioning bodies (in England) and LHBs (in Wales) so that they can work closely with NHS clinical governance teams to establish whether patterns or clusters of deaths give any cause for concern, and to improve medical provision in the area. All medical examiners will complete training based on a curriculum developed by an intercollegiate group established by the Academy of Medical Royal Colleges and, if successful, will be accredited to act as medical examiners. The Coroners and Justice Act 2009 includes provision for the Secretary of State to appoint a National Medical Examiner (NME) to provide professional leadership to medical examiners.

At the time of writing, regulations had not yet been prepared in relation to appointment and training as well as details as to the functions that the medical examiners will be expected to carry out but it was envisaged the main responsibilities of medical examiners would be as follows:

- provide advice to the attending doctor, coroner and/or coroner's officer at different stages of the death certification process (this might include providing general advice to the attending doctor on completing the MCCD or giving more specialised advice to the attending doctor or the coroner where there are questions relating to the cause of death or the medical conditions associated with reportable deaths)
- scrutinise the MCCD while seeking information from the bereaved families and others where necessary
- authorise burial or cremation or refer the case to the coroner
- provide a liaison role between the bereaved families and the coroner where the cause of death may require further investigation
- obtain and consider the deceased's medical records where necessary.

Death certification process in Northern Ireland

The system of death certification in Northern Ireland has not been subject to statutory change and the certification and coronial processes are separate from each other. Different certification requirements apply depending on whether the body is to be buried or cremated. Following completion of the MCCD and delivery of this to the local registrar who issues an authority for the disposal of the body, the body can be buried. If the body is to be cremated, a 'three-tier' process involving three certifying doctors takes place. The final approval is given by the medical referee at the crematorium.[63] (See above for details on the common law duty to report certain deaths to a coroner.) The coroner's service in Northern Ireland has essentially been unchanged since the enactment of the Coroners Act (Northern Ireland) 1959. However, both the death certification and coronial processes are under review with the intention of modernising the system in line with the recommendations arising from the Luce Review.[64]

Death certification process in Scotland

As in the rest of the UK, after death, the MCCD is completed by the doctor to enable the body to be buried and the death registered. If the body is to be cremated the 'three-tier' certification process applies (see above). Scotland's burial and cremation and death certification legislation is under review with the aim of modernising the Cremation Acts of 1902 and 1952 (and the Cremation (Scotland) Regulations 1935, as amended) and the Registration of Births, Deaths and Marriages (Scotland) Act 1965. It has been recommended that all current primary and secondary legislation be repealed and consolidated into a single Act covering burial, cremation and other forms of disposal. It is proposed that the role of the medical referee be replaced by either a medical investigator or medical examiner function.[65] The role of the Procurator Fiscal Service is unlikely to change but will be integrated into the relevant legislation.[66]

Summary – certifying and confirming death

- The law requires a doctor who attended a patient during his or her last illness to certify the cause of death.
- From April 2013, doctors will have a statutory duty to report certain deaths to the coroner in England and Wales.
- Death certificates will be subject to independent scrutiny from April 2013.
- Doctors who are unsure as to what to write as the cause of the death on the MCCD can seek advice from the medical examiner.

Post-mortem examinations

This section summarises the key points relating to consent (authorisation in Scotland) for post-mortem examination but more detailed advice about consent, licensing and standards for those in England, Wales and Northern Ireland is provided in the HTA's code of practice on post-mortem examinations.[67] This section also highlights the importance of post-mortem examinations and the benefits they can bring to living individuals.

Coroner or procurator fiscal post-mortem examinations

The coroner or procurator fiscal may order a post-mortem examination in order to clarify the cause of death where the death is sudden or unexpected. Consent (authorisation) is not required for coroner or procurator fiscal post-mortem examinations. Respectful and sensitive communication with bereaved families is essential. Those close to the patient should understand the reasons for the investigation, even though they have no power to prohibit the examination from taking place. If it is known that the deceased had specific cultural or religious objections to post-mortem examination, this should be made known to the coroner or procurator fiscal.

Hospital post-mortem examinations

Hospital post-mortem examinations are undertaken to investigate the cause of death or to improve knowledge of the disease or effectiveness of the treatment given. These examinations are optional and appropriate consent or authorisation is always required. (For information on who may authorise a hospital post-mortem examination see pages 523–526.)

Discussing post-mortem examinations with families

The way the family is approached about post-mortem examination is clearly important and good, sensitive communication skills are essential. The HTA advises that families should be given:

'i.   honest, clear, objective information
i.   the opportunity to talk to someone of whom they feel able to ask questions
ii.   reasonable time to reach decisions (for example, about the retention or donation of tissue)
iii. privacy for discussion between family members if applicable
iv.   emotional or psychological support if they need and want it.'[68]

For hospital post-mortem examinations, the family should also be given the opportunity to change their minds within an agreed time limit of preferably not less than 12 hours.[69]

The individual providing information and seeking consent must have relevant experience and a good understanding of why the examination is being requested, what the post-mortem examination involves and how it will be undertaken. This person should also have received training in bereavement support and, ideally, have an established relationship with the family.

Retention and use of organs and tissue removed at post-mortem examination

In England, Wales and Northern Ireland any retention or use of organs or tissue for a 'scheduled purpose' following a post-mortem examination requires appropriate consent. Scheduled purposes are defined in Schedule 1 of the Human Tissue Act 2004 and include storage and use of retained material for activities such as quality assurance, education or research. More information about the scheduled purposes, and who may give consent, is set out on pages 523–526.

Amendments to the Coroner's Rules[70] introduced in June 2005 require coroners to notify the appropriate relative about any material that has been retained as part of the post-mortem examination and to invite them to state what should happen to the tissue once the coroner's investigation is complete. With hospital post-mortem examinations, consent for subsequent retention and use may be sought at the same time as consent is sought for the examination.[71]

In Scotland, a distinction is made between whole organs and tissues, blocks and slides. Tissue samples, blocks and slides (including samples taken from organs) automatically become part of the deceased person's medical record and may be used for diagnostic and audit purposes without the need for specific authorisation. Retention and use for other purposes, such as research, requires authorisation. Any retention or use of whole organs after the conclusion of the post-mortem examination also requires explicit authorisation. Information about who may give authorisation is set out on pages 524–526.

Existing holdings

The above rules do not apply to the use of material that was collected before 1 September 2006 when the legislation came into force. This material – known as 'existing holdings' – may continue to be used without the need for consent or authorisation. As a matter of good practice, however, existing collections should be reviewed at regular intervals to ensure that the material has continuing value and, if it is unlikely to serve any useful purpose, it should be respectfully disposed of.[72]

Regulatory action within the post-mortem sector

The Human Tissue Act 2004 carries criminal penalties of up to 3 years in jail and a substantial fine. The HTA carried out an inspection of post-mortem examination facilities at University Hospital of Wales in Cardiff on 30 July 2009 which raised serious concerns about the procedures relating to post-mortem examinations and poor compliance with HTA standards. As a result, the HTA suspended its licences meaning that post-mortem examinations could not legally take place at the hospital mortuary. The Designated Individual, responsible for ensuring compliance with the necessary standards, was replaced. Further inspections took place in September 2009, which found that there had been significant improvements, and the suspension was subsequently lifted.[73] In addition a copy of the HTA's inspection report was referred to South Wales Police.[74] They undertook a full criminal inquiry, although in February 2010 it was announced that no grounds for criminal prosecution had been found.

When the HTA published its compliance report for the post-mortem sector for 2008–09[75] it was clear that this was not an isolated incident and there were wider concerns about compliance within the post-mortem sector. In particular, the HTA reported that in some cases tissue blocks and slides had been retained without consent and, since April 2008, it had been notified of five incidents in which brains had been kept without consent following forensic post-mortem examination, due to failures of communication between mortuaries and the criminal prosecution agencies.

As a result, the HTA issued General Directions in April 2010 requiring all premises licensed for post-mortem examination to:

- complete annual compliance assessment reports against core HTA standards,[76] and
- complete an audit of all whole organs and wet tissue and a representative sample of tissue blocks where material was removed from a body after September 2006 and was stored on the premises at the time of the audit.[77]

Importance of post-mortem examinations

While the implementation of the Human Tissue Act 2004 and Human Tissue (Scotland) Act 2006 have clarified the need for consent or authorisation for post-mortem examinations, the consent process is now used less and less. The rate of hospital post-mortem examinations, carried out with consent, had been falling for many years, but since the publicity around organ retention most hospitals report rates of less that 1 per cent of deaths in hospital. Some report none. This has often been attributed to a loss of public confidence in autopsy practices following intense adverse publicity over retained organs but it has been suggested that most of the fall is attributable to a change in the attitudes of health service staff.[78] An audit undertaken at a hospital in Leicester showed that of those who were asked for consent, 51 per cent gave consent to a hospital post-mortem examination before the adverse publicity on organ retention and 49 per cent gave consent afterwards, indicating that fewer relatives are approached about consent.[79] The reason for this change in staff attitude is unclear. A number of possible factors have been put forward including a perception that the bereaved may be distressed by having to consider the possibility of a post-mortem examination; the time taken to complete the lengthy new consent processes; and the possibility that a post-mortem examination will reveal errors in diagnosis in an increasingly litigious environment.[80]

Consent for post-mortem examination rates in paediatric practice have also fallen, although less precipitously. Research carried out by the Confidential Enquiry into Maternal and Child Health (CEMACH) in 2007 found that the percentage of hospital post-mortem examinations in England, Wales and Northern Ireland involving stillbirths had declined from 54.7 per cent in 2000 to 45 per cent in 2007.[81] The data from CEMACH also show that, despite an increase in the number of parents or guardians who were offered post-mortem examinations by health professionals, there has been a rise in the number declining the examination for neonatal deaths, from 33.1 per cent in 2000 to 47.1 per cent in 2007.[82] The increased intensity of media interest from 1999 onwards has also been associated with a downturn in registrations of tissues in a national tumour bank, although there is evidence that numbers are now beginning to recover.[83]

The decline in the number of post-mortem examinations is a matter of concern as these examinations can bring huge benefits to living people. Even in the setting of an intensive care unit, comparison between pre-mortem and post-mortem diagnoses has resulted in rates of 'major missed diagnoses' as high as 39 per cent.[84] In addition, research has found that the number of post-mortem examinations on children is only half what experts believe is ideally needed to gain a better understanding of why some infants die, or are born with conditions such as cerebal palsy.[85] Post-mortem examinations are important for informing relatives and healthcare professionals about the cause of death; however, they may also inform individuals about possible acquired or genetic diseases that may need treatment and care. Without a post-mortem examination, it is estimated that the cause of death can be wrong in up to one-third of cases.[86] The HTA stresses the importance of post-mortem examination in improving clinical care, maintaining clinical standards, increasing understanding of disease, identifying the spread of infectious diseases and supporting research and training.[87] Post-mortem examinations have a valuable role in medical research and it is generally acknowledged that much of modern medical knowledge would not have been discovered without their use. Laing and Bercher have suggested that the reduction in the number of neonatal post-mortem examinations has meant many families may have suffered because of the decrease in information available to them. They recognise neonatal post-mortem examinations as being of great value when counselling families after the loss of a child by improving understanding about the circumstances surrounding the life and death of their child.[88] Furthermore, if parents experience the loss of their baby, a post-mortem examination may be able to provide information about whether it is safe to try to conceive again, and possibly prevent complications in any future pregnancy. The above-mentioned CEMACH research suggests that post-mortem examinations may be crucial to gaining a full understanding of the true cause of death for babies that have died during pregnancy or in the neonatal period.[89] This is reinforced by Elder and Zuccollo's previous study of necropsy reports for 29 infants born at less than 28 weeks' gestation which found new diagnoses following autopsy in 79 per cent of cases.[90] There is a need to increase general public awareness about the importance of post-mortem examinations and the enhanced knowledge they can bring both to families and to the benefit of wider society.

Concern for justice and the public good

There are various ways in which post-mortem examinations promote the concept of justice. They help to identify, for example, when patients' disease has not been treated correctly and can also contribute evidence to the legal system. Correcting previous miscarriages of justice in homicide cases often depends upon the evidence obtained by pathologists. The responsibilities of doctors involved in such inquiries may extend beyond the provision of evidence at the time to include alerting the courts to any important and relevant information they subsequently obtain.

Provision of evidence in legal cases

Sally Clark was convicted in 1999 of murdering her two baby sons but was released in 2003 when the post-mortem evidence was re-examined. The children died in 1996 and 1998. Post-mortem examinations were carried out on both. It was reported that microbiological tests at the time of the post-mortem examination showed the presence of *Staphylococcus aureus* infection in eight sites of the second child's body, but the pathologist judged the infection to be irrelevant to the legal case and failed to disclose it at the trial.[91] In 2000, the evidence was re-evaluated and Sally Clark's conviction was subsequently quashed after it was revealed that the Home Office pathologist had not disclosed such vital information to other doctors prior to the trial or later.

In September 2004, following the acquittal of Sally Clark, the Royal College of Pathologists and Royal College of Paediatrics and Child Health published a joint report, *Sudden unexpected death in infancy*.[92] The stated aims were to prevent miscarriages of justice and to protect the welfare of infants. It contained a national investigation protocol and specific recommendations for various professionals, including for ambulance staff, GPs, health visitors, accident and emergency department staff, pathologists, social services and the police.

Maximising useful knowledge in an ethical manner is an obligation of doctors. This means, for example, that when a post-mortem examination is carried out, it should be done in a manner that is technically adequate to yield accurate information that is useful to relatives and to the way that future patients are managed. Among its purposes are the following:

- the need to ascertain or confirm the cause of death
- the classification of disease or condition so as to explain biological behaviour to relatives
- the collection of information about the extent of the disease or condition in the patient's case
- to contribute to a better understanding of the disease and the biological responses to it
- the assessment of the patient's response or otherwise to the treatment provided
- the detection of other relevant pathology not established in life
- the need to contribute to audit of patients' medical management, including the value of investigations and treatment and the accuracy of diagnosis
- the detection of genetic or other heritable conditions relevant to other family members
- the provision of reliable data on which to base death certification.

Learning from deaths: example of positive change triggered by coroner post-mortem examination

In 2005, a national patient safety alert was issued by the National Patient Safety Agency (NPSA) for adults and children following the outcome of an inquest at Sheffield Coroners Court (a similar alert was issued for neonates in 2006). The coroner's report in this case had indicated possible risks associated with the existing method of testing the positioning of nasogastric feeding tubes. As a result of the information contained in the coroner's report, an investigation by the NPSA (and other national and international experts) culminated in new national guidance and recommendations regarding the placement of nasogastric feeding tubes in order to reduce risk to patients. The guidance was subsequently adopted internationally.[93]

Is there a role for minimally invasive autopsies?

Among some patient groups there is strong religious or cultural opposition to the performance of invasive post-mortem examinations. Nevertheless, there is still a long way to go before less invasive autopsy can be implemented.[94] In such circumstances, doctors must be frank about the limitations of any investigation that relies on the external examination of a body or circumstantial evidence.

However, there has been an increased interest in imaging post-mortem examination techniques in recent years and several studies have shown the potential value of the imaging process as well as its difficulties;[95] for example, it has been noted that there is sufficient evidence to recommend routine use of magnetic resonance imaging (MRI) in fetuses with suspected brain malfunctions.[96] Under the Coroners and Justice Act 2009, coroners will have the option to consider non-invasive examinations for those who oppose the conventional post-mortem examination. This might include, for example, using MRI scans, which may be useful for identifying problems within the brain of the deceased person. Clearly, the precise purpose of the post-mortem examination is relevant. Although literature indicates minimally invasive autopsy has a high diagnostic performance for detection of common causes of death such as pneumonia, it has also demonstrated significant error rates such as failure to establish cardiac diseases as the underlying cause of death.[97]

Pathologists point out that one of the significant benefits of full autopsies is the number of unexpected findings made that are unrelated to the initial question that the procedure set out to answer. Although there may be limited circumstances in which minimally invasive examinations are of use, the general view among practitioners appears to be that minimally invasive examinations are unlikely to be a valid alternative to a conventional autopsy. As evidence accumulates, it is possible that a new medical speciality of 'death investigation' may develop, where an expert decides what techniques can best be used to investigate the unique circumstances of each death, bearing in mind the requirements of the state and the wishes of the bereaved.

Summary – post-mortem examinations

- Consent is required for hospital post-mortem examinations but not for those authorised by the coroner or procurator fiscal.
- The general rule is that consent is needed for the use or storage of human materials removed after death.

- Doctors must provide honest and clear information in order to allow families to make informed decisions.
- When post-mortem examinations are legally required, people close to the patient should be kept informed.
- Society expects an environment of openness and honesty in relation to interventions on deceased people.
- The public needs more information about how data from post-mortem examinations can bring huge benefits for living people.

Organ and tissue transplantation

Organ and tissue donation for transplantation may proceed only with the explicit consent (authorisation in Scotland) of the donor, given during his or her lifetime, or someone else legally empowered to give it (see pages 523–526). In addition, if it may be necessary for a coroner or procurator fiscal to carry out a post-mortem examination, organs or tissues may be removed only with the specific authorisation of those authorities. More detailed information for those in England, Wales and Northern Ireland can be found in the HTA's code of practice on transplantation.[98]

The Human Tissue Act 2004 and Human Tissue (Scotland) Act 2006 clarified the law around the use of procedures shortly after death to preserve the organs, and thus the possibility of donation, while consent or authorisation is being sought. Throughout the UK it is now clearly lawful to take the minimum steps necessary to preserve the organs after death has been confirmed. This usually involves making a small incision in the groin, inserting a cannula and using a cooling fluid to perfuse the organs. All such activity must stop, however, if it becomes clear that consent (authorisation) for donation cannot or will not be obtained.

Increasing the number of donors

For at least the last 20 years concerns have been expressed about the lack of organs available for donation and the increasing gap between the number of organs needed to meet demand and the number available for transplantation. Although public opinion surveys in the UK consistently report that around 70–90 per cent of those interviewed support organ donation only around 28 per cent have made their wishes known by signing up to the NHS Organ Donor Register.[99] Where their views are not known, relatives are asked about donation when they have just been told their relative is dying or has died. Not surprisingly, a high number (around 40 per cent) opt for the default position which is not to donate.[100] It is much easier for relatives to address the issues around donation when they are aware of what the deceased person wanted. The importance of making known one's views about organ donation cannot therefore be overstated and, where feasible, health professionals should sensitively encourage people to talk to those close to them about their wishes. GPs can have an important role in raising the issue of donation and encouraging those who want to donate to register their views and discuss their wishes with their families and those close to them. Other mechanisms for joining the Organ Donor Register, such as on passport or driving licence applications, should also be more widely promoted in order to maximise the number of potential donors on the register. From 2011, those applying for a driving licence have been required to complete the questions on organ donation rather than being able to skip over them.

In 1999, the BMA undertook a review of the organ donation system in the UK and the range of factors that could lead to improved donation rates. At its annual meeting the BMA voted to support a shift to an opt-out system for organ donation (see below) as one part of a broader strategy to improve donation rates. The BMA recognised, however, that changing the law on consent, by itself, would not have the desired effect and that major changes and investment were also required to develop the infrastructure within which donation took place. The BMA has been campaigning on these two issues since 1999.

Organ donation taskforce

In 2006, the Labour Government set up an organ donation taskforce to identify the obstacles to organ donation and suggest solutions that would deliver an increase in the number of transplants carried out within the existing legal structure. The Taskforce reported in January 2008[101] with 14 recommendations which, it believed, would lead to a 50 per cent increase in donation rates by 2013. All of the recommendations were accepted by UK health ministers and significant funding was allocated to implementing the recommendations.[102] The Taskforce focused on investment and coordination to improve the infrastructure, including the following:

- the need for a UK-wide organ donor organisation to be established as part of NHS Blood and Transplant
- a strengthened network of dedicated organ retrieval teams working with critical care teams in hospitals
- the appointment of a senior clinician as a 'donation champion' (subsequently renamed clinical lead for organ donation), and the establishment of a donation committee, in each NHS trust
- a doubling of the number of transplant coordinators (subsequently renamed specialist nurse, organ donation)
- additional training for hospital staff and formal monitoring of donation activity within trusts
- the establishment of a UK Donation Ethics Committee to resolve some outstanding legal, ethical and professional issues in order to facilitate donation.

The Department of Health set up a Programme Delivery Board to manage and over-see implementation of the recommendations which published its first annual report in October 2009.[103] The report states that '[e]ach individual should be given the choice and opportunity to offer their organs for the purposes of transplantation after their death. This choice should not be denied by the assumptions of NHS staff or a lack of facilities and infrastructure.'[104] The BMA supports this view and has long advocated that part of the healthcare team's duty of care to dying patients is to seek to ascertain and fulfil their wishes regarding organ donation. In January 2011, NHS Blood and Transplant reported that the number of donors had increased by 28 per cent since implementation of the Taskforce's recommendations began.[105] (Up-to-date information on the implementation of the Taskforce's recommendations can be found on the transplantation pages of the Department of Health's website.[106])

Opt in or opt out?

The BMA believes that changing the default position in support of donation, by introducing an opt-out system – in addition to the type of changes set out above – would maximise donation from willing individuals while providing additional protection for those who do not wish to donate organs after their death. The system would work as follows.

- Before the new system is introduced there would be extensive and high profile publicity to ensure all members of society are aware of the forthcoming change and to encourage them to consider their own wishes about donation.
- A database would be established with mechanisms for people to easily and quickly opt out if that is their wish.
- Once implemented, when someone dies and donation is a possibility, the opt-out register must, by law, be checked and if the individual had opted out donation could not proceed.
- As an extra safeguard, if the individual had not opted out, their family would be asked if they were aware of any unregistered objection.
- If they were not aware of any objection, they would be informed that donation would proceed. There would, however, be discretion not to proceed if it became evident that this would cause serious distress to the family.

Following support for an opt-out system being expressed by the Chief Medical Officers in England[107] and Scotland[108] and the then Prime Minister Gordon Brown,[109] the Organ Donation Taskforce was invited to carry out a review of the potential impact of introducing such a system for organ donation in the UK. Its report, published in 2008, acknowledged that the issue was very finely balanced and that moving to an opt-out system 'may deliver real benefits' but also carried some risks.[110] It concluded that the recommendations made in its first report (see above) – which it believed could deliver a 50 per cent increase in donation over 5 years – may make a change in the law unnecessary. It preferred therefore to adopt a 'wait and see' approach, with the option of revisiting the issue if the proposed strategy did not meet the target set. The BMA supports the changes proposed by the Taskforce, considering them to be essential to the improvement of the organ donation system. For the first time, there has been a significant investment of funds into organ donation and a coordinated approach to address some of the problems, which should improve donation rates. Whether the increase of 50 per cent put forward by the Taskforce is achievable, however, only time will tell; even it if is, it will still be insufficient to meet demand and people will still be dying who might have lived had an organ been available.

The BMA believes that an opt-opt system operated within a well-organised and well-funded system would increase the number of donors available but the area is complex. It is not possible to extrapolate directly from one country's experiences to another and there are a number of factors that impact on donation rates, so a causal effect between rates and any single factor is difficult – if not impossible – to prove. Nonetheless, there appears to be growing evidence that there is a positive correlation between opt-out systems and higher donation rates around the world.[111] The Taskforce commissioned an independent systematic review of the evidence from the University of York.[112] The review identified eight studies comparing donation rates in countries with opt-out systems and ones without, four of which were methodologically sound. All of these found that opt-out law or practice was associated with increased rates of organ donation (of up to 30 per cent) and three of the four were statistically significant. It also identified five studies comparing donation rates before and after the introduction of an opt-out law all of which reported an increase in donation rates following the introduction of opt out.

Of course, just because opt out can lead to higher donation rates does not necessarily mean it will. Clearly, if large numbers of the population opt out of donation any increase would be lost. Understandably, there are concerns about a public backlash – with people opting out in protest at the change. But the overwhelming experience of other countries that have implemented such a change is that this has not happened. The exception is Brazil, where an opt-out system was imposed on an unwilling and unsupportive population and had to be reversed.[113] This is not an argument against opt out but an argument for ensuring, before its introduction, that there is public support for such a change. Although there has so far been little coordinated public debate about opt out in the UK, surveys have found 64 per cent of the public in favour of such a change.[114] The Taskforce's own deliberative events with the public found 65 per cent support for a shift to opt out before the event, rising to 72 per cent once more information had been received.[115] There is, however, a need for more informed public debate. In Wales, the majority of responses to a 2009 consultation on changes to the organ donation system supported the introduction of an opt-out system.[116] (More information about opt out can be found on the BMA's website.)

Summary – organ and tissue transplantation

- Organ and tissue donation may only proceed with the consent (authorisation in Scotland) of the individual before death or of someone else legally empowered to give it.
- Throughout the UK it is lawful to take the minimum steps necessary, after death, to preserve organs for donation while consent is sought.
- There is a large, and increasing, gap between the number of organs needed to meet demand and the number available for donation.
- The Organ Donation Taskforce made a number of recommendations to improve the infrastructure and coordination of organ donation.
- The BMA supports the introduction of an opt-out system for organ donation as one way of addressing the shortage of organs.

Organ and tissue donation for research and teaching

During their lifetime, people can give advance permission for tissue samples, organs or their entire body to be kept and used for research or teaching purposes. Some support groups or organisations supporting a particular condition, such as Parkinson disease, campaign for people to sign up during their lifetime to donate their organs or tissue for research after their death and hold a register of willing donors.[117] With this exception, there are few formal mechanisms for people to record their views about research and teaching in advance and consent (authorisation in Scotland) is usually provided by the individual's relatives. Where a post-mortem examination is being carried out, the relatives should be informed of the possibility of donation for research after the examination is complete and their agreement should be sought. Where a woman who has died was pregnant, the fetal tissue is considered, in law, to be her tissue and its use is therefore covered by the consent or authorisation provided for the use of material removed from the deceased woman. The Human Tissue Act and Human Tissue (Scotland) Act make it a criminal offence to use tissue removed after death for research or teaching purposes without the necessary consent or authorisation.

More information about the use of tissue for research is provided in Chapter 14 and, for those in England, Wales and Northern Ireland, in the HTA's code of practice on research.[118]

Anatomical examination

The written, witnessed consent (authorisation in Scotland) of the deceased person, given during his or her lifetime, is required for donation for anatomical examination,[119] which involves the use of whole bodies to teach students or trainees about the body and how it works (including dissection). Nobody else may give consent on behalf of the individual. This means that the bodies of babies or young children cannot be used under any circumstances. The BMA has expressed concern in the past about the shortage of people donating their bodies for anatomical examination and the effect this might have on the training of future doctors. One of the problems has been that those wishing to donate their bodies for anatomical examination have found it difficult to access information and did not know how to go about implementing their wish. The HTA has subsequently produced a leaflet for potential donors providing advice about how to contact a local medical school[120] and has produced a model consent form for body donation.[121] In Scotland, those wishing to enquire about donating their body for anatomical examination should contact their nearest medical school. There is still a need to publicise the importance of body donation and encourage more people to think about this option.

In all cases, the altruism and generosity of those who donate their bodies for anatomical examination should be appropriately recognised and their remains treated with respect by those who make use of them. Public confidence that bodies will be treated with due respect is vital in encouraging people to volunteer. The HTA's code of practice on anatomical examination[122] (which establishments in England, Wales and Northern Ireland, licensed to conduct such examinations, are expected to follow) puts great emphasis on the need to treat bodies with dignity and respect.

Use of bodies or body parts for public display

As with anatomical examinations, the written, witnessed consent (authorisation in Scotland) of the donor is required for the public display of human material and nobody else may authorise such use. This means that the bodies, or human material, from babies or young children may not be used for public display under any circumstances.

The HTA defines public display as: 'an exhibition or display in which the body of a person, or relevant material which has come from the body of a person, is used for the purpose of being exposed to view by the public'.[123] Two activities are specifically exempt from the Human Tissue Act: display for the purposes of enabling people to pay their final respects or which is incidental to the funeral of the deceased; and display in places, and for the purpose, of religious worship. Consent is also not required where more than 100 years have elapsed since the death of the person whose body, or human material, is on display or when the bodies, or material, are imported from another country. Although consent is not a legal requirement for imported material, the HTA's code of practice advises that consent should be in place and this is taken into consideration when deciding whether to issue a licence. A number of examples are provided in the HTA's code of practice on public display[124] to illustrate when consent and an HTA licence is required. These include, for example, some cases where people wish to witness a post-mortem examination or anatomical examination and whether this would be classed as public display requiring a licence. Where, however, there is any doubt about whether an activity would be classified as public display, or whether consent and/or a licence is required, advice should be sought from the HTA.

Both the HTA's code of practice and guidance produced by the Department for Culture, Media and Sport[125] emphasise the importance of ensuring that human bodies are treated with respect and dignity.

In Scotland, a licence is required from Scottish ministers for the public display of the bodies of people who have died or material taken from the bodies of those who have died (certain museums are exempt from this requirement). Before issuing a licence, Scottish ministers must think it is desirable in the interests of education, training or research, to do so. The requirement for public display to be in the interests of education, training or research is not present in the English legislation, or in the HTA's code of practice,[126] where the focus is on ensuring proper consent to the activity and that bodies or body parts are not subjected to undignified or disrespectful treatment.

Use of skeletons for private study

The BMA occasionally receives enquiries from its members who have a skeleton that they have used for private study and are concerned about how, if at all, the human tissue legislation affects this. Most skeletons are over 100 years old and so fall outside the scope of the legislation. Those that are less than 100 years old and were already held when the legislation came into force, in September 2006, are classed as 'existing holdings' (see page 508). Existing holdings can also continue to be kept and used without the need for consent from the deceased person.

In England, Wales and Northern Ireland, if a skeleton is being held privately, and is not being used for a scheduled purpose (such as formal education and teaching), neither the consent nor the licensing requirements of the 2004 Act apply.

There is a restriction on commercial dealings under both the 2004 and 2006 Acts, but these provisions apply only to material for transplantation. There is, therefore, no restriction on people selling skeletons. Those who wish to dispose of skeletons need to be mindful of the method of disposal. Given that skeletons are human material, they should be disposed of respectfully and in accordance with official guidance.[127] Local hospitals may be willing to provide assistance with this.

Testing for communicable diseases

It is an offence to remove any material from a deceased person to ascertain the cause of death unless there is appropriate consent or the authority of a coroner or procurator fiscal. Therefore, testing deceased people for communicable diseases should be done only when it is likely to be relevant to the cause of death and a post-mortem examination has been authorised or ordered. Clearly, in many instances testing is necessary for these purposes. If this is not the case, the testing should not be performed routinely simply to protect healthcare workers. Pathology teams often have only imprecise information about the deceased individual and so this means they should take full precautions on every occasion that an invasive procedure is carried out.

It may be useful to consider the moral reasons why we seek to apply the same rules about testing to the dead as we do to the living. Clearly, for living patients there can be serious personal and financial implications in having a communicable disease such as HIV and, as a result, individuals often take steps to avoid knowing their own infection status. This is not true for dead people and, even if information about them was discovered through testing, which might impinge on their posthumous reputation, it would still be governed by the ethical obligation of confidentiality. It can be argued that obtaining some tangible benefit in terms of protecting living people should take precedence over notions of symbolic harm to dead individuals. To sustain such an argument, however, would require evidence that the difficulties involved in protecting the health team were great and the risk of infection to them serious. There would also need to be societal consensus that the aim of protection is more important than the privacy of deceased persons. At present, there is no such consensus.

Some patients who have died can be assessed as suitable organ donors if consent or authorisation has been obtained. It should be explained to the family or nominated representatives, who need to be aware that assessment includes testing for certain infections, including HIV. Health professionals and people close to the deceased person need to consider in advance how the resulting information should be handled, as there is no current legislation regarding the breach of confidentiality when disclosing positive virology results after death. The view of the Department of Health and that of the BMA is that the decision to disclose information regarding positive virology results should be made by balancing the benefits and harms of disclosure. In other words, concern for the interests of others who may be affected must be weighed against the duty of confidentiality owed to the deceased patient. In the BMA's view, information about a living or dead patient may be disclosed to protect a person from death or serious harm but it should not normally be disclosed to relatives who are not at risk. Therefore, it could be appropriate to disclose the deceased's positive HIV status to a spouse or partner, for example, but not to parents or siblings. In its guidance on the management of potential organ and tissue donors with positive virology results, NHS Blood and Transplant (NHSBT), describes the notification process of next of kin and significant others once a decision has been taken to disclose information.[128] This involves discussion between the specialist nurse and the clinician in charge of the potential donor's care about what information should be disclosed, how it will be disclosed and by whom. NHSBT guidance states that a meeting with the next of kin and/or significant others should take place after the confirmatory results have been received and expert advice sought. This meeting should involve no less than two appropriate healthcare professionals. The information discussed at this meeting should include the following:

- a detailed discussion of the positive result and the implications for the next of kin and/or significant other
- an offer to screen all those who may be at risk
- the need for precautions to be taken until their own results are confirmed – if testing is declined then advice should be given on prevention of transmission
- approval should be sought and encouraged for permission to disclose the findings to the GPs of those who are at risk
- contact numbers for local clinics and support groups.[129]

Post-mortem DNA testing

With specific exceptions (see below and Chapter 9, page 373) it is unlawful under the Human Tissue Act 2004 to have 'human bodily material' with the intention of testing the human DNA within it without consent. Curiously, the offence refers specifically to having bodily material with the intention of analysing its constituent DNA, not the DNA itself. 'Bodily' material is defined as consisting of or including human cells, so once a collection of cell-free DNA samples has been prepared for legitimate purposes the Act contains no prohibition on its further use. However, this does not negate the ethical duty to study DNA responsibly.

The offence applies to the whole of the UK. When an adult dies, the HTA code of practice on consent states that an individual (such as a relative or friend) who was close to the adult at the point of death, may give consent for a DNA test.[130] In cases relating to DNA analysis, the hierarchical ranking applicable for most activities under the Human Tissue Act (discussed on page 523) does not apply; however, the HTA advises that the individual giving consent should be encouraged to discuss the decision with other family members.[131] The HTA also points out that at the time of discussing consent, it should be raised with the family whether they wish to know of any results that may have potential significance, such as a genetic condition.[132]

It is not an offence to analyse DNA without consent if the results of the analysis are intended to be used for 'excepted' purposes. These include the following:

* for the purposes of the coroner (England, Wales and Northern Ireland) or procurator fiscal (Scotland)
* prevention or detection of crime, or prosecution
* national security
* court or tribunal order or direction.[133]

In its published advice[134] on diagnostic genetic testing after death, the BMA notes that this may occur when it is suspected that death was caused by a genetic disorder or if it is thought that an unborn fetus died from a genetic or chromosomal disorder. In either case, a post-mortem examination (either with the family's permission or at the behest of the coroner or procurator fiscal) may be carried out to clarify the cause of death, but the results can have profound implications for other family members. It should not be assumed that a coroner will necessarily authorise genetic testing to clarify a natural cause of death. For example, some coroners may consider 'cardiac dysrhythmia' to be an adequate conclusion from a post-mortem examination, without authorising investigations to identify the underlying cause, even if that investigation is of benefit to the family. In such circumstances it would be unlawful to investigate the cause further, or even to take samples to facilitate investigation, unless consent had been obtained.

Prior to testing, thought should be given to how the results will be handled and who should have access to them, including the fact that some family members may not want to know. When a test is proposed for a deceased child or fetus, the issues should be discussed in advance with the parents, whose agreement should be sought.

Internationally, guidance has been produced by organisations such as the International Committee of the Red Cross to identify remains of 'the missing' in conflict situations or through the excavation of mass graves.[135] Ethical aspects in such cases include ensuring that relatives who donate DNA are not given unrealistic expectations about what is achievable in individual cases, and consideration of how data will be made public.[136]

Practising procedures on newly deceased people

It is unlawful to carry out training procedures such as intubation on deceased people unless consent (or authorisation) has been received. As discussed on pages 515–516, the

HTA regulates the donation of bodies by individuals while still alive for education and training purposes.

Dealing with unusual requests

The BMA is occasionally asked about the acceptable limits of what may be done to a deceased person's body in order to conform with their advance wishes. Typical of this type of enquiry are concerns about the deceased person's former fear of being inadvertently buried alive or cremated while still living. In such cases, deceased patients may have left instructions that a vein should be opened or their heart removed prior to disposal of the body. In the past, such requests have sometimes been stimulated by media coverage of a misdiagnosis of death and 'recovery' of a patient in the mortuary. While alive, patients can be counselled about the improbability of this happening, but if such instructions have been left by a person now deceased, health professionals are often unsure how to handle them. In the past, complying with the patient's wish was not seen as problematic. Nevertheless, health professionals are more likely to have reservations after the impact made by the Shipman case (see page 496). Doctors who are willing to implement such wishes should take legal advice.

Cryonics is the practice of freezing the body of a deceased person in the belief that possible resuscitation might occur in the future when a cure has been found for the disease that caused the individual's death. This procedure is dependent upon unpredictable future technology and its history in the USA has been tainted by fraud and mismanagement. (One of the first organisations promoting the practice in the 1960s froze and stored a number of corpses underground but owing to financial mismanagement failed to keep them in a frozen condition.) Biological death is a process rather than a single event, which causes particular problems for this type of preservation. Deterioration at cellular level occurs in the hours after cessation of the heartbeat. People wishing to be preserved for possible reanimation request that cryopreservation procedures be initiated as soon as possible after the legal declaration of death to minimise deterioration of cells. Previously, all the organisations offering cryonic suspension services were in the USA; however, a Russian firm now offers cryonics services, reporting that, in 2005, it had two corpses in neurosuspension in storage.[137] Some European countries have legislation restricting the preservation of bodies, so some people make arrangements directly with American companies to circumvent such restrictions.

Legality of cryonics in Europe

In France in February 2002, Remy Martinot froze his father when he died at the age of 80. The father, Dr Raymond Martinot, had been a pioneer in the field of cryonics and had previously frozen his wife when she died of cancer in 1984. At that time, he had permission to bury her at the family's chateau but he had in fact injected anticoagulants into her veins and placed her body in a refrigerator. In March 2002, a French court ruled it illegal for bodies to be frozen for later reanimation and ordered that the frozen cadavers must be removed from their refrigerated chambers and either buried or cremated. In January 2006, France's highest administrative court, the Council of State, ordered M Martinot to either bury or cremate his parents. He had planned to take his case before the European Court of Human Rights before a technical fault in the freezer caused temperatures to rise and the bodies to thaw. Both bodies were removed and cremated.[138]

Ownership and trade in human bodies, body parts and tissue

While the Human Tissue Act 2004 and Human Tissue (Scotland) Act 2006 have provided legal clarity around the control and use of human tissue, neither Act directly addresses the question of ownership of the human body or whether a person owns bodily material once it has been removed. This legal debate is ongoing and an extensive literature exists on the subject. The common law does not recognise a notion of ownership of bodies or of human material as property, known as the 'no property in a corpse' principle, although relatives or executors and administrators of an estate have limited possessory rights to a corpse, mainly related to its burial or disposal.[139] Nevertheless, it is interesting to note that whole bodies or body parts that have been modified in some way may constitute property. The case of *R v Kelly* indicates at least that 'parts of a corpse are capable of being property . . . . if they have acquired different attributes by virtue of the application of skill, such as dissection or preservation techniques, for exhibiting or teaching purposes'.[140]

Limitations to the 'no property in a corpse' rule

In this case the Court of Appeal had to consider whether it was theft for a technician of the Royal College of Surgeons to remove body parts for use, and ultimately disposal, by an artist who wished to use them as moulds for his sculptures. The technician and the artist were charged with theft but argued that they could not be guilty because corpses, or parts of corpses, could not be property. However, as work had been carried out on the body parts in question, in that they had been preserved and used as specimens, the Court ruled that to remove them from the College, without authority, was theft. The Court went on to suggest that if body parts attracted a 'use or significance beyond their mere existence' they could become property.[141]

Herring and Chau suggest that the case law indicating that a part of the body can become property if it is subject to the exercise of work or skill will presumably apply to whole bodies. Otherwise, it would be difficult to explain why skilful preservation of a part of a body turns it into property, while that is not the case if the same thing is done to a whole corpse.[142]

Further confirmation of the limitations to the 'no property in a corpse' rule

In 2004, parents of three children brought legal proceedings against Leeds Teaching Hospital NHS Trust after it had emerged that the hospital removed and retained organs from their deceased children. The parents complained that the hospital improperly retained possession of the organs and also had failed to inform them of this possibility. The Court held that the parents could claim no possessory interest in the organs removed from their children. Following the *R v Kelly* case (see above), Mr Justice Gage confirmed that parts of a body may give rise to rights of possession provided sufficient skill and labour had been employed. It was stated that: '. . . .to dissect and fix an organ from a child's body requires work and a great deal of skill. . . . The subsequent production of blocks and slides is also a skilful operation requiring work and expertise of trained scientists.' In the case of each child, it was held that the post-mortem examinations were capable of generating rights of possession, on the part of the pathologist, to retained samples, rather than the parents of the deceased children.[143]

The ruling from Mr Justice Gage clarifies the existence of property rights in cadavers at common law, although it was made clear that it may have been different had the parents expressly requested the return of an organ when consenting to post-mortem examination.[144]

Trade in organs and tissue

In England, Wales and Northern Ireland, the Human Tissue Act 2004 prohibits 'trafficking' of human organs and tissue for transplantation.[145] It has been suggested that, with this exception, there is no reason in principle why human tissue could not be sold, or otherwise transferred in ownership, for activities such as research. The question also arises as to whether tissue samples can be sold for profit. Provision to prohibit any commercial use of tissue for research was initially included in the Human Tissue Bill. However, during the passage of the Bill it was decided that this would be impossible to implement and, as it did not appear to be a problem, the relevant clause was removed. The concerns expressed during the parliamentary debate on this clause centred on the fact that certain clinical research activities, such as indemnity payments to participants in clinical trials and payments to companies that sourced tissue for research projects legitimately carried out for profit, would become unlawful if the clause remained in the Bill.[146] Therefore, in order to avoid interference with commercial activities that had been lawfully carried out for many years, offences connected with the supply of human tissue for reward were confined to transplantable material only.

Although there is no legal restriction on the sale of tissue for research, there is good practice guidance which prevents it. Guidance from the Medical Research Council (MRC) states that neither donors nor researchers should sell samples for either cash or benefits in kind.[147] Although this is not binding on researchers, anyone who receives funding from the MRC is expected to comply with this guidance.

The law

Human Tissue Act 2004

The Human Tissue Act 2004 covers England, Wales and Northern Ireland and regulates the removal, storage and use of human material after death and the storage and use of human tissue from living individuals. It replaced, in England and Wales, the Human Tissue Act 1961, Anatomy Act 1984 and Human Organ Transplants Act 1989. In Northern Ireland it replaced the Human Tissue Act (Northern Ireland) 1962, Human Organ Transplants (Northern Ireland) Order 1989 and Anatomy (Northern Ireland) Order 1992. The Act also established the HTA to issue guidance about the legislation, to ensure best practice and to regulate, through a system of licensing, the following activities:

- both hospital post-mortem examinations and those carried out under the authority of a coroner
- the removal, use and storage of material, organs or tissue after death (except for whole and part organs for transplantation)
- anatomical examinations
- with some specific exceptions, storage of human bodies, body parts or human tissue;
- public display of bodies or human tissue removed after death.

At the time of writing, the Government was seeking to reallocate the functions of the HTA and abolish the regulatory body as part of its plan to reduce the number of arm's-length bodies. Up-to-date information on this can be found on the BMA website.

The Human Tissue (Quality and Safety for Human Application) Regulations 2007 made procurement, testing, processing, storage, import/export and distribution of tissues or cells for transplantation licensable activities. This applies, for example, to establishments that are collecting cord blood at birth, procuring bone marrow or developing stem cells for human application. (Detailed advice about the role of the HTA and more information about licensing can be found at: www.hta.gov.uk.)

The Human Tissue Act directly affects post-mortem services, anatomy schools, the transplant community, establishments storing tissue and sites displaying human material such as museums or exhibitions.

Consent

Consent is the central focus of the legislation and carrying out any of the activities covered by the legislation, without appropriate consent, is a criminal offence punishable by imprisonment, or a fine or both. Details of the specific requirements for consent in relation to different activities are covered earlier in this chapter (for material removed after death) and in Chapter 2 (living organ donation) and Chapter 14 (use of tissue from living individuals for research). The BMA also has separate guidance on the human tissue legislation.[148]

For anatomical examination and public display the individual's own written and witnessed consent is required and nobody else has the authority to give consent. For other uses of material removed after death, appropriate consent means:

- the individual's own consent given before death, or
- if the individual did not make a decision (to consent or not to consent) any person nominated by an adult to make decisions after death or, for a child, someone with parental responsibility, or
- if the adult did not nominate anyone and there is nobody with parental responsibility for a deceased child, someone who was in a 'qualifying relationship' with the individual before death.

The qualifying relatives ranked in order of priority are:

- spouse or partner, including civil partner
- parent or child
- brother or sister
- grandparent or grandchild
- niece or nephew
- stepfather or stepmother
- half-brother or half-sister
- friend of long-standing.

Relatives should be approached in order of priority. When there is more than one individual within a category, the consent of only one individual is required to proceed. The HTA's codes of practice make clear that the known wishes of the deceased individual take precedence over the views of relatives. Those nominated by, or who are close to the deceased, have no legal right of veto over the known wishes of the person who has died.[149]

There are some exceptions where the general rules on consent do not apply. Consent is not required where:

- an investigation into the cause of death is carried out under the authority of a coroner
- material removed from a person after death is stored for coroners' or criminal justice purposes
- the material used is classed as 'existing holdings' in that it was already in storage for a scheduled purpose on 1 September 2006, when the Act came into force
- residual tissue from living individuals is used anonymously for research that has approval from a research ethics authority or approval is pending
- the tissue has been imported or comes from a body that has been imported
- the tissue comes from the body of a person who died before 1 September 1906.

Human Tissue (Scotland) Act 2006

The Human Tissue (Scotland) Act 2006 replaced the provisions of the Human Tissue Act 1961 and amended the Anatomy Act 1984 as they applied to Scotland. It regulates the removal, storage and use of material removed from bodies after death. Unlike the English equivalent, the Act does not apply to the storage or use of material removed from living people (except for transplantation). The Scottish legislation did not set up a regulatory body to regulate this area. Under Regulations made under the Act, however, two tasks are delegated to the HTA (see above): regulation of the procurement, testing, processing, storage, import/export and distribution of tissue for human use (in order to comply with the EU Human Tissues and Cells Directive)[150] and living organ donation.[151]

The Act impacts upon the donation of material after death for transplantation, research, education or training and audit, the removal, retention and use following a post-mortem examination as well as anatomical examination and public display.

Authorisation

The Human Tissue (Scotland) Act focuses on authorisation (rather than consent) and carrying out any of the activities covered by the legislation, without the necessary authorisation, is a criminal offence punishable by imprisonment, or a fine or both. Details of the specific requirements for authorisation in relation to different activities are covered earlier in this chapter. The rules for living organ donation are the same throughout the UK and are covered in Chapter 2. The BMA also has separate guidance on the human tissue legislation.[152]

For anatomical examination and public display the individual's own written authorisation is required and nobody else can give authorisation. For other uses of material removed after death, the following rules apply.

Adults (over the age of 16):

- the adult's own authorisation given before death
- for hospital post-mortem examinations (and subsequent retention and use of organs), an individual may nominate one or more person to give authorisation after the individual has died
- if the individual has not given authorisation before death, or nominated an individual to authorise a post-mortem examination, the adult's nearest relative (see below) may give

authorisation provided he or she has no knowledge that the individual was unwilling for any part of the body to be used for the purposes proposed.

Children aged 12–16 years old:

- the child's own authorisation given before death
- for hospital post-mortem examinations (and subsequent retention and use of organs), a child may nominate one or more persons to give authorisation after the child has died
- if the child has not given authorisation before death or nominated an individual to authorise a post-mortem examination, a person with parental rights or responsibilities (but not a local authority) may give authorisation provided he or she has no knowledge that the child was unwilling for any part of the body to be used for the purposes proposed
- if the child had not given authorisation before death or nominated an individual and there is nobody with parental rights and responsibilities at the time of the child's death, the organs and tissue may not be removed, stored or used because nobody has the power to give authorisation.

Children under 12 years of age:

- a person with parental rights and responsibilities (but not a local authority)
- if there is nobody with parental rights and responsibilities at the time of the child's death the organs and tissue may not be removed, stored or used because nobody has the power to give authorisation.

The nearest relatives ranked in order of priority are:

- spouse or civil partner
- partner living with the adult in a relationship resembling a spouse or civil partner for at least 6 months
- child
- parent
- brother or sister
- grandparent
- grandchild
- uncle or aunt
- cousin
- niece or nephew
- friend of long-standing.

(This list is extended in relation to authorisation of the use of material removed at a post-mortem examination authorised by the procurator fiscal, to include 'a person who had a long-standing professional relationship with the adult'.)

The authorisation of only one person is required to proceed. The legislation explicitly states that nominated individuals or relatives cannot give authorisation if they know the individual was unwilling for any part of the body to be used for that purpose. It also states that priority should be given to transplantation and so, for example, an individual's authorisation for transplantation will override his or her expressed wish to donate his or her body for anatomical examination.

There are some exceptions where the general rules on authorisation do not apply. Authorisation is not required for:

- a post-mortem examination or any other activity carried out under the authority of the procurator fiscal
- retaining, as part of the medical record, tissue blocks and slides (not organs) following post-mortem examination and their use for diagnostic and audit purposes
- use of organs or tissues following post-mortem examination carried out before 1 September 2006 for diagnosis, audit, education and training and for existing research that has research ethics committee approval
- use of material in a collection that was held before 1 September 2006 for audit, education, training or research
- the use of material that was removed from the body of a person who died before 1 September 1906.

Anatomy Act 1984 (as amended)

In England, Wales and Northern Ireland, the Anatomy Act has been repealed and replaced by the Human Tissue Act 2004 (see above). In Scotland, the Act has been amended but remains in place enabling those over the age of 12 to bequeath their bodies for anatomical examination by dissection for teaching, study or research purposes. The request to donate must be made by the individual, in writing and witnessed. Establishments in Scotland undertaking anatomical examinations are licensed by HM Inspector of Anatomy.

Coroners and Justice Act 2009

The Coroners and Justice Act 2009, expected to come into force in April 2013, is divided into nine parts and covers a variety of different reforms. Part 1 reforms the law in relation to coroners and to the certification and registration of deaths. It replaces the existing framework for the investigation of certain deaths by coroners in the Coroners Act 1988 (the 1988 Act); that Act was a consolidation of existing coroner legislation, dating back to the early 1900s. In replacing the 1988 Act, Part 1 introduces a number of new concepts, the majority of which are contained within Chapter 2 of Part 1 of the Act, 'Notification, Certification and Registration of Deaths', where the following key changes are to take place over the coming years:

- requirement of medical practitioners to notify certain categories of death to a senior coroner
- introduction of the role of the medical examiner who will authorise burial or cremation
- regulations with regard to independent scrutiny and confirmation of MCCD
- unified certification process for both burial and cremation
- removal of cremation certification processes and associated forms
- removal of the role of the Cremation Referee
- introduction of a charter for the bereaved.

Access to Health Records Act 1990, Access to Health Records (Northern Ireland) Order 1993 and Data Protection Act 1998

Statutory rights of access to relevant parts of the deceased patient's health record by those with a claim arising out of the death are contained in the Access to Health Records Act 1990 and the Access to Health Records (Northern Ireland) Order 1993 (see Chapter 6, pages 259–260). The Data Protection Act 1998 does not extend to data relating to deceased people, although the BMA, the GMC and the Department of Health emphasise that the ethical obligation of confidentiality endures beyond the patient's death (see Chapter 5, pages 221–223).

Summary – the law

- In most circumstances, the law requires consent or authorisation for activities around the removal, use and storage of material from the deceased.
- Consent is not required for post-mortem examinations ordered by a coroner or procurator fiscal.
- MCCD are subject to scrutiny by the medical examiner (from April 2013).
- From April 2013, medical examiners provide authorisation for burial or cremation (unless further investigation is required).
- Those with a claim arising out of the death have a statutory right to access relevant parts of the medical record.

References

1   The Shipman Inquiry (2003) *Third Report: Death Certification and the Investigation of Deaths by Coroners*, The Shipman Inquiry, London.
2   Independent Review Group on Retention of Organs at Post Mortem (2001) *Retention of organs at post mortem: final report*, SEHD, Edinburgh, p.16. Brazier M. (2003) Organ retention and return: problems of consent. *J Med Ethics* **29**, 30–3.
3   Human Tissue Authority (2009) *Code of Practice 1: Consent*, HTA, London.
4   Human Tissue Authority (2009) *Code of Practice 1: Consent*, HTA, London, paras 97–100.
5   Human Tissue Authority (2007) *Code of Practice 8: Import and export of human bodies, body parts and tissue*, HTA, London.
6   Scottish Executive Health Department (2006) *Human Tissue (Scotland) Act 2006: A guide to its implications for NHS Scotland*, NHS HDL 46, SEHD, Edinburgh.
7   Human Tissue Authority (2009) *Code of Practice 1: Consent*, HTA, London, para 83.
8   Human Tissue Authority (2009) *Code of Practice 1: Consent*, HTA, London, paras 84–7.
9   Harris J. (2002) Law and regulation of retained organs: the ethical issues. *Legal Studies* **22**(4), 527–49, p.535.
10 McHaffie HE. (2001) *Crucial decisions at the beginning of life: Parents' experiences of treatment withdrawal from infants*. Radcliffe Medical Press, Oxford, p.409.
11 Anon. (2001) Hospital chapel used as mortuary for years. *BBC News Online* (31 January). Available at: www.bbc.co.uk/news (accessed 22 February 2011).
12 Jones DG. (2009) *Speaking for the dead: cadavers in biology and medicine*, Ashgate Dartmouth, Aldershot, p.22.
13 Richardson R, Hurwitz B. (1995) Donors' attitudes towards body donation for dissection. *Lancet* **346**, 277–9.
14 Brazier M. (2002) Retained organs: ethics and humanity. *Legal Studies* **22**, 550–69, p.561.
15 Lyon A. (2004) Perinatal autopsy remains the 'gold standard'. *Arch Dis Child Fetal Neonatal Ed* **89**, F284.
16 Richardson R. (2001) *Death, dissection and the destitute*, University of Chicago Press, Chicago.
17 Anon. (2002) Police report on public autopsy. *BBC News Online* (21 November). Available at: www.bbc.co.uk/news (accessed 2 February 2011).

18 Anon. (2005) Bill to clarify organ retention. *BBC News Online* (7 June). Available at: www.bbc.co.uk/news (accessed 2 February 2011).

19 Anon. (2009) Paris appeal court upholds ban on body parts show. *France24 Online* (1 May). Available at: www.france24.com (accessed 2 February 2011).

20 Jones DG. (2009) *Speaking for the dead: cadavers in biology and medicine*, Ashgate Dartmouth, Aldershot, p.22.

21 Jones DG. (2009) *Speaking for the dead: cadavers in biology and medicine*, Ashgate Dartmouth, Aldershot, p.4.

22 Jones DG. (2009) *Speaking for the dead: cadavers in biology and medicine*, Ashgate Dartmouth, Aldershot, p.53.

23 The Bristol Royal Infirmary Inquiry (2001) *The Report of the Public Inquiry into children's heart surgery at the Bristol Royal Infirmary 1984–1995: learning from Bristol*, (Cm 5207 (I)), The Stationery Office, London. The Royal Liverpool Children's Inquiry (2001) *The Royal Liverpool Children's Inquiry Report* (HC12-II), The Stationery Office, London. Independent Review Group on Retention of Organs at Post Mortem (2001) *Retention of organs at post mortem: final report*, Scottish Executive, Edinburgh. The Human Organs Inquiry (2002) *The human organs inquiry report*, DHSSPS, Belfast.

24 The Royal Liverpool Children's Inquiry (2001) *The Royal Liverpool Children's Inquiry report* (HC12-II), The Stationery Office, London.

25 Milburn A. (2001) Royal Liverpool Children's Inquiry. *House of Commons official report (Hansard)*, 30 January, col 175.

26 Department of Health (2001) *Report of a census of organs and tissues retained by pathology services in England*, The Stationery Office, London.

27 The Bristol Royal Infirmary Inquiry (2001) *The Report of the Public Inquiry into children's heart surgery at the Bristol Royal Infirmary 1984–1995: learning from Bristol*, (Cm 5207 (I)), The Stationery Office, London. The Royal Liverpool Children's Inquiry (2001) *The Royal Liverpool Children's Inquiry Report* (HC12-II), The Stationery Office, London. Independent Review Group on Retention of Organs at Post Mortem (2001) *Retention of organs at post mortem: final report*, Scottish Executive, Edinburgh. The Human Organs Inquiry (2002) *The human organs inquiry report,* DHSSPS, Belfast.

28 The Bristol Royal Infirmary Inquiry (2001) The Report of the Public Inquiry into children's heart surgery at the Bristol Royal Infirmary 1984–1995: learning from Bristol, (Cm 5207 (I)), The Stationery Office, London. The Royal Liverpool Children's Inquiry (2001) *The Royal Liverpool Children's Inquiry Report* (HC12-II), The Stationery Office, London. Independent Review Group on Retention of Organs at Post Mortem (2001) *Retention of organs at post mortem: final report*, Scottish Executive, Edinburgh.

29 Milburn A. (2001) Royal Liverpool Children's Inquiry. *House of Commons official report (Hansard)*, 30 January, col 177.

30 The Redfern Inquiry (2010) *The Redfern Inquiry into human tissue analysis in UK nuclear facilities*, The Stationery Office.

31 Department of Health, Welsh Assembly Government (2002) *Human bodies, human choices: the law on human organs and tissue in England and Wales: consultation report,* DH, London. Scottish Transplant Group (2002) *An organ donation strategy for Scotland. Scottish Transplant Group Report*, The Stationery Office, Edinburgh.

32 The Shipman Inquiry (2005) *Sixth Report – Shipman: The Final Report*, The Shipman Inquiry, London.

33 The Shipman Inquiry (2005) *Sixth Report – Shipman: The Final Report*, The Shipman Inquiry, London.

34 Department for Constitutional Affairs (2006) *Coroner Reform: The Government's Draft Bill: Improving death certification in England and Wales*, (Cm 6849), The Stationery Office, London.

35 Harris J. (2002) Law and regulation of retained organs: the ethical issues. *Leg Studies* **22**(4), 527–49.

36 Harris J. (2002) Law and regulation of retained organs: the ethical issues. *Leg Studies* **22**(4), 527–49, p.530

37 Human Tissue Authority (2009) *Code of Practice 1: Consent*, HTA, London, para 74.

38 Human Tissue Authority (2009) *Code of Practice 1: Consent*, HTA, London, para 76.

39 Brazier M. (2002) Retained organs: ethics and humanity. *Legal Studies* **22**, 550–69.

40 Cremation (England and Wales) Regulations 2008. SI 2008/2841, regulation 22.

41 General Medical Council (2009) *Confidentiality*, GMC, London, para 70.

42 Ministry of Justice (2009) *Charter for Bereaved People*, MoJ, London, para 10.

43 Cremation (England and Wales) Regulations 2008. SI 2008/2841, regulation 22.

44 World Health Organization (1999) *Ethical practice in laboratory medicine and forensic pathology*, WHO, Geneva.

45 General Medical Council (2006) *Good Medical Practice*, GMC, London, para 69.

46 The Coroners (Amendment) Rules 2008. SI 2008/1652. The agency receiving such a report will be required to give the coroner a written response stating what action has been taken, or an explanation of no action taken. Coroners must also provide the Lord Chancellor with a copy of the report and the response.

47   General Medical Council (2009) *Confidentiality*, GMC, London, para 71.
48   Office for National Statistics (2008) *Guidance for doctors completing Medical Certificates of Cause of Death in England and Wales*, ONS, Newport.
49   Nursing and Midwifery Council (2008) *Confirmation of death for registered nurses, Topic Advice Sheet*, NMC, London.
50   British Medical Association (2009) *Confirmation and certification of death: Guidance for GPs in England and Wales*, BMA, London.
51   Academy of Medical Royal Colleges (2008) *A code of practice for the diagnosis and confirmation of death*, AoMRC, London.
52   The Review of Coroner Services (2003) *Death Certification and Investigation in England, Wales, Northern Ireland: The report of a fundamental review 2003*, The Stationery Office, London, p.32.
53   The Review of Coroner Services (2003) *Death Certification and Investigation in England, Wales, Northern Ireland. The report of a fundamental review 2003*, The Stationery Office, London, p.10.
54   This is a condition of registration with the Care Quality Commission under the Health and Social Care Act 2008. Care Quality Commission (Registration) Regulations 2009. SI 2009/3112, regulation 17.
55   The doctor may certify death if he or she has seen the patient during the 14 days before death (28 days in Northern Ireland) or if he or she has seen the body after death. The Review of Coroner Services (2003) *Death Certification and Investigation in England, Wales, Northern Ireland: The report of a fundamental review 2003*, The Stationery Office, London, p.10.
56   The Review of Coroner Services (2003) *Death Certification and Investigation in England, Wales, Northern Ireland: The report of a fundamental review 2003*, The Stationery Office, London, pp.32–3.
57   Regulations and guidance are yet to be produced clarifying which deaths should be reported to the coroner. The national guidance will form the basis of the list of reportable deaths, and will be framed in secondary legislation and associated guidance under the Act.
58   Crown Office and Procurator Fiscal Service (2008) *Death and the procurator fiscal: Information and guidance for medical practitioners*, Crown Office and Procurator Fiscal Service, Edinburgh.
59   Crown Office and Procurator Fiscal Service (2008) *Death and the procurator fiscal: Information and guidance for medical practitioners*, Crown Office and Procurator Fiscal Service, Edinburgh, pp.4–6.
60   Further information on the process of death certification is available on the Department of Health website: www.dh.gov.uk (accessed 21 April 2011).
61   Department of Health (2010) *Improving the process of death certification in England and Wales: overview of programme*, DH, London.
62   Cremation (England and Wales) Regulations 2008. SI 2008/2841, regulation 22.
63   The cremation process involves forms being completed by the treating doctor, a second (independent) medical practitioner and a third medical practitioner (medical referee) based at the crematorium.
64   The Review of Coroner Services (2003) *Death Certification and Investigation in England, Wales, Northern Ireland (2003), The Report of a Fundamental Review 2003*, The Stationery Office, London.
65   Scottish Government (2008) *Burial and Cremation Review Group: Report and Recommendations*, Scottish Government, Edinburgh.
66   Scottish Government (2008) *Burial and Cremation Review Group: Report and Recommendations*, Scottish Government, Edinburgh, para 17.
67   Human Tissue Authority (2009) *Code of Practice 3: Post-mortem examination*, HTA, London.
68   Human Tissue Authority (2009) *Code of Practice 3: Post-mortem examination*, HTA, London, para 32.
69   Human Tissue Authority (2009) *Code of Practice 3: Post-mortem examination*, HTA, London, paras 32 and 97.
70   Coroners (Amendment) Rules 2005. SI 2005/420.
71   Human Tissue Authority (2009) *Code of Practice 3: Post-mortem examination*, HTA, London, para 87.
72   Human Tissue Authority (2009) *Code of Practice 5: Disposal of human tissue*, HTA, London, paras 57–85. Scottish Executive Health Department (2006) *Human Tissue (Scotland) Act 2006: A guide to its implications for NHS Scotland*. *NHS HDL (2006) 46*, SEHD, Edinburgh, paras 54–5.
73   Human Tissue Authority (2009) *HTA regulatory action at University Hospital Wales. Information for members of the public*, HTA, London.
74   Human Tissue Authority (2009) *Mortuary facilities at the University Hospital of Wales*. Press release, 18 August.
75   Human Tissue Authority (2009) *Summary of Compliance 2008/09. Regulating the post-mortem sector*, HTA, London.
76   Human Tissue Authority (2010) *Directions relating to the making of a post-mortem examination; the removal from the body of a deceased person (otherwise than in the course of carrying out an anatomical examination or making a post-mortem) of relevant material, for use for a Scheduled Purpose other than transplantation; and the storage of the body of a deceased person, or relevant material which has come from a human body, for use for a Scheduled Purpose. Ref 001/2010*, HTA, London.

77 Human Tissue Authority (2010) *Directions relating to the making of a post-mortem examination; the removal from the body of a deceased person (otherwise than in the course of carrying out an anatomical examination or making a post-mortem) of relevant material, for use for a Scheduled Purpose other than transplantation; and the storage of the body of a deceased person, or relevant material which has come from a human body, for use for a Scheduled Purpose. Ref 002/2010*, HTA, London.

78 National Confidential Enquiry into Patient Outcome and Death (2006) *The Coroner's Autopsy: Do we deserve better?*, NCEPOD, London. Statement by Peter Furness. Available at: www.ncepod.org.uk (accessed 2 February 2011).

79 National Confidential Enquiry into Patient Outcome and Death (2006) *The Coroner's Autopsy: Do we deserve better?*, NCEPOD, London. Statement by Peter Furness. Available at: www.ncepod.org.uk (accessed 2 February 2011).

80 National Confidential Enquiry into Patient Outcome and Death (2006) *The Coroner's Autopsy: Do we deserve better?*, NCEPOD, London. Statement by Peter Furness. Available at: www.ncepod.org.uk (accessed 2 February 2011).

81 Confidential Enquiry into Maternal and Child Health (2007) *Perinatal Mortality 2007*, CEMACH, London, p.46.

82 Confidential Enquiry into Maternal and Child Health (2007) *Perinatal Mortality 2007*, CEMACH, London, p.46.

83 Seale C, Kirk D, Tobin M. *et al.* (2005) Effect of media portrayals of removal of children's tissue on UK tumour bank. *BMJ* **331**, 401–3.

84 Perkins GD, McAuley DF, Davies S. *et al.* (2003) Discrepancies between clinical and post-mortem diagnoses in critically ill patients: an observational study *Critical Care*. **7**, R129–32.

85 Murphy C. (2009) Organ scandal legacy lives on. *BBC News Online* (23 June). Available at: www.bbc.co.uk/news (accessed 22 February 2011).

86 National Institute for Health and Clinical Excellence. *NHS Clinical Knowledge Summary: Postmortems.* Available at: www.cks.nhs.uk (accessed 2 February 2011).

87 Human Tissue Authority (2009) *Code of Practice 3: Post-mortem examination*, HTA, London, para 13.

88 Laing I, Becher JC. (2006) The Role of Neonatal Necropsy Today: A Scottish Perspective. *NeoReviews* **7**, e177–e182.

89 Confidential Enquiry into Maternal and Child Health (2007) *Perinatal Mortality 2007*, CEMACH, London, p.44.

90 Elder D, Zuccullo J. (2005) Autopsy after death due to extreme prematurity. *Arch Dis Child* **90**, F270–F272, p.F270.

91 Dyer C. (2005) Pathologist in Sally Clark case suspended from court work. *BMJ* **330**, 1347.

92 Royal College of Pathologists, Royal College of Paediatrics and Child Health (2004) *Sudden unexpected death in infancy*, RCPath, London.

93 National Patient Safety Agency (2005) *Reducing the harm caused by misplaced nasogatric feeding tubes: Patient safety alert 0180*, NPSA, London.

94 Thayyil S. (2011) Less invasive autopsy: an evidence based approach. *Arch Dis Child* **96**, 681–7. A recent study in the *Lancet* also confirms that the traditional autopsy should be encouraged. Whitby E. (2009) Minimally invasive autopsy. *Lancet* **374**, 432–3.

95 For example, Thayyil S, O'Cleary J, Sebire N. *et al*. (2009) Postmortem examination of human fetuses: a comparison of whole-body high-field MRI at 9.4 T with conventional MRI and invasive autopsy. *Lancet* **374**, 467–75.

96 Thayyil S. (2011) Less invasive autopsy: an evidence based approach. *Arch Dis Child* **96**, 681–7.

97 Weustink A, Hunick MG, van Dijke CF. *et al*. (2009) Minimally invasive autopsy: an alternative to conventional autopsy? *Radiology* **250**, 897–904.

98 Human Tissue Authority (2009) *Code of practice 2: Donation of solid organs for transplantation*, HTA, London.

99 For more information and up-to-date statistics see: NHS Blood and Transplant, www.organdonation.nhs.uk (accessed 18 May 2011).

100 Murphy C, Carter C. (2009) *Potential donor audit: summary report for the 24 month period 1 April 2007–31 March 2009*, NHS Blood and Transplant, Bristol.

101 Department of Health (2008) *Organs for Transplants: a report from the Organ Donation Taskforce*, DH, London.

102 Keogh B. (2008) *Letter to all Trust Chief Executives – Organ Donation Taskforce – "Organs for Transplants" Implementation of the Organ Donation Taskforce Recommendations (Gateway Ref: 9693)*, DH, London.

103 Department of Health (2009) *Working together to save lives: The Organ Donation Taskforce Implementation Programme's Annual Report 2008/09*, DH, London.

104 Department of Health (2009) *Working together to save lives: The Organ Donation Taskforce Implementation Programme's Annual Report 2008/09*, DH, London, p.3.

105 NHS Blood and Transplant (2011) *Major milestone in organ donation*. Press release, 21 January.

106   One of the recommendations of the Taskforce was to provide guidance for coroners to strengthen local protocols and optimise organ donation. The guidance for England and Wales, published in 2010, was developed with stakeholders including the Human Tissue Authority, NHS Blood and Transplant, coroners and the transplant community. Department of Health (2010) *Organ and Tissue Donation. An aide memoire for coroners*, MoJ, London.

107   Donaldson L. (2007) *2006 Annual Report of the Chief Medical Officer: On the state of Public Health*, DH, London, pp.26–33.

108   Foster K. (2007) Chief medic backs our campaign for new organ donor law. *The Scotsman* (7 October). Available at: news.scotsman.com (accessed 18 May 2011).

109   Brown G. (2008) Organ donations help us make a difference. *The Telegraph* (13 January). Available at: www.telegraph.co.uk (accessed 18 May 2011).

110   Organ Donation Taskforce (2008) *The potential impact of an opt-out system for organ donation in the UK: An independent report from the Organ Donation Taskforce*, Organ Donation Taskforce, London, p.5.

111   Gimbel RW, Strosberg MS, Lehrman SE. *et al.* (2003) Presumed consent and other predictors of cadaveric organ donation in Europe. *Progress in Transplantation* **13**, 17–23. Abadie A, Gay S. (2006) The impact of presumed consent legislation on cadaveric organ donation: a cross-country study. *J Health Economics* **25**, 599–620.

112   Rithalia A, McDaid C, Suekarran S. *et al.* (2008) A systematic review of presumed consent systems for deceased organ donation. In: Organ Donation Taskforce *The potential impact of an opt-out system for organ donation in the UK: A report from the Organ Donation Taskforce – Supporting Information*, Organ Donation Taskforce, London, Annexes A–N: Annex I.

113   Rithalia A, McDaid C, Suekarran S. *et al.* (2008) A systematic review of presumed consent systems for deceased organ donation. In: Organ Donation Taskforce *The potential impact of an opt-out system for organ donation in the UK: A report from the Organ Donation Taskforce*, Organ Donation Taskforce, London, p.64.

114   British Medical Association (2007) *Support grows for presumed consent*. Press release, 19 October.

115   Organ Donation Taskforce (2008) *The potential impact of an opt-out system for organ donation in the UK: An independent report from the Organ Donation Taskforce*, Organ Donation Taskforce, London, p.26.

116   Welsh Assembly Government (2009) *Options for changes to the organ donation system in Wales: Consultation report*, WAG, Cardiff.

117   Anon. (2009) Parkinson's plea for brain donors. *BBC News Online* (20 April). Available at: www.bbc.co.uk/news (accessed 2 December 2009).

118   Human Tissue Authority (2009) *Code of Practice 9: Research*, HTA, London.

119   Human Tissue Act 2004, s 3(3)-(5). Human Tissue (Scotland) Act 2006, s 53(5).

120   Human Tissue Authority, *How to donate your body*. Available at: www.hta.gov.uk (accessed 25 May 2011).

121   Human Tissue Authority (2011) *Model consent forms*. Available at: www.hta.gov.uk (accessed 25 May 2011).

122   Human Tissue Authority (2009) *Code of Practice 4: Anatomical examination*, HTA, London.

123   Human Tissue Authority (2009) *Code of Practice 7: Public display*, HTA, London, para 18.

124   Human Tissue Authority (2009) *Code of Practice 7: Public display*, HTA, London.

125   Department for Culture, Media and Sport (2005) *Guidance for the Care of Human Remains in Museums*, DCMS, London.

126   Human Tissue Authority (2009) *Code of Practice 7: Public display*, HTA, London.

127   Human Tissue Authority (2009) *Code of practice 5: Disposal of Human Tissue*, HTA, London.

128   NHS Blood and Transplant (2004) *UK policy for management of potential organ/tissue donors with confirmed positive virology results*, NHSBT, Bristol, paras 8.1–8.4.

129   NHS Blood and Transplant (2004) *UK policy for management of potential organ/tissue donors with confirmed positive virology results*, NHSBT, Bristol, para 8.4.

130   Human Tissue Authority (2009) *Code of Practice 1: Consent*, HTA, London, para 155.

131   Human Tissue Authority (2009) *Code of Practice 1: Consent*, HTA, London, para 155.

132   Human Tissue Authority (2009) *Code of Practice 1: Consent*, HTA, London, para 155.

133   Human Tissue Authority (2009) *Code of Practice 1: Consent*, HTA, London, para 154.

134   British Medical Association (1998) *Human genetics: choice and responsibility*, Oxford University Press, Oxford.

135   International Committee of the Red Cross (2009) *Missing people, DNA analysis and identification of human remains*, ICRC, Geneva.

136   British Medical Association (2001) *The medical profession and human rights: handbook for a changing agenda*, Zed Books, London, ch 6.

137   Saxer M. (2006) *A Cryonics Society News Brief: May 2006*, Cryonics Society. Available at: www.cryonicssociety.org (accessed 9 February 2011).

138   Anon. (2006) Frenchman cremates frozen parents. *BBC News Online* (16 March). Available at: www.bbc.co.uk/news (accessed 2 February 2011).

139   *Dobson v North Tyneside Health Authority* [1996] 4 All ER 741.
140   *R v Kelly* [1998] 3 All ER 741:749.
141   *R v Kelly* [1998] 3 All ER 741: 750.
142   Herring J, Chau PL. (2007) My body, your body, our bodies. *Med Law Rev* **15**, 34–61.
143   *AB v Leeds Teaching Hospital NHS Trust* [2005] Q.B. 506: para 135.
144   *AB v Leeds Teaching Hospital NHS Trust* [2005] Q.B. 506: para 161.
145   Human Tissue Act 2004, s 32.
146   Winterton R. (2004) Human Tissue Bill Report Stage. *House of Commons official report (Hansard)*, 28 June, col 115.
147   Medical Research Council (2001) *Human tissue and biological samples for use in research*, MRC, London, p.3.
148   British Medical Association (2009) *Human Tissue Legislation: Guidance from the BMA Medical Ethics Department*, BMA, London.
149   Human Tissue Authority (2009) *Code of Practice 1: Consent*, HTA, London, para 75. Human Tissue Authority (2009) *Code of Practice 2: Donation of solid organs for transplantation*, HTA, London, para 100.
150   The Human Tissue (Quality and Safety for Human Application) Regulations 2007. SI 2007/1523.
151   The Human Organ and Tissue Live Transplants (Scotland) Regulations 2006. SI 2006/390.
152   British Medical Association (2009) *Human Tissue Legislation: Guidance from the BMA Medical Ethics Department*, BMA, London.

13: Prescribing and administering medication

The questions covered in this chapter include the following.

- Who is ultimately responsible for shared prescribing decisions?
- How should doctors respond to patients' requests for particular medication?
- What, if any, hospitality may be accepted from pharmaceutical companies?
- Should doctors prescribe for patients they have not seen?
- Should doctors inform patients about medication that could help them but is not available within the NHS?

The challenges and dilemmas

Changes within the doctor–patient relationship, in the health service and in knowledge and technology, continue to lead to new challenges and dilemmas in relation to prescribing. The traditional dilemmas – conflicts of interest, resource allocation, relations with pharmaceutical companies and pressures on doctors' independence in prescribing – remain, but many of these have taken on increased importance or greater prominence. This has been partly the result of patients becoming more informed, sometimes asking doctors to prescribe particular drugs or treatments, the rise of so-called 'lifestyle drugs', and the increasingly consumerist attitude towards healthcare. Changes in the role of pharmacists and nurses have not only required modifications in traditional methods of working, but have also increased the frequency of shared prescribing, which can cause tension and raise questions of responsibility and liability for prescribing decisions.

Prescribed medicine is the most common form of NHS intervention. In recent years, there has been a significant shift towards prescribing preventative treatments and in managing long-term conditions with medication. The rising prescription bill across the UK means that supporting patient adherence in taking medicines remains important, not only for individual health but also for economic reasons. The cost of providing access to the latest medicines within such limited resources means that rationing decisions will increasingly shape which treatments are made available within the NHS in the future.

The rapid increase in knowledge and technology over the last decade has affected not only the range of products available, but also the way in which they are provided. Developments in information technology have offered an alternative to the traditional face-to-face consultation by introducing consultations and prescribing via the internet so that the doctor and the patient may never meet and may be in different towns, or even in different countries. Increasingly, patients are also able to obtain access to prescription-only medication over the internet, sometimes without a valid prescription, which can raise a number of challenges for doctors. Further changes are expected as knowledge develops

Medical Ethics Today: The BMA's Handbook of Ethics and Law, Third Edition. Sophie Brannan, Eleanor Chrispin, Martin Davies, Veronica English, Rebecca Mussell, Julian Sheather and Ann Sommerville.
© 2012 BMA Medical Ethics Department. Published 2012 by Blackwell Publishing Ltd.

of the part that genetic factors play in the success or otherwise of particular medicines. Pharmacogenetics may change significantly the way in which medication is prescribed in the longer term and it is important for doctors to be aware of the type of dilemmas that may arise. This chapter discusses the issues raised by such changes and offers practical advice.

General principles

The following general principles apply in relation to prescribing.

- The doctor who signs a prescription accepts clinical and legal responsibility for the decision.
- Doctors should prescribe medication only when they have sufficient knowledge and experience to be satisfied that it is appropriate for the patient.
- If the prescribing doctor is not the patient's GP, he or she should communicate with the GP, unless the patient objects, in order to avoid any conflict with existing treatment.
- Doctors must not ask for or accept any inducement, gift or hospitality from pharmaceutical companies or others that may affect, or be seen to affect, their judgement.
- It is generally unwise for doctors who prescribe to form business connections with companies that produce, market or promote pharmaceutical products.

Responsibility for prescribing

A major part of medical practice is prescribing medicines, products and treatments. Deciding which medication to prescribe for which patient and in what dose is a matter of clinical judgement based on training, experience and published guidance, which reflect the evidence base on factors such as efficacy, safety and cost. Decisions are made on the basis of appropriateness, effectiveness, safety and economy. The range of drugs available is constantly changing, so it is important that doctors keep up to date with new products and guidance through regularly updated resources, such as the latest available edition of the *British National Formulary (BNF)*,[1] and authoritative guidance from national advisory bodies (where available) and other organisations, such as the National Prescribing Centre.

Prescribing doctors accept absolute clinical and legal responsibility for their prescribing decisions and must be prepared to justify them if called upon to do so. Doctors should therefore prescribe medication only when they have sufficient knowledge and experience to be satisfied that it is appropriate for the patient, and where they are willing to accept this responsibility. This can sometimes prove difficult when prescribing is shared between a GP and a specialist (see pages 557–562) or when a patient requests a particular form of medication that is unfamiliar to the doctor. If the prescribing doctor is not the patient's GP, he or she should ensure that the prescription does not conflict with any other treatment provided to the patient. In some cases this may involve liaison with the patient's GP, with the patient's consent. If the patient refuses consent to the GP being consulted, then this should be respected. Whether the doctor should go on to prescribe in the absence of that information is a matter of clinical judgement and is likely to depend on the risks of the particular drug to be prescribed. If patients have not been referred by a GP, doctors should ask for patients' consent to inform their GP before starting treatment, except in emergencies or when this is impractical.[2] Prescribing out of hours can present problems to doctors because of a lack of access to patient records.

Prescribing and pandemic flu

In national emergencies, the normal routes through which patients access treatment and medication can come under severe pressure. During the 2009 H1N1 pandemic, there was a significant increase in demand for primary care services throughout the UK and particularly in England, as surgeries coped with high numbers of patients presenting with influenza-like symptoms. In response to this demand, the Government in England introduced the National Pandemic Flu Service (NPFS) which was designed to relieve the pressure on primary care services and ensure that patients were able to access both assessment and medication quickly. The service represented a radical departure from normal prescribing practice. Where previously patients would be prescribed antiviral drugs following assessment by a clinician, typically a GP, under the NPFS patients were assessed either over the phone or online using an algorithm. Patients assessed as suffering with pandemic flu were allocated a unique identifying number with which they could acquire antiviral medication at one of the 2000 collection points set up throughout the country. In England, the NPFS ran for roughly 6 months. Over the course of the outbreak, over 2 million assessments were completed and over a million courses of antiviral treatments were distributed.[3]

The devolved administrations in Wales and Northern Ireland relied on public messaging and national helplines to relieve the burden on services and medication was distributed following consultation with a patient's GP. Similarly in Scotland, the Scottish Flu Response Centre was set up to provide advice and guidance to the public and health professionals. The majority of cases were handled through normal primary care routes, although some health boards did set up collection points to deal with large increases in numbers and the pressures on services this created. The methods of accessing medication implemented through the NPFS were controversial. A year after the outbreak, the Patients Association raised concerns about the service after figures, obtained through a freedom of information request, indicated that a significant proportion of patients who accessed antiviral medication did not test positive for the virus.[4]

In addition to the clinical and legal responsibilities of prescribing, doctors are also under a professional duty to prescribe in an appropriate and responsible manner. The General Medical Council (GMC) sets out the standards expected of doctors in relation to prescribing in *Good Medical Practice*[5] and supplementary guidance, *Good Practice in Prescribing Medicines*.[6] The GMC states that doctors should only prescribe drugs or treatment when they have 'adequate knowledge of the patient's health, and are satisfied that the drugs or treatment serve the patient's needs'.[7]

Failings in relation to prescribing

In 2002, a doctor was found guilty by the GMC of serious professional misconduct for a series of failings in relation to his prescribing of phentermine (the licence for which had been withdrawn in May 2001) to three women attending his private slimming clinic. It was found that his decision to prescribe this drug had been inappropriate, unjustified, not in the best interests of the patients and contrary to accepted medical practice. In addition, it was found that he had failed to:

- adequately, or at all, warn of the dangers of taking phentermine, in particular when it was an unlicensed drug
- take and record an adequate physical examination
- properly or adequately discuss the nature of obesity, its dangers or levels of severity
- enquire as to the identity of the patients' GPs and/or advise the patients of the benefits and importance of keeping their GPs informed of the treatment and seeking their agreement to do so
- properly discuss or make arrangements for adequate follow-up review or treatment
- record the dosage of phentermine.

The doctor's registration was restricted to practice within the NHS, and not in a single-handed general practice either as a principal or a locum, for a period of 3 years.[8]

Prescribing off-label and unlicensed drugs

Doctors have long had the clinical freedom to prescribe unlicensed drugs or drugs for use outside the terms of their license (off-label). Prescribing in these circumstances, however, can carry additional risks. The licensing process, carried out by the Medicines and Healthcare Products Regulatory Agency (MHRA) in the UK or Europe-wide by the European Medicines Agency (EMA), tests the safety, efficacy and quality of drugs for a specific indication and ensures that they are manufactured to appropriate quality standards. Doctors therefore arguably take on greater responsibility when prescribing drugs that have not undergone these rigorous checks. Prescribing drugs off-label is relatively common and often necessary in certain specialities, such as paediatrics (see pages 543–544). The level of risk involved can depend on whether the prescription constitutes established practice and how it deviates from the terms of the licence (different indication, changes to dose, formulation, etc.).

GMC guidance[9] emphasises that decisions to prescribe off-label or unlicensed medicine should be based on sufficient evidence and/or experience of using the medicine that demonstrates its safety and efficacy, taking into account the availability of alternative, appropriately licensed medication. Doctors must take responsibility for the prescription and for overseeing the patient's care, including monitoring and follow-up treatment. Where a prescription deviates from established practice, doctors should record in the patient's notes the reasons for choosing the medication.

Given the potential risks involved in prescribing in these circumstances, doctors are, in most cases, required to explain to patients the reasons behind the decision and obtain and document their consent. GMC guidance advises that doctors 'must explain the reasons for prescribing a medicine that is unlicensed or being used outside the scope of its licence where there is little research or other evidence of current practice to support its use, or the use of the medicine is innovative'.[10] Where drugs are used routinely outside the scope of their licence it may not be necessary to draw attention to the licence when obtaining consent, but doctors should ensure they provide patients or their proxies with as much information as they want or may see as significant to enable them to make an informed decision.

Prescribing drugs off-label for economic reasons

Although prescribing off-label is typically done when there is no suitably licensed alternative, there are cases where doctors may have a choice between prescribing a drug off-label or prescribing an appropriately licensed alternative for the same indication. As there can sometimes be large differences in price between the two, there is the potential for cost to become a factor in determining which drug to prescribe. Although a doctor's primary duty is to individual patients, doctors also have a responsibility to use NHS resources cost-effectively across the whole population of patients they treat. Prescribing a drug off-label over a licensed alternative based in part on economic considerations, however, has the potential to raise ethical issues, because the best interests of the patient are no longer motivating the decision. Patients typically expect to be prescribed the safest and most clinically effective treatment available within the NHS for their condition. It could be argued that a drug prescribed off-label is a suboptimal product when compared with an approved drug that has undergone the rigorous tests involved in the licensing process.

There are several examples of off-label prescribing in current medical practice that are motivated in part by the savings that can be made compared with prescribing a licensed alternative. These arise either as the result of the recommendations of guidance from advisory bodies, such as the National Institute for Health and Clinical Excellence (NICE), or from existing practice (see box below). Ideally, all drugs would go through the licensing process for all possible indications and, where needed, be evaluated via a NICE technology appraisal or similar (see pages 552–554). Only companies that market a drug can apply for it to be licensed however, and the cost and time involved in the process can mean that often there is insufficient commercial incentive for companies who market a particular drug to extend the licence for a different indication.

Avastin and Lucentis

A high-profile example of prescribing off-label for cost reasons is the reported off-label use of Avastin (bevacizumab) in the treatment of wet age-related macular degeneration (wet AMD) in preference to Lucentis (ranibizumab), which is licensed to treat the condition. Bevacizumab is approved for the treatment of certain cancers. However, before the licensing approval of ranibizumab, it was used off-label to treat wet AMD. NICE and the Scottish Medicines Consortium (SMC) technology appraisals both recommend the use of ranibizumab in the NHS, therefore removing any restrictions from commissioning bodies on the availability of the drug. However, the practice of prescribing bevacizumab for wet AMD continued overseas, in private practice and reportedly by some NHS trusts,[11] due to the considerable differences in the cost of treatment for the two drugs; £750 per dose for ranibizumab compared with just £50 per dose for bevacizumab.[12] In 2009, the Royal College of Ophthalmologists stated that, because of the lack of data regarding the dose, dose frequency and the medium to long-term safety and efficacy for the drug, it could not recommend the routine use of intravitreal bevacizumab for wet AMD while other licensed and NICE-approved medicines were available.[13]

In 2010, NICE, which rarely conducts single technology appraisals of unlicensed drugs, carried out a stakeholder review into the feasibility of conducting an appraisal of bevacizumab for wet AMD.[14] Roche, who own Genentech, the company that devloped both Lucentis and Avastin, confirmed in its evidence submission that the decision not to develop bevacizumab in wet AMD was taken on the basis of 'corporate considerations' and that there were no plans to apply for a licence in the future. Despite concerns that a licence holder would not be involved in the process, the report concluded that there was support for an appraisal of intravitreal bevacizumab for eye conditions, dependent on regulatory involvement in assessing its safety and quality.

The British Medical Association (BMA) advises that doctors should only prescribe off-label in preference to an appropriately licensed alternative medication, on cost grounds, where authoritative clinical guidance, such as that from NICE for example, exists.

Prescribing errors

Medication errors can occur in all areas of medical practice and different healthcare settings. In 2007, there were 86,085 medication incidents reported to the National Patient Safety Agency (NPSA) in England and Wales.[15] The incidents occurred at the prescribing, dispensing and administration stages of the process and the majority resulted in clinical outcomes of low harm or no harm. Of the 100 serious incidents reported to the NPSA – those involving serious harm or death – 32 per cent were caused by errors in prescribing.

Common prescribing errors

In a survey of 1000 clinical negligence claims against GPs, 193 prescribing errors were identified.[16] The four most common errors were:

- a failure to warn about or recognise drug side effects
- errors in medication or prescribing
- a problem associated with an injection
- incorrect or inappropriate medication.

In 2006, senior pharmacologists raised concerns that changes to the way pharmacology was taught in medical schools and a reduction in the number of teaching hours dedicated to the subject, had led to an increase in the number of prescribing errors made by junior doctors.[17] The complexity of modern pharmacology and system failures, such as the lack of a universal nationwide inpatient prescribing sheet, were also highlighted as contributory factors to the high prevalence of prescribing errors.

The GMC commissioned an in-depth study into the prevalence of medication errors which focused on foundation trainees and the potential link between the errors and failings within undergraduate medical education.[18] The study found that trainees reported deficiencies in their medical education with respect to prescribing and clinical pharmacology, and particularly with respect to linking theory with practice. However, the study also found that prescribing errors were the result of a range of interconnected factors including the complexity of the system in which prescribing errors were made, issues related to the working environment and the interaction and communication within the medical team. Although foundation year two doctors had the highest rates of prescribing errors, the study found that medication errors occurred across all grades, including consultants. The study recommended a number of changes to undergraduate medical training, foundation year one education and higher specialist training, but also suggested ways to improve the clinical working environment to help reduce prescribing errors in the future.

Although the primary responsibility for ensuring prescriptions are correct lies with the prescriber, nurses and pharmacists also have a vital role in checking prescriptions and picking up errors. Electronic prescribing systems, used mostly in primary care, can also help reduce errors at all stages of the prescribing process by, for example, giving doctors access to Clinical Decision Support systems to help identify potential drug interactions or patient allergies.

Summary – responsibility for prescribing

- Doctors who prescribe accept full clinical and legal responsibility for any prescribing decisions.
- Where doctors do not feel they have sufficient knowledge or experience to be satisfied that the treatment is appropriate they should not prescribe.
- Doctors can prescribe unlicensed medicines and drugs to be used outside the terms of their licence but take on greater responsibilities when doing so, particularly when a course of treatment is innovative or there is little evidence to support its use.

- Prescribing off-label where alternative licensed medication exists for economic reasons should only be done when recommended by authoritative guidance from bodies such as NICE.

Providing information to patients about medication

Patients should be offered sufficient information about any products they are prescribed to enable them to make informed decisions. Doctors should offer patients information about the benefits and risks of the medication prescribed – including any side effects, complications or potential that the medication will fail to achieve the desired aim – and inform the patient of any alternatives available. Where medication is administered to patients, as with other forms of treatment, valid consent is required (consent issues are covered in more detail in Chapter 2). The amount of information patients need depends upon a range of factors including the diagnosis, prognosis, the type of medication proposed, the level of risk associated with it and the amount of information the patient is willing and able to accept. Doctors need to have up-to-date knowledge of effectiveness, safety and cost, and possess good communication skills in order to assist individual patients in making informed choices about treatment. (Communication with patients is discussed in greater detail in Chapter 1, pages 33–39.)

Information should be comprehensible to individual patients, with special attention given to the needs of those who may require particular assistance, such as older people with hearing difficulties and people for whom English is not their first language. If serious doubts exist over a patient's capacity to understand a prescription or significant information relating to it, a mental capacity test should be carried out. (For general discussion of mental capacity, see Chapter 3.) Written patient information leaflets must be provided for all marketed medication. Where the product is prescribed and dispensed as an original pack, then this is not a problem but, when the dispensing requires the pack to be split, it is sometimes difficult in practice always to supply either an original information leaflet or a copied version. Medicines used in hospitals fall into a special category and so medication dispensed for inpatients does not require an information leaflet to be provided, but one should be held either in the pharmacy or on the ward.[19] This is also a problem for GPs who are administering medication out of hours. Even when written information is given to patients, this does not diminish the duty of doctors to discuss the medication with them and to answer any questions except in emergencies when this may not be feasible. The primary responsibility for informing patients about prescribed medicines and how they are to be taken rests with the prescribing doctor. Pharmacists also have a role in providing information to patients about prescription drugs as well as over-the-counter medicines.

Medicines adherence and involving patients in 'concordance'

Medicines adherence is defined as the extent to which a patient's behaviour matches agreed recommendations from the prescriber. Patient non-adherence is common, with many patients either not taking a course of treatment as directed, failing to complete the full course of treatment or not taking their medication at all. There are various estimates as to the extent of the problem, but it is thought that between one-third and half of medication for long-term conditions is not taken as recommended.[20] It can affect all therapy areas, from treatment for asthma to post-transplantation care, and levels of adherence can vary between treatment types and different patient groups. Serious health problems can result from patients not taking their medication correctly or consistently and this can impact on NHS resources. A significant proportion of avoidable medicine-related illnesses treated in UK hospitals are the result of patients not using their medications as recommended. NICE estimated that in 2006–2007 the cost of these admissions to the NHS was between £36 million and £196 million.[21]

Historically, a key factor in non-adherence has been the unpleasant side effects and complications associated with different drugs, which can discourage patients from keeping up with their drug regimen. Despite advances in pharmacology and the subsequent availability of new drugs that have significantly reduced the number of side effects and improved the convenience of medicine taking, patients still do not take their medicine as advised, even where there may be life-threatening consequences.[22] Patients can have complex but coherent sets of beliefs about medicines and illnesses and it is recognised that a number of factors can lead to a patient not taking their medicines as directed. These can be said to fall into two interconnected categories: intentional non-adherence and unintentional non-adherence.[23] Unintentional factors involve practical difficulties patients can have with their medication, such as confusion over how or when to take their medication, or unwelcome side effects. Significant intentional factors include the value patients place on the appropriateness of taking medication and their own perceptions as to the threat they face from their illness.

'Concordance' describes the process of discussion and negotiation that should take place between a doctor and patient regarding their medication. The aim of concordance is to involve patients in decisions about prescribed medicines and to reach an agreement that takes into account the beliefs and wishes of the patient in determining whether, when and how medicines are to be taken. It is based on the concept of partnership and highlights not only patients' rights but also their responsibilities for maintaining their own health and not burdening the NHS unnecessarily. Its central themes are also echoed in the GMC's prescribing guidelines.

Prescribing medicines in the best interests of the patient – GMC guidance[24]

To ensure that prescribing is appropriate and in the best interests of patients the GMC advises that doctors should seek to reach an agreement with a patient on the use of any proposed medication and the management of the condition by exchanging information and clarifying any concerns. As part of this consultation, doctors should, where appropriate:

- establish the patient's priorities, preferences and concerns and encourage the patient to ask questions about medicine taking and the proposed treatment
- discuss other treatment options with the patient
- ensure that the patient has been given appropriate information, in a way he or she can understand, about:
  - any common adverse side effects
  - potentially serious side effects
  - what to do in the event of a side effect
  - interactions with other medicines
  - the dosage and administration of the medicine
- ensure that the patient understands how to take the medicine as prescribed and is able to take the medicine as prescribed.

Both doctors and patients need to have a say and reach agreement in any discussion on how medicines should be used to control the problem under discussion.

Interventions should not consist of information provision alone but should respect patient autonomy and support informed choice through education and practical, emotional and behaviourally supportive interventions.[25] It is well recognised that, in many senses, the most influential person in any prescribing consultation is ultimately the patient. Doctors should be non-judgemental in discussing non-adherence and encourage patients to be open about their medicine taking. Some patients, after weighing up the benefits and drawbacks, will decide not to start or to stop taking a course of medication. Providing patients with more information and involving them in the decision-making process will not necessarily result in more patients taking their medicines as directed. If patients have capacity and the doctor is satisfied that they are making an informed decision, this choice should be respected, even if the doctor believes it could be detrimental to the patient's health. Doctors should make a note of the patient's decision in the medical record along with any discussions that took place and the information that was provided to the patient. It is important that doctors regularly review such decisions, however, making a note of any further discussions that take place, as motivating factors in non-adherence can change over time. If doubts exist over a patient's capacity to understand a prescription or significant information relating to it, doctors should conduct a mental capacity test. (For general discussion of mental capacity, see Chapter 3.)

Supporting adherence is important, particularly given the focus in modern healthcare on preventative medicines and the long-term management of chronic conditions, which can require a high degree of commitment from patients. NICE has published clinical guidelines on best practice in involving patients in discussions about prescribed medicines and supporting adherence.[26] The National Prescribing Centre also has a range of resources and learning materials to help doctors involve patients in the decision-making process about prescribed medication.[27]

Summary – providing information to patients about medication

- Patients must be offered sufficient information about any medication prescribed, including details about known side effects, to enable them to make informed decisions.
- Written information for patients is provided with all medication, but this does not diminish the duty of doctors to discuss the medication with patients and answer any questions.
- Doctors should discuss with patients the importance of taking the medication and should encourage them to ask any questions. Efforts should be made to work towards agreeing a plan with the patient about how the medication will be taken.
- Where patients decide not take a particular course of medication, doctors should make a note of the discussion, and any information provided to the patient, in the medical record and should review the decision on a regular basis.

Prescribing for different patient groups

Prescribing and providing information for older people

Challenges in prescribing for older people

Older people receive more prescriptions than any other age group. In 2007, people over 60 accounted for more than 59 per cent of the prescriptions dispensed by community pharmacists in England.[28] Prescribing for older people can be problematic and present a number of different challenges for doctors. Physiological changes associated with ageing can have effects on both pharmacokinetics and pharmacodynamics in older people. Changes to renal clearance, liver size and body mass can all affect how drugs are distributed, metabolised and cleared from the body, while older people are also more sensitive to the effects of drugs and so are more susceptible to idiosyncratic and adverse reactions. Polypharmacy is also common in older people with patients often requiring a number of prescriptions to address co-morbidities, which can leave them at greater risk of adverse drug interactions.[29]

The difficulties that doctors can face when prescribing for older people can be contributory factors to the high prevalence of drug errors that occur amongst this age group. However, there are a number of other factors related to the settings in which older people are cared for, which can exacerbate the problem. A study into the use of medicines in residential and nursing homes found that over two-thirds of residents were exposed to one or more forms of medication error.[30] These errors were found to occur at all stages of the process, including the prescribing, monitoring, administration and dispensing of drugs. The study found that communication problems and systemic problems, such as a lack of integration and coordination between the different elements of care, were factors in the errors made at the care homes featured in the study.

Involving older people in concordance

There is conflicting evidence as to whether older people are more or less likely to be non-compliant than other age groups.[31] A 2009 survey conducted by the Royal Pharmaceutical Society of Great Britain (RPSGB) however, showed that nearly half of over-65 s take more than five medicines at any one time, and 1 in 5 do not take these medicines as prescribed.[32] As in other age groups, some older people will make intentional decisions to not take or to stop taking a course of medication. There are a number of factors, such as physical and cognitive impairment, that are more likely to affect older people than other groups and which can impact on medicine-taking behaviour. The fact that older people are taking multiple medications can also lead to confusion, for example due to complicated drug regimens or adverse side effects, which can result in patients not following their treatment regimen as directed.

There can sometimes be an assumption in the treatment of older people that they have less desire for information or that they may be overwhelmed or confused by receiving too much, even if they have mental capacity. Older people in care homes and hospitals often complain that they are not told the reason behind their medication and had no choice or active involvement in the prescribing decision.[33] It is not necessarily the case that information has been withheld deliberately. Some older patients may only want to receive certain aspects of information while others may prefer to let the treating physician make decisions on their behalf. Although this may suggest a high level of trust in the doctor–patient relationship, it may also be symptomatic of attitudes held by those in older generations who are not accustomed to the levels of autonomy and patient involvement that are often seen in modern medical practice. These attitudes are likely to become less common as individuals who are used to being involved in decisions relating to their care grow older. Doctors should ensure that all patients receive at least a minimum amount of information about their medication, including what it is used for and what side effects patients may experience. Where any information is provided, it should be in a form best suited to accommodate the needs of individual patients.

Elder abuse and over-medication

In 2004, the House of Commons Health Committee published its report on the prevalence and causes of elder abuse. One of the main types of physical abuse the report focused on was the over-medication of older people in care homes. The committee heard evidence from the Alzheimer's Society that the over-prescription of neuroleptics or antipsychotics were often used to sedate people with dementia in care homes as a management tool to prevent residents wandering, becoming agitated or to deal with uncooperativeness. In its recommendations, the committee concluded that 'the incorrect prescription of medication is a serious problem within some care homes, and that medication is, in many cases, being used simply as a tool for the easier management of residents'.[34]

In 2009, Professor Sube Banerjee published a review of the use of antipsychotic medication for patients with dementia.[35] The report highlighted that the current systems of care in the UK deliver a largely antipsychotic-based response to deal with the behavioural and psychological symptoms that are common in dementia. Evidence detailed in the report, however, showed that the drugs appear to have only a limited positive effect and can cause significant harm to patients with dementia. Of the 180,000 dementia patients estimated in the report to be treated by the NHS using antipsychotics per year, only up to 36,000 may actually derive benefit from the treatment. The report recognised that the problem of inappropriate prescribing for patients with dementia is a consequence of a failure within the structure of dementia care as a whole. It set out 11 recommendations for change across all care settings with the aim of reducing the rate of use of antipsychotic medication by two-thirds. Although acknowledging that there will be a continued need to prescribe antipsychotic medication in some cases, the report recommends that it should only be prescribed when patients really need it and should not be used where alternative approaches can be employed.

Over-medication or covert administration of medication to patients with capacity is unethical. It violates the fundamental principle of informed choice and breaks the trust that should be at the heart of the doctor–patient relationship. Doctors should not write prescriptions for their convenience or that of the medical or care team. There may be exceptional occasions when it is in the best interests of patients who lack capacity to administer medication covertly; however, this practice should not become routine (see page 573).

Prescribing for children

One of the key challenges that doctors face when prescribing for children is the lack of drugs that are licensed for use in this age group. As the majority of medicines used in the UK are licensed for adults only, in paediatric care doctors are often forced to prescribe drugs off-label or prescribe unlicensed medicines. Such prescriptions may or may not be appropriate for the child, but doctors can have limited evidence available to them on which they can base their decisions. Children are very different to adults when it comes to the development and prescription of drugs. The range of factors that need to be taken into consideration across this group, for example different ages, weights and changes in pharmacokinetic and pharmacodynamic maturity, mean that 'standard doses' rarely exist as they do with adults.[36]

The lack of available medicines licensed specifically for children was historically due in part to ethical reservations associated with involving children and babies in clinical trials. There has also been reluctance in the pharmaceutical industry to develop and test medicines specifically for children, as the market for paediatric medicines is relatively small and not commercially profitable. Although European regulations have been introduced to address this problem and facilitate the development of new medicines for children (see Chapter 14, pages 599–601), in the short term at least, doctors may still face difficulties prescribing for children in their everyday practice and, in the absence of an alternative, prescribing off-label will often be necessary. In 2005, the first *British National Formulary for Children (BNFC)*[37] was launched in the UK. In addition to providing information and guidance on prescribing for children of all ages, the *BNFC* also includes advice on prescribing outside of a medicine's product licence.

As with all prescribing, doctors should provide patients or their proxies with as much information as they require regarding the proposed course of treatment. In the case of prescribing for children this may involve informing patients or people who make decisions for them that a drug is being prescribed off-label or is unlicensed. As indicated above (see page 536), the GMC advises that where the off-label use of a medicine is supported by current practice, it may not be necessary to draw attention to the licence when seeking consent, although it is good practice to provide patients or their carers with as much information as they require or may see as significant. If concern is expressed that the medication a child has been prescribed is not licensed, or is not licensed for children, doctors should explain in broad terms the reasons why medicines are not licensed for their proposed use. The Royal College of Paediatrics and Child Health (RCPCH), Neonatal and Paediatric Pharmacists Group (NPPG) and WellChild have together developed a series of online patient information leaflets for a range of medicines, which are specifically related to their use in children and may be useful in supporting explanations. The leaflets give parents and carers information regarding dosage, side effects, the different formulations available and how the medicine should be taken.[38]

Religion, belief and prescribing

Sensitivity to the religious faith and beliefs of patients is a core element of medical practice and it is important that doctors consider such beliefs, when possible, in their prescribing practice. Religious law in a number of faiths forbids the consumption of certain products used in the manufacture of some medicines, for example alcohol or animal derivatives. The issue as to whether a particular form of medication is acceptable under religious law in different faiths can be complicated and, in some cases, religious leaders may exempt some prohibited medicines if there is no alternative available and medical need exists.[39]

Whether a patient belonging to a particular faith would object to taking certain drugs is not straightforward, as people often take a personal view on adherence to different religious laws. The threat of ill health can also influence the observance of religious practices. Some individuals for example may place a greater emphasis on religious practices at times of illness, while for others medical need may take precedence. It is important that doctors treat patients as individuals and do not make assumptions regarding their religious beliefs.

The Medicines Partnership, working with the Muslim Council of Britain and members of the Jewish community, has produced guidance for patients and carers on the issue of informed choice in relation to drugs of porcine origin.[40] The guidance recommends that patients should be proactive in making members of a healthcare team aware of any objections they may have to taking medicines that contain products that would be unacceptable because of their beliefs and should do so during their initial assessment. Clearly, doctors cannot be expected to know the constituents of all drugs they may need to prescribe, but, where the doctor knows the product contains ingredients to which the patient has expressed an objection, this should be discussed with the patient. In some circumstances it may be appropriate for the doctor to check the ingredients of a particular medication before prescribing to patients who have a known objection, where this can be achieved easily and quickly. Patients can also be advised to check the patient information leaflet, although this will not always detail all components. As with any form of medication, patients have the right to refuse treatment. If this is the case, doctors should satisfy themselves that the patient has capacity and is fully aware of the risks associated with the decision. Where patients decide to refuse a particular type of medication, a record of this decision and any discussion held with the patient should be recorded in the patient's notes.

Summary – prescribing for different patient groups

- Over-medication and covert administration of medication to patients with capacity is unethical.
- Prescribing off-label is often necessary in paediatric care. If the use of a medicine off-label is supported by current practice, it may not be necessary to draw attention to the scope of the licence when obtaining consent.
- Where parents or carers express concern that medicine prescribed for a child is unlicensed or to be used off-label, doctors should explain the reasons why this is the case in broad terms, using written information to support the explanation where appropriate.
- Where possible, doctors should take the religious faith and beliefs of their patients into account when prescribing.

Pressure from patients

Although doctors' prescribing decisions can be informed by colleagues, medical literature and established guidelines, patient preference must also be considered. Ethical dilemmas may arise, however, when substantial additional expenditure for the NHS results from acceding to such preferences, thus affecting the resources available for other patients, or when patients request particular drugs.

Requests for particular medication

Increasing public access to medical information, particularly on the internet, has empowered patients and enabled them to participate to a greater extent in medical decision making. The availability of this information has led to patients asking their GPs to prescribe particular drugs or treatments, some of which may be of unproven efficacy or may be requested outside the scope of the drug's licence. Doctors faced with such requests are not obliged to comply and should do so only if they are satisfied that the treatment requested is the most appropriate option for the particular patient. If the doctor is concerned about the safety or efficacy of the drug, this should be explained to the patient and the doctor should refuse to prescribe and offer an alternative to the patient where available. It is always important to explain the reasons for refusing to comply with the patient's request. This can be because the patient has obtained inaccurate or misleading information about his or her illness or medication and doctors may find it useful to use clinical knowledge summaries[41] or patient information leaflets (PILs) to support their consultations.

There are also websites, such as NHS Choices,[42] which aim to provide patients with access to reliable and authoritative information and advice on a range of different health conditions and treatments. The MHRA website also includes information on the safety of herbal medicines and their interaction with other medication.[43] Patients who present with inaccurate information can be encouraged to access these websites where there is a higher degree of control over the accuracy of the material published.

Pressure can also arise from inaccurate or incomplete information that patients have received from the media. A particular problem has arisen in England and Wales from the way in which the decisions of NICE have sometimes been reported. Headlines stating that a particular medication has been 'approved' by NICE have resulted in all patients assuming they have an immediate and automatic right to that particular product within the NHS. In reality, NICE guidance may only recommend that a treatment is used for certain categories of patients and commissioning bodies may be disinclined to fund it for other groups of patients.

The BMA considers that it is the doctor's ethical duty to use the most economical and clinically effective treatment available when the patient is receiving treatment within the NHS. Therefore, choosing a more costly product is unethical unless it can be expected to produce a superior outcome. Patient preference and adherence may be elements that contribute to a superior outcome. Implicit in this view is the assumption that objective assessment should be made of the factors that could justify prescribing the more expensive product. When patients are being treated privately, there can be no objection to them choosing a more expensive option that they prefer and are prepared to pay for, provided the doctor is willing to accept clinical responsibility for the prescription requested. However, private insurance companies are very unlikely to be willing to cover options that are more expensive than they consider necessary.

Dealing with patient expectations

A common problem, particularly for GPs, is dealing with patients' expectation that they will leave the surgery with a prescription for some form of medication irrespective of the nature of their complaint. Some doctors may opt for the easier option of writing a prescription rather than spending time assessing the root of the problem or explaining why medication is not the answer. Patient demand and the placebo effect have been put forward as a justification for prescribing drugs acknowledged by the doctor to be pharmacologically ineffective for the condition diagnosed. This is not good practice and undermines the ideal of a doctor–patient relationship based on honesty and trust. In its guidance on the core principles of prescribing, the GMC states that 'you should only prescribe drugs to meet identified needs of patients and never for your own convenience or simply because patients demand them'.[44]

A good example of patient expectation affecting prescribing is the inappropriate use of antibiotics. Although public education campaigns have been helpful in addressing patient misconceptions in relation to antibiotics and in reducing the demand for prescriptions, doctors frequently report coming under pressure from patients to prescribe antibiotics for self-limiting illnesses against which antibiotics are ineffective, such as the common cold. Prescribing antibiotics inappropriately may contribute to the growing problem of antibiotic resistance but may also lead to repeat consultations and reinforcement of the belief that antibiotics are effective in these circumstances. As with all medicines, doctors should prescribe antibiotics only when they are clinically indicated and not just to satisfy the expectations of their patients.

Requests to continue medication

Other dilemmas arise from patients insisting on the continuation of a prescription that the doctor feels can no longer be justified. Common examples include hypnotics and anxiolytics, which may have been prescribed to enable the patient to deal with a painful situation such as bereavement. Similarly, centrally acting appetite suppressants are often sought by patients who want to lose weight. Patients may underestimate or disregard the possibility of creating a physical or psychological dependence, particularly when they are feeling in control of their drug use. Dealing with the situation requires time for doctors to listen to patients' views and for doctors to explain their clinical understanding of the situation.

Repeat prescriptions

Repeat prescribing has now become an essential NHS service and accounts for the majority of prescriptions written by GPs. It offers benefits to both patients and doctors by removing the need for unnecessary consultations and providing a more convenient service. Although repeat prescribing is an established part of everyday healthcare, pressure from patients for continuous repeat prescriptions, without a consultation, must not be permitted to undermine the quality of care that patients receive. The importance of regular clinical assessment for those taking ongoing medication should be explained to patients, and doctors must resist pressure from patients to prescribe larger doses of medication than they consider clinically appropriate or for repeat prescriptions to be issued repeatedly without clinical review. The National Prescribing Centre has published guidance, *Saving time, helping patients,* which provides advice on best practice in repeat prescribing.[45]

In an attempt to tackle the problem of medicines wastage, some commissioning bodies have introduced policies to limit the length of prescribing periods to 28 days. Such policies have attracted criticism from doctors, pharmacists and patients, particularly those with long-term conditions on stable medication, who argue that strict adherence to short prescribing periods can inconvenience patients and raise dispensing costs for people who pay for their prescriptions.

Medicines wastage is a problem within the NHS. An independent report commissioned by the Department of Health estimated that the gross annual cost of prescription medicine wastage in NHS primary and community care in England was £300 million; however, it also stated that less than 50 per cent of medicine waste is likely to be cost-effectively preventable.[46] In discussing the issue of 28-day prescribing periods, the report acknowledged that these policies can help tackle medicines wastage in some cases and should be used where they benefit patients, but that a 'one size fits all' approach will not be universally successful. According to the report findings, the available literature indicated that 'achieving optimum economy in areas such as prescribing and dispensing must involve informed health professionals being enabled to practice in an intelligently flexible manner, which is responsive to individual service user requirements'.[47]

Requests for 'lifestyle drugs'

It is generally accepted that doctors should prescribe medication only if they consider it necessary for the patient, but views of what is 'necessary' differ. More frequent requests from patients for what have been termed 'lifestyle drugs', such as anti-obesity drugs and hair loss treatments, illustrate the way in which perceptions of 'clinical need' have changed. Although there are certainly those for whom drugs such as appetite suppressants are clinically indicated and cannot be considered as lifestyle drugs, for many others they are seen as a quick and easy solution when compared with, for example, spending time and energy on diet and exercise.

What constitutes a lifestyle drug has been the subject of debate in the medical literature. It is defined in the *Concise Oxford Dictionary* as: 'a pharmaceutical product characterised as improving quality of life rather than alleviating or curing disease'. Improving quality of life is, however, a legitimate aim of the health service, so the fact that products such as oral contraceptives fall within this definition does not mean they should not be prescribed within the NHS. Where the boundary lies between what is and what is not acceptable to prescribe with NHS funding, however, is a matter for debate and, unless clear guidance exists, cases should be considered on an individual basis. An analysis of the prescribing of norethisterone in Oxford over a 3-year period identified clear peaks during the holiday seasons (a similar pattern was found throughout England), which the researchers concluded was most likely to be caused by patients wishing to delay menstruation during their holidays. The researchers questioned whether this meant that norethisterone was a lifestyle drug, or was being used as such, and whether such 'lifestyle or convenience prescribing' was appropriate for the NHS.[48] This suggestion was challenged by many of those who responded to the article arguing, for example, that 'health is not merely the absence of disease, but a positive concept of wellbeing. Norethisterone used to delay a period is no more a "lifestyle treatment" than other activities of the NHS aimed at promoting health.'[49]

It is important that doctors should give some thought to how to respond to requests for medication intended to be used in a way that could lead to them being described as lifestyle drugs. Guidance from national advisory bodies may be available, and access to some of these drugs within the NHS may be either prohibited or restricted.[50] In other cases, it is for the individual doctor to decide whether it is appropriate to prescribe as requested. In addition to the financial considerations, there are also questions of safety. There are inherent risks with virtually all medication and part of the doctor's role is to balance those risks against the anticipated benefits for the patient. When the drug is not clinically indicated, the benefits the patient will, or believes he or she will, derive need to be weighed against the risks. Doctors must be willing to justify their decisions to prescribe in these circumstances and should not prescribe based on patient demand or preference alone.

Prescription drugs for cognitive enhancement

Along with the growth in demand for lifestyle drugs, there is also an increasing trend in people buying prescription-only medication without a valid prescription from online pharmacies (see pages 570–571). Often, these drugs are obtained for the performance-enhancing effect they can have on healthy people. One of the more high-profile examples of this trend is the off-label use of drugs such as modafinil (Provigil) and methylphenidate (Ritalin) to improve elements of cognition. These drugs alter the chemical balance of neurotransmitters in the brain and are typically used to treat narcolepsy and attention-deficit hyperactivity disorder (ADHD), but have also been shown to improve concentration and alertness for people with otherwise normal cognitive functioning.

The potential beneficial effects of 'smart drugs' have made them popular with students as study aids and reports suggest that demand is growing quickly in this demographic. This raises a number of ethical questions regarding whether students who take enhancing drugs have an unfair advantage over others and the degree to which other students may feel coerced into taking such drugs to remain competitive with their peers. Although much of the debate has focused on using 'smart drugs' to improve academic performance, the issues raised could have much wider ethical and practical implications for society. On the one hand, for example, it has been argued that cognitive enhancement could potentially help tackle the inequalities that exist within society, counteracting the disadvantages many face in learning and development as a result of environmental and economic factors beyond their control. Widespread use of psycho-pharmaceuticals could also negatively impact on the psychological and physical health of society and reinforce a culture of competiveness and individualism.[51]

There are also safety concerns associated with people buying medication over the internet from unknown sources and without appropriate medical advice. The drugs obtained may be counterfeit or of substandard quality and doctors may be called upon to treat patients who have are suffering from side effects or adverse reactions. The long-term effects on the brain of sustained use of 'smart drugs' are also unknown.

Summary – pressure from patients

- When faced with patients' requests for particular medication, doctors are not obliged to comply and should do so only if they are satisfied that the treatment requested is the most appropriate option for the particular patient.
- Doctors have an ethical duty to use the most economic and efficacious treatment available when the patient is receiving treatment within the NHS.
- Doctors must resist pressure from patients to prescribe larger doses of medication than they consider clinically appropriate or for prescriptions to be issued repeatedly without clinical review.
- 'Lifestyle drugs' should be prescribed only when the doctor considers them clinically appropriate for the patient and where the actual, or perceived, benefits outweigh any risks.

Pressure from employers

A doctor employed by a private organisation bears responsibility for prescribing and must be able to exercise independent clinical judgement, regardless of the policies of the organisation's management. In the past a practice developed whereby some establishments, particularly slimming clinics, appeared to have a predefined policy concerning the product and dose that doctors should supply to all patients. Prescriptions must not be influenced by factors such as the convenience of a clinic or hospital management, and any pressure from employers for doctors to practise according to such predefined prescribing policies must be resisted.

Clinical freedom and resources

Doctors can prescribe whatever approved medicine they consider appropriate for a patient but, in practice, clinical autonomy is not absolute. Within the NHS, the state takes an interest in prescribing habits and studies have identified tremendous variations in the volume and cost of prescribing between different geographical areas and between individual prescribers. Inevitably, resources are limited and there are various ways in which this can create ethical dilemmas for doctors.

Explicit rationing within the NHS

The prescribing of sildenafil (Viagra) was the first time the NHS refused to fund a licensed drug with proven benefits to a large number of people.[52] Sildenafil was licensed
in the UK on 15 September 1998, for use by patients with erectile dysfunction. The
Government anticipated a huge demand for the drug and was fearful of the financial
implications of making it freely available within the NHS. It had been estimated that
the annual drug bill for Viagra would exceed £1 billion a year if all men who might
benefit were prescribed the drug.[53] As a result of these fears, the Standing Medical
Advisory Committee of the Department of Health advised doctors not to prescribe the
drug until definitive guidance had been drawn up.

After many months of intense debate, both in the media and among professional
groups, and a 6-week period of formal consultation, final guidance was issued. For
the first time the Government was rationing access to a drug explicitly, not on the
basis of clinical need or through the use of the waiting list system, but on the basis of
the aetiology of the condition. From 1 July 1999 the availability of sildenafil and other
treatments for impotence within the NHS was restricted, by extending schedule 11 of
the GMS Regulations, to patients who:

- were receiving NHS treatment for impotence on 14 September 1998
- were suffering from: diabetes, multiple sclerosis, Parkinson disease, poliomyelitis,
  prostate cancer, severe pelvic injury, single gene neurological disease, spina bifida
  or spinal cord injury
- were receiving treatment for renal failure by dialysis, or
- had undergone the following surgery: prostatectomy, radical pelvic surgery, renal
  failure treated by transplant.[54]

In addition, treatment was to be made available, in exceptional cases of severe distress, through specialist care.

At the time, the BMA opposed this form of rationing – on the basis of the cause
of the underlying condition rather than on the basis of clinical need – which, it argued, makes 'a cruel, unethical, and inequitable distinction between "acceptable" and
"unacceptable" forms of impotence'.[55]

Truth telling and resources

Although truth telling is generally advocated, some doctors have expressed concern
about the implications of telling patients that there is medication available that could
potentially help them, but that it is not available within the NHS or in the area in which
they live. Under GMC guidelines, doctors have a duty to provide patients with as much
information as they need or want about treatments that could have greater potential
benefit than those available within the organisation in which they work.[56] Where a doctor
believes that paying for the treatment privately would be beyond the financial means of
the patient, however, this can be problematic. Doctors have raised concerns for example,
that discussing the option of private treatment could simply add to the patient's burden,
raise unreasonable hopes that treatment is available and put pressure on the patient and
his or her family somehow to find the money to pay for the treatment.

In the BMA's view, part of the role of doctors is to ensure that decision making
is returned as much as possible to the patient, rather than pre-empting the choice by
withholding potentially important information. The BMA therefore believes that, as a
general rule, patients should be given information about other treatment options that may
benefit them, even if the doctor does not believe that the patient could afford to pay for
the treatment. There may be rare cases, however, in which such information would clearly
be unwelcome, when doctors should take their cue from patients as to the amount of

information to impart. When information is to be provided, the manner and timing of its provision needs to be carefully considered and may need to be supported by professional counselling. If the treatment cannot be funded, patients should have access to information about the factors leading to the rationing decision and it should be made clear whether the treatment is unavailable because it is unproven or because it provides only minimal benefit relative to the cost of the drug.

Top up fees

Arrangements in place in England and Scotland allow patients to supplement or 'top up' the care they receive in the NHS with treatment or medication in the private sector. The arrangements in both countries give patients the option of purchasing drugs to supplement their care, which were rejected by the relevant health advisory bodies on the grounds of clinical, or cost-effectiveness. The Department of Health and Scottish Government have issued guidance for health authorities in their respective countries on the circumstances in which it is acceptable to combine NHS and private healthcare services.[57] Both English and Scottish arrangements are based on several fundamental principles.

- All possibilities of NHS funding for a particular medicine should be considered and exhausted.
- NHS resources should never be used to subsidise private treatments and the patient must bear the full cost of any private treatment.
- There must be a clear distinction between the NHS and private care provided to a patient.
- Patients who combine NHS and private care are fully entitled to the NHS care they would otherwise be given.
- Such patients are entitled to NHS services on the same basis of clinical need as any other patient.
- Patients should not be disadvantaged in relation to the NHS care they receive.

Doctors should inform patients about the possibility of topping up their care, where such arrangements are in place and where circumstances indicate it may be appropriate.

Where patients decide to supplement their NHS care with medicines not available within the NHS, GPs may be asked to prescribe medication, either directly by the patient or by the consultant providing the private care, that they are not familiar with or have no experience of prescribing. GPs should not prescribe if they feel they do not have sufficient expertise or experience in prescribing a particular drug. Where prescribing is shared between a GP and consultant, GPs should ascertain who retains overall clinical responsibility for prescribing in these circumstances (see pages 557–562).

Summary – pressure from employers

- The BMA believes that, as a general rule, patients should be given information about treatment options that are not available within the NHS but which may benefit them, even if the doctor does not believe that the patient could afford to pay for the treatment.

- If treatment cannot be funded by the NHS, patients should be informed whether it is not available because it is unproven or because it provides only minimal benefit relative to the cost of the drug.
- Where patients have the option to 'top up' their care, they should be informed of this.

Clinical freedom and official guidance

Since the late 1990s, new and some established treatments, devices and drugs have been subject to formal assessment for clinical efficacy and cost-effectiveness. Different national bodies are responsible for this role in England and Wales, Scotland and Northern Ireland.

National Institute for Health and Clinical Excellence

NICE aims to provide health professionals, patients and the public with authoritative, robust and reliable guidance on current best practice. Although the remit of NICE extends only to England and Wales (see box below), NICE guidelines are clearly influential throughout the UK. The main function of NICE is to create consistent clinical standards across the NHS. Guided by evidence-based practice, NICE is responsible for collecting and evaluating all relevant evidence and considering its implications for clinical practice, with reference to both clinical and cost-effectiveness.

NICE produces technology appraisals, primarily of pharmaceutical products but also of medical devices, diagnostic techniques, health promotion and surgical procedures. These result in recommendations in the form of guidance as to whether, and, if so, in what circumstances, it would be appropriate to use the technology in the NHS. There are two types of technology appraisal. Single technology appraisals evaluate an individual drug for a particular condition whereas in a multiple technology appraisal NICE compares several different types of treatment resulting in more detailed and lengthy guidance.

The role of NICE has undergone considerable change since it was established in 1999. In addition to evaluating newly licensed drugs, NICE produces clinical guidelines, which although not binding on health professionals, give recommendations on the management of particular diseases and clinical conditions based on the best available evidence. The remit of NICE has also expanded over the years to include guidance on cancer services, diagnostic technologies, interventional procedures, medical technologies and public health issues, such as the prevention of sexually transmitted infections, smoking cessation and the promotion of physical activity. In its first 10 years NICE published over 580 individual pieces of guidance across all the areas within its scope.[58] In 2010, NICE published the first set of approximately 150 Quality Standards on stroke, dementia and venous thromboembolism prevention.

Where NICE guidance applies in the UK[59]

England	Wales
- Clinical guidelines - Single and multiple technology appraisals - Interventional procedures - Public health guidance - Medical technologies guidance	- Clinical guidelines - Single and multiple technology appraisals - Interventional procedures

Northern Ireland	Scotland
• Clinical guidelines (subject to general review) • Single and multiple technology appraisals (subject to local review) • Interventional procedures • Public health guidance (subject to local review)	• Multiple technology appraisals (with advice on implementation from Healthcare Improvement Scotland) • Interventional procedures • Public health guidance (subject to local review)

Since its inception, one of the main aims of NICE has been to evaluate the cost-effectiveness of new treatments in the context of the significant pressures that exist on NHS resources. In the past, where NICE approved the use of a drug as part of its appraisal process, commissioning bodies were required to provide funding for the drug in the NHS within 3 months. Its role in rationing the availability of new drugs was, however, controversial. Decisions not to fund or to restrict access to drugs were subject to intense scrutiny in the media, with NICE facing public criticism and pressure from both pharmaceutical companies and groups advocating on behalf of patients. (The ethical issues associated with rationing are discussed in more detail in Chapter 20, pages 835–847.)

While the decisions of NICE have in the past been binding on commissioning bodies, in 2010 the Government outlined its intention to make a number of significant changes to the role of NICE in its wide-reaching white paper, *Equity and Excellence: Liberating the NHS*.[60] At the time of writing these changes were under review, but it is foreseeable that NICE will continue to have a significant and possibly expanded role in the way different medications and treatments are assessed and delivered in England and Wales in the future. Updates on any developments regarding NICE will be available on the BMA website.

Scotland, Wales and Northern Ireland

In Scotland, Healthcare Improvement Scotland (HIS) is responsible for providing advice to health boards about new and existing technologies. This guidance is sometimes based on a review of the recommendations of NICE and sometimes on separate health technology assessments. HIS also supports the Scottish Medicines Consortium (SMC), which advises NHS boards about the efficacy of all newly licensed medicines, all new major formulations of existing medicines and any major new indications of established medicines.

HIS evaluates the multiple technology appraisals published by NICE for their applicability in Scotland. Where HIS validates a positive NICE multiple technology appraisal, NHS boards in Scotland are required to make these medicines available. Single evaluations of newly licensed drugs are performed by the SMC. Health boards in Scotland are expected to ensure that the drugs or treatments recommended by the SMC are made available to meet clinical need, but doing so is not mandatory. Doctors in Scotland also have the benefit of guidance from the Scottish Intercollegiate Guidelines Network (SIGN), which also comes under the remit of HIS. The aim of SIGN is to improve the quality of healthcare for patients in Scotland, by reducing variation in practice and outcome, through the development and dissemination of national clinical guidelines containing recommendations for effective practice.

Although NICE technology appraisals apply in Wales, the All Wales Medicines Strategy Group (AWMSG) also has a role in the approval of high cost cardiac and cancer medicines either ahead of NICE guidance or in its absence.[61] AWMSG appraisals are intended to complement those from NICE, which remain the primary source of guidance on new medicines and ultimately take precedence should the two differ. Local health boards and trusts are required to follow the recommendations of AWMSG within 3 months.

In Northern Ireland, a formal link exists between the Department of Health, Social Services and Public Safety and NICE through which guidance produced by NICE is subject to either general or local review before its implementation in Northern Ireland.

Summary – clinical freedom and official guidance

- Different national bodies in the UK are responsible for assessing new and some established treatments, devices and drugs for clinical and cost-effectiveness.
- The remit of NICE covers England and Wales, but NICE guidelines are influential throughout the UK and can be implemented following review in Scotland and Northern Ireland.

Conflicts of interest in prescribing matters

Prescribing decisions should be made on the basis of the individual needs of the patient. Doctors must not be, or be seen to be, influenced in prescribing matters by the offer of any pecuniary or other incentives, or any personal financial interests. It is important therefore for doctors to be alert to any actual, or perceived, conflicts of interest and to take steps to avoid them. The types of situation in which a conflict of interest could arise in relation to prescribing are discussed below.

Gifts or hospitality from pharmaceutical companies

The offer of financial or other incentives from the manufacturers of particular drugs would clearly raise questions about the motivation of a doctor who prescribed that drug in preference to one produced by a competitor. Even if the doctor sincerely believed the former drug to be the best option for the patient, it would be difficult to prove that his or her judgement had not been affected by personal gain. For this reason, doctors are not permitted to accept gifts or hospitality from pharmaceutical companies, and representatives of pharmaceutical companies are not permitted to offer them. The Medicines (Advertising) Regulations 1994 specifically forbid the offer or acceptance of 'any gift, pecuniary advantage or benefit in kind, unless it is inexpensive and relevant to the practice of medicine or pharmacy'[62] although industry guidelines further restrict what can be offered to doctors (see below). Along with this legal duty, doctors also have a professional obligation to avoid conflicts of interest in any dealings with pharmaceutical companies. The GMC's guidelines advise that 'you must act in your patients' best interests when making referrals and providing or arranging treatment or care. So you must not ask for or accept any inducement, gift or hospitality which may affect or be seen to affect your judgment.'[63] Doctors who have financial or commercial interests in pharmaceutical or other biomedical companies must not let these affect how they prescribe for, treat or refer patients.[64]

The Association of the British Pharmaceutical Industry (ABPI) Code of Practice sets out standards for all types of promotion of prescription-only medicines to doctors and health professionals and sets out the requirements that must be met for industry sponsorship of meetings and any hospitality provided.[65] Changes to the code in 2011 prohibit the provision of any promotional aids, such as pens, pads and mugs, to healthcare professionals and administrative staff. Inexpensive items that are to be passed onto patients as part of a formal patient support programme, and which directly benefit patient care, are permitted. Medical and educational goods and services may also be provided, but not for the personal benefit of individuals and only when it is in the interests of patients or will benefit the NHS while maintaining patient care.[66] In 2011, the BMA signed a joint letter with other key stakeholders, including the ABPI, the Department of Health and the RPSGB, supporting these changes to the code of practice, which aim to support greater openness and transparency in the relationship between the industry and healthcare professionals.

There is nothing to prevent a doctor accepting travel costs for attendance at a meeting, or accepting hospitality at a meeting or event hosted or sponsored by a pharmaceutical company provided that:

- the meeting has a clear scientific or educational content
- the meeting is held at an appropriate venue and the hospitality offered is reasonable in level, the cost of which does not exceed what the recipients would normally choose when paying for themselves
- the hospitality is subordinate to the main purpose of the meeting, and
- it applies only to those qualified to attend the meeting and does not, for example, extend to their spouses or other accompanying person.[67]

Meetings that are wholly or mainly centred around sporting or social events are prohibited. Where meetings are organised by pharmaceutical companies which take place outside the UK, while not necessarily deemed unacceptable, they must meet the criteria listed above for any meeting involving the industry. There must also be valid reasons for the meeting to take place in that particular location which itself should not be seen as an incentive for doctors to attend, over and above the purpose and content of the meeting.[68] The ABPI code permits companies to use health professionals as consultants and advisors for various purposes, including speaking at or chairing meetings, providing they meet certain criteria. Under the code, doctors who act as consultants must be contractually obliged to declare the arrangement whenever they write or speak in public on any issue relating to the company.[69]

Pharmaceutical companies sometimes offer to provide a nurse or other member of staff to a general practice or hospital to undertake audit or a review of prescribing. It has been suggested that acceptance of such an offer could be interpreted as a gift or benefit in kind, because the company is effectively giving the practice the cost of the staff member's time. Concerns have also been expressed about the motivations of companies making such offers, with fears that there could be implicit pressure on the practice to change its prescribing patterns to the benefit of the company. The extent to which such concerns are justified is likely to depend upon the individual circumstances, but doctors must ensure that they are able to defend any decision to accept such offers and can show that their prescribing decisions have not been affected. Any practice planning to accept the offer of such assistance should ensure that there is a detailed written protocol specifying the terms of the agreement. The ABPI code of practice states that therapeutic reviews, which seek to ensure a patient receives optimum treatment following clinical assessment, are a legitimate activity for pharmaceutical companies to either support or assist with, providing they do not solely serve the interests of the company and its products and they ultimately enhance patient care and benefit the NHS.[70]

Payments for meeting pharmaceutical representatives

It is unacceptable for doctors to demand payment for meeting and listening to pharmaceutical representatives or to charge a fee for the use of a room for such a meeting. It is also contrary to the ABPI's code of practice for industry representatives to offer any inducements in return for an interview.[71]

Financial involvement of doctors in external health-related services

With some types of financial interest in health-related services, such as doctors having a stake in private nursing homes or clinics, it is considered sufficient for the doctor to make the patient aware of his or her financial interest in the matter, and of any suitable alternatives. The declaration of a financial interest, however, does not provide sufficient safeguard in the case of prescribing, because the patient is usually not in a position to exercise an informed choice about other medicines available as suitable alternatives to the one in which the doctor has a financial interest.

Common enquiries in this area concern the propriety of prescribing medicines marketed by companies in which the doctor or the doctor's family has a significant financial interest. Sometimes the financial interest is acquired after patients have been prescribed a long-term course of a drug that suits them. In such cases, it has been thought unlikely that any objection would be raised to the doctor maintaining a patient's prescription. On the other hand, it would be questionable to consider changing a patient's medication from an already established pattern to a new medicine in which the doctor has a financial interest. It would certainly be unethical to do so if the doctor's decision was influenced by any financial benefit. Dilemmas arise, however, if doctors become convinced of the superiority of the product in which they have a financial interest. Genuine concern for the patient's benefit can easily be confused with self-interest. For such reasons, the BMA believes it is generally unwise for doctors to form a business connection with companies producing, marketing or promoting such products.

Participation in market research

Doctors are sometimes invited to participate in market research, carried out by an independent organisation on behalf of a pharmaceutical company. This can include questionnaires, interviews or focus group work to ascertain doctors' views and practices in relation to certain generic drugs. Usually, the doctor participating does not know which company has sponsored the research. The ABPI code of practice makes it clear to pharmaceutical companies that market research simply involves the collection and analysis of information and must be unbiased and non-promotional.[72] There is no problem with doctors participating in such research provided that the personal health information of individual patients is not disclosed without their consent. Doctors must also be able to demonstrate that their participation, and any remuneration received, has not in any way influenced, or could be perceived as influencing, their prescribing decisions. The British Healthcare Business Intelligence Association publishes legal and ethical guidelines on the appropriate remuneration of healthcare professionals for participating in market research.[73]

Ownership of pharmacies

The BMA does not object to doctors owning pharmacies; however, as with all potential conflicts of interest, doctors should ensure that any commercial or financial interests they or their employers have in pharmacies do not influence the advice they give to patients. Patients should be free to choose which pharmacy they wish to use and should not be directed to use a particular pharmacy during the course of a consultation. The GMC advises that patients should have access to information about any financial or commercial interests that either their doctor or their employer has in a pharmacy they are likely to use.[74]

GPs who practise in rural or semi-rural areas, where there are few, if any, pharmacies in the locality, have long been able to dispense prescription medication to patients. Dispensing doctors are under the same ethical obligations as all doctors to act in the best interests of patients and to use NHS resources cost-effectively. The freedom of patients to choose where they have their medicines dispensed should be respected and doctors should not prescribe differently for patients to whom they dispense for commercial or financial benefit.[75]

Summary – conflicts of interest in prescribing matters

- Doctors must not be, or be seen to be, influenced in prescribing matters by the offer of any pecuniary or other incentives or any personal financial interests. They should be alert to any actual or perceived conflicts of interest and take steps to avoid them.
- Doctors are not permitted to accept gifts from pharmaceutical companies and under the ABPI Code of Practice, companies are not permitted to provide branded promotional aids to health professionals.
- Subject to certain conditions doctors may accept hospitality to attend meetings or events hosted by pharmaceutical companies.
- The BMA believes it is generally unwise for doctors to form business connections with companies producing, marketing or promoting pharmaceutical products.

Shared prescribing

It is preferable for one doctor, usually the GP, to be fully informed about, and be responsible for, the overall management of a patient's healthcare. When different doctors prescribe a patient medication, or if patients obtain medication over the internet, it is particularly important that one doctor is fully aware of the range of medication being taken, in order to advise on any contraindications or adverse reactions. When more than one health professional is involved in aspects of the patient's care, effective liaison and communication is essential. All doctors should help to facilitate effective communication and should encourage patients to allow information about their treatment, and any medication prescribed, to be passed to others involved in their care. If patients refuse to allow information to be shared, for example with their GP, this should be respected, but the implications of their decision should be explained to them and, depending upon the level of risk, doctors may decide not to prescribe.

Prescribing shared between GPs and hospital doctors

There is a range of situations in which prescribing is shared between GPs and hospital doctors. GPs may be asked to take over the prescribing of long-term medication or to continue ongoing medication after a patient's discharge from hospital. It is not unusual for a patient to present his or her GP with a list of medication recommended by the treating specialist with the expectation that the GP will issue a prescription. If GPs prescribe this medication they accept full clinical responsibility for the decision. This means that GPs should comply with such requests only if they are satisfied that the recommended course of treatment is the correct medication and dose for the individual patient and they are willing to accept ongoing responsibility for monitoring the drug regimen. Shared prescribing happens quite frequently, but all parties, including patients, need to be happy with the situation and the decisions made in each particular case. Sometimes this arises from the GP receiving a full and detailed report, which enables him or her to confirm that the drug recommended is appropriate. On other occasions, the hospital doctor discusses the case with the GP (with the patient's consent) and agreement is reached on the most appropriate course of action. Decisions about who should take responsibility for continuing treatment should be based on the best interests of the patient and not convenience or cost.[76] Where there is disagreement about the appropriate medication, or dose, which cannot be resolved through discussion, the GP should refuse to participate in a shared prescribing arrangement and explain the reasons for this to both the requesting doctor and the patient.

Guidance on the transfer of prescribing responsibility between hospitals and GPs was issued in 1991 by the Department of Health.[77] This guidance can help GPs to decide under what circumstances to accept prescribing responsibility, and hospital consultants to assess whether transfer of responsibility is appropriate. The following basic points should be borne in mind.

- Legal responsibility for prescribing rests with the doctor who signs the prescription.
- Hospital consultants have full responsibility for prescribing for inpatients and for specific treatments administered in hospital outpatient clinics.
- Responsibility for prescribing should rest with the consultant if the drugs are included in a hospital-based clinical trial and when it is more appropriate for the consultant to monitor the medication because of the need for specialised investigations, or where there are supply problems with the drugs.
- When a consultant considers that a patient's condition is stable, he or she may seek the agreement of the GP concerned to share the care. In proposing a shared care arrangement, a consultant may advise the GP which medicine to prescribe. When a new or rarely prescribed medicine is being recommended, its dosage and administration must be specified and any potential adverse drug reactions to watch out for identified by the consultant so that the GP is properly informed and can monitor and adjust the dose if necessary. When a treatment is not licensed for a particular indication, full justification for the use of the drug should be given by the consultant to the GP. Where a hospital drug formulary is in operation and a recommended treatment is not included, the GP must be informed and given the option of prescribing alternatives.

- When an inpatient is discharged from hospital, sufficient drugs should be prescribed and dispensed by the hospital pharmacy for at least a 7-day period. For outpatients, a minimum 14 days' supply should be prescribed and dispensed. The GP to whose care the patient is transferred should receive notification in good time of the patient's diagnosis and drug therapy in order to maintain continuity. If that information cannot be transferred to the GP within the timescale, drugs should be prescribed by the hospital for as long a period as is necessary.
- When clinical, and therefore prescribing, responsibility for a patient is transferred from hospital to GP, it is of the utmost importance that the GP feels fully confident to prescribe the necessary drugs. It is essential that a transfer involving drug therapies with which GPs would not normally be familiar should not take place without full agreement between the hospital consultant (or any transferring doctor) and the GP, who must have sufficient information about the drug therapy. When drawing up shared care protocols, or when there is a professional disagreement over who should prescribe, it may be necessary for local discussion to take place between hospital managers and medical staff and the relevant local medical committee as a prelude to establishing agreement with individual GPs. A GP is obliged only to provide treatment that is consistent with GPs' terms of service.
- When a GP takes responsibility for prescribing or dispensing drugs that have not normally been dispensed in the community, there should be liaison between the transferring hospital and the community pharmacist to ensure continuity of supply.

The BMA's General Practitioners Committee has produced guidance on the role of GPs when prescribing is shared between primary and secondary care, which provides an overview of common problems and gives examples of best practice.[78]

Across Northern Ireland[79] and in individual areas of Scotland, England and Wales, a traffic light system has been introduced locally, which classifies different medicines to help identify where responsibility for prescribing different drugs should lie. Under this system, medicines are divided into 'red list drugs', for which prescribing responsibility should remain with the consultant, and 'amber list drugs' for which responsibility may be transferred to primary care with the agreement of the individual GP. 'Green list drugs' are those commonly prescribed by GPs and feature in local formularies. Shared care arrangements are developed locally, in collaboration with GPs and consultants, for amber listed medicines.

Prescribing shared between the private sector and the NHS

In addition to questions of clinical responsibility, a frequent enquiry concerns the acceptability of a patient seeking private treatment but requesting that any medication recommended is supplied by the NHS. Even though individuals opt for private treatment or assessment, they are still entitled to NHS services. If the GP considers that the medication recommended is clinically necessary, he or she would be required under the terms of service to prescribe that medication within the NHS, even if the assessment from which the need was identified was undertaken in the private sector. This is subject to the comments above about whether the GP has sufficient information and is willing to accept clinical responsibility for the prescribing decision recommended by another doctor.

The same obligation to prescribe does not arise if the medication recommended is not clinically necessary or if it is generally not funded within the NHS. A common example is fertility treatment, where patients seek *in vitro* fertilisation in the private sector and ask their GP to issue NHS prescriptions for the drugs. The decision about whether to comply with such requests rests with the individual GP or, where the medication is not generally funded on the NHS, the commissioning body. In the past, these requests have caused some concern amongst GPs, who felt they were being placed in the invidious position of either appearing unsupportive of their patients or accepting legal, financial and ethical responsibility for a course of medication that they had not initiated and which, in some cases, they may not consider to be clinically necessary. When the product is of a very specialised nature, requiring ongoing monitoring, some GPs may feel they have insufficient expertise to accept responsibility for the prescription and so refuse such requests. Others initiate discussions with the relevant specialists to reach a position with which all parties are content.

Many of the problems and concerns that arise in relation to prescribing shared between the private sector and the NHS can be avoided by improved communication between the parties concerned. Consultants who want GPs to prescribe medication for patients should avoid simply informing patients that GPs will be willing to prescribe and consider either recommending that patients ask their GP if he or she would be willing to prescribe or, preferably, contact the GP in question directly. This is not simply a matter of etiquette. If the GP does not feel able to accept clinical responsibility or, in the case of medication that is not clinically necessary, financial responsibility for the recommended medication, this could cause difficulties for the doctor–patient relationship. Those requesting GPs to take over prescribing should bear these points in mind when discussing the matter with patients.

Patient group directions

Patient group directions (PGDs) are drawn up by multi-disciplinary groups and signed by a senior doctor and a senior pharmacist and must meet certain legal requirements. They permit certain named health professionals to supply medicines to patients but without the need for an individual prescription. The traditional form of prescription, where the doctor prescribes to a patient on an individual basis and retains clinical responsibility for the decision, should always be the preferred method of providing patients with the medicines they need. The supply and administration of medicines under PGDs are reserved for those limited situations where this method offers a distinct advantage for patient care and where it is consistent with appropriate professional relationships and accountability;[80] the provision of emergency hormonal contraception provides a good example of their use (see Chapter 7, page 276). PGDs can be used in the NHS or for services funded by the NHS but provided by the private, voluntary or charitable sector. Independent hospital agencies and clinics registered under the Care Standards Act 2000 are also permitted to use PGDs, as are prison healthcare services, police services and defence medical services. As with individual prescriptions, doctors should not sign PGDs if they have any doubts about the safety or efficacy of the medication, or uncertainties about the ability of the named health professional adequately to assess the patient's suitability for the treatment. The BMA has published guidance on the use of PGDs within general practice[81] and the National Prescribing Centre also has guidance for all health professionals and organisations that work with and devise PGDs.[82]

Supplementary prescribing and independent non-medical prescribers

The prescribing role of health professionals other than doctors has expanded over time. Prescribing arrangements now often seek to utilise the skills of different members of the healthcare team more effectively, in order to provide more convenient access to medicines for patients and to help reduce the prescribing burden on doctors. Certain groups of health professionals can undertake training enabling them to operate as either independent or supplementary prescribers within the NHS. Although medicines legislation allows the extension of prescribing responsibilities across the UK, administrations in the devolved nations are responsible for deciding whether and how the legislation is implemented in their respective countries.

Supplementary prescribing involves a voluntary partnership between a doctor and another member of the healthcare team who can be a registered nurse, podiatrist or chiropodist, optometrist, physiotherapist, radiographer or pharmacist who has completed approved training to carry out the role. The aim of supplementary prescribing is to implement a clinical management plan (CMP) drawn up by the doctor and agreed with the patient following a medical assessment. Supplementary prescribers can prescribe any licensed or unlicensed medicine detailed on the CMP including controlled drugs.

After completing specialised training, nurses and pharmacists are able to become independent prescribers and are permitted to prescribe any licensed drug for medical conditions that fall within their level of competence and area of expertise, including, for nurses, some controlled drugs for specified medical conditions. Optometrists are also able to become independent prescribers after specialist training and can prescribe any licensed drug for ocular conditions affecting the eye and surrounding tissue with the exception of controlled drugs and medicines for parenteral administrations. Community Practitioner Nurse Prescribers have more limited prescribing responsibilities and are only permitted to prescribe the specific preparations listed in the Nurse Prescribers' Formulary for Community Practitioners.[83]

Where prescribing is shared between different health professionals, collaborative working is essential to ensure patient safety. Prescribing activity should be recorded such that it is easily accessible to all prescribing members of the healthcare team who can review any relevant information before prescribing themselves.

Practitioners of complementary therapies

An area of concern about shared prescribing arises in connection with the treatments recommended by complementary practitioners to whom patients frequently self-refer. Anxiety is often expressed by doctors about patients' decisions to suspend or postpone orthodox treatments while they explore other remedies. Often, patients will use complementary and orthodox medicine simultaneously. There is a wide range of complementary therapies and the evidence base for these can vary (see Chapter 19, pages 786–788). Where treatment is being provided by more than one practitioner, it is important that patients keep both informed to ensure that any risk of harmful interaction between the preparations recommended is identified and avoided. It is important that complementary therapists encourage patients to inform their GPs about any medication prescribed. Doctors who are registered with the GMC and who provide complementary therapies are obliged to share with a patient's GP 'the results of any investigations, the treatment provided and any other information necessary for the continuing care of the patient, unless the patient objects'.[84]

However, some patients are reluctant to discuss complementary therapies with their GPs, fearing that their decision to seek alternative remedies may be derided or perceived as a lack of faith in the doctor's skills. Research on the attitudes of health professionals to herbal medicines, showed that a significant proportion (73 per cent) of those surveyed were worried that their patients would take herbal medicines and not inform them.[85] GPs should adopt a non-judgemental approach to their patient's choices and should encourage the sharing of relevant information about the patient's treatment. Where the doctor considers the complementary therapy to be potentially harmful, however, either because of the treatment itself or the qualifications and experience of the practitioner, this should be sensitively explained to the patient. (For more information on liaison with complementary therapists, see Chapter 19, pages 786–788.)

Summary – shared prescribing

- Where a patient may be prescribed medication by different doctors, each doctor should be fully aware of the range of medication being taken in order to advise on any contraindications or adverse reactions. Ideally, one doctor should take overall coordinating responsibility.
- If patients refuse to allow information to be sought from their GP, this should be respected but the implications of the decision should be explained and, depending upon the risks and the seriousness of the condition, other doctors may decide not to prescribe.
- GPs should prescribe medication at the request of another doctor only if they are satisfied that the recommended course and dose of medication is appropriate for the individual patient and if they are willing to accept full clinical responsibility for the prescribing decision.
- Patients sometimes ask their GPs for NHS prescriptions for medication recommended during private consultations. If the GP believes the medication to be clinically necessary (and it is medication for which the GP is willing to accept clinical responsibility) the GP would be required to comply. This does not apply if the medication recommended is not considered clinically necessary, or if the medication is generally not provided within the NHS.
- Doctors should not sign PGDs if they have any doubts about the safety or efficacy of the medication or doubts about the ability of the named health professional adequately to assess patients' suitability for the treatment or to provide any necessary supervision.
- Doctors should adopt a non-judgemental approach to their patient's choices regarding complementary therapies and encourage the sharing of relevant information; where doctors consider the complementary therapy to be potentially harmful, however, this should be sensitively explained to the patient.
- Doctors who are registered with the GMC and who provide complementary therapies are obliged to share relevant information about treatment with a patient's GP, unless the patient objects.

Referrals and discharge summaries

It is important that there is prompt exchange of information about patients' medication when they transfer from one clinical setting to another to ensure continuity of care. Hospitals need to be aware of any existing medication that patients are taking on admission, as this could be incompatible with treatment or any new prescriptions that may be provided while they are in hospital. Similarly, when the patient is discharged, GPs need to be informed of any new medicines the patient has been prescribed and any medicines that have been changed during the patient's stay in hospital, unless the patient objects. Any changes need to be reviewed and incorporated into the patient's record to avoid patients receiving inappropriate repeat prescriptions.

A 2009 report from the Care Quality Commission looked at the issue of medicines management with respect to the information shared both on admission to, and discharge from, hospital.[86] Although the report found there were generally good systems in place to ensure the quality of repeat prescribing and medication reviews of high-risk patients, it also raised some concerns over specific parts of the process. With respect to information shared on admission, the study found that 24 per cent of GPs surveyed did not systematically provide information on co-morbidities, allergies and drug reactions, and that the approach to providing information to hospitals in an emergency tended to be too slow and informal. However, it did highlight a number of initiatives introduced in some parts of the country, such as 'patient's own drug' (POD) and 'green bag' schemes, which encourage patients to bring their existing medication with them into hospital and can be especially beneficial when admitted in an emergency. Deficiencies were also found in the quality of information provided in discharge summaries, particularly with respect to medicines prescribed on discharge, with over 80 per cent of GPs surveyed reporting that the details of prescribed medicine were incomplete or inaccurate in the majority of cases. Among the report's recommendations were the use of standard referral forms to cover elective and emergency admissions; that GPs should carry out a higher proportion of medication reviews with the patient present; and that acute trusts should ensure that their clinicians were aware of their responsibilities regarding the timely completion of discharge summaries including full information on medication changes.

Doctors who prescribe complementary and alternative medicine

Many patients wish to explore different treatment options that are available and some look to complementary therapies such as homeopathy, herbal medicine and acupuncture as an alternative to the treatments offered in conventional medicine. Patients access complementary medicines through various routes. Many self-refer for private treatment or ask their GP for a referral to a complementary and alternative medicine (CAM) practitioner. (Chapter 19, pages 786–788 discusses the issues associated with referring patients and the regulation of CAM in more detail.) Some GPs offer CAM services to their patients themselves or through CAM practitioners employed within their practice. Where registered medical practitioners prescribe CAM medicines, they are accountable to the GMC for their actions. As with all prescriptions, irrespective of whether they are for alternative therapies or orthodox medication, doctors should base their decisions on the best available evidence and ensure that the treatment is in the patient's best interests. Where doctors discuss the option of prescribing CAM therapies with patients they must ensure they maintain clinical objectivity and do not allow their personal beliefs to interfere with the treatment offered to patients. If invited to do so, doctors may suggest options such as complementary or alternative therapies if they consider them to be appropriate for a particular patient. Information must, however, be provided objectively, giving a balanced view of the options available and the evidence for the efficacy of different treatments. Doctors should ensure that, as with all other interventions, they do not place any pressure on patients to accept their advice regarding CAM treatments.

Failing to obtain consent for homeopathic treatment

In 2003, a GP was found guilty by the GMC of serious professional misconduct for failing to obtain the informed consent of patients before prescribing homeopathic or natural remedies for them. None of the patients had specifically requested homeopathic treatment. The GP also failed to explain the rationale for using dowsing in the process of the selection of a remedy. In addition, the GP was found to have put pressure on the mother of a young child to accept the services of a geopathic stress consultant (and did not inform her that the consultant was not medically qualified) by indicating that geopathic stress gridlines in the vicinity of her house could cause cot death.

The GP was suspended from the medical register for 3 months. The GMC's Professional Conduct Committee strongly recommended that she used the opportunity, during her suspension, to consider the effect on her patients of her use of alternative medicine, in order to ensure that, in future, her personal beliefs did not prejudice her patients' care.[87]

The NHS funds some CAM therapies and decisions regarding availability are made at a local level. The issue can be controversial though and one of the key debates has centred on the provision of homeopathy. Much of the debate has focused on whether there is sufficient evidence of efficacy to justify using public resources to fund homeopathic treatment. Proponents of homeopathy, including doctors who use it as part of their medical practice, argue that many patients benefit from homeopathic treatments and allowing access to homeopathy is in line with maximising patient choice in the NHS. Critics claim that, as there is insufficient scientific evidence for its efficacy, homeopathy should not be funded using scarce NHS resources. The House of Commons Science and Technology Committee investigated the evidence base for homeopathy in 2010 and discussed the issue of whether it should be funded using NHS money. In its report, the Committee argued that the theoretical basis for homeopathy was 'weak' and 'scientifically implausible', and that the evidence from systematic reviews and meta-analyses showed that homeopathic products are non-efficacious and perform no better than a placebo.[88] The Committee argued that providing homeopathy constituted NHS endorsement and as a result, patients may reasonably form the view that homeopathy is an evidence-based treatment. The report concluded that the Government should stop funding homeopathy and that NHS doctors should not prescribe placebo treatments or refer patients to homeopaths. The Government at the time responded to the report acknowledging some of the Committee's arguments, but rejecting the main recommendations, stating that decisions on what treatment is most appropriate and should be provided for patients, including complementary therapies, should be made by the local NHS and clinicians and not by the Department of Health.[89] In 2010, the BMA's annual representatives meeting voted against the provision of homeopathy on the NHS.

Prescribing placebos

The House of Commons Science and Technology Committee report on homeopathy reignited the long-standing and controversial debate over whether it is ethical to prescribe a placebo in a clinical setting. In concluding that homeopathic treatments are non-efficacious and produce no better results than a placebo, the Committee stated that it was important for the Government to understand the power of the 'placebo effect' and to have clear policy on prescribing placebos in the NHS.

Placebos are commonly referred to as 'dummy' pills or treatments which, unknown to the patient, have no active pharmacological or physiological properties, or at least have none specific to the condition for which they are prescribed. The term can also apply to a much broader range of therapeutic interventions, including non-pharmacological and non-surgical elements of care, which have an effect on a patient that is not specific to the procedure carried out. The placebo effect is the change this intervention causes to a patient's illness which is 'attributable to the symbolic import of a treatment rather than a specific pharmacologic or physiologic property'.[90]

There is evidence of the placebo effect manifesting itself in many different ways. A common example is where a placebo provides relief from chronic pain despite the treatment administered containing no analgesic properties. It has been argued that doctors should be able to harness the power of the placebo effect; if prescribing a placebo can have a positive impact on a patient's symptoms it may have a place within medical practice as a legitimate form of treatment. It is not known exactly how common placebo prescribing is amongst doctors. Research carried out in the USA into the attitudes of physicians practicing internal medicine and rheumatology found that around half of those surveyed reported prescribing placebos on a regular basis and 62 per cent believed that the practice was ethically permissible.[91] A report commissioned by the German Medical Association also found similar levels of placebo prescribing, with half of doctors in the study stating they had prescribed placebos for patients.[92]

There are fundamental problems associated with doctors prescribing placebos within a clinical setting and, in the BMA's view, the unacknowledged use of placebos for patients with capacity is unethical. Prescribing and administering a placebo must entail some degree of patient deception because to maximise the placebo effect, a patient needs to believe that the 'dummy' treatment administered is real. Deceiving a patient, even where the doctor is acting in his or her best interests, obviously undermines trust and risks damaging the doctor–patient relationship. Depriving a patient of the opportunity to exercise informed choice does not respect patient autonomy and runs contrary to the concordant model of prescribing and the principles of shared decision making. These arguments, however, may not have the same weight in cases where patients have diminished capacity. Commentators have also argued that prescribing placebos is not good medical practice.[93] The placebo effect is unpredictable and a doctor can never be sure whether it will manifest itself in a particular patient or know the extent to which placebo treatments will affect different patients. The majority of medical science is based on the diagnosis and treatment of the underlying biological processes that cause illness, whereas placebos can only treat the symptoms of illness. There is a danger therefore that in prescribing placebos to treat a particular symptom, serious underlying conditions may be left untreated or undiagnosed which may risk patient safety.

Controlled drugs

The fourth report of the Shipman Inquiry (see Chapter 12, page 496), *The Regulation of Controlled Drugs in the Community*,[94] set out a number of recommendations to improve the way in which controlled drugs were prescribed, dispensed and stored. The report specifically identified the monitoring and collection of information relating to private prescriptions for controlled drugs as a key area that needed strengthening to prevent similar abuses of the system occurring again.

Following the recommendations of the report, a number of legislative changes and best practice requirements were introduced including the following:

- special forms for private prescriptions of schedule 2 and 3 controlled drugs
- requirement that patients or individuals who collect prescriptions on their behalf, must sign for private or NHS prescriptions for controlled drugs on collection
- the validity of prescriptions for schedule 2, 3 and 4 controlled drugs limited to 28 days
- private prescribers of controlled drugs must be issued with a unique identifying number
- prescriptions for controlled drugs written by private prescribers in a certain area should be subject to external monitoring
- prescriptions for controlled drugs can be typed but must be signed by the prescriber
- strong recommendation that prescriptions for schedule 2, 3 and 4 drugs are limited to a quantity necessary for up to 30 days' clinical need
- all healthcare providers who keep controlled drugs on site must comply with the terms of a standard operating procedure.

The changes sought to implement the tighter controls recommended by the report without compromising access to controlled drugs for patients who need them and without adversely affecting the prescribing practices of doctors. In the wake of the Shipman Inquiry, media reports suggested that some doctors were reluctant to prescribe opioids for pain relief, which was affecting patient care at the end of life. (Pain relief for patients at the end of life is discussed in more detail in Chapter 10, pages 434–435.) There are also anecdotal reports to suggest that post-Shipman some doctors had reservations about carrying controlled drugs in their medical bags. It is important that doctors carry controlled drugs in environments or for situations where they may be required.

Prescribing for addicts

Doctors who are responsible for prescribing to drug addicts must be familiar with the relevant regulations and guidance,[95] and ensure that their actions comply with the law. The role of doctors who work with addicts often extends beyond simply prescribing and may include health promotion, harm minimisation and treatment or rehabilitation.

GPs should not refuse to accept patients on to their list solely on the grounds of their addiction, although they are not required to provide specialist treatment for a patient's drug addiction. To prescribe, administer or supply diamorphine, dipipanone or cocaine in the treatment of drug addiction, doctors must hold a general licence that is issued by their relevant health department. Other practitioners must refer addicts requiring these drugs to a treatment centre.

Controlled drugs that are commonly prescribed to addicts, such as methadone, have a potential street value and there is a danger that such drugs could be fraudulently obtained and diverted into the community. Under legislation in England, Scotland and Wales, dispensers are required to ascertain the role of the person who is collecting a prescription for a schedule 2 controlled drug and, although it is not a legal requirement, they have the discretion to request proof of identity. The legislation permits the dispenser to refuse to supply the drugs if they are not satisfied as to the person's identity. Guidance from the Department of Health states that dispensers also retain the discretion not to request proof of identity if they have concerns that doing so would compromise patient confidentiality.[96]

Self-prescribing and prescribing for family members

The BMA and the GMC advise doctors against prescribing for themselves or for family, friends or colleagues. There are clearly some cases, such as in an emergency situation, in which such action would be reasonable, but as a general rule it should be avoided. There is a risk that doctors who self-treat may ignore or deny serious health problems or may simply treat symptoms without taking steps to identify the underlying cause. There have also been occasions in the past where self-prescribing has lead to drug abuse or addiction.

Treating family, friends or colleagues could raise questions about the objectivity of the advice provided and, although the same duty of confidentiality would apply, raises issues of privacy for the family members and friends. One-off prescribing for family and friends, other than in exceptional circumstances, is also to be avoided because this could interfere with care or treatment being provided by the patient's usual doctor. There is also a risk that, if the patient is harmed by the medication, the doctor's motives could be called into question.

One of the recommendations of the Shipman Inquiry was that the GMC should 'make plain that it will be regarded as professional misconduct for a doctor to prescribe controlled drugs for anyone with whom s/he does not have a genuine professional relationship'.[97] In its prescribing guidance the GMC states that doctors should not prescribe controlled drugs for themselves or anyone close to them, unless:

- no other person with the legal right to prescribe is available to assess the patient's clinical condition and to prescribe without a delay which would put the patient's life or health at risk, or cause the patient unacceptable pain, and
- that treatment is immediately necessary to:
  - save life
  - avoid serious deterioration in the patient's health, or
  - alleviate otherwise uncontrollable pain.

Where doctors need to prescribe controlled drugs to someone close to them, the GMC states that they must be able to justify their actions and record the relationship the doctor has with the patient and the reasons why it was necessary to prescribe.[98]

Prescribing at a distance

Consulting by internet, email or telephone

Developments in information technology and increased customer demand for more convenient ways to access health services have seen a growth in the availability of email consultations and internet prescribing. Individual, face-to-face interaction between patient and doctor remains the 'gold-standard' of medical consultations. In some circumstances though, providing medical advice and treatment over the telephone or by email can be a useful addition to the services offered to patients. As with all consultations, doctors need to satisfy themselves that patients have capacity and that they have given consent for the consultation to take place. Doctors also need to ensure that they are able to provide patients with sufficient information for them to make informed decisions. Standards of record keeping should be maintained and doctors should be conscious of security considerations and patient confidentiality when using electronic means of communication (see Chapter 6, pages 243–245).

Consultations conducted remotely have significant limitations when compared with a consultation conducted in person. Doctors are obviously unable to conduct a physical examination of a patient and, depending on the medium used, may not be able to hear, see or speak directly with the patient they are consulting with. The distance between the doctor and patient imposed by different technologies, particularly with respect to text-based communication such as email and online consultations, may also make it difficult to convey the correct tone to the patient compared with face-to-face interaction. The BMA General Practitioners Committee's guidance, *Consulting in the modern world*, discusses the various advantages and disadvantages of using a range of electronic means of communication and offers advice on how doctors should approach remote consulting.[99]

The limitations inherent to various forms of remote consultation inevitably have an impact on the advisability of doctors prescribing for patients through such media. Repeat prescribing through remote means may be less problematic than other forms of prescribing and can be convenient for both patient and doctor. There may also be a more limited number of occasions where doctors feel that it is appropriate to prescribe for their patient outside normal face-to-face consultations. The GMC suggests that such occasions are most likely to occur if doctors have sole responsibility for a patient, are deputising on behalf of another doctor who does or where a doctor has prior knowledge of a patient's condition and has the authority to access his or her medical record. Where this is the case, the GMC advises that doctors must ensure that they:

- establish the patient's current medical conditions and history and concurrent or recent use of other medications including non-prescription medicines
- carry out an adequate assessment of the patient's condition
- identify the likely cause of the patient's condition
- ensure that there is sufficient justification to prescribe the medicines or treatment proposed and discuss other treatment options with the patient where appropriate
- ensure that the treatment and/or medicines are not contraindicated for the patient
- make a clear, accurate and legible record of all medicines prescribed.[100]

Doctors should be especially cautious with respect to remote prescribing if they do not have prior knowledge of the patient in the ways described above. Doctors should consider very carefully whether prescribing in this way can be done safely and whether it would be in the best interests of the patient in question. Doctors should bear in mind that they may not be able to verify who the patient is or whether their medical complaints are genuine. Although the GMC does not rule out prescribing remotely in such situations, it specifies that doctors must provide the patient with their name and GMC number and take the following steps in addition to those listed above:

- give an explanation to the patient of the processes involved in remote consultations
- establish a dialogue with the patient, using a questionnaire, to ensure that sufficient information about the patient can be ascertained to enable safe prescribing
- make appropriate arrangements to follow the progress of the patient
- monitor the effectiveness of the treatment and/or review the diagnosis
- inform the patient's GP, providing that the patient gives consent to the information being shared.[101]

If doctors cannot satisfy these requirements, the GMC advises that doctors should not prescribe remotely.

Failings in internet prescribing

In 2009, a GMC fitness to practise panel found a doctor guilty of serious professional misconduct for prescribing medication to patients through his online company in a way that was judged 'irresponsible, not in the best interests of patients and below the standard expected of a registered medical practitioner'.[102] The panel heard that the doctor had prescribed the powerful analgesic dihydrocodeine to a patient remotely but had failed to:

- conduct an examination of the patient
- take an adequate history from the patient
- contact the patient's GP regarding the prescriptions or take adequate steps to ascertain whether the patient had a GP at the time or previously
- inform the patient that her GP should be made aware of the prescription.

The panel decided the doctor had put the patient at risk by not putting himself in a position where he could assess the patient's condition or judge whether the patient was misleading him in any way. The doctor continued to provide the patient with repeat prescriptions for dihydrocodeine over a period of around 16 months without examining her, monitoring her condition or contacting her GP. The patient was later arrested for attempting to copy and forge the doctor's prescriptions and admitted during her police interview that she was addicted to the drug. The doctor was also found guilty of involvement in the inappropriate prescribing of Viagra and the weight loss pill, Reductil, to two different patients.

The hearing followed an earlier appearance before the panel in 2007 where the doctor was described as having a cavalier attitude to prescribing after being found guilty of serious errors of conduct in relation to prescriptions made out to five persons. One of the patients was a 16-year-old who was receiving psychiatric treatment at the time and had informed the doctor of previous suicide attempts and current suicidal thoughts. He later took an overdose of the beta-blocker, propranolol, which the doctor had prescribed.

The GMC panel found that the doctor had put his business interests ahead of the safety of his patients and had not met the standards of prescribing expected of a competent medical practitioner. Given his conduct, the panel decided that the doctor should be erased from the medical register.

Prescribing for patients in other countries

A very difficult question concerns prescriptions for patients who live in other parts of the world. Relatives in this country sometimes approach their own GP with a request for medication for a seriously ill patient living abroad where appropriate drugs are unobtainable. As with any other prescription, the prescribing doctor would retain full clinical responsibility for prescribing such medication and this can prove particularly difficult when he or she cannot examine the patient personally, but is relying on information obtained from others. There is no obligation on doctors to comply with such requests and many refuse because of the obvious risks of prescribing for a patient they have not seen. However, some doctors feel impelled by humanitarian considerations to look into the case and to offer some assistance if they can. Such situations are fraught with difficulty, but if doctors wish to pursue the matter, after considering the risks for the overseas patient, and for themselves if harm to that patient should result, the BMA gives the advice below.

Doctors should not rely solely on relatives' accounts of the patient's condition. Often the patient's own doctor abroad is willing to give a clinical report of the condition and recommendations for medication, as well as confirming that the medication is necessary and unobtainable by other means. Such cases virtually amount to a situation of shared prescribing, with the doctor who writes the prescription relying heavily on the medical opinion of the examining doctor. Some lives are probably saved by this arrangement and this is usually the factor that persuades the prescribing doctor to cooperate, on the grounds that in the particular situation the risks of not obtaining treatment at all are likely to be greater than the risks of prescribing error. The BMA has not heard of any cases in which a prescribing doctor subsequently suffered legal repercussions, although the possibility of erroneous prescribing in such situations cannot be ruled out.

Even when the prescribing doctor is willing to participate in such an arrangement, there are a number of further hurdles to be overcome and these may influence the doctor's view of the practicality of the proposal. For example, relatives have to consider how the drugs will be transported, including the rules governing the export and import of drugs that are not for their personal use. Many countries have their own restrictions on the drugs that can be taken into the country; even some that are available over the counter in the UK cannot be taken into other countries. Advice will need to be sought in individual cases from the relevant embassy for the country concerned. Before prescribing for patients who are overseas, doctors should also ensure that they have adequate indemnity cover.[103] Any drugs posted overseas are subject to customs labelling and postage regulations and any such prescriptions must, of course, be paid for privately as they are not covered by the NHS.

Availability of prescription-only medication on the internet

The adoption of an increasingly consumerist attitude towards healthcare in the UK has seen patients requesting easier and more convenient methods of obtaining medication. The expansion of the internet has precipitated a rapid growth in online pharmacies to meet this demand and many companies now offer over-the-counter and prescription-only medications direct to patients via the internet. Internet pharmacies offer a number of significant benefits to patients including greater convenience and more choice and control over where and how medication can be obtained. Online providers also offer greater accessibility to pharmacy services for people who are house bound or have limited mobility. However, there are also a number of potential risks involved in buying pharmaceuticals online.

The RPSGB has estimated that over 2 million people regularly purchase medication via the internet.[104] While some online pharmacies are legitimate and provide a valuable service to patients, there are a growing number of websites, often based outside of the UK, which offer prescription-only drugs direct to patients without requiring a valid prescription. A key motivation for people buying pharmaceuticals online is the level of privacy this method of purchase provides. The RPSGB reports that the most popular prescription medicines bought online are so-called 'lifestyle drugs', such as Viagra, and other medicines such as Prozac, Ritalin and Provigil, which are often obtained for off-label use. Research into online pharmacies that supply UK customers has also found that a number of prescription-only analgesics, including controlled opioids, can be obtained easily without prescription.[105]

There are a number of significant risks associated with purchasing potent medication from unregulated suppliers. The quality of the drugs people obtain may be substandard, out-of-date, not licensed for use or banned in the UK. Consumers may receive counterfeit drugs which can contain toxic substances and unknown amounts of active ingredients.

Medication may also be supplied to the customer without the necessary information regarding, for example, the correct dosage or potential side effects. It is the BMA's view that patient safety in relation to prescription drugs can only be assured if a full medical consultation takes place. Patients who do not consult with their doctor before taking certain medications put themselves at risk from contraindications and adverse reactions. Even where prescription medications are obtained to address genuine medical complaints, without clinical assessment individuals may be self-medicating for the wrong diagnosis. Doctors have also voiced concerns that the availability of prescription drugs online could have a negative effect on the doctor–patient relationship and threaten patient safety in prescribing. As a key motivation for online purchasing of pharmaceuticals is privacy, patients may be reluctant to speak with their GP about the medicines they have obtained online. There is a danger therefore that doctors may prescribe medication without knowing whether the patient is taking any other products.[106]

The scale of the harm caused by the availability of prescription medicines on the internet is unknown. The Nuffield Council on Bioethics, in its 2010 report, *Medical Profiling and Online Medicine*, found there was little systematic evidence of widespread harms resulting from people purchasing pharmaceuticals from the internet, although the report suggested that this may be because individuals are reluctant to report adverse reactions, even in the face of significant health problems.[107] A survey of GPs carried out in 2009, however, found that one in four doctors had treated patients for adverse reactions relating to medicines bought over the internet, which suggests that doctors are seeing the impact of patients obtaining medication through this method in their everyday practice.[108] Beyond the individual risks associated with internet pharmacy, the availability of antibiotics over the internet could also have a serious long-term negative impact on public health by increasing antibiotic resistance.[109]

The MHRA regulates the safety, efficacy and quality of medicines in the UK, and all pharmacies in England, Scotland and Wales, including internet pharmacies, are required to register with the General Pharmaceutical Council (GPhC). To help members of the public identify safe, legitimate online sites, the GPhC runs an Internet Pharmacy Logo scheme. To display the logo on their site, internet pharmacies must be registered with the GPhC and meet the Council's *Standards for pharmacy owners and superintendent pharmacists of retail pharmacy businesses*.[110] By clicking on the logo, members of the public can verify if a particular pharmacy is registered on the GPhC website.

Regulation of pharmacies in Northern Ireland is the responsibility of the Pharmaceutical Society of Northern Ireland (PSNI). The PSNI document, *Professional Standards and Guidance for Internet Pharmacy Services*, outlines how internet pharmacies registered in Northern Ireland must operate.[111] At the time of writing, the PSNI did not run an internet pharmacy logo scheme similar to that in place in the rest of the UK.

Summary – prescribing at a distance

- Prescribing by email or over the telephone could seriously compromise the standard of care provided to patients. Doctors should think carefully about whether prescribing in this way is in the best interests of their patients.
- There are serious safety risks of prescribing in cases where the patient is unknown to the doctor, there is no opportunity for examination and the arrangements for monitoring and follow up are limited.
- Doctors are not obliged to comply with requests from patients to prescribe drugs for relatives in another country. Those who wish to assist, however, must be aware of

the possibility of liability arising and should seek information from the patient's own doctor whenever possible in order to verify the information provided. They also need to give consideration to the practicalities of such an arrangement.

Drug administration

Although there are restrictions on who can train to become a prescriber and administer medicines using a PGD, any suitably trained member of staff within health or social care can administer medicines prescribed by an authorised prescriber that are to be given to an individual named patient.

Doctors who are responsible for administering drugs must ensure that they have the necessary knowledge and expertise to do so safely and effectively. Those who are responsible for training doctors have an ethical responsibility to ensure that medical students are adequately supervised and trained in any procedures they may be required to undertake. Any doctor who is in doubt about the method of administration of a particular drug, or the correct procedures to be followed, should seek advice from a more senior member of the team or from a pharmacist. Similarly, the advice of a pharmacist should be sought if there is uncertainty about the appropriate dosage of a drug for a particular patient.

Protocols should be in place in all hospitals, setting out clearly the checking procedures that must be followed to ensure that the dose and strength of a drug are those prescribed and that the drug is administered to the correct patient in the correct way. It is important that adequate training, supervision and safeguards are in place, as far as possible, to guard against potential medication errors. Doctors should not feel pressured to carry out procedures they feel are beyond their training or capability, and it is their responsibility to speak out about any concerns.

Error in drug administration

On 4 January 2001, a young male patient, WJ, attended Queen's Medical Centre, Nottingham, for the administration of chemotherapy as part of his medical maintenance programme after successful treatment of leukaemia. He was to receive cytosine by intrathecal (spinal) injection and, on the following day, he was to receive vincristine intravenously. Owing to a series of errors and the lack of training and experience of the doctors concerned, the vincristine was administered on the same day and also by intrathecal injection. This error is almost always fatal and, despite emergency treatment being provided, WJ died on 2 February 2001.

An external inquiry was carried out, which concluded that the death 'was not caused by one or even several human errors but by a far more complex amalgam of human, organisational, technical and social interactions'.[112] Among the failings highlighted in the report were the lack of explicit written protocols, the lack of formal training for the doctors concerned and the unwillingness of the senior house officer to mention his doubts about the treatment to his senior colleague.

Special safeguards

Some drugs carry significant risks, require particularly rigorous safeguards and should be administered according to standard operating procedures. Because of the potency of the drugs involved in chemotherapy, for example, a set protocol should exist for their use and the drugs should be administered only by those who have received specific training.

This should include how to make up the drugs, the nature of the agents, including their danger to the administering health professional and other employees, and their administration. The individual administering the drug should also be aware of the appropriate procedures to follow in the event of spillage or a failure in clinical technique during administration, as well as procedures for the safe disposal of any unused drugs and the containers and instruments used in administration. Where necessary, supervision and advice should be available from a more senior colleague and doctors must not be afraid to seek help. Doctors have an ethical responsibility to be satisfied that they have the necessary competence and support to undertake these procedures.

Covert administration of medication

Patients with capacity have the right to refuse medication, as well as any other treatment, and must not be given medication against their wishes. When patients lack capacity to take decisions about their healthcare, they should be treated with the authorisation of an appointed healthcare proxy or in their 'best interests' or, in Scotland, under the general authority to treat (see Chapter 3). There may be exceptional cases in which doctors take the view that a patient who lacks capacity requires medication and his or her interests would be best served by giving this in the least distressing manner, which could include covert administration. Any such decision must be made on an individual basis, and blanket rules must not be applied to particular categories of patient. Covert administration of medication is never justified for the convenience of those providing treatment (see Chapter 1, pages 39–40).

Summary – drug administration

- Doctors who are responsible for administering drugs must ensure that they have the necessary knowledge and expertise to do so safely and effectively.
- Doctors should not feel pressured to carry out procedures they feel are beyond their training or capability, and it is their responsibility to speak out about any concerns.
- Patients with capacity have the right to refuse medication and must not be given medication against their wishes.
- In exceptional cases where a patient who lacks capacity requires medication, it may be acceptable to administer the medicine covertly if this is in the best interests of the patient. Any such decision must be made on an individual basis, and blanket rules must not be applied to particular categories of patient.
- Covert drug administration is never justified for the convenience of those providing treatment.

Reporting adverse drug reactions

The Yellow Card Scheme is run by the MHRA and the Commission on Human Medicines (CHM) and helps to monitor and investigate adverse drug reactions. This UK-wide scheme invites spontaneous reporting of suspected adverse drug reactions and relies on information supplied on a voluntary basis by doctors, dentists, pharmacists and coroners, and by pharmaceutical companies under statutory obligations.[113] Doctors should be alert to the possibility of side effects and are strongly encouraged to participate in this scheme, which provides pseudonymised information to the MHRA or CHM, which can be traced back to an identifiable individual if necessary. Patients can also report any suspected adverse reaction to a drug using the scheme. Health professionals and patients are particularly encouraged to report all suspected reactions to drugs that are newly licensed for use in the UK, known as 'Black Triangle' medicines, which are closely monitored for any rare or long-terms adverse effects that may not be identifiable during clinical trials. The MHRA and CHM produce a monthly drug safety update that provides health professionals with the latest drug safety information and guidance.[114]

The NPSA manages a National Reporting and Learning System in England and Wales through which adverse incidents and near misses, including those involving medication, are collected.[115] NHS staff are encouraged to report all patient safety incidents irrespective of whether they result in harm. Using these data the Agency seeks to develop solutions to try to ensure that the same errors are not repeated. (In 2010, it was proposed that the NPSA be abolished as part of the Government's plan to reduce the number of arms-length bodies; for up to date information see the BMA website.)[116]

Generic prescribing

Prescribing figures for England, Wales and Scotland show that over 80 per cent of prescriptions written are for generic medicines.[117] As prescribing generic drugs is considerably cheaper than branded drugs, doctors are encouraged to prescribe generic alternatives wherever possible. Ethical issues can arise, however, in changing a patient's prescription from a branded to a generic drug.

Drug switching

Given that there can be significant price differences between branded drugs and their generic counterparts, pressure on limited drug budgets has meant that health managers as well as individual practitioners have sometimes reduced costs by switching patients from proprietary drugs to generic substitutes. Individual practitioners have also come under pressure to switch drugs in this way and have also been offered incentives to do so. Although with some drugs, such as statins, the savings in drug costs have been significant, the practice nonetheless raises a number of ethical concerns, particularly in relation to wholesale switching where, for example, all patients at a particular practice are switched from a specific branded drug to a generic.

Ordinarily drug switching takes one of two forms. Either the drug is switched to a generic substitute containing the same active ingredient, or it is switched for a 'therapeutic substitute', one with a different active ingredient but with a similar therapeutic purpose. Clearly, therapeutic substitutes can have different biological pathways and different side-effect profiles. There is also at least anecdotal evidence to suggest that generic substitutes can still act in subtly different ways because of variations in bioavailability and dosage strengths. Although, where possible, a less expensive product is to be preferred to a more expensive equivalent, the process by which patients might be transferred should be carefully considered. It can, for example, take some time to stabilise patients on particular drugs, and variations in bioavailability in generics may have an impact on patient tolerance of the active ingredient. Where dosages or packaging differ, or the drugs seem very unlike those with which they have become familiar, some patients may struggle with the new regime and this clearly raises the possibility of negative outcomes. In relation to therapeutic substitution, given that the active ingredient is different, and that the side effects are likely to be different, a failure to discuss directly with the individual any intended change in regime could potentially leave doctors open to claims of negligence if harm results.

In the BMA's view, best practice in relation to drug switching should involve informed discussion with individual patients. In this way doctors can fully enrol patients in the decision-making process, can discuss in advance any problems that might occur and can also identify those patients who may need more support, or whose medical history indicates that they may be likely to respond with more difficulty to any change. Where doctors believe that the overall best interests of a patient suggests that he or she should not be switched, then pressures to change should be resisted. In the BMA's view, the wholesale switching of an entire cohort of patients to an equivalent drug without discussion with patients is unlikely to constitute best practice.

In relation to the payment of incentives to doctors to undertake drug switching, the Association of the British Pharmaceutical Industry brought an action to the European Court of Justice questioning its lawfulness under Article 94(1) of European Directive 2001/83 relating to medicinal products for human use. The Court held that the use of such incentives was lawful.[118]

Supply of drugs into the UK

The majority of doctors will have little direct involvement in the medicines supply chain. Issues that affect the flow of drugs into and out of the UK, however, can cause shortages of vital prescription medication that can impact on doctors' practice and have serious consequences for patient safety. Under European[119] and UK law,[120] market authorisation holders and distributors are obligated to ensure a continued supply of their products to pharmacies and individuals or bodies who supply drugs. This legislation is designed to prevent medicine shortages by protecting the levels of drugs imported into the country and ensuring they are sufficient to meet patient need. The UK still experiences significant drug shortages of branded prescription medicines and in recent years there have been reports of shortages for drugs to treat conditions such as epilepsy, cancer and schizophrenia. Since November 2009, the Pharmaceutical Services Negotiating Committee (PSNC) has published an official list of branded drugs that are in short supply.[121] One of the main causes of these shortages is the export and 'parallel trading' of medicines from within the UK, which can threaten the country's stock levels of prescription drugs.

Parallel trading

Parallel trading involves intermediaries buying drugs cheaply in one country and exporting them to other countries for profit. Drug prices are negotiated between companies and governments and parallel trading exploits the price differences that can exist between countries. In the UK, pharmacists, NHS trusts and dispensing doctors are all in a position to take advantage of parallel trading and can be attracted by the short-term financial gains on offer. In 2009, the *Health Service Journal* (*HSJ*) reported that the Royal Surrey County Hospital Foundation Trust had sold millions of pounds worth of drugs over a 10-month period making £300,000 profit in the process.[122] The Trust insisted that none of the drugs they had sold were in short supply. Further investigation by the *HSJ* found that of the 33 product lines sold by the Trust, 13 were cancer drugs and four were drugs to treat HIV.[123] One of the cancer drugs sold, imatinib (Glivec), was placed on the list of drugs in short supply during the period the Trust was trading; however, it insisted it did not export imatinib after this point.

Exporting medicines in this way is legal, providing that the exporter holds a wholesaler's licence, but remains highly controversial. Governments, who may have satisfied themselves that they have imported sufficient levels of prescription medicines to serve the country's healthcare needs, can find that these drugs are subsequently exported and therefore diverted away from patients. Guidance from the Department of Health, endorsed by the BMA, MHRA, ABPI and other stakeholders, outlines the ethical and legal obligations of different parties within the medicines supply chain.[124] Dispensing doctors are advised that 'in exporting medicines or selling stock for exportation by others, dispensing doctors should carefully consider their ethical responsibilities to their patients and the public . . . Patient care must never come second to business considerations.'[125]

Importing cheap drugs from overseas can also give rise to patient safety issues. Parallel traded medicines often carry instructions printed in a foreign language, which can be confusing for patients and lead to poor adherence to a drug regimen. The process of repackaging medicines also increases the risk of counterfeited medicines entering the UK drug supply, which could represent a serious threat to public health.

Pharmacogenetics

It is well known that individuals respond in different ways to medication: some patients do not respond at all to a particular drug, others require a higher than the usual dose to be effective and some people develop adverse effects. It is also known that some of this difference is due to genetic variation. Pharmacogenetics offers the potential to identify how individual patients will respond to certain types of medication, based on differences in their genetic make-up, which can then be taken into account in prescribing decisions. This could lead to a form of individualised treatment regimen for some conditions whereby prescribing would be preceded by a genetic test to ascertain whether a particular drug will be effective, the appropriate dose to administer and whether the individual is likely to suffer adverse effects, avoiding a trial and error approach that may expose patients to unnecessary harm.

While having huge potential benefits, pharmacogentics raises a number of ethical issues, which were explored in detail by the Nuffield Council on Bioethics in 2003.[126] Many of the issues at stake are similar to those discussed in Chapter 9 about the implications of genetic information being available and, in particular, issues around consent, confidentiality and privacy. There are some aspects, however, that are novel to pharmacogenetics. In addition to identifying those who are likely to experience side effects, testing the individual's response to a drug would also identify a group of patients for whom the treatment may not be effective. In most cases this would not give a certain answer about whether the drug will work or not, but is more likely to offer a probability of success. This leads to questions about where to draw the line in terms of prescribing and, in particular, when to restrict the use of public funds. If a genetic test indicates that an individual has only a very low chance of the drug being successful, it may be questionable to provide it within the NHS. These decisions clearly depend partly on other factors such as the risks or side effects of the medication, the seriousness of the condition and whether other treatments are available that may be more successful. As with other forms of treatment, however, ultimately some judgement is needed about what anticipated level of success is sufficient to justify providing the treatment.

One likely effect of the development of pharmacogenetics would be an increase in the number of people having genetic tests. This could lead to new dilemmas. If, for example, a test carried out to assess drug response was also capable of providing evidence of a high genetic risk of a serious disease, this would need to be explained carefully to the patient who would need to take that into account when deciding whether to consent to the test. Problems could arise if the information available to assess drug response was later found to have relevance in terms of the risk of developing another condition, because the individual would be given no choice about whether to receive that information. It cannot be assumed that patients would be willing to consent to testing and this raises the question of whether a patient can have the option to receive treatment without taking an associated pharmacogenetic test.[127] The requirement for testing may be included in the licence conditions of a medicine. Although doctors can prescribe off-label, they have the responsibility to ensure that a patient will, on balance, benefit from the treatment. If there is a significant chance that a patient could suffer adverse reactions from the treatment, or there is significant doubt that the treatment will work, it is unlikely a doctor would agree to prescribe without the patient first taking a test. Where a genetic test could be used, but was not part of the licensing conditions, it would be down to doctors' clinical judgement, taking into account factors such as the potential side effects and availability of alternative treatments, as to whether to prescribe the drug without the patient being tested.

There is a possibility that the application of pharmacogenetics, and therefore its benefits, will be limited because of economic considerations. By identifying those patients for whom the drugs would not be effective, pharmaceutical companies would reduce the market for their products. This could lead to a reduction in the development of drugs that would be suitable for only a small group of the population unless incentives were provided for research into those conditions. Another possibility is that, by reducing the market for particular products, pharmacogenetics could lead to inexorable rises in the price of some medicines, which would raise serious questions about affordability within the NHS. Pharmacogenetics also offers the potential for information about the genetic characteristics of some diseases, such as cancer, to inform drug design, as seen with the development of Herceptin (trastuzumab). However, while greater understanding of the genetic characteristics of different diseases may lead to the development of more efficacious drugs, it may also result in greater stratification of patient groups and the classification of more diseases as 'rare' based on their genomic profile. This could significantly disadvantage some patients, as the limited commercial market could act as a disincentive for pharmaceutical companies to develop drugs for these disease types or, if treatments were developed, the cost of supplying the drugs may be prohibitively expensive, again raising questions about provision within the NHS.

References

1   Joint Formulary Committee (published biannually) *British National Formulary*. British Medical Association and Pharmaceutical Press, London.
2   General Medical Council (2006) *Good Medical Practice*, GMC, London, paras 52–3.
3   Hine D. (2010) *The 2009 Influenza Pandemic: An independent review of the UK response to the 2009 influenza pandemic*, Cabinet Office, London, p.101.
4   Triggle N. (2010) Swine flu drug hand-out service raises concerns. *BBC News Online* (July 5). Available at: www.bbc.co.uk/news (accessed 1 November 2010).
5   General Medical Council (2006) *Good Medical Practice*, GMC, London.
6   General Medical Council (2008) *Good Practice in Prescribing Medicines*, GMC, London. At the time of writing the GMC was in the process of updating this guidance for publication in late 2011. Up-to-date information can be found on the BMA and GMC websites.

7   General Medical Council (2006) *Good Medical Practice*, GMC, London, para 3b.

8   GMC Professional Conduct Committee hearing, 23–25 September 2002.

9   General Medical Council (2008) *Good Practice in Prescribing Medicines*, GMC, London, paras 18 and 20.

10 General Medical Council (2008) *Good Practice in Prescribing Medicines*, GMC, London, para 23.

11 Boseley S. (2011) Firms fight move to obtain cheap anti-blindness drug Avastin. *The Guardian* (January 2). Available at: www.guardian.co.uk (accessed 15 February 2011). The article reports that Stockport and Bury PCT offered patients the choice of Avastin at a private hospital with shorter waiting lists, or Lucentis in the NHS.

12 National Institute for Health and Clinical Excellence (2010) *Eye conditions – bevacizumab (Avastin): report of findings from a workshop held at NICE on 13 July 2010*, NICE, London, p.6.

13 Royal College of Ophthalmologists (2009) *The intravitreal use of bevacizumab (Avastin) in age related macular degeneration*, RCOphth, London, p.4.

14 National Institute for Health and Clinical Excellence (2010) *Eye conditions – bevacizumab (Avastin): report of findings from a workshop held at NICE on 13 July 2010*, NICE, London.

15 NHS National Patient Safety Agency (2009) *Safety in doses: Improving the use of medicines in the NHS*, NPSA, London, p.1.

16 Medical Protection Society (2008) *GP Registrar: Prescribing* (Autumn 2008), MPS, Leeds, p.6.

17 Aronson JK, Henderson G, Webb DJ. *et al.* (2006) A prescription for better prescribing. *BMJ* **333**, 459–60.

18 Dornan T, Ashcroft D, Heathfield H. *et al.* (2009) *An indepth investigation into the causes of prescribing errors by foundation trainees in relation to their medical education – Equip study*. Available at: www.gmc-uk.org (accessed 5 July 2010).

19 Department of Health (2002) *Provision of patient information with dispensed medicines: guidance note*. Available at: www.dh.gov.uk (accessed 5 March 2011).

20 National Institute for Health and Clinical Excellence (2009) *Medicines adherence: involving patients in decisions about prescribed medicines and supporting adherence CG76*, NICE, London, p.4.

21 National Institute for Health and Clinical Excellence (2009) *Costing statement: Medicines adherence – involving patients in decisions about prescribed medicines and supporting adherence*, NICE, London.

22 Carter S, Taylor D, Levenson R. (2005) *A question of choice: compliance in medicine taking*, 3rd edn, Medicines Partnership. Available at: www.keele.ac.uk/pharmacy/npcplus (accessed 31 May 2011), p.7.

23 National Institute for Health and Clinical Excellence (2009) *Medicines adherence: involving patients in decisions about prescribed medicines and supporting adherence CG76*, NICE, London, p.4.

24 General Medical Council (2008) *Good Practice in Prescribing Medicines*, GMC, London, para 5c.

25 Carter S, Taylor D, Levenson R. (2005) *A question of choice: compliance in medicine taking*, 3rd edn, Medicines Partnership. Available at: www.keele.ac.uk/pharmacy/npcplus (accessed 31 May 2011), p.8.

26 National Institute for Health and Clinical Excellence (2009) *Medicines adherence: involving patients in decisions about prescribed medicines and supporting adherence CG76*, NICE, London.

27 The National Prescribing Centre learning resources are available at www.npci.org.uk (accessed 31 May 2011).

28 NHS Information Centre (2008) *Prescriptions dispensed in the community statistics for 1997–2007: England*. Available at: www.ic.nhs.uk (accessed 7 March 2011).

29 British Medical Association (2007) *Evidence-based prescribing*, BMA, London, p.10.

30 Barber ND, Alldred DP, Raynor DK. *et al.* (2009) Care homes' use of medicines study: prevalence, causes and potential harm of medication errors in care homes for older people. *Qual Saf Health Care* **18**, 341–6.

31 Carter S, Taylor D, Levenson R. (2005) *A question of choice: compliance in medicine taking*, 3rd edn, Medicines Partnership. Available at: www.keele.ac.uk/pharmacy/npcplus (accessed 31 May 2011), p.94.

32 Royal Pharmaceutical Society of Great Britain (2009) *Royal Pharmaceutical Society calls for older people to review their medicine with a pharmacist*. Press release, 29 July.

33 British Medical Association (2009) *The ethics of caring for older people*, Wiley-Blackwell, Chichester, p.15.

34 House of Commons Health Committee (2004) *Elder Abuse: Second report of Session 2003–04*, Vol. 1, The Stationery Office, London, para 65.

35 Banerjee S. (2009) *The use of antipsychotic medication for people with dementia: time for action*, DH, London.

36 Sammons H, Conroy S. (2008) How do we ensure safe prescribing for children? *Arch Dis Child* **93**, 98–9.

37 Paediatric Formulary Committee (published annually) *BNF for Children*, BMJ Publishing Group, Pharmaceutical Press and Royal College of Paediatrics and Child Health Publications, London.

38 For more information see: www.medicinesforchildren.org.uk (accessed 31 May 2011).

39 Robinson K, Hoey M. (2009) Religion and drugs. *Student BMJ* **17**, b4453.

40   Mynors G, Ghalamkari H, Beaumont S. *et al. Informed choice in medicine taking: drugs of porcine origin and their clinical alternatives*, Medicines Partnership. Available at: www.keele.ac.uk/pharmacy/npcplus (accessed 31 May 2011).

41   For more information see: www.cks.nhs.uk (accessed 31 May 2011).

42   For more information see: www.nhs.uk (accessed 31 May 2011).

43   Medicines and Healthcare Products Regulatory Agency (2011) *Herbal Medicines: Advice to consumers*. Available at: www.mhra.gov.uk (accessed 7 March 2011).

44   General Medical Council (2008) *Good Practice in Prescribing Medicines*, GMC, London, para 3.

45   National Prescribing Centre (2004) *Saving time helping patients: a good practice guide to quality repeat prescribing*, NPC, Liverpool.

46   York Health Economics Consortium and The School of Pharmacy, University of London (2010) *Evaluation of the scale, causes and costs of waste medicines*, YHEC and School of Pharmacy, University of London, p.5.

47   York Health Economics Consortium and The School of Pharmacy, University of London (2010) *Evaluation of the scale, causes and costs of waste medicines*, YHEC and School of Pharmacy, University of London, p.24.

48   Shakespeare J, Neve E, Hodder K. (2000) Is norethisterone a lifestyle drug? Results of a database analysis. *BMJ* **320**, 291.

49   Bryant G, Scott I, Worrall A. (2000) Is norethisterone a lifestyle drug? Health is not merely the absence of disease. *BMJ* **320**, 1605.

50   Schedule 1 of the National Health Service (General Medical Services Contracts) (Prescription of Drugs etc.) Regulations 2004. SI 2004/629, N.629 provides for a list of drugs and other substances that are not to be prescribed within the NHS, also frequently referred to as the 'blacklist'. Schedule 2 drugs are a small list within the drug tariff of drugs to be prescribed within the NHS only in certain circumstances.

51   For a detailed discussion of different forms of cognitive enhancement and the issues it raises, see British Medical Association (2007) *Boosting your brainpower: ethical aspects of cognitive enhancement*, BMA, London.

52   Brooks V. (1998) Viagra is licensed in Europe but rationed in Britain. *BMJ* **217**, 765.

53   Brooks V. (1998) Viagra is licensed in Europe but rationed in Britain. *BMJ* **217**, 765.

54   NHS Executive (1999) *Treatment for impotence* HSC 1999/115, DH, Leeds.

55   Chisholm J. (1999) Viagra: a botched test case for rationing. *BMJ* **318**, 273–4.

56   General Medical Council (2008) *Consent: patients and doctors making decisions together*, GMC, London, para 9 l.

57   Department of Health (2009) *Guidance on NHS patients who wish to pay for additional private care*, DH, London. Scottish Government Health Directorates (2009) *Arrangements for NHS patients receiving healthcare services through private healthcare arrangements*, SGHD, Edinburgh.

58   National Institute for Health and Clinical Excellence (2009) *Annual Report 2008/9*, Vol. 1, NICE, London, p.3.

59   National Institute for Health and Clinical Excellence (2010) *Nice and the NHS*. Available at: www.nice.org.uk (accessed 18 January 2011).

60   Department of Health (2010) *Equity and Excellence: Liberating the NHS*, The Stationery Office, London.

61   All Wales Medicines Strategy Group (2010) *Appraisals*. Available at: www.wales.nhs.uk (accessed 18 January 2011).

62   The Medicines (Advertising) Regulations 1994. SI 1994/1932, s 21(1).

63   General Medical Council (2006) *Good Medical Practice*, GMC, London, para 74.

64   General Medical Council (2006) *Good Medical Practice*, GMC, London, paras 75–6.

65   Association of the British Pharmaceutical Industry (2011) *Code of Practice for the pharmaceutical industry 2011*, ABPI, London.

66   Association of the British Pharmaceutical Industry (2011) *Code of Practice for the pharmaceutical industry 2011*, ABPI, London, clause 18.

67   Association of the British Pharmaceutical Industry (2011) *Code of Practice for the pharmaceutical industry 2011*, ABPI, London, clause 19.

68   Association of the British Pharmaceutical Industry (2011) *Code of Practice for the pharmaceutical industry 2011*, ABPI, London, clause 19.

69   Association of the British Pharmaceutical Industry (2011) *Code of Practice for the pharmaceutical industry 2011*, ABPI, London, clause 20.

70   Association of the British Pharmaceutical Industry (2011) *Code of Practice for the pharmaceutical industry 2011*, ABPI, London, clause 18.4.

71   Association of the British Pharmaceutical Industry (2011) *Code of Practice for the pharmaceutical industry 2011*, ABPI, London, clause 15.3.

72   Association of the British Pharmaceutical Industry (2011) *Code of Practice for the pharmaceutical industry 2011*, ABPI, London, clause 12.2.

73   British Healthcare Business Intelligence Association (2009) *The Legal and Ethical Guidelines for Healthcare Market Research*, BHBIA, St Albans.
74   General Medical Council (2008) *Good Practice in Prescribing Medicines*, GMC, London, para 10.
75   General Medical Council (2008) *Good Practice in Prescribing Medicines*, GMC, London, para 17.
76   General Medical Council (2008) *Good Practice in Prescribing Medicines*, GMC, London, para 27.
77   NHS Management Executive (1991) *Responsibilities for prescribing between hospitals and GPs (EL(91)127)*, Department of Health, London.
78   British Medical Association (2007) *Prescribing and the primary and secondary care interface*, BMA, London.
79   Department of Health, Social Services and Public Safety (2003) *The regional group on specialist drugs – implementation of red/amber lists – 1 May 2003 (*HSS(MD)16/2003). Available at: www.dhsspsni.gov.uk (accessed 7 March 2011).
80   General Medical Council (2008) *Good Practice in Prescribing Medicines*, GMC, London, para 28.
81   British Medical Association (2010) *Patient Group Directions and Patient Specific Directions in General Practice*, BMA, London.
82   National Prescribing Centre (2009) *Patient Group Directions: a practical guide and framework of competencies for all professionals using patient group directions*, NPC, Liverpool.
83   Nurse Prescribers' Formulary Subcommittee (published biannually) *Nurse prescribers' formulary for community practitioners*, British Medical Association and Royal Pharmaceutical Society of Great Britain in association with Community Practitioners' and Health Visitors' Association and the Royal College of Nursing, London.
84   General Medical Council (2006) *Good Medical Practice*, GMC, London, para 52.
85   Anon. (2010) Herbal medicines: what do clinicians know? *Drug Ther Bull* **48**, 4.
86   Care Quality Commission (2009) *Managing patients' medicines after discharge from hospital*, CQC, London.
87   GMC Professional Conduct Committee hearing, 13–17 January 2003.
88   House of Commons Science and Technology Committee (2010) *Evidence check 2: Homeopathy – Fourth Report of the Session 2009–10*, The Stationery Office, London.
89   Department of Health (2010) *Government Response to the Science and Technology Committee report 'Evidence Check 2: Homeopathy'*, The Stationery Office, London.
90   Quoted in: House of Commons Science and Technology Committee (2010) *Evidence check 2: Homeopathy – Fourth Report of the Session 2009–10*, The Stationery Office, London, p.10.
91   Tilburt J, Emanuel E, Kaptchuk T. *et al.* (2008) Prescribing 'placebo treatments': results of a national survey of US internists and rheumatologists. *BMJ* **337**, a1938.
92   d'Arcy Hughes A. (2011) Half of German doctors prescribe placebos, new study shows. *The Guardian* (March 6). Available at: www.guardian.co.uk (accessed 8 March 2011).
93   House of Commons Science and Technology Committee (2010) *Evidence check 2: Homeopathy – Fourth Report of the Session 2009–10*, The Stationery Office, London, p.11 and pp.27–8.
94   Smith J. (2004) *The Shipman Inquiry, Fourth Report: The Regulation of Controlled Drugs in the Community*. Available at: www.the-shipman-inquiry.org.uk (accessed 2 November 2010).
95   Department of Health (England) and the devolved administrations (2007) *Drug Misuse and Dependence: UK Guidelines on Clinical Management*, Department of Health (England), the Scottish Government, Welsh Assembly Government and Northern Ireland Executive. Available at: www.dh.gov.uk (accessed 31 May 2011).
96   Department of Health (2008) *Safer Management of Controlled Drugs: Changes to Record Keeping Requirements*, DH, London, p.8.
97   Smith J. (2004) *The Shipman Inquiry, Fourth Report: The Regulation of Controlled Drugs in the Community*. Available at: www.the-shipman-inquiry.org.uk (accessed 2 November 2010), p.16.
98   General Medical Council (2008) *Good Practice in Prescribing Medicines*, GMC, London, paras 13–5.
99   British Medical Association (2001) *Consulting in the modern world: guidance for GPs*, BMA, London.
100   General Medical Council (2008) *Good Practice in Prescribing Medicines*, GMC, London, para 40.
101   General Medical Council (2008) *Good Practice in Prescribing Medicines*, GMC, London, para 41.
102   General Medical Council, Fitness to Practise Hearing, 24 August – 2 September 2009.
103   General Medical Council (2008) *Good Practice in Prescribing Medicines*, GMC, London, para 43.
104   Royal Pharmaceutical Society of Great Britain (2008) *Millions risk health buying drugs online*. Press release, 10 January.
105   Raine C, Webb DJ, Maxwell SRJ. (2008) The availability of prescription-only analgesics purchased from the internet in the UK. *Br J Clin Pharmacol* **67**(2), 250–4.
106   Nuffield Council on Bioethics (2010) *Medical Profiling and Online Medicine: the ethics of 'personalised healthcare' in a consumer age*, NCB, London, p.108.
107   Nuffield Council on Bioethics (2010) *Medical Profiling and Online Medicine: the ethics of 'personalised healthcare' in a consumer age*, NCB, London, p.109.
108   Moberly T. (2009) 1 in 4 GPs report online drug concerns. *GP* (17 April), p.4.
109   Nuffield Council on Bioethics (2010) *Medical Profiling and Online Medicine: the ethics of 'personalised healthcare' in a consumer age*, NCB, London, pp.120–1.

110   General Pharmaceutical Society (2010) *Standards for pharmacy owners and superintendent pharmacists of retail pharmacy businesses*, GPhC, London.

111   Pharmaceutical Society of Northern Ireland (2009) *Professional Standards and Guidance for Internet Pharmacy Services*, PSNI, Belfast.

112   Toft B. (2001) *External inquiry into the adverse incident that occurred at Queen's Medical Centre, Nottingham, 4 January 2001*, DH, London.

113   Medicines for Human Use (Marketing Authorisations, etc.) Regulations 1994. SI 1994/3144, Regulation 7.

114   For more information see the MHRA website: www.mhra.gov.uk (accessed 31 May 2011).

115   For further information see the National Reporting and Learning Service website at: www.nrls.npsa.nhs.uk (accessed 31 May 2011).

116   Department of Health (2010) *Liberating the NHS: report of the arms-length bodies review*, DH, London.

117   NHS Information Centre (2010) *Prescriptions Dispensed in the Community, England – Statistics for 1999 to 2009*. Available at: www.ic.nhs.uk (accessed 7 April 2011), p.8. Statistics for Wales (2010) *Prescriptions by General Medical Practitioners in Wales 2009–10*. Available at: wales.gov.uk (accessed 7 April 2011), p.20. Information Services Division Scotland (2010) *Generic Prescribing*. Available at: www.isdscotland.org (accessed 5 November 2010).

118   *R (on the application of the Association of the British Pharmaceutical Industry) v Medicines and Healthcare Products Regulatory Agency* [2010] EUECJ C-62/09_O.

119   European Directive 2001/83/EC on the Community code relating to medicinal products for human use, Article 81.

120   The Medicines (Marketing Authorisations etc.) Amendment Regulations 2005. SI 2005/2759 and The Medicines for Human Use (Manufacturing, Wholesale Dealing and Miscellaneous Amendments) Regulations 2005. SI 2005/2789.

121   For more information see the Pharmaceutical Services Negotiating Committee (PSNC) website: www.psnc.org.uk (accessed 31 May 2011).

122   Gainsbury S. (2010) Royal Surrey sold millions of pounds of NHS drugs in unacceptable export trading. *Health Service Journal* (February 16). Available at: www.hsj.co.uk (accessed 5 August 2010).

123   Gainsbury S. (2010) FT admits selling low stock drugs. *Health Service Journal* (14 April). Available at: www.hsj.co.uk (accessed 5 August 2010).

124   Department of Health (2010) *Trading Medicines for Human Use: Shortages and Supply Chain Obligations*. Available at: www.dh.gov.uk (accessed 8 March 2011).

125   Department of Health (2010) *Trading Medicines for Human Use: Shortages and Supply Chain Obligations*. Available at: www.dh.gov.uk (accessed 8 March 2011).

126   Nuffield Council on Bioethics (2003) *Pharmacogenetics: ethical issues*, NCB, London.

127   Nuffield Council on Bioethics (2003) *Pharmacogenetics: ethical issues*, NCB, London, p.xxii.

14: Research and innovative treatment

The questions covered in this chapter include the following.

- How does innovative treatment differ from research?
- Why have issues of consent been perceived as particularly crucial in this area?
- Is it ever acceptable not to tell patients about a research project that involves them?
- How can patients who cannot consent personally be involved in research?

This chapter discusses research ethics and some of the problems associated with innovative or experimental therapy. The same principles about truth telling, informed consent, the patient's interests and minimising harm are pertinent to both. A large amount of published guidance on these topics is already available. Rather than attempt to duplicate it here, sources of relevant advice are flagged up, not least because guidance by regulators on the issues covered is subject to periodic review and it is anticipated that various aspects of research governance may undergo significant change following the publication of this book. The focus here is particularly on those areas of medical research and experimental treatment that give rise to most queries to the British Medical Association (BMA). These tend to concentrate on issues of valid consent, the inclusion of children and other vulnerable people in medical and pharmaceutical trials and the use of stored human material. BMA policy on less common but potentially controversial issues such as embryo and stem cell research is also set out in this chapter.

Definitions

Questions sometimes arise about the boundary between research and innovative treatment or between research and audit. New treatments almost inevitably involve an element of both research and audit so that their efficacy and risks can be properly assessed. In all cases, the safeguards to be applied must be commensurate with the risks involved. 'Research' and 'experimentation' are sometimes used interchangeably but there are significant differences. Research follows a predetermined course of action set out in a protocol with which researchers have to comply until a defined endpoint is reached. Experimental therapy involves a more speculative approach to the patient's care and may be modified to take into account that individual's response.[1] Innovative or experimental therapy is devised to try and help a particular patient or group of patients whereas the aim of research is to acquire knowledge rather than to benefit participants.

Research

'Research' is the attempt to derive generalisable new knowledge by addressing clearly defined questions using systematic and rigorous methods. It includes studies that generate

Medical Ethics Today: The BMA's Handbook of Ethics and Law, Third Edition. Sophie Brannan, Eleanor Chrispin, Martin Davies, Veronica English, Rebecca Mussell, Julian Sheather and Ann Sommerville.
© 2012 BMA Medical Ethics Department. Published 2012 by Blackwell Publishing Ltd.

hypotheses as well as those that test them. Among the aims of research are an increased understanding of the biology of diseases so that preventive measures, as well as diagnostic and therapeutic interventions, can be developed and the safety and efficacy of such interventions can be tested. All research must meet defined minimum standards. It must have a well-designed protocol, constitute a well-conducted project, involve statistically appropriate participant numbers, not unnecessarily duplicate previous research and be subject to external review. Ideally, research projects should also have continuing surveillance. Research involving people who are dependent or particularly vulnerable must take special account of their interests and priorities. Research aims to produce new knowledge, not to benefit participants. They may accrue some incidental benefit from their involvement but, above all, they must be protected from harm. Future patients are the real beneficiaries of research. Whenever the intention is to acquire new knowledge rather than solely to care for individuals, the constraints applicable to research apply. When doctors propose a treatment that diverges from normal medical practice in order to gain information (this could be research or innovative treatment), patients must be informed about this and about the alternatives open to them.

A distinction can be drawn between the involvement of individual patients in research and the use of their data when the patient him or herself has no actual involvement. (Use of data for research is discussed later in this chapter and in Chapter 5, pages 207–211.) In this chapter, we focus mainly on the involvement of research participants themselves and also the use of their bodily material, such as DNA or human tissue.

Therapeutic and non-therapeutic research

From the 1960s to 2000, research was often divided into two categories. Research combined with trying to improve patient treatment was termed 'therapeutic' or 'clinical' research. In many cases, this was what we now call 'innovative treatment' although there is still a strong research element. Research that simply sought knowledge without claiming to benefit its participants was termed 'non-therapeutic'. The key early guidance on research ethics, the World Medical Association's Declaration of Helsinki[2] (first adopted in 1964 and regularly updated since then) perceived a fundamental distinction between the two. So-called 'therapeutic' research is that involving patients who already have a diagnosed condition, such as cancer, and for them the standard treatment is also likely to carry some risks or side effects. In cancer research, for example, clinical trials may use agents with a high potential for toxic effects and volunteer patients rather than healthy volunteers are involved in the first-in-human tests. They are usually more appropriate participants, based on a risk–benefit assessment. Higher risk drugs are targeted at serious diseases, where all existing therapeutic options for the patient have been exhausted. In 'non-therapeutic' research, no direct benefit is expected for participants and only minimal risk is acceptable.

'Therapeutic research' was often seen in the past as requiring less stringent scrutiny and safeguards than was necessary for projects that were pure research, because its aim was to ensure that patients could access experimental procedures, in the absence of any proven 'best treatment'. Although sounding reassuring, however, the 'therapeutic' label reflected the intention of the researcher rather than the effectiveness of the intervention. By 2000, it was agreed that this therapeutic/non-therapeutic categorisation was outmoded and that all research should be assessed according to the same criteria of risks and benefits. In 2000, the World Medical Association, which had originally introduced the terms to a wide audience, deleted them from its guidance. It also reversed the previous expectation that more allowance should be made for research combined with patient care by insisting that *extra* safeguards be applied in such cases. Seriously ill people and parents of sick children were thought more likely than healthy volunteers to be tempted into risky innovative treatments and research, or to misunderstand the extent to which they personally could expect to benefit.

Innovative treatment

Doctors have always modified methods of investigation and treatment in the light of experience and so innovative therapy is a standard feature of care. In some cases, however, it is the same thing as what used to be called therapeutic research. In particular, innovative treatments can differ little from research when they involve an unknown or increased risk for the patient. The aim of innovative treatment is to achieve the best outcome for the individual patient when standard treatment options have no, or only limited, success. The usual process of seeking patient consent should be followed so that the individual is aware of how and why the proposed treatment differs from the usual measures and has an opportunity to consider the risks involved. The degree of digression from usual practice is an important consideration for patients and the healthcare team. Conclusions reached from the implementation of changes in treatments should be shared with others as a step towards improving care for subsequent patients.

Nowadays, it would be unacceptable for unproven remedies or new surgical techniques to be applied without ethical overview or independent assessment. New medicinal products require research ethics approval and innovations such as new surgical techniques should also undergo ethical review. Traditionally, the monitoring of new treatment was part of the profession's own responsibility, but the importance of external, independent review became increasingly recognised at the end of the twentieth century. In 2001, the report of the public inquiry into children's heart surgery at the Bristol Royal Infirmary between 1984 and 1995 (the Bristol Report) recommended that any new, untried, invasive, clinical procedure should be subject to ethical review.[3] The Government's response was to require that new interventional procedures should be overseen by the National Institute for Health and Clinical Excellence (NICE) which assesses the efficacy of both existing and innovative therapies. (The role of NICE is covered in Chapter 13, pages 552–553 and Chapter 20, pages 837–838.) In Scotland, Healthcare Improvement Scotland carries out some of the same functions and the Scottish Medicines Consortium approves drugs and carries out rapid technology appraisals. In addition, research ethics committees (RECs) scrutinise studies of new procedures, as advised by NICE.

Audit

Audit is a means of assessing whether clinical performance conforms to good clinical practice. It is defined by the General Medical Council (GMC) as the 'evaluation of clinical performance against standards or thorough comparative analysis, to inform the management of services'.[4] Research adds to the knowledge base and routine audit ensures that the knowledge base is used, by observing what has been done and assessing the degree to which predetermined standards for any given healthcare activity are met. If they are not met, the reasons should be identified and changes implemented prior to re-audit. Audit methods can be similar to research. Like records-based epidemiology, audit does not require patient involvement beyond what is necessary for normal clinical management. If patients are involved in audit by the use of questionnaires or interviews, advance ethical scrutiny of the questions is desirable to minimise the possibility of distressing topics being raised without appropriate support. As with research, patient consent and confidentiality are issues for consideration. The use of medical records for audit by the clinical team managing the patient's care does not require explicit patient consent; implied consent is generally sufficient. Patients should be aware that audit is carried out but the GMC makes a distinction between local clinical audit, which does not need patients' express consent, and other uses of identifiable information, such as financial audit, which does.[5] (Use of data in audit is discussed in more detail in Chapter 5, page 188.) Nor is consent normally needed for any audit using anonymised data. (Chapter 5, pages 193–194 also has more discussion of anonymous information.)

Assessing benefit, harm and risk in research and innovative treatment

General concepts of 'benefit' and 'harm' are discussed in the introductory chapter (see page 2) but the terms apply in a slightly different way to research and innovative treatment. As with other areas of treatment, the potential benefits of any intervention must outweigh any inherent risks of harm but the individuals who agree to undertake the potential risks in research and innovative treatment are not the ones who ultimately benefit most. Healthy volunteers and patients involved in research help to secure improvements for later patients and for society as a whole. When innovative treatment is subjected to ethical review, the risks associated with it are compared with those of the standard option. Patients should face no greater risk from being included in a trial of new treatment than they would encounter in standard care. According to the principle of equipoise, the expected benefits for them should also be commensurate to, not less than, the benefits of standard treatment. The researcher has a duty to consider this and, if necessary, consult other colleagues in the field. Although patients with a diagnosed condition may be seen as more appropriate research participants than healthy volunteers in Phase 1 trials, if the drug or procedure being tested for their condition has some potentially harmful effect, healthy volunteers are generally more appropriate if patients' concurrent medication might skew the interpretation of results. (But see also pages 596–597 on inclusiveness and the importance of developing proven remedies for patients who have multiple morbidity.) The safety and well-being of patients and healthy volunteers are the primary concerns but not all risks of harm can be fully identified in advance. Some risks can be reduced if information with implications for safety is shared between developers of new medicines, research funding bodies and regulatory authorities worldwide. This was one of the practical recommendations from the expert scientific group established in 2006 to look at the TGN1412 trial (see pages 588–589) and to devise ways of improving safety, particularly in Phase 1 trials.[6] The group suggested that regulatory bodies worldwide should facilitate information sharing, based on the existing EU model for reporting suspected unexpected serious adverse reactions (SUSARs). These are unexpected events whose nature or severity is not consistent with existing information about the product. Serious adverse reactions are defined as 'any untoward medical occurrence or effect that at any dose results in death, is life-threatening, requires hospitalisation or prolongation of existing hospitalisation, results in persistent or significant disability or incapacity, or is a congenital anomaly or birth defect'.[7]

When assessing potential disadvantages of research projects or innovation, it is also essential to avoid too narrow a definition of 'harm' or one that relates only to physical damage. Less tangible harms, such as loss of trust arising from deception, need to be considered. In failing to assess these risks, research and innovative treatment have sometimes run into trouble. Developing new techniques and gaining knowledge should be subordinate to the main aim of medicine, which is to enhance the welfare of individual patients. Those who agree to participate in research must not be seen as merely a means to an end. There is wide agreement that, for their part, the public needs to be much better informed about research generally and about the benefits that can be obtained through small, incremental steps as well as by major scientific advances. In 2009, the NHS Constitution for England emphasised the need to ensure that patients are made aware of research projects relevant to them, in which they might wish to participate.[8] The BMA strongly encourages feedback from researchers and clinicians to participants on the general findings and implications of the research and new therapies in which they have been involved. Clearly, in some contexts this may involve giving bad news and needs to be done very carefully, ideally after seeking advice from any patient representatives who were involved in the research design at the outset.

General principles

In the BMA's view, the key principles applicable to research and innovative treatment include the need for:

- informed consent and voluntary participation of research subjects who have capacity
- additional safeguards when research involves individuals who cannot give consent or refusal
- primary consideration to be given to the safety and welfare of the individual participants
- truth telling, effective communication and clarity of information, including about uncertainties
- safeguards in proportion to the known or expected risks of harm
- inclusiveness and fairness in recruiting participants
- adherence to the law and governance arrangements
- careful independent scrutiny of research and experimental treatment
- the confidentiality of participants to be maintained.

Consent

The principles underpinning the need for consent and the degree of information required to make it valid are discussed in more detail in Chapter 2. Valid and unpressured consent is even more vital when the procedure is not intended to benefit the individual undergoing it, as is the case with research and innovative treatment. Participants need to have information in order to be engaged as voluntary partners in the project.

GMC guidance on information giving[9]

'You must give people the information they want or need in order to decide whether to take part in research. How much information you share with them will depend on their individual circumstances. You must not make assumptions about the information a person might want or need, or their knowledge and understanding of the proposed research project.'

'You must make sure that people are given information in a way that they can understand. You should check that people understand the terms that you use and any explanation given about the proposed research method. If necessary, you should support your discussions with simple and accurate written material or visual or other aids.'

Discussing the risks

Assessment of risk is an important part of any decision in healthcare and is notoriously difficult to explain to patients. The increasing emphasis on both training and evaluation of doctors' communication skills seeks to address problems such as this. The GMC provides advice about the discussion of side-effects, complications and risks.[10] It emphasises the importance of not only assessing carefully the patient's condition, but ascertaining what individual patients want to know and how much information they require. Information about risk must be given in a balanced way, without bias.

GMC guidance on discussing risk

'In order to have effective discussions with patients about risk, you must identify the adverse outcomes that may result from the proposed options. This includes the potential outcome of taking no action. Risks can take a number of forms but will usually be side effects, complications or failure of an intervention to achieve the desired aim. Risks can vary from common but minor side effects to rare but serious adverse outcomes possibly resulting in permanent disability or death.'[11]

'You should do your best to understand the patient's views and preferences about any proposed investigation or treatment, and the adverse outcomes they are most concerned about. You must not make assumptions about a patient's understanding of risk or the importance they attach to different outcomes.'[12]

'You must use clear, simple and consistent language when discussing risks with patients. You should be aware that patients may understand information about risk differently from you. You should check that the patient understands the terms that you use, particularly when describing the seriousness, frequency and likelihood of an adverse outcome. You should use simple and accurate written information or visual or other aids to explain risk, if they will help the patient to understand.'[13]

When patients are told that the treatment or research involves some uncertainty, the issue about which they most often seek reassurance is the degree of risk of harm involved. Despite the existence of some guidelines, no generally applicable categorisation of 'risk' is available and so it needs to be discussed on a case-by-case basis. Clinicians need to ensure that there is systematic review of the evidence base for the procedures they offer, so that the information they provide reflects accurately what is currently known about the risks and relative merits. Sometimes the risks in research projects are unknown to experts, particularly in Phase 1 'first-in-human' pharmaceutical studies. This was highlighted in an extreme form in 2006 by the trial of TGN1412 (see below) which drew attention to the difficulty of accurately assessing the risks associated with new drugs when making the transition from animal to human studies.

Trial of TGN1412

On 13 March 2006, six healthy male volunteers received TeGenero's drug, TGN1412, which was a monoclonal antibody that stimulates T cells and was being developed to treat leukaemia and auto-immune diseases such as rheumatoid arthritis. Two other volunteers received a placebo in the Phase 1, first-in-human clinical trial run by Parexel, a contract research organisation. The research had been approved by two European Regulatory Agencies and a local REC. It was a randomised, placebo-controlled trial to assess the safety of the drug and carried out in a private laboratory at the Northwick Park Hospital site in London.

Within 90 minutes of receiving the drug intravenously, the six volunteers experienced symptoms, including headaches, nausea, diarrhoea, erythema and vasodilatation. Within hours, they developed a severe systemic inflammatory reaction with multi-organ failure. They were transferred to the Intensive Therapy Unit (ITU) at

Northwick Park Hospital.[14] All needed assisted ventilation and three of the volunteers needed a prolonged stay in ITU. They were supervised for 3 months after the event when all were still experiencing health problems, such as memory loss, headaches and inability to concentrate. The drug had previously been tested on monkeys, rats and rabbits in higher doses without ill effect and the unexpected reaction in human volunteers generated uncertainty over the entire class of monoclonal antibodies that alter the behaviour of the immune system. One of the issues highlighted in the media reporting of the health problems suffered by the participants was the amount that they had been paid for acting as healthy volunteers (see below). This was reported to be £2000 each which was considered normal for the number of hours for which they had to be present and undergo tests. Contrary to expectations, recruitment companies reported a surge in applications following the TGN1412 trial as the public began to realise how lucrative participation could be.

The trial was immediately suspended. The documentation relating to it was made publicly available on the website of the Medicines and Healthcare Products Regulatory Agency (MHRA) which also issued an interim report in April 2006. This found no evidence to suggest there had been any problem with the drug manufacture nor any contamination. Nor did anything in the running of the trial contribute to the adverse reaction in the volunteers, which appeared to be species-specific. The MHRA gave assurances that future trial applications for biological agents would be subject to higher levels of scrutiny by the Commission on Human Medicines as well as the MHRA itself.

In the wake of the TGN1412 incident, an expert scientific group was established to look at the lessons to be learned and make recommendations to increase safety in similar trials. Among the practical lessons learned were that recruits for a Phase 1 study on a new drug should be dosed sequentially, not together and that the starting dose should be lower than had been used previously on animals; with the benefit of hindsight, it was unsurprising that a human antibody failed to show effects in mice. Other recommendations included better global sharing of information about potential risks, including the establishment of an open access database with preclinical reports of results which signal potentially dangerous medicines.[15]

The TGN1412 trial was exceptional. The vast majority of research and innovative treatment does not involve risks of such magnitude. When innovative treatment is considered, the potential risks have to be assessed both in terms of the likely effects of the new procedure and the risks to the patient if it is not carried out. In all cases, the degree of risk must be in proportion to the expected benefit. In the past, health professionals were criticised for minimising or poorly communicating the risks of innovative treatment, so that patients or families lacked adequate explanations.[16] Doctors must make clear which aspects of a proposed treatment are innovative and answer honestly any questions about their own success rate. If new treatment involves significant risk, an independent and objective second opinion should be sought so that clinicians can be confident that they are not putting too positive a gloss on it. Patients should be informed if procedures are not standard treatment in other comparable hospitals or clinics. It is not acceptable to rely on the concept of implied consent on the grounds that an innovative treatment is 'standard' if this view is not supported by other colleagues in the field. Consent can never be implied or taken for granted in this situation. (The distinction between express or explicit consent and implied or implicit consent is discussed in Chapter 2, page 61.)

Consent and financial incentives

Consent may be influenced by various factors, including financial or other incentives to participate. In 2010, the existence of diverse attitudes to payment were among the issues that the Nuffield Council on Bioethics raised for debate in a public consultation.[17] The Council had established a working party to look at a range of topics related to donation and volunteering in different settings, including remuneration for participation in research or for donating bodily material. It noted the continuing controversy about whether cash payments or other financial benefits constitute a form of undue influence, invalidating consent or act simply as an incentive which increases the individual's options. Its consultation drew attention to the inconsistency of permitting payment for clinical trial participants but not for organ or gamete donors.[18] The findings from the consultation were due for publication in late 2011.

Although attention often focuses on financial payment, patients' strong desire to try to access new treatment and their expectation that they will get better care and attention can also tempt them to participate in research, as can their wish to please a doctor to whom they feel indebted. The term 'inducement' implies a more calculated act on the part of the person recruiting participants and may be seen as offering a temptation for people in need of money to act contrary to their better judgement. The GMC tells doctors involved in research that they must not allow their judgement to be influenced, or be seen to be influenced, by any financial, personal, political or other external interests. Furthermore, they must declare any actual or potential conflicts of interests that arise to the REC, other appropriate bodies and the participants.[19]

In practice, a distinction is drawn between the participation of patients and healthy volunteers. In research on new drugs and surgical procedures, patients are often willing to participate without reward and those who are already undergoing treatment are perceived as less inconvenienced by additional examinations than volunteers who attend solely for research purposes. Patients tend to be paid only expenses. Healthy volunteers are usually more generously rewarded because they give their time and undergo procedures that offer no benefit to them, apart from the satisfaction of having helped others. Payment is usually the only way to recruit them but there have been persistent worries about very large cash payments.

Incentives exist in other spheres of healthcare to encourage people to do what is considered to be the right thing, by making it easy for them or providing them with some tangible benefit. (See the discussion in Chapter 20, pages 832–833 on offering patients incentives to make good health choices.) For patients, research participation can provide early access to new procedures, better monitoring or more frequent attention from health professionals. These kinds of non-monetary incentives are well established and uncontroversial. 'Inducements' imply the temptation to take risks or act contrary to one's own interests. Where altruism fails to meet demand, large financial payments might be seen as coercive since their purpose is to overcome the reticence of people to participate. Most anxiety about 'undue inducements' is generated by practices such as the recruitment of some vulnerable groups, such as homeless or unemployed people, to test drugs. Various general concerns arise.

- People who need money may give less attention to understanding the risks. Their consent may be less voluntary or less informed.
- Economically disadvantaged populations bear the brunt of the risks and burdens of research.
- Money as a recruitment tool attracts people who do not care about the research goals.
- Payment can be seen as undermining the ethical norms of the doctor–patient relationship.

Despite this, payment is the norm for research involving healthy volunteers. Recruitment websites set out the advantages of trial participation, focusing not only on cash payment, but also on benefits such as free meals, accommodation and medical care during the trial period. Some portray participation in research as an easy way of earning money, as an alternative to part-time jobs. RECs need to assess what constitutes an unacceptable level of financial inducement, as opposed to an acceptable incentive. Most guidance simply stresses that participants are not paid to take risks and should not be persuaded against their better judgement but that any expenses they incur should be reimbursable. Guidance within the pharmaceutical industry recommends payment based on the minimum wage. Transparency about payments and independent scrutiny of them are key issues in all research.

BMA advice on payment to research participants

- RECs should look closely at the level of financial and non-monetary incentives when scrutinising the way research participants are recruited, in each individual protocol.
- Payment should not constitute an 'inducement'. Financial incentives should not be of a level as to encourage people to act against their own better judgement.
- The sum paid should be commensurate with the amount of time and inconvenience involved.
- Payments must never be for undergoing risk.
- Participants need to have accurate information about the risks and inconveniences involved.

Donation of bodily material and issues of payment

When malignant tissue is excised or bodily samples, such as blood or urine, are no longer needed, patients are generally willing for them to be used in research and, when relevant, should be made aware of that option. Consent to donate surplus tissue for the purposes of future research, audit and education should be separate to their consent for surgery or other treatment. Specific consent is needed if tissue is taken in excess of what is required for the patient's healthcare with a view to undertaking research, but where the tissue has been removed as part of the patient's therapy and will be used anonymously in research approved by an REC consent is not required (see also pages 615–616). Consent can also be generic and enduring. When patients do not wish the material to be used for such purposes after its diagnostic value for themselves is exhausted, their wishes regarding disposal should be respected. The Medical Research Council (MRC) points to a lack of legal clarity about whether human biological material can be 'owned' or whether donors have property rights over it.[20] It recommends that tissue samples for research be treated as a gift, thus promoting the 'gift relationship' and altruistic motivation of the research participant. This bypasses the problem about ownership and transfers any property rights that might exist to the researcher.

The MRC guidance declares payment for donation of tissue or samples unethical. It says that neither donors nor researchers should be able to sell samples, either for cash or benefits in kind, but donors can be reimbursed reasonable expenses. Nevertheless, payment remains a topic of debate, partly due to the previously mentioned inconsistencies in attitudes. (See also Chapter 8, pages 333–336 on assisted reproduction, which sets out arguments for and against the payment of gamete and embryo donors.) Scrutiny to ensure that no 'undue inducements' or 'undue influences' are involved in the donation of human material is left to RECs.

Families authorising the use of cadaveric material in research should be offered information about the purpose, the anticipated time span and the eventual manner of disposal. Discussing such issues with bereaved relatives is universally acknowledged to be a difficult and challenging task that requires appropriate training. Face-to-face discussion with families can be usefully augmented with written information. Guidance on consent issues has been published by the Royal College of Pathologists[21] and advice for families asked to donate a child's tissue for research is available from organisations such as the Child Bereavement Charity.[22] (See also pages 615–616 on the human tissue legislation.)

People in a dependent situation

In the past, researchers often involved people who were in a dependent position, such as their students or employees, as a potential pool of healthy volunteers. From the 1990s, reservations were increasingly expressed about this practice. Consent is dubious when the person's 'willingness to volunteer in a clinical trial may be unduly influenced by the expectation, justified or not, of benefits associated with participation or of a retaliatory response from senior members of a hierarchy in case of refusal to participate'.[23] Organisations with a hierarchical structure, such as laboratories and pharmaceutical companies, should not recruit volunteers for research from their own staff. Some companies prohibit the involvement of their employees in research projects. Medical, pharmacy, dental and nursing students may also feel under pressure if asked to participate. The BMA emphasises that the recruitment of students and junior staff from the same department as the researcher should be avoided. The GMC also tells doctors involved in research to make sure that safeguards are in place to protect anybody who may be vulnerable to pressure.[24]

While people living in institutions might be seen as a captive pool of potential research participants, they are often excluded. The reasons include anxiety about possibly exploiting a vulnerable group and the practical difficulties of carrying out a trial involving people with impaired mental capacity or multiple morbidity. Older people, for example, face a deficit of evidence-based research for some conditions they suffer. They should neither be automatically excluded from research nor coerced to participate. As for all other research participants, they need to be offered clear information about the options and implications.

Detainees

People in prison and in other places of compulsory detention should be involved only in projects that specifically address the health problems experienced in that setting, such as the physical and psychological effects of imprisonment, impact of detention on different minority groups or nutrition in custodial settings. Careful consideration needs to be given by the relevant REC if incentives or special privileges are proposed to attract volunteers in such contexts. (General advice about care in detention settings is given in Chapter 17.)

Can people be obliged to participate in research or innovative treatment?

Normally, no-one can be obliged to participate in either research or new therapies against their will but there are some exceptional instances in which people are acknowledged to have little or no choice. Those who join the armed forces, for example, may forfeit their rights to opt out of some medical interventions, such as vaccination programmes. Where such programmes have not already been rigorously tried out on other volunteers, there is an element of both research and innovative therapy in their use. The ethical justification given is the obligation to protect individuals against infection and their duty, in turn, to protect the welfare of the unit. Doctors still have a responsibility to maximise benefit and minimise risk but, clearly, this can be problematic in the absence of reliable evidence about potential risks and benefits. They also have duties to the individuals they treat and, wherever possible, should be willing to offer them whatever information they can. It is also important that there is ethical oversight of such programmes, for example, by Ministry of Defence RECs.

Case example of experimental treatment

In preparation for the first Gulf War in 1990, the requirement for informed consent for experimental vaccination was removed for American personnel who could be facing chemical or biological weapons. The US Department of Defense said that informed consent was important in peacetime but that different considerations applied in a combat situation. Thousands of army personnel were given pyridostigmine bromide and a botulism toxoid vaccination, although both drugs had some known problems. The aim was to use them therapeutically. It was subsequently argued that their use blurred the distinction between treatment and research, because the drugs had not been established to be either effective or safe. Some British service personnel were also similarly vaccinated.[25]

Consent, placebos and patient preferences

Randomised controlled trials (RCTs) are the most widely known method of comparing treatment options and obtaining an objective answer. The prerequisite for them is the lack of a recognised optimum treatment for the condition, or the presumption that a new product may be more effective than existing therapies. Thus, randomisation is ethical only if there is substantial uncertainty about the best treatment for that patient. New treatments are tested against an existing treatment, a placebo or no treatment at all. Participants consent to participate but cannot choose which option they receive. Patients are sometimes alarmed at the prospect of deliberate randomisation and those who have particular treatment preferences should not participate in RCTs. Where therapies with established effectiveness exist they, rather than placebos, should be the comparator for new treatments. If the doctor considers that one of the treatments in the study is appropriate or inappropriate for a particular patient for any reason (including that patient's irrational fears or subjective preferences), then randomisation would be unethical. In such cases, the responsible clinician should talk to the patient about the options that are available outside the RCT and seek to identify those likely to reflect the patient's preferences.

Welfare of individuals as a primary consideration

Important among the core principles and duties is the responsibility to protect the welfare of research participants, minimise risks for them and ensure that these are offset by any expected benefits. Research guidelines, including GMC advice[26] and the World Medical Association's Declaration of Helsinki, emphasise that the welfare of the research participant must be a primary concern.[27] It is unacceptable to prioritise the expected benefits for society over the welfare of individual people. In the history of research, however, there have been many examples of abusive research and of treatments being withheld from patients in order for researchers to assess the effects of leaving diseases untreated.[28] Both breach ethical standards and human rights. Participants' consent to being involved does not diminish the responsibility of researchers and RECs to ensure that all foreseeable risks are minimised. Assessment of risk may extend beyond a particular study to take account of the background context. Patients with rare conditions, for example, may be repeatedly asked to participate in research where the risks of serial involvement differ from the risks of involvement in just one study. Recommended minimum periods between research projects should be specified for such patients and this is among the factors that RECs should consider.

Patient welfare is equally crucial in the development and implementation of innovative treatments. All doctors should be assiduous in monitoring outcomes from their treatment patterns and investigate the reasons if their success rates fall below those achieved by other practitioners in similar circumstances. The emphasis on both self-monitoring and peer review is increasing. All doctors should collect audit results and be open with patients in a sensitive manner if it is revealed that errors have been made (see Chapter 1, pages 36–38). If standard treatment is adapted for a particular patient and seems successful, a formal research protocol should be drawn up for appraisal by an REC. All doctors have a duty to know their own limitations and not exceed their knowledge or competence. Innovative medical and surgical techniques are constantly developing and specialists need to learn to use them safely and, if necessary, adapt them for specific patients, including for children and babies. It is unethical for doctors who are on a steep learning curve to fail to monitor their own mastery of a new technique and their own success rate in performing it in comparison with national rates or those of colleagues. Regular appraisal, audit and external scrutiny by means of clinical governance and revalidation make it less likely that serious errors in practice will remain undetected. Nevertheless, the primary responsibility to ensure that their treatment is safe and ethical rests with doctors themselves.

The possibility of harm cannot be entirely eliminated from research or from new treatments but patients often find it hard to resist agreeing to a therapy – even an unproven treatment – when they have few other treatment options. By ensuring that participants have adequate information and a choice about taking part, the possibility of exploiting them is reduced. By their nature, innovative treatments have less evidential support than conventional regimens. The benefit for the patient is harder to predict. At the same time, there is likely to be an intuitive wish to try anything that may help to save or improve a life. Clinicians may be more tempted to be over-optimistic and to recommend treatment, especially if the patient is a young person who potentially has a long life ahead but they must ensure that they avoid discrimination in their decision making. It would be unethical to base choices or treatment recommendations on factors such as the patient's age or perceived quality of life rather than the likely benefit for that patient.

Truth telling and effective communication

Consent is a key concept in both research and innovative treatment. An essential prerequisite for valid consent is for participants to have access to accurate and relevant information that is provided in ways that are appropriate for their general level of knowledge (and language skills, if relevant). People must be told when a proposal would involve them in research or innovation. The options and alternatives must be effectively explained in ways they can readily grasp. It is unacceptable, for example, to recall patients for what they assume to be health monitoring for their own benefit when the actual intention is to carry out research on some aspect of their condition. What is adequate information varies according to the requirements of the individuals involved and the complexity of the procedures proposed. (Chapters 2 and 4 discuss consent and refusal in more detail.)

Patient information sheets are a useful way of providing reference material but these cannot replace discussion and the opportunity for patients to pose questions. Potential participants in research or innovative treatment need to know the likely benefits and risks involved, why the options are proposed and what alternatives exist. They should know that they can withdraw at any stage without detriment to the provision of medical care and treatment (unless the specific treatment they would like is only available as part of a research trial). If asked to participate in research, they need to know how the project is expected to advance knowledge and the researcher's own stake (if any) in proposing it. Much routine research, including in primary care, involves testing new variants of existing drugs, so it is important that patients have an accurate perception of their contribution. The potential significance of the research should not be exaggerated when recruiting participants and when the findings are reported.

Some innovative treatments and research involve discomfort or pain. It is important that this fact is not omitted from information sheets for volunteers. Participants should have a realistic impression of what is involved or their consent is likely to be invalid. Opinions frequently differ about how pain should be defined, especially in relation to research or innovative treatment involving children. From a child's perspective, routine procedures such as venepuncture can seem frightening[29] and there need to be opportunities to discuss the patient's own perspective. The BMA's recommendations about the kinds of information that people involved in research or innovative treatment need to be given are set out below.

Research participants need to know:

- why they have been asked to participate
- the purpose of the research and confirmation of its ethical approval
- whether the individual (if a patient) stands to benefit and, if so, the difference between research and treatment
- the risks and arrangements for reporting adverse events
- the meaning of relevant research terms (such as placebos and randomisation)
- the nature of each procedure, and how often or for how long each may occur
- the rights and safeguards for participants, including compensation if harm occurs
- how their health data will be stored, used and published
- if samples of human material are donated, what they might be used for
- the names of the researcher and the doctor responsible for their care
- that they can withdraw from the project and that such a decision will not affect their healthcare.

Patients involved in innovative therapies need to know:

- why the therapy is proposed in their case
- the evidence to support its use and the areas of uncertainty about it
- what ethical review it has received
- the clinician's experience with it
- the alternatives and how the new procedure differs from standard treatment
- the likely risks and benefits for themselves
- the measures for safety monitoring and support that will be provided if things go wrong.

Is it ever acceptable not to inform patients?

As a general principle, failure to inform participants that their treatment involves research is unacceptable. One of the few circumstances in which patients cannot be properly informed that their treatment is innovative or part of research occurs when the patient lacks mental capacity. In such cases, the safeguards set out in the Mental Capacity Act 2005, Adults with Incapacity (Scotland) Act 2000 and clinical trial regulations come into play. This includes research in the contexts of emergency treatment, resuscitation and intensive care (see pages 598–599 and Chapter 3, page 102).

Research involving adults with mental capacity in which the patient's awareness of it could itself significantly affect the outcome poses a particular challenge. In each case where it is being argued that specific patient consent need not be sought, it is important that health professionals and local RECs are clear about the robustness of the justification. As part of that assessment, consideration needs to be given to the wider harms to public confidence if research or innovative therapy is carried out in what appears to be a clandestine manner or if research participants find out subsequently that they have been deceived.

Proportionate safeguards

Safeguards need to be proportionate to the risks involved in the research and take account of factors such as the vulnerability of the participant. Overly strict regulation can mean that some populations, such as older people or patients lacking mental capacity, are effectively excluded. (See also the section on inclusiveness below.) In 2011, the Academy of Medical Sciences strongly criticised the EU Clinical Trials Directive, which is reflected in UK Regulations (see pages 612–613), for placing unnecessary burdens on clinical trials of new and established products in an attempt to standardise procedures rather than adopting a proportionate approach.[30] Partly as a result of such criticisms, the European Commission announced a review of the Directive scheduled for the end of 2011.

Inclusiveness

In the ethics literature, attention is traditionally given to the potential harms for the people who take part in research but the harms of being excluded from research feature less. Some patient groups are disadvantaged by being excluded. The age range of potential participants who could benefit is sometimes ignored and 'protective ageism' means that older people, in particular, are frequently excluded. They may be ruled out because they have multiple morbidities but this results in a lack of data about the effects of new treatments for patients who have multiple conditions for which they already take commonly prescribed medications. In 2010, a Europe-wide project[31] reported specifically on the under-representation of older people in clinical trials of treatments for conditions common to their age group, such as coronary heart disease, hypertension, Alzheimer disease and Parkinson disease, depression and colorectal cancer. Although some people over the age of 60 were included in research on these conditions, the mean age tended to be much lower than would be expected in a representative population. A *Charter for the Rights of Older People in Clinical Trials* was published with a parallel version for older patients themselves, emphasising that regulators should require the inclusion of people with multiple morbidities in trials on treatments intended for people in later life.[32] Improved recruitment of such groups and people living with disabilities could be achieved by positively addressing the well-recognised barriers to involving them and taking practical steps to making participation easy for them.

People who have limited English language skills are also often excluded even though information about health research is increasingly translated into other languages. Owing to the rightly heavy emphasis on autonomy and individual consent, there is a reluctance to conduct research on young children and on adults with impaired capacity. (These populations are discussed on pages 597–604.) This research deficit can result in a lack of proven treatments for some patient populations. In 2010, the GMC issued supplementary guidance on good practice and research and, among the key principles, drew attention to the need for researchers to be free from discrimination when recruiting participants. It said that they should 'take all reasonable steps to ensure that people eligible to participate in a project are given equal access to take part and the opportunity to benefit from the research'.[33]

Summary – general principles

- Opportunities to participate in research and innovative procedures should be offered without discrimination to potentially eligible groups.
- Participants should have access to detailed information according to their requirements, including information about the hazards, pain or inconveniences involved.
- Precautions to avoid coercion or inducement of vulnerable people must be given particular attention by researchers and RECs.
- Consent must be voluntary and attention needs to be given to issues such as excessive financial payments or the dependent situation of the participant.
- Participants should know that they can withdraw without prejudice to future treatment (unless the treatment in question is only available in a research trial).

People who cannot consent to research or innovative therapy

Special rules apply when the individual cannot consent personally to participation in research or innovative therapy. Whenever possible, research and innovative therapy should involve consenting adults with capacity rather than patients whose mental capacity is impaired. Excluding them completely, however, makes it impossible to develop proven therapies for the conditions that specifically affect them. Drug trials on antidepressants need to involve people experiencing depression and the same applies to other debilitating mental conditions. Many people with a mental impairment can give valid consent or refusal, if the issues are explained carefully. Legal rules governing research on people with impaired capacity, including unconscious patients, are discussed below in the section on law and regulation.

In some exceptional cases the patient's chances of recovery with an unproven treatment are better than with standard therapies. In very serious situations with few other options there may be a justification for exposing people to some risk if they potentially have much to gain. In such cases, it is essential that the patient (where possible), families and the healthcare team give careful consideration to all the evidence. In other cases, the prospect of success may be relatively low, but the value of attempting a new treatment may be high for the patient and the family. Care is needed not to overstate the possible benefits unless there is evidence to support them. Clearly, very sick people should not be exposed to experimental treatment if there is significant doubt about either the likelihood of success or the value of attempting it. In some cases advice may need to be sought from the courts.

Simms v Simms

In December 2002, the High Court was asked to decide whether it would be lawful to provide treatment that had not been tested on humans to two patients with new variant Creutzfeldt–Jakob disease (vCJD). Both patients, aged 18 and 16, lacked capacity to make the decision but their parents argued that it would be in their interests to try the therapy. It involved intraventricular administration of pentosan polysulphate, which had been tested in Japan on rodents and dogs infected with scrapie. Although not expected to provide a cure, it was hoped that the treatment would improve the patients' lives. The judge said that, although the patients would not recover, the concept of 'benefit' to a patient suffering from vCJD would encompass the possibility of an improvement from the present state of illness, a continuation of the existing state of illness without deterioration for a longer period than might otherwise have occurred or the prolongation of life for a longer period. Given the possibility of some benefit and the lack of other alternatives, it was held that this treatment would be in the best interests of both patients and it could lawfully be provided. Jonathan Simms became the first victim of vCJD to be given the drug pentosan polysulphate, by direct infusion into his brain in 2002. This produced some small but significant improvements. In 2009, he was the longest recorded survivor in the world. He was occasionally able to try speaking and could swallow. He stopped experiencing uncontrollable jerking movements linked with his disease and was free from the chest infections he previously suffered.[34]

General ethical guidance on consent and impaired capacity

- Individuals should be positively involved in decision making to the maximum of their ability.
- If apparently unwilling, potential participants should not be included in research or new treatment.
- Any competent advance refusal made by the individual must be respected.
- Extra safeguards must be in place when participants cannot consent.
- Assurances must exist that the research cannot feasibly be carried out by involving a less vulnerable group.
- The research must relate to the participant's condition and be expected to involve no risks to the participant or the benefits to the participant are expected to outweigh any foreseeable risk of harm.
- Information for proxy decision makers must be as detailed as for other persons.

(See also pages 612–616.)

Participation of adults who lack capacity

Fluctuating capacity and dementia research

In 2009, the Nuffield Council on Bioethics published guidance, *Dementia: the ethical issues*, which pointed to the growing worldwide prevalence of this condition and the increasing need for more research on it, including on the effectiveness and transferability of different models of care and support for people with dementia.[35] It highlighted the low priority given to research on preventive strategies and to non-Alzheimer dementia. It recognised the challenge of trying to convey effectively to patients with dementia the distinction between participating in research that might benefit them, by early access to new therapy, and that which would only benefit other people with the same condition. The report emphasised the importance of seeking personal consent on their 'good' days from people with fluctuating mental capacity or offering patients the opportunity, while they have mental capacity, to make advance decisions about future participation in research. The option of proxy consent by a relative or welfare attorney was covered in the report, which noted that some people have particular concerns about a proxy's ability to second-guess the wishes of the person with dementia. (Proxy consent is discussed in the section on the law and regulation of research on pages 612–614.)

The PREDICT project (see page 596) also looked closely at the involvement of older people in research when they might have cognitive or communication problems. It recommended specific training for researchers undertaking trials with an older population so that extra time and support would be given to such participants.[36]

Emergency research

Research and innovation in the context of emergency care have long posed an ethical challenge. In this setting, there is no time to contact families or proxy decision makers if the patient is incapable of communication. Similarly, few patients in intensive care wards can give valid consent. In 2004, when the UK implemented the Medicines for Human Use (Clinical Trials) Regulations, which cover only clinical trials of investigational medicinal products (CTIMPs) (see pages 612–613), it was made clear that these were not intended to hamper research in emergency situations. The regulations required that consent be provided in advance of the incapacitated person being involved but the impossibility of obtaining such advance consent was highlighted by international trials on conditions such as cardiac arrest. It became increasingly clear that a change was required to make an exception to the requirement for prior proxy consent in emergency situations. In December 2006, the regulations were amended to allow CTIMPs on incapacitated adults in emergency situations without prior consent, as long as REC agreement had been obtained. Proxy consent is still needed for continuing participation in the trial of emergency measures but, in the absence of such consent at the start, patients can be initially entered. All trial protocols – including those for emergency care – should be scrutinised by RECs which consider whether the exception should apply to individual emergency trial protocols. The amendment applied to CTIMPs in emergency situations throughout the UK and required an amendment to the Adults with Incapacity (Scotland) Act 2000.

Summary – participation of adults who lack capacity

- Research or innovative treatment should ideally involve adults with capacity but, in order to develop safe and effective remedies for the conditions experienced by people with impaired capacity, they also need to be involved in appropriate research.
- Many people with impaired capacity can consent to involvement in research or innovative treatment if the issues are explained in an appropriate way. Researchers should have special training in how to do this and be prepared to provide extra time and support to such participants.
- Special attention must be given by the REC to how consent is to be obtained and from whom if the individual cannot consent or refuse personally.
- Any apparent objection displayed by the participant should be seen as refusal.

Research and innovative treatment involving children and young people

Children and babies should be eligible for inclusion in research and innovative therapy, with appropriate safeguards. As with other vulnerable population groups, it is argued that it would be unethical not to carry out clinical research on newborn babies and infants as this would lead to stagnation and the continuation of unproven remedies. On the other hand, in terms of risk, neonates and premature babies are often seen as the most vulnerable group of all in research. Protocols involving them require particularly thorough scrutiny from ethics committees and investigators.

The need for pharmaceutical products specifically designed for children has long been recognised. These need to be developed with the involvement of children and young people once initial studies involving adults have proved the safety and efficacy of the product. The final decision about participation normally rests with young people (when competent) and with their parents. For CTIMPs (see above), consent comes from a person with parental responsibility or a legal representative, although the explicit wish of a competent child to refuse participation or to be withdrawn must be taken seriously by the investigator. (Parental responsibility is discussed in Chapter 4, pages 160–161). For children who are not competent, parents can give their agreement which should represent the child's presumed will (see also pages 602–603). The child's will should generally be respected, without reasons having to be given, for withdrawal from research, unless that would be detrimental to the child's health. Families need clear and candid explanations of the purposes, risks and expected benefits of the research and they may also need independent support when making decisions. It has been suggested, for example, that a 'cultural mediator' might be involved in seeking consent from families of a different cultural background to that of the researcher.[37] Particular attention needs to be given to parents being clearly told which procedures are standard care and which are specific to research or innovative care. It is unethical to replicate trials unnecessarily in any patient group and so information gained in any trial should be made available to other researchers and the public. Systematic registration of paediatric trials and publication of results, including unfavourable ones, should take place and the public should be able to access an international database to ensure against replication. (For the EU database, EudraCT, which contains information about all CTIMP research, including paediatric research, see page 601.)

The GMC has some general advice on the involvement of children and young people in research. This emphasises that for patients, the potential therapeutic benefits for them should outweigh the foreseeable risks and, for healthy volunteers, the research should carry only minimal risk and not be against their best interests.[38] The Royal College of Paediatrics and Child Health (RCPCH) publishes more detailed advice on the involvement of children in research, pointing out that because children are not small adults, they have an additional, unique set of interests.[39] Research involving them should not only meet the minimum standards set for research on adults but also take account of children's special interests and perspectives. Researchers need to bear in mind that many children are easily bewildered and unable to express their needs. 'Potentially with many decades ahead of them, they are likely to experience, in their development and education, the most lasting benefits or harms from research.'[40]

Development of a paediatric formulary

For many years, the lack of drugs developed specifically for children, or an evidence-based paediatric formulary, created dilemmas for health professionals. Doctors had little choice but to administer to children reduced dosages of adult medicines, without knowing whether they were effective or whether the side effects in children would differ. The relative lack of information on safe paediatric prescribing (off-label use) meant that children sometimes experienced adverse reactions that were more severe or different from those associated with adult use. Some medicines used in paediatric care are still not specifically licensed for use in children. Traditionally, there were disincentives for pharmaceutical companies to invest in researching children's medicines, because the market is relatively small and not commercially profitable. It is difficult to recruit children and babies to studies and children who are recruited risk being exposed to multiple research projects if they have a rare condition. Without specific studies in the paediatric population, however, important information on matters such as dosage and efficacy was unavailable and sick children were left more vulnerable than they needed to be.

A paediatric formulary was originally produced by the RCPCH and the Neonatal and Paediatric Pharmacists Group. This was superseded in 2005 when the BMA, in partnership with the Royal Pharmaceutical Society of Great Britain, the Royal College of Paediatrics and Child Health and the Neonatal and Paediatric Pharmacists Group, published the first *British National Formulary for Children (BNFC)* (this is also discussed in Chapter 13, pages 543–544).[41] The Formulary represents the gold standard in terms of advice to prescribers and dispensers of medication. Both published evidence and the accumulated experience of experts informed its advice but it could not cover all areas of paediatric prescribing.

Internationally, in 2004, the European Commission proposed regulation for medicinal products for paediatric use to support and fund research into off-licence drugs. This resulted in the Paediatric Regulation[42] which, in 2007, introduced a number of practical changes into the regulation of children's medicines. The objective was to produce evidence-based treatment by giving pharmaceutical companies incentives to produce relevant data for paediatric formulations, ideally without subjecting children to unnecessary clinical trials. It sought to strike a balance between targeted investment in children's health and commercial reward for pharmaceutical companies. This copied the USA where similar rules were introduced in 1998 to encourage paediatric research by making it mandatory for paediatric studies to accompany adult studies for conditions in which significant paediatric use was expected.

Companies wishing to obtain marketing authorisation for new drugs for adults in the EU after January 2007 have to include the results of studies that have been conducted on children, in compliance with an agreed paediatric investigation plan (PIP), unless the European Medicines Agency (EMA) grants them a deferral or gives them a waiver. The PIP is agreed in advance and is binding on the pharmaceutical company. It sets out the timing and the measures needed to produce an age-appropriate product for children. Funding, provided through the EU Framework Programmes, covers the development of off-patent medical products and, in order to ensure that funds go into the research that is most urgent for the paediatric population, the EMA publishes a priority list, for which studies are needed. Waivers are given when a paediatric equivalent of the adult drug is not needed or not appropriate. A list of medical conditions that occur only in adults is given on the EMA website[43] and treatments for these are exempt from the requirement for a paediatric investigation plan. The Agency also provides free advice on paediatric research issues, including on the design and conduct of trials.

As part of the EMA's implementation of the 2007 Paediatric Regulation, a Paediatric Committee was created. This is responsible for providing opinions within the EU on the development of medicines for use in children. It assesses the data generated in accordance with agreed PIPs and provides opinions on the quality, safety or efficacy of any medicine for use by children. It also advises Member States on the type of data to be collected for a survey on all existing uses of medicinal products in the paediatric population. It keeps and regularly updates an inventory of paediatric medicinal product needs. February 2009 saw the creation of a European network of organisations and experts on paediatric studies. All clinical trials carried out in the EU are registered on a database (EudraCT) and this also holds the results of paediatric clinical trials that take place in and outside the EU and makes them publically available. The Commission is bound to publish a report by January 2013 on the implementation of the regulation and experience gained.

Consent by competent young people and by parents

For research involving them, competent children should be consulted. As for adults, minors' consent should be voluntary and based on adequate knowledge and understanding of the information relevant to the research. The Gillick case established the common law in England, Wales and Northern Ireland in relation to the ability of competent young people to consent to treatment (see Chapter 4, pages 149–150).[44] In Scotland, statute makes legal provision for competent young people to consent to medical procedures or treatment.[45] In the past, it was sometimes queried whether the legal principles relating to minors' consent to medical treatment applied equally to their consent to participate in medical research. This was clarified by the Medicines for Human Use (Clinical Trials) Regulations which define a minor as someone under the age of 16 and stipulate that, for under-16s, consent for research participation is also needed from parents or the patient's legal representative.[46] Although the regulations apply to clinical trials, it is generally seen as good practice to apply them to other forms of research, unless other rules already are in operation for the specific project.

Therefore, when competent under-16s consent to research or innovative treatment, it is also necessary to obtain consent from someone with parental responsibility. Competent children and young people should also be given appropriate information and can refuse to be involved unless there is evidence that it would be in their best interests and consent has been provided by a person with parental responsibility. It is hard to imagine that a non-therapeutic procedure that the child rejects could be in the child's interests. If the procedures are more intrusive than those required for ordinary clinical care, a child's refusal is usually good reason not to proceed even if parental consent has been obtained.

Assent from minors who lack competence

Wherever possible, children should still be included in discussion about the decision even if they lack the ability to understand fully what the research involves. 'Consent' reflects a positive agreement by individuals who do understand whereas 'assent' is more passive and refers to the patient's acquiescence. While it is far from being the same as informed consent, assent may be a relevant consideration when recruiting children to research projects. Children or young people who are not judged to be capable of giving properly informed consent on their own behalf may still be deemed capable of giving assent, indicating general agreement or lack of any objection to it. Assent can be a contentious issue as questions sometimes arise as to whether the child's apparent assent is agreement to participate or is simply ill-informed compliance. For that reason, properly informed consent would still be required from someone with parental responsibility.

> ### Guidance on assent from the Medical Research Council
>
> If the child is deemed incompetent to consent to participate in research, then he or she should normally not participate without the consent of a person with parental responsibility. A person with parental responsibility may legally consent to treatment on an incompetent child's behalf. If the child is able to give assent to decisions about participation in research, the investigator must obtain that assent in addition to the consent of the legally authorised representative. If the child does not assent, this should be respected.[47]

In some situations, parents may disagree about whether a child, who cannot express a view, should participate in research or experimental therapy. Legally, the consent of one person with parental responsibility should suffice if the intervention is not contrary to the child's interests. There are obvious circumstances when the consent of one parent has to be sufficient because, for example, the child is in contact with only one parent. If parents disagree and one is opposed to the child's involvement, the reasons for that would need to be taken very seriously. The MRC advises that if agreement cannot be reached in such cases, the child should be excluded from the research study unless a treatment option that the child needs is only available as part of the research programme. In the latter case, every effort should be made to overcome the disagreement without having to refer to the courts.[48]

As is discussed in Chapter 4, parents and those with parental responsibility can consent on behalf of a child who lacks competence if the procedure is judged to be in the child's interests but not if it is likely to be against the child's interest in some way. Much research on babies and young children involves relatively routine interventions such as the taking of blood samples. Where these are additional to the blood tests required for the child's own medical treatment, it is important that parents (or those with parental responsibility) are fully aware that the samples are for research purposes and that they can refuse such procedures without any detriment to the child's treatment.

Emergency research involving children and babies

The RCPCH grappled in the 1990s with the dilemmas inherent in any effort to develop new therapies for children who cannot give consent. In 1999, it suggested a compromise in the form of 'provisional' consent when research is needed on the emergency treatment of newborn babies.[49] It suggested that parents, confronted by the possibility of a future emergency in which they would have no time to reflect on their decision, might be willing to agree in principle to an unproven intervention if it were likely that such emergency care would be needed and clinicians were unsure of the best option. For example, parents of babies or children who were likely to require resuscitation would be asked to agree in advance to allowing one of several methods of resuscitation or ventilation, in conditions where the best method was unclear. The proposal attempted to deal with the unsatisfactory situation when parental decision making is under intense time pressure, and the even less satisfactory alternative of seeking only retrospective consent. The proposal was eventually overtaken by formal regulations. In August 2007, the MHRA issued a consultation, proposing that the same rules applying to emergency research on adults without prior consent be extended to minors in emergency situations. The proposal was to allow a child to be entered into an emergency research trial, without prior consent by parents or guardians, as long as REC approval had been granted. In 2008, the Medicines for Human Use (Clinical Trials) and Blood Safety and Quality Amendment was passed, amending the regulations to enable children to take part in emergency care trials where there would be no time to seek initial consent before administering the medicine.[50]

Summary – research and innovative treatment involving children and young people

- Consent from a parent or person with parental responsibility should be obtained for the involvement of people under the age of 16 in research or innovative treatment.
- Parents cannot agree on a child's behalf to anything that is contrary to the child's interests.

- If competent, the child or young person should be provided with information and give voluntary and informed consent, but for those under 16, the consent of someone with parental responsibility is also required.
- Children who are not judged to be capable of giving properly informed consent on their own behalf, may still be deemed capable of giving assent.
- Children can be entered into research on emergency care, without prior consent, where there is uncertainty about the best option and the trial has REC approval.

Confidentiality

The importance of protecting individuals' confidentiality in all healthcare contexts, including medical research, is discussed in Chapter 5. Patients and healthy volunteers who agree to participate in research projects have a right to expect that their personal health information will be securely protected throughout the trial and any disclosures only take place on pre-agreed terms. (Disclosure of some information is essential if an adverse event occurs, for example, or publication of the research findings may indirectly identify someone if the condition being researched is a rare one, but research participants should be aware of such possibilities in advance.) People with impaired mental capacity (see pages 598–599) may also be involved in some kinds of research and their confidentiality needs to be taken as seriously as that of other participants. Confidentiality is one of the key ethical issues that RECs scrutinise when considering a protocol.

Confidentiality and records-based research

As well as individuals physically participating in clinical trials, their data may be used for research purposes and RECs need to carefully scrutinise the proposed provisions for confidentiality and disclosure. Wherever possible, research should use anonymised or de-identified data. At the time of writing it was proposed that identifiable data could be anonymised or aggregated to de-identify them by 'honest brokers' in 'safe havens' which are designated physical or electronic areas that provide the most appropriate level of security for the use of the most sensitive and confidential information.[51] The concept of honest brokers and safe havens, in order to process and manage the disclosure of identifiable data, including its anonymisation or coding, was approved by the GMC in its guidance on confidentiality.[52] (Honest brokers and safe havens are discussed in Chapter 5, page 209.)

Where the use of identifiable information is essential, patients should be asked to consent to the research use of their medical records. Many are happy for their identifiable information to be used for research but they still generally want to be asked. The Data Protection Act 1998 requires the fair and lawful processing of information, so patients should be aware about which organisations may process their data and why.

In England and Wales, disclosure of identifiable information without consent has been possible in certain circumstances. This required the research protocol having approval from an REC and the National Information Governance Board (NIGB) under the Health Service (Control of Patient Information) Regulations 2002 to support 'medical research'. Such use has to be in the interests of improving patient care or the public interest, and is only acceptable when seeking consent is not practicable and where anonymised information would not suffice (see Chapter 5, pages 209–210). In 2011, the Health and Social Care Bill was introduced into Parliament and contained a proposal to abolish NIGB and transfer its statutory functions to the Care Quality Commission (CQC).[53] (Up-to-date information can be found on the BMA website.)

Disclosure of identifiable patient data is permitted in some circumstances without the subject's consent if it is in the public interest (see Chapter 5, pages 207–208). In 2009, the GMC published guidance on such disclosure for research purposes.[54] It advises doctors that, if identifiable information is needed for research it will often be perfectly practicable to get patients' express consent.[55] Under the GMC guidance, identifiable data can be used in some cases for research in the public interest *without* the individual's consent but only when it would be impracticable to attempt to gain consent and when the research could not be carried out using anonymised information. Where identifiable data are requested, attention needs to be given to why anonymised data could not be used and whether patient consent could practicably be sought. In some cases, the age of the records, poor traceability of them or the sheer number of records may make obtaining express consent impracticable. In any situation, where a judgement needs to be made between the public interest in disclosure and the patients' interest in keeping information confidential, the GMC advises that a number of factors must be taken into account.

GMC advice on disclosure in the public interest for research

The GMC sees medical research as a justifiable reason for a public interest disclosure without consent if:

- it is essential to use identifiable information, or
- it is not practicable to anonymise the information
- and not practicable to seek consent.[56]

The GMC also lists the factors that must be explained to an REC when it has to decide whether a breach of confidentiality in the public interest would be justified:

- the nature of the information involved
- the use that will be made of it
- how many people will have access to it
- the security arrangements to protect further disclosure
- the advice of an independent expert advisor
- the potential for harm or distress to patients.[57]

Some records-based research is carried out in parallel with the provision of treatment by health professionals who already have access to the records as part of their duty of care for that patient. Nevertheless, when it was provided by patients, the information was given for treatment purposes and so patients need to be made generally aware that it may be used by their own health team for research and audit connected with their care. Explicit consent for clinical audit purposes undertaken by the team that provided care is not legally required.

In other cases, research is carried out by researchers who are not involved in the patient's care but want access to records. In such circumstances, the advice from the GMC and other relevant bodies should be followed and express consent be sought from the participants wherever that is legally required and practicable. Identifiable information can be disclosed without consent if it is approved by NIGB (in England and Wales) or if disclosure can be justified in the public interest. In Northern Ireland the Privacy Advisory Committee can advise on some aspects of disclosure but lacks statutory powers. In Scotland, the Privacy Advisory Committee has a different role and BMA advice to doctors there has been that they should seek guidance from an expert such as a Caldicott Guardian. In 2011, however, as part of a range of proposals for reform of research governance, the Academy of Medical

Sciences recommended that Caldicott Guardians should not be involved in the approval of research studies but rather facilitate them when approval had been granted by other bodies.[58] (Up-to-date information can be found on the BMA website.) Authorisation for the detailed research protocol should be obtained from an appropriately constituted REC. The fact that a research project is solely records based does not mean that it is exempt from the requirement for review.

Confidentiality and research involving children

Long-term issues of confidentiality can be rather different in respect of research on children and young people, partly because their health information, typically collected with the agreement of parents when the patients are young, may be stored for a long time and used for projects that cannot currently be predicted. The potential retention of tissue samples and the need to consider consent for their future use may need to be discussed in the research protocol (see also pages 615–616). The trial documents for paediatric research should be archived for a duration that takes into consideration the potential need for long-term review of safety in trials carried out with children.

Children and young people may be unaware of the information kept about them and researchers have a duty to consider the long-term implications of future access to it. Protocols should specify the level of protection of educational records, for example, when studies are performed in schools and the information given to parents or legal representatives. This is particularly important when the information is very sensitive, such as that including issues of sexuality, illicit drug use or violence. Where personal information on a child is collected, stored, accessed, used or disposed of, a researcher should ensure that the privacy, confidentiality and cultural sensitivities of the subject are protected, subject to the usual exemptions (such as where there is a statutory duty to disclose or a public interest in doing so).

Confidentiality and publication

Researchers should publish results whenever possible, including adverse findings, preferably through peer-reviewed journals and on relevant shared databases. Patient consent must be sought for publication of case studies where individuals who have participated in research or innovative treatment could be identified by themselves, or by people close to them. With research on rare conditions, patients may be identifiable even if the obviously identifying details are removed. Aggregated data do not usually pose the same problems.

Summary – confidentiality

- Where possible, research should use de-identified data and individuals should be aware of the research use of their medical records.
- If identifiable information is needed for research it will often be perfectly practicable to get patients' express consent.
- As part of the ethical scrutiny of the research protocol, the REC and any other relevant authorising body should consider the issues of confidentiality raised by the research.
- When it is feasible neither to use de-identified information nor to obtain subject consent to disclosure for research, doctors need to satisfy themselves that the GMC's advice on disclosure in the public interest is followed.

Research governance

A very substantial amount of guidance on research governance is available. As there is broad consensus about best practice, the main points tend to be reiterated and echo the principles set out at the beginning of this chapter. Research guidance and regulations are also updated periodically and so this chapter mentions some of the main bodies providing advice so that readers can review the latest versions for themselves. First, we set out the background to the development of research governance in the UK which underwent much change at the end of the twentieth century and start of the twenty-first. In 2010–2011, there was further debate about reforming the system to minimise delays and bureaucracy and, at the time of writing, it is unclear if some proposed changes will be implemented. (Information about recent developments is available on the BMA's website.)

Background to research regulation

It has long been agreed that the use of new or unproven interventions, either in research or therapy, needs special care. Traditionally, in the UK, good practice in both research and innovative treatment was defined by guidance from professional bodies rather than law (although embryo research has been an exception). The way in which research is regulated began to change when the European Parliament agreed in 2001 to implement uniform rules on clinical trials of medicinal products[59] and the UK drafted specific regulations to do this.[60] Prior to this, the International Conference on Harmonisation Guidance on good clinical practice[61] set the standards for research projects in Europe. These were generally followed in the UK even when not formally binding on researchers. In 2001, the Department of Health's research governance framework for health and social care[62] (and the parallel document in Wales,[63] Scotland[64] and Northern Ireland[65]) formalised the requirement that all research involving patients, service users, care professionals or volunteers, or their organs, tissue or data, be reviewed independently to ensure that it met ethical standards. A quality and accountability framework for research in health and social care was set out. It emphasised the principles that were widely regarded as crucial in research, such as the importance of obtaining informed consent from participants. It also included issues such as the need for research to involve a diversity of participants in terms of ethnicity, gender, disability, age and sexual orientation and the need for clear agreements detailing the respective responsibilities and rights of all those involved. The document spelled out the accountability of investigators, employers and sponsors. The Clinical Trials Directive required all European countries to harmonise their legislation on clinical trials of medicinal products.[66] The UK's Medicines for Human Use (Clinical Trials) Regulations 2004 implemented the EU rules and made it obligatory, for example, to obtain a favourable opinion from an ethics committee prior to starting a research trial on any medicine.

In 2010, the European Commission announced a further overhaul of the rules governing medical research as a result of criticisms that had been made about the Clinical Trials Directive and the fact that there were inconsistencies in how member states were applying it. A project sponsored by the Commission to assess the effect of the Directive on the pharmaceutical industry, academics, RECs and regulators had found that it had increased researchers' workloads unnecessarily. For example, researchers had previously reported all 'serious adverse events' (SAEs) but the Directive only required EU researchers to report 'suspected unexpected serious adverse events' (SUSARs): that is to say, only side-effects directly relevant to the medicine used in the trial had to be notified to the authorities.

Although this should have lightened the workload of EU researchers, the fact that outside the EU it was still obligatory to report SAEs meant that international trials had to comply with two sets of reporting – doubling researchers' work. The scientific community, particularly academic researchers, complained that the European rules significantly increased costs and bureaucracy: previously feasible low budget trials became prohibitively expensive with increased insurance and administration costs. This coincided with the rapid development of the clinical trials infrastructures in non-EU countries such as Brazil, Russia, India and China, making it more difficult to attract research to Europe. To deal with such problems, the European Commission announced it would put forward new legislative proposals on clinical trials in late 2011.

Role of research ethics committees

Concern existed about the system for monitoring research prior to the 1990s. Anxieties focused on the apparently erratic monitoring of research projects and variations in training and membership of the committees supervising them. Researchers were frustrated in multi-centre projects, if one committee approved the research and another rejected it. RECs were established in the NHS in the mid-1960s, when they were voluntary. The system was reorganised by the Department of Health in 1991 in England and Wales and in 1992 in Scotland. Two kinds of RECs were set up: Local Research Ethics Committees (LRECs) and, in 1997, Multi-centre Research Ethics Committees (MRECs), but dissatisfaction remained. Some researchers were unhappy about the LRECs' treatment of the scientific aspects of research but thought that issues relating to consent and protection of patients' welfare were generally well handled.[67] In 2000, the Central Office for Research Ethics Committees (COREC) was established and worked until 2004 to coordinate the work of RECs whose procedures were described in *Governance arrangements for NHS research ethics committees* (GAfREC).[68] This gave health authorities the responsibility of setting up such committees and detailed the duties of committee members. The *Standard Operating Procedures* set out the factors they must consider.

In November 2004, the REC system again came under scrutiny. Lord Warner established a group to examine its operation resulting in a report in 2005[69] when the National Patient Safety Agency (NPSA), which had responsibility for the National Research Ethics Service (see below), also took over responsibility for COREC. The Warner Report noted improvements that had occurred but also listed ongoing concerns, criticisms and frustrations within the research community. More changes were needed. Inconsistency amongst RECs was still evident and the report called for more training and better dissemination of good practice guidelines. It said that RECs should focus on the ethics, not the science, of research and should not be involved in scrutinising projects that did not raise genuine ethical questions – these could be handled by screeners. In 2006, the NPSA consulted on the future of the REC service, with a view to implementing the recommendations of the Warner Report, most of which were subsequently put into practice. In 2010, however, it was proposed that the NPSA itself be abolished as part of a further reform of research governance.[70] The proposals for reform are discussed further on pages 609–610.

One of the problems in authorising research has long been the range of guidance available and lack of consistency in some aspects of it. Attempts have been made to standardise it. In 2009, for example, the four UK Health Departments consulted on an updated version of GAfREC, intended to harmonise the guidance across the UK, replacing the versions that had been issued separately in England and Scotland in 2001. It also applied in Wales and Northern Ireland and took account of legal, policy and operational developments since the previous guidance in 2001. The revised version of GAfREC, agreed by the four UK Health Departments, was published in 2011, with an implementation date of 1 September 2011.[71] Nevertheless, inconsistencies persisted in other aspects of research guidance and the way in which projects were scrutinised which led to the suggestions for reform in 2010 and 2011, which are discussed later in the chapter.

Factors to be considered by RECs include:

- whether the chief investigator in the trial is competent and has adequate facilities
- possible hazards to trial participants and precautions taken to deal with them
- measures for providing information and seeking appropriate consent
- whether adequate compensation arrangements are in place in case of any harm arising from the trial
- methods of recruitment and any payments to participants
- payments to investigators
- storage and use of subject identifiable information.

Centralised bodies involved in regulation and governance

UK Ethics Committee Authority

In 2004, regulations made provision for a new statutory system throughout the UK for establishing and recognising RECs. A supervisory body, the UK Ethics Committee Authority (UKECA) was set up under the Medicines for Human Use (Clinical Trials) Regulations 2004. UKECA was established solely to comply with EU legislation requiring the existence of a body to coordinate national activity.

National Institute for Health Research

Most health research takes place in the NHS. The NHS Research and Development network was set up to support research and development projects in health and social care, by facilitating the sharing of best practice. The National Institute for Health Research, and similar initiatives in the devolved nations, worked to create the infrastructure and facilities for research in which the NHS is a partner.

Health Research Agency

In 2010, the Department of Health in England published a report[72] proposing a number of reforms, including the abolition of the National Patient Safety Agency, which had responsibility for the National Research Ethics Service (NRES; see below) and the establishment of a new Health Research Agency (HRA) as a single regulator for research. Such a single body would take on responsibility for overseeing general ethical approval via the NRES, as well as providing specialist approvals and licences for research involving patient data, human tissue and stem cells and gene therapy. In March 2011, the Treasury confirmed that it would proceed to set up the HRA to streamline regulation and improve the cost effectiveness of clinical trials. The plan undertook to remove outdated regulations and ensure that future funding by the National Institute for Health Research (NIHR) to providers of NHS services would be conditional on meeting specified benchmarks, such as a 70-day benchmark to recruit first patients for trials.[73]

Early in 2011, as part of these broader reforms, the Academy of Medical Sciences (AMS) published a report on research regulation. It expressed anxiety about the fall in the UK's global share of clinical trials which it partly attributed to the costs and delays incurred by the UK's existing complex research approval process.[74] The AMS urged that the proposed HRA be established promptly to facilitate a streamlined UK-wide regulatory system, together with a new National Research Governance Service (NRGS) in England. It recognised that regulatory and governance arrangements still varied across the four UK administrations but said that this could be overcome by the HRA working with its counterparts in the devolved nations.

The AMS report said that the NRGS would facilitate approval of research studies conducted in single or multiple NHS sites by taking responsibility for all study-wide checks that have been duplicated by each participating NHS Trust. The AMS also defined the functions of the HRA as providing a national research governance service and a single system for ethical approval. It argued this would:

- eliminate inefficiency, provide support and a single system of checks, ensure common standards and consistent interpretation of the requirements
- oversee arrangements enabling trusts to determine local research feasibility within agreed timescales and allow trusts to focus on monitoring local issues of capacity, conduct and performance
- establish a single ethical approval system, with a single source of advice, for general and specialist research, with clear interpretation of legislation
- enable the pooling of resources and ensure greater transparency and accountability.

National Research Ethics Service

The role of the NRES includes the following:

- ensuring robust ethical review of research by RECs
- providing ethical guidance and management support to RECs
- delivering a quality assurance framework for the research ethics service
- providing training programmes
- working with colleagues across the UK to maintain a UK-wide framework for ethical review
- working with colleagues in the wider regulatory environment to streamline the processes for approving research
- working with colleagues to promote transparency in research.

The NRES has worked to standardise and harmonise procedures and has sought to reduce delay in the approval of protocols. In 2009, following up the recommendations of the Warner Report (see page 608), the NRES introduced a scheme to divert studies that raise no clear ethical issues, such as questionnaires for NHS staff, to a small subcommittee for scrutiny and free up RECs to concentrate on ethically challenging studies. The review of research by the Academy of Medical Sciences in 2011 recommended that the NRES should continue to provide centralised, coordinated ethical guidance, working in future with the proposed HRA.[75]

In 2009, the Social Care Institute of Excellence (SCIE) appointed a Social Care Research Ethics Committee (SCREC), operating within the framework of the NRES to provide ethical review of social care research in England. Social care research in Northern Ireland involving health and social care staff, service users or carers as research participants, or which requires access to their tissue or data, continued to be reviewed by the Health and

Social Care Research Ethics Committees, managed by the Office for Research Ethics Committees Northern Ireland.

Specialist bodies providing ethical review

Research governance has hitherto been managed by RECs, plus some specialist bodies which scrutinise single areas of potentially contentious research where specialised knowledge is needed, such as that involving human embryos and gene therapy. In 2010, as part of a wide programme of proposed reforms, it was suggested that some of the specialised bodies could be abolished and their functions transferred elsewhere to streamline the system. Included in this proposal were the Gene Therapy Advisory Committee (GTAC), Human Tissue Authority (HTA) and Human Fertilisation and Embryology Authority (HFEA).[76] The abolition was also proposed of the National Information Governance Board for Health and Social Care (NIGB), whose role it has been to consider uses of confidential patient information in research when it would be impractical to seek subject consent. The Public Bodies Bill introduced into Parliament in January 2011 contained proposals to abolish all of these regulators and transfer their research scrutiny functions to the proposed HRA or other regulators. It was suggested that as an interim measure the functions of NIGB be transferred to the CQC, with the CQC being required to appoint a National Information Governance Committee until March 2015. (Up-to-date information can be found on the BMA website.)

Medicines and Healthcare Products Regulatory Agency

Under the Medicines Act 1968, all trials of new medicinal products on people had to be notified to the Medicines Control Agency, which became the Medicines and Healthcare Products Regulatory Agency in April 2003. The MHRA regulates a wide range of materials, such as medicines, medical devices, blood and therapeutic products and services such as those that are derived from tissue engineering.

General Medical Council

The GMC regulates all facets of doctors' behaviour, including their involvement in research. In 2009, the GMC published guidance on confidentiality, including for secondary uses such as medical research, and the following year it issued two pieces of supplementary guidance on consent in research and good practice in research.[77] The former explains how the core principles set out in the GMC guidance on consent[78] apply specifically to research, including research involving people and human tissue. The good practice guidance sets out a series of principles, such as the duty of honesty and integrity and provides advice on confidentiality and use of health records in research.

Guidance from other UK bodies

A large amount of expert guidance on the conduct of research has been published by UK bodies. The MRC, for example, provides advice on implementing statutory and good practice standards for research, including on personal information and human tissue samples. Early MRC guidance pre-dated most other national and international ethical guidelines.[79] The Council aims to support research across the biomedical spectrum, from fundamental lab-based science to clinical trials, and in all major disease areas. It publishes a range of material to assist medical researchers, including on relevant primary legislation regarding adults who cannot give consent for themselves and children and covers the differences across the UK.[80] The Royal College of Physicians also has a long and highly respected tradition of publishing detailed ethical guidance for research and has traditionally been at the forefront of standard setting in this area.[81] The RCPCH produces specific guidance for research involving children and young people.[82] The Wellcome Trust is another source of guidance, including on allegations of research misconduct.[83] Patient organisations, such as the Alzheimer's Society, also publish guidance intended to inform the public.[84] The UK Research Integrity Office provides advice to research organisations and individual researchers. It aims to share best practice about identifying misconduct and publishes a code on dealing with questionable practices.[85]

International guidance

Since the 1960s, a significant amount of international and national ethical guidance has been published about the supervision that should be applied to research. It is impossible to do full justice here to this literature. Internationally, the first set of ethical guidelines was much earlier: the Nuremberg Code set standards which arose out of the Nuremberg trials of Nazi doctors, following the Second World War.[86] Similar standards were echoed by the World Medical Association's Declaration of Helsinki,[87] adopted in 1964 and regularly updated since then. This became the foundation of most subsequent guidance. United Nations agencies, including the World Health Organization[88] and the Joint United Nations Programme on HIV/AIDS (UNAIDS),[89] built upon the Helsinki Declaration. At European level, the European Forum for Good Clinical Practice (EFGCP) is a respected source of practical guidance. It is a non-profit organisation which aims to encourage common, high-quality standards in all stages of biomedical research throughout Europe. An example of its work is its report identifying how aspects of the ethical review process, embodied in the 2001 EC Directive on Clinical Trials, are interpreted and applied in different European countries.[90] All European counties adopted the Directive but, until the EFGCP's report, it was often difficult for researchers wishing to conduct a project in Europe to find out how precisely the rules are applied in a particular EU jurisdiction. Although the UK is not a signatory to it, the European Convention on Human Rights and Biomedicine also set standards for research in the European Union.[91] International guidance is also available for trials or joint projects in developing countries: core documents include those from the Council for International Organizations of Medical Science,[92] and the Nuffield Council on Bioethics.[93]

Law and regulation

Medicines for Human Use (Clinical Trials) Regulations 2004

In 2003, the Government published draft legislation on clinical trials of investigational medicinal products for human use, including placebos. Its aim was to incorporate into UK law the European Clinical Trials Directive. The Regulations came into force in the UK in May 2004 and the main points include:

- the foreseeable risks and inconveniences must be weighed against the anticipated benefit for each participant in the trial, and other present and future patients
- there must be provision for indemnity

- the rights of each participant to physical and mental integrity, privacy and protection of personal data must be safeguarded
- provision is made for involvement of individuals who cannot consent
- a statutory system for establishing and recognising RECs was set in place.[94]

The provisions apply only to clinical trials of medicinal products and not to other forms of research or experimental therapy but some see the European Directive's requirement for new regulations in member states as the trigger for the British Government's wider overhaul of research regulation.[95] The UK Regulations cover the participation in research of incapacitated adults specifying that there should be grounds for expecting that administering the medicinal product to be tested in the trial will produce a benefit to the subject outweighing the risks, or produce no risk at all. Any advance refusal of the treatment made by the person prior to the onset of incapacity must be respected. In the absence of such evidence about the patient's views, provision was made for two types of legal representative who could consent to interventions in the patient's interests. Close relatives can act as 'personal legal representatives' and provide proxy consent for the patient. Health professionals (if not connected with the research) can act as a 'professional representative' for patients lacking close family members. In December 2006, the Regulations were amended to allow CTIMPs on adults without prior consent in emergency situations where proxy consent was unavailable (see page 599). In 2008, the regulations were further amended to allow CTIMPs in emergency situations on children without prior consent. The 2004 Regulations already allowed consent by a legal representative if the emergency meant that a person with parental responsibility could not be contacted prior to the minor's inclusion. The 2008 amendment allowed inclusion without a legal representative's prior consent.

Mental Capacity Act 2005

The Mental Capacity Act 2005 applies in England and Wales. As yet, there is no comparable legislation in Northern Ireland (but see the BMA website for further information) and the provisions of the Scottish legislation are set out below. The Act has a clear statement on the legality of enrolling incapacitated adults in some closely regulated medical research. This clarified an area of concern and confusion among researchers. Excluded from the Act are clinical trials, regulated under the Medicines for Human Use (Clinical Trials) Regulations 2004 (see above). In keeping with established international norms in medical ethics, research involving incapacitated adults *must* be related to the condition that contributes to the impairment of the mind or brain from which the incapacitated person suffers. This includes research into the impact of the impairment on the person's day-to-day health and welfare, as well as into the causes of the impairment and any possible treatments. The research must be approved by an REC and it must not be possible to conduct the research involving individuals who retain the capacity to consent.

Where the research is expected to benefit the individual, that anticipated benefit should outweigh any risks. Where the patient is not expected to benefit, the risk to that person must be negligible. Any intrusion or restriction on the patient's basic rights must be kept to a minimum, thus permitting observational research, projects solely using medical notes or investigations into the provision of services.

Before an incapacitated person can be enrolled in a research project, researchers must identify an appropriate person close to the subject who is willing to be consulted about the acceptability of the patient's involvement. If no such person can be found, an independent person, unconnected with the research, can be asked to make that judgement. RECs closely scrutinise this aspect of research protocols. Additional safeguards are in place once the research is underway. If the incapacitated person shows signs of reluctance to be involved, he or she must be withdrawn from the research. Some people give valid consent to participate in research but subsequently become mentally impaired before the research is completed. Regulations drawn up under the Act catered for the management of such an adult enrolled with consent in a research project prior to the Act coming into force but who lost capacity after the research had commenced.[96] Guidance from the Department of Health for England and from the Welsh Assembly explains where consent given prior to the loss of capacity can be relied upon.[97] In the absence of consent, the requirements of the Mental Capacity Act must be fulfilled, including obtaining agreement from a personal or professional representative and obtaining REC approval. The Mental Capacity Act also covers the removal of tissue from incapacitated individuals for purposes scheduled under the Human Tissue Act 2004.

Adults with Incapacity (Scotland) Act 2000

In Scotland, the Adults with Incapacity (Scotland) Act 2000 empowers proxy decision makers to make a range of decisions for incapacitated adults as long as the proposed intervention meets the criteria set out in the Act. These are that surgical, medical, nursing, dental or psychological research can involve incapacitated people only if it could not be carried out equally well on adults with capacity. The purpose of the research must be to obtain knowledge of the causes, diagnosis, treatment or care of the adult's incapacity or to understand the effect of treatment that has been provided for it. Such research should generally be expected to produce some benefit for the participant but, even when it cannot, it may still be carried out if it meets the other requirements and is likely to benefit other people who have the same cause of their incapacity. Participation in the research project must reflect the incapacitated person's wishes as far as these can be ascertained and take account of the views of other relevant people close to that person. It must have REC approval, involve no more than minimal risk or minimal discomfort, and cannot proceed if the person indicates unwillingness to participate.

Human Rights Act 1998

The Human Rights Act 1998 is relevant to consent to, or refusal of, involvement in research. If appropriately informed participant consent is not sought for research or experimental treatment, this failure could raise issues under the Human Rights Act. In the case of *X v Denmark*,[98] the European Commission of Human Rights concluded that medical treatment of an experimental character and without the consent of the subject may, under certain circumstances, be a breach of human rights under the prohibition on torture and inhuman or degrading treatment. Similarly, the use of personal health information without permission could be a breach.[99] The Act imposes duties on public authorities and RECs are likely to fall into that category, which means that they need to ensure that all their decisions are compatible with human rights legislation.

Data Protection Act 1998

The Data Protection Act 1998 is a complex piece of legislation which is discussed in detail in Chapter 5. It sets legal limits on the use of identifiable personal information but gives some exemptions for data used in research, if certain criteria are met. These are set out in Section 33 of the Act which is commonly known as 'the research exemption'. It specifies the following criteria which must be met for research to be permissible:

- the data cannot also be used in connection with measures or decisions relating to particular individuals
- the use of the data must not cause damage or distress to the data subject
- the data cannot be published in a way which allows identification of the subject.

The data processing must meet the common law requirements for consent and the data controller must ensure that the data subject is aware of what is intended for the data. That is to say, at the time of giving the information, the individual providing it should be made aware of how it will be used in research. If the person holding the information would subsequently like to use it for further research, not envisaged when the data were collected, the 'fair processing' requirements of the Act (see Chapter 5, page 190) still need to be met. This involves providing general information to data subjects about future intended research uses. The research exemption cannot be used to justify the retention of records longer than normal simply because they could be useful in future research. This means that the exemption applies only if research is actually about to be carried out or there is a firm intention to use the records for that purpose.

Human Tissue Legislation

Following revelations in the early 1990s of the unauthorised retention of human organs and tissue following post-mortem examination (see Chapter 12, pages 494–495), there were widespread calls for the Human Tissue Act 1961 to be repealed and replaced with a clear, modern legislative framework. This resulted in the Human Tissue Act 2004 (covering England, Wales and Northern Ireland) and the Human Tissue (Scotland) Act 2006. Both pieces of legislation cover the removal, storage and use of tissue after death but the 2004 Act went further and also regulated some aspects of the storage and use of tissue from living individuals. The 2004 Act also established the Human Tissue Authority (HTA) to oversee implementation of the legislation and to regulate the storage and use of human tissue (see Chapter 12, pages 522–523). (In 2010, the Government announced plans to abolish the HTA and transfer its functions to other bodies – for up-to-date information see the BMA's website.) Prior to the revised legislation, there was considerable sensitivity about the notion of retaining samples from deceased people for the purposes of research and much of this was due to the general lack of openness about such practices in the past. A consistent message in all current published advice is the need for transparency and authorisation. The main provisions of the legislation that are relevant to research are summarised below; more information is provided in Chapter 12, pages 522–526 and in the BMA's separate guidance.[100]

England, Wales and Northern Ireland

- Consent must be obtained for any storage and use of tissue removed after death for research purposes.
- Storage of material removed after death, for research purposes, requires a licence from the HTA unless it is stored for use in a particular project that already has research ethics authority approval or approval is pending. (A 'research ethics authority' is a UKECA recognised ethics committee or a person or committee recognised for the purpose by

the Secretary of State, the National Assembly of Wales or the Department of Health, Social Services and Public Safety in Northern Ireland.)
- Consent is required for the storage and use of tissue from living individuals for research unless the material has been anonymised, such that the researcher cannot know the identity of the donor (there may still be a link to the donor via a third party) and the project has research ethics authority approval or approval is pending.
- Where tissue removed from living individuals is stored for future research that does not have ethics authority approval (ie tissue banks) a licence is required from the HTA.
- In very exceptional circumstances, such as an extreme public health emergency, the Secretary of State may make regulations to allow tissue from the living or the dead to be used for research without consent.

For further information see the HTA's research Code of Practice.[101]

Scotland

In Scotland, a distinction is made between whole organs and tissues, blocks and slides. Tissue samples, blocks and slides (including samples taken from organs) automatically become part of the deceased person's medical record and may be used for diagnostic and audit purposes without the need for specific authorisation. Retention and use for research, however, requires authorisation. Any retention or use of whole organs after the conclusion of a post-mortem examination also requires explicit authorisation. The use of tissue from living individuals for research is not covered by the Human Tissue (Scotland) Act 2006.

Specialised areas of research

Highly specialised areas of research and innovative therapy involve only a small proportion of doctors on a day-to-day basis, but this section sets out BMA policies on issues that are frequently raised in debate.

Human embryo research

Human embryo research has been exceptional as an area in which there is clear legislation. There is also a statutory regulatory body to monitor research, the HFEA, but this is one of the bodies whose abolition was proposed in 2010.[102] In future, therefore, its functions may be transferred to other regulators. (See the BMA's website for up-to-date information.)

After the recommendation of the Warnock Committee (see Chapter 8, page 312) that research involving human embryos should be permitted up to 14 days after fertilisation, there followed nearly a decade of fierce debate on the subject. The Human Fertilisation and Embryology Bill was published in 1989 with alternative clauses either allowing or prohibiting embryo research. The parliamentary vote was overwhelmingly in support of the use of human embryos for certain categories of research, with strict controls. The Human Fertilisation and Embryology Act 1990 required that a licence must be issued for every research project in the UK that involves the creation or use of human embryos. A list of all licensed research projects is available on the HFEA's website.[103]

Human embryos used in research come from two sources. They may have been created as part of the research process or as part of an *in vitro* fertilisation (IVF) procedure, to which they are now surplus (and would otherwise be donated to other infertile people or allowed to perish). Those who believe that embryos have, or should have, equal moral status to that of living people believe that research on them can never be ethically acceptable. Others accept research on 'spare' embryos but not the creation of embryos for research purposes. Adherents of this latter view assume that the creation of more embryos than is strictly necessary for IVF is unavoidable for medical reasons and argue that to use them for research is no worse than destroying them and may bring about some good. Both sources of embryos for research are permitted under the Human Fertilisation and Embryology Act.

In the mid-1980s, there was extensive discussion within the BMA about the ethics of research involving human embryos. Opinions were sharply divided on the question of whether human life could be created for the purposes of research, although there was wide acceptance of the need for such research into contraception and the diagnosis and treatment of infertility and inherited diseases. There was less objection to research on 'spare' embryos and, despite some concerns, it was recognised that there are some areas of research in which embryos must be created as part of the research process. For example, when new methods of infertility treatment are being developed, it is an essential part of the research carefully to assess the effect of the treatment on the development of the embryo, to ensure that the embryo itself is not damaged.

This type of research was particularly important for the development of new techniques, such as intracytoplasmic sperm injection (ICSI), in which a single sperm is injected into the centre of an egg as a means of overcoming severe male infertility. Before embryos created using this new technique were replaced in the uterus for development, it was necessary to assess the embryos for any damage caused by the procedure itself. The process of checking the development of the embryo meant that they were no longer suitable for replacement. A failure to permit this type of research would have resulted either in embryos created in this way being replaced without proper checks on their safety or an end to the development of such new treatments for infertility. After debate, the BMA confirmed its belief in the need for research involving embryos and refused to rule out the possibility that embryos could be created for this purpose, although it also stressed that 'the prime objectives' of IVF concerned the provision of infertility treatment for those who are unable to have children naturally.

Embryonic stem cell research

In 1998, stem cells from human embryos were isolated and cultured in a laboratory for the first time. The ability of embryonic stem cells to develop into almost any body cell type meant that this development raised the possibility of a new source of tissue for the treatment of diseased or damaged tissues or organs. Combined with the technique of cell nuclear replacement this could lead to the development of compatible tissue for transplantation, which would involve transferring the nucleus – containing the genetic material – from one of the patient's own cells into a donor egg that has had its own nucleus removed. The egg would then be stimulated so that it begins to divide, but it would be allowed to develop only to the stage needed to separate and grow embryonic stem cells. It was believed that these embryonic stem cells could then be stimulated to develop into whatever tissue was needed by the patient, such as:

- neural tissue for the treatment of degenerative diseases such as Parkinson disease
- bone marrow for leukaemia patients

- muscle tissue for the repair of a damaged heart, or
- skin for treating burns.

The BMA welcomed these developments, recognising the potential to benefit vast numbers of people with disorders that threaten or impede their lives. They could potentially offer a means of overcoming the severe shortage of tissue available for transplantation. In addition, the generation of tissue using the patients' own genetic material would remove the need for them to take the strong immunosuppressive drugs that can be harmful when taken over a long period of time.

In 2000, an expert group was set up by the Chief Medical Officer to review the potential for developments in stem cell research and cell nuclear replacement to benefit human health.[104] Noting that this work did not fall within any of the categories of research permitted under the Human Fertilisation and Embryology Act, this group recommended that embryo research in this area should be permitted. It therefore recommended that the categories of research that could be licensed should be expanded to bring embryonic stem cell research within the scope of the Act. Although it had been suggested that major advances could be made by the use of adult stem cells, the expert group concluded that the use of human embryos was justified. By January 2001, both Houses of Parliament had voted to extend the purposes for which embryo research may be undertaken to include this work.[105]

The BMA has taken the view that, if a similar level of success could be achieved, the use of adult, rather than embryonic, stem cells would be preferable because of the special status of human embryos. Experts in the field, however, believe that there are likely to be limitations to the types of tissue that could be derived from adult stem cells, thus limiting the potential benefits. Research aimed at the development of methods to reprogramme adult human cells to a pluripotent state (induced pluripotent stem (iPS) cells) appears promising[106] but until such time as there is clear evidence for the safety and efficacy of the use of adult stem cells, the BMA strongly believes that research using both adult and embryonic stem cells should progress in parallel.

Cell nuclear replacement embryos

The Chief Medical Officer's expert group had concluded that the research use of embryos created by cell nuclear replacement was not prohibited by the Human Fertilisation and Embryology Act, but would be subject to the same restrictions as other embryo research. Shortly after the Regulations were passed, however, the Pro-life Alliance challenged this interpretation and was granted a judicial review, arguing that the definition of 'embryo' in the Act did not include an organism created by cell nuclear replacement. It therefore argued that both reproductive cloning (with the intention of creating genetically identical individuals) and research on embryos created by cell nuclear replacement were completely unregulated in the UK. The definition of 'embryo' in the 1990 Act was: 'a live human embryo where fertilisation is complete' and included 'an egg in the process of fertilisation' and stated that 'for this purpose, fertilisation is not complete until the appearance of a two cell zygote'.[107] The Pro-life Alliance argued that, with cell nuclear replacement, fertilisation does not take place and so the organism created cannot possibly be an 'embryo where fertilisation is complete'. The Government, although accepting that fertilisation does not take place, argued for a purposive rather than a literal interpretation. In November 2001, Mr Justice Crane accepted 'with some reluctance' the Pro-life Alliance's arguments and concluded that to accept the Government's approach would involve an unacceptable extension of the definition.[108]

The Government responded by passing the Human Reproductive Cloning Act 2001. Although this put beyond doubt the illegality of reproductive cloning, it did not, as some had anticipated, extend the definition of 'embryo' in the Act to incorporate those embryos created by cell nuclear replacement. Instead, the Government launched an appeal against the decision of Mr Justice Crane, arguing that the Act was clearly intended to provide comprehensive control of human reproduction by either prohibiting or licensing particular activities. The Court of Appeal agreed and reversed the earlier decision.[109] The Pro-life Alliance was denied leave to appeal to the House of Lords, but announced that it would submit a petition to the House of Lords. This petition was rejected.[110]

After the Regulations were passed, the House of Lords Select Committee on Stem Cell Research was established. Its report, published in 2002, concluded that there were strong arguments for research to continue with both embryonic and adult stem cells in order to maximise the chance of medical benefit.[111] The Select Committee also recommended the establishment of an embryonic stem cell bank to ensure their purity and provenance, and to monitor their use. This led directly to the establishment of the UK Stem Cell Bank. The HFEA announced that it would be a condition of the research licence that any cell line derived from human embryos must be deposited in the Stem Cell Bank.

In August 2004, the HFEA issued the first licence to create human embryonic stem cells using cell nuclear replacement for research. The Government used the Human Fertilisation and Embryology Act 2008 to amend the definition of 'embryo' in the 1990 Act to put it beyond doubt that embryos created by cell nuclear replacement were covered by the legislation. Also in 2008, the remit of GTAC (see Chapter 9, pages 405–406) was extended to include the ethical oversight of clinical trials involving therapies derived using stem cell lines. (In 2010, however, it was announced that GTAC was to be abolished and its ethical review work transferred to the National Research Ethics Service – see the BMA's website for more information.)

The regulatory framework for stem cell research is complex, potentially involving the HFEA, HTA, GTAC and MHRA. An online resource has been developed to help researchers to navigate their way through this complex regulatory landscape and to identify all of the regulatory steps needed to take their ideas for a new treatment from the laboratory to patients.[112]

Human admixed embryos

Subsequent research developments also focused attention on the need to reassess the definition of 'embryo' in the 1990 Act. In 2006, the HFEA received two applications for research projects involving the use of animal eggs for cell nuclear replacement to create human embryonic stem cells. The researchers wished to create 'cytoplasmic hybrid embryos' and use them for research. Although the principal reason for this move was to overcome the severe shortage of human eggs donated for research, some commentators argued that the use of animal eggs was morally preferable given the small but inherent risks of ovarian stimulation and egg collection procedures. In line with its standard model for handling difficult and controversial new areas, the HFEA published a consultation document setting out the scientific background to the creation of these and other types of inter-species embryos and considering the ethical issues raised. In its response the BMA argued that the use of animal oocytes as a 'vessel' in which to develop human embryonic stem cells provided an acceptable alternative to the use of human oocytes. The BMA also questioned the rationale for affording greater status and protection to a hybrid embryo than to embryos created using human oocytes and cell nuclear replacement (CNR) when, in fact, it could be argued that they should have less status and protection because that they are not 'human'.

In September 2006, the HFEA decided, in principle, that it would consider applications for the use of cytoplasmic hybrid embryos. At that time, the HFEA decided that it would not consider the use of other types of inter-species embryos (such as chimeras and true hybrids) because there was no pressing need to do so and the issue was due to be debated in Parliament as part of the review of the Human Fertilisation and Embryology Act. Detailed reports on these broader issues were published by the House of Commons Science and Technology Committee[113] and by the Academy of Medical Sciences[114] in advance of parliamentary debate. When the issue was debated by Parliament during 2007 there was overwhelming support for the use in research of what the Government had called 'human admixed embryos'. The 1990 Act was therefore amended to permit the use in research of human admixed embryos.[115]

Drafting a definition that would cover future as well as current scientific developments and possibilities was problematic and so the Act also contains provision for the definition to be amended (but not repealed), by regulations, if necessary.

Research involving fetuses or fetal material

In law, fetal tissue is regarded as the tissue of the mother. Its use and storage is therefore covered, in England, Wales and Northern Ireland, by the terms of the Human Tissue Act 2004. Although legally tissue removed from living individuals may be used anonymously for research without the need for consent, the HTA's Code of Practice states that it is good practice to always obtain consent for the use or storage of fetal tissue.[116] Because the Human Tissue (Scotland) Act 2006 does not regulate the use of tissue from living individuals, the legislation only applies where fetal tissue is removed after the death of the mother.

In the past, research involving fetuses has been governed by guidance rather than the law. The guidance on the research use of fetuses and fetal material (the Polkinghorne Report[117]) set out the expected standards in 1989. Much of this guidance is now outdated however and was superseded, in England, Wales and Northern Ireland, by guidance from the HTA. For example, the Polkinghorne Report had, as one of its central recommendations, that women should give general consent but should not be given details about the specific research to be undertaken. This does not reflect contemporary societal expectations, or current practice, under which individuals are given specific information in order to make informed choices. The HTA has made clear that consent must be based on the person's understanding of what the activity involves.[118]

Genetic research

There is considerable guidance on genetic testing and screening for health care and research. (The ethical issues around genetic testing and screening are discussed in detail in Chapter 9.) In addition, stored human material is sometimes used in genetic research projects and would be covered by the consent provisions of the human tissue legislation discussed above. In 2001, the MRC published detailed advice on the use in research of samples from both living and dead donors, including guidance on genetic research on archived samples.[119] It stated that when a genetic test is of known predictive value or gives reliable information about a known heritable condition, samples must be anonymised before testing. Where the research requires the use of identifiable individuals and involves tests of known clinical or predictive value, explicit consent should be obtained and participants should be given the option of whether to know the result.

Gene therapy

In the UK, all clinical trials of gene therapy have been assessed, approved and monitored by the GTAC (see Chapter 9, pages 405–406). In 2010, however, the Government announced plans to abolish this body and transfer its functions to the NRES. (Up-to-date information can be found on the BMA's website.)

Fraud and misconduct in research and innovative treatment

By its nature, research fraud is difficult to detect. It involves the generation of false data with the intention to deceive. Classic examples include fabrication, falsification and plagiarism. Cases may be invented or some relevant data missed out when research findings are made public. The established peer review system for publication was not set up to detect fraudulent work although expert reviewers sometimes identify grounds for suspicion. Some misconduct stems from ignorance of accepted standards or lack of awareness of changing expectations. In the past, for example, it was considered acceptable when publishing research findings to include as named authors senior colleagues who had not been involved in the project. Senior clinicians were automatically invited to add their name to research papers published by members of their team, even when they did not meet the criteria for authorship (which include having made a substantive intellectual contribution) of the International Committee of Medical Journal Editors (ICMJE).[120] This practice is now seen as unacceptable unless they have verified the results for themselves, have been closely involved and are prepared to be accountable for the findings. Traditionally too, there was no clear obligation to disclose any potential conflicts of interest when publishing. Due to the pressure on researchers to have significant publications to their name, redundant publication also often occurred. Such practices have now long been seen as unacceptable.

Clinical trials, including those sponsored by the pharmaceutical industry, are subject to the principles of good clinical practice which includes regular audit throughout the study. Nevertheless, it is claimed that pharmaceutical companies are likely 'to get the results they want from the clinical trials they sponsor' and 'positive results are likely to be published more than once, whereas negative results may not be published at all'.[121] Fraudulent research data are dangerous as they provide misleading information upon which later treatment options may be decided, risking harm to patients and wasting healthcare resources. It is sometimes argued that failure to publish research results is also a form of misconduct as it deprives decision makers of all the available information.[122] Because negative findings about a product are least likely to be published, this can lead to bias in prescribing patterns.

Misconduct is not only about the way data are presented but can also include failure to get approval from an REC (or other appropriate authority), omitting to obtain proper consent from research participants or failing to gain their consent to publish their cases anonymously. Publication of any personal information about a patient normally requires that person's consent, even if obvious identifying details are removed. (Confidentiality issues are discussed in more detail in Chapter 5.) When exposed, fraud also undermines public confidence.

Measures to improve research practice

- The values of responsible research conduct should be instilled in staff at an early stage by all institutions engaged in research. New researchers should be required to read and sign off the institution's guidance documents.[123]
- New researchers should receive training in UK legislation as well as the principles of research practice.
- Regular audit should occur throughout the conduct of a study and a culture of routine self-audit should be developed among research teams.
- Research should be recorded in logs, which include details of the research, the achievement of targets and specified responsibilities of the researchers. The log book should be in the public domain.
- The senior academic or consultant who is conducting the research, or in whose name the research is conducted, should take personal responsibility for the supervision and management of the project.
- Research projects should be subjected to rigorous scientific evaluation and all but the simplest should undergo external peer review.
- Consideration should be given to the use of independent third parties to obtain consent to research, particularly where this involves vulnerable groups of patients or especially stressful situations when anxious patients and/or relatives may rely heavily on medical staff involved in the research.
- Journal editors have an important role in ensuring that publication is declined for research that does not meet standards set out by bodies such as the ICMJE.
- Editors may also check with the named REC that approval was obtained or, if anomalies are apparent, with the university or other employing body of the researcher.

Whistleblowing

It is essential that people who become aware of unethical activities in any sphere are able to ask questions and, if unsatisfied by the answer, report their concerns to an appropriate body, such as senior members of the research team, employers, contracting bodies, the GMC or other regulators if the researchers are not doctors. The general issues for whistleblowers are discussed in more detail in Chapter 21, but the main point is that they should not be silenced by fear for their own career prospects, or erroneous or misplaced notions of loyalty to colleagues. Speaking out can be immensely difficult, but bodies such as the GMC have shown themselves ready to act against senior clinicians who attempt to threaten or bully potential whistleblowers. On the other hand, if health professionals who are aware of misconduct or fraudulent research fail to take action, they may themselves be considered to be guilty of a culpable omission.

Committee on Publication Ethics

One of the mechanisms for identifying fraud and misconduct in medical research is the Committee on Publication Ethics (COPE), which was established in 1997 by the editors of several British journals, including the *British Medical Journal* and *The Lancet*. Its establishment reflected a growing anxiety about the integrity of papers submitted to medical journals. Its aims were:

- to advise on cases raised by editors
- to publish an annual report describing those cases
- to produce guidance on good practice
- to encourage research
- to offer teaching and training.

COPE also acts 'as an editors' self-help group', providing a forum in which difficult cases can be considered anonymously. It identified over 100 cases of possible misconduct in its first 3 years and led commentators to believe that existing UK procedures for dealing with misconduct were inadequate.

The prevalence of fraud and misconduct in research and innovative treatment in the UK is unknown and depends on the particular definition adopted. In the first 103 cases considered by COPE, 80 contained some evidence of misconduct. The kinds of problems highlighted were:

- undeclared redundant submission or publication (29 cases)
- disputes over authorship (18)
- falsification (15)
- failure to obtain informed consent (11)
- performing unethical research (11)
- failure to gain approval from an REC (10).[124]

Summary

As is emphasised throughout this chapter, research and innovative treatment need to be open, accountable and involve patients and the public. Patients and healthy volunteers need to be engaged in research and innovative therapy as real partners and this means that the public generally need to be made more aware of the benefits to society of well-conducted research and their own possible role in it. Often, this may only mean agreeing to the use of their medical records, subject to appropriate safeguards. In the past, much research was carried out without informed consent and without proper regard to the welfare of the participants. Much effort has been made in recent years in the UK to create a more professional and accountable system of monitoring research. As a result a vast amount of guidance has been published to govern specific aspects of it. A potential problem for some members of RECs is the vast amount of published ethical guidance of which they are expected to be aware.

References

1   Mason JK, Laurie GT. (2011) *Mason & McCall Smith's Law and Medical Ethics*, 8th edn, OUP, Oxford, pp.612–3.
2   World Medical Association (1964) *Declaration of Helsinki: ethical principles for medical research involving human subjects*. Available at: www.wma.net (accessed 16 May 2011).
3   The Bristol Royal Infirmary Inquiry (2001) *Learning from Bristol: the report of the public inquiry into children's heart surgery at the Bristol Royal Infirmary 1984–1995*, Cm 5207 (I), The Stationery Office, London, recommendation 100.
4   General Medical Council (2009) *Confidentiality*, GMC, London, p.31.
5   General Medical Council (2009) *Confidentiality*, GMC, London, paras 30–2.
6   Department of Health (2006) *Expert Group on Phase One Clinical Trials: Final Report*, The Stationery Office, London.
7   Directive 2001/20/EC of the European Parliament and of the Council of 4 April 2001 on the approximation of the laws, regulations and administrative provisions of the member states relating to the implementation of good clinical practice in the conduct of clinical trials on medicinal products for human use, Article 2.
8   Department of Health (2009) *The NHS Constitution for England*, DH, London.
9   General Medical Council (2010) *Consent to research: supplementary guidance*, GMC, London, paras 4 and 7.

10 General Medical Council (2008) *Consent: patients and doctors making decisions together*, GMC, London, paras 28–36.
11 General Medical Council (2008) *Consent: patients and doctors making decisions together*, GMC, London, para 29.
12 General Medical Council (2008) *Consent: patients and doctors making decisions together*, GMC, London, para 31.
13 General Medical Council (2008) *Consent: patients and doctors making decisions together*, GMC, London, para 34.
14 Suntharalingam G, Meghan RP, Ward S. *et al.* (2006) Cytokine storm in a Phase I trial of the anti-CD28 monoclonal antibody TGN1412, *N Engl J Med* **355**, 1018–28.
15 Department of Health (2006) *Expert Group on Phase One Clinical Trials: Final Report*, The Stationery Office, London.
16 West Midlands Regional Office (2000) *Report of a review of the research framework in North Staffordshire Hospital NHS Trust (Griffiths inquiry)*, NHS Executive, Birmingham, para 10.2.
17 Nuffield Council on Bioethics (2010) *Give and take? Human bodies in medicine and research*, NCB, London.
18 Nuffield Council on Bioethics (2010) *Give and take? Human bodies in medicine and research*, NCB, London, p.32.
19 General Medical Council (2010) *Good practice in research: supplementary guidance*, GMC, London, para 27.
20 Medical Research Council (2001) *Human tissue and biological samples for use in research: operational and ethical guidelines*, MRC, London.
21 The Royal College of Pathologists has several guidance notes on consent, see: www.rcpath.org (accessed 23 May 2011).
22 Child Bereavement Charity, *Paediatric post mortem examination (autopsy)*. Available at: www.childbereavement.org.uk (accessed 23 May 2011).
23 European Medicines Agency (2002) *Note for guidance on good clinical practice* (CPMP/ICH/135/95), EMA, London, para 1.61.
24 General Medical Council (2010) *Good practice in research: supplementary guidance*, GMC, London, para 17.
25 Annas GJ. (1992) Changing the consent rules for desert storm. *N Engl J Med* **236**, 770–3.
26 General Medical Council (2010) *Good practice in research: supplementary guidance*, GMC, London, paras 15–20.
27 World Medical Association (2008) Declaration of Helsinki. Available at: www.wma.net (accessed 1 June 2011).
28 British Medical Association (2001) *The Medical Profession and Human Rights*, Zed Books, London, pp.205–40.
29 Royal College of Paediatrics and Child Health (2000) Guidelines for the ethical conduct of medical research involving children. *Arch Dis Child* **82**, 177–82.
30 Academy of Medical Sciences (2011) *A new pathway for the regulation and governance of health research*, AMS, London, p.3.
31 'Increasing the PaRticipation of the ElDerly in Clinical Trials' (PREDICT) was an EU project in nine countries. The PREDICT charter, coordinated by the Sheffield Medical Economics and Research Centre, was launched at the BMA in February 2010. Available at: www.predicteu.org (accessed 23 May 2011).
32 Medical Economics and Research Centre (MERCs) UK (2010) A *Charter for the Rights of Older People in Clinical Trials*. Available at: www.predicteu.org (accessed 23 May 2011).
33 General Medical Council (2010) *Good practice in research: supplementary guidance*, GMC, London, para 10.
34 *Simms v Simms, A v A* [2002] 2 WLR 1465; [2003]1 All ER 669.
35 Nuffield Council on Bioethics (2009) *Dementia: the ethical issues*, NCB, London, p.136.
36 Medical Economics and Research Centre (MERCs) UK (2010) A *Charter for the Rights of Older People in Clinical Trials*. Available at: www.predicteu.org (accessed 23 May 2011), para 3.1.2.
37 European Commission (2006) *Ethical Considerations for Clinical Trials Performed in Children*, European Commission, Brussels. Available at: ec.europa.eu (accessed 1 June 2011).
38 General Medical Council (2007) *0–18 years: guidance for all doctors*, GMC, London, para 37.
39 Royal College of Paediatrics and Child Health (2000) Guidelines for the ethical conduct of medical research involving children. *Arch Dis Child* **82**, 177–82, p.177.
40 Royal College of Paediatrics and Child Health. (2000) Guidelines for the ethical conduct of medical research involving children. *Arch Dis Child* **82**, 177–82, p.177.
41 Paediatric Formulary Committee (published annually) *BNF for Children*. BMJ Publishing Group, Pharmaceutical Press, and RCPCH Publications, London.
42 European Medicines Agency (2007) The Paediatric Regulation comprising Regulation (EC) No 1901/2006 of the European Parliament and Regulation (EC) No 1902/2006 is available at www.ema.europa.eu.

43   European Medicines Agency, *Class Waivers*. Available at: www.ema.europa.eu (accessed 1 June 2011).

44   *Gillick v West Norfolk and Wisbech AHA*, 3 All ER 402.

45   Age of Legal Capacity (Scotland) Act 1991.

46   Medicines for Human Use (Clinical Trials) Regulations 2004. SI 2004/1031, sch 1, part 1(2).

47   Medical Research Council (2004) *Medical Research Involving Children*, MRC, London, p.28.

48   Medical Research Council (2004) *Medical Research Involving Children*, MRC, London, p.28.

49   Royal College of Paediatrics and Child Health (1999) *Safeguarding informed parental involvement in clinical research involving newborn babies and infants*, RCPCH, London.

50   The MHRA published an explanatory memorandum which is available on its website at: www.mhra.gov.uk (accessed 23 May 2011).

51   Care Record Development Board (2009) *Report of the Care Record Development Board Working Group on the Secondary Uses of Patient Information*, DH, London, para 5.1.3.

52   General Medical Council (2009) *Confidentiality*, GMC, London, para 49.

53   Health and Social Care Bill 2011, clause 260 and sch 19, part 3.

54   General Medical Council (2009) *Confidentiality*, GMC, London.

55   General Medical Council (2009) *Confidentiality*, GMC, London, para 41.

56   General Medical Council (2009) *Confidentiality*, GMC, London, para 45.

57   General Medical Council (2009) *Confidentiality*, GMC, London, para 44.

58   Academy of Medical Sciences (2011) *A new pathway for the regulation and governance of health research*, AMS, London, p.102.

59   Directive 2001/20/EC of the European Parliament and of the Council of 4 April 2001 on the approximation of the laws, regulations and administrative provisions of the member states relating to the implementation of good clinical practice in the conduct of clinical trials on medicinal products for human use.

60   Medicines for Human Use (Clinical Trials) Regulations 2004. SI 2004/1031.

61   European Agency for the Evaluation of Medicinal Products (1996) *Note for guidance on good clinical practice* (CPMP/ICH/135/95), EMA, London.

62   Department of Health (2008) *Research governance framework for health and social care*, DH, London.

63   Welsh Assembly (2001) *Research governance framework for health and social care*, Wales Office of Research and Development, Cardiff.

64   Scottish Executive Health Department, Chief Scientist's Office (2006) *Research governance framework for health and community care*, Scottish Executive, Edinburgh.

65   Department of Health, Social Services and Public Safety (2002) *Research governance framework for health and social care*, Office of Research and Development, Belfast.

66   Directive 2001/20/EC of the European Parliament and the Council of 4 April 2001 on the approximation of the laws, regulations and administrative provisions of the member states relating to implementation of good clinical practice in the conduct of clinical trials on medicinal products for human use.

67   Foster C, Holley S. (1998) Ethical review of multi-centre research: a survey of multi-centre researchers in the South Thames region. *J R Coll Physicians Lond* **32**(3), 242–5.

68   Department of Health (2001) *Governance arrangements for NHS research ethics committees*, DH, London.

69   Department of Health (2005) *Report of the Ad Hoc Advisory Group on the Operation of NHS Research Ethics Committees* (Warner Report), DH, London.

70   Department of Health (2010) *Liberating the NHS: report of the arms-length bodies review*, DH, London.

71   Department of Health (2011) *Governance arrangements for research ethics committees: a harmonised edition*, DH, Leeds.

72   Department of Health (2010) *Liberating the NHS: report of the arms-length bodies review*, DH, London.

73   HM Treasury, Department for Business, Innovation and Skills (2011) *The Plan for Growth*, The Stationery Office, London, p.8.

74   Academy of Medical Sciences (2011) *A new pathway for the regulation and governance of health research*, AMS, London.

75   Academy of Medical Sciences (2011) *A new pathway for the regulation and governance of health research*, AMS, London, p.82.

76   Department of Health (2010) *Liberating the NHS: report of the arms-length bodies review*, DH, London.

77   General Medical Council (2010) *Good practice in research and consent to research: supplementary guidance*, GMC, London.

78   General Medical Council (2008) *Consent: patients and doctors making decisions together*, GMC, London.

79   Medical Research Council (1963) *Responsibility in investigations in human subjects, MRC annual report*, MRC, London.

80   See, for example: Medical Research Council, *Data and Tissues Toolkit*. Available at: www.dt-toolkit.ac.uk (accessed 18 May 2011).

81   Royal College of Physicians (2007) *Guidelines on the practice of ethics committees in medical research with human participants*, RCP, London.

82   Royal College of Paediatrics and Child Health (2000) *Guidelines for the ethical conduct of medical research involving children*, RCPCH, London.

83   Wellcome Trust (2005) *Statement on the handling of allegations of research misconduct*, Wellcome Trust, London.

84   For more information see the Alzheimer's Society website at: www.alzheimers.org.uk (accessed 1 June 2011).

85   UK Research Integrity Office (2009) *Code of Practice for Research: Promoting good practice and preventing misconduct*, UKRIO, Brighton.

86   British Medical Association (2001) *The Medical Profession and Human Rights: Handbook for a Changing Agenda*, Zed Books, London, ch 9.

87   World Medical Association. *Declaration of Helsinki: ethical principles for medical research involving human subjects* adopted in Helsinki in June 1964 and updated by WMA General Assemblies since then see: www.wma.net (accessed 23 May 2011).

88   See, for example: World Health Organization (1995) *Guidelines for good clinical practice (GCP) for trials on pharmaceutical products*, WHO, Geneva. World Health Organization (2000) *Operational guidelines for ethics committees that review biomedical research*, WHO, Geneva.

89   Joint United Nations Programme on HIV/AIDS (2000) *Ethical considerations in HIV preventive vaccine research*, UNAIDS, Geneva.

90   European Forum for Good Clinical Practice (2010) *The Procedure for the Ethical Review of Protocols for Clinical Research Projects in the European Union*. Available at: www.efgcp.eu (accessed 16 May 2011).

91   Council of Europe (1999) The convention on human rights and biomedicine also known as the Oviedo Convention (ETS 164), Council of Europe, Brussells.

92   See: www.cioms.ch (accessed 16 May 2011).

93   Nuffield Council on Bioethics (2002) *The ethics of research related to healthcare in developing countries*, NCB, London.

94   Medicines for Human Use (Clinical Trials) Regulations 2004. SI 2004/1031.

95   Mason JK, Laurie GT. (2011) *Mason & McCall Smith's Law and Medical Ethics*, 8th edn, OUP, Oxford, p.612.

96   Mental Capacity Act 2005 (Loss of Capacity During Research Project) (England) Regulations 2007. SI 2007/679. Mental Capacity Act 2005 (Loss of Capacity During Research Project) (Wales) Regulations 2007. SI 2007/837, W.72.

97   Department of Health, Welsh Assembly Government (2007) *Mental Capacity Act and consent for research*, DH, London.

98   *X v Denmark* (1983) Application No. 9974/82 32 DR282.

99   British Medical Association (2007) *The impact of the Human Rights Act 1998 on medical decision-making*, BMA, London.

100   British Medical Association (2009) *Human Tissue Legislation: Guidance from the BMA Medical Ethics Department*. BMA, London.

101   Human Tissue Authority (2009) *Code of Practice 9: Research*, HTA, London.

102   Department of Health (2010) *Liberating the NHS: report of the arms-length bodies review*, DH, London.

103   For more information see HFEA website at: www.hfea.gov.uk.

104   Department of Health (2000) *Stem cell research: medical progress with responsibility. A report from the Chief Medical Officer's expert group reviewing the potential of developments in stem cell research and cell nuclear replacement to benefit human health*, DH, London.

105   Human Fertilisation and Embryology (Research Purposes) Regulations 2001. SI 2001/188.

106   Blow N. (2008) Stem Cells: A new path to pluripotency. *Nature* **451**, 858.

107   Human Fertilisation and Embryology Act 1990, s 1(1).

108   *R (on the application of Quintavalle) v Secretary of State for Health* [2001] 4 All ER 1013: 1024.

109   *R (on the application of Quintavalle) v Secretary of State for Health* [2002] 2 All ER 625.

110   *R (on the application of Quintavalle) v Secretary of State for Health* [2003] 2 All ER 113.

111   House of Lords (2002) *Stem cell research. Report from the Select Committee* (HL Paper 83(1)), The Stationery Office, London.

112   Department of Health, *UK stem cell tool kit*. Available at: www.sc-toolkit.ac.uk (accessed 4 March 2011).

113   House of Commons Science and Technology Committee (2007) *Government proposals for the regulation of hybrid and chimera embryos* (HC 272-1), The Stationery Office, London.

114   Academy of Medical Sciences (2007) *Inter-species embryos: a report by the Academy of Medical Sciences*, AMS, London.

115   Human Fertilisation and Embryology Act 1990 (as amended), s 4A(6).

116   Human Tissue Authority (2009) *Code of Practice 1: Consent*, HTA, London, paras 157–61.

117   Committee to Review the Guidance of the Research Use of Fetuses and Fetal Material (1989) *Review of the guidance on the research use of fetuses and fetal material* (Cmnd 762), HMSO, London.

118   Human Tissue Authority (2009) *Code of Practice 1: Consent*, HTA, London, para 160.

119   Medical Research Council (2001) *Human tissue and biological samples for use in research: operational and ethical guidelines*, MRC, London.
120   The International Committee of Medical Journal Editors defines authorship and also provides other guidance in relation to the publication of research, see: www.icmje.org (accessed 16 May 2011).
121   Smith R. (2008) Ethical issues in the publication process. In: Wells F, Farthing M. (eds.) *Fraud and misconduct in biomedical research*, 4th edn, Royal Society of Medicine Press, London, p.14.
122   Chalmers I. (1990) Underreporting research is scientific misconduct. *JAMA* **263**, 1405–8.
123   Farthing M. (2008) The role of national advisory bodies. In: Wells F, Farthing M. (eds.) *Fraud and misconduct in biomedical research*, 4th edn, Royal Society of Medicine Press, London, p.279.
124   The Committee on Publication Ethics has more information and sample cases on its website, see: www.publicationethics.org (accessed 31 May 2011).

15: Emergency situations

The questions covered in this chapter include the following.

- Is a refusal of treatment following attempted suicide ever valid?
- Should relatives be encouraged or allowed to witness resuscitation attempts?
- Is it ever appropriate to carry out forensic tests that have no therapeutic benefit on incapacitated adults?
- Are doctors obliged to provide 'Samaritan' care in an emergency?
- Is it reasonable for doctors to exceed their competence to help an injured person?

This chapter considers ethical dilemmas in emergency care, including those that arise in emergency departments and with urgent impromptu treatment outside hospitals, such as at the site of a disaster, in aircraft and at road accidents. We aim to show how core ethical principles apply equally in emergency care as in other branches of medicine, but with some differences in emphasis.

General principles

The general principles applicable to emergency care include:

- the duty to promote patient autonomy and patient-centred services
- the protection of patient confidentiality, privacy and dignity
- the duty of care both for patients and, in some cases, families
- a recognition of the abilities of others in the healthcare team to work across traditional boundaries
- the obligation to act within one's sphere of competence.

Consent and refusal

The majority of patients attending hospital emergency departments do not require urgent life-saving treatment. In these cases there is time for discussion about the treatment proposed and to seek appropriate consent or to make a best interests judgement for adults who lack capacity. For these patients the usual rules apply and the guidance set out in Chapters 2, 3 and 4 should be followed.

Providing information and seeking consent

It should not be assumed that patients requiring even urgent interventions are incapable of discussing treatment options. In one study, the majority of patients undergoing urgent surgery for acute abdominal conditions felt capable of assimilating information and deciding on options.[1] Over 80 per cent were in pain and 70 per cent had already

Medical Ethics Today: The BMA's Handbook of Ethics and Law, Third Edition. Sophie Brannan, Eleanor Chrispin, Martin Davies, Veronica English, Rebecca Mussell, Julian Sheather and Ann Sommerville.
© 2012 BMA Medical Ethics Department. Published 2012 by Blackwell Publishing Ltd.

received analgesia, but many claimed this did not interfere with their decision. Only a minority, however, felt that they had received a proper explanation of the side effects and complications of surgery. Where there were competing options for treatment with differing side effects and complications, the study found that these were discussed differently between urgent and elective patients.

Nevertheless, the delivery of emergency care sometimes involves situations in which immediate and irreversible decisions have to be made without being able to discuss the implications or knowing the patient's preferences. In such cases, essential treatment should be provided without delay unless the patient is an adult with capacity who is refusing the treatment proposed (see Chapter 2, pages 75–80) or there is clear evidence of a valid and applicable advance refusal of treatment (see Chapter 3, page 96).

Where there is doubt about the patient's capacity and treatment is required urgently, such that consent cannot be sought, immediately necessary treatment that is in the person's best interests should be provided. Both the Mental Capacity Act 2005 and the Adults with Incapacity (Scotland) Act 2000 give protection from liability for doctors who provide life-saving treatment where they have a 'reasonable belief' that a patient lacks capacity to refuse treatment and the act is in the patient's best interests, or, in Scotland, provides a benefit. Where doubts exist over a patient's capacity or the validity of an advance refusal (see below), or where disputes exist between a proxy decision maker and the treating clinician on the best course of action, a doctor should take whatever steps are necessary to prevent the patient's condition deteriorating before resolving any issues associated with his or her capacity.

Suicide attempts and self-harm

A significant number of admissions to emergency departments in the UK are after an episode of self-harm with an estimated 150,000 cases reported every year.[2] These cases raise specific practical and ethical dilemmas for emergency medicine and at the heart of these is the mental capacity of patients to give or withhold consent to treatment. Patients who present at the emergency department after an episode of self-harm may be in serious pain or have limited consciousness depending on the severity of their injuries or degree of intoxication.

Some patients presenting after an episode of self-harm are conscious and able to communicate, but refuse urgent medical treatment. Such cases can be particularly problematic as decisions about how to proceed often need to be made quickly by the emergency department doctor on duty. Where an adult suffering from a mental disorder has seriously self-harmed and retains the capacity to refuse treatment for the consequences of that harm, the option still remains to provide treatment under mental health legislation where the relevant criteria are met. Wherever possible therefore, in such cases, a specialist psychiatric assessment should be obtained as a matter of urgency, both to assess the individual's capacity and also to determine whether mental health legislation can, and should, be invoked. In its report on the standards for assessment following self-harm, the Royal College of Psychiatrists (RCPsych)[3] states that all hospital attendance following self-harm should result in a specialist psychosocial assessment. The emergency department staff should therefore have access to a psychiatrist, or designated self-harm mental health specialist, who can undertake psychosocial assessment and management. Where emergency department medical staff undertake such assessments themselves, the RCPsych recommends that they should undergo appropriate training. Emergency departments should have facilities, such as an interview room, in which assessments can take place in a safe setting that preserves privacy and confidentiality.

If, after assessment, it is determined that the patient has the capacity to refuse treatment, is informed and determined, the refusal must be respected unless treatment has been authorised under mental health legislation. The decision not to proceed should be taken by a senior doctor. The patient should still be offered other treatment, information and support. If the patient agrees to a health professional calling relatives or friends, they may be able to persuade the patient to accept treatment. In such circumstances, health professionals must have due respect to confidentiality, however, and only discuss the details of the patient's condition and treatment with consent from the patient. If such patients discharge themselves it should be made clear that the hospital healthcare team remains ready to offer treatment should they change their minds. In difficult borderline cases, legal advice should be sought and an application may need to be made to the courts where time permits.

Kerrie Wooltorton

In 2007, 26-year-old Kerrie Wooltorton took a fatal dose of antifreeze and then telephoned for an ambulance. She was taken to Norfolk and Norwich University Hospital and carried with her an advance statement she had written 3 days before that expressed her wish not to receive life-saving treatment. In the letter she explained that she understood the consequences of this decision but did not want to die alone or in pain. Ms Wooltorton had been diagnosed previously as having an emotionally unstable personality disorder. She had attempted suicide a number of times before but had accepted life-saving treatment. On this occasion though, she refused medical treatment and was assessed as having the mental capacity to do so by the hospital's consultant renal surgeon. After seeking a second opinion and taking advice from the hospital medical director, the consultant respected Ms Wooltorton's wishes and no interventions were made to save her life. She died the next day. At the inquest into her death the coroner ruled that the treating doctor's actions were lawful and the hospital was not responsible for her death.

The circumstances of Kerrie Wooltorton's suicide (see box) received considerable media attention when the inquest into her death gave its verdict in 2009. Much of the coverage was misleading, with many reports claiming that this was the first time an advance decision refusing treatment (ADRT) had been used to prevent treatment in a suicide attempt.[4] In fact, as the coroner stated at the inquest, Kerrie Wooltorton had made a contemporaneous decision to refuse medical treatment and was assessed as having the mental capacity to do so.[5] Any doctor who provided medical treatment in the face of such a refusal (which had not been authorised under mental health legislation), would have been liable for assault. If Kerrie Wooltorton had arrived at the hospital unconscious with a valid ADRT, any attempt to save her life would be similarly unlawful. On this occasion, however, the ADRT was not a factor in the doctors' decision not to treat as she was conscious and deemed to have capacity.

If a patient brought into hospital following a suicide attempt or self-harm is thought to lack capacity, a contemporaneous refusal of treatment will be invalid (see Chapters 3 and 4). Any refusal of treatment by a child or young person who has attempted suicide, or is admitted to hospital following self-harm, is likely to be invalid and treatment that is immediately necessary and in the young person's best interests should be provided without delay.

Advance decisions refusing treatment following a suicide attempt or self-harm

Doctors sometimes ask whether a suicide note refusing life-saving treatment is legally binding. In the view of the British Medical Association (BMA), this is highly unlikely. For an advance decision refusing life-saving treatment to be legally binding it must meet the criteria laid out in the Mental Capacity Act 2005. These include that:

• the person making the ADRT was over 18 years old and had the necessary capacity to make the decision at the time the decision was made
• an ADRT must specify the treatment to be refused in the particular circumstances
• it must be in writing, signed and witnessed, and
• it must contain a statement that it is to apply even where life is at risk.

Similar criteria for validity are likely to apply in other parts of the UK (see Chapter 3).

Given that questions of capacity always arise when patients have attempted suicide or self-harmed, the usual presumption that patients had capacity at the time an advance decision was made (see Chapter 3, page 115) would normally be set aside. In emergency care the normal assumption, when faced with unconscious or incapacitated people who have self-harmed, is that death was not their true intention or that their capacity to decide in a valid way was likely to have been impaired. Certainly, when doctors have reasonable doubt about an individual's prior capacity, necessary emergency treatment should be provided.

Arguably, however, a distinction can be made between cases in which the self-harm is associated with a history of psychiatric disturbance or erratic behaviour, and treatment refusals that individuals have clearly thought about for a long time, discussed with other people and where their capacity has been assessed. Such cases are likely to be rare.

Potentially binding advance refusal of resuscitation

In a case prior to the Mental Capacity Act 2005, W was a prisoner who refused potentially life-prolonging treatment and this was discussed with him on numerous occasions. In April 2002, the High Court ruled that he had the mental capacity to make a valid refusal even if this resulted in death. He had previously attempted suicide, but the Court deemed this to have been a facet of his need to command public attention. Nevertheless, W said that he did not wish to be resuscitated in future if he were at the point of death as a result of trying to hang himself, cutting his throat or inducing blood poisoning. In the light of these comments, the judge was asked to say what should happen if he attempted suicide. She suggested that W draw up a statement clarifying his verbal refusal of resuscitation if he were to attempt suicide by any means. Prison service rules required him to be cut down if he again attempted to hang himself, but not necessarily to attempt resuscitation. The judge made clear that the onus was on W to say precisely whether he was serious in refusing all medical help in that situation. In such cases, where there was clear forewarning of the patient's wish, the judge said that authorities could risk litigation against them if they resuscitated a person contrary to an express wish.[6]

This case is also discussed in Chapter 17, pages 695–696, where it is noted that W is exceptional in having discussed his intentions with lawyers and other people in advance and having had his mental capacity assessed. In most situations, there is not clear evidence of capacity and informed intention. In an emergency setting, there is also unlikely to be time to make enquiries about the existence of a valid ADRT if it is not immediately available. The responsibility for ensuring that the existence of an ADRT is known rests with the patient.

As indicated in the case of Kerrie Wooltorton (see page 631), if a person refused treatment following a suicide attempt, and it was deemed that the refusal was valid and binding on health professionals, the refusal would continue to apply once capacity was lost.

Summary – consent and refusal

- The majority of patients attending hospital emergency departments do not require urgent life-saving treatment and the usual rules on consent apply.
- Where urgent treatment is required, and there is no time to seek consent, essential treatment should be provided without delay unless the patient is an adult with capacity who is refusing the treatment proposed or there is clear evidence of a valid and applicable advance refusal of treatment.
- Where patients are admitted after a suicide attempt or self-harm, questions of capacity will arise and specialist assessment will be required as a matter of urgency, both to determine capacity and to assess whether mental health legislation can and should be invoked.

Confidentiality

All patients are entitled to confidentiality of their personal health information, although this right is not absolute and information may be disclosed where there is an overriding public interest (see pages 639–641 and Chapter 5). In an emergency, people who are emotionally close to the patient expect to act as advocates and be consulted about decisions when time permits. Sharing general information with families should be with the patients' permission where they have capacity. Where patients lack capacity, it is normally seen as in the patients' interests to provide information to those close to the patient unless this would be contrary to the patient's previously expressed views.

Information sharing within the healthcare team

Effective and prompt sharing of essential information is vital for assessment, diagnosis and treatment in emergency departments. Good links with primary care services are also important. Information obtained at each stage of the patient's transit through the system should be available to other professionals seeing that person, subject to patient consent and to the introduction of appropriate safeguards to preserve confidentiality.

Confidentiality after death

The medical duty of confidentiality extends beyond the death of the patient, but this must be balanced with other moral imperatives. Relatives and people who are close to the deceased patient want information and reassurance about what has occurred, and need to be consulted about procedures such as post-mortem examinations. These issues are discussed in detail in Chapters 5 and 12.

Duties to families

In the hospital situation, teams working in emergency care often have to help relatives as well as patients. Care of people who have been suddenly bereaved is part of the responsibility of emergency departments, but has not always received sufficient attention. The Department of Health, in its document, *When a Patient Dies: advice on developing bereavement services in the NHS,* highlights the need for specialist bereavement nurses in emergency departments and named bereavement lead nurses in each emergency department's team.[7]

Witnessed resuscitation

The BMA is sometimes asked about its views on whether people who are emotionally close to the patient should be invited to remain in the room when resuscitation is attempted in hospitals. This is not an issue upon which the Association has a firm policy, but some general factors for consideration can be set out.

Witnessed resuscitation

The following factors should be considered:

- whether additional people in the vicinity would hamper the resuscitation efforts
- whether their presence would be what the patient would have wanted
- whether witnessing a resuscitation attempt is likely to have a bad effect on the witnesses or leave them with very disturbing memories
- whether being present would reassure them that everything possible has been attempted
- whether the family needs to express emotions physically or vocally at such a time and, if so, whether this can be accommodated in a manner that does not distract the resuscitation team
- whether there are appropriately trained staff available to concentrate just on looking after relatives
- whether there is time to provide a proper explanation and choice for those who may want to be present.

If having additional people present would hamper the patient's treatment, or would be contrary to the patient's known wishes, families should be excluded.

In cases of terminal illness, it is common for family members to stay with their loved one at the end of that person's life, but this has not generally been the case when patients die in emergency departments during attempted cardio-pulmonary resuscitation (CPR). A 2004 study found that 79 per cent of UK emergency departments allowed family-witnessed adult resuscitation, and 93 per cent allowed it in the resuscitation of a child.[8] Generally, health professionals seem to have little objection to bringing in people who are close to the patient once resuscitation efforts are being scaled down, either because the process has been unsuccessful or when the patient appears to have survived the worst. Health professionals have concerns, however, if family members are exposed, without appropriate preparation and support, to the team's efforts to revive a patient.

An early report by the UK Resuscitation Council found that the majority of relatives or friends of deceased people who had been present during attempts to resuscitate their loved one preferred to be there and believed that it helped in coping with their bereavement when the patient died.[9] Some saw it as a last opportunity to communicate and be heard by the dying person, and thought that it was important both for the patient and themselves to be together in the final moments. The Council also cited anecdotal evidence that the presence of a loved one could be beneficial to some patients with fleeting consciousness, increasing their will to live. It noted that patients undergoing resuscitation after cardiac arrest may retain some awareness. The report concluded that attitudes about the presence of families were changing and that 'for many relatives it is more distressing to be separated from their loved one during these critical moments than to witness attempts at resuscitation'.[10] The positive benefits were especially felt by younger adults (under the age of 40).

Summary of Resuscitation Council guidance

- Acknowledge the difficulty of the situation. Ensure that relatives understand that they do not have to be present and should not feel guilty about declining.
- Relatives should be accompanied by staff to care specifically for them and should know who these staff are. They should be introduced and know each other's names.
- Relatives should be given a clear explanation of what to expect to see, the nature of the illness or injury, and the procedures they will witness.
- Relatives should know that they can leave the room and will be accompanied.
- Relatives should be aware that they cannot intervene or touch the patient until they are told this is safe. They should be given opportunities to touch the patient when it is safe to do so.
- Procedures should be explained to relatives as they occur. This includes telling them when resuscitation is not succeeding and will be abandoned, and when the patient has died.
- They should be advised that if resuscitation is unsuccessful and the person has died, there may be a brief interval during which the equipment is removed, after which they can have time alone with the deceased person. They need to know if the coroner is likely to require certain tubes to be left in place.
- Relatives should be offered time to think about the situation and ask questions.[11]

More recent guidance from the Resuscitation Council – in conjunction with the Royal College of Anaesthetists, Royal College of Physicians and Intensive Care Society – has specified that when resuscitating a child 'consideration should be given to the presence of relatives. A member of staff should be delegated to stay with them and liaise with the team on their behalf.'[12]

The issue of witnessing attempted resuscitation was debated at the 2000 Congress of the Royal College of Nursing, where there was overwhelming support for relatives being present. The College published detailed guidance on the subject in 2002, which also included a model hospital policy for witnessed attempted resuscitation.[13] The College thought that, among other benefits, witnessed resuscitation was likely to reduce complaints from relatives and lawsuits because families would see for themselves that all reasonable steps had been taken.

Asking families about research and education

One of the difficult issues that may have to be raised with the families of incapacitated people in the emergency care setting is that of the possible involvement of their loved one in research initiatives, innovative treatment or medical education. All doctors have general obligations to maximise useful knowledge and make appropriate efforts to improve care.

Treatment should be evidence-based, but in emergency and acute care there are few opportunities to carry out research on potential treatment options with properly informed patient consent. For example, it may be important to research different modes of cardiac compression to ascertain what is most effective in cardiac arrest or to compare different possible ways of attempting to resuscitate babies.

To introduce changes in practice without evidence of efficacy and research data is likely to be unethical. These kinds of dilemmas are discussed in Chapter 14 where the importance is emphasised of involving patients or people close to them, wherever possible, in any discussion of experimental procedures. In particular, the parents of children must be involved in deciding whether they wish the child to be involved in any research or innovative treatment. In December 2006, the Medicines for Human Use (Clinical Trials) Regulations 2004 were amended to allow research on incapacitated adults in emergency situations without prior consent, as long as research ethics committee (REC) agreement has been obtained. Proxy consent is still needed for continuing participation in the trial of emergency measures but in the absence of such consent at the start, patients can be initially entered. All trial protocols – including those for emergency care – should be scrutinised by RECs which consider whether the exception should apply to individual emergency trial protocols. The amendment applied to emergency research throughout the UK. In 2008, Regulations extended these provisions to emergency research involving children, permitting a child to be entered into an emergency research trial, without prior consent by parents or guardians, as long as REC approval had been granted (see Chapter 14, page 603).[14]

As well as research and innovative treatment, another extremely sensitive issue that may need to be raised in the emergency care setting is the fact that medical education occurs there and needs support from patients and their relatives. Seeking consent for patient involvement in education is discussed in Chapter 18.

Asking families about organ and tissue donations

Raising the option of organ and tissue donation when an unexpected death occurs in an emergency department can be difficult although, in the long term, many families derive comfort from the knowledge that other lives have been saved or transformed. The BMA also believes it is part of the duty of care to dying patients to determine and, as far as possible facilitate, their wishes regarding donation. Whenever donation is likely to be an option, this should be raised with the family. (General issues concerning organ donation and discussion with relatives are covered in Chapter 12, pages 512–515.)

Summary – duties to families

- Where family members wish to be present during attempted resuscitation a member of staff should be available to provide information and support.
- If having family members present during attempted resuscitation would hamper the patient's treatment, or would be contrary to the patient's known wishes, this should not be permitted.
- All doctors have general obligations to maximise useful knowledge and, in emergency departments, this may include asking families about participation in research, innovative treatment and education.
- When a patient has died and donation is likely to be an option, this should be raised with the family.

Treating the victims or perpetrators of crime or abuse

Some of the patients seen in emergency departments are the victims, or possible perpetrators, of crime. These cases can raise particular issues such as whether procedures may be carried out for forensic, rather than therapeutic, purposes and the limits of confidentiality where a crime has, or may have been, committed. Emergency departments frequently deal with the effects of abuse or neglect and those working in such settings are often faced with difficult decisions about whether, in what circumstances, and to whom, to report any such suspicions.

Forensic testing of unconscious victims of crime

Diagnostic testing in patients' interests is uncontentious, but decisions may also have to be made about whether forensic testing should be allowed. Wherever feasible, it is best to wait for an unconscious patient to recover consciousness and be able to give consent if this would not prejudice the reliability of the test. When a fatality or serious crime has occurred, however, and forensic information from an unconscious patient could provide vital evidence, there may be a strong public interest in carrying out such tests. If an unconscious patient has been a victim of serious crime, such as an assault or rape, it may also be what the patient would want. Although doctors must act in patients' best interests, such interests are not necessarily confined to purely medical matters. The facts of each case should be considered to determine whether testing would be in the patient's best interests. Doctors should be prepared to justify their decisions.

Where samples are to be taken, this should be by a forensic physician rather than the treating doctor. The treating doctor should object, however, if any proposal to take forensic samples could be harmful to the patient's care and treatment. Patients' clinical needs should be of paramount importance and doctors must err on the side of caution if they feel that any intervention is likely to jeopardise recovery.

The Faculty of Forensic and Legal Medicine has issued guidance specifically on consent in relation to complaints of serious assault, including sexual assaults.[15] Regarding patients who lack capacity, it states that the forensic physician should:

- inform the consultant responsible for the patient's care of the proposed examination and ensure that the consultant has no objections
- inform any contactable people close to the patient about the purpose of the proposed examination so that they can say whether the patient previously held strong views about such tests (care must be taken to respect the patient's confidentiality)
- document such enquiries clearly in the patient's medical record
- consider whether to hand forensic samples to the police or to store them securely for testing with patient consent when the patient regains capacity or on the order of a court
- ensure that the patient is informed about what has been done, and why, as soon as the patient has recovered sufficiently to understand.

Testing incapacitated drivers for blood alcohol levels

The possibility of taking and testing blood samples that may not be in an incapacitated patient's interests, but could be in the public interest, was debated by the BMA for many years. Although, in some cases, prompt testing of incapacitated drivers who have been in accidents may exonerate them from any blame, it is a non-therapeutic intervention carried out without consent. In 2002, the Police Reform Act made such testing lawful, without consent, in specific circumstances in England, Wales and Scotland; Northern Ireland subsequently passed similar provisions in the Criminal Justice (Northern Ireland) Order 2005. The Act allows for a police constable to ask a doctor to take a specimen of blood from an incapacitated person who has been involved in a road traffic accident. Samples should not be taken by any doctor involved in the care of the patient, but rather by a forensic physician.

Taking blood specimens from incapacitated drivers

A blood sample may be taken for future testing for alcohol or other drugs from a person who has been involved in an accident and is unable to give consent when:

- a police constable has assessed the person's capacity and found him or her to be incapable of giving valid consent for medical reasons
- the forensic physician taking the specimen is satisfied that the person is not able to give valid consent (for whatever reason)
- the person does not object to or resist the specimen being taken, and
- in the view of the doctor in immediate charge of that patient's care, taking the specimen would not be prejudicial to the proper care and treatment of the patient.

The specimen taken must not be tested until the person regains capacity and gives valid consent for it to be tested.

Although it would be lawful for a forensic physician to take a blood sample in the circumstances covered by the legislation, the police cannot require a doctor to take a specimen. Legally, doctors taking blood specimens in these circumstances can do so as long as they are satisfied that the patient lacks capacity to give valid consent. Clearly, any doctor involved in taking samples specifically for forensic use must be appropriately trained so that the sample is forensically useful. The BMA and the Faculty of Forensic and Legal Medicine (FFLM) believe that doctors should not take samples if the patient refuses or resists and consider it ethically unacceptable to use force or restraint. It is also unlikely to be appropriate to take a specimen without consent if the person is expected to recover capacity within a very short period of time. The BMA and the FFLM have produced joint guidance for those involved in taking blood specimens from incapacitated drivers.[16]

Treating detained people in the emergency department

Communication can be difficult with patients who are brought to an emergency department by prison staff or police officers. The BMA receives many queries about the use of handcuffs or shackles in such situations, and the fact that accompanying prison staff or police officers can make difficult any confidential discussion with the patient. Risk assessment procedures should have been used by the prison, detention centre or police officers prior to transferring the detainee so that hospital staff can be guided by the officers. Clearly, the medical condition of the detainee is also likely to be a factor to take into account when considering whether there is a risk of violence or attempted escape. However, emergency department doctors occasionally report that their requests to assess in private a patient who very clearly poses no threat are sometimes refused. The general rules on these issues are set out in detail in Chapter 17.

Disclosure of information in the public interest

The general rules about disclosure are discussed in Chapter 5. In emergency departments there are some categories of patients that give rise to particular concern and questions about disclosure may arise. For example, emergency staff often come into contact with patients who feign pain or illness to obtain prescription medicine or narcotics under false pretences. They also see patients with Munchausen disease and may embark on lengthy and expensive diagnostic and treatment initiatives for them. Once identified by one emergency team, the question sometimes arises about whether identifying information can be passed to other hospitals in the locality where the same patient is likely to present. Arguably, it is in the public interest that abuse or fraudulent use of the system be addressed, even at the cost of the individual's confidentiality. As a general principle, the BMA has recommended that patients be told in advance of disclosure. In addition, general notices about such information sharing should be displayed in hospital facilities, so that everyone is aware that attempts to obtain drugs or unnecessary treatment will be made known to other medical facilities in the area.

Confidentiality and disclosure to the police

Emergency health teams are often approached by the police and other authorities, such as the courts, about patients who have been treated after an assault or other violent incident, where there may be a strong public interest in ensuring that the perpetrators are identified. Such requests should be directed to the consultant in charge of the patient's care, who should ascertain what kind of information is sought and why. Wherever possible, consent should be sought prior to disclosure. When consent is refused, or it proves impossible to contact the patient concerned, doctors should consider their duty of confidentiality and disclose information only if there is an overriding public interest. If the injured person is a suspect hurt in the course of committing a serious crime, the public interest is likely to override the medical duty of confidentiality owed to that person. Further guidance on confidentiality and disclosure in the public interest, and disclosures required or permitted by law, is provided in Chapter 5.

The General Medical Council (GMC) has specific guidance on the reporting of gunshot and knife wounds,[17] which outlines a two-stage process when a patient arrives at an emergency department with such injuries.

> ### GMC guidelines on the reporting of gunshot and knife wounds
>
> The GMC stipulates the following.
>
> (a) You should inform the police quickly whenever a person arrives with a gunshot wound or an injury from an attack with a knife, blade or other sharp instrument. This will enable the police to make an assessment of risk to the patient and others, and to gather statistical information about gun and knife crime in the area.
> (b) You should make a professional judgement about whether disclosure of personal information about a patient, including their identity, is justified in the public interest.[18]
>
> Disclosure of personal information should only be made with consent or where there is an overriding public interest in disclosure (see Chapter 5).

It is also likely that some patients attending emergency departments are illegal immigrants, who are seldom registered with primary care services. The BMA has firmly rejected any role of doctors in denouncing such patients to the authorities and decisions about disclosure should be made on the same basis as any other patient.

Domestic violence

In 2007, the BMA issued advice concerning the management of the sequelae of domestic violence.[19] Over 1 per cent of emergency department visits are due to domestic violence. There are also strong links between domestic violence and child protection issues. Traditionally, emergency staff believed that the high turnover of such patients, and difficulties with follow up, meant that any intervention with the patient would be unlikely to effect any change in the abusive situation. Nevertheless, studies have shown that the process of empowerment for many victims is a gradual one, and over time health professionals can play an important part in reinforcing basic messages.[20] A vital first step is to question patients who are likely to be in this category, including attempting to discover whether other people are at risk of harm. The fact that an adult may refuse to allow disclosure of information about an abuser does not mean that health professionals do not continue to have some duty to other vulnerable persons, such as children or elderly people, who may be caught up in an abusive situation.

Multi-Agency Risk Assessment Conferences (MARACs) have been established in England and Wales to try to help individuals who are at high risk of domestic abuse. MARACs are voluntary meetings between representatives from local police, health, child protection, housing practitioners, Independent Domestic Violence Advisors (IDVAs) and other specialists from the statutory and voluntary sectors. A coordinated safety plan for each referred victim is created. Health professionals can make referrals to MARACs using the Coordindated Action Against Domestic Abuse (CAADA) risk assessment tool which helps referring agencies determine the level of risk.[21] Disclosure of information to MARACs or to any other agencies should be made with the consent of the patient. The exceptions to this are where confidentiality can be overridden either by a court order (or other legal requirement) or in the public interest. Public interest justifications in such cases usually relate to disclosures to prevent significant harm to third parties or to prevent or prosecute a serious crime (see also Chapter 5, pages 199–206).

Domestic abuse in the emergency setting

- While routine enquiry for domestic abuse is not recommended in emergency departments, it is still important that emergency doctors know how to create the opportunity and environment for a patient to disclose domestic abuse, so that self-reported victims can be offered help.
- Following a disclosure of domestic abuse a healthcare professional should carry out specific enquiries into drug and alcohol use, the presence of children in the home and any suicidal ideation.
- The first priority with a patient who has suffered from domestic abuse would be to treat the physical injuries. It is crucial that these are meticulously recorded and photographs taken if appropriate. It must be explained to victims that domestic abuse is unacceptable and against the law.
- While police contact must be offered, the healthcare professional must not put pressure on the patient to make any decisions about disclosure.[22]

Suspected child abuse or neglect

When children come into emergency care in situations in which non-accidental injury, other abuse or neglect is suspected, a meticulous record must be made and as thorough an explanation as possible sought from carers. Competent children should be sensitively encouraged to talk through what has happened without the involvement or presence of accompanying persons. Specialist staff need to be involved at an early stage with a view to possibly initiating child protection procedures and interagency cooperation. Where any doubt exists about the safety of a child who is due to be discharged back to family care, specialist advice should be taken. Keeping families together is an important goal, but the safety of the child must be the paramount consideration. Child protection issues are discussed in more detail in Chapter 4, pages 174–180.

Summary – treating the victims or perpetrators of crime or abuse

- Where a patient who is unconscious has been the victim of a serious assault or rape, it may be in that person's best interests to have forensic samples taken to identify the assailant.
- The law permits the taking of samples from incapacitated drivers to test for blood alcohol levels in some circumstances.
- The GMC states that the police should be informed without delay if a patient is admitted with a gunshot wound or an injury from a knife attack.
- In some circumstances where a crime has been committed, there will be an overriding public interest in disclosing information to the police or other authority.

Recognising skill and competence levels

Effective use of resources is an ethical issue and includes using appropriately the skills of all members of the healthcare team. Just as team working has assumed greater importance in other spheres of medicine, similar developments have occurred in emergency care. Nurse practitioners have a growing role in treating patients rather than simply assessing them. Increasingly, they request diagnostic procedures, interpret results, give medication and discharge patients. Although consultants spend more time on the most complex cases, greater responsibility is given to physiotherapists, radiographers and paramedics to deal with straightforward cases. As in all other spheres of medicine, good communication and teamwork are vital. Effective teamwork recognises the skills of various professionals and encourages good communication between them. Emergency departments particularly illustrate how beneficial this can be for patient care. More information about team working is provided in Chapter 19.

Challenging rigid professional roles

Experienced nurses in one Trust were guiding senior house officers in the treatment of minor injuries, but their role expansion had not been formally recognised. Staff could see that there were problems with strict demarcation of roles and restricted boundaries of practice. A need was identified for developing autonomous practice consistent with ensuring patient safety. The minor injury nurse treatment service was established, whereby nurses could work at three levels, developing their skills within a competency framework and moving up the levels as their skills increased.

- Level 1 nurses work under the supervision of a level 2 or 3 practitioner and can initiate certain investigations.
- Level 2 nurses work with minimal supervision and peer support from a level 3 practitioner. They initiate and interpret some investigations, but do not refer or discharge patients.

- Level 3 are senior nurses working without direct supervision. They interpret the results of investigations, assimilate those into the overall clinical picture, and can treat and discharge patients.

The effect was to challenge the traditional role of emergency nurses, develop their skills and improve patient flow.[23]

Acting within the limits of competence

Within hospital settings critical situations can sometimes arise when doctors have to balance the likely harms and benefits and may need to act to the limits of their capacity and training rather than await the arrival of a more specialised colleague. For example, career emergency doctors (as opposed to specialty trainees) receive training in anaesthesia, but current practice in most emergency departments is for all anaesthetics to be provided by qualified anaesthetists or anaesthetists in training. Nevertheless, urgent situations can arise when an anaesthetist is unavailable and an emergency doctor has to weigh up the comparative risks of proceeding with or delaying treatment. There are also some situations in which a trained emergency doctor who knows the procedure that is required, but has not actually carried it out, may be required to do so.

In addition, as doctors become more senior, working fewer clinical hours, their exposure to certain clinical techniques may decline, with consequent deskilling, and they need to decide whether to cease carrying out certain procedures at all. Ideally, general advice should be sought in advance of an emergency from colleagues and from trust lawyers. Conceivably, however, there may be rare occasions when they should carry out a procedure they rarely do if the choice is genuinely between that and risking serious harm to the patient through a delay in intervening. In all such cases, judging what is 'reasonable' and most likely to preserve life or reduce harm needs to be considered on a case-by-case basis. Clearly, doctors should be well aware of their own limitations and never act beyond their competence if there is a viable alternative. The need for such emergency interventions should be audited and steps taken to minimise their occurrence. If inadvertent harm is caused to a patient by a doctor acting at the limits of his or her competence, this should be discussed with the patient at the earliest appropriate opportunity.

Emergency care outside healthcare establishments

The 'duty to help'

In some countries, and in some US states, there are 'Good Samaritan' or 'failure to stop' laws obliging any passing health professional to offer assistance in an emergency. There are no parallel legal obligations in the UK, although doctors may be considered to have special obligations to people with whom they already have a therapeutic relationship. Nevertheless, the GMC advises doctors that 'in an emergency, wherever it may arise, you must offer anyone at risk the assistance you could reasonably be expected to provide'.[24] The BMA's general advice is also that doctors should be willing to identify themselves in such cases and offer help in a road traffic accident or aircraft emergency, for example.

For doctors not specialised in emergency care, there may be a difficult decision about whether to intervene in emergencies for which they are ill equipped. When there is likely to be a long delay in obtaining specialised help, however, immediate non-specialised medical assistance can make the difference between life and death. How much to intervene or whether to risk acting beyond one's competence must be considered within the context of the case. Doctors dealing with an aircraft emergency on a long flight are more likely to need to intervene to the very limits of their competence than a doctor coming across a traffic accident to which an ambulance is on its way. Doctors are normally advised to restrict themselves to interventions well within their competence. In an emergency far from a hospital, however, they may well be justified in going beyond what they would normally attempt, as a last resort when no other help is at hand. As a general principle, in an emergency, health professionals do not have the option of non-involvement and they may not have the choice of waiting for someone better qualified to handle the situation. Doctors who have a conscientious objection to abortion, for example, can generally opt out of participating except in an emergency when they must do what they can to assist the pregnant woman (see Chapter 7, pages 288–289).

Liability

Doctors frequently worry that they may exceed their competence and incur litigation if they embark upon an intervention outside their normal sphere of practice in an emergency situation. Fear of liability has traditionally been cited as the common reason for doctors' reluctance to offer help in an in-flight emergency.[25] As far as can be ascertained, however, there is no evidence that litigation has ever been brought in the UK against a doctor who rendered assistance during such an emergency.[26] In general terms, the law expects doctors to do what appears most reasonable in the circumstances and the Medical Defence Union says that 'if you are trying to do the right thing by using your professional expertise to help a fellow human continue to live ... the chances of you facing legal action are so low they are almost non-existent'.[27] In respect of errors, 'judges have recognised that in an emergency responsible professionals may be more prone to errors' and 'the fact that a mistake is made should not lead lightly to a finding of negligence'.[28] Such situations are said to reflect 'battle conditions'.[29]

Advice from an indemnifying body

'The fact that you are not a consultant in emergency medicine, have never been trained in advanced trauma life support (ATLS), and do not have a fully equipped crash trolley should not be a barrier to helping someone to the best of your ability. However, you should remember that whatever you do would be classed as a clinical intervention. You must therefore, record the name of the patient, make a clinical record of what you are doing and give your name and address to a suitable official such as a member of the aircraft cabin crew. Remember to take appropriate precautions with infectious diseases although advance airline permission may be required for doctors to take needles, syringes or other equipment for their use. Remember also the duty of confidentiality to patients, which continues beyond death, especially if there is media interest subsequently.'[30]

In-flight emergencies

In-flight medical events are relatively common on some airlines – one airline reported 1 per 12,000 passengers and another, 1 per 1,400 passengers[31] – but most incidents are not serious. Nevertheless, serious cardiac, neurological and respiratory emergencies do occasionally occur and these account for the majority of instances in which airlines have to make unscheduled landings.[32] There do not appear to be standard international guidelines on the management of in-flight medical events, but each airline has its own policy. Several companies provide continuous ground to air medical advice and employ doctors trained in emergency and aviation medicine.[33] Airline staff are trained to use the first aid equipment on board the aeroplane and can also follow instructions provided by the ground-based doctor. Most of the major airlines, and many of the smaller airlines, carry automated external defibrillators (AEDs).[34] The role of medical passengers who volunteer help is not to take sole control but to assist the flight crew, who remain responsible for the patient. The BMA advises doctors who are frequent flyers and who are often asked to intervene to check their indemnity situation with their defence body. The Medical Defence Union, the Medical Protection Society and the Medical and Dental Defence Union of Scotland insure all their members for Good Samaritan acts where they are a bystander, anywhere in the world.[35]

Although it is not strictly a matter of medical ethics, some doctors object to volunteering help for airline emergencies without some form of reimbursement because they sometimes feel that advantage has been taken by the airline. If no thorough checks are made prior to embarking sick passengers, the likelihood of an emergency is increased. Doctors can ask for payment, but none of the major airlines has a policy of hourly rates for Good Samaritan acts, although some offer upgrades or free flight vouchers as tokens of gratitude. Doctors asking for payment may also be exposing themselves to a legal claim as insurance may specify cover only for Good Samaritan acts.[36]

Care at accident and disaster sites

Pre-hospital emergency care in the UK developed after a major rail disaster at Harrow station in the early 1950s drew attention to the field hospital techniques used by US military medical units. Such units based nearby attended the crash and provided stabilising care in situ to crash victims. Immediate and pre-hospital care then developed significantly as a specialist area of medicine from the 1970s. The British Association for Intermediate Care (BASICS), established in 1977, continues as a voluntary organisation, providing volunteer medical help. BASICS doctors often work with pre-hospital paramedic teams and can make critical on-the-spot decisions to assist paramedics who have to work strictly to protocols. In the past, perceived role divisions sometimes hampered cooperative work between doctors and paramedic teams, or between volunteers and professionals. Part of the important contribution of BASICS has been to foster good teamwork across such barriers.

Triage

Triage is essential when there are multiple casualties and may occur both at the scene of a disaster and in the emergency department. Medical assessment and pain relief are vital for all the injured, but most attention has to be centred on those with the best chance of survival and recovery. Therefore, in disasters, the common sense rule of triage is to attend to people whose condition does not appear to be fatal but requires immediate attention, without which they will deteriorate seriously. The most severely injured people may simply be made as comfortable as possible but left untreated if their care would mean that people with better chances of recovery are left to deteriorate. Utilitarian considerations about saving the greatest number tend to come to the fore rather than focusing on doing the best for a particular individual.

Teamwork

Mobile specialist care is delivered in various ways, ranging from a motorcycle paramedic to a mobile coronary unit or helicopter emergency team. It can be provided by a single emergency expert or a team including appropriately trained technicians. Paramedics have an ever-growing role in emergency care and are increasingly developing their own codes of ethics that reflect changing practice. In the past, paramedics and ambulance staff were expected to work to fairly inflexible guidelines in which all decision making was left with doctors. In the 1980s and 1990s, the BMA received queries, for example, from ambulance staff who had been instructed always to attempt resuscitation unless directly instructed to the contrary by a doctor, generally a GP. This caused dilemmas when they were faced by patients who collapsed at home having clearly made an advance refusal of such treatment, but when the GP was not immediately contactable. In such cases, a lack of preparation for such eventualities meant that emergency workers were caught in the middle between relatives supporting non-resuscitation on the basis of an advance refusal of treatment and rules requiring a doctor to make a judgement. Gradually, more attention has been given to the need for emergency workers, like all other health professionals, to take account of patient autonomy and abide by evidence of patients' refusals of treatment. Although bound by certain widely agreed protocols, emergency healthcare workers are independently responsible for decision making within their sphere of competence. They must also treat in accordance with mental capacity legislation when an adult patient lacks capacity (see Chapter 3).

Ambulance paramedics have extended training in advanced life support skills. Despite this, there are some procedures and emergency decisions that protocols decree should be undertaken only by doctors. Dilemmas can arise, however, if no doctor is immediately available and another health professional is faced with the choice of breaching protocols and attempting a procedure normally outside his or her competence, or risking the patient's death. Paramedics' training should prepare them for such dilemmas before they arise.

Patients refusing to attend hospital

Some patients refuse to attend hospital for examination after an accident or injury and a significant number of these have a serious health condition.[37] Emergency teams in the community are advised to persist in trying to persuade patients to go to hospital if certain clinical criteria are met, such as indications of a history of drug ingestion, head injury, disorientation or chest pains, but treatment cannot be forced upon patients with capacity. Even if refusing hospitalisation, patients should be strongly encouraged to allow their GP to be informed and it should be stressed that they should seek medical help immediately if their condition worsens. Patients should be advised that they are entitled to change their mind about treatment without prejudice. Efforts should also be made to find a responsible adult to stay with the patient and call for help if necessary.

Dealing with stress and trauma

A difference between emergency medicine and most other spheres of treatment concerns the impact on the health professionals involved. All medicine requires health staff to deal with tragedy and grief in some form, but emergency care at a disaster site, such as a major crash or bombing, can be particularly dangerous and traumatic. The risks of post-traumatic stress disorder for health staff after major disasters have to be taken into account and plans devised. Emergency care can involve exposure to sudden large numbers of deaths, horrific injuries and mutilation, the effects of which can be extremely stressful for health professionals. The option for health staff who are faced with these situations to obtain support and counselling without adverse career implications is essential. Some of the effects of persistent stress on doctors are discussed further in Chapter 21.

Summary – emergency care outside healthcare establishments

- Although there is no legal obligation to do so, the GMC states that doctors are expected to give whatever assistance they can in an emergency.
- Doctors should not normally intervene beyond or at the limits of their competence, but in an emergency situation this may be the only alternative to permitting serious harm to occur.
- In emergency settings, doctors may have to make difficult decisions about which patients to treat first.
- Health professionals need to bear in mind their own need for support in order to continue providing care effectively.

References

1 Kay R, Siriwardena AK. (2001) The process of informed consent for urgent abdominal surgery. *J Med Ethics* **27**, 157–61.
2 National Institute for Clinical Excellence (2004) *Self Harm CG16*, NICE, London, p.27.
3 Royal College of Psychiatrists (2004) *Assessment following self-harm in adults*, Council Report CR122, RCPsych, London.
4 Gabbatt A. (2009) Doctors acted legally in 'living will' suicide case. *The Guardian* (October 1). Available at: www.guardian.co.uk (accessed 3 March 2011). Smith R, Laing A, Devlin K. (2009) Suicide woman allowed to die because doctors feared saving her would be assault. *The Telegraph* (September 30). Available at: www.telegraph.co.uk (accessed 3 March 2011).
5 Gabbatt A. (2009) Doctors acted legally in 'living will' suicide case. *The Guardian* (October 1). Available at: www.guardian.co.uk (accessed 3 March 2011).
6 *Re W (adult: refusal of treatment)* (2002) MHLR 411.
7 Department of Health (2005) *When a Patient Dies: advice on developing bereavement services in the NHS*, DH, London, p.26.
8 Booth MG, Woolrich L, Kinsella J. (2004) Family witnessed resuscitation in UK emergency departments: a survey of practice. *Eur J Anaesthesiol* **21**, 725–8.
9 Resuscitation Council (UK) (1996) *Should relatives witness resuscitation?* Resuscitation Council (UK), London, p.5.
10 Resuscitation Council (UK) (1996) *Should relatives witness resuscitation?* Resuscitation Council (UK), London, p.6.
11 Resuscitation Council (UK) (1996) *Should relatives witness resuscitation?* Resuscitation Council (UK), London, p.9.
12 Resuscitation Council (UK), Royal College of Anaesthetists, Royal College of Physicians, Intensive Care Society (2008) *Cardiopulmonary Resuscitation: standards for clinical practice and training*, Resuscitation Council (UK), London, p.14.
13 Royal College of Nursing (2002) *Witnessing resuscitation: guidance for nursing staff*, RCN, London.
14 Medicines for Human Use (Clinical Trials) and Blood Safety and Quality (Amendment) Regulations 2008. SI 2008/941.
15 Faculty of Forensic and Legal Medicine (2008) *Consent from patients who may have been seriously assaulted*, FFLM, London.
16 British Medical Association, Faculty of Forensic and Legal Medicine (2010) *Taking blood specimens from incapacitated drivers*, BMA, London.
17 General Medical Council (2009) *Confidentiality: reporting gunshot and knife wounds*, GMC, London.
18 General Medical Council (2009) *Confidentiality: reporting gunshot and knife wounds*, GMC, London, para 3.
19 British Medical Association (2007) *Domestic abuse*, BMA, London.
20 Stevens KLH. (1997) The role of the accident and emergency department. In: Bewley S, Friend J, Mezey G. (eds.) *Violence against women*, RCOG Press, London.

21   The Co-ordindated Action Against Domestic Abuse (CAADA) risk assessment tool is available at: www.caada.org.uk (accessed 3 March 2011).
22   British Medical Association (2007) *Domestic abuse*, BMA, London, p.7.
23   Emergency Services Collaborative (2002) *Improvement in emergency care: case studies*, NHS Modernisation Agency, London, case study 1c.
24   General Medical Council (2006) *Good Medical Practice*, GMC, London, para 11.
25   Rayman RB. (1998) Inflight medical kits. *Aviat Space Environ Med* **69**, 1007–10.
26   Genreau MA, DeJohn C. (2003) Responding to medical events during commercial airline flights. *N Engl J Med* **346**, 1067–73, p.1070.
27   Kirkpatrick A. (2002) Come join the good samaritans. *Student BMJ* **10**, 89–130.
28   Montgomery J. (2002) *Health care law*, 2nd edn, Oxford University Press, New York, pp.179–80.
29   *Wilsher v Essex AHA* [1986] 3 All ER 801, 812.
30   Kirkpatrick A. (2002) Come join the good samaritans. *Student BMJ* **10**, 89–130.
31   British Medical Association (2004) *The impact of flying on passenger health: a guide for healthcare professionals*, BMA, London, p.26.
32   Genreau MA, DeJohn C. (2003) Responding to medical events during commercial airline flights. *N Engl J Med* **346**, 1067–73, p.1067.
33   British Medical Association (2004) *The impact of flying on passenger health: a guide for healthcare professionals*, BMA, London.
34   British Medical Association (2004) *The impact of flying on passenger health: a guide for healthcare professionals*, BMA, London.
35   British Medical Association (2004) *The impact of flying on passenger health: a guide for healthcare professionals*, BMA, London, p.28.
36   Shepherd B, Macpherson D, Edwards CMB. (2006) In-flight emergencies: playing The Good Samaritan. *J R Soc Med* **99**, 628–31.
37   Forster J. (2008) Tributes to nurse who died after refusing to go to hospital. *Sunderland Echo* (26 December) www.sunderlandecho.com (accessed 3 March 2011). Cooke MW. (1999) *Churchill's pocket book of pre-hospital care*, Churchill Livingstone, Edinburgh.

16: Doctors with dual obligations

The questions covered in this chapter include the following.

- How does the nature of the doctor–patient relationship change when doctors have contractual obligations to third parties?
- What rights of confidentiality do patients have when reports are being written about them by independent medical examiners?
- Should doctors act as referees for firearms licences?
- Can information about genetic tests be put into medical reports for third parties?
- How should occupational physicians balance their duty of confidentiality to their patients with their obligations to management?
- What duties of confidentiality do sports doctors owe to players and athletes?

When do dual obligations arise?

Much of medical practice, and much of its attendant ethical discussion, is based on a direct relationship between doctors and patients (see Chapter 1) and, although the impact of decisions on both other people and the wider public interest is important, there are usually only two main parties to the relationship. (Public health practice is covered separately in Chapter 20). This chapter concerns situations in which there is an identifiable third party, such as an insurer or employer, to whom the doctor has contractual responsibilities, or a court for which a doctor is acting as a witness. Obligations to third parties may be express or implied, real or perceived. The common factor is that the doctor–patient relationship cannot be reduced to the usual model of a therapeutic partnership and this has implications for both the doctor and the patient. While ongoing changes to the context in which healthcare services are delivered in the UK are leading to a greater awareness among doctors that they can have multiple obligations, this chapter focuses on those situations where doctors have a clear obligation to a third party that can be in tension with the obligation to the patient. Doctors who have dual obligations as a result of working in detention settings or as part of criminal proceedings are dealt with separately in Chapter 17.

Implications of having dual obligations

Traditionally, codes of medical ethics have centred on the notion that a doctor's primary loyalty is to the welfare of the patient. International codes such as the World Medical Association's Declaration of Geneva (the modern restatement of the Hippocratic Oath) emphasise that the health of the patient must be a doctor's primary obligation.[1] Whereas all doctors have multiple professional loyalties, such as those to colleagues, health

Medical Ethics Today: The BMA's Handbook of Ethics and Law, Third Edition. Sophie Brannan, Eleanor Chrispin, Martin Davies, Veronica English, Rebecca Mussell, Julian Sheather and Ann Sommerville.
© 2012 BMA Medical Ethics Department. Published 2012 by Blackwell Publishing Ltd.

service employers and society at large, these are generally in the background. The duties at the forefront of doctors' concern are normally those owed to individual patients. When loyalties conflict, doctors have to be prepared to support their patients by, for example, reporting poor practice by colleagues or employers that has put their patients at risk (see Chapter 21).

In the doctor–patient relationship, decision making is usually a joint process, with the patient's health and well-being as the primary concern. In the situations covered in this chapter, however, the welfare of individual patients may not be the main focus, although all doctors have some responsibility for the people they see or advise professionally. Dual obligations are a live issue in any debate about civil and political rights because it is generally recognised that doctors with pronounced dual obligations can be at risk of subordinating the rights of patients to other interests. Although this is particularly true for doctors working in detention settings, who have become increasingly attuned to these pressures (see Chapter 17), it can also be true, for example, of occupational health physicians whose responsibilities are divided between protecting the health of workers and advising management on all aspects of occupational health.[2] Doctors employed by benefit agencies can also have conflicting loyalties where clinical objectivity and compassion can at times be in tension with duties toward their employer and, by extension, public finances.

Dual obligations and medical assessment for sickness benefits – a case study

One area where doctors can experience dual obligations is in relation to medical assessments for sickness benefit. In 2009, the Government introduced a more stringent medical assessment – the Work Capability Assessment (WCA) for a new sickness-related benefit, the Employment and Support Allowance (ESA). The new WCA focused on the work claimants could do rather than what they are unable to do. The explicit goal of the new assessment was to reduce the number of people claiming incapacity benefit, which had risen by more than 1 million during the 1980s. Given the goal of the assessment, doctors employed by the benefit agencies are clearly subject to dual obligations. Government targets to reduce the numbers of claimants could potentially put pressure on the findings of assessors. Doctors working in these situations need to ensure that their employers are aware of the need for scrupulous clinical independence in each individual assessment.

Many of the issues covered in this chapter are drawn from the cases that doctors bring to the British Medical Association (BMA) for advice. Although doctors in these situations recognise that they may have some therapeutic role, they also acknowledge that they have a strong obligation to another party or a wider population, such as an employer, insurer or court of law. In many cases, this duty to another may appear to come into conflict with the patient's usual rights, particularly the right to confidentiality. In these circumstances, doctors often feel that their responsibilities towards the patient are vague and unspecified, while their duties to their employer or the body paying for the medical report are more clearly defined. There is also a risk that they will assimilate the norms and values of the third party rather than acting in accordance with their professional standards. A central argument in this chapter is that, although doctors may be acting outside the normal therapeutic relationship, the usual ethical standards still apply. In particular, they have a duty to inform their patients of the nature of their obligations to any third party and the effect those obligations may have on the patient.

Circumstances in which dual obligations arise

This chapter focuses on three areas. Within each there are a number of different examples. These are given below.

- Doctors providing medical reports for third parties: doctors write medical reports for the immigration service, employers, insurers, the courts and others. A common factor is that the medical report serves a purpose other than facilitating treatment. Reports for third parties are often carried out by a patient's own GP, although sometimes an independent expert is commissioned to examine a patient and write a report.
- Doctors who are employed by third parties: this includes occupational physicians, doctors in the armed forces and sports doctors employed by, for example, professional football clubs.
- Doctors whose role does not focus on individual patients: in this final category we consider the work of doctors in the media and those with business interests.

General principles

The following principles should inform doctors' actions where they have dual obligations.

- Doctors acting for a third party must ensure that the patient understands that fact, and its implications.
- Doctors appointed and paid by a third party still have a duty of care to the patient whom they advise, examine or treat, and must abide by professional guidelines on ethics and law.
- Medical reports must be truthful and objective.
- Consent is as important as it is in other areas of medical practice, although in the armed forces there may be some additional constraints on individuals.
- Doctors have a duty of confidentiality, and information should not normally be disclosed without the patient's knowledge and consent (see Chapter 5).

Providing reports for third parties

This section outlines some general points that are common to all situations in which doctors write reports for non-medical purposes. Specific advice about the most common areas can be found on pages 654–673.

When doctors are called upon to write medical reports, they should ensure that they are factual, detailed and carefully worded, avoiding assertions that cannot be defended. They should also bear in mind who will be reading the report. Responsibility for assessing medical reports for insurance rests with the insurance company's chief medical officer. In contrast, medico-legal reports are mainly read by non-medical officials, so unnecessarily complex medical terms should be avoided or, where used, they should be defined. Colloquial terms that lack precision should also be avoided.

Confidentiality

All the health information that doctors obtain about identifiable individuals and which they learn in a professional capacity is subject to the duty of confidentiality. It follows that all doctors who write reports about patients need consent for the report to be released. They should be prepared to discuss the contents of reports with patients, and be aware of patients' statutory rights of access to reports. Care must also be taken to ensure that where the release of medical information is a condition of access to certain goods, such as social security benefits, patients understand as fully as possible the nature of the personal data likely to be disclosed (see Chapter 5).

General Medical Council advice on confidentiality and medical reports

'If you are asked to provide information to third parties, such as a patient's insurer, employer or a government department or an agency assessing a claimant's entitlement to benefits, either following an examination or from existing records, you should:

(a) be satisfied that the patient has sufficient information about the scope, purpose and likely consequences of the examination and disclosure, and the fact that relevant information cannot be concealed or withheld

(b) obtain or have seen written consent to the disclosure from the patient or a person properly authorised to act on the patient's behalf; you may accept an assurance from an officer of a government department or agency or a registered health professional acting on their behalf that the patient or a person properly authorised to act on their behalf has consented

(c) only disclose factual information you can substantiate, presented in an unbiased manner, relevant to the request; so you should not usually disclose the whole record, although it may be relevant to some benefits paid by government departments and to other assessments of patients' entitlement to pensions or other health-related benefits, and

(d) offer to show your patient, or give them a copy of, any report you write about them for employment or insurance purposes before it is sent, unless:
   i. they have already indicated they do not wish to see it
   ii. disclosure would be likely to cause serious harm to the patient or anyone else
   iii. disclosure would be likely to reveal information about another person who does not consent.'[3]

Doctors who are writing independent reports sometimes think that the very fact that a patient has cooperated with an examination, and volunteered information about health, means that the patient gives consent for the disclosure of information. This does not automatically follow, and doctors should ensure that they have written consent to disclosure once the examination is completed. This can also reduce the likelihood of reports containing factual errors.

Breach of confidentiality for disclosure of a report

Pamela Cornelius was a schoolteacher who felt that her mental health was being affected by difficulties at school which she blamed on the head teacher. She was considering resigning and bringing a claim for constructive dismissal, and therefore approached a solicitor. Her solicitor advised that they should seek a report from a consultant psychiatrist to ascertain whether Mrs Cornelius's health problems could properly be attributed to her conditions of employment. Dr Taranto was commissioned to write a report.

Mrs Cornelius was seen by Dr Taranto, and a report prepared. Dr Taranto wanted to refer Mrs Cornelius to another consultant psychiatrist, and claimed in court that she had consented to do so. As part of the referral, she sent a copy of the report to a psychiatrist and Mrs Cornelius's GP.

Mrs Cornelius claimed that she had neither given consent for the referral to be made, nor for the report to be sent to another psychiatrist or her GP. As such, her confidentiality had been breached. Dr Taranto, on the other hand, argued that Mrs Cornelius had agreed to being referred for treatment and that sending the report to the other doctors was a consequence of that. The medical records showed no note of a discussion about consent for the referral or disclosure of the report.

The judge in the Court of Appeal upheld Mrs Cornelius's claim and said that her express consent for the report's transmission to a third party was necessary, even if she had agreed to the referral.[4]

Access to reports

The BMA strongly supports openness between doctors and patients, and encourages doctors to share the reports they write with patients whenever possible. Reports written for insurance or employment purposes by a doctor with whom the patient already has a therapeutic relationship are covered by the Access to Medical Reports Act 1988 and Access to Medical Reports (Northern Ireland) Order 1991. The legislation gives specific rights to be informed when a report is sought, to be offered the opportunity to see the report before it is sent, and to have any inaccuracies amended. Detailed advice is given in Chapter 6, pages 260–261, and in separate guidance available via the BMA's website.[5]

In addition, all health records, including, in the view of the BMA and the Information Commissioner, reports written by independent medical examiners, are covered by the subject access provisions of data protection legislation. Detailed advice is given in Chapter 6, pages 255–258 on health records and in separate guidance available via the BMA's website.[6]

Truthfulness

Doctors must not allow the requirements of a third party who is commissioning a report, or their sympathies for the individual being examined, to deflect them from accurate and truthful reporting. They should not be drawn into speculation if asked, for example, to offer an expert opinion on insufficient or flawed evidence, or on something outside their area of expertise. In such cases, it is important to state clearly either the limits of what can be deduced or the extent of the doctor's expertise.

The need for honesty can create dilemmas for doctors, such as GPs, who have developed a professional relationship with a patient over a period of time, and who see their role as the patient's advocate. It is important therefore that doctors who have a prior relationship with a patient, and are called upon to provide a report relating to that patient, should ensure that he or she understands the nature of the relationship and that the doctor is under an obligation to provide an honest report.

Patients sometimes try to persuade doctors to change a report or to omit relevant information to make it more favourable from their perspective. It is important that the doctor should correct any errors, and that a patient's disagreement with any part of a report should be noted and explained. The report must, however, be truthful and must not omit information that the doctor believes to be relevant.

General Medical Council advice on report writing

'• You must be honest and trustworthy when writing reports, and when completing or signing forms, reports and other documents.
• You must always be honest about your experience, qualifications and position, particularly when applying for posts.
• You must do your best to make sure that any documents you write or sign are not false or misleading. This means that you must take reasonable steps to verify the information in the documents, and that you must not deliberately leave out relevant information.
• If you have agreed to prepare a report, complete or sign a document, or provide evidence, you must do so without unreasonable delay.
• If you are asked to give evidence or act as a witness in litigation or formal inquiries, you must be honest in all your spoken and written statements. You must make clear the limits of your knowledge or competence.'[7]

Medical reports for insurance

One of the most common situations in which doctors have a duty to another party is when they are completing medical reports about patients who want insurance cover. Patients are under no obligation to accept either an examination or the release of personal medical information, although the fact that a refusal is likely to render an application for insurance unsuccessful does put pressure on patients to agree to examination and disclosure. However, there is little that doctors can do in such situations after impartially counselling the patient. Ultimately, it is for the patient to decide whether or not to accept the terms laid down by the insurance company or to consider other alternatives. Detailed advice about the use of medical information in insurance can be found in joint guidance from the BMA and the Association of British Insurers (ABI).[8] The release of information about deceased patients to insurance companies is covered on page 660.

How is medical information for insurance collected?

Insurance companies gain information about their applicants' health in a number of ways. The most common is direct from the applicant. Applicants have a legal duty to reveal all information that is material to the insurer's actuarial decisions, whether or not it is specifically requested. Failure to do so could invalidate a policy. Doctors are not experts in insurance, however, and may not always be aware of whether information is actuarially relevant.

Where more detailed information is needed, insurers sometimes seek a report from the applicant's GP (see pages 655–656) or an independent medical examiner (see page 656). Occasionally, applicants will be asked to undertake specific screening or blood tests. Frequently, more than one source of information is used. Provided applicants have given valid consent, doctors' responsibilities in all these situations are to respond to the questions they are asked based on information they have acquired in a professional capacity. Their role is to provide factual information about the applicant's health. Doctors should not express opinions, for example about whether an applicant's condition merits the application of a 'normal' or 'increased' rate of insurance. If they are asked questions that they consider are inappropriate for them to answer, such as speculative questions about lifestyle or other non-factual matters, they should indicate this on the form.

Medical reports

Insurance companies generally prefer to ask the applicant's GP to write a report based on the medical notes rather than arrange an independent examination. A GP is likely to be able to provide an overall picture of the applicant's health instead of just the snapshot seen by an independent examiner. A GP's report (GPR) can, for example, validate the information that the applicant has provided or clarify whether an applicant's condition is being controlled. Some applicants also prefer this option as it may be more convenient than having an independent examination.

Some GPs have expressed concerns about this process, as they believe that it endangers the open, trusting nature of the doctor–patient relationship. There is anecdotal evidence to suggest that some patients do not share information with their GP or avoid going to their GP for advice or treatment because they think the information will not be kept confidential. They may believe that it will jeopardise their chances of obtaining insurance at standard rates or of obtaining insurance cover at all. In fact, if they subsequently develop an illness of which they would have had symptoms at the time of application, the policy may be invalidated, even if they withheld that information from the GP. The BMA is concerned about the effects on the health of individuals, and the public, of information being withheld from doctors who are providing care. The scale of this problem is not known, but the ABI and the BMA suggest that, should such fears arise, insurers should explain to their clients the reasons why the information is needed, their confidentiality safeguards and applicants' rights under the Data Protection Act 1998 and the Access to Medical Reports Act 1988. In the BMA's view it would be helpful if insurance companies offered applicants a choice between a GPR and an independent examination.

BMA policy states that doctors should refuse to complete insurance reports about their patients unless a copy of the applicant's written consent has been provided for the doctor's retention. The consent form should make it clear that the applicant understands the nature and purpose of the report and any examination, and to whom information will be disclosed. Legal rules governing the sending of medical reports to insurers give patients rights of access to them. These are covered in detail in Chapter 6, pages 260–261. Some GPs prefer to send copies of medical reports to their patients first, asking them to forward them to their insurers if they are happy that they are accurate or to discuss them with the doctor if they are not.

GP reports

The BMA and the ABI have jointly developed a standard GPR package which is available on both the ABI's and the BMA's website and is widely used.[9] The package contains:

- a standard covering letter for insurers to send to GPs, together with an overview of the types of information that are relevant to different types of insurance policy
- a standard GPR form, and
- a standard consent declaration for patients.

When providing a report, doctors should only provide relevant information. Doctors should not send the original records, nor should they send photocopies or printouts of the full medical record in lieu of the report. GPs should also be careful only to include information gained from the patient's medical record, and not information gained, for example, solely from the doctor's knowledge of other family members or via hearsay or as a result of living in the same community.

Independent medical reports

Instead of seeking a GPR, or sometimes as well as, insurance companies may ask applicants to be seen and examined by an independent doctor. Doctors undertaking these examinations must be satisfied that the company has explained the nature and purpose of the examination, together with the necessary practical details. The examining doctor also has responsibilities to ensure that the applicant gives valid consent to the examination, and understands the nature and implications of any tests involved. Consent is also needed before information about the applicant may be disclosed to the insurance company.

Occasions arise where the examining doctor detects some significant abnormality or other feature of the applicant's health that requires investigation or treatment, and of which the applicant may not be aware. In such cases, the examining doctor has an ethical responsibility to inform the patient, and encourage him or her to consent to the GP being informed. If the patient is unwilling for the examining doctor to write directly to the GP, it might be possible to agree a way for the patient to pass on the information. Examining doctors may find it helpful to ascertain the applicant's views on disclosure to the GP before the examination, and to obtain permission to liaise with the GP, should the need arise.

Rights of access to independent medical reports are discussed in Chapter 6, pages 260–261.

Consent for disclosure

Doctors' professional, ethical and legal duties require them not to disclose information about patients without their consent. This is true in all but the most exceptional circumstances, such as where a risk of serious harm to another person can be averted by disclosure (see Chapter 5).

When seeking a medical report, the insurance company or agent is responsible for ensuring that the consent is competently given and is based on a proper understanding of the nature and scope of the information requested. There is anecdotal evidence that, in the past, the subjects of GPRs have not always been aware of the extent of the information that is requested. In the BMA's view, it would be helpful if insurance companies or their agents could, as part of the application process, give applicants a copy of the questions the doctor will be asked, with time for the information to be read and understood. In this way, misunderstanding is likely to be minimised and any consent to disclosure more likely to be valid.

If doctors are in any doubt about whether valid consent has been given, they should check with the applicant. The General Medical Council (GMC) requires doctors to:

'• be satisfied that the patient has sufficient information about the scope, purpose and likely consequences of the examination and disclosure, and the fact that relevant information cannot be concealed or withheld
• obtain or have seen written consent to the disclosure from the patient or a person properly authorised to act on the patient's behalf.'[10]

Where there has been a significant lapse of time between signing the initial consent and the forwarding of the report, doctors should consider confirming that the individual still consents to the disclosure.

Content of reports

There are some restrictions on the use of medical information in insurance. Data protection legislation prohibits insurers from having more information about applicants than is relevant for the insurance product being sought. The doctor therefore needs to be aware of what the product is, and what information is relevant to it, before completing a report. A brief explanation of different insurance products, and the information insurers need in relation to each, is given in joint guidance from the BMA and ABI.[11]

The sections that follow highlight some specific areas where special rules apply.

Sexually transmitted infections

The possibility that information about sexually transmitted infections (STIs) will be revealed to another party, such as an insurance company, might discourage some people from approaching their GP about this aspect of their health. The problem of information being withheld from the GP is particularly pronounced in this area because genitourinary medicine is a field of specialist medical care that patients can access without a referral from their GP. Anecdotal evidence suggests that patients sometimes seek services direct from genitourinary medicine clinics because they prefer to retain their anonymity or privacy, or in order to conceal from their GP information that they believe may affect their chance of obtaining insurance at the standard rate, or of obtaining it at all.

Both the BMA and the ABI believe that insurers should not request, and doctors should not reveal, information about an isolated incident of an STI that has no long-term health implications, or even multiple episodes of non-serious STIs, again where there are no long-term health implications. Other incidents of STIs that are likely to have long-term health implications, and will therefore be actuarially relevant, should be revealed in accordance with the consent guidelines in this chapter.

HIV, and hepatitis B and C

In the view of the BMA and the ABI, insurance companies should not ask whether an applicant has had a HIV or a hepatitis B or C test, received counselling in connection with such a test, or received a negative test result. Doctors should not reveal this information when writing reports and insurance companies do not expect it to be provided. Insurers may ask only whether someone has had a positive test result, or is receiving treatment for HIV/AIDS, or for hepatitis B or C.

For large value policies or when there is a need to clarify the level of risk, insurers may send applicants a supplementary questionnaire and/or request that they are tested for HIV, or for hepatitis B or C. A test should only be administered, with appropriate pre- and post-test counselling, after the applicant has given valid consent in writing and nominated a doctor or clinic to receive the results if the test is positive. Ordinarily, unless there are clinical indications suggesting the patient might be at risk of having contracted HIV, the test should be organised privately and paid for by the patient or insurer.

In the rare cases of a positive test result it is important that the nominee is told the result as quickly as possible so the applicant can be informed and arrangements made for future care. Existing life insurance policies will not be affected in any way by undergoing a HIV test, even if the result is positive. Providing that the applicant did not withhold any material facts when the life policy was taken out, life insurers will meet all valid claims whatever the cause of death, including AIDS-related diseases. Material facts that the applicant may need to reveal include information about activities that increase the risk of HIV infection.

The ABI has produced a statement of best practice on HIV and insurance for under-writers as well as a consumer guide.[12]

Lifestyle questions

Clinicians are expert in clinical matters and can give professional advice only about issues in which they have expertise. They should refuse to answer questions that invite speculation about a patient's lifestyle. Although doctors often do hold some information about certain 'lifestyle' issues, such as smoking, alcohol intake, eating habits or sexual behaviour, it is, of course, only the individual himself or herself who has accurate, up-to-date information about these things, and applicants should consider providing such information themselves. Medical conditions that have arisen as a result of a patient's lifestyle choices are legitimate areas for doctors to comment on, with appropriate consent.

Genetic information

The use of the results of genetic tests by insurers is tightly controlled. A genetic test is defined as:

'[a] test that examines the structure of chromosomes (cytogenetic tests) or detects ab-normal patterns in the DNA of specific genes (molecular tests). A genetic test can be predictive or diagnostic.

- A predictive genetic test is taken prior to the appearance of any symptoms of the condition in question.
- A diagnostic genetic test is taken to confirm a diagnosis based on existing symptoms.'[13]

The ABI's Code of Practice on genetic testing incorporates a moratorium on the use of unfavourable predictive test results to certain levels of insured benefits.[14] This moratorium is effective until 2017 although it will be reviewed in 2014. Key points in the Code of Practice include the following.

- Applicants must not be asked or put under any pressure to undergo a predictive genetic test in order to obtain insurance.
- Insurance companies may not ask for predictive genetic test results from applicants for insurance policies up to limits specified by the ABI.
- Above these levels, insurers may only take into account the results of genetic tests which have been approved for this purpose.
- Applicants may wish to volunteer favourable genetic test results that demonstrate that they have not inherited a condition in their family. Insurers may take these into account in underwriting. In this case an insurer may wish to seek confirmation from the GP, or geneticist, of the interpretation of the test result, with the patient's consent.
- Insurance companies have been asked to publicise their policies on the use of favourable genetic test results on their websites.

Doctors should not, therefore, disclose unfavourable genetic test results in insurance reports for policies up to the limits set out in the Code of Practice, and insurance companies should make it clear that such information is not required. Information about a family history of a genetic disease is not covered by the moratorium. The use of this information is discussed in more detail below. (Further discussion of the use of genetic information by insurance companies can be found in Chapter 9, pages 396–398.)

Family history information

Information about a patient's family history of disease is not covered by the moratorium on the use of genetic information in insurance. Many companies ask an applicant to provide details if parents or siblings have suffered from, or died of, conditions with an inherited component. These usually include heart disease, stroke, multiple sclerosis, diabetes and cancer. GPR forms also often ask doctors to provide any information from the applicant's own medical record which shows that the applicant is aware of a family history of inherited conditions.

Requesting information about family history from an applicant's doctor presents ethical and practical difficulties. Information on GP records about a genetic risk may have come from a number of sources, including direct from the patient or from the GP's knowledge of other family members, and it is not always apparent which. Where disclosure would involve breaching a GP's duty of confidentiality to a family member, it should not be done without consent, but if the information has come from the patient, it is legitimate for the GP to report it with the patient's consent. Clearly, patients can only give valid consent for the disclosure of information when they are aware of the nature and extent of the information being disclosed. Where there is reasonable doubt about where the information came from, in order to ensure that there is no breach of family members' confidentiality, in the BMA's view, doctors may choose not to complete this section of the GPR if they wish. Doctors should, however, report the results of any tests or investigations they have undertaken on applicants because of their family history that fall outside the moratorium on the use of genetic information in insurance (see above). This information may be useful in confirming or counteracting information about family history provided by the patient. No information should be included in a patient's insurance report that is known solely as a consequence of another family member also being a patient.

Explanations

On request, insurance companies must provide applicants or insured people with written reasons for any higher than standard premium, the rejection of an application, any exclusion or the rejection of a claim or the cancellation of a policy. They must not ask applicants' doctors to explain their actuarial and underwriting decisions. If the company is concerned that the applicant is not aware of a health condition that has influenced the underwriting, or, if it believes that further care or treatment may be beneficial, a medical officer of the company should promptly discuss with the applicant's GP the best way to proceed. Any health concerns that the insurance company has brought to the attention of the GP should be discussed, if the GP feels it to be necessary, in a normal NHS consultation.

Release of information to verify claims

Insurance companies will frequently seek medical information to verify claims, for example before a company organises the repatriation of an insured person taken ill abroad. Where the patient has capacity, consent is required for any such disclosure, and it is for the company concerned to approach the insured person for permission for the doctor to release sufficient information to verify the claim. Where the patient has capacity, doctors cannot release such information without evidence, usually in writing, that the individual has given his or her valid consent.

Sometimes, insurance companies need information about people other than the holder of the policy. This is most often the case with travel insurance, for example where a close relative of the insured person becomes ill and the insured person has to curtail a holiday and return home urgently. In such cases, insurance companies will want to confirm that the seriousness of the condition was such that the insured person was urgently required to attend the relative. Ordinarily, it should be possible for a doctor to confirm the seriousness of a relative's health problem without disclosing confidential information, but if such information is required, the sick relative's consent is required before doctors can release information to verify the claim.

Adults who lack capacity

Although ordinarily disclosures of health information require consent, where adults lack the capacity to consent on their own behalf to disclosures of their information, in certain circumstances, disclosure can still take place. Both the Adults with Incapacity (Scotland) Act 2000 and the Mental Capacity Act 2005, for England and Wales, provide for the nomination of individuals to make health and welfare decisions on behalf of adults lacking the capacity to make specified decisions. These are discussed in more detail in Chapter 3. Where these proxy decision makers require access to health information that is necessary to carry out their functions, that information should ordinarily be provided. These individuals can also be asked to consent for disclosure to third parties. Where there are no nominated individuals, requests for access to information relating to adults lacking the capacity to consent to disclosure can usually be granted where there is both a legitimate need for the information and releasing the information would be in the best interests of the adult. In all cases, only such information as is necessary to achieve the purpose or purposes for which disclosure has been requested should be released. Where the information relates to a third party who lacks capacity to consent to the disclosure, doctors may disclose relevant information provided this is not contrary to the interests or previously known wishes of the patient lacking capacity. Important questions here will be whether information can be disclosed in a non-identifiable way, and whether the request is sufficiently serious to make disclosure of information a proportionate response.

Deceased patients

The ethical obligation to respect a patient's confidentiality extends beyond death. In 2006, the Information Commissioner ruled that, other than the limited rights of access set out under access to health records legislation (discussed in more detail below) a duty of confidence attaches to the medical records of deceased people under section 41 of the Freedom of Information Act 2000. Insurance companies will, at times, however, request information relating to deceased patients in order to assess claims arising from their death. The Access to Health Records Act 1990 and the Access to Health Records (Northern Ireland) Order 1993 state that a personal representative, or anyone who may have a claim arising out of the patient's death, has a right of access to information directly relevant to the claim. Disclosure may take place unless it contains information that:

- the patient indicated before death the he or she did not want released
- identifies a third party who is not a health professional who has been directly involved in caring for the patient
- is likely to cause serious mental or physical harm to somebody's health.

Summary – medical reports for insurance

- Insurers and their agents have responsibility for ensuring that applicants give valid consent to the release of information, although, if there is any doubt, doctors should check with the patient.
- Patients have a right of access to reports provided by their GP before they are sent.
- Doctors need to be aware of the type of information that is relevant to the insurance report, and of any rules that apply to special categories of information, such as genetic test results.

Expert witnesses

Following a number of high-profile cases in which expert medical evidence from doctors has been linked to miscarriages of justice, anecdotal evidence suggests that many doctors may be unwilling to act as expert witnesses. Partly as a result, the Government initiated a review of the delivery of expert witness evidence, initially in the Family Court although it is anticipated that the review will extend more widely. (This is discussed in more detail on page 663.) However, doctors can act as various types of witness during their professional career, entering court as either ordinary, professional or expert witnesses. Ordinary witnesses in court are asked to report what they have seen or heard. Doctors acting as professional witnesses are called upon to comment on matters of medical fact, usually in relation to patients they have seen or treated. Experts, on the other hand, are invited to say not only what they have seen and heard, but also to express an opinion, and this section concentrates on doctors acting in this capacity.

When doctors are instructed as expert witnesses, their primary duty is to assist the court on specialist or technical matters within their expertise and, it follows, to remain independent of the parties, regardless of who called the doctor to court. Detached objectivity is required of medical experts at all times and it is not the role of doctors to plead the case of either the patient or the side paying the fee. Expert witnesses are not advocates and should not have, or be seen to have, an interest in the outcome of the case. The weight of a doctor's opinion is clearly likely to be diminished if it appears biased. Doctors should bear in mind that their opinion may be challenged in court, and that their evidence and their reasoning may be subject to intensive and searching cross examination. One useful indicator of the independence of the opinion offered is whether or not the doctor would express the same opinion if given the instructions by an opposing party.

Experts may be asked to prepare a report outlining what, if any, injury has been sustained, the role of pre-existing or coincidental factors, the likely causation, and prognosis. Because solicitors must represent their client's best interests, they are concerned to present such evidence as will assist in advancing the client's case. Solicitors are under no obligation to inform doctors from whom they are commissioning a report of any facts adverse to the case. Doctors cannot therefore assume that they have been given all the material facts. In such a situation, the onus is upon doctors to ensure that they request all relevant information such as any pleadings, witness statements, investigation reports, incident or accident reports, and previous medical records. When doctors are drawing up their reports they must address themselves to any material features whether they consider these may be adverse to the case of the party instructing them or not.

Submission of an expert report in the context of litigation

Unless instructed otherwise, a report to a court should be addressed to the court and it must:

- give details of the expert's qualifications
- give details of any literature or other material that the expert has relied on in making the report
- contain a statement setting out the substance of all facts and instructions given to the expert that are material to the opinions expressed in the report or upon which those opinions are based
- make clear which of the facts stated in the report are within the expert's own knowledge
- say who carried out any examination, measurement, test or experiment that the expert has used for the report, give the qualification of that person and say whether or not the test or experiment has been carried out under the expert's supervision
- where there is a range of opinion on the matters dealt with in the report, summarise the range of opinion and give reasons for the conclusion the expert reached
- if the expert is not able to give an opinion without qualification, the qualification should be stated
- contain a statement that the expert understands his or her duty to the court, and has complied and will continue to comply with that duty
- be verified by a 'statement of truth' which confirms that the expert believes that the facts he or she has stated are true, and that the opinions expressed are correct.[15]

If individuals are medically examined for a report, doctors need to check that the solicitor has properly communicated to the client the exact reason for the medico-legal appointment. Doctors should normally reiterate the fact that it is not a therapeutic exchange and information will be disclosed in the doctor's subsequent report. Consent should be sought for both the examination and subsequent disclosure of information. When writing reports, it is important that doctors restrict comments to relevant clinical issues and do not ask questions that lead the report towards unnecessary or inappropriate assumptions of potential liability. Nor should doctors get drawn into commenting on the standard of care the patient has received unless specifically invited to do so. Where expert witnesses are asked to give an opinion about individuals without having had the opportunity to examine them, they should explain the impact that this is likely to have on the report. When writing reports, doctors should bear in mind that they will be read by all parties involved in the action, as well as the presiding officer of the court. Doctors should also consider that the report will be read by people who have no medical training. Wherever possible, doctors should use clear non-technical language that can be understood by an intelligent lay person. Technical terms, abbreviations or other unfamiliar terms should be explained.

As a general principle, an expert should not accept instructions in any matter in which there is an actual or potential conflict of interest. If doctors are acquainted with the person, or if they stand to benefit from the case, they need to consider seriously whether it is appropriate to give evidence as an expert. In exceptional cases, if full disclosure of the nature of the conflict is made by the medical expert and acknowledged by those commissioning the report, it may be acceptable to take instructions. If an actual or potential conflict of interest arises only in the course of preparing the report, the doctor must notify all concerned of this and, if appropriate, return the instructions and resign from the case. In addition, doctors must not be offered, or accept, instructions where payments will be linked to the nature of the evidence given or to the outcome of the case.

In order to provide constructive feedback for medical experts, some judges arrange for their judgments to be provided to the experts at the end of the case, and recommend that they are given debriefing letters from the instructing solicitors. This can clearly assist experts in their practice, and doctors offering expert witness services should consider requesting such feedback as a routine part of their work. Many courts also provide witness training days, which offer an opportunity to develop the skills necessary to become a good expert witness.

The GMC has a guidance note for doctors acting as expert witnesses.[16] The BMA's Medico-legal Committee also publishes detailed advice on a variety of aspects of medico-legal work, including for both professional and expert witnesses.[17]

Reforming the delivery of expert opinion in health

In 2006, the Chief Medical Officer (CMO) published a report into the delivery of medical expert evidence in family law cases.[18] The report was produced in response to a small number of high-profile criminal court cases that threw doubt on the quality of medical expert witnesses, in particular the evidence of a small number of paediatricians relating to cases where mothers were accused of killing or seriously harming their children. In these cases, serious concerns arose as to whether disputed medical evidence had led to a miscarriage of justice. At the same time, the Family Justice Council received reports that there was a severe shortage of clinicians prepared to give evidence in the family courts. The CMO's report, *Bearing Good Witness*, outlined a number of proposals for reforming the delivery of medical expert evidence. The report recommended that the provision of expert witnesses in family law cases should no longer be based on informal and ad hoc local arrangements between solicitors and doctors. It should be replaced by publicly commissioned multi-disciplinary teams of health professionals from the NHS and other public, private or voluntary sector organisations.

In 2009, the Legal Services Commission (LSC) set up a pilot to explore the feasibility of the CMO's key recommendation.[19] The LSC set out to contract with and pay directly a number of NHS and private organisations in order to ensure the provision of high quality expert opinion within court timescales and based on agreed rates of pay. Although the pilot initially related to the provision of medical expertise in family law cases, it is intended that the system will be extended more widely. The pilot concluded in 2010, and once the evaluation of the pilot has been published, the LSC will develop recommendations for future development, including the potential for the approach to be rolled out to other types of proceedings. (Further information is available on the LSC website.[20])

Summary – expert witnesses

- The primary duty of the expert witness is to assist the court.
- The impartiality of expert witnesses is essential.
- If individuals are medically examined for a report, doctors need to check that the solicitor has properly communicated to the client, and that the client has understood, the reason or reasons for the medico-legal appointment and that the client consents both to the examination and disclosure of information.

Refereeing firearms licences

Doctors are sometimes asked to act as referees or countersignatories for people wanting to own firearms or shotguns and this has been a source of concern for some doctors, believing it to involve them to some extent in making judgements about likely future risk. There is nothing to prevent doctors from countersigning shotgun certificate applications when they are simply acting as a person of good standing. In the same circumstances there is no bar to them acting as a referee for a firearm certificate application. Where the applicant is a patient, however, doctors are advised not to endorse such applications unless they believe that they have sufficient knowledge about the individual to justify a judgement that the individual could safely possess and control such firearms or shotguns. In the BMA's view, such occasions will probably be rare. Doctors must make it clear that they are in no position to judge the 'future dangerousness' of any applicant.

Current legal situation

Application forms for firearms and for shotguns are different. Applicants for both need to provide a number of medical details, including whether they suffer from any 'medical condition or disability including alcohol and drug related conditions'. They also have to make a declaration as to whether or not they have ever suffered from epilepsy or been treated for 'depression or any other kind of mental or nervous disorder'.[21]

An application for a firearm requires two referees. They must have known the applicant personally for 2 years, be 'of good character' and be resident in Great Britain. They cannot be members of the applicant's immediate family. An application for a shotgun, by contrast, requires the endorsement of a single countersignatory in place of the referees. Countersignatories are required to confirm that they know of no reason why the applicant should not be permitted to possess a shotgun and to 'bear in mind the character, conduct and mental condition of the applicant in so far as they are relevant'.[22] At the time of writing, the Home Office was considering replacing the countersignatories for shotgun certificates with a single referee.

Medical information

Application forms for both firearm and shotgun certificates require the applicant to give permission for the police to approach the applicant's GP in order to obtain factual details of the applicant's medical history. In 2010, following discussion between the Association of Chief Police Officers and the British Medical Association, agreement was reached that where an individual applied for a firearms' certificate, or for a renewal of an existing certificate, his or her GP would automatically be informed. Should the GP have any concerns, then these should be raised in a return letter. In addition to this, the police may request details from the GP on other occasions where genuine doubts arise about the applicant's medical history that may have a bearing on the applicant's suitability to possess firearms. Where police do require additional information, requests should be limited to specific factual issues, and requests for access to the entire medical record should not normally be agreed to.

Any requests for the release of further information require consent from the applicant. If the applicant does not give consent, the information should not be provided unless the doctor has reason to believe that the applicant may pose a risk to themselves or others if the request for a licence were granted. (For applicants who may pose a risk to themselves or others, see section below.)

Role of the referee or countersignatory

The decision as to whether an individual is fit to hold firearms or shotguns rests in law with the police and, ultimately, the courts. Under the Firearms Act 1968, the onus is therefore on a chief officer of the police, not the countersignatory or referee, to be satisfied that the applicant has a good reason for acquiring a shotgun or firearm and that its acquisition would not be prejudicial to public safety or peace. It is also the responsibility of a chief officer to ensure that applications for firearms or shotgun certificates by anyone of 'intemperate habits or unsound mind' are refused.[23]

According to Home Office guidelines for the police,[24] the role of the countersignatory or referee is to provide information and opinions that the police can take into account when making a judgement. Neither are expected to offer an 'expert' opinion, regardless of their backgrounds. In particular, doctors acting as referees or countersignatories should do so on a personal basis rather than as medical professionals, and they should not therefore be expected to offer any medical opinion as to the applicant's mental state or likely future behaviour. It is open to the police to contact the referee or countersignatory to discuss the information provided on the reference form or any other matter relating to the application.

In its previous guidance on firearms, the BMA expressed concern that doctors were being asked to make predictions about an applicant's 'future dangerousness'. The BMA believes that doctors are not in a position to make such a judgement. The guidance from the Home Office therefore makes it clear that doctors should not, and should not be called upon, to offer such an opinion.

Issues for concern

Although the BMA welcomes the Home Office guidance relating to countersignatories and referees, it still has some concerns about the weight placed on their endorsement. Although the guidance suggests that countersignatories and referees are not called upon to offer a medical opinion, the Association is concerned that excessive emphasis may still be given to an endorsement by a doctor, because of the specialist nature of his or her expertise. Doctors who have contacted the BMA have pointed out that they very rarely have sufficient knowledge of the mental stability of an individual to certify that he or she has not suffered from any mental disorder, nor will they be able to give a meaningful medical opinion on more general issues such as the character, conduct and mental condition of the applicant.

The doctor is only one of a number of people 'of good standing' or 'good character' who can be asked to act as a countersignatory or referee for a shotgun or firearm certificate application. When the doctor is simply acting in this capacity – that is, where the applicant is not a patient – then the Association believes that there is nothing to prevent doctors from endorsing the application, as long as this is made clear. Where the applicant is a patient, however, the Association believes that doctors are not seen by the public as solely persons of good standing but are still considered to be making a medical assessment and therefore have a greater responsibility. In these circumstances, the Association advises doctors not to endorse applications unless they have a sufficiently detailed knowledge of the patient's mental and physical health to be confident that the individual can safely possess and control firearms without endangering themselves, their families or the public. The BMA expects that very few doctors will be this confident about their knowledge of a patient.

Applicants who may present a risk

In the majority of cases, individuals obtain firearm or shotgun certificates with the assistance of people of good standing, and no problems arise. In exceptional circumstances, however, a doctor may have good reason to believe that an individual either applying for a firearm or shotgun certificate, or already in possession of one, may represent a danger either to themselves or to others. In these circumstances doctors should strongly encourage the applicant to reconsider or revoke their application. If the applicant refuses, the doctor should consider breaching confidentiality and telling the police firearms licensing department of their concerns. Consent should initially be sought from the applicant for contacting the police, but if it is not possible to obtain consent, the doctor should consider making his or her concerns known without consent. Where possible, the doctor should discuss the reasons for this with the applicant beforehand. The GMC's guidelines on consent in these circumstances state:

> [p]ersonal information may … be disclosed in the public interest, without patients' consent, and in exceptional cases where patients have withheld consent, if the benefits to an individual or to society of the disclosure outweigh both the public and the patient's interest in keeping the information confidential.[25]

'Tagging' medical records

During 2009 the BMA was involved in discussions concerning the desirability of GPs placing electronic tags in medical records to indicate that the patient either held a firearm or shotgun certificate or had applied for one. The Information Commissioner has indicated, however, that the use of tags in medical records for this purpose would be in contravention of the Data Protection Act.[26]

Objections to signing firearms certificates

The BMA has received enquiries in the past from doctors who do not wish, on grounds of conscience, to sign firearm or shotgun certificate applications. Doctors are under no obligation to sign these certificates and the BMA would support any doctor who refuses such a request.

Summary – refereeing firearms licences

- Any person of good standing may act as a referee on firearms licence applications although doctors should be aware that his or her reference may be seen to reflect a medical opinion.
- Doctors need to be clear if they are being asked to comment on an applicant's 'future dangerousness'. In the BMA's view, very few doctors are likely to be in a position to do this.
- Doctors who are in a professional relationship with the applicant should not act as referees unless they are satisfied that the individual can safely possess a firearm.
- If a doctor has reason to believe that an individual either in possession of a firearms licence, or applying for one, may represent a danger to themselves or others, doctors

should strongly encourage the applicant to reconsider or revoke their application. If the applicant refuses, the doctor should consider breaching confidentiality and informing the police firearms licensing department.

• Doctors are under no obligation to sign firearm certificates.

Doctors examining asylum seekers

Individuals who arrive in the UK claiming that they have suffered torture or ill-treatment in their country of origin are ordinarily offered an examination by port medical officers employed by the Department of Health. Some of these new arrivals will apply for asylum. The BMA recognises that the identification of torture sequelae requires particular expertise and training, and cannot be done quickly. Nevertheless, brief but adequate notes and, where possible, photographs, of abnormalities taken by port medical officers, or any other doctor seeing the patient, could be crucial in the later assessment of the validity of an asylum seeker's case. It is helpful if any record made by port of entry medical officers is made available, with the patient's consent, to other doctors who examine the same individual later in connection with an asylum application. In the past, independent doctors providing reports at a later date have been unable to gain access to medical records made at the time of entry to the country. The use of hand-held records, or the provision of copies to the individual claiming asylum should be considered where appropriate.

As with the provision of all medical reports, doctors who are assessing asylum seekers must be accurate and truthful. Doctors who undertake this form of work normally build up expertise in the patterns of maltreatment or torture common to the region of the applicant's origin. They may offer an opinion about the most likely aetiology of the asylum applicant's condition, but should be able to support such an opinion on the basis of evidence or their clinical experience.

People who have suffered torture, ill-treatment and related psychological trauma in their country of origin rely partly upon medical documentation of the detectable sequelae to substantiate their claim for asylum. This can be an emotive area, and doctors asked to provide a medical report for asylum seekers must ensure both the accuracy and truthfulness of their report and that each application is subject to careful and objective scrutiny. The doctor's role is to discover and report on any material features that he or she considers relevant, even if these may adversely affect the case of the instructing party. It is no part of an examining doctor's role to give an opinion as to whether asylum should or should not be granted.

Expert assessment

Asylum seekers may be housed in the community pending adjudication, or they may be detained. (For more detailed information on the ethical implications of doctors treating detained asylum seekers, see Chapter 17, pages 724–728.) Asylum seekers do not form a homogeneous group, but some common health problems have been identified by experienced doctors working with torture survivors' rehabilitation organisations.[27] These draw attention to the fact that the full effects of any ill-treatment that the applicant may have suffered are unlikely to be immediately evident upon initial examination. Although conclusive physical signs are apparent in only a minority of cases, predictable patterns of psychological sequelae are nevertheless common. It should be noted, however, that medical opinion varies concerning the extent to which such sequelae may be categorised as exclusive to survivors of certain types of trauma. Earlier trauma can also be complicated by subsequent traumatic experiences, such as those encountered in transit.

Psychological sequelae of torture can also take a long time to emerge, which can be problematic given the time limits imposed upon asylum applications. Discussing past physical abuse, particularly if it involved cultural taboos such as sexual humiliation, is likely to be extremely difficult for the applicant. Doctors must also recognise that there are often cultural differences in the way in which patients present medical symptoms and the importance they accord to different types of injury. Doctors should bear in mind when examining asylum seekers that it is not part of their function to give an opinion on whether asylum should be granted.

In recent years the BMA has been concerned about the possible involvement of health professionals and health technology in the age assessment of young asylum seekers. Local authorities have different statutory responsibilities in relation to minors, and age assessment can have a significant bearing on the nature of the support offered to the asylum seeker. There has been considerable controversy over the use of bone X-rays, for example, to identify the age of asylum seekers. In the BMA's view, given the unreliability of bone age assessment, the small but definite levels of risk involved in using ionising radiation and the absence of any clinical justification, it would be inappropriate for doctors to be involved in this practice.

The London-based organisations, the Medical Foundation for the Care of Victims of Torture and the Helen Bamber Foundation, provide volunteer doctors experienced in documenting evidence of torture, who can give a medical assessment. The BMA also publishes a separate guide to the health needs of asylum seekers.[28]

Language services

Finding appropriate interpretation services for asylum seekers can sometimes present a problem. In some cases, other members of the patient's family or cultural group offer to interpret. This raises potential problems with confidentiality and should be avoided unless there is an emergency and no other interpreter can be found. Confidentiality issues can be particularly acute if patients want to discuss sensitive information or need to access services such as family planning, abortion or HIV testing. Some UK commissioners of health services, including most of those in London, provide interpretation services, although paying for them can present problems. Wherever possible, sensitivity should be exercised in selecting interpreters, with regard to factors such as gender and political or cultural background. This is particularly important in cases where patients need to discuss very personal issues such as sexual health or traumatic experiences. Health services should not rely on embassies or official agencies of the patient's home country if the patient claims to have been persecuted or tortured because information may be collected that puts patients at risk and may jeopardise the safety of their relatives. Where possible, professional interpreters experienced at working with asylum seekers should be used. Untrained third parties should ordinarily be avoided, unless there is no alternative.

Summary – doctors examining asylum seekers

- When preparing reports for asylum applications accuracy and truthfulness are essential.
- Identifying the sequelae of torture requires specialist knowledge and sensitive interaction with patients.

- Doctors are advised not to involve themselves in the use of X-rays to establish the age of young asylum seekers.
- Where interpreters are used, doctors need to give particular consideration to issues of confidentiality.

Pre-employment reports and testing

Employers sometimes need to confirm prospective employees' medical fitness for the job. They can also have duties to third parties that require them to assess whether their employees pose any threat to others. NHS trusts, for example, owe a clear duty of care to their patients and, if they fail to undertake suitable vetting procedures for prospective employees, they may be failing in this duty. This was highlighted by the Clothier Report, which examined the deaths and injuries caused by nurse Beverly Allitt and put forward the following recommendations for the screening of people entering the nursing profession.[29]

- For all those seeking entry into nursing, in addition to routine references, the most recent employer or place of study should be asked to provide at least a record of sick leave.
- Nurses should undergo formal health screening when they obtain their first post after qualifying.
- The possibility should be explored of making available to occupational health departments any records of sickness absence from any institution that an applicant for a nursing post has attended or where he or she has been employed.
- Consideration may be given to how GPs could, with the consent of candidates, be asked to certify that there is nothing in the medical history of candidates for employment in the NHS that would make them unsuitable for their chosen occupation.

More recently, following on from the inquiry into Beverly Allitt, a rigorous system of employment checks, both for those seeking to work in the NHS and for those already employed, have been put in place. These include those checks required by law, by DH policy and for the purposes of gaining access to the NHS Care Record Service.

Pre-employment assessments

Where employers are intending to use pre-employment assessments, the purpose of the system must be clearly established, and any assessment must be proportionate to the goal it is seeking to achieve. Health screening, even by means of a questionnaire, is an invasion of privacy, and, as the Data Protection Act 1998 lays out, the information that is sought must be 'adequate, relevant and not excessive in relation to the purpose.'[30] Occupational health advisers should bear in mind that, under equality legislation, it is unlawful for an employer to treat a disabled job applicant or employee less favourably because of their disability, unless that disability has a direct bearing on their ability to perform the task, even after appropriate adjustments have been made.

Employers sometimes seek to obtain information about the impact of health conditions on the ability of employees to perform their roles by commissioning GP reports or independent examinations. Consent is always needed in these cases. Those applying for jobs may effectively bar themselves from that particular post if they do not agree to information being disclosed, but the BMA does not believe that pressure of that nature necessarily invalidates their consent, provided that they are properly informed and only relevant information is sought. It helps if prospective employers provide clear detailed criteria of the conditions that are being looked for and why.

If potential employees prohibit doctors from disclosing information to the employer, doctors must respect their decision. The fact of refusal must be made clear to the employer, taking care to avoid revealing any details. However, there may be exceptional circumstances, such as where the prospective employee may put individuals at risk of significant harm, in which confidentiality may be breached and information disclosed to a potential employer or appropriate agency (see Chapter 5).

Patients have statutory rights of access to reports written about them for employment purposes. Detailed advice is given in Chapter 6, pages 260–261.

When doctors are involved in designing pre-employment medical questionnaires, they should encourage employers to limit the information requested to that which is directly relevant to an individual's fitness for the particular work concerned. Health problems that do not affect their ability to perform the tasks they will be employed to undertake are not relevant. The doctor involved should be familiar with both the workplace and the types of employment involved. Wherever possible, specific information should be requested and 'catch all' type questions should be avoided. Doctors need to be aware that claims of racial, sexual or disability discrimination could arise from the collection of irrelevant medical data. It could also breach the third data protection principle referred to above, that information 'shall be adequate, relevant and not excessive in relation to the purpose or purposes for which they are processed'.[31] The NHS Employers website contains extensive information about pre-employment checks.[32] The Information Commissioner's Office has also produced a detailed employment practice code concerning the data protection responsibilities relating to the requesting, processing and retention of health and related data for employment processes.[33]

Pre-employment testing for HIV, drugs and alcohol

When any pre-employment testing is carried out, it must be done to the highest clinical and ethical standards, and the consent of the individual must be obtained. Employers should only be testing for conditions relevant to employment. In relation to blood-borne viruses for example, screening can be relevant for clinicians carrying out exposure-prone procedures, but it will not be necessary to test someone for HIV for a job that does not involve such procedures, and the individual's HIV status is not otherwise relevant.

Employers who require testing should inform people of the precise nature of the tests and to whom the results may be disclosed. The Faculty of Occupational Medicine publishes guidance on the ethics of drug testing in the workplace, which sets out good practice for testing both job applicants and current employees for illicit substances.[34] When employers wish to use pre-employment testing, a clear explanation must be given to potential employees so that they can make an informed choice about whether or not to undergo that test. Pre-employment testing of health professionals is covered in more detail in Chapter 21.

Consent for pre-employment testing

When applying for a temporary position with the European Commission as a typist, Mr X had a medical examination but refused to be screened for HIV antibodies. During the examination, a blood sample was taken and the medical officer ordered blood tests in order to determine the T4 and T8 lymphocyte counts. When these were below the normal ratio, the medical officer concluded that Mr X was suffering from a significant immunodeficiency constituting a case of AIDS. He was thus rejected on the grounds of his physical condition. Mr X brought a legal case on the grounds that he had been effectively subjected to an AIDS screening test without his consent.

Although the court of first instance supported the employer's decision, the European Court of Justice held that the manner in which Mr X had been medically examined and declared physically unfit constituted an infringement of his right to respect for his private life as guaranteed by Article 8 of the European Convention on Human Rights. The court said that:

> [t]he right to respect for private life, embodied in Article 8 and deriving from the common constitutional traditions of the Member States is one of the fundamental rights protected by the legal order of the Community. It includes in particular a person's right to keep his state of health secret.

It went on to say that:

> although the pre-employment medical examination serves a legitimate interest of the Community institutions, which must be in a position to fulfil the tasks required of them, that interest does not justify the carrying out of a test against the will of the person concerned ... If the person concerned, after being properly informed, withholds his consent to a test which the medical officer considers necessary in order to evaluate his suitability for the post for which he has applied, the institutions cannot be obliged to take the risk of recruiting him.[35]

GP involvement in pre-employment assessments

Some of the same concerns that arise with reports for insurance are evident in queries from BMA members about pre-employment reports. GPs sometimes question the extent of medical information that potential employers seek. They point out that, although the patient gives consent, in areas of high unemployment, for example, the individual has little free choice in the matter. There are also concerns that patients may decline to inform their doctors of certain episodes of illness if they believe that they may need a pre-employment report at a later date.

Some argue that this pressure on patients to agree means that any consent cannot be valid. The BMA is concerned about anecdotal evidence that patients do withhold information, but considers that it would be incorrect for doctors to pre-empt patient choice and to assume it is necessarily contrary to the patient's interest to provide information. The decision about whether to authorise disclosure must ultimately rest with the patient. Patients should be encouraged to see the report before it is sent if GPs believe that there is information that may affect their chances of getting the job, so that patients are forewarned. Although at this stage patients may choose to withdraw their consent for the report to be sent, they cannot demand that information that the doctor believes to be relevant is withheld. If asked to do this, doctors should explain that they must be honest and, in accordance with the guidance from the GMC,[36] must not deliberately leave out relevant information.

In a similar vein, patients may give consent for the release of information to a potential employer because if it is withheld the employer will draw adverse conclusions. The BMA believes that it is not for the doctor to enquire into the motives that underlie a consent freely given in full knowledge of the implications. Therefore, provided the statutory requirements relating to consent for reports have been met, doctors should accept the consent given. As with insurance reports, doctors should retain a copy of the letter of consent and, if they have any concerns about its validity, they should check with the patient.

In their reports, GPs should limit themselves to statements of fact. Commenting on whether they are aware of any health reason why a patient would be unsuitable for a job is acceptable, but they should be wary of making more general judgements about suitability for employment or to make value judgements about previous periods of absence through sickness. It is not the role of the GP to predict future actions by patients, or to try to judge the likelihood of future health problems. GPs should limit themselves to certifying whether there is anything in the medical record that raises concerns about the suitability of the person for the job or activity in question. It is then for the prospective employer to make a judgement about suitability for employment. Clearly, GPs should have sufficient relevant knowledge of the nature and context of the job for which the person has applied before making any assessment about fitness for work or related matters.

Genetic screening for employment purposes

Although it has been predicted that employers may wish to use genetic screening of employees and prospective employees, there is very little evidence that this is happening. Although employers are not asking specific questions about existing genetic tests, doctors sometimes ask the BMA about their responsibility to disclose such information in response to general health questions. These can include whether there is anything in the medical record that raises concerns about the individual's current or future health or ability to meet the requirements of the job, or about recent referrals to specialists. Clearly, a positive predictive genetic test result, or a referral to a geneticist because of a family history of a late onset genetic disorder, falls into that category and doctors may be obliged to release the information in order to answer the question truthfully. There are a number of difficulties with this information being requested in this indirect manner. First, the patient may not be aware that the information will be provided if there is no specific question about genetic tests, so the consent obtained may not be valid. Secondly, the employer or occupational health department receiving the information may not have the necessary expertise to interpret it accurately. There is therefore a risk that all people who have had a positive genetic test, or those with a family history of a genetic disorder, may be excluded from employment even though they may not be affected by the disorder for many years, or possibly at all. Although people with disabilities have some protection under disability discrimination legislation, those who have had an unfavourable genetic test do not, if they are asymptomatic, because they would not fall within the definition of a person with a 'disability'. A further problem with such indirect requests is that the true extent to which employers are using genetic information is hidden. This presents difficulties for those who are responsible for monitoring the situation and deciding whether additional safeguards are needed.

If sensitive information is required to answer questions on the report accurately, doctors must ensure that the patient is aware of any such information that may be revealed, and has given consent on that basis. Even when patients have chosen not to see the report before it is sent, it would be a sensible precaution for the doctor to discuss its content with the patient in these circumstances. Doctors presenting genetic information in reports also have a responsibility to see that it is both accurate and fair, and provides sufficient detail to put it in context. This could include providing information about the meaning of a particular genetic test and possibly suggesting that additional specialist advice should be sought. Occupational health doctors receiving such information, in turn, have a responsibility to respond fairly and, where necessary, to seek more specialist advice. More information about genetics and employment can be found in Chapter 9.

Information about occupational hazards

Genetic testing may also be suggested as a way of identifying those who are more susceptible to the occupational hazards of a particular type of employment. In theory, this information could help people to make informed decisions about their choice of employment, although it needs to be recognised that, in some areas of high unemployment, such choices may be constrained. Employers could use screening to help them to fulfil their duties under health and safety legislation, to provide a safe working environment, without making themselves liable under current anti-discrimination legislation. A common concern is that, rather than improving the working environment, employers could simply exclude from employment anyone who represents a higher than the average risk. This would save the employer the cost of making improvements to the working environment and may also save them from paying out compensation for work-related injuries at a later stage.

To an extent these concerns are speculative. There is a lack of certainty about the genetics of susceptibility to hazardous substances in the workplace and there is no evidence that such screening is being used. It is possible, however, that such screening could be developed in the future.

Summary – pre-employment reports and testing

- Pre-employment medical reports should be restricted to information that is relevant to the job.
- Patients must be properly informed about the nature and purpose of any disclosure to a potential employer.
- Patients have a right of access to pre-employment reports prepared by their GP.
- Consent for disclosure of reports is essential, and doctors should not assume that simply because patients are under pressure to give consent that this is necessarily invalid.
- If a report contains information that is sensitive or likely to be prejudicial to the patient's interests then even when patients have chosen not to see the report before it is sent, it would be a sensible precaution to discuss its content with the patient.

Occupational health physicians

Occupational medicine deals with the effects of work on health and the impact of the employee's health on his or her performance and that of others in the workforce. The objectives of an occupational health service can be summarised in five points:

- to promote and maintain the health and safety of employees
- to provide emergency treatment for sick and injured employees
- to advise on rehabilitation and suitable placement of employees who are temporarily or permanently disabled by illness or injury
- to promote safe and healthy conditions by informed assessment of the working environment and by providing advice or educative material
- to promote research into causes of occupational diseases and the means of their prevention.[37]

Occupational health physicians must act as impartial professional advisers, concerned with the health of all those employed in the organisation. Such responsibilities can, however, lead to very real dilemmas such as when the doctor believes that the working environment may exacerbate health problems for certain employees or applicants for employment. Statutory and other periodic medical examinations may also identify health problems that may have an impact on continued employment. Pilots, workers in the atomic energy industry and individuals who develop allergies to products that they are required to handle are examples of difficult cases. Here, occupational health physicians must be careful not to take over the role of the line manager in deciding whether such an individual should be offered employment or dismissed. The patient must be reminded that the doctor's role, as the agent of a third party in such cases, is to advise the employer, with the individual's consent, of possible health problems that could arise.

Pre-employment assessment

When occupational health physicians undertake pre-employment assessments, their primary responsibility is to the employer, although there is still a duty of care owed to the applicant to conduct a clinically sound examination that is appropriate for the job in question. Generally speaking, a medical examination is normally justified only when the job involves working in hazardous environments, requires high standards of fitness, is required by law or when the safety of other workers or of the public is concerned. Usually, a health assessment by questionnaire should suffice, and occupational health physicians have an important role in advising about what standards of mental and physical health are necessary for a particular job. In relation to health professionals, both the Department of Health and the BMA, have further guidance on pre-employment testing.[38] This issue is also covered in more detail in Chapter 21.

Confidentiality

Although paid by the management, the occupational health physician's duties concern the health and welfare of the whole workforce, both individually and collectively. They have similar duties of confidentiality as other doctors. The fact that a doctor is a salaried employee gives no other employee of that company any right of access to medical records or to the details of examination findings. With the employee's consent, the employer may be advised of any relevant information relating to a specific matter on a strictly need to know basis, the significance of which the employee clearly understands. If an employer explicitly or implicitly invites an employee to consult the occupational health physician, the latter must still regard such consultations as strictly confidential. It is also important to recognise that managers and human resources staff are seldom qualified to interpret medical details. It is unlikely therefore that there will be many occasions when they need direct access to confidential medical information. Instead, occupational health physicians should provide information on the likely impact of any underlying medical conditions on the worker's ability to perform his or her tasks, or the effect working conditions might have on an individual's health. If this does require the disclosure of confidential information, consent is required. The Court of Appeal has ruled that employers have no rights of access to occupational health records and are not presumed to know information held only by their occupational health physician.

Confidentiality of occupational health records

In 2005, the Court of Appeal simultaneously heard several cases involving claims for psychiatric damages arising from stress at work. In the case of Mrs Hartman, the court of first instance held that the employing Trust should have known, on the basis of information held by the Trust's occupational health department (OHD), that she was suffering from a stress-related psychological disorder. Overturning the judgment, the Court of Appeal cited BMA guidance and held that 'it was not right to attribute to the Trust in their capacity as employers, knowledge of confidential medical information disclosed by Mrs Hartman to the OHD'.[39] The Court established that employers have no rights of access to occupational health records and are not presumed to know information held only by their occupational health physician.

Occupational health professionals should bear in mind that both employees and employers can have a poor understanding of the kinds of health information that can be both held, and disclosed, by occupational health services. It can be helpful if occupational health practitioners develop clear guidelines on confidentiality and the recording and disclosure of health information in the work setting. Employees should be informed at the earliest opportunity if clinical records are being created, by, for example, including a statement to that effect on any pre-employment health questionnaire. The Faculty of Occupational Medicine also recommends that an explicit policy on confidentiality is developed, which should include details of who, within the occupational health team, can access the information and for what purpose.[40]

The occupational health physician and nurse are responsible for ensuring the confidentiality of clinical records. The arrangements for custody of the records should be defined in the occupational health physician's contract of employment. Under the supervision of the occupational health team, clerical support staff may see clinical records in the same way as staff in a GP's surgery; that is, when they have a legitimate 'need to know' the information for the purposes of providing support to the occupational health clinician. The occupational health physician must ensure that such staff understand the need for confidentiality and have a contractual obligation to preserve it.

Although individual clinical findings are confidential, their significance may be made known to an appropriate third party, such as the employer or health and safety representatives. Thus, while the reading of a laboratory result is confidential to the individual tested, it is nonetheless proper to disclose to those with a responsibility for overseeing safety that a group, or an individual, shows, for example, a significant degree of exposure to a potentially toxic hazard. Similarly, although a report of being 'fit' or 'unfit' for work can be made known to the employer, the clinical details cannot be disclosed unless the individual gives consent.

Where occupational physicians believe that a process or product in the workplace constitutes a risk to health, they should try to persuade the employer to take action. Even when there are issues of commercial secrecy, the doctor's responsibility for the health of workers exposed to the hazard takes precedence over the obligations to management. If employers fail to take necessary action, doctors should take urgent advice from their professional, regulatory or indemnifying bodies. Alternatively, the Health and Safety Executive is also able to offer impartial and, if necessary, anonymous advice. More detailed information on the use of health data in the workplace is available from the Information Commissioner.[41]

Consent to examination

In some companies, employees are required by statute or their contracts to undergo medical examinations. Examples of examinations of fitness required by statute include drivers of heavy goods or public service vehicles, workers in the atomic industry and airline pilots. Industries that involve food handling frequently impose contractual obligations on employees to undergo examination after sickness absence or where they have been in contact with anyone with a gastrointestinal infection or virus. Examinations are also required under legislation regulating hazardous substances. Doctors working in this field will be aware of these requirements, and advice is given by the BMA's Occupational Health Committee.[42]

It is important not to infer from an employee's attendance at a contractually imposed health assessment that the person agrees both to the examination and to the disclosure of the result. Doctors should ensure that employees understand the context in which the examination takes place, the nature of the examination, the need for disclosure of the significance of the findings and what, if any, clinical information is to be disclosed. Employees should be informed of these things in their contract of employment or corresponding reference documents, and consent forms specifying both examination and disclosure of relevant findings should be signed by the employee on each occasion that a medical examination is required by the employer. One-off or 'blanket' consent for examination or subsequent disclosure at the start of the contract is not sufficient.

Random drug testing

The BMA is sometimes asked to comment on schemes for doctors to conduct random drug or other testing among both applicants for employment and current employees. Such testing, although not widespread in the UK, is sometimes justified by the argument that the employee or applicant may endanger the lives of others if impaired by drugs or alcohol.

The BMA believes that job applicants and employees should be informed explicitly, and in advance, for example via clauses in the contract of employment to which their attention should be drawn, that testing is required on a regular or random basis. General advice about drug misuse should also be provided. When employers are considering implementing drug testing, it is important that the tests used are proportionate and appropriate to the risk that has been identified. Drug testing should only be used where less intrusive tests are not sufficient to address the risk.

When employees provide samples to be tested for other purposes, it is not acceptable for them to be tested for drugs without these individuals being told of this possibility and giving consent. Seeking to use samples for other purposes could breach employees' rights to privacy as enshrined in Article 8 of the European Convention on Human Rights and given effect in UK domestic law by the Human Rights Act 1998.

Clinical tests for alcohol or drugs are subject to the same degree of confidentiality as any other medical examination. However, where the results indicate that the person is affected by drugs or alcohol and is, as a result, putting others at risk, doctors may need to consider whether it is appropriate for information to be passed to management. A line may need to be drawn between intoxication at work, for which there should be appropriate disciplinary procedures, and, where they can be identified, the health effects of chronic misuse, although this is more likely to be a management than a medical issue. In some cases it may be sufficient for the doctor to declare that the individual is unfit for work without specifying the reasons. When disclosure is necessary, voluntary disclosure should be the aim. Circumstances in which it may be necessary to override confidentiality in the public interest are discussed in Chapter 5, pages 199–206. Advice about what to do if you have health concerns about members of the health team is given in Chapter 21, pages 879–883.

The introduction of a policy of random drug testing is unlikely to be controversial where the use of drugs or alcohol could lead to a risk of serious harm to either the individual, fellow workers or members of the public. More problematic is the use of such policies to promote a drug-free working environment for the sake of a positive corporate image. In these circumstances, legal advice should be taken as such policies could be in breach of human rights legislation.

The involvement of health staff in the 'policing' of employment procedures should be avoided. It is not a legitimate role for them to adopt and it may also undermine their status as confidential medical advisers.

Sickness absence

Occupational physicians do not usually become involved in confirming or refuting that an individual employee's absence from work is due to sickness or injury, but can sometimes assist in the management and analysis of sickness absence. In such cases, it is crucial to separate out the roles and responsibilities of managers and occupational physicians, and for employees to be aware of these different roles.

On an employee's return to work, the occupational physician is responsible for advising management on the worker's fitness for the job and may be asked to assess whether temporary or permanent modifications to the work are necessary. Doctors should inform employees of the advice they intend to give management and seek the employee's consent to discuss with the employer any important changes required by the employee's present health state.

In order for occupational health physicians to be able to give informed advice to an employer about a member of staff who has had long or frequent sick leave, they need to be able to see and examine the employee and, if necessary, to contact the relevant GP or hospital consultant, with the written consent of the employee. The importance of good communication between the occupational health physician and the GP or hospital consultant cannot be overstated. This is vital in helping the occupational health physician to give well-informed advice to both employer and employee. If the occupational health physician examines a worker who is or has been absent for health reasons, the GP should, with the patient's consent, be informed of any conclusion reached.

If an employee's record of sickness absence is very prolonged, the occupational health physician may be asked to advise both employee and employer about future employability. Although the employer has no right to clinical details of sickness or injury, it is reasonable for employers to expect the doctor to give an opinion about the anticipated date of the employee's return to work, the employee's work capacity, the likely degree and duration of any disability and the likelihood of future absences. If employees request that doctors do not release this information to their employers, doctors should take advice from their professional, regulatory or indemnifying body. In general, medical information should not be released without the patient's or client's consent. Employees should be aware, however, that it is the prerogative of management to take action against an employee who has been sick long term or is too frequently absent from work, even if the employee refuses to authorise a medical report. In any cases where the dismissal is challenged by the individual as unfair or discriminatory under disability discrimination legislation, the occupational health physician may be called upon by either party to give evidence as a professional witness to the employment tribunal. Again, honesty and impartiality are crucial.

Occupational health records

Occupational health records provide a factual record of employees' health status for the purposes of workplace risk management and safety. In addition, they can be a very powerful tool in research into work-related diseases. The usual rules about patient consent for the use of records in research apply, and any research using occupational health records should have the approval of an appropriately constituted research ethics committee (see Chapter 14). Access to occupational health records is governed by the Data Protection Act 1998 (see Chapter 6, pages 255–258).

If an employee has incurred injury or illness at work and is taking legal action against the employer, the occupational health physician may, with the individual's written informed consent, provide the legal advisers of both sides with factual information about attendance at medical departments, first aid and other treatment. In all questions of litigation, clinical records or abstracts from them should not be released without the individual's written consent. However, a court or employment tribunal may order disclosure.

If a particular document or set of documents is ordered to be disclosed, then the doctor or nurse has a duty to disclose them or to challenge the disclosure in the court or tribunal. However, if the nurse or doctor is to challenge the disclosure, then he or she must bring the originals to court in case the order is upheld. It is also important that written consent is obtained for records to be released to trade union representatives.

Transfer of records

Arrangements must be made for the proper transfer of health records to another doctor or occupational health nurse when the occupational health physician leaves the company or when an occupational health facility is closed down. It follows therefore that records should be kept in such a way as to facilitate either transfer, or, if appropriate, destruction (see below). Where records are being transferred, occupational health professionals should, in accordance with responsibilities under the Data Protection Act, make arrangements to inform the data subjects that their information is being transferred. Where the doctor does not have a clear contract or agreement, supervision of the records can be left in doubt when the doctor moves on. In some cases, doctors have attempted to take records with them in the belief that they own them, but the position in law is not clear. Although it is likely to be the case that the employer owns the material in or on which the data is stored, in these circumstances the data itself is usually considered to be the property of its author. The BMA believes that if no other doctor or nurse has been appointed to succeed the occupational health physician, the latter retains responsibility for the custody of those records. If an occupational health department closes, the medical records should be transferred to the care of medical staff on another site in that organisation. Alternatively, the records may be offered to a part-time doctor if there is one, or to a suitably qualified nurse who has responsibility for workers. In the absence of occupational health staff, it is acceptable for medical records to be kept securely locked, within the organisation, as long as they can be accessed only by a registered medical practitioner. If the employer's business closes down, the clinician who was in charge of occupational health should take advice from the regional Health and Safety Executive officer about appropriate retention or disposal. Doctors may also contact the BMA's Occupational Health Committee for advice. When the continued security of medical records cannot be guaranteed, the records may be offered to the patients or, if the patients decline or cannot be traced, destruction of the records may be considered (but see below).

Occupational health records should normally be retained for at least 10 years after the termination of an employee's service. Records of significant exposures, episodes or accidents should, however, be retained for at least 30 years. There are also statutory requirements relating to the retention of records that relate to exposure to ionising radiation and other substances that may be hazardous to health.[43] In order to save space or to improve clerical efficiency, old records may be stored electronically. If external contractors are used to assist in the archiving process, their contract must contain a confidentiality clause. (Further information on health records is available in Chapter 6.)

Liaison with colleagues

The occupational health practitioner deals constantly with the patients of other doctors and, in order to ensure the best management of these patients, should generally provide treatment only in cooperation with the patients' own doctors, except in an emergency. Similarly, in an emergency, the occupational health physician may refer a patient to a hospital or to a specialist, but thereafter they should inform the patient's usual doctor of the action taken. Patient consent must be obtained for liaison between the occupational physician and the GP. Where there is a work-related health problem that is not an emergency, the occupational health physician should seek consent to write to the patient's GP if a referral is necessary, or arrange referral in agreement with the GP.

Summary – occupational health physicians

- Occupational health physicians must act as impartial professional advisers and this should be made clear to both employers and employees.
- Occupational health physicians have the same duty of confidentiality as other doctors. Rarely, it may be necessary to reveal information without consent; when this is necessary, employees should be informed and clinical details kept to a minimum.
- The involvement of health staff in the 'policing' of employment procedures should be avoided.
- Patients must be reminded of doctors' obligations to third parties and the impact of such obligations on the patient.
- Consent is required every time an employee undergoes an examination or test.
- Occupational health records provide a factual record of employees' health status for the purposes of workplace risk management and safety. They can also be a powerful tool for research into work-related diseases.

Doctors in the armed forces

All members of the armed forces are subject to both civil and military law. A doctor in the armed forces must obey any lawful command; disobedience is punishable by means of various sanctions including those determined by court martial. In addition, however, like all doctors, those serving in the forces must behave in accordance with professional ethics.

Doctors working in the armed forces are responsible for their professional actions to the same extent as any other doctor, and are expected to work to the same ethical standards. It follows therefore that it would be unethical for a medical officer to be required to treat a patient under the constraint of non-medical orders when the doctor believes that treatment is not in the individual's best interests.

When doctors in the armed forces believe that the medical resources available to them are substandard, it is important that they discuss this with their commanding officers. If this fails to remedy the situation, doctors need to consider whether the best interests of their patients would be served by 'blowing the whistle'. Advice can be sought from the BMA's Armed Forces Committee. (See also Chapter 21 for further information on whistleblowing.)

Another ethical issue sometimes facing doctors serving in the armed forces relates to individuals asking to be declared unfit for active service after receiving notification that they are to be sent to a war zone, or upon learning that war has been declared. Here, doctors must be particularly vigilant to ensure that they make a dispassionate, impartial and independent evaluation of the individuals concerned on the basis of sound medical principles.

Confidentiality

Doctors working in the armed forces may at times need to balance the interests of the individual patient's confidentiality and the interests of the unit of which he or she is a part. It follows therefore that there will be occasions when a medical officer is required to discuss the personal health information of patients with a commanding officer. Wherever possible, they should do this with consent. Although doctors working in the armed forces have the same duty of confidentiality as other doctors, the extreme situations in which they often work means that information needs to be shared much more often than in civilian life. Ill health of service personnel can put the lives of others at risk and jeopardise military goals, so circumstances are likely to arise where, even if the patient refuses, the 'public interest' in disclosure overrides confidentiality (see Chapter 5, pages 199–206). When a doctor in the armed forces feels that it is appropriate that information is disclosed to a commanding officer, he or she should notify the patient of the information that is to be released and the reasons for its disclosure. Doctors should ensure that only information that is necessary to the issue at hand is released. Additional details that do not have a bearing on the health of the individual patient or are not relevant to the issue for which disclosure is required (such as his or her sexual orientation) should not be released.

In many cases, the liberties that people in the armed forces have given up are also lost to other members of their families, who may find that, in practice, they have no choice of medical practitioner and have reduced rights of confidentiality, because it is assumed that the health of the families may affect the service personnel and the unit. This raises some very difficult issues for such families. If, for example, a child is suspected of having suffered abuse, it would be customary for the officer in charge of welfare to attend the case conference. In effect, this is involving a representative of the employer, and would be unacceptable in other situations. It is a matter for the judgement of the individual doctor to decide how much information to disclose in these circumstances.

Consent

To a certain extent, individuals who join the armed forces freely revoke some of their freedoms for the duration of their term of service. They are expected to follow orders issued for the benefit of the unit, platoon, ship or squadron of which they are part and to the interests of which they subject their own. Discipline is an essential part of the effective functioning of the services, which must inevitably set greater than normal limits to the exercise of freedom of choice. This extends to some degree to consent for certain medical procedures. When there may be doubt, for example about an individual's fitness for combat, or if it is believed that his or her mental or physical health presents a threat to others, he or she may be ordered to submit to appropriate medical testing, or, exceptionally, to certain forms of treatment such as vaccination. A refusal to obey a direct order in this context may well be dealt with by means of the ordinary disciplinary procedures that would apply to any refusal to obey an order.

Disciplinary or forensic procedures

The BMA has received several enquiries relating to potential conflicts where doctors with clinical responsibility for members of the armed forces are called in to administer blood tests to assess whether individuals are, for example, under the influence of drugs or alcohol. In the BMA's view such requests can undermine the doctor–patient relationship and should be avoided wherever possible. The appropriate route is for local forensic physicians to carry out this work, as they will not only be trained to do so, but are also highly unlikely to have any existing therapeutic relationship with the patient concerned.

Boxing

One matter that has been raised with the BMA on several occasions concerns armed forces doctors who object to boxing matches. These doctors, who do not agree with boxing as a sport, have been required to carry out pre-bout medical examinations. The BMA has advised that a full explanation of the doctor's objections to boxing as a sport should be given to the commanding officer and that the matter should be handled through the recognised appeals procedure. Doctors may also wish to refer to the BMA's objections to boxing.[44] Some doctors who feel strongly on the matter have considered resigning from the forces, rather than having anything to do with boxing matches. Some doctors have also complained that they had insufficient examination time and facilities to assess adequately the potential risk to each participant. Where doctors believe that the examination facilities or the way in which the sport is practised do not minimise the risk of severe injury, they should report these dangers to the commanding officer, making clear the distinction between these concerns and any conscientious objection they may have.

Summary – doctors in the armed forces

- Doctors in the armed forces must strive to work to the same ethical standards as other doctors.
- Doctors should raise concerns about medical standards with their commanding officer in the first instance.

- Although there are likely to be more circumstances in which confidential health information should be disclosed than in civilian life, this should be with the patient's cooperation and consent whenever possible.
- Doctors who provide care and treatment for members of the armed forces should avoid being involved in taking samples for forensic purposes.

Sports doctors

Doctors can be asked to perform a number of roles for sports clubs and teams. Where they are asked to conduct a medical assessment, for example when a player transfers between football clubs, their responsibilities and obligations are similar to those of a doctor writing a medical report for employment, discussed earlier in this chapter. Where acting in a more therapeutic role, however, doctors may find themselves subject to further conflicting loyalties. On the one hand, they are agents of the team or club with the contractual obligations of an employee, and, on the other, as doctors they are advocates for the individual athletes or players who are their patients.

Pressures on best practice in sports medicine

An extreme illustration of the ethical conflicts doctors can experience within sports medicine came when the conduct of a sports doctor hit the headlines in 2009 as part of the 'bloodgate' scandal. During a Rugby Union cup match, one of the players simulated an injury by biting a fake blood capsule, enabling the team to bring on a specialist penalty kicker as a blood replacement and therefore give them an advantage in the last few minutes of the game. It emerged later that the player, after realising that match officials suspected that his injury was not real, had asked the team doctor to cut his lip in order to cover up the deception. The doctor reluctantly agreed to the request and subsequently described how she had succumbed to 'huge pressure' from the player.

At a GMC fitness to practise hearing into her conduct in 2010, the doctor admitted that she had deliberately cut the lip of the player and that she failed to inform a European Rugby Cup disciplinary hearing that she had caused the injury. The GMC panel found no evidence that the doctor had prior knowledge of the deception. It stated that because the player was a patient to whom the doctor had a duty of care, irrespective of the pressure she was put under, the doctor had not acted in the best interests of her patient. During the hearing, it emerged that the doctor was suffering from depression at the time of the incident. The panel stated that, while the doctor's misconduct would normally be expected to result in a finding of impaired fitness to practise, the doctor's depression constituted exceptional circumstances as it had affected her judgement. The doctor was issued with a formal warning, but the panel decided that her fitness to practise was not impaired.[45]

The most obvious area in which problems may arise is in relation to confidentiality. This can be particularly true in the case of high-profile teams or clubs, such as in professional football. Managers and coaches, often under considerable pressure to succeed, can claim to require information about the fitness of players to plan and prepare teams successfully and often players have contractual obligations to pass relevant information on to their managers. Additional pressure from officials, from the media, or even from sponsors, can also be exerted on doctors to release confidential information.[46] Medical staff in sports teams can therefore be placed in the difficult position where they are contractually obliged to disclose information about an athlete to their employer, but where doing so would override patient confidentiality and breach the professional codes of conduct laid down by the GMC. The BMA advises that doctors should not sign contracts that would obligate them to act outside of the conduct expected of them in respect to confidentiality by the GMC. It is important that an athlete can have confidence in the therapeutic relationship with medical staff employed by a team or club. Erosion of trust could lead to an athlete withholding information during a consultation in fear that it will be disclosed to a manager or coach without their consent. This could prevent effective diagnosis and treatment and could endanger the health either of an individual athlete or that of others within a team, for example in the case of a blood-borne infection.[47]

Ethically, a sports doctor's chief loyalty is to their patients and the duty of medical confidentiality doctors have under GMC guidance remains unchanged (see Chapter 5). Doctors should only disclose confidential information with the express consent of the patient and breaches of confidentiality can be justified only when there is a risk of serious harm either to the patient or to a third party. If an athlete is contractually obliged to release medical information, but refuses to give consent for disclosure, the doctor should respect the athlete's decision. Any potential breach of contract between an athlete and a club should not override the duty of confidentiality a doctor has to a patient.

Individuals who have sustained injuries may come under pressure from managers or may themselves want to continue to play, particularly in team sports where the outcome of a match is crucial for the team's long-term success. This may be the case even when continuing to play may exacerbate injuries or incur risks of long-term damage. Further-more, there is evidence to suggest that in professional football there can be a presumption that players will continue to play with pain and injury.[48] Here, the doctor's chief obligation must be to the long-term health and well-being of individual players. In such a situation, doctors must inform both player and manager of the risks involved so that both parties can make an informed decision about whether play should continue. A note of any such discussion should be recorded in the relevant health record. Where there is a long-term risk to the health of a sportsperson, local anaesthetic injections or other treatments producing an analgesic effect, which are aimed at enabling the sportsperson to continue to practise a sport with an injury, should not be given.[49]

The Faculty of Sport and Exercise Medicine (FSEM) publishes a professional code for doctors who work within the field.[50] The Code emphasises the professional and ethical obligations doctors have to patients under GMC guidelines and provides supplementary guidance on issues specific to sports medicine, including drug testing, assessing an athlete's fitness to practise a sport and the relationship with third parties, such as managers and coaches, in the management of an athlete's health.

Drugs and sport

Doctors may from time to time be asked by players or athletes to provide performance-enhancing drugs such as anabolic steroids. Not only must doctors clearly operate, and be seen to operate, within the law, but also the long-term health interests of their patients must be their primary concern. GMC advice on prescribing performance-enhancing drugs in the *British National Formulary* states that:

> [d]octors who prescribe or collude in the provision of drugs or treatment with the inten-
> tion of improperly enhancing an individual's performance in sport would be contravening
> the GMC's guidance, and such actions would usually raise a question of a doctor's con-
> tinued registration. This does not preclude the provision of any care or treatment when
> the doctor's intention is to protect or improve the patient's health.[51]

Doctors should be aware when treating athletes that drugs used in everyday practice or that are available over the counter may contravene anti-doping regulations. Where there is the potential for this to happen, doctors should either avoid prescribing or talk through the issue with the athlete in question. UK Anti-Doping is responsible for the implementation and management of the UK's anti-doping policy and more information can be found on its website.[52] A BMA book, *Drugs in sport: the pressure to perform,*[53] provides further advice on this issue and the BMA internet resource, *Doctors providing medical care at sporting events,*[54] provides general guidance for sports doctors and doctors working at sporting events.

Summary – sports doctors

- Ethically, a sports doctor's chief loyalty is to their patients and the duty of medical confidentiality doctors have under GMC guidance remains unchanged.
- Doctors should not sign contracts that would oblige them to act outside of the conduct expected of them in respect to confidentiality by the GMC.
- Doctors should not prescribe drugs or treatment with the intention of improperly enhancing an individual's performance in sport.

Media doctors

Some doctors choose to work partly or exclusively in the media, for example by editing medical journals or commenting on health issues for newspapers and television. Their role is often to provide general medical advice or background commentary on medical issues in a form that lay people find accessible. When providing commentary about specific cases or individuals, doctors must distinguish between the legitimate provision of background information – for example, commenting, in a general way on the ordinary nature and prognosis of a disease – and the far more questionable practice of speculative diagnosis. Doctors should also resist any temptation to comment on information that they think may have been improperly released into the public domain. The issues of confidentiality that arise when doctors working in clinical practice are asked to release information about patients to the media are discussed in Chapter 5, pages 216–217.

Many areas of the media offer discussion with doctors about health issues, often in the form of a helpline, where callers discuss problems with a health professional by telephone or email. Phone-in programmes and helplines that attempt to provide individual advice to people, however, may create problems. To supply detailed and specific medical advice of the nature usually provided by the patient's own GP is not appropriate in these circumstances. It must be made clear that the information provided by the telephone advice line or website is designed to support, not replace, the relationship between patients and their GPs.

Where websites or advice lines are supported by commercial organisations, this support must be clearly identified. If advertising is a source of funding, this must also be stated and any advertising or promotional material must be presented in a manner that makes it easily distinguishable from the advice on offer. Any claims relating to the benefits of particular treatments or services, particularly those in which the individual or group running the service has a financial interest, must be supported by appropriate, balanced clinical evidence, and the nature of the financial interest must be clearly acknowledged. As with advertisements published in practice leaflets (see Chapter 19, page 795), the BMA recommends that doctors do not advertise health-related products and services. It is also inappropriate for sites to carry advertisements for products that clearly affect health adversely.

Doctors with business interests

Traditionally, guidance to doctors relating to business interests has tended to focus on conflicts of interest that have arisen where patient care could be, or could be seen to be, in tension with the financial interests of doctors. This would arise where, for example, doctors were treating patients in institutions in which they, or members of their families, held a financial interest. Increasingly, the delivery of healthcare in the UK is becoming more mixed, both in terms of the increased involvement of commercial providers, and in terms of the use of commercially orientated mechanisms, such as incentives, in the delivery of NHS care. Recognising that potential conflicts of interest are an established feature of health delivery, in the BMA's view, doctors should ensure that, where such conflicts of interest are unavoidable, they are managed appropriately and patients are informed about any factors likely to have an impact on their care. Where doctors have financial interests that may be, or may be seen to be, in tension with the best interests of their patients, the following broad principles should be considered.

- Conflicts of interest should be avoided where possible.
- Clinical decisions, such as prescribing or referral, must be made on the basis of an assessment of the best interests of the individual patient.
- Patients should be informed of any conflicts of interest that may have an adverse impact on their care.
- Where conflicts of interest arise in relation to work carried out under contract to the NHS, mechanisms should be put in place both to minimise conflicts of interest and to ensure transparency.
- Where conflicts of interest cannot be avoided, financial or other incentives must not interfere with objective clinical judgement.

References

1 World Medical Association (2006) *International code of medical ethics (Declaration of Geneva)*, WMA, Geneva.
2 International Dual Loyalty Working Group (2002) *Dual loyalty and human rights in health professional practice: proposed guidelines and institutional mechanisms*, Physicians for Human Rights, Boston.
3 General Medical Council (2009) *Confidentiality*, GMC, London, paras 33–4.
4 *Pamela Cornelius v Dr Nicola de Taranto* [2002] 68 BMLR 62.
5 British Medical Association (2009) *Access to health records*, BMA, London.
6 British Medical Association (2009) *Access to health records*, BMA, London.
7 General Medical Council (2006) *Good Medical Practice*, GMC, London, paras 63–7.
8 British Medical Association, Association of British Insurers (2008) *Medical information and insurance: joint guidelines from the British Medical Association and the Association of British Insurers*, BMA, London.
9 British Medical Association and Association of British Insurers (2011) *General practitioner's report (GPR)*. Available at: www.bma.org.uk (accessed 19 May 2011).
10 General Medical Council (2009) *Confidentiality*, GMC, London, para 34.
11 British Medical Association, Association of British Insurers (2008) *Medical information and insurance: joint guidelines from the British Medical Association and the Association of British Insurers*, BMA, London.
12 Association of British Insurers (2008) *ABI statement of best practice for insurers*, ABI, London. Association of British Insurers (2008) *HIV and life insurance: a consumer guide for gay men*, ABI, London.
13 Association of British Insurers (2008) *Genetic testing: ABI code of practice*, ABI, London, p.2.
14 Association of British Insurers (2008) *Genetic testing: ABI code of practice*, ABI, London, p.2.

15   In England and Wales, the rules for submission of an expert report are contained in: Ministry of Justice (2005) *Civil Procedure Rules. Practice Direction. Part 35: experts and assessors*, MoJ, London. The Civil Justice Council has also developed guidance for expert witnesses in civil claims. Civil Justice Council (2005) *Protocol for the Instruction of Experts to give Evidence in Civil Claims*. CJC, London. In Northern Ireland it is governed by Order 25 of the Rules of the Supreme Court (Northern Ireland) 2009, as amended by Amendment No.2. In Scotland, information about expert witnesses and the submission of medical evidence can be found in: Ross ML, Chalmers J. (2009) *Walker and Walker: The Law of Evidence in Scotland*, 3rd edn, Bloomsbury Professional, Hayward Heath, paras 16.3.1–16.3.16.

16   General Medical Council (2008) *Acting as an expert witness*, GMC, London.

17   British Medical Association (2007) *Expert witness guidance*, BMA, London.

18   Department of Health (2006) *Bearing Good Witness: Proposals for reforming the delivery of medical expert evidence in family law cases*, DH, London.

19   Legal Services Commission (2009) *Reforming the delivery of health expert witnesses*, LSC, London.

20   www.legalservices.gov.uk (accessed 13 February 2011).

21   The law relating to certification for firearms and shotguns in England and Wales is contained in the Firearms Acts 1968 to 1997 and the Firearms Rules 1998. SI 1998/1941, s 3–7. In Scotland, the law is contained in the Firearms (Scotland) Rules 1989. SI 1989/889, s 3–7. In Northern Ireland, certification for firearms and shotguns is contained in the Firearms (Northern Ireland) Order 1981, part 3.

22   Firearms Acts 1968 to 1997. Firearms form 103: part D.

23   Firearms Acts 1968 to 1997. Firearms form103: notes to part D.

24   Home Office (2002) *Firearms law: guidance to the police 2002*, HMSO, Norwich, p.47.

25   General Medical Council (2009) *Confidentiality*, GMC, London, para 37.

26   Personal communication regarding memorandum from the Information Commissioner, 16 February 2011.

27   See, for example: Forrest D, Hinshelwood G, Peel M. (2000) The physical and psychological findings following the late examination of victims of torture. *Torture* **10**(1), 12–5.

28   British Medical Association (2002) *Asylum seekers: meeting their health care needs*, BMA, London. See also: British Medical Association (2011) *Access to health care for asylum seekers and refused asylum seekers*, BMA, London.

29   Clothier C, Macdonald CA, Shaw DA. (1994) *The Allitt inquiry: independent inquiry relating to the deaths and injuries on the children's ward at Grantham and Kesteven General Hospital during the period February to April 1991*, HMSO, London. For further information about pre-employment testing in the NHS in England and Wales, see: www.nhsemployers.org (accessed 13 February 2011). For further information about pre-employment checking in Scotland, see: www.disclosurescotland.co.uk (accessed 13 February 2011). Information on pre-employment checking in Northern Ireland can be found at: www.accessni.gov.uk (accessed 13 February 2011).

30   Data Protection Act 1998, Sch 1, Part 1.

31   Data Protection Act 1998, Sch 1, Part 1.

32   www.nhsemployers.org (accessed 13 Febuary 2011).

33   Information Commissioner (2005) *The Employment Practices Code*, ICO, Wilmslow.

34   Faculty of Occupational Medicine (2006) *Guidance on ethics for occupational physicians*, FOM, London.

35   *X v The European Commission* [1995] IRLR 320, 321.

36   General Medical Council (2006) *Good Medical Practice*, GMC, London, para 63.

37   For further information on the role and responsibilities of occupational health physicians, see: www.facoccmed.ac.uk (accessed 13 February 2011).

38   Department of Health (2007) *Health clearance for tuberculosis, Hepatitis B, Hepatitis C and HIV; new healthcare workers*, DH, London. British Medical Association (2007) *Testing medical students for blood borne viruses*, BMA, London.

39   *Hartman v South Essex Mental Health and Community Care NHS Trust* [2005] EWCA civ 6, para 33.

40   Faculty of Occupational Medicine (2006) *Guidance on ethics for occupational physicians*, FOM, London, p.8.

41   Information Commissioner (2005) *The Employment Practices Code*, ICO, Wilmslow.

42   British Medical Association (2009) *The Occupational Physician*, BMA, London.

43   The Ionising Radiation Regulations 1999. SI 1999/3232.

44   See: www.bma.org.uk (accessed 13 February 2011).

45   General Medical Council, Fitness to Practise Hearing, 23 August–1 September 2010.

46   Waddington I, Roderick M. (2002) Management of medical confidentiality in English professional football clubs: some ethical problems and issues. *Br J Sports Med* **36**, 118–23.

47   Anderson L. (2008) Contractual obligations and the sharing of confidential health information in sport. *J Med Ethics* **34** e6, 115–20, p.119.

48   Waddington I, Roderick M. (2002) Management of medical confidentiality in English professional football clubs: some ethical problems and issues. *Br J Sports Med* **36**, 118–123.

49   Faculty of Sport and Exercise Medicine (2010) *FSEM Professional Code*, FSEM, London, para 8.4.

50   Faculty of Sport and Exercise Medicine (2010) *FSEM Professional Code*, FSEM, London.

51 Joint Formulary Committee (2010) *British National Formulary*, 59th edn, British Medical Association and Royal Pharmaceutical Society, London, p.29.
52 See: www.ukad.org.uk (accessed 19 May 2011).
53 British Medical Association (2002) *Drugs in Sport: the pressure to perform*, Wiley-Blackwell, Chichester.
54 British Medical Association (2009) *Doctors providing medical care at sporting events*. Available at: www.bma.org.uk (accessed 6 October 2009).

17: Providing treatment and care in detention settings

The questions covered in this chapter include the following.

- Do doctors' ethical obligations differ significantly in detention settings?
- Can detainees refuse essential medical treatment?
- Can detainees make advance decisions refusing treatment, including prior to commencing, or during, a hunger strike?
- What rights to confidentiality do detainees have?
- Do different rules about consent apply if the detainee is a minor or has a history of mental illness?
- Is it acceptable for health professionals to be involved in the restraint of detainees?
- What special considerations should be given to the rights of children and young people in detention?

Doctors' duties in detention settings

Chapter 16 discussed fundamental aspects of dual loyalties; this chapter considers the specific issue of divided loyalties in detention settings. The chapter discusses the general principles and issues common to any form of detention setting, as well as the ethical issues that arise in five particular types of establishment: prisons; young offender facilities and those accommodating children and young people; immigration removal centres (IRCs); and police stations.

Since April 2006, the NHS has commissioned health services in public sector prisons in England and Wales, thereby fully transferring responsibility for prison healthcare from the Prison Service to local commissioning bodies. In those prisons where healthcare is commissioned privately, common NHS standards are now applied. As a result, NHS, Department of Health and Welsh Assembly Government provisions and policies[1] are equally applicable across the entire prison estate, as they are throughout the wider health sector. This represents a significant step towards ensuring 'equivalence' of healthcare services available to individuals in prison with those available to all other NHS patients in the community. (In early 2011, the Government was seeking to implement wide-ranging changes to the healthcare system in England. These changes were likely to impact on the commissioning of health services for prisons; however, at the time of writing, the specific implications were not known. Up-to-date information on this can be found on the BMA website.) In Northern Ireland, direct responsibility for prison healthcare provision was transferred away from the Prison Service significantly earlier, in 1974, and now lies with the Department of Health, Social Services and Public Safety. Responsibility for healthcare provision was due to be transferred from the Prison Service in Scotland to the NHS in October 2011. Equivalence is therefore an important principle of good practice across the UK.

Medical Ethics Today: The BMA's Handbook of Ethics and Law, Third Edition. Sophie Brannan, Eleanor Chrispin, Martin Davies, Veronica English, Rebecca Mussell, Julian Sheather and Ann Sommerville.
© 2012 BMA Medical Ethics Department. Published 2012 by Blackwell Publishing Ltd.

In spite of developments towards replicating NHS standards of care in the prison system, prison health services across the UK remain under considerable pressure and, although often acute in prisons, this pressure reflects problems that are encountered in all detention settings. The recruitment and retention of suitable doctors continues to pose difficulties. There are a number of different models of commissioning offender healthcare services, but none are able to recruit sufficient experienced healthcare staff to provide the services required to meet the particular needs of the detained population. This problem is likely to become more acute where budgets continue to be cut. In the past, reports critical of prison health services have focused on the lack of adequate training for prison doctors and the fact that some doctors worked beyond the limits of their ability.[2] Indeed, specific training in prisoner health, apart from substance misuse training, remains largely absent. A welcome development has been the growing role of appropriately trained nurse practitioners, although similar recruitment and retention problems are experienced across the healthcare professions.

The British Medical Association (BMA), in its 2007 dossier of case studies documenting first-hand accounts of prison and police doctors working in the English and Welsh penal system, stressed that prison doctors lacked the resources, infrastructure and time to treat and assess the large numbers of detainees with severe mental health and drug addiction problems.[3] It noted that detainees' health was being put at risk by a system that failed to address the causes of criminal activity, which, in many cases, led to re-offending after release. The dossier drew attention to concerns that failure to provide effective treatment in prison meant that newly released individuals had drug addiction and mental health problems which could affect public health. In addition, the persistent problem of prison overcrowding was cited as having a significant impact on healthcare, for example by leading to unacceptable delays in assessing and treating patients, and stretching mental health and substance misuse services beyond their capacity. More recently, a joint Care Quality Commission and Her Majesty's Inspectorate of Prisons' (HMIP) study, published in 2010, concluded that prison healthcare still failed to match NHS standards.[4] The regulators acknowledged that improvements had been made: governance arrangements were more robust, investment had driven up overall standards and staff training had improved. Significant concerns over continuity of care between detention and release were highlighted, however, and drug misuse services followed a best practice model in only six of the 21 commissioning bodies surveyed.[5]

While the amalgamation of prison healthcare into the NHS in England and Wales has strengthened expectations of parity, it also highlights a question fundamental to the practice of doctors working in any detention setting: how successfully can the same *ethical* standards be maintained in these settings as across the rest of the health service? The BMA recognises that, while it is essential to strive for parity in standards of care, healthcare professionals face significant difficulties in achieving this, not least as mental health disorders, substance misuse, smoking rates and many chronic physical health conditions are all substantially more prevalent in the detainee population than in the general population. Health professionals are therefore constrained in what services they are able to deliver and standards of care may suffer.

In all of the situations discussed in this chapter, doctors have a normal therapeutic role, and the associated ethical obligations, in relation to the patients they see and treat. As well as their obvious responsibilities for patients' welfare, doctors also have obligations to other parties, including employers, non-medical colleagues and the public. The establishments in which they work are concerned with public security, law enforcement and the containment of those detained. Clinicians work in close proximity to punitive activity with vulnerable individuals who, on entering custody, have lost aspects of their autonomy and independence and, as a result, may have limited capacity to make choices. At the same time, doctors often exercise less direct control over their physical environment and are dependent on working with prison management to achieve many health objectives. The pronounced nature of these dual loyalties inevitably gives rise to professional and ethical tensions which can be problematic for health professionals.

At the beginning of the twenty-first century, international events heightened awareness of these conflicting obligations. In November 2004, US and international media reported allegations concerning the possible use, in detainee interrogation, of the medical information of American-held detainees in Guantánamo Bay. The US Defense Department argued that, where health professionals were not employed in a therapeutic capacity, they were not bound by conventional medical ethical standards. This represented a challenge to international ethical norms as set out in the United Nations principles of medical ethics. As a result, amendments were made to the World Medical Association (WMA) Declarations of Tokyo[6] and Geneva,[7] and its Regulations in Times of Armed Conflict,[8] prohibiting the use of medical notes in detention settings for this purpose.

The BMA has consistently stressed that the general ethical principles regarding the duties of doctors working in detention settings be upheld at all times; the guidance contained in this chapter aims to assist doctors working in these settings to maintain the highest ethical standards, while taking account of the manifest pressures brought to bear upon them by their dual obligations. For many of the practical problems raised in this chapter, guidance has already been developed and we point out where guidelines designed for one specific setting have wider utility.

General principles

The General Medical Council's (GMC) *Good Medical Practice* is the basis on which *all* doctors should practise, including those working in detention settings.[9] In addition, the following principles are important. All health professionals working in detention settings should:

- remember their duty of care for individuals, even when health assessments occur for other purposes than the provision of treatment, such as for forensic purposes
- provide healthcare that is at least of a comparable standard to that provided in the community
- seek informed consent, even if the law does not oblige consent to be obtained, such as for intimate body searches
- provide information to patients about treatment options
- respect patient confidentiality – patients should be aware at the time they provide information if it will be used for purposes other than their care, and they should know what those purposes are likely to be and whether they can opt out
- facilitate good cooperation and communication between all members of the health team and work to ensure continuity of care between different detention establishments and community health teams on release
- be continually aware of the obligation to respect patients' human rights and be sensitive to the ways in which those rights may be compromised
- use opportunities to encourage patients to pursue choices that will promote their health, especially for those who have had no past experience of accessing the NHS or health facilities

- assert, to the maximum extent possible, clinical independence in referral and prescribing decisions
- speak out when services are inadequate or pose a potential threat to health
- audit their own expertise and know their limitations.

General issues of consent, confidentiality and choice within detention settings

There should be no need for separate codes of medical ethics specifically for use in detention establishments, because the general principles that apply are the same as those underpinning all other healthcare situations. The principles and best practice outlined in this section relate to a range of detention settings including, but not limited to, prisons.

In all interventions, doctors should seek consent if the patient has capacity (see Chapters 2 and 4). All patients are owed a duty of confidentiality, but this is never absolute (see Chapter 5). It is particularly limited in relation to forensic examinations (see the discussion of confidentiality in relation to forensic physicians on pages 731–732). Situations may arise in all healthcare settings in which other considerations override the individual patient's rights, but where confidential information is to be disclosed without consent, this should ordinarily be discussed with patients in advance of any disclosure wherever possible. Good communication with patients and with colleagues is a key requisite in all healthcare settings, and is equally applicable to practice in a detention context (see Chapters 1 and 19).

All health professionals have duties to draw attention to inadequacies in the service that pose a hazard to health and so need to be wary of employment contracts that seek to limit their ability to do so. (BMA members can obtain advice on this from the BMA.) Doctors working in establishments have a duty to ensure that treatment guidelines are observed and that any signs of neglect or maltreatment are properly investigated. Normally, these issues can be raised through a monitoring system. Internal procedures for reporting suspicions should be followed, but if health professionals are unable to obtain a satisfactory answer through such mechanisms, they need to consider other action. This is often a very difficult and isolating decision; health professionals can seek support from professional bodies such as the BMA (whistleblowing is discussed in Chapter 19, page 778 and Chapter 21, pages 878–879).

Some practical differences clearly exist between the provision of healthcare in the community and healthcare in detention. In the latter situation, patients are ordinarily more vulnerable due to loss of autonomy and choice, and it may be problematic for them to complain effectively. Although there are several complaint mechanisms within the NHS and prison services, detainees may not understand the most effective route available, and literacy and language difficulties can create barriers to access. The media and the public are often indifferent to the treatment of detainees or are unsympathetic to their situation. On the other hand, some individuals in custody are adept at manipulating the healthcare system. Prescription medication, for example, is often misused and bartered with other detainees.[10] Health services for this population have been significantly underresourced, which has affected the efficacy of treatment. Although these distinctions can present doctors working in detention establishments with very particular challenges, all individuals deserve equivalent care, regardless of the setting in which they receive it, and doctors should endeavour to maintain ethical standards of practice that apply more generally, as set out in the GMC's *Good Medical Practice*.[11]

Seeking consent

In terms of consenting to treatment or refusing it, the same general rules apply to those in detention as to those in the community. Adult detainees can accept or refuse treatment as long as they have capacity and are informed of the implications (see Chapter 2), unless compulsory treatment is required under mental health legislation. Mental health legislation specifically excludes compulsory treatment in prison. Although some mental health problems can be treated in detention settings, it is inappropriate to provide treatment to individuals with very serious mental disorders outside of a hospital and, where necessary, a secure setting. Where mental health needs would otherwise be treated in hospital if the patient were in the community, treatment must be given in a secure psychiatric facility.

Minors can also consent if they are competent and informed. If aged over 16, they are assumed to be competent to consent unless there is evidence to the contrary. Alternatively, consent can be provided on their behalf by someone with parental responsibility or by the courts. Minors cannot always refuse treatment, however (see pages 722–723 below and Chapter 4 for further discussion). In relation to young people who are detained, a local authority, court-appointed proxy or authorised person with an emergency protection order may have been awarded parental responsibility, in addition to parents. The fact of detention in custody does not in itself remove the ability of parents to consent to treatment on behalf of their children (see Chapter 4).

The fundamental principles relating to patient consent are summarised in the box below.[12]

Summary of guidance on patient consent

- Respect for people's rights to determine what happens to their own bodies is a fundamental aspect of good medical practice.
- Valid consent requires that the individual patient has capacity, is informed and is not acting under duress.
- Adults should be assumed to have capacity unless the opposite is proved, although it is difficult to ensure that detainees do not feel coerced, even when they are not, in fact, being pressurised to make particular choices. Special effort may be needed to explain treatment decisions to people with learning disabilities or who do not have English as a first language.
- Seeking consent is a process. Patients must be aware that they can change their minds.
- Verbal consent is as valid as written consent, but it is good practice to use consent forms for treatments that are complex, or involve significant risk or side effects.
- Adults with capacity can refuse any treatment and cannot be treated against their will unless they require compulsory mental health treatment.
- Competent minors can consent to treatment, but may have less option to refuse it.

In prisons, all detainees, including those held on remand, are routinely asked to undergo a medical examination, generally carried out by a nurse, on reception into custody. This is intended primarily to identify symptoms of physical illness, communicable diseases, mental illness or suicide risk, and to ensure that prisoners continue to receive medication previously prescribed. European guidelines emphasise the importance of undertaking this examination within 24 hours of the prisoner's arrival.[13] The fact that this has generally been an automatic and routine procedure does not mean that properly informed consent can be forgone. If detainees refuse to be examined, their refusal should be recorded and respected, unless it is judged that the patient is likely to have a serious mental illness. When this is the case, assessment under mental health legislation can be carried out.

Assessment of capacity

In order to give valid consent to examination or treatment, or to make a valid refusal contemporaneously or to cover future treatment, patients must have capacity. The terms mental 'capacity' and 'competence' are often used interchangeably, although the former is most often used in law and is used throughout this text when referring to adult patients (those 18 years old and over in England, Wales and Northern Ireland, and 16 years old and over in Scotland).

Adult patients are presumed to have the capacity to make treatment decisions unless there is evidence to suggest otherwise. Where there are reasons to doubt that an adult patient has such capacity, an individual assessment must be carried out (see Chapter 3). Such assessment is a matter for clinical judgement, guided by professional practice and subject to legal requirements, and the key points set out below should be considered.

- Capacity is not usually something that patients either definitively have or lack. It depends on the nature of the decision to be made and individuals' capacity can fluctuate.
- Most people, including those with mental health problems or learning disabilities, have the capacity to make some decisions. A mental health problem or learning disability is not of itself proof of incapacity; a lack of capacity should not be assumed on the basis of these or other factors, such as age or appearance, alone.
- When detainees have a serious mental disorder, for which they require compulsory treatment, they must be transferred out of the prison or other detention setting as soon as possible; the Mental Health Act 1983, as amended, in England and Wales specifically excludes compulsory treatment in prison, as does the Mental Health (Care and Treatment) (Scotland) Act 2003 and the Mental Health (Northern Ireland) Order 1986.
- When patients are highly disturbed or violent, it may be very difficult to assess their capacity. Even in such cases, unless doctors have a reasonable belief that an individual may be incapacitated, they should never simply assume incapacity.
- Patients who lack capacity can be treated in their 'best interests', under the Mental Capacity Act 2005 in England and Wales and the common law in Northern Ireland (at the time of writing, mental capacity legislation for Northern Ireland was being drafted; see Chapter 3, pages 140–141); meanwhile, issues of capacity in Northern Ireland are governed by common law provisions), or for their 'benefit' under the Adults with Incapacity (Scotland) Act 2000. Decisions made in a patient's best interests or overall benefit should follow the least restrictive option and should take account of the patient's own wishes, where these can be identified. Ascertaining such wishes may involve discussion with those close to the individual. Patients cannot be given treatment for which they have made a valid advance decision refusing it, unless it is compulsory treatment given under mental health legislation. Patients given emergency psychotropic medication on the basis of best interests or overall benefit must be transferred out of prison to an appropriate psychiatric facility as a matter of urgency.
- In order to assess the best interests of, or what may be for the overall benefit to, a patient lacking capacity, doctors should review the patient's medical history and seek views from colleagues who know the person, including prison officers, other healthcare

staff and probation officers. In doing so, doctors should always bear in mind the duty of confidentiality to the patient.

- People who are close to the patient may also have helpful views. Again, issues of confidentiality should be considered before discussing medical details with a patient's relatives or close friends. In England and Wales, a welfare attorney, and in Scotland any proxy appointed for an incapacitated person, should be consulted (this is discussed in Chapter 3).
- Doctors are accountable for their decisions and, as with other clinical assessments, must be able to justify decisions relating to the assessment of capacity.
- Monitoring of decision-making capacity is required so that, if the patient regains capacity at any point during the treatment, consent to continue it can be discussed.[14]

Respecting refusal

An adult patient with capacity has a right to refuse any medical treatment (except under mental health legislation), for any reason, rational or irrational, or for no reason at all, even where the decision could lead to the patient's death. Adults with capacity can refuse contemporaneously or in advance of losing their mental capacity. (For a discussion of treatment refusal by adults with capacity, see Chapter 2, pages 75–80 and for further information on advance decisions, see Chapter 3, page 96.)

Detainees can therefore refuse medication if they have decision-making capacity. They should not be pressured into accepting treatment by, for example, implying that a refusal could affect their privileges or remission of sentence. As with other areas of medical practice, it is important to seek consent and explain the implications of medication in an unbiased way, which patients, including non-English speakers and those with learning difficulties or who cannot read, are able to understand. Wherever possible, patients should be given opportunities to be cooperatively involved in their treatment.

Occasionally, doctors have expressed concern to the BMA that the prevailing culture in certain detention settings results in some patients not receiving an appropriate explanation that they can refuse referral, examination or treatment in situations that do not require treatment under mental health legislation. In particular, sex offenders and prisoners with a history of violent behaviour need to be aware when they have a choice about being referred for treatment, including that relating to their offending behaviour. Doctors can be placed in a difficult position here because, while some patients prefer to avoid confronting their past behaviour, they are also under a degree of pressure to accept treatment because parole is considered on the basis of the risk they present to others. Therefore, there is pressure on patients to accept treatment in order to be eligible for early release, although such treatment is normally seen as being both in the patient's best interests and those of society. Many patients are well aware of this, but it is still important that doctors do not contribute to the pressure by directly or indirectly implying that the acceptance of treatment is obligatory.

Scope and limits of detainees' choice

W was a high security prisoner, convicted of murder in 2000. He was assessed as having a severe psychiatric disorder and was initially sent to Broadmoor Hospital, where doctors found him extremely difficult to treat because of his aggressive behaviour.

After being transferred to a prison segregation unit, he began to mutilate his right leg in protest at what he perceived to be a denial of his right to be treated in a special hospital. He said that he wished to receive mental healthcare, but not treatment for his leg, and that he was willing to die if kept in the prison unit. He was told that continuing to mutilate his leg would result in blood poisoning, septicaemia and death.

In April 2002, the High Court ruled that W had the mental capacity to decide whether or not to accept medical treatment for his leg. The judge was satisfied that, although W was suffering from a psychopathic disorder, his capacity to understand, retain, weigh and use the information relevant to the decision to refuse medical treatment was unimpaired. He understood that he would die if he continued his protest and refusal of medical help for his leg wound. The judge upheld his right to refuse treatment and also made clear that transfer to a mental health unit would be dependent upon his doctor's recommendation, rather than his own choice or that of the Prison Service. She also drew comparisons with prisoners' suicide attempts when they had made a clear advance decision refusing cardio-pulmonary resuscitation. In such cases, the judge said that prison authorities could risk litigation against them if they resuscitated a prisoner against his or her express advance decision.[15]

Advance decisions and suicide attempts

In the legal case described above, attention was drawn by the judge to the theoretical possibility of a person attempting suicide after having made a clear and informed advance decision refusing treatment. The dilemmas arising in such a circumstance are particularly pertinent to the detention setting and are discussed in Chapter 3, page 96 and Chapter 15, pages 632–633.

Health professionals find it counter-intuitive and contrary to their training to refrain from all life-saving efforts when suicide is attempted. This is especially so in the context of the enormous efforts that have been made to reduce the level of self-harm and suicide in custody. In the BMA's opinion, a distinction can be drawn between a demonstrably well-reasoned, sustained, informed and documented advance decision refusing treatment made by a person with capacity, and a refusal for which there is no clear evidence of such validity. In the case of W, there were opportunities to discuss with the patient the implications of his choice and assess his ability to make it. Other examples where a person with capacity may refuse life-saving treatment include the refusal of antiretroviral drugs to treat HIV and AIDS, insulin to treat diabetes or of food and drink (see pages 713–716 on the management of hunger strikes). These situations can be distinguished from most attempted suicides or impulsive acts of self-harm, where the patient is very rarely able to express a competent, clear and settled refusal of treatment, and where doctors lack firm evidence of whether or not the individual was in a disturbed or reasonable frame of mind when initiating the suicide attempt. In any case of doubt, and when there is a possibility of reviving the person, the BMA strongly recommends that appropriate emergency treatment should be started and when the patient is stabilised, further investigation into the patient's capacity should be initiated.

Respecting confidentiality

All patients have a right of confidentiality, but this right is not absolute. In some cases disclosure without consent may be necessary on public interest grounds, or required by statute or by a court.[16] The general principles concerning confidentiality and disclosure in the public interest, as well as the relevant legislation, are discussed in detail in Chapter 5. Individuals should be made aware of the foreseeable use of their information when they provide it. Helpful general information about confidentiality and inter-agency information sharing is available from the Department of Health.[17] Although designed for use in the prison system in England and Wales, the guidance could be useful in other, similar contexts.

In particular, it stresses the importance of appropriate inter-agency information sharing, with the individual's consent, and according to locally agreed protocols. The prison services in England, Wales, Scotland and Northern Ireland have moved towards a system of keeping multi-disciplinary healthcare records, which are accessible to all members of the healthcare team. This facilitates good communication between professional groups. Patients have rights of access to their own medical records so that they can see what information may be shared among those who are treating them. Ensuring continuity of care after release is emphasised in the guidance and this is particularly important for patients with mental health problems.

National prison healthcare IT system

By April 2011, a national prison healthcare IT system had been installed in all prisons and young offender institutions, and three immigration removal centres providing NHS-commissioned care, in England. It was hoped that, by giving all clinicians ready access to individual patients' up-to-date medical information, including medical history and current conditions, using a single system across multiple sites, the system would:

- support team working
- facilitate early intervention and preventative care
- make it less likely that the physical and mental health needs of prisoners and young offenders go undetected
- improve the security of patient information, with tightly controlled user access rights
- ensure greater equivalence, in terms of the quality and range of healthcare available in the community
- facilitate staff training to support standardised ways of working and the sharing of good practice
- allow for effective audit of healthcare activity across the prison estate.

The Department of Health also stressed that patients would benefit from improved continuity of care as they move between prisons, with medical records immediately and securely transferred from one prison to another.[18]

Achieving a good balance between patients' confidentiality and the legitimate security interests of the establishment can sometimes be problematic, as highlighted by the case discussed below. The fundamental presumption, however, should be that detainees see health personnel in a confidential setting. In some cases, the risk-assessment process indicates the advisability of using a chaperone, including another member of the healthcare team or arranging other supervision. All non-medical staff should have contractual obligations to maintain confidentiality. When patients attend hospital appointments outside of the detention setting, wherever possible accompanying staff should not be in a position to overhear the consultation. Where detainees remain handcuffed during consultations, doctors are presented with very difficult scenarios (see page 712). The security implications of such a situation have to be balanced carefully against the implications for the patient, in terms of his or her right to confidentiality. Details of treatment can be passed between the hospital and prison medical team via the accompanying staff, but must be in sealed envelopes.

Confidentiality of prisoners' medical correspondence

Mr Szuluk was sentenced in November 2001 to 14 years' imprisonment for drugs offences. In April 2001, while on bail pending trial, he suffered a brain haemorrhage for which he received surgery. Following his discharge back to prison, he was required to attend hospital every 6 months for a specialist check up. The governor of the prison in which Mr Szuluk was detained granted his request for a confidentiality order for his medical correspondence with his neuro-radiology specialist, provided that it was marked 'medical in confidence' and that inward letters carried identifying franking stamps. This permission was later withdrawn on security grounds and a prison medical officer monitored correspondence between Mr Szuluk and his treating doctor.

After his challenge of this decision failed in the domestic courts, Mr Szuluk took his claim to the European Court of Human Rights, on the basis that the interception and monitoring of his medical correspondence was disproportionate and amounted to interference with his rights under Article 8 (right to respect for private and family life) of the European Convention on Human Rights.

The Court held that, although the reading of his medical correspondence had been in accordance with law and directed to the prevention of crime and protection of the rights and freedoms of others, there had been interference with Mr Szuluk's Article 8 rights. Some measure of control of correspondence was not incompatible with Convention rights. Medical information was, however, of fundamental importance in the exercise of an individual's rights under Article 8 and was crucial to preserving patients' confidence in the health services and ability to convey their medical information honestly and fully. It was significant that Mr Szuluk was suffering from a life-threatening condition, which made him vulnerable to abuse. As the prison medical officer was a prison officer, and was likely to encounter criticism of his own performance in Mr Szuluk's correspondence with his doctor, this could lead to negative consequences for Mr Szuluk. In addition, there was nothing to suggest the initial confidentiality regime had been abused, or that it would be, for example by communicating information that would otherwise be subject to interception. The state had failed to give sufficient reasons as to why the risk of abuse in correspondence with named doctors, where there was no reason to question their integrity, was a greater risk than that taken with confidential correspondence between prisoners and lawyers or MPs. It was therefore disproportionate to refuse Mr Szuluk's confidentiality and the monitoring of his medical correspondence had not struck a fair balance with his right to respect for his confidentiality. Accordingly, there had been a breach of Article 8.[19]

Doctors who work in detention facilities are sometimes faced with a conflict between maintaining patients' confidentiality and the obligation to assist in ensuring the safe and proper management of the establishment. When governors or managers need information in order to protect the security or safety of prisoners, doctors have an obligation to divulge it. Nevertheless, only relevant health information should be divulged in such circumstances and disclosure should be made only on the strictest 'need to know' basis unless, for example, the patient requests disclosure to a solicitor or other advocate. Guidance can also be sought from senior colleagues where there is any doubt as to whether disclosure should be made. The reasons for disclosing should be documented. Doctors working in prisons must be able to keep confidential records and the health records system used must be secure. In the course of their duties, doctors may make written or verbal reports to courts, adjudication boards, prison governors or other authorities. Detainees should be told when there is an obligation to pass medical information to other people and its purpose. On transfer from police to prison custody, patient information provided by a forensic physician should be made available only to the prison health team and transferred immediately to the prison medical record. It is not acceptable for medical details to be included in the detainee's main prison or other record, with the exception of opinions about his or her fitness for detention or interview, or matters directly affecting a detainee's management by staff.

Disclosures in connection with crime

One of the issues raised by doctors with the BMA and medical defence bodies is that of confidentiality in cases where a patient apparently confesses to previous crimes or denounces other people during counselling or therapy sessions. Ideally, patients should be aware in advance that absolute confidentiality cannot be guaranteed in all circumstances, and that doctors have a duty to consider the public interest and the interests of justice as well as the confidentiality owed to patients. Where information could prevent serious harm or injustice, or solve a serious crime, it is clearly important to bring it to the attention of the police or other professionals able to act upon it. More difficult to assess are cases where the information is unverifiable or likely to be unreliable. Professional judgement is required to assess such statements. In some cases, the individual may be deluded or deliberately seeking to mislead or wrongly incriminate others. It is helpful to collect details and clarify inconsistencies. Nevertheless, doctors are not able to investigate such claims and need to bring allegations of substance to the attention of the relevant authorities. This, and general issues of disclosure in the public interest, are discussed in Chapter 5.

Translation and interpretation

Detainees are a diverse population. This diversity is not only apparent within the immigration detention setting; many establishments have increasing numbers of foreign national detainees. The need for competent and independent interpretation and translation services in detention settings is well recognised. The Office for Criminal Justice Reform, in consultation with criminal justice system agencies, has produced a national agreement on arrangements for the use of interpreters, which provides detailed guidance for all agencies on the procedures to follow at each stage of the criminal justice process where an interpreter is required.[20] It highlights the requirement for the use of interpreters from the National Register of Public Service Interpreters. This is ideal, and should certainly be attainable in metropolitan areas, but may not always be practical in urgent medical cases where interpreters are not immediately available, for example in rural settings. It may therefore be necessary to use telephone interpretation. Information supplied by the Prison Service to foreign national prisoners states that every establishment has access to Language Line, a 24-hour telephone interpreting service that covers over 100 languages, as well as access to a variety of other interpreting services.[21] The best alternative to such services would be to use a clinical colleague who speaks the relevant language. Where no one speaking the required language is available, however, and the patient requests that another individual, for example a friend of the patient who is not a prisoner but who speaks the required language, be permitted to interpret, this should normally be agreed to. In this situation, health professionals must be absolutely confident that there is no coercion. Using other detainees as translators is likely to undermine the notion of medical confidentiality and could give other detainees information about the particular vulnerabilities or anxieties of the patient, which could subsequently be misused. However, doctors should use their discretion carefully in situations where using a fellow detainee may be the only option available to avoid serious harm to the patient in question.

In Scotland, a code of practice for working with interpreters in the Scottish criminal justice system has been developed, which sets out the responsibilities of those providing interpreting services and those working with interpreters at police stations, at precognition interviews and in court.[22] Although there is no national register in Scotland, the Scottish Translation, Interpreting and Communication Forum aims to promote good practice in these services by bringing together a range of public sector providers of translation and interpretation services.[23] The Northern Ireland Prison Service's foreign national prisoner strategy included recommendations for the use of accredited translation and interpretation services for the communication of confidential information.[24] In addition, the Regional

Health Interpreting Service provides face-to-face interpreting services in prison healthcare centres in Northern Ireland, as in the community.

In all cases, contractors must make the confidentiality requirements clear to all employees, including interpreters and translators of medical records.

Choice of doctor

People who are detained in police custody have the right to request examination by their own doctor, at their own expense. GPs attending police stations at the request of their patients do so at their own discretion. They should be made aware of the special procedures that apply to treating patients in custody and, where time permits, should be given a copy of the Police and Criminal Evidence Act Code of Practice C (which is available in all police stations).[25] Advice may also be sought from a forensic physician, who will be familiar with the terms of the legislation and guidance. If the police initiate a medical assessment or if the patient has been injured, or claims to have been injured, while in custody, then the examination should be carried out by a forensic physician or other appropriate healthcare professional, rather than the patient's own GP. Further detailed advice for GPs attending police stations at the request of their patients is available from the BMA.[26]

Individuals held on remand have a right to consult a doctor or dentist of their own choice, although this appears to be rarely exercised. Consultations should be arranged through the individual's solicitor. If clinical facilities are required, special arrangements need to be made with the Head of Healthcare at the establishment concerned. Although the doctor or dentist of the individual's choice can make recommendations regarding treatment, the final decision about the treatment offered rests with the prison doctor or dentist.

Once convicted and sentenced, prisoners in detention lose their right of access to a doctor of their choice. Legally, convicted prisoners have no freedom of choice regarding the doctor they see, but in practice if a request is made for a consultation with a prisoner's own doctor, and the doctor is willing to attend, it would be unusual for this to be refused. In most establishments, more than one GP will provide GP services and therefore prisoners do retain some choice over which of these doctors they see, just as a patient in the community would choose to see a particular doctor within a practice.

Summary – general issues of consent, confidentiality and choice within detention settings

- The general ethical principles that apply in detention settings are the same as those underpinning all other healthcare situations and all individuals deserve equivalent care, regardless of the setting in which they receive it.
- The distinctions between the detention context and the community do present doctors working in detention establishments with particular challenges.
- Doctors should seek consent for all interventions if the patient has capacity.
- An adult patient with capacity has a right to refuse any medical treatment (except under mental health legislation), for any reason, even where the decision could lead to the patient's death.
- It is unlawful to give compulsory mental health treatment in a setting other than a hospital. Where mental health needs would otherwise be treated in a hospital if the

patient were in the community, it is inappropriate to treat patients in the detention setting.

- All patients are owed a duty of confidentiality, but this is never an absolute duty.
- When governors or managers need information in order to protect the security or safety of other detainees or patients, doctors have an obligation to divulge it, but only relevant health information should be disclosed.
- People detained in police custody have the right to request examination by their own doctor, and individuals held on remand have a right to consult a doctor of their choice, but convicted prisoners have no general freedom of choice regarding the doctor they see.

Practical issues common to various detention settings

Although all doctors have to balance their various responsibilities to patients, relatives and the community, particular dilemmas arise when dual loyalties are in sharp focus and are an integral feature of daily work. In detention settings, doctors can find that their ethical duties towards their patients involve a different framework to that of colleagues, for example prison managers, whose main focus is on the management and control of those detained. All staff within the detention context need to work cooperatively to promote a safe and orderly environment, but doctors must also ensure that their patients' rights are respected with regard to confidentiality and self-determination on questions of medical treatment. Best practice guidance given here is relevant to a range of detention settings and where it refers to prisons or prisoners specifically, it can also be applied more widely.

Doctors working in various detention settings often deal with transient populations of patients who have pre-existing health problems. People detained within the criminal justice system are not generally from a healthy population prior to their detention. Many are not registered with a doctor or dentist, and a high proportion comes from socially excluded sections of society. Some detainees do not live in one place long enough for all, or even some, of their health problems to be addressed effectively. Ensuring aftercare can be difficult. Health professionals also need to be aware of those aspects of cultural diversity that impact on the health of their patient population and to be knowledgeable about laws that are applicable to the healthcare of detainees.

The prison population: a medical student's perspective

A final year medical student who undertook her elective at Holloway, a women's prison and young offenders institution in North London, described her experience in 2010.

The GPs at Holloway dealt with the usual range of ailments, but an extraordinary group of patients. For instance, there were the women who welcomed a prison term because it was better than life outside: it meant regular meals, a guaranteed bed, access to a doctor and the means to keep clean. One woman I met had 'deliberately' come to prison. Frustrated with waiting times and overstretched services outside, she believed that only behind bars would she receive the psychiatric care she needed. She had been attempting suicide when she was arrested for a minor criminal offence. Every woman had a tale to tell. Some had fled to the UK in desperation, escaping rape, beatings and imprisonment, only to be imprisoned here for having no documentation. Most of the British women had equally heart-rending stories – tales of deprived childhoods, and sexual and emotional abuse leading to self harm and drug misuse; many had children scattered across the country. I saw prisoners and doctors alike tortured with the knowledge that the cycle was starting again with another shattered family. The doctors were unable to make the usual assumption that patients would tell the truth. Many prisoners would tell tales of severe pain in order to gain opioids – if not for themselves, then as valuable currency. Any drug was better than nothing. One entirely well woman lied repeatedly to get hold of an antipsychotic, something that most patients outside would be desperate to avoid. A visit to the doctor was a break from the monotony of prison life, and the real reason for the consultation might be simply to have someone new to talk to.[27]

In detention situations, health teams can come under exceptional stress. They face a difficult task in maintaining patient trust due to tensions resulting from reduced patient autonomy and a high proportion of patients who have never trusted authority figures. In many establishments, there is a high turnover of detainees, making it difficult to establish a therapeutic relationship. Many establishments rely heavily on locum and agency healthcare staff, which increases the difficulties experienced by health professionals who have less chance to build sustained team relationships as a result. Verbal abuse and threats of harm directed at healthcare staff are common and may arise from mental health problems experienced by those detained. Doctors working in detention settings may also need greater peer support, for example from their colleagues in the community, than other doctors because of the complexity of their caseload; such support is not always available. In places of detention, doctors may be faced with fatalities resulting from suicide, hunger strike and other circumstances arising in custody. Despite following good practice guidance, health professionals cannot always predict these outcomes.

Suicides in prison

In March 2002, fatal accident inquiries were held concerning two deaths at Cornton Vale Prison in Scotland. There was considerable discussion of the efficacy of the suicide risk management strategy in the prison because, between April 1995 and October 2001, 10 women at Cornton Vale had taken their own lives by hanging. In respect of the two deaths reviewed in March 2002, however, the sheriff concluded that risk assessments had been carried out appropriately and society had to accept that not all suicides were preventable.

Michelle McElver had been admitted to Cornton Vale late on 23 October 2001 and assessed as not presenting a suicide risk. She was experiencing heroin withdrawal symptoms and was given medication for these, as well as being assessed independently by a doctor and a nurse. By 5 o'clock in the evening on 24 October, however, she was found dead, hanging by her shoelaces on a hook in a bathroom after a visit to the nurse. The sheriff was satisfied that the assessments of risk had been carried out appropriately and there was no obvious way in which the death could have been avoided.[28] In the same prison, 2 days later, another woman, Frances Carvill, who had a history of self-harm, hanged herself from the bars at a bathroom window at Cornton Vale and died in hospital on 29 October. In both of these cases, there was no criticism of the health professionals involved, but rather a recognition by the sheriff that such cases raised hugely difficult issues of patient management, in which it would always be difficult to strike the right balance.[29]

While the need to promote a good doctor–patient relationship in detention establishments is paramount, the detained population is a challenging patient group, many of whom regard the medical profession with suspicion. Some asylum seekers and other foreign nationals, for example, have had little previous interaction with health professionals or may associate doctors with previous bad experiences at the hands of the authorities in their country of origin. Health teams looking after them may have to deal with distressing accounts of torture or other trauma and need to be aware of their own need for support.

Ensuring good communication with patients

Good communication depends on trust, but also on health professionals having sufficient time to explain to patients their rights of confidentiality and choice. Lack of time in some establishments is one of the problems doctors raise with the BMA. The detained population presents other difficulties in terms of communication. High rates of learning disability and illiteracy limit the usefulness of text-based patient information leaflets or health promotion materials. While working to maintain the trust of their patients, doctors should be aware of the risks of detainees becoming institutionalised in their approach to life. Doctors have a vital therapeutic and advocacy role in relation to their patients and should also avoid coming to be seen as just another part of the punitive process. The additional tension in the doctor–patient relationship resulting from these factors, and from the patient's reduced autonomy, means that it is important that doctors should, as far as possible, actively promote their patients' interests, including by encouraging choices that will promote general health and well-being.

Ensuring good communication with other health professionals

It is important that health professionals working in detention settings keep themselves informed about developments in best practice, so as to maintain high standards and avoid professional isolation. It may also help to facilitate continuity of care of patients once they have left detention. Contacting previous treatment providers and obtaining accurate medical information about an individual's previous history can be challenging to healthcare teams in detention settings. The health team often has to rely initially upon information provided by patients when they come into detention, which may be inaccurate, incomplete or deliberately misleading. Transfer of health records between prisons has also been problematic and has hampered continuity of care, although, in England, this is improving with the implementation of a common information technology system (see page 697). Detainees have a right to withhold medical details. Some do not know details of their medical history, having not had any contact with the health service. Some detainees are suspicious of the purposes for which information is required or are not convinced that it will be kept confidential. Where they have been registered with a GP, detainees should be asked to provide details and to allow the health team to contact that doctor to obtain confirmation of the medical history. In such cases, detainees need to be made aware that liaison with their doctor is important in helping to determine appropriate medication to prescribe. If they have been previously assessed by a forensic physician, that assessment should be made available to the prison health team. The importance of providing such information cannot be overemphasised.

The importance of good communication

At a fatal accident inquiry in Glasgow in 1999, the sheriff drew particular attention to the need for any report made by a forensic physician while an individual is in police custody to be made promptly available to those subsequently responsible for the individual's care. In this case, a 21-year-old man who had previously been assessed by a forensic physician later died by hanging in Barlinnie Prison. In Scotland, the legislation requires the sheriff to consider whether such deaths could have been avoided and whether any defects in the system of working contributed to the death.[30] As part of his duty to identify defects in the system, the sheriff highlighted the importance of good communication in respect of individuals going through the custodial system. He recommended that 'if a forensic physician's report is prepared when an accused is in police custody, a copy of that report should accompany the accused if he/she is committed to prison'.[31]

Where prison healthcare is the responsibility of the NHS, it is not appropriate for NHS GPs in the community to request fees, or to delay, before agreeing to provide access to information in a patient's GP medical record. As a general point, NHS bodies should not normally charge each other and information needed for the purposes of continuing patient care should certainly not be delayed; a community GP requiring a fee would effectively be creating a situation whereby one NHS practitioner was asking another for a fee as part of patient care.

GPs in the community report delays in receiving medical information from the prison health team after patients' release. There is an ethical duty for doctors promptly to provide clinical information, such as a disease and drug summary, with the patient's consent. In emergencies, information should be provided by fax or secure email. If the release is planned, the patient should be given a summary of his or her notes and sufficient medication for a few days. Sometimes, however, detainees are released at very short notice and this is not always possible; in addition, some individuals destroy their medical records rather than pass them on (for example, if they document a steady dose reduction of prescribed benzodiazepines). Prompt liaison is particularly important when a detainee has a psychiatric illness or is being treated for substance misuse, and information about past medication needs to be available to current health staff. Such cases highlight the imperative need for information systems that facilitate effective and timely communication between healthcare professionals and establishments.

Ensuring access to appropriate care

All detainees are entitled to a standard of medical and nursing care equivalent to that which is available in the community. This includes prompt access not only to primary care services, but also to psychiatric services, physiotherapy, rehabilitation services, dietetics, dentistry, optician and genitourinary-medicine services.

Healthcare is subject to resource limitations within the general community and this can affect the delivery of services to those who are detained. However, detainees should not be subjected to lower levels of care. Health professionals have an obligation to draw attention to poor quality care. Under the Human Rights Act 1998, each individual has the rights set out in the European Convention on Human Rights (ECHR), such as the right to life (Article 2). The state is under a positive obligation to take adequate measures to protect life and thus Article 2 may be engaged if medical treatment were so deficient as to put detainees' lives at risk. Similarly, Article 3 (prohibition of torture and of inhuman or degrading treatment or punishment) could be invoked if there is a failure to provide proper treatment that results in suffering. Also, Article 14 (freedom from discrimination in respect of Convention rights) could be relevant if detainees receive treatment that is inferior to that provided to other sectors of society, and their rights under another ECHR Article are engaged. In some exceptional circumstances, it may be possible that detainees who would otherwise be deported, but need continuing medical care, can claim this under human rights legislation.

Claim to treatment under human rights legislation

D was born and spent most of his life in St Kitts. On arrival in the UK in 1993, seeking permission to enter for 2 weeks, he was found to be in possession of a substantial quantity of cocaine and was sentenced to 6 years' imprisonment. While in prison, D was found to be HIV positive and developed AIDS for which he received medical treatment. On his release on licence, D applied to remain in the UK on compassionate grounds, so that he could continue to receive the level of medical care he needed. This request was turned down by the immigration authorities. Following the dismissal of his claim at judicial review and subsequent appeal, he took his case to the European Court of Human Rights.

D's solicitor argued that D's removal to St Kitts would entail the loss of the medical treatment he was currently receiving, thereby shortening his life expectancy. Furthermore, such action would condemn him to spend his remaining days in pain and suffering in conditions of isolation, squalor and destitution. The Court held that, although it could not be said that the conditions that would confront him in the receiving country were themselves a breach of the standards of Article 3 (prohibition of torture and of inhuman or degrading treatment or punishment), D's removal to St Kitts would expose him to a real risk of dying in distressing circumstances and would thus amount to inhuman treatment in violation of Article 3. Although released foreign national prisoners did not normally have the right to remain so as to continue to receive medical or welfare services, D's case was exceptional and involved compelling humanitarian factors.[32]

Limited resources can result in pressure on doctors not to refer patients outside the establishment for treatment owing to the cost of an escort and the attendant risk of escape. A related problem has involved last minute cancellation of outpatient appointments because of a lack of escorts. The Chief Inspector of Prisons in England and Wales, in her 2008–2009 annual report, noted that hospital appointments were often cancelled and rescheduled, thereby delaying treatment, and that some prisons fail to monitor cancellations and re-bookings, making it impossible to identify whether prisoners are being seen within target waiting times.[33] Cancellation of outpatient appointments disadvantages detained patients and wastes NHS resources, but is not always easily preventable. Where prison staff are absent due to, for example, illness, hospital escorts can be used to cover the gaps in prison staffing. Although the deployment of staff in this way may sometimes be appropriate, this will not always be the case. If outpatient appointments need to be cancelled due to staffing problems, the prison healthcare team should be involved, for example, in deciding which patient is the most appropriate to defer and liaising with the hospital to minimise the negative impact of the cancellation on both the patient and the clinic.

Recruitment of prison health managers with an NHS background should help to improve the use of resources in relation to healthcare delivery. Doctors cannot ignore the cost implications of their recommendations but, by measures such as regular audit of their own referral and prescribing practice, should be able to demonstrate that their practice reflects the standards applied in the community. Their referral rates should be comparable with those in society at large for similar medical conditions.

Studies have revealed that the rates of illness in older prisoners are higher than in younger prisoners and in the general population of a similar age.[34] In 2009, the over-60s were reported to be the fastest growing age group in the prisoner population; from 1996 to 2006, prisoner numbers for those aged under 60 increased by one and a half times, while numbers for those aged 60 and over rose threefold during the same period.[35] Older patients may present with multiple morbidities and debilitating conditions, posing a significant challenge for prison healthcare services. Patients with limited mobility, requiring the use of mobility aids, such as wheelchairs or walking frames, can struggle with the lack of space available in prison buildings not generally adapted for people with chronic health or mobility problems. Older prisoners are often more vulnerable than younger ones, and elder abuse has been identified as a problem.[36] The Department of Health and Nacro have issued guidance on care for older prisoners,[37] but limited resources mean that their multiple needs may not be met. Healthcare professionals should promote the interests of older patients in detention, just as they would for those in the community.

The fact that detainees are entitled to an equivalent standard of care as is available in the community does not mean that they have a right to every possible medical intervention. Clearly, it would be inappropriate for prisoners to have special access to interventions that are unavailable or very scarce for others in society. A more unusual example of this issue was the legal judgment in the case of convicted murderer Gavin Mellor, who requested assisted reproduction as part of his claimed right under Article 12 (the right to marry and found a family) of the ECHR. This case is discussed in detail in Chapter 8, pages 316–318.

Prisoners' right to assisted reproduction

Mr Mellor's imprisonment made it impossible for his wife to conceive his child naturally, but his application for fertility treatment was refused. At judicial review, the refusal was upheld and the judge made clear that it was for the Secretary of State to formulate a policy for dealing with such requests by prisoners and to decide particular cases. In upholding the decision, the Court of Appeal emphasised that, although it will not always be justifiable to prevent a prisoner from inseminating his wife, in this case, there were no exceptional circumstances, for example to demonstrate that a refusal would prevent the founding of a family altogether, rather than merely delaying it.[38]

The 'exceptional circumstances' referred to in this case were present in a subsequent case which had a different outcome. Kirk and Lorraine Dickson had also been refused permission to use artificial insemination while Mr Dickson was serving a life sentence for murder. They applied to the European Court of Human Rights on the grounds that the Secretary of State's decision breached their Article 8 (right to respect for private and family life) and/or Article 12 rights. In December 2007, the Grand Chamber held that there had been a violation of Article 8 because insufficient account had been taken of the fact that, due to the woman's age (43 years when the application was originally made in 2001) and the term of imprisonment, fertility treatment represented the couple's only chance to have their own child.[39]

Minimising harm

Assessment of potential for self-harm

Prisoners have a much higher than average history of self-harm as well as psychological needs that are not easily met by offender healthcare teams. The prevalence of survivors of childhood sexual abuse, who may require psychological support, is much higher than in the general population. A 2005 research study on suicide rates among male prisoners found that they were five times more prone to suicide than men in the general population, and that young men in prison aged 15–17 were 18 times more likely to take their own lives.[40] Undiagnosed, undeclared and unrecognised mental illness and a lack of detoxification services for drug addiction were seen as important contributing factors.[41]

The National Suicide Prevention Strategy for England, launched in 2002, set out targets for 2009–2011 for reductions in the suicide rate. In 2008, a Ministerial Council on Deaths in Custody was established to consider how to prevent deaths in all forms of custody. By 2010, it was reported that good progress had been made in preventing suicide in prisons.[42] After a rise in the number of self-inflicted deaths in prisons in 2007, the number fell to

61 in 2008, a 34 per cent decrease on the previous year.[43] This was the lowest number of self-inflicted deaths in prisons since 1995.

Despite these improvements, the number of suicides in British prisons continues to be a matter of grave concern. Assessing each detainee's risk of suicide and self-harm is a key part of the role of health professionals working in all detention settings.

Measures to provide emergency attention

A crisis card scheme was introduced at Moorland Prison whereby prisoners with mental health problems could have access to a mental health professional within 30 minutes, day or night. Prisoners who have been assessed as likely to benefit from the reassurance provided by immediate access are issued with a card, which, if they wish, they can show to prison officers, who will call the health team. Prison officers know which individuals have a card but have no other details of prisoners' health status.[44]

Prisoners trained by the Samaritans to act as listeners and to support other prisoners who are at risk of self-harm are perceived to be an extremely valuable resource by both staff and detainees. They provide essential human contact and a sounding board for fellow prisoners. According to the Howard League for Penal Reform, trained listeners are one of the best defences against suicide and self-injury, especially when there is also provision of special rooms for use by listeners, where efforts are made to create a more relaxed atmosphere than in normal cells.[45]

Prompt assistance should be available in advance of, during and after a crisis. Healthcare teams need to have training in recognising and dealing with self-harming behaviour. Detailed strategies have been developed in establishments around the UK to reduce the occurrence of self-harm. The Prison Service in England and Wales uses a care-planning system called ACCT (Assessment, Care in Custody, and Teamwork), which has been in place in all establishments since April 2007. ACCT was designed to provide more flexible multi-disciplinary support to prisoners at risk of harming themselves, by encouraging staff to work together to provide individual care to prisoners in distress, to help defuse a potentially suicidal crisis or to help individuals with long-term needs, such as those with a pattern of repetitive self-injury, to better manage and reduce their distress.[46] A Prison Service Order (PSO) on suicide prevention and self-harm management was issued in 2007,[47] setting out mandatory requirements and specific approaches for establishments holding women and young people, as well as those dealing with detainees who regularly self-harm and at-risk individuals whose behaviour is particularly challenging. It provides instructions on identifying prisoners at risk of suicide and self-harm, and on providing the subsequent care and support for such prisoners, and support for the staff who care for them.

Role of healthcare in the prevention of self-harm, as outlined by the Prison Service Order on suicide prevention and self-harm management[48]

- Common risk factors include mental illness, serving a life term, drug and alcohol problems, experience of abuse, bereavement and, especially for women, the loss of children to the care system. Staff need to be aware of these issues and be vigilant, both in terms of the related risks of self-harm in individual prisoners, and in order to identify the specialist support that should be made available to them.
- Healthcare staff should share relevant risk and basic care information with other prison staff who manage prisoners who are at risk of self-harm or suicide, while ensuring that patient confidentiality is maintained.

- Mental health services should be well integrated into the mainstream prison to allow patients to benefit from care provided by mental health specialists, primary mental health staff and prison staff.
- At-risk prisoners benefit from mental health workers working with those with lower levels of mental health problems, rather than exclusively with those with severe problems.
- 'Dual diagnosis' covers a wide range of problems, incorporating mental health disorders and substance misuse, and should be considered by healthcare staff when treating prisoners with either issue.
- It is not expected that prisoners in a low category establishment at risk of suicide or self-harm will automatically be transferred to a higher security establishment. Consideration needs to be given to what access to health services, including mental health services, and other support can be provided at the current establishment, and the impact of transfer on the prisoner.
- The quality of the prison establishment and local commissioning body partnership is crucial to success in developing an effective suicide prevention and self-harm management strategy.

Communicable diseases

Healthcare services in detention settings should ensure that information about transmissible diseases (including tuberculosis, hepatitis and HIV/AIDS) is available to detainees, who need to be aware of preventive strategies as part of general information to improve their health. Some conditions that are eradicated from the general UK population may be present among immigration detainees, if they come from a country or region where, for example, hepatitis is endemic. The Health Protection Agency's (HPA) Prison Infection Prevention Team coordinates the surveillance of infectious diseases affecting the prison population, monitors hepatitis B vaccine coverage and aims to improve vaccine uptake and reporting of notifiable diseases in prisons. The team also provides regular information to prison healthcare staff on infectious diseases affecting the prison population through a quarterly bulletin on infectious disease.[49] (At the time of writing, the Government was seeking to reallocate the functions of the HPA and abolish the authority as part of its plan to reduce the number of arm's-length bodies. Up-to-date information on this can be found on the BMA website.) The World Health Organization's *Declaration on Prison Health as Part of Public Health* strongly emphasises the importance of close links and integration between public health services and prison healthcare (see also Chapter 20). As well as the duties owed to detained people, the document highlights the risks to civil society if detainees' communicable diseases are not promptly diagnosed and treated.[50]

Tuberculosis and public health dimensions of prison healthcare

Guidance for prison officials,[51] published in 2006, cited the increase in tuberculosis (TB) rates in the UK and the risks posed to vulnerable groups, such as those in prisons. Late diagnosis, due to the masking of TB symptoms (for example, by the symptoms of smoking or drug abuse, such as coughing or weight loss), inadequate treatment, overcrowding, poor ventilation and repeated prison transfers of infectious individuals, are all highlighted as factors encouraging the spread of TB infection within the prison population. This, in turn, can result in infection among the general population on the release of infected individuals who remain untreated.

The HPA has collaborated with the Department of Health to develop information resources to increase awareness among prisoners and prison staff, including non-clinical staff, about TB. These resources provide information about testing, treatment and support for patients who have been diagnosed with the disease in prisons.[52]

> The most challenging obstacle to TB control is ensuring that those with TB take the full, 6-month (or longer) course of treatment necessary to cure the disease. Patients receiving treatment for TB in prison are strongly recommended to have directly observed therapy where each dose of medication is personally supervised. Adequate release planning is also essential for these patients. The available guidance highlights the wider public health and health promotion implications of TB screening and treatment, by suggesting that all prison staff can support screening by reassuring prisoners and motivating people to get checked.

The provision of condoms in prison to reduce the transmission of sexually transmitted infections has long been a matter of debate. Since 1988, BMA policy has been that condoms and health education, including information about HIV infection, should be freely available in prisons.[53] The United Nations Office on Drugs and Crime has recommended that prison rules should 'recognize that consensual sexual activity occurs in prisons, and ensure that consensual sexual activity is not penalised as this will discourage prisoners accessing condoms'.[54] It has also addressed the issue of condom provision in the context of equivalence of care, suggesting that the measures available outside of prisons to prevent transmission of HIV are also available in prisons, for example through the provision of condoms and sterile needles and syringes. In turn, HIV prevention measures should be accessible in a confidential and non-discriminatory way.[55] Condoms are available on request from any member of the healthcare team in prisons in England and Wales. Legitimate concerns still exist among prison doctors and prison authorities, however, that condoms can be used to conceal illicit drugs, which have profoundly negative health consequences for detainees, and that, in distributing condoms, healthcare staff may be perceived to be complicit in sexual coercion.

The BMA has also long argued for effective measures to minimise needle sharing among detained individuals, given that it appears impossible to eliminate illegal drug use completely.[56] Common arguments against the provision of needle exchange are that it may appear to endorse illegal activity, encourages drug use or increases the risk of needles being used as weapons. In the BMA's view, however, such fears are not necessarily borne out in practice. In addition, while the vast majority of health authorities in England and Wales provide needle exchange programmes to injecting drug users in the community setting, a lack of provision of sterile needles in prisons can be seen to undermine the commitment to provide prisoners with healthcare services equivalent to those available in the community. Therefore, while recognising the drawbacks of needle exchange programmes, the Association has supported the concept of pilot schemes as part of broader strategies of education and risk reduction. By 2010, needle exchange was not available in UK prisons, although the policy had been under review and had come under legal scrutiny.

Legal review of government decision on needle exchange programmes

Mr Shelley, a prisoner at Whitemoor Prison, believed that the Government was obliged to conduct a trial of needle exchange programmes (NEPs) in prisons in England and Wales, and, in 2004, sought judicial review of the decision not to do so.[57] He based his claim on an alleged breach of his rights under Article 2 (right to life), Article 3 (prohibition of inhuman and degrading treatment and torture) and Article 8 (right to respect for private and family life) of the European Convention on Human Rights. As the use of illicit drugs in prison is a criminal offence, Mr Shelley refused to say whether or not he was a user; nevertheless, he claimed that non-users could also be adversely affected by the state's breach of its obligation under human rights legislation, as non-injecting prisoners and staff were put at risk from contracting HIV and hepatitis B and C from used needles.

Mr Shelley's application for judicial review was refused on two occasions and the Secretary of State defended the policy on a number of grounds, most of which centred on the harm that could arise from the likely increase in drug use that would follow from the increase in the number of syringes in prisons, and the possibility of syringes being used as weapons.

After these decisions, a Scottish report[58] found that with the implementation of NEPs in prisons, drug prevention programmes remained equally effective, drug use and the number of users did not rise, and the transmission rates of HIV and hepatitis decreased. On this basis, Mr Shelley renewed his application for judicial review, but was again refused. The Court of Appeal was satisfied that the Government's policy was justified, provided that it was kept under review. Mr Shelley then took his case to the European Court of Human Rights.

The obligations to provide equivalent health services to prisoners as to members of the wider community, and the responsibility of the Prison Service to provide preventive medicine, were highlighted by the case. However, the Court did not consider Articles 2 or 3 had been engaged. Given that Mr Shelley would not say whether he was an intravenous drug user, it was not clear that the risk to which he was exposed had sufficient weight to ground a claim. The Court did consider the arguments under Article 8. There was a lack of authority for an Article 8-based state obligation to implement a specific preventive healthcare policy. Although the Court accepted that, in principle, positive obligations could arise, in its view:

> matters of healthcare policy, in particular as regards general preventive measures, are in principle within the margin of appreciation of the domestic authorities who are best placed to assess priorities, use of resources and social needs.[59]

As there were preventive measures in place, and the Government continued to review its policy, in this instance the Court found that the state was behaving in a justified manner. Mr Shelley's case was therefore rejected and his complaint deemed inadmissible.[60]

The BMA also considers it important to make available to detainees guidance about decontaminating injection equipment. Sterilising or cleansing tablets to clean injecting equipment and information about how to use them are available in prisons. They have been freely available in all Scottish prisons, for example, since 1993 and accessible in all prisons in England and Wales from 2005.[61]

Clearly, patients with communicable diseases need not only appropriate medication but also living conditions that allow them to benefit from it. They need to be able to take their medication at the correct time, for example, regardless of normal prison timetables, and any associated dietary requirements need to be met. Interruptions to treatment need to be avoided by means of good liaison when detainees are transferred between prisons. Guidance for health professionals working in detention settings generally emphasises the opportunities that detention can bring, not just to try to tackle existing health problems and addiction, but also to attempt to engage detainees in health promotion. Doctors working in detention settings will also be aware that many detainees are resistant to accepting treatment and healthcare advice. While realising this, the healthcare team should work to ensure that such advice and treatment is available and well publicised.

Solitary confinement, segregation and separation

The term 'solitary confinement', or 'segregation', implies no contact with other prisoners. 'Separation and care units', as they are sometimes known within the prison setting, are used to segregate prisoners who have encountered problems due to their behaviour, although some detainees are, or ask to be, segregated for their own protection. Solitary confinement should be distinguished from situations in which detainees are accommodated in individual cells; in many establishments the majority of prisoners share a cell, often with a bunk bed in a cell originally designed for single occupancy, and being in a single cell is, by and large, seen as a privilege. The BMA considers that therapy or counselling should be an integral part of the care and treatment pattern for at-risk detainees and supports the move away from solitary confinement for those who are perceived to be potentially suicidal. A prisoner with his or her own cell may be locked away alone for long periods of time, but he or she should be able to socialise with others at appropriate times and such a situation cannot be called 'solitary confinement' in the sense in which it is discussed below.

The European Committee for the Prevention of Torture and Inhuman or Degrading Treatment or Punishment (CPT) has published guidance on the use of solitary confinement, stating that the principle of proportionality requires that a balance be struck between the requirements of the case and the use of solitary confinement.[62] This type of regime can have harmful consequences for the individual and according to the CPT can, in certain circumstances, amount to inhuman and degrading treatment. The CPT stresses that all forms of solitary confinement should be as short as possible. It identifies access to a doctor, without delay, on request, as an essential safeguard during a period of solitary confinement. In addition, detainees in solitary confinement must be seen daily by a mental health professional in order to identify any deterioration in mental health. The CPT recommends that doctors forward the results of any medical examination, including the foreseeable consequences of continued isolation, to the appropriate prison authorities. In the BMA's view, when sharing such information, doctors should only include specific medical details where the patient consented to the disclosure of health information.

The CPT has been 'particularly concerned about the placement of juveniles in conditions resembling solitary confinement' and stresses that, if held separately from others, they should be guaranteed appropriate opportunities for human contact and outdoor exercise, as well as access to reading materials.[63] In England and Wales, the Chief Inspector of Prisons has reported that, although all segregation units accommodating children and young people have been relabelled as 'care and separation', 'reorientation' or 'intensive supervision' units, they often operate as traditional segregation units, with the emphasis on separation rather than care.[64]

The medical role in restraint and control

When restraint is essential in dealing with detainees' health needs, health professionals need to be involved. However, if restraint or control measures are invoked for the purposes of maintaining order or discipline, this should not involve health staff. The BMA has published advice on the medical role in the use of restraint in detention settings.[65] It makes clear that restraint should only ever be used as an act of care and control, not as punishment or a convenience. The use of restraint can result in physical injury, psychological morbidity, demoralisation and feelings of humiliation. Advice specifically to forensic physicians emphasises that rapid tranquillisation should be performed only where equipment for cardio-pulmonary resuscitation is present and there are trained staff to use it.[66] Authoritative guidance on the appropriate conditions in which restraint may be used is available from the CPT.

European Committee for the Prevention of Torture and Inhuman or Degrading Treatment or Punishment guidelines on the use of force and restraint[67]

- The use of force or physical restraint against violent prisoners requires specific safeguards.
- Prisoners who are subjected to physical restraint should be kept under constant and adequate supervision, and the restraint should be removed at the earliest possible opportunity.
- Restraint should never be prolonged or applied as a punishment.
- A record should be kept of every use of restraint or force against prisoners.
- Prisoners who have been subjected to any means of force should be immediately offered a medical examination by an appropriate healthcare professional and, if necessary, treated by a doctor.
- If possible, medical examination should be conducted out of sight and hearing of non-medical staff; a record should be made of the findings of the examination, including any relevant statements by the prisoner and the doctor's conclusions, and this should be available to the prisoner.
- Effective inspection and complaints procedures must be in place. Prisoners should be aware of the avenues of complaint open to them.

Restraint of detained patients in NHS facilities

Detainees may need treatment in NHS hospitals and other healthcare facilities. From the perspective of prison staff, hospitals are sometimes seen as the 'weak link' in the chain of secure custody where detainees may try to give a false impression of their medical condition in order to attempt to escape. Health professionals are often unsure about whether they are entitled to ask for handcuffs to be removed during assessment and treatment, or if they can ask accompanying guards to leave the room. They should certainly do so if the method of restraint interferes with treatment or if the detained person is clearly too incapacitated either to threaten others or to abscond. The general advice given to prison staff around the UK is to comply, where feasible, with such requests and that restraints must not be used to attach any prisoner to furniture, fixtures or fittings. Advance risk assessment procedures should have already clarified, prior to the consultation in the outside healthcare facility, the potential threat of escape or violence. Whether or not restraint is advisable should be discussed between health professionals and the detaining authorities, and judgements made on a case-by-case basis. In some cases, it is unnecessary and humiliating for the detainee to be shackled and closely attended by guards. Ideally, restraints should be removed from pregnant women attending hospital for antenatal care and those in labour (see pages 718–720). Where there is a risk of escape or violence to others, the safeguards employed should be commensurate with the risk. Some hospitals located near to prisons have special secure areas for the treatment of detainees.

Prison Service Order on the use of force[68]

Prison Service Order 1600 emphasises that the use of force by one person on another without consent is unlawful unless it is justified; the use of force will be justified, and therefore lawful, only if:

- it is reasonable in the circumstances
- it is necessary
- no more force than necessary is used
- it is proportionate to the seriousness of the circumstances.

Restraint in transit

An issue previously raised with the BMA relates to the role of in-flight nurses and doctors who are escorting asylum seekers who have been refused residence in the UK and are deported either to the first country they passed through on their entry to the European Union, or their country of origin. Concerns were expressed about the use of both physical and chemical restraints in situations in which a doctor and a nurse were accompanying 50–100 people at a time, with a private security organisation managing the process. In the BMA's view 'the involvement of doctors in the forcible removal of refugees or illegal immigrants constitutes an inappropriate use of medical skills'.[69] It supports the WMA's view that health professionals should not become involved in providing medication that cannot be medically justified. In 2008, the WMA reaffirmed a resolution stating that doctors 'cannot be compelled to participate in any punitive or judicial action involving refugees or IDPs [internally displaced persons] or to administer any non-medically justified diagnostic measure or treatment, such as sedatives to facilitate easy deportation from the country or relocation'.[70] The BMA makes a distinction between health professionals being available to provide necessary medical attention to the passengers and being there as part of an 'enforcement' procedure. It recognises that people whose appeals have been heard fairly should be returned to their first port of entry, but the BMA would be greatly concerned if it were seen to be the role of doctors to keep deportees passive.

In 2009, the Chief Inspector of Prisons for England and Wales published a report on escorted removals. This found a number of weaknesses in the systems for monitoring, investigating and complaining about incidents where force had been used or where abuse was alleged. Reasons for the use of force were not always clear and medical examinations were not routinely carried out afterwards. Its recommendations included that detainees subject to the use of force, including handcuffing, be promptly medically assessed, that detention and escorting staff use professional interpretation when communicating key information to detainees, including about journeys and medication, and whenever necessary to alleviate anxiety. In addition, detention and escorting staff should check that detainees have access to all prescribed medication at appropriate times.[71]

Health professionals need to make sure that their presence is primarily to deal with complications that may arise during repatriation of deportees. Nevertheless, it can be difficult to separate necessary medical attention from enforcement procedures. Their conditions of employment and the circumstances in which they are expected to use their skills should be made clear at the outset. They should act with the deportees' health needs foremost in their minds and keep a focus on treatment and care. The BMA also recommends that agencies involved in deportations should be informed that this is the only appropriate role of health professionals.

Health professionals need to speak out if they are aware of any breaches of established guidance in relation to restraint. Any means of restraint can be dangerous if improperly applied. Methods whose level of risk has not been thoroughly investigated should not be used. In 1998, the BMA objected to the use of CS spray in confined spaces such as police vans. It argued that there was a lack of data about the full effects of the interaction of the CS and the carrier spray, especially on people who were already taking medication. Subsequent research has indicated that CS spray used by the police is more harmful than had previously been thought.[72]

Management of hunger strikes

Hunger strikes are a form of protest used in detention settings. The Department of Health has produced comprehensive guidelines for the clinical management of people refusing food in these settings, which includes information on both the legal aspects and the physical effects of food and fluid refusal.[73] In addition, a revised Declaration of Malta, including a glossary and background guidance paper, on the ethics of the medical management of hunger strikes was adopted by the WMA in 2006.[74] Principles for their management remain the same in each setting and involve ascertaining as far as possible the individual's wishes and intention. A psychiatric assessment may be required in order to clarify a detainee's ability to make a valid refusal. Patients who do not appear to have capacity, for example because they have a serious mental disorder for which they require treatment, should be transferred to a hospital setting.

Forcible feeding

In March 2000, the High Court decided that convicted murderer, Ian Brady, could not make a valid and binding decision to starve himself to death. Brady's lawyers argued that Ashworth Hospital had exceeded its powers in tube feeding Brady against his will and attempted to obtain the Court's authority to prevent further artificial feeding. Despite the fact that Brady claimed not to be suffering from a mental illness, for which artificial feeding could constitute a medical treatment, and a forensic psychiatrist said his decision was a rational one, the judge was swayed by medical arguments that Brady was psychopathic and prone to need to control others. His attempts to prevent feeding were a manifestation of his personality disorder and accordingly his force feeding had constituted necessary medical treatment for his mental disorder under the Mental Health Act 1983. Brady's refusal of food was seen as part of his psychological condition because he had previously employed hunger strikes as a tactic, which he claimed gave him a 'massive psychological boost', in what he perceived as a battle of wills with the hospital authorities, rather than an intent to starve himself to death.[75]

Doctor–patient discussion

At the start of a hunger strike, detainees should be offered a medical examination and accurate clinical information about the foreseeable effects of fasting. They need to be aware that underlying health problems are likely to come to the fore and should indicate whether they accept treatment or pain relief for these. Doctors should discuss what the patient intends and whether health staff are expected to intervene with emergency treatment before permanent damage occurs. Patients need to be aware that resuscitation attempts, particularly at a late stage, may not be successful and that, even when they are, residual neurological problems may persist. In the absence of such detailed advance discussion, it is likely to be difficult for health staff to judge later what the individual would want if concessions are achieved after the patient has lost mental capacity. If, for example, a significant concession is made, doctors may feel justified in intervening on the grounds that the current situation differs substantially from that envisaged by the patient when the treatment refusal was made. Where mass hunger strikes occur, detainees are often under considerable peer pressure to participate. Even solitary hunger strikes can be the result of certain individuals being chosen by the peer group. Medical staff must have opportunities to speak to patients privately about their decision and, if it is clear that the fast is non-voluntary, efforts should be made to remove the pressures on the detainee.

Hunger strikes and advance decisions

In England and Wales, the Mental Capacity Act 2005 imposes particular legal requirements and safeguards on making an advance decision refusing life-sustaining treatment, which must be met in order for such a decision to be valid and binding. (For detailed guidance on advance decisions refusing treatment in all UK jurisdictions, see Chapter 3.) The decision must be written, signed and witnessed, and must include a clear, specific statement from the person making the advance decision that it is to apply to the specific treatment, even if life is at risk. In the BMA's view, it is important for a person making an advance decision to refuse life-sustaining treatment to discuss it with a healthcare professional in order to explain what type of treatment may be life-sustaining and in what circumstances, and the implications and consequences of refusing treatment. Clinicians are advised to refer to detailed advice on the use of advance decisions in these circumstances, which has been issued by the Department of Health.[76]

In the community, it is acceptable to record the outcome of discussions regarding advance decisions refusing treatment in the medical records. However, advice from the Ministry of Justice Legal Directorate is that, in detention settings, it is preferable to have an advance decision recorded in a separate document used solely for that purpose. It is sensible to have at least one witness for such discussions, but preferably two. The existence of such a document should not be public knowledge among other detainees. Witnesses should be independent to avoid detainees being pressured by others into making an advance decision refusing life-sustaining treatment. The discussion should ascertain that the individual understands the situation and the consequences of their actions. This document should record that their judgement is not impaired through lack of mental capacity.[77]

As with any form of advance decision, patients may want to change their mind later, which, of course, they are entitled to do while they retain capacity. At the time treatment is required, the healthcare professional must try to find out if the patient has withdrawn the advance decision refusing life-sustaining treatment.[78] In most situations in the community, a change of decision is unproblematic. In the context of a hunger strike undertaken in a detention setting, a documented advance decision can potentially deprive patients of an opportunity to retract their refusal without losing face, for example among their peers who are also involved in the protest. If freely made by a person with capacity who is informed, however, advance decisions are as binding in detention as in other settings.

Advance decision refusing nutrition

In November 2001, Barry Horne died in hospital of liver failure resulting from a hunger strike in Long Lartin High Security Prison in Worcestershire. He was an animal rights activist, serving an 18-year sentence, and had carried out many hunger strikes, previously narrowly avoiding death on a 68-day strike in 1998. During his last hunger strike, he signed an advance decision refusing medical intervention, at a time when he was declared to have capacity. The prison and hospital authorities were therefore bound to abide by his refusal.[79]

Respecting treatment refusal

Respecting the voluntary refusal of patients with capacity who are informed accords with the principles set out in the WMA's Declaration of Tokyo.[80] This affirms that, when patients with capacity refuse nourishment in full knowledge of the consequences, they should not be fed artificially. Doctors sometimes take over care only when it is too late to be certain about the individual's real intention. If there is good reason to believe that death was not intended, emergency treatment should be started. Patients should be transferred to appropriate hospital care. If cardio-pulmonary resuscitation is likely to be needed, the hospital or medical room should be suitably equipped. When it is clear that detainees intend to continue the strike until death, they must be allowed to die with dignity. It should be decided at a relatively early stage whether they will die in the detention setting, where the staff know them, or be transferred to an NHS hospital. Transfer to a hospital may be easier for the individual's family, but should be arranged in time for some rapport to develop between the patient and staff before the patient loses capacity (see also Chapter 10).

Summary – practical issues common to various detention settings

- As well as working cooperatively with other staff to promote a safe and orderly environment, doctors must primarily promote the interests and rights of their patients in detention settings.
- In order to facilitate the work of health professionals in detention settings, strategies need to be in place to:
    - ensure that health professionals have sufficient time to facilitate good communication with both patients and colleagues
    - ensure prompt patient access to care in detention and continuity of care after release
    - offer patients health protection and disease prevention advice
    - prevent the misuse of medication
    - identify detainees' risk of, and prevent opportunities for, self-harm and suicide
    - use restraint appropriately
    - establish the medical role in the management of hunger strikes
    - address the exceptional stress on health professionals.

Healthcare in prisons

Improvements have undoubtedly been made as a result of prison health reform (see pages 689–691), however, providing healthcare in prisons will always be a complex task.

Challenges of healthcare delivery in prisons

Summarising the findings of her eighth and final annual report in 2010, the outgoing Chief Inspector of Prisons for England and Wales, Anne Owers, commented that health had improved and the number and rate of self-inflicted deaths in prison had declined. However, concerns remained about the prevalence of self-harm, especially in women's prisons, insufficient primary mental health services and the lack of focus on work with alcohol misusers.[81]

She captured, in stark terms, some of the key challenges that the prison environment presents to those delivering healthcare services:

> . . . in spite of the progress made, prisons remain caught between the irresistible force of an increasing population and the immovable object of budget cuts. Population pressure affects the whole system – stretching resources, keeping in use buildings that ought to be condemned, doubling up prisoners in cramped cells. Prisons are larger and more complex. Resource pressures are at present being contained, but should not be underestimated. There are two risks: of increased instability in inherently fragile environments and of reducing prisons' capacity to rehabilitate those they hold.[82]

These pervading pressures can have a manifestly negative impact on the health of those detained, as well as on the attainment of successful health outcomes within the prison setting.

From a health perspective, detention represents an opportunity to address neglected health problems and doctors working in secure settings are generally aware of the possibility for influencing patients' attitudes positively. While for some detainees it is possible to identify and address chronic health problems, for many health is a low priority. It can take time and significant input from a range of multi-disciplinary services to address healthcare needs, to promote health and, even then, efforts may not always be productive.

Mental health services

Prisoners have significantly higher rates of mental health problems than the general population, with a higher prevalence of behavioural disorders, history of violence, personality disorder, psychosis, history of self-harm and other mental health problems. Among prisoners, the range of conditions and illnesses that fall into the 'mental health problems' category is broad. It represents a similar range to that experienced by people living in the community (although the proportions are different) and so requires similar services to treat them effectively. Evidence gathered for Lord Bradley's 2009 review of people with mental health problems and learning disabilities in the criminal justice system suggests that prisons are currently struggling to provide such services. In particular, the report identified that certain elements of the prison population are not receiving any treatment at all.[83] Problems experienced by prison doctors in obtaining prompt and appropriate mental health services for patients have been consistently highlighted. These include: delays in the assessment of prisoners' mental health needs; the conviction and imprisonment of mentally ill people due to failures in community mental health provision; and offenders who become mentally ill in prison but are not transferred to specialist units when appropriate.[84] There is also a lack of resources to manage those who have complex mental health problems but are not considered sufficiently 'severe' to be transferred.

In England and Wales, under the Mental Health Act 1983, prisons, including healthcare wings, are specifically excluded as places where patients can be given compulsory treatment. In Scotland, the Mental Health (Care and Treatment) (Scotland) Act 2003, and in Northern Ireland, the Mental Health (Northern Ireland) Order 1986, also exclude the delivery of compulsory mental health treatment outside of a hospital setting. When a patient has a mental illness that is so severe that, if living in the community, he or she would be sectioned, the patient must be transferred to a psychiatric hospital.[85] However, a frequent problem for doctors has been the difficulty in transferring mentally ill prisoners who need specialised care to a hospital.[86] This can be a particularly stressful situation for prison doctors, who are limited in the amount they can do to prevent patients' mental health deteriorating while they await transfer. The CPT has previously stated that the transfer of mentally ill patients to adequately equipped and properly staffed psychiatric facilities should be treated as a matter of the highest priority. It reiterated concerns about this issue in the report of its 2008 visit to the UK, which noted that the transfer of mentally ill patients usually took months rather than weeks to complete.[87] Indeed, the Bradley report suggested that the Department of Health should develop a new minimum target for the NHS of 14 days to transfer a prisoner with acute, severe mental illness to an appropriate healthcare setting.[88]

By 2009, several practical initiatives had been implemented to try to address the problems of mental healthcare provision in prisons. Mental health in-reach teams were established alongside the transfer of health services from the Prison Service to the NHS in England and Wales. Although originally designed to treat patients with severe and enduring mental illness, practice has in fact broadened to include a whole range of mental health problems.[89] The first formal national evaluation of in-reach services indicated that, as a result of this development, only 14 per cent of prisoners studied with a current severe and enduring mental illness were accepted onto in-reach caseloads. Furthermore, 85 per cent of in-reach team leaders stated that their teams were not sufficiently staffed to meet the needs of patients.[90] The evaluation report seems to suggest that the poor resourcing of other mental health services in prison, and poor links to drug and alcohol services, have prevented in-reach teams from focusing on those with severe and enduring mental illnesses, as originally intended. Yet, at the same time, prison doctors report that there remain limited resources for doctors to manage jointly, with a community mental health team, conditions such as moderate to severe depression.

Despite these initiatives, other barriers to the early identification and assessment of mental health problems exist, some of which are more difficult for prison doctors to overcome than others. Examples include inadequacies in the transfer of health information throughout the criminal justice system; on entering prison, information on an individual patient's health from community, police or court assessments is often not readily available.[91] Balancing patient confidentiality with efforts to improve information flow between prisons, GP practices, social services, probation officers, police and courts, is potentially problematic. In addition, many GPs who are responsible for primary care in prison lack specialist training in the care of prisoners and their complex mental health needs.[92]

A 2008 thematic report by HM Chief Inspector of Prisons identified that many of the barriers discussed above also applied to the prison estate in Scotland.[93] In Northern Ireland, an independent review of mental health services and legislation was undertaken, in which the Prison Service was a partner.[94] This was followed by a commitment by the Northern Ireland Government to place the legal provisions surrounding mental capacity and mental health on a statutory footing, with the introduction of new legislation, which, at the time of writing, was being drafted.

Substance misuse services

Substance misuse and drug addiction have been cited by both clinicians and policy makers as a major cause of reoffending. The majority of prisoners are said to have a diagnosable mental illness, alcohol or drug misuse problem, or both. In addition, mainstream mental health services may refuse to address mental health problems until the substance misuse issues have been resolved. In 2007, the All-Party Parliamentary Group on Prison Health noted that dealing with drugs is the area where conflict between prison policy and public health policy is most acute, and that despite the fact that local commissioning bodies had taken over commissioning prison healthcare in England, prisoners were still not receiving a level of care comparable with that delivered by community NHS services. Their report drew links between the impact of addiction in prisons upon public health and the wider community, and gave a number of recommendations concerning detoxification programmes and maintenance therapy (the prescribing of heroin substitutes such as methadone or buprenorphine), which have subsequently been implemented.[95]

Management of pregnancy and childcare

The number of pregnant women held in prisons is not routinely collated, but information contained in a 2008 answer to a parliamentary question indicated that between April

2005 and July 2008, 283 children were born to women in prison.[96] Prison Service figures indicate that, in England and Wales, around 120 women in custody give birth each year.[97] An important issue here is the ability of women to attend routine antenatal care sessions and give birth without being handcuffed or constantly monitored by accompanying prison personnel.

In the 1990s, the Howard League for Penal Reform publicised a number of cases of women who were allegedly handcuffed while being given an antenatal examination, while giving birth and while trying to breastfeed.[98] The CPT asserts that restraint of pregnant women during gynaecological examinations or delivery is completely unacceptable and identifies such practice as inhuman and degrading treatment.[99] Prison Service guidance acknowledges that restraint may be used, but only where the woman's behaviour is unmanageable or there are indications that she presents a significant risk of escape.[100]

Management of pregnancy and healthcare: advice from the Prison Service

- Pre-natal and post-natal care for pregnant women, including ongoing support to breastfeed, where appropriate, should be available in all women's prisons.
- Pregnant women and nursing mothers should receive a suitable diet based on Department of Health guidelines.
- The location and management of a pregnant woman must be risk assessed and her views taken into account.
- Pregnant women are not to be handcuffed after arrival at a hospital or clinic. Restraints should not be used unless the woman's behaviour is unmanageable or there are indications that she may escape.
- Women in labour should not be handcuffed either en route to, or while in, hospital.
- Pregnant women must not be transferred between prisons or court in a cellular vehicle except in exceptional circumstances, or with the agreement of the healthcare manager following a full risk assessment.[101]

The Children's Commissioner for England, in a 2008 report, recommended an end to the routine use of custody for women who are pregnant, or mothers of very young children, other than in exceptional circumstances where they represent a danger to society.[102] (For a discussion of the welfare of children in immigration detention, see pages 726–727.) In 2010, however, there were seven mother and baby units in prisons across England. Prison Service standards emphasise the importance of an open and equitable system for prisoners to acquire information about mother and baby units and to apply for a place, with an appropriate appeals process.[103] The standards stress the interests of the child as the basis for decision making. A full range of health services for mothers and babies must be available, equivalent to what is provided in the community, and services must meet the needs of women and children from all backgrounds. Separation plans must be drawn up and discussed with the mother when her application for a child place is refused, and aftercare support should be offered to women who are not permitted to keep their babies with them. Childcare plans for those admitted to a unit should also include consideration of arrangements for possible future separation where that may be necessary for the child's development needs, or in case of emergency. Alternative carers for babies need to be identified at the earliest opportunity when separation is judged to be in the babies' best interests.

In addition to the women who give birth while imprisoned, many women in jail have dependent children at home. Although data are not routinely collected, Home

Office research has indicated that 66 per cent of the female prison population have dependent children.[104] Nevertheless, childcare arrangements are not necessarily taken into consideration when women are allocated to a prison, with the result that women can be serving their sentence hundreds of miles away from their children, making visits impossible. Clearly, when their families are a source of anxiety for prisoners, there needs to be appropriate liaison between the relevant agencies.

Independence of health professionals

Health professionals should not have a disciplinary or punitive role in any establishment, although they must be aware of the need for order and discipline to be maintained. They are primarily responsible for the physical and mental health of prisoners and should not be expected to fulfil both clinical and disciplinary roles. However, some confusion about role identity can arise.

Doctors must be able to make independent clinical and ethical judgements concerning patients' healthcare. A problem in the past has been the wide variation in prescribing practice in prisons. Clearly, clinical decisions in any context should be evidence-based and all health professionals should have regard to equitable use of resources. For example, in prisons, doctors may be asked to prescribe from a limited drug list, with medicines not on the list requiring special justification. As this is intended to reduce costs in an equitable manner, without damaging the health of individual patients, the principle of using prescribing protocols is ethically acceptable; such protocols are also common outside prison settings. Doctors sometimes object, however, that they cannot prescribe what they judge to be the most appropriate treatment for individuals and feel that patient trust can be undermined as a result. Doctors are accountable to the GMC for their standard of care, including the medications they prescribe, but they also have to work within budgetary constraints. The Department of Health states that they must 'only prescribe treatments which make an effective contribution to the patient's overall management' and 'take resources into account when choosing between treatments of similar effectiveness'.[105] Pharmacy protocols should contribute to better standardisation. Prescribing issues more generally are discussed in depth in Chapter 13.

Independence and the duty to speak out

The BMA has received enquiries from doctors working in prisons regarding whether they are prevented from speaking out about poor conditions or evidence of abuse. The Association's advice is that health professionals must not be prevented from taking appropriate action when detainees appear to be subject to abuse or brutality by prison staff or other prisoners. Suspicions should be reported to the governor of the establishment and, if this appears to have no effect, advice should be sought from the relevant area manager and medical director of prison health. In this situation, doctors need to obtain objective clinical evidence and reflect critically on the situation in which they find themselves to ensure that they have not been manipulated by their patients. There must be accurate clinical recording of findings.

Where doctors are employed to provide medical services to prisoners detained by British or allied armed forces in other countries, the duties of health professionals to speak out about abuse remain the same.[106] (For guidance on doctors working in the armed forces, see Chapter 16, pages 679–682.)

Diversion from prison: drug treatment and testing orders and drug rehabilitation requirements

The diversion of some categories of offender away from custodial sentencing can blur the distinction between therapeutic and judicial strategies and, in turn, can raise dilemmas for health professionals because medical treatment in the community could be seen as part of the criminal justice system. Conflict has arisen in the past in relation to drug treatment and testing orders (DTTOs), whereby patients are 'sentenced' to take part in a specified treatment regimen as an alternative to a prison sentence. Legislation for DTTOs was first introduced in the UK in 1998 and is still in force in both Scotland[107] and Northern Ireland.[108] In England and Wales, from 2005, DTTOs were renamed Drug Rehabilitation Requirements (DRRs) and subsumed under a single community order along with 11 other possible requirements or conditions around which the community sentence is based, such as mental health treatment, curfew or compulsory (unpaid) work.[109] DTTOs and DRRs can be imposed only if the court is satisfied that the offender is dependent on drugs or has a propensity to misuse them. The dependency or propensity must not only require treatment, but also be treatable, and the patient must be willing to give consent. Orders include both a treatment and a testing requirement, and specify whether treatment should be on a residential or non-residential basis.

An inherent problem with such orders is the different perspectives, aims and objectives of the various parties involved. One key concern is the potential conflict between the ethical responsibilities treatment providers have to patients and the obligations they have to the criminal justice system.[110] This tension can manifest itself in a number of ways. Some health professionals have concerns about providing treatment when the patient has effectively been coerced to consent. As mentioned throughout this book, however, there are other circumstances in which there are pressures on consent, but where the consent is nonetheless considered to be valid. Ultimately, the decision of whether to accept the treatment regimen that is offered to them as an alternative to prison rests with individual patients. They must understand their options and the implications of their choices in order to give valid consent but, provided this information has been given, it is for each individual to decide whether treatment is the best option. This must include an awareness and acceptance that the usual rules of confidentiality do not apply and that information must be provided to other agencies.

For both DRRs and DTTOs, although the treatment provider is involved with drawing up the treatment schedule, this must be within the general framework set out in national standards. For DRRs, where assessment takes place in the community, Probation Service guidance states it may be good practice for a dual assessment to take place involving the treatment team and probation services, but this is not essential. Where the DRR involves substitute prescribing, the patient should be assessed by relevant clinical personnel for his or her suitability for treatment.[111]

Some doctors report that they do not always believe that a treatment order, along the lines of the national standards, is in the best interests of a particular patient, but they are concerned that changing the programme could lead to difficulties for that patient. In the past some doctors complained to the BMA about the requirement in the national standards for urine samples to be produced under direct observation. They considered that, despite the punitive aspect to such treatment orders, patients should be entitled to the maximum amount of dignity and privacy consistent with the aims of the testing. Advances in technology have seen the accuracy of other testing methods improve and oral fluid testing is now considered to be a viable alternative to urine testing and is permitted on both DRR and DTTO schemes.

When doctors have concerns about any aspect of the treatment proposed, they should discuss them with the named treatment provider and others involved in supervising the treatment orders, with a view to maximising the likelihood of the patient succeeding in the programme. Although only the court has the power to amend any of the order's specific requirements or provisions, in practice the court is likely to depend on advice from the treatment provider or supervising officer about any necessary amendments. The aim should be to find a balance between the treatment needs of the patient and the aims of the court to enforce the terms of the order and to prevent the patient from reoffending.

As with other cases in which doctors are prescribing, it is important, with the patient's consent, to keep the GP informed of any medication prescribed and of the progress of treatment.

Facilities accommodating young adult offenders, children and young people

When offenders under the age of 21 are sentenced to a custodial term, they may be sent to one of two types of Prison Service-run establishment, dependent upon their age; young offender institutions (YOIs) accommodate 18- to 20-year-olds, while secure accommodation for young people (formerly referred to as 'juvenile offenders') accommodates 15- to 17-year-olds. Other facilities include privately run secure training centres and local authority secure children's homes, run by social services. Many reports have criticised youth detention facilities and drawn attention to the problems of child detention. In 2008, the Scottish Justice Secretary announced a decision to end the use of custodial remand for children under the age of 16;[112] in 2009, HM Chief Inspector of Prisons for Scotland stated that 'prison is no place for a child'.[113] Others have drawn particular attention to problems of self-harm and bullying.[114] Drug dependency, alcohol misuse and mental health problems lie behind many of the vulnerabilities of young detainees in addition to their youth. While children and young people are detained there is the opportunity to detect, diagnose and treat health problems in a group that is often not engaged with health services.

Clearly, many of the same issues arise with young offenders as with the care of adult detainees, with the additional vulnerability that is likely to be experienced by a young person in detention. The population in this group is diverse. As with adult prisoners, an important factor directly affecting the quality of care for young detainees has been the role confusion within the health service offered in those detention settings accommodating this group. In 2008, the CPT drew particular attention to the fact that healthcare staff at Huntercombe YOI regularly carried out custodial officer tasks, for example taking part in strip searches when detainees were admitted. The CPT's report stressed that this was inappropriate and that healthcare services in facilities for young offenders should be discrete and independent.[115]

Children and young people's consent and refusal of treatment

The general rules on consent relating to children and young people are set out in detail in Chapter 4 and summarised on page 693. Legally, competent young people are able to consent on their own behalf, but may not always be able to refuse an intervention that is deemed to be in their best interests if people with parental responsibility, or the courts, consent on their behalf. Where the relationship between parents and the young person is strained, as is often the case for detainees, parents still have a legal right to consent, but this does not necessarily mean that doctors are obliged to carry out their wishes. It is always important to listen to the views of young people and try to understand why they object. Health professionals are very reluctant to impose a medication or treatment that a competent young person refuses because this is likely to undermine their relationship with that patient. Moreover, any use of restraint in order to impose treatment would raise additional ethical issues (see pages 711–713). Doctors should seek legal advice if a competent young person refuses essential medical treatment, although emergency treatment should not be delayed. Chapter 4 provides advice on the action to be taken when a young person refuses a procedure that has been validly authorised by those with parental responsibility.

Child protection in detention

The prevalence of psychiatric disorder among young people and children in detention is even higher than that among the adult prison population; 95 per cent of the detained population aged under 21 suffer from a mental disorder, substance misuse problems, or both.[116] Institutionalisation when young can cause some types of personality disorder. The vulnerability of detained children and young people raises substantial and complex protection issues.

In a High Court ruling in 2002,[117] the judge held that the Children Act 1989 applies to people under the age of 18 held in custody. Mr Justice Munby noted that 'bullying, self harm and suicide remain serious and in some instances untackled problems' for this group.[118] His judgment means that local authorities in England and Wales have a legal duty to promote the welfare of detained minors. Local authorities have to undertake a needs assessment if the young person falls within the statutory criteria set out in the Children Act and develop a care plan that meets those needs. This obviously has huge resource and staffing implications for services that are already stretched.

Self-harm and assessing suicide risk

Young people (18–20 years) in prison are more likely to have mental health problems and are more likely to commit or attempt suicide than both younger and older prisoners.[119] Behavioural and mental health problems are particularly prevalent among children in prison, with 85 per cent of those detained showing signs of a personality disorder and one in 10 showing signs of a psychotic illness.[120] There are established links between mental health problems and self-harm.

It is particularly important that training in assessment of detainees takes account of the differing needs of young people and adult prisoners. Detention facilities should have a comprehensive vulnerability assessment procedure, rather than relying upon evidence of previous attempts to self-harm, and staff should be trained in the particular problems of young people.

Good practice: peer mentoring[121]

In an effort to tackle the connected issues of suicide and self-harm prevention, and bullying and violence reduction, Thorn Cross YOI has developed a peer mentor scheme in cooperation with the National Society for the Prevention of Cruelty to Children, Samaritans and ChildLine. The collaboration was the first peer mentor scheme of its kind in a YOI.[122]

Within 2 years of its establishment, the scheme had proved to be successful, with the mentors giving information, advice and support to new prisoners and those who may be vulnerable due to bereavement, relationship issues or because they have been the target of bullying. The mentors themselves reported gaining in self-confidence and self-esteem. It was hoped that a formal qualification would eventually be available for the mentors.

In addition, at Thorn Cross, violence reduction workshops were offered to all prisoners receiving adjudications for assaults, fights or using threatening or abusive behaviour. A survey by the psychology unit into bullying at Thorn Cross showed that more prisoners felt safer there than in closed prisons and, while verbal bullying was still prevalent, it was less than had been reported previously.[123]

Immigration removal centres (IRCs)

In the BMA's view, the detention of people who are not convicted of a criminal offence should be a measure of last resort, used only in exceptional circumstances. In such cases, the detainees should be informed, in a language they understand, of their rights and the procedures applicable to them, in line with guidance from the CPT.[124] The lack of understandable information about the reasons and likely duration of detention can obviously contribute to anxiety and depression in this patient group. Detainees should also receive accessible information relating to the provision of healthcare.

Duty of care for detainees held in immigration detention

In 2002, the Government proposed to establish a system of induction and accommodation centres for fast tracking some asylum seekers' claims.[125] The power to detain foreign nationals is exercised by officials of the UK Border Agency (UKBA), formed in 2008, and such detention is not subject to any time limit. In 2010, there were 12 IRCs across the UK; in addition, a number of short-term holding facilities operate at major ports and other points of entry. Healthcare services at IRCs are not routinely commissioned by local commissioning bodies and links with such bodies can be variable.

During the first 6 months of 2009, nearly 14,000 men, women and children entered immigration detention.[126] The Chief Inspector of Prisons, who had previously levelled criticism at IRCs for asylum seekers in England,[127] noted in her 2008–2009 report that detention is not predominantly a short-term phenomenon, and commented on the subsequent pressure placed on the IRC estate.[128] For example, mental health provision was unable to meet need in most centres inspected.

Pressures on immigration detention healthcare services: a case example

In November 2006, much of the living accommodation at Harmondsworth Immigration Removal Centre (IRC), near Heathrow Airport, was destroyed in a serious disturbance. Riots were apparently triggered by a highly critical inspection report by Anne Owers, Chief Inspector of Prisons for England and Wales. The report on Harmondsworth was described by the Chief Inspector herself as 'undoubtedly the poorest report we have issued on an IRC'. It said the regime there was as strict as that at a high security prison and that detainees were victimised by staff; some were strip searched and temporarily locked in solitary confinement. Since a riot had taken place there in 2004, after a detainee committed suicide, the centre had, according to the report, slipped into 'a culture wholly at odds with its stated purpose'.

The recommendations of this inspection report, concerning healthcare at the Centre, serve to highlight the pressures to which healthcare services and professionals in this particular detention context are subject, as well as establishing a framework for best practice within the immigration detention setting. Examples of the recommendations are set out below:

- The contract for primary care services should be revised to ensure there is an appropriate balance between GP and nurse-led sessions so that resources are used appropriately to meet all health needs.
- Centres should be given sufficient notice of detainee movement to enable healthcare staff to make the necessary preparation, including the transfer of medical notes and appropriate discharge arrangements on release.
- Specialist nursing staff, such as registered mental health nurses, should be recruited to develop a primary mental health service, so that detainees with identified mental health needs are cared for appropriately.
- Nurses should be trained in the treatment of minor illnesses.
- A counselling service should be available to all detainees.
- Healthcare staff should receive specific training in the identification and management of detainees who have been tortured. Such training should be part of the induction programme and updated regularly.
- Patients transferred to hospital following an emergency call should only be handcuffed following an individual risk assessment determining that this is necessary and taking into account the views of medical staff.
- Professional interpreters should be used whenever there is a clinical need.[129]

During its 2008 inspection visit to Harmondsworth, the European Committee for the Prevention of Torture and Inhuman or Degrading Treatment or Punishment (CPT) acknowledged the generally relaxed atmosphere at the centre, but noted in particular the need for attention to be paid to the mental health and psychological state of those in immigration detention.[130] The CPT stressed that the indefinite nature of detention could lead to a deterioration in mental health. It commented on the number of detainees who had spent more than a year in immigration detention, and that in certain cases it had seemed there was little prospect of the people concerned being sent back to their countries of origin.

All detainees are entitled to the same range and quality of services as the general public. In addition, immigration detainees and asylum seekers may need extra services to address their own specific health problems.[131] Access to a second opinion and out-of-hours care should be available according to the same criteria used by GPs in the community, rather than decided solely on management priorities. The BMA has particular concerns about the mental health impact of detention on asylum seekers, some of whom are likely to have previously been the victims of abuse or violence in detention in their own countries. Various studies have highlighted the multiple traumatic experiences which many detained asylum seekers have suffered, as well as the deleterious effects of subsequent detention upon their health.[132] These problems have been compounded by inadequate assessment prior to detention, which means that individuals' health problems are often not monitored while they are detained. In the past, detainees received little information about the reasons for detention or its likely duration, which is always unpredictable.

If patients in immigration detention are to have timely access to hospital services on the same basis as patients in the community, it is obviously important that referrals are not delayed merely for administrative convenience. As with prisoners, the BMA has received reports of access to hospital being denied or postponed because of the costs of providing escorts for patients in immigration detention.

The provision of medication to this patient group should be in line with that for comparable conditions in the community.

Healthcare for detainees in immigration removal centres

The BMA supports the principles of good practice documented in the Detention Centre Rules 2001, which deal with the provision of healthcare to detainees in IRCs and set out the following rules for every IRC.

- A fully registered GP shall be available.
- A healthcare team will be responsible for detainees' physical and mental health.
- Healthcare team members should be able to recognise medical conditions in a diverse population and be culturally sensitive.
- Professional guidelines on confidentiality will be observed.
- Requests to see the doctor will be recorded and passed on.
- The doctor has discretion to consult other doctors.
- Detainees can request a doctor and dentist of their own choice if:
  o they pay the costs incurred
  o the request is reasonable
  o attendance is in consultation with the IRC doctor.
- As far as possible, the doctor will obtain detainees' previous medical records.
- Medical records will be passed on appropriately when the detainee leaves detention.
- Doctors must ensure that detainees know they can request a doctor of their own sex.
- Any doctor chosen by a detainee who is facing legal proceedings must have reasonable access to examine the detainee in connection with the proceedings.[133]

Welfare of children in immigration detention

Of the 14,000 people entering immigration detention during the first 6 months of 2009, 470 were children; almost half of the children entering detention were under 5 years of age.[134] The detention of children has been a considerable cause for concern and a range of reports on the effects of detention on the well-being of children have been produced.[135] A briefing paper from the Royal College of Paediatrics and Child Health, Royal College of General Practitioners, Royal College of Psychiatrists and the Faculty of Public Health stressed that '[a]ny detention of children for administrative rather than criminal purposes causes unnecessary harm and further blights already disturbed young lives'.[136] In addition, the Chief Inspector of Prisons for England and Wales has observed that, in spite of the fact that the UK has agreed to remove its immigration reservation to the International Convention on the Rights of the Child, which would prevent the detention of children for immigration purposes, there is little evidence that decisions to detain or to maintain detention fully take account of the needs and welfare of children. There is also no specific guidance within the detention standards on the circumstances in which force can be used, or the methods that can be deployed, on infants and children.[137] (For specific guidance on pursuing child protection concerns, see Chapter 4, pages 174–180.)

The UK Government, as part of the 2010 Conservative–Liberal Democrat coalition agreement, indicated its commitment to bring an end to the detention of children for immigration purposes and subsequently pledged to implement the change by May 2011.[138]

Unaccompanied child migrants are particularly vulnerable. Disputes about whether a young person is a 'child' are common where unaccompanied young asylum seekers arrive in the UK with no documentary proof of age and there has previously been concern about the way in which the age of young asylum seekers is assessed. Medical methods of age assessment, including the use of X-rays, have limited reliability, due to wide variations, both within and across racial groups, in physiological characteristics as a result of nutrition, culture and genetic background. Exposing individuals to ionising radiation for non-clinical reasons has also been controversial.[139] A 2007 report recommended that the process of age assessment should be holistic and take into account a range of social, emotional and psychological indicators of age and need, and should not rely solely or primarily on physiological characteristics or factors.[140] In the BMA's view, given the unreliability of bone age assessment, the small but definite levels of risk involved in using ionising radiation, and the absence of any clinical justification, it would be inappropriate for doctors to be involved in this practice.

Consent in immigration detention

Detainees must be offered a physical and a mental health examination within 24 hours of admission. This cannot proceed if the detainee refuses. In such cases, the detainee is nevertheless entitled to an examination upon request. Under the Immigration and Asylum Act 1999,[141] however, the manager of the centre can require that a detainee be medically examined in the interests of other people in order to ascertain if he or she has a transmissible disease. In such cases, doctors must still seek consent, explain the nature of the suspected disease and tell the patient that refusal, without reasonable excuse, is an offence. If the doctor cannot exclude a serious communicable disease, the patient may have to be isolated to protect others.

Examination for the purposes of providing an independent report for the immigration services or courts is discussed in Chapter 16, pages 667–669.

Confidentiality in immigration detention

Interpretation and translation are particularly important in the care of this population. The BMA has been concerned about the reported use of fellow detainees as interpreters, or of other people who happen to speak the same language as the patient (see also pages 699–700). Family members and friends, however, are not generally appropriate to use to interpret. People who have survived torture, for example, are often unwilling to disclose the details in front of people they know. In some cases, however, finding an interpreter would involve a significant delay in treating the patient. With consultations involving routine health problems it may be necessary to use family members, but this should only be done where the patient is happy for a relative to interpret. Asylum seekers can also be greatly concerned if interpreters appear to represent officialdom or are recommended by embassies that they fear will filter back information to the authorities in their own country or cause problems for their relatives.

The Detention Centre Rules 2001 require doctors to report to the centre managers any detainee whose health is likely to be adversely affected by continued detention and any person at risk of suicide.[142] The same general advice, discussed previously, about providing a supportive environment for people who are likely to harm themselves is equally valid here (see pages 706–708). The Detention Centre Rules also require the reporting to managers of detainees believed to be torture survivors. This is usually in the detainee's interests. Most torture survivors want that information known, as it is likely to support their case, and they also may need treatment. The fact that doctors believe an individual to have been subjected to abuse should be noted appropriately, although managers do not necessarily need any detail. Patients should be aware of how their information will be used and their agreement to any disclosure should be sought, as would be common practice in any other setting. Doctors working with immigration detainees and asylum seekers have sometimes expressed concern to the BMA that, although such information is passed on to the Home Office, it is not acted upon. It is important, therefore, that detainees or their authorised representative can access their own health record to see, and if appropriate challenge, what has been written and passed on in reports about their health. Access to health records by patients and their representatives is discussed in Chapter 6, pages 255–259.

Detainees have also alleged that their medical reports have sometimes been improperly transcribed by detention staff. In October 2001, the BMA expressed concerns to the Home Office about allegations by detainees that the recommendations for release or specialist treatment submitted by community psychiatrists had been toned down. The BMA strongly emphasises the importance of accuracy and transparency in passing on the recommendations made by consultants in such cases. One option is for patients to access their records under the provisions of the Data Protection Act 1998 in order to address the problem of improper transcription or inadvertent error. Clearly, medical reports and assessments should not be altered unless shown to be inaccurate in some way and then the alteration should be clearly marked and the reasons for it given. As in all other cases, health professionals are accountable for what they write and should be able to show proper justification for their decisions, including a decision not to act upon views provided by specialists.

Summary – healthcare in prisons, facilities accommodating young adult offenders, children and young people, and immigration removal centres

- Specific training for health professionals should be available and properly resourced.
- Good contact with community services needs to be preserved.
- Independence and a clear sense of the medical role need to be maintained.
- Doctors should not be involved in disciplinary issues.
- Strategies are needed to ensure prompt access to care, including mental health care.
- All detainees should be aware of their rights regarding consent to or refusal of treatment.
- The need for appropriate liaison and prevention of self-harm should be balanced with prisoners' rights to confidentiality.

Police stations and forensic physicians

Forensic physicians can have both forensic and therapeutic roles. They examine, on behalf of the police, victims and suspected perpetrators of crime, as well as examining and treating people who are taken ill while in custody. They see detained people to determine their fitness for custody or interview, and may examine people, detained or otherwise, for forensic purposes or to obtain forensic samples. In all cases, forensic physicians should identify themselves to the person to be examined and explain how their role differs from that in the usual doctor–patient relationship. Although complicated by the fact that the examinations they carry out have both therapeutic and forensic content, forensic physicians still have obligations to respect patient consent and confidentiality. In general terms, therapeutic information is subject to the same degree of confidentiality accorded to other patients, bearing in mind that no patient's right to confidentiality is absolute. However, forensic information is likely to have greater implications for the public interest and the need to ensure justice. The BMA and the Faculty of Forensic and Legal Medicine (FFLM) have produced joint guidance on the healthcare of detainees in police stations.[143]

Forensic physicians and consent

Consent for examination of victims of crime

Evidential examination is different in aim, and procedure, from clinical examination. Its purpose is to elicit material evidence regarding a possible criminal charge. Although the police sometimes ask GPs or hospital doctors to provide a report of injuries sustained in an alleged criminal act, documenting those injuries for forensic purposes is a specialised task requiring a trained forensic physician.

When a serious crime, such as rape or assault, has occurred there is inevitable pressure to act quickly to protect others. The time limits for obtaining supporting evidence, and full information on the alleged crime, dictate that examinations be carried out promptly. This has to be explained to the victim. The police have done much work to address sensitive issues surrounding sexual crimes and generally have specially trained officers to provide counselling and support. Nevertheless, the doctor cannot assume that the person's presence by itself implies consent. In order for consent to be valid, the individual needs to know what is entailed by the examination and understand that forensic information will be passed to the police. Everyone involved should be sensitive to patients' preferences regarding the gender of the examining doctor. Consent to treatment from adults with capacity is discussed in detail in Chapter 3.

In cases of suspected child sexual abuse, it is important that children are not subjected to repeated examination. It is good practice for one examination to be carried out jointly by a forensic physician and a paediatrician. Children's consent to examination and treatment is discussed in Chapter 4.

Consent for examination of those held in custody

If detainees have capacity, their consent for medical examination must be sought (see Chapter 2). The purpose of examination may be to look for evidence of involvement in a crime or to deal with any illness or injury. In either case, the individual has the right to refuse to be examined or treated, or to provide specimens, but must be informed that the refusal to consent will be documented and that fact itself may be used in evidence. (It is lawful for an intimate body search to be undertaken without consent, although the BMA and FFLM consider that doctors should participate only with the individual's consent, see page 730.) In order for consent to be valid, the detainee should have capacity, be informed of the purpose of the examination, or which specimens are to be taken, and not be subject to coercion. The ability of detainees to give consent can obviously be compromised by factors such as illness, distress or the effects of alcohol or drugs, and their situation is also likely to make them feel a certain degree of pressure. Nevertheless, most people can make decisions about whether or not to consent even in difficult situations.

Consent should be written or, if verbal, witnessed and recorded in the medical notes. A police officer may have to be present for the examination but should be out of immediate earshot. This is not always attainable and depends on the circumstances. Assaults on forensic physicians are not uncommon and unfounded allegations are also sometimes made against them. The FFLM strongly recommends the presence of a chaperone when doctors examine a detainee. If detainees agree, their solicitor can attend the examination. An informed refusal to be examined or treated must be respected. If consent for examination is unobtainable because the detainee is incapacitated at the time, information should not generally be passed to the police until the person can consent (for information on incapacitated detainees, see below).

Problems can arise when the examination begins with one purpose, which is explained to the individual, but the information obtained is later wanted for another purpose, which has not been mentioned. Patients with minor injuries, for example, are examined to ascertain their fitness for custody, but their injuries may be the result of assaulting another person. Therefore, detainees should be made aware that information obtained from the examination may be requested by the police or by lawyers. Where there is doubt about the validity of the original consent, the consent should be obtained expressly for the purposes of disclosure that later become apparent.

Consent by minors

When the detainee is a minor, relatives or friends may be present at the examination if the young person agrees. For people aged under 16, it is good practice to obtain both the consent of the young person and someone with parental responsibility, where reasonably practicable, before undertaking forensic examination or taking samples. In addition to ensuring that valid consent has been obtained, the forensic physician also needs to ensure that the relevant legal considerations are met regarding the admissibility in court of any forensic evidence obtained.[144]

Incapacitated detainees

As with any other patients, when those detained by the police lack the capacity to consent, treatment should be provided in accordance with relevant capacity legislation (see Chapter 3). Where an intervention is deemed to be either in an incapacitated adult's best interests (in England, Wales and Northern Ireland) or is expected to provide a benefit (in Scotland), it would ordinarily be lawful to proceed. In these circumstances, specimens can also be taken for diagnostic purposes. They should not be taken or used for forensic purposes, however, except where a blood sample is taken from a driver who lacks capacity under the terms of the Police Reform Act 2002 or the Criminal Justice (Northern Ireland) Order 2005 (see below).

Acting without consent

Intimate body searches

Intimate body searches without consent are lawful, provided that appropriate authorisation has been received.[145] Nevertheless, the ethical obligation to seek consent applies. The BMA and the FFLM have produced joint guidance setting out their policy that doctors should *not* carry out intimate body searches without consent.[146] This view has been supported by the GMC's Standards Committee. Detainees faced with the prospect of an intimate search often request that a doctor undertakes it rather than a police or prison officer. Doctors working in an environment in which intimate searches are likely should seek agreement that they are always called when an intimate search is proposed. This does not commit them to carrying out searches, but allows doctors to ascertain the detainee's wishes and establish whether consent has been given. When detainees refuse to be searched, this should be recorded in the notes. The BMA and the FFLM advise doctors not to participate, although in rare circumstances an intimate search may be justified in order to save the individual's life. Where there is such a risk, doctors should take advice from their medical defence organisation.

Taking blood samples to test for alcohol and drugs

Forensic physicians may be asked by the police to take a blood sample from an incapacitated driver to test for alcohol or drugs. In the limited circumstances set out in the Police Reform Act 2002 and the Criminal Justice (Northern Ireland) Order 2005, this would be lawful in the UK, and, in the BMA's view, would also be ethically acceptable. The BMA and the FFLM have produced joint guidance for those involved in taking blood specimens from incapacitated drivers (further information is provided in Chapter 15, pages 637–638).[147]

Confidentiality and forensic physicians

The primary purpose of most examinations conducted by forensic physicians is to obtain evidence for a possible prosecution. Confidentiality is a difficult issue in this regard and people who are examined – both victims and suspects – should be clear about the use that will be made of their medical information. Forensic physicians should say explicitly at the outset that part of their job is to collect evidence for the police and therefore that no assurances about confidentiality can be given. They should also explain that they are required to disclose information obtained during the examination that might affect the outcome of the case.

There has been some confusion in the past about potential conflicts between forensic physicians' duty to disclose information to the police and their duty of confidentiality. The situation was clarified for England, Wales and Northern Ireland in parliamentary debate on the Criminal Procedure and Investigations Act 1996. It was made clear that the reports forensic physicians prepare for criminal proceedings must be given to the police, but any information obtained for therapeutic purposes would be subject to the usual rules of confidentiality.[148] In order to fulfil this requirement, however, forensic physicians need to separate out the forensic evidence (and any other information obtained that is likely to affect the outcome of the case) from information that is not germane to the case and was provided solely in a therapeutic context. Only forensic information and other information likely to affect the case should be included in the statement prepared for the police. If the police or the Crown Prosecution Service request access to the therapeutic information, the individual's written consent should be sought. If the individual refuses or consents only to partial disclosure, that decision must be respected unless a judge orders full disclosure or exceptionally where there is a public interest in disclosure (see Chapter 5). In court, forensic physicians should state why the information should not be disclosed or why they think it would not affect the outcome of the case. However, if a court order is issued, the patient should be told of this and the information must be disclosed. (See Chapter 5 on general issues of confidentiality.)

Patient confidentiality in the police station setting

- Careful attention must be given to ensuring that people who are being examined understand the role of the forensic doctor.
- Before any information is volunteered, doctors should state explicitly that part of their role is to collect evidence for the prosecution. They should make clear that any information given may be so used and that confidentiality cannot be guaranteed. The patient should understand and agree to this prior to examination or to the collection of the information.

- Doctors should explain that, in addition to forensic evidence, they are required to provide to the police any information obtained during the examination that may affect the outcome of the case.
- Before an examination takes place, doctors should ensure that the patient has consented to the forensic examination, the provision of medical care and the disclosure of forensic evidence and any other information likely to affect the outcome of the case.
- While carrying out the examination, doctors should consciously attempt to separate out forensic evidence, other information obtained that is likely to affect the outcome of the case and information that is not germane to the case but is given solely in the therapeutic context.
- A statement should be provided for the police, giving all the forensic evidence and any other information obtained that is likely to affect the outcome of the case.
- If the police request further information about the medical examination that was not included in the report, the specific consent of the patient should be sought before this is disclosed.
- If the patient refuses to consent, or consents only to partial disclosure, the doctor should abide by that decision unless, exceptionally, disclosure can be justified by the potential for serious harm to others or a likely miscarriage of justice, or by a court order.

Information to be included in police station records

Full contemporaneous notes of any assessment and examination undertaken by a forensic physician must always be kept. Any notes made in station records should be relevant to the care of the detainee, or briefly describe the relevant injuries in the case of a victim. Doctors must be aware that, as such police station records are widely accessed, they should contain a minimum of clinical information. As far as the person's health is concerned, only the information necessary to enable the police to take proper care of the individual should be disclosed. In the case of serious illness in a person in custody, information relevant to supervision may be given to the police. Worries are sometimes expressed that forensic physicians document details such as the HIV status of detainees in police records without the person's consent. Unless this information is necessary for the provision of appropriate care, this would be a breach of confidentiality.

A confidential record of any medical treatment provided or requested by the forensic physician while the individual is in police custody should accompany the person when transferred elsewhere. It should accompany detainees when they first appear in court, in a sealed envelope marked 'confidential', or be transmitted electronically. This information may be relevant to the granting or refusal of bail and may be used by court forensic psychiatrists or other doctors who later become responsible for the care of the detainee. When the care of a patient is passed over from one forensic physician to another, all relevant information must be provided to ensure continuity of care.

Detainees held without charge

The passing of the Terrorism Act 2006 extended from 14 to 28 days[149] the period that suspects can be held without charge, prompting concerns from some forensic physicians that this may result in suspects being detained for longer periods in police cells not designed for protracted detention. (In February 2011, the Government published the Protection of Freedoms Bill, which proposed to reduce the maximum period of pre-charge detention for terrorist suspects to 14 days. At the time of writing, the maximum period of detention for suspects held without charge was still 28 days.) It was originally expected that suspects would be moved out of police stations into more appropriate facilities with exercise, dietary and psychiatric provision, but as yet no such provision seems to exist and so some detainees are likely to be kept inappropriately in police cells. The BMA's publication, *Health care of detainees in police stations,*[150] points out the unsuitability of police cells for detention lasting more than a few days, as facilities in police stations are only designed to hold detainees for short periods. In the absence of alternative secure accommodation, it seems likely that individuals may be held without exercise, catering or washing facilities for much longer. The Home Office Codes of Practice set standards for the treatment of those detained under terrorism legislation.

Home Office Codes of Practice on the care and treatment of those detained under terrorism legislation[151]

- Detainees held for more than 96 hours must be visited by a healthcare professional at least once every 24 hours.
- If a complaint is made by a detainee about a possible assault or the use of unnecessary or unreasonable force, an appropriate healthcare professional must be called as soon as possible.
- When arrangements are made for a detainee to receive clinical attention, the custody officer must make sure all relevant information which might assist in the treatment of the detainee's condition is made available to the responsible healthcare professional.
- If a detainee requests a clinical examination, an appropriate healthcare professional must be called as soon as possible. Detainees may also be examined by a medical practitioner of their choice, at their own expense.
- If a detainee is required to use any medication in compliance with clinical directions prescribed before detention, the custody officer must consult the appropriate healthcare professional before the use of the medication.
- If a detainee has or needs medication for a heart disorder, diabetes, epilepsy or a condition of comparable potential seriousness then the advice of a healthcare professional must be obtained.
- Whenever a healthcare professional is called to examine or treat a detainee, the custody officer is advised to ask for their opinion about any risks or problems which the police need to take into account when making decisions about the detainee's continued detention, when to carry out an interview and the need for safeguards.

Summary – police stations and forensic physicians

- Doctors should seek consent from individuals with capacity, even when it is not a legal requirement.
- People who are examined in custody may want their lawyer to be present.
- People who are examined for forensic purposes need to be aware that any information obtained may be used as evidence in court.
- Confidentiality cannot be guaranteed, but a distinction should be made between information obtained for therapeutic and forensic purposes.
- Forensic physicians should make every effort to ensure continuity of care by passing on medical information to health professionals who subsequently provide care.
- Special attention should be paid to the healthcare needs of those kept in police custody for extended periods.

References

1   Offender Health, a joint Department of Health/ Ministry of Justice National Offender Management Service unit, produces guidance and other information relevant to doctors working across the range of detention settings discussed in this chapter, available at: www.dh.gov.uk (accessed 18 February 2011).

2   Royal College of Physicians, Royal College of General Practitioners, Royal College of Psychiatrists (1992) *Report of the working party of three medical royal colleges on the education and training of doctors in the Health Care Service for prisoners*, Home Office, London.

3   British Medical Association (2007) *Crisis in the cells: Doctors reveal the problems gripping prisons in England and Wales*, BMA, London.

4   Care Quality Commission, HM Inspectorate of Prisons (2010) *Commissioning healthcare in prisons 2008/09: Key findings from our analysis of primary care trusts as commissioners of prison health care*, CQC and HMIP, London.

5   Care Quality Commission, HM Inspectorate of Prisons (2010) *Commissioning healthcare in prisons 2008/09: Key findings from our analysis of primary care trusts as commissioners of prison health care*, CQC and HMIP, London, p.11.

6   World Medical Association (2006) *Declaration of Tokyo: Guidelines for Physicians Concerning Torture and other Cruel, Inhuman or Degrading Treatment or Punishment in Relation to Detention and Imprisonment*, WMA, Divonne-les-Bains.

7   World Medical Association (2006) *Declaration of Geneva*, WMA, Divonne-les-Bains.

8   World Medical Association (2006) *Regulations in Times of Armed Conflict*, WMA, Divonne-les-Bains.

9   General Medical Council (2006) *Good Medical Practice*, GMC, London.

10 NHS National electronic Library for Medicines (2007) *Prescribing in a Secure Environment*. Available at: www.nelm.nhs.uk (accessed 18 February 2011).

11 General Medical Council (2006) *Good Medical Practice*, GMC, London.

12 Further guidance can also be found in: Department of Health (2002) *Seeking Consent: Working with People in Prison*, DH, London.

13 European Committee for the Prevention of Torture and Inhuman or Degrading Treatment or Punishment (2010) *CPT standards*, Council of Europe, Strasbourg, p.28, para 33. International standards also provide for a medical examination 'as promptly as possible after [the detainee's] admission to the place of detention or imprisonment': United Nations General Assembly (1988) *Body of Principles for the Protection of All Persons under Any Form of Detention or Imprisonment*, UN, New York, principle 24.

14 The BMA and the Law Society have issued detailed guidance on assessing mental capacity: British Medical Association, The Law Society (2010) *Assessment of Mental Capacity*, 3rd edn, The Law Society, London. This book covers the law in England and Wales, but the medical aspects of assessment are relevant to good practice throughout the UK.

15 *Re W (adult: refusal of medical treatment)* (2002) MHLR 411.

16 For a discussion of the sharing of criminality information, see: Magee I. *The Review of Criminality Information*. Available at: www.statewatch.org (accessed 18 February 2011).

17 Department of Health, HM Prison Service (2002) *Guidance on the protection and use of confidential health information in prisons and inter-agency information sharing* (PSI 25/2002), DH, London.

18 Department of Health (2011) Prison health to improve as result of national IT system. Press release, 12 April. NHS Connecting for Health (2011) *Prison Health IT*. Available at: www.connectingforhealth.nhs.uk (accessed 26 April 2011).

19 *Szuluk v United Kingdom* (2010) 50 EHRR 10.

20 Office for Criminal Justice Reform (2007) *National agreement on arrangements for the use of interpreters, translators and language service professionals in investigations and proceedings within the criminal justice system*, Office for Criminal Justice Reform, London.

21 HM Prison Service, Prison Reform Trust, London Probation (2004) *Information and advice for foreign national prisoners*, HMPS, London, p.10.

22 The Working Group on Interpreting and Translation (2008) *Code of practice for working with interpreters in the Scottish criminal justice system*, Crown Office and Procurator Fiscal Service, Edinburgh.

23 The Scottish Translation, Interpreting and Communication Forum website can be accessed at www.stics.org.uk (accessed 18 February 2011).

24 Northern Ireland Prison Service (2008) *Foreign national prisoner strategy (draft 2008–2010)*, NIPS, Belfast, p.12.

25 Home Office (2008) *Police and Criminal Evidence Act 1984 (PACE). Code C. Code of Practice for the detention, treatment and questioning of persons by police officers*, The Stationery Office, London.

26 British Medical Association, Faculty of Forensic and Legal Medicine (2009) *Healthcare of detainees in police stations*, BMA, London, p.9.

27 Mansell A. (2010) Medic cell block H. *Student BMA News* (3 July), p.8.

28 Determination by Robert Alastair Dunlop, QC, Sheriff Principal of the Sheriffdom of Tayside Central and Fife following an Inquiry held at Stirling on 4, 5, 6 and 7 March 2002 into the death of Michelle McElver. Available at: www.scotcourts.gov.uk (accessed 19 May 2011).

29 Determination by Robert Alastair Dunlop, QC, Sheriff Principal of the Sheriffdom of Tayside Central and Fife following an Inquiry held at Stirling on 8, 12 and 13 March 2002 into the death of Frances Carvill, p.6. Available at: www.scotcourts.gov.uk (accessed 19 May 2011).

30 Fatal Accidents and Sudden Deaths Inquiry (Scotland) Act 1976, s 6(1)(c) requires the sheriff to determine whether reasonable precautions were taken that might have avoided the death, and s 6(1)(d) requires the sheriff to determine whether any defect in the system of working contributed to the death.

31 Determination by TA Kevin Drummond, Sheriff of the Sheriffdom of Glasgow and Strathkelvin following an inquiry held at Glasgow on 17 February 1999 into the death of Daniel Lynch, p.1. Documentation provided by the Medical and Dental Defence Union of Scotland.

32 *D v United Kingdom* (1997) 24 EHRR 423.

33 HM Chief Inspector of Prisons for England and Wales (2010) *Annual report 2008–09*, HMIP, London, p.29.

34 Fazel S, Hope T, O'Donnell I. *et al*. (2001) Health of elderly male prisoners: worse than the general population, worse than younger prisoners. *Age Ageing* **30**, 403–7.

35 James E. (2009) No place to grow old. *The Guardian* (6 July). Available at: www.guardian.co.uk (accessed 18 February 2011).

36 Stojkovic S. (2007) Elderly prisoners: a growing and forgotten group within correctional systems vulnerable to elder abuse. *J Elder Abuse Neglect* **19**, 97–117.

37 Department of Health, Nacro (2009) *A resource pack for working with older prisoners*, Nacro, London. See also: Department of Health, Prison Reform Trust (2009) *Information book for prisoners with a disability*, PRT, London.

38 *R (on the application of Mellor) v Secretary of State for the Home Department* [2001] 3 WLR 533.

39 *Dickson v United Kingdom* (2008) 46 EHRR 41.

40 Fazel S, Benning R, Danesh J. (2005) Suicides in male prisoners in England and Wales, 1978–2003. *Lancet* **366**, 1301–2, p.1301.

41 Fazel S, Benning R, Danesh J. (2005) Suicides in male prisoners in England and Wales, 1978–2003. *Lancet* **366**, 1301–2.

42 HM Government (2009) *New Horizons: a shared vision for mental health*, DH, London, p.48.

43 National Mental Health Development Unit (2009) *National Suicide Prevention Strategy for England: Annual Report on Progress 2008*, NMHDU, London, p.7.

44 Department of Health, HM Prison Service, the National Assembly for Wales (2001) *Changing the Outlook: A Strategy for Developing and Modernising Mental Health Services in Prisons*, DH, London, p.17.

45 The Howard League for Penal Reform (2003) *Suicide and self-harm prevention: the management of self-injury in prison*, The Howard League for Penal Reform, London.

46 HM Prison Service Safer Custody Group. *The ACCT Approach: Caring for People at Risk in Prison*. Available at: www.hmprisonservice.gov.uk (accessed 18 February 2011).

47 HM Prison Service (2007) *Suicide Prevention and Self-Harm Management* (PSO 2700), HMPS, London.

48 HM Prison Service (2007) *Suicide Prevention and Self-Harm Management* (PSO 2700), HMPS, London.

49 Health Protection Agency (2011) *Prison Infection Prevention Team*. Available at: www.hpa.org.uk (accessed 18 February 2011).

50 World Health Organization (2003) *Moscow Declaration on Prison Health as Part of Public Health*, WHO, Moscow.

51 Health Protection Agency, HM Prison Service (2006) *Tuberculosis (TB): Guidance for prison officials*, HPA, London.

52 Health Protection Agency (2010) *Information resources for TB in prisons*. Available at: www.hpa.org.uk (accessed 21 February 2011).

53 British Medical Association Annual Representatives Meeting 1988: 'That this Meeting believes that condoms and health education on the risks of HIV infection should be freely available in prisons.'

54 United Nations Office on Drugs and Crime, World Health Organization, Joint United Nations Programme on HIV/AIDS (2006) *HIV/AIDS Prevention, Care, Treatment and Support in Prison Settings: A Framework for an Effective National Response*, UN Office on Drugs and Crime, Vienna, p.19.

55 United Nations Office on Drugs and Crime, World Health Organization, Joint United Nations Programme on HIV/AIDS (2006) *HIV/AIDS Prevention, Care, Treatment and Support in Prison Settings: A Framework for an Effective National Response*, UN Office on Drugs and Crime, Vienna, p.24.

56 British Medical Association (2001) *The medical profession and human rights: handbook for a changing agenda*, Zed Books, London, p.113.

57 *Shelley v United Kingdom* (2008) 46 EHRR SE16.

58 Scottish Prison Service (2005) *The direction of harm reduction in the SPS: from chaotic drug use to abstinence*, SPS, Edinburgh.

59 *Shelley v United Kingdom* (2008) 46 EHRR SE16:207.

60 *Shelley v United Kingdom* (2008) 46 EHRR SE16:207.

61 HM Prison Service (2007) *Re-introduction of Disinfecting Tablets (PSI 34/2007)*, HMPS, London.

62 European Committee for the Prevention of Torture and Inhuman or Degrading Treatment or Punishment (2010) *CPT standards*, Council of Europe, Strasbourg, p.18, para 56.

63 European Committee for the Prevention of Torture and Inhuman or Degrading Treatment or Punishment (2010) *CPT standards*, Council of Europe, Strasbourg, p.76, para 35.

64 HM Chief Inspector of Prisons for England and Wales (2010) *Annual report 2008–09*, HMIP, London, p.67.

65 British Medical Association (2009) *The medical role in restraint and control: custodial settings*, BMA, London.

66 Faculty of Forensic and Legal Medicine (2010) *Acute behavioural disturbance: guidelines on management in police custody*, FFLM, London, p.2.

67 European Committee for the Prevention of Torture and Inhuman or Degrading Treatment or Punishment (2010) *CPT standards*, Council of Europe, Strasbourg, p.17, paras 53–4.

68 HM Prison Service. *Use of Force* (PSO 1600), HMPS, London. Available at: pso.hmprisonservice.gov.uk (accessed 19 May 2011).

69 British Medical Association (2001) *The medical profession and human rights: handbook for a changing agenda*, Zed Books, London, p.408.

70 World Medical Association (2008) *WMA Resolution on Medical Care for Refugees and Internally Displaced Persons*, WMA, Seoul.

71 HM Inspectorate of Prisons (2009) *Detainee escorts and removals: a thematic review*, HMIP, London.

72 Euripidou E, MacLehose R, Fletcher A. (2004) An investigation into the short term and medium term health impacts of personal incapacitant sprays: a follow up of patients reported to the National Poisons Information Service (London). *Emergency Med J* 21, 548–52.

73 Department of Health (2010) *Guidelines for the clinical management of people refusing food in immigration removal centres and prisons*, DH, London.

74 World Medical Association (2006) *WMA Declaration of Malta on Hunger Strikers*, WMA, Pilanesberg.

75 *R v Collins, ex parte Ian Stewart Brady* [2001] 58 BMLR 173.

76 Department of Health (2010) *Guidelines for the clinical management of people refusing food in immigration removal centres and prisons*, DH, London, pp.20–2.

77 Department of Health (2010) *Guidelines for the clinical management of people refusing food in immigration removal centres and prisons*, DH, London, p.22.

78 Department of Health (2010) *Guidelines for the clinical management of people refusing food in immigration removal centres and prisons*, DH, London, p.22.

79 Anon. (2001) Animal activist dies on hunger strike. *BBC News Online* (5 November). Available at: www.bbc.co.uk/news (accessed 21 February 2011).

80 World Medical Association (2006) *Declaration of Tokyo: Guidelines for Physicians Concerning Torture and other Cruel, Inhuman or Degrading Treatment or Punishment in Relation to Detention and Imprisonment*, WMA, Divonne-les-Bains.

81 HM Chief Inspector of Prisons for England and Wales (2010) *Annual report 2008–09*, HMIP, London.

82 HM Inspectorate of Prisons (2010) *Prison improvements made, but risks lie ahead, says Owers*. Press release, 23 February.

83 Bradley K. (2009) *The Bradley Report: Lord Bradley's review of people with mental health problems or learning disabilities in the criminal justice system*, DH, London, p.98.

84 House of Commons Home Affairs Committee (2005) *Rehabilitation of prisoners: First Report of Session 2004–2005*, Vol. I, The Stationery Office, London, pp.103–5.

85 Bradley K. (2009) *The Bradley Report: Lord Bradley's review of people with mental health problems or learning disabilities in the criminal justice system*, DH, London, p.105.

86 Department of Health (2011) *Good Practice Procedure Guide: The transfer and remission of adult prisoners under s47 and s48 of the Mental Health Act*, DH, London.

87 European Committee for the Prevention of Torture and Inhuman or Degrading Treatment or Punishment (2009) *Report to the Government of the United Kingdom on the visit to the United Kingdom carried out by the European Committee for the Prevention of Torture and Inhuman or Degrading Treatment or Punishment (CPT) from 18 November to 1 December 2008*, Council of Europe, Strasbourg, p.36, para 69.

88 Bradley K. (2009) *The Bradley Report: Lord Bradley's review of people with mental health problems or learning disabilities in the criminal justice system*, DH, London, p.106.

89 Bradley K. (2009) *The Bradley Report: Lord Bradley's review of people with mental health problems or learning disabilities in the criminal justice system*, DH, London, p.103.

90 As reported in: Bradley K. (2009) *The Bradley Report: Lord Bradley's review of people with mental health problems or learning disabilities in the criminal justice system*, DH, London, p.104.

91 Bradley K. (2009) *The Bradley Report: Lord Bradley's review of people with mental health problems or learning disabilities in the criminal justice system*, DH, London, p.101.

92   HM Inspectorate of Prisons (2007) *The mental health of prisoners: a thematic review of the care and support of prisoners with mental health needs*, HMIP, London, p.11, para 1.18.

93   HM Chief Inspector of Prisons for Scotland (2008) *Out of Sight: Severe and Enduring Mental Health Problems in Scotland's Prisons*, Scottish Government, Edinburgh.

94   The Bamford Review of Mental Health and Learning Disability (Northern Ireland) (2007) *A comprehensive legislative framework*, DHSSPS, Belfast. Available at: www.rmhldni.gov.uk (accessed 22 February 2011).

95   All-Party Parliamentary Group on Prison Health (2007) *Tackling the Drug Problem in UK HM Prisons: A Report from the All-Party Parliamentary Group on Prison Health*, APPGPH, London.

96   Reported in: Prison Reform Trust (2009) *Bromley Briefings Prison Factfile*, PRT, London, p.20.

97   HM Prison Service (2008) *Women Prisoners* (PSO 4800), HMPS, London, p.51.

98   The Howard League for Penal Reform (1995) *Prison Mother and Baby Units*, Howard League, London.

99   European Committee for the Prevention of Torture and Inhuman or Degrading Treatment or Punishment (2010) *CPT standards*, Council of Europe, Strasbourg, p.81, para 27.

100   HM Prison Service (2008) *Women Prisoners* (PSO 4800), HMPS, London, p.51.

101   HM Prison Service (2008) *Women Prisoners* (PSO 4800), HMPS, London, p.51.

102   Children's Commissioner for England (2008) *Prison Mother and Baby Units: do they meet the best interests of the child?* 11 MILLION, London, p.10.

103   HM Prison Service (2008) *Mother and baby units* (Performance standard 35), HMPS, London.

104   Home Office (2000) *Home Office Research Study 208. Women prisoners: a survey of their work and training experiences in custody and on release*, HO, London, p.9.

105   Department of Health (2003) *Good Medical Practice for Doctors providing Primary Care Services in Prison*, DH, London, p.24.

106   British Medical Association (2001) *The medical profession and human rights: handbook for a changing agenda*, Zed Books, London, ch 4.

107   Crime and Disorder Act 1998, s 89–95 and Sch 6.

108   Criminal Justice (Northern Ireland) Order 1998, article 8.

109   Criminal Justice Act 2003, s 177–80.

110   Walsh C. (1999) Sentenced to treatment. *Web Journal of Current Legal Issues* 5, 5. Available at: webjcli.ncl.ac.uk (accessed 22 February 2011).

111   National Probation Service (2005) *Effective management of the drug rehabilitation requirement (DRR) and alcohol treatment requirement (ATR)* (PC57/2005), NPS, London, p.5.

112   The Scottish Government (2008) *Keeping children out of prison*. Press release, 21 February.

113   HM Chief Inspector of Prisons for Scotland (2009) *Annual Report 2008–2009*, Scottish Government, Edinburgh, p.5.

114   See for example: Davies R. (2003) Children locked away from human rights in the UK. *Lancet* **361**, 873.

115   European Committee for the Prevention of Torture and Inhuman or Degrading Treatment or Punishment (2009) *Report to the Government of the United Kingdom on the visit to the United Kingdom carried out by the European Committee for the Prevention of Torture and Inhuman or Degrading Treatment or Punishment (CPT) from 18 November to 1 December 2008*, Council of Europe, Strasbourg, p.47, para 98.

116   Bradley K. (2009) *The Bradley Report: Lord Bradley's review of people with mental health problems or learning disabilities in the criminal justice system*, DH, London, p.97.

117   *R (on the application of the Howard League for Penal Reform) v Secretary of State for the Home Department (No.2)* [2003] 1 FLR 484.

118   *R (on the application of the Howard League for Penal Reform) v Secretary of State for the Home Department (No.2)* [2003] 1 FLR 484:526.

119   Lader D, Singleton N, Meltzer H. (2000) *Psychiatric morbidity among young offenders in England and Wales*, ONS, London.

120   Social Exclusion Unit (2002) *Reducing re-offending by ex-prisoners*, Social Exclusion Unit, London, p.158.

121   Independent Monitoring Board HMYOI Thorn Cross (2009) *Annual Report, May 2008–April 2009*, IMB, London, p.10.

122   National Offender Management Service (2008) Thorn Cross anti-bullying conference success. *Safer Custody News* (January/February), p.3.

123   Independent Monitoring Board HMYOI Thorn Cross (2009) *Annual Report, May 2008–April 2009*, IMB, London, p.10.

124   European Committee for the Prevention of Torture and Inhuman or Degrading Treatment or Punishment (1997) *7th General Report on the CPT's activities covering the period 1 January to 31 December 1996*, Council of Europe, Strasbourg, para 30.

125   Home Office (2002) *Secure Borders, Safe Haven: Integration with Diversity in Modern Britain*, The Stationery Office, London.

126   HM Chief Inspector of Prisons for England and Wales (2010) *Annual report 2008–09*, HMIP, London, p.71.

127 HM Inspectorate of Prisons (2002) *An Inspection of Campsfield House Immigration Removal Centre*, HMIP, London. HM Inspectorate of Prisons (2002) *An Inspection of Haslar Immigration Removal Centre*, HMIP, London. HM Inspectorate of Prisons (2002) *An Inspection of Lindholme Immigration Removal Centre*, HMIP, London. HM Inspectorate of Prisons (2002) *An Inspection of Oakington Reception Centre*, HMIP, London. HM Inspectorate of Prisons (2002) *An Inspection of Tinsley House Immigration Removal Centre*, HMIP, London.

128 HM Chief Inspector of Prisons for England and Wales (2010) *Annual report 2008–09*, HMIP, London, p.71.

129 HM Chief Inspector of Prisons (2006) *Report on an unannounced inspection of Harmondsworth Immigration Removal Centre*, HMIP, London, pp.61–9.

130 European Committee for the Prevention of Torture and Inhuman or Degrading Treatment or Punishment (2009) *Report to the Government of the United Kingdom on the visit to the United Kingdom carried out by the European Committee for the Prevention of Torture and Inhuman or Degrading Treatment or Punishment (CPT) from 18 November to 1 December 2008*, Council of Europe, Strasbourg, p.55.

131 British Medical Association (2002) *Asylum seekers: meeting their healthcare needs*, BMA, London, pp.5–10.

132 See, for example: Bail for Immigration Detainees (2005) *Fit to be detained? Challenging the detention of asylum seekers and migrants with health needs*, BiD, London. Prisons and Probation Ombudsman (2004) *Report of the inquiry into the disturbance and fire at Yarl's Wood Removal Centre*, The Stationery Office, London. Fazel M, Silove D. (2006) Detention of refugees. *BMJ* **332**, 251–2.

133 Detention Centre Rules 2001. SI 2001/238, rules 33–7.

134 HM Chief Inspector of Prisons for England and Wales (2010) *Annual report 2008–09*, HMIP, London, p.71.

135 Children's Commissioner for England (2009) *The Arrest and Detention of Children Subject to Immigration Control: A report following the Children's Commissioner for England's visit to Yarl's Wood Immigration Removal Centre*, 11 MILLION, London. Children's Commissioner for England (2010) *The Children's Commissioner for England's follow up report to: The arrest and detention of children subject to immigration control*, 11 MILLION, London.

136 Royal College of Paediatrics and Child Health, Royal College of General Practitioners, Royal College of Psychiatrists, Faculty of Public Health (2009) *Intercollegiate Briefing Paper: Significant Harm: the effects of administrative detention on the health of children, young people and their families*, RCPCH, RCGP, RCPsych, FPH, London, p.1. Available at: www.rcpsych.ac.uk (accessed 19 May 2011).

137 HM Chief Inspector of Prisons for England and Wales (2010) *Annual report 2008–09*, HMIP, London, p.72.

138 Gower M. (2010) *Ending child immigration detention*, House of Commons Library, London. Available at: www.parliament.uk (accessed 28 February 2011).

139 British Medical Association (2001) *The medical profession and human rights: handbook for a changing agenda*, Zed Books, London, p.404.

140 Immigration Law Practitioners' Association, Crawley H. (2007) *When is a child not a child? Asylum, age disputes and the process of age assessment*, ILPA, London, pp.197–202.

141 Immigration and Asylum Act 1999, Sch 12.

142 Detention Centre Rules 2001. SI 2001/238, rule 35.

143 British Medical Association, Faculty of Forensic and Legal Medicine (2009) *Health care of detainees in police stations*, BMA, London.

144 Faculty of Forensic and Legal Medicine (2008) *Consent from children and young people in custody in England and Wales*, FFLM, London.

145 Police and Criminal Evidence Act 1984 (as amended), s 55 (England and Wales). Police and Criminal Evidence (Northern Ireland) Order 1989, art 56 (Northern Ireland). In Scotland, 'proper authorisation' is the authority of a sheriff's warrant.

146 British Medical Association, Faculty of Forensic and Legal Medicine (2010) *Recommendations for healthcare professionals asked to perform intimate body searches*, BMA, London.

147 British Medical Association, Faculty of Forensic and Legal Medicine (2010) *Taking blood specimens from incapacitated drivers*, BMA, London.

148 Blatch B. (1996) *House of Lords official report (Hansard)*, February 5, col 50.

149 After the suspect has been arrested under s 41 of the Terrorism Act 2000.

150 British Medical Association, Faculty of Forensic and Legal Medicine (2009) *Health care of detainees in police stations*, BMA, London, p.6, para 2.1.

151 Home Office (2006) *Police and Criminal Evidence Act 1984 (PACE). Code H. Code of Practice in connection with the detention, treatment and questioning by police officers of persons under section 41 of, and schedule 8 to, the Terrorism Act 2000*, The Stationery Office, London, pp.116–8.

18: Education and training

The questions covered in this chapter include the following.

- Why and how should medical students learn about medical ethics and law?
- Is patient consent needed for medical students to be present during consultations?
- Should patients be told if a medical student is to carry out part of their treatment?
- What is the 'hidden curriculum'?
- Are there ethical dilemmas that are particular to medical students?
- What should medical students do if they witness unethical practice?

The ethical practice of medicine

The aim of medical education is to provide doctors with the knowledge and skills needed to practise medicine within an ethical and legal framework. As discussed in the introductory chapter, doctors are confronted by ethical issues every day of their working lives; the medical training they receive must equip them with the skills and confidence needed to deal with these situations in an appropriate manner and to seek advice when appropriate. In this chapter we examine the contribution that the teaching of medical ethics and law makes to medical education. This is a contribution that extends well beyond the provision of a body of knowledge about ethics and law, to the teaching of analytical and communication skills, and appropriate attitudes and behaviour towards patients. As the object of medicine is to maximise the health and well-being of patients; however, technically proficient or knowledgeable doctors may be, if their practice is unethical, they are failing to fulfil this objective. An understanding of ethics, and of the ethical practice of medicine, is therefore essential to being a good doctor.

This chapter considers several distinct but related areas. It begins by considering the way in which medical education has changed, introducing a greater emphasis on medical ethics as a core part of the medical curriculum. This part of the chapter focuses primarily on the teaching of medical ethics and law in the medical undergraduate curriculum, but recognises the increasing role of continuing professional development throughout a doctor's career. The chapter goes on to look at the ethical issues that arise specifically in medical education, focusing on the ethics of teaching and ways of ensuring that medical students can gain the experience they need without risk to patient safety or undermining patient choices and preferences. Finally, the chapter considers those ethical issues that arise for medical students in particular.

General principles

The following general principles apply in education and training.

- An understanding of medical ethics and law, and the ethical practice of medicine, is essential to being a good doctor.

Medical Ethics Today: The BMA's Handbook of Ethics and Law, Third Edition. Sophie Brannan, Eleanor Chrispin, Martin Davies, Veronica English, Rebecca Mussell, Julian Sheather and Ann Sommerville.
© 2012 BMA Medical Ethics Department. Published 2012 by Blackwell Publishing Ltd.

- A primary aim of the teaching of medical ethics is to develop within students a questioning, enquiring and analytical mind.
- In addition to knowledge of medical ethics and law, teaching should aim to provide medical students with the skills and confidence necessary to address difficult ethical dilemmas and to seek advice when necessary.
- Education and training is a necessary, ongoing process throughout a doctor's career.
- Tutors must ensure that teaching, both formal and informal, complies with good ethical practice; careful attention should be paid to consent and confidentiality when medical students are present during consultations.
- Medical students who witness unethical practice have a responsibility to make their concerns known.
- Teaching institutions have a responsibility to establish accessible mechanisms for students to raise ethical concerns about aspects of their training without fear of repercussions.

Medical education: the changing landscape

The General Medical Council (GMC) has statutory responsibilities for regulating all stages of medical education in the UK. This includes responsibility for undergraduate medical education; the GMC determines the knowledge and skills to be taught and the standard of proficiency required at qualifying examinations. In the later years of the twentieth century, and on into the twenty-first, the educational landscape over which the GMC exercises regulatory control has experienced a significant period of change. In early 2011, it was suggested that aspects of the education and training of doctors should undergo further change.[1] (Up-to-date information is available via the British Medical Association (BMA) website.) As medical education has continued to develop, so too has the place of medical ethics and law within its ambit. One feature of this evolving landscape has been the appearance of new ethical dilemmas driven by changes in technology and medical practice.

The GMC's *Tomorrow's Doctors* guidance sets the standards expected of medical schools for the delivery of teaching, learning and assessment, and lists the outcomes that medical students must demonstrate before graduation.[2] It explicitly states that medical graduates 'will be able to behave according to ethical and legal principles'[3] and will know about and follow the GMC's ethical guidance and standards.[4] Since its original publication in 1993, when it addressed problems resulting from the 'gross overcrowding of most undergraduate curricula' and a process of medical education that 'taxed the memory but not the intellect',[5] it has been revised several times to take account of major developments. These include the publication of *Good Medical Practice*,[6] the merger of the Postgraduate Medical Education and Training Board (PMETB) with the GMC in 2010, and the creation of the Foundation Programme, the 2-year generic training programme which forms the bridge between medical school and specialist or general practice training.

Tomorrow's Doctors acknowledges the following as an overarching outcome for medical graduates:

> Medical students are tomorrow's doctors. In accordance with *Good Medical Practice*, graduates will make the care of patients their first concern, applying their knowledge and skills in a competent and ethical manner and using their ability to provide leadership and to analyse complex and uncertain situations.[7]

The pace of change looks set to continue. The 2010 Lord Naren Patel review made a number of recommendations for the future of medical education, training and regulation, identifying areas where regulation might be enhanced and options for how this might be achieved. These recommendations included the need for regulation to reach across and link the various stages of doctors' education and learning, to support their transition from one stage to another and, ultimately, to minimise risk.[8]

Since the mid-1990s, the BMA has also paid significant attention to the perceived short-comings in medical education. The Association established a medical education working party in response to a number of resolutions passed at its annual representatives meetings, calling for complete reform of the undergraduate curriculum. In its recommendations for all professional training, the BMA has recognised that, although educational structures may be formal, teachers should be seen as facilitators of learning, rather than providers of information, and they should help students to see their own role as an active one.[9]

British Medical Association recommendations for undergraduate medical education

In its detailed recommendations, the BMA stressed that medical undergraduates should:

- have well-developed skills of thinking and reasoning
- have skills for personal development and self-criticism
- be taught and understand the ethical principles underpinning medical practice
- know their limitations and when to call for help
- have good communication skills
- develop attitudes appropriate to the practice of medicine
- be given support at all levels
- have interactive teaching to encourage them to reflect on, and critically evaluate, their own work
- be encouraged to define educational objectives to meet their personal learning needs
- have teachers who are kind and thoughtful towards them
- have access to a confidential advice and counselling service separate from any academic support.[10]

The BMA has continued to develop policy focusing on improving the strength of medical education. At its 2010 annual representatives meeting, policy was passed stressing the importance of regular and constructive formative feedback, as well as the benefits for all doctors of being involved in teaching and medical education, whether or not via a formal teaching role.[11]

Selection for medical schools

The traditional prioritisation, within the medical curriculum, of technical and rational skills above capacities such as compassion, respect and intuition, has inevitably been reflected in the type of students selected for medical school. Indeed, anecdote has it that in the 1960s intending medical students were advised *against* stating that one of the reasons they wished to become a doctor was to help sick people and that having a parent who was a doctor greatly boosted an applicant's chances of selection. The BMA has previously considered the appropriateness of the selection techniques used by medical schools and, in order to develop a more diverse student body, concluded that there should be greater emphasis on graduate entry, the social basis of medicine should be widened and information about the variety of non-standard entry requirements should be distributed more widely.[12]

Selection for medical school

In March 2010, the Medical Schools Council (MSC) published a set of nine guiding principles for the admission of medical students to medical school. The principles identify the interplay of academic abilities and personal attributes required to make a successful doctor. They stress that selection for medical school implies selection for the medical profession, and in turn emphasise that the highest standards of professional and personal conduct are required of those undertaking the study of medicine. Among the principles is the recognition that medical students' primary duty of care is to patients and that honesty and integrity, as essential attributes of the practising doctor are, by extension, essential qualities for the medical student. The principles also stress the need for medical schools to select those with the greatest aptitude for medical training from those with high academic ability, thereby acknowledging that, although they may have attained the necessary academic standards to study medicine, some students will nevertheless not be suited to a medical career.[13]

The MSC principles are consistent with guidance from the GMC, which recognises the importance of considering applicants' capacity for ethical practice, as well as the personal and academic qualities needed in a doctor, from the outset of the selection process.[14]

Debate about fair access to medical education and initiatives to promote it have remained prominent in the discourse surrounding selection for medical schools. In 2009, the UK Government appointed a panel of experts and representatives of the professions, including medicine, to examine the best ways to increase social mobility into the professions. The report of the panel's findings highlighted that members of the professions, particularly medicine and law, grew up in families with an income well above the average and that the professions themselves need to take the lead so that 'opportunities [become] available to more people more of the time'.[15] In the same year, the BMA published a report focusing on equality and diversity in medical schools, which similarly noted that, despite demographic changes in medical schools, the majority of medical school students are still drawn from professional and managerial family backgrounds.[16] The report also highlighted that, as well as socio-economic background, the age, ethnicity and gender profile of medical school students continue to raise important questions, both about the structure of medical education and the future composition of the profession. The 2009 version of the GMC's *Tomorrow's Doctors* guidance places greater emphasis on equality and diversity than previous versions, stating that medical schools 'will have policies which are aimed at ensuring that all applicants and students are treated fairly and with equality of opportunity, regardless of their diverse backgrounds and needs'.[17]

The BMA is opposed to all forms of inappropriate discrimination in the selection of candidates to study medicine and supports efforts to attract medical students from a broader range of social backgrounds. This position is formally expressed in a wide range of policy statements drawn up at the BMA's annual representatives meetings, including the statement, from 2000, that 'racism and discrimination in any form must be eliminated in the NHS'.

The teaching of medical ethics and law

Although the introduction of medical ethics and law as a core part of the undergraduate medical curriculum is a relatively recent development,[18] the notion that practical expertise should be accompanied by an awareness of certain moral standards goes back to the beginning of medicine. A surprisingly consistent set of values and standards is reflected in all codes of medical ethics, regardless of their cultural, geographical or historical context. The teaching of medical ethics was traditionally intended to pass on these professional values to future generations of practising doctors, but in the past such teaching was often sparse and formulaic. In many medical schools, medical ethics was either barely mentioned or was chiefly taught through the observation of senior doctors and as a measure to protect medical staff against potential litigation.

As the teaching of ethics has become more formal, both in the UK and elsewhere, its aims, methodology and content have changed; as it has become established as a necessary element of the curriculum, the extent and substantive content of medical ethics teaching remains a subject of debate. The Institute of Medical Ethics (IME), having advocated the introduction of formal medical ethics teaching in UK medical schools in its 1987 Pond Report,[19] was subsequently involved, in cooperation with most UK teachers of medical ethics and law, and others, in developing a model core curriculum for teaching these subjects within medical education. This core curriculum was described in the 1998 *Consensus statement by teachers of medical ethics and law* (for a summary of the updated core curriculum, see pages 746–747) and demanded 'a balanced, sustained, academically rigorous and clinically relevant presentation of both ethics and law in medicine, and of the relationship and tensions between them'.[20] Later work highlighted the continuing variations in both the time allocated to the subject and the depth in which ethical issues are explored. The BMA and the IME have continued to focus on undergraduate teaching in ethics and law, in particular on what and how teaching is carried out and assessed. A nationwide survey of medical schools, funded by the IME, was carried out by Peninsula Medical School and reviewed the current status of medical ethics in undergraduate education. The findings were published in the *Journal of Medical Ethics*[21] and discussed at a joint IME/BMA conference in 2006.[22] The main findings of this study were as follows:

- significant progress had been made to establish the place of ethics within undergraduate courses in medicine
- there was still much that needed doing to ensure that ethics learning is adequate across the board, in particular:
  - staffing and curricular involvement varied very widely
  - relevant academic posts were precariously funded
  - teaching, learning and assessment methods varied greatly.

It was suggested that medical ethics and law were at risk of marginalisation within the medical undergraduate curriculum. A further joint conference, in 2008,[23] initiated the IME's 3-year programme of work to promote best practice in the integrated teaching, learning and assessment of medical ethics and law, and in 2009 the IME published an updated version of its core content of learning (see pages 746–747).[24]

Educational goals of teaching ethics and law

The teaching of medical ethics is sometimes criticised for being insufficiently practical. There is no place, it is argued, for philosophical abstractions amidst the messy contingencies of day-to-day medical practice and cumbersome philosophical theories are more of a hindrance than a help to busy doctors. As discussed in the introductory chapter, however, a practical approach to resolving ethical dilemmas does not demand a detailed understanding of, or agreement about, the philosophy underpinning discussion about medical ethics. In some cases, reaching a reasoned decision may demand little more than attentiveness to norms of good medical practice, the dignity and autonomy of patients, together with knowledge of the relevant laws and guidance. Inevitably, difficult dilemmas arise that require a more formal critical analysis of, for example, the conflicting duties owed to different people. Training in and understanding of medical ethics equips doctors to deal with these situations.

Research ethics teaching in practice[25]

Experienced researchers struggle with the research ethics approval process[26] and the problem extends to students.[27] Worryingly, a study of postgraduate research students has indicated that those with prior experience of applying for ethical approval for research were, in fact, more resistant to training in research ethics than those who had no such prior experience.[28] Incorporating the teaching of research ethics methodology into the undergraduate curriculum is one way this problem has been addressed.

At the University of East Anglia, medical students are taught ethics as a fundamental element of research design. As part of a course on research methods, students identify a suitable research question and apply their knowledge of research methodology, ethics and bureaucracy in order to draft a research protocol. Students learn that only where ethical considerations are fully integrated into a research project will a research proposal be sufficiently robust.

Students are also taught about the importance of external research ethics review and the function of research ethics committees (RECs). Working in problem-based learning groups they discuss ethical aspects of research protocols using the same approach as an REC. Experienced members of local National Research Ethics Service committees and university RECs are recruited to facilitate dedicated meetings of the groups. Here students present a research project protocol they have reviewed in depth, highlighting ethical and scientific concerns.

Following this teaching session, students are asked to provide a written piece of coursework that summarises their ethical review of the protocol and takes into account the group discussion. They then complete a summary that is assessed as part of their degree programme.

Overall, this aspect of the course has been well received by students, whose comments have included, 'the peer review sessions were extremely helpful, not only for personal feedback on my own project but also to learn how to feedback on other projects'.

The BMA and other bodies have come increasingly to recognise the fundamental importance of good communication skills and an emphasis on patient-centred care to medical practice.[29] Many complaints of unethical practice would never have arisen but for a breakdown in dialogue between doctors and patients. Good communication is critical to ethical practice and is an area of education in which a small amount of attention reaps considerable benefit.

Objectives of teaching medical ethics and law

In the British Medical Association's view, teaching should ensure that students develop:

- an ability to identify the morally relevant issues, values and principles at stake in particular dilemmas
- the skills to analyse these in order to reach a morally justified decision about how to proceed
- an awareness of their legal and professional obligations to patients, employers and the community
- the competence to communicate well with patients and professional colleagues

- an understanding of the generally complementary nature of ethics and law
- an overview of the implications for medical practice of ethical principles and law
- skills in communicating ethical concepts in a professional environment
- an attitude of respect for patients' rights as an integral part of medical ethics and law.

In the UK, the last decades of the twentieth century saw a rapid development in legal aspects of medical practice, both through new statutes and developments in case law (see introductory chapter). Although some study of law has always been advisable for medical students, and is particularly relevant to certain medical specialties such as forensic medicine, it was often seen as a precautionary measure to help doctors to avoid litigation and raise their awareness of potential liability. Increasingly, the courts have become involved in deciding about the legal scope within which doctors may decide to give or withhold treatment, as well as in determining the reasonableness of medical opinion. In some cases, sophisticated, imaginative and complex ethical debates have taken place in the courts about, for example, the purpose of medical treatment, the limits of individual choice and definitions of life and death. In the BMA's view, it is important that doctors should understand the key principles of law that affect medical practice and have knowledge of their legal obligations and duties, including when to seek legal advice in relation to more complex cases. Students also need to be introduced to the nature of legal reasoning and exposed to the reality that definitive legal answers to some questions may constrain their actions in some circumstances, while in others such definitive answers may not be available.

General Medical Council recommendations on the ethical and legal principles graduates must uphold

'[Medical graduates] will be able to:

- Know about and keep to the GMC's ethical guidance and standards including *Good Medical Practice*, the 'Duties of a doctor registered with the GMC' and supplementary ethical guidance which describe what is expected of all doctors registered with the GMC.
- Demonstrate awareness of the clinical responsibilities and role of the doctor, making the care of the patient the first concern. Recognise the principles of patient-centred care, including self-care, and deal with patients' healthcare needs in consultation with them and, where appropriate, their relatives or carers.
- Be polite, considerate, trustworthy and honest, act with integrity, maintain confidentiality, respect patients' dignity and privacy, and understand the importance of appropriate consent.
- Respect all patients, colleagues and others regardless of their age, colour, culture, disability, ethnic or national origin, gender, lifestyle, marital or parental status, race, religion or beliefs, sex, sexual orientation, or social or economic status. Graduates will respect patients' right to hold religious or other beliefs and take these into account when relevant to treatment options.
- Recognise the rights and equal value of all people and how opportunities for some people may be restricted by others' perceptions.
- Understand and accept the legal, moral and ethical responsibilities involved in protecting and promoting the health of individual patients, their dependants and the public – including vulnerable groups such as children, older people, people with learning disabilities and people with mental illness.
- Demonstrate knowledge of laws, and systems of professional regulation through the GMC and others, relevant to medical practice, including the ability to complete relevant certificates and legal documents and liaise with the coroner or procurator fiscal where appropriate.'[30]

Academic and professional misconduct

Patterns and habits of conduct learnt at medical school can clearly set the basis for ethical practice throughout a doctor's career. As it is vital that doctors are honest and trustworthy, the ethical conduct of students during the academic parts of their training, when they will have no direct contact with patients, is also of primary importance. Reported problems with the academic conduct of medical students include plagiarism and fraud.[31] It is clear that students need to be aware that the ethical practice of medicine extends beyond the doctor–patient relationship and incorporates all aspects of their working lives, and indeed certain aspects of their personal lives; for example, the misuse of alcohol or drugs can lead to concerns relating to student fitness to practise. Similarly, where caution is not exercised, the use of social media can expose students to risk of legal complaint or challenges over their fitness to practise. (For further discussion of doctors' use of social media, see Chapter 1, pages 52–53.)[32] Furthermore, as medicine is widely seen as a career that entails lifelong learning, the need for scrupulous academic honesty throughout both undergraduate and postgraduate training is essential.

As noted at the beginning of this chapter, the ability to become a successful doctor relies on more than academic aptitude alone. Medical students must demonstrate fitness to practise medicine from the outset of their medical studies, and this includes showing an awareness of ethical issues in their professional behaviour with patients.[33] Students must keep to the guidance *Medical students: professional values and fitness to practise*, developed by the GMC and the MSC, which stresses that they:

> [h]ave certain privileges and responsibilities different from those of other students. Because of this, different standards of professional behaviour are expected of them. Medical schools are responsible for ensuring that medical students have opportunities to learn and practise the standards expected of them.[34]

Commentators have suggested that medical schools can struggle to deal with students whose unsuitability for a career in medicine is not reflected in academic difficulty.[35] This would indicate that fitness to practise should be determined by both academic and non-academic ability if medical students at risk of subsequent misconduct are to be identified and supported early on in their careers. It is vital that medical schools have systems for documenting concerns, identifying problem students and supporting and managing these students, so as to attribute equal value to both the academic and non-academic aspects of fitness to practise.[36]

A core curriculum for teaching ethics and law

In 2010, the *Journal of Medical Ethics* published an updated version of the 1998 consensus statement by teachers of medical ethics and law in the UK. (For discussion of the IME's work on the development of ethics teaching in undergraduate medical education, see pages 742–743.[37]) This outlined a model core curriculum for the UK, which is summarised below.

Core content of learning for medical ethics and law: a summary

The core content recommends that students demonstrate a critically reflective understanding and, where relevant, appropriate attitudes and practical skills in the areas listed below.

- *Foundations of medical ethics and law:* including methods of ethical reasoning; the legal and professional frameworks within which medicine is practised in the UK; the importance, scope and implications of the doctor's duty of care.
- *Professionalism: 'Good Medical Practice':* including the importance of trust, integrity, honesty and good communication; the need to accept personal responsibility and be aware of limitations in practical skills or knowledge; the need to maintain professional boundaries.
- *Patients: their values, narratives, rights and responsibilities:* including the differences between moral, legal and human rights; the importance of the patient's dignity, narrative and perspective; the rights and responsibilities of patients.
- *Informed decision making and valid consent/refusal:* including informed consent, voluntariness and disclosure of diagnosis; patient refusal of treatment; the significance and limits of respect for patient autonomy.
- *Capacity and incapacity:* including ethical and legal aspects of treatment for patients who lack capacity or who have capacity but are otherwise vulnerable; the legal criteria for establishing that a person lacks capacity; the ethical challenges and legal requirements of determining and acting in the best interests of patients who lack capacity.
- *Confidentiality:* including when it is legally, professionally and ethically justifiable or mandatory to breach confidentiality; how to share confidential information within clinical teams; good practice in sharing information with relatives and carers.
- *Justice and public health:* including legal and ethical issues in balancing individual and community interests in accessing healthcare resources; principles and criteria for just distribution of finite healthcare resources; the role of the doctor as patient advocate.
- *Children and young people:* including the duty to respect the rights and interests of children and young people; the legal and ethical aspects of the capacity of young people to consent to and refuse treatment; the respective roles of parents/guardians, healthcare professionals and the courts in decisions about the treatment of children.
- *Mental health:* including the implications of mental capacity legislation for clinical practice; mental health legislation relating to compulsory detention and treatment; the ethical and legal issues of restraint.
- *Beginning of life:* including ethical and legal issues surrounding the status of the embryo and fetus; concepts of personhood; ethical, legal and professional aspects of contraception, artificial reproductive technologies, termination of pregnancy and neonatal care.
- *Towards the end of life:* including dignity, patient choice, limits on respect for patient autonomy; 'ageism', 'futility', sanctity and quality of life; withdrawing and withholding treatment and advance decisions about treatment.
- *Medical research and audit:* including the importance of trust and integrity in research and audit; the situations when research ethics committee approval may be required and how to seek it; potential conflicts of interests in relationships with pharmaceutical and medical equipment industries.[38]

The consensus group concluded that the standards expected of students by the GMC can only be achieved when the teaching and learning of medical ethics, law and professionalism are fundamental to and thoroughly integrated throughout the curricula of all medical schools, from the outset and reinforced throughout the course, as a shared obligation of all teachers. Its findings stressed that the adequate provision and coordination of teaching and learning of medical ethics and law required at least one full-time equivalent senior academic in ethics and law with relevant professional and academic expertise.[39]

Graduation oaths

Studies have shown that about half of all UK medical schools and almost all medical schools in the USA ask students to make a formal and ceremonial commitment to various ethical precepts of good medical practice, either on graduation or at the beginning of their medical studies.[40] Texts vary; some use a version of the Hippocratic Oath (see Appendix a), while others use the World Medical Association's Declaration of Geneva (see Appendix b), or an oath formulated by the institution itself, including those drawn up by students (see Appendix c as one example). Some are applicable only to doctors; others reflect the reality of multi-disciplinary practice.

One of the strengths of the 'Hippocratic tradition', asking that doctors pledge themselves to demanding ethical standards, has been its contribution to the understanding of the unique position, and the unique powers and responsibilities, of members of the medical profession; the ethical standards are demanding in proportion to doctors' potential to act for good or bad in their patients' lives. Views differ about the benefits and drawbacks of such ceremonies.[41] Those who support them focus on their perceived benefits, including the development of ethical sensitivity, the promotion of professional bonding and responsibility, and the recognition by students of the gravity of their undertaking. Those who oppose their use draw attention to their potential drawbacks, including their promotion of cultural and professional isolation, the confusing number of oaths available and reservations about whether medical students are yet sufficiently experienced to understand the ramifications of the oath or the commitment they make.

The BMA supports the practice of health professionals making some formal commitment to ethical standards as an awareness raising act at the beginning of their careers.

Postgraduate training in ethics

Although most of this chapter focuses on the training of undergraduate medical students, medical education generally, and training in medical ethics specifically, are ongoing processes throughout a doctor's career. Continuing education and professional development is not an optional extra; they are part of the professional obligations of all doctors, the assessment of which forms part of the revalidation process and an important aspect of the cultural orientation of doctors who have trained overseas and practise in the UK. For example, the Professional and Linguistics Assessment Board (PLAB) test, by which international medical graduates demonstrate that they have the necessary skills and knowledge to practise medicine in the UK, assesses doctors' ability to practise ethically and lawfully via various practical clinical scenarios.[42] The BMA[43] and GMC[44] have undertaken work aimed at tackling disparities between the culturally influenced expectations and behaviours, in terms of ethical decision making, of doctors who have trained overseas and come to work in the UK, and those who have completed their undergraduate training in the UK.

In addition to their own educational needs, doctors are also involved in teaching more junior colleagues, both formally and informally. The GMC, which, since April 2010, regulates all stages of medical education, including at postgraduate level, advises doctors:

> You must keep your knowledge and skills up to date throughout your working life. You should be familiar with relevant guidelines and developments that affect your work. You should regularly take part in educational activities that maintain and further develop your competence and performance.[45]

Examples of ways in which qualified doctors might ensure that their knowledge and skills in relation to medical ethics are kept up to date include becoming a member of a research or clinical ethics committee and undertaking various postgraduate refresher courses or higher degrees in medical ethics and related subjects.

The GMC, Department of Health and the BMA, via its website, can provide more detailed information on licensing, revalidation and appraisal.[46]

From theory to practice

One of the consistent problems raised by junior doctors with the BMA has been that, although as students they learn the importance of medical ethics and law, once graduated they are often expected by other professionals to conform to accepted custom and practice. The force of tradition is hard to resist and is compounded by younger doctors' anxieties that their career prospects can easily be jeopardised by questioning or objecting to the instructions of senior health professionals.

This issue is brought into sharp focus where a junior member of the healthcare team is tasked with obtaining patient consent, but may be unable to answer patient questions or does not have the experience properly to convey information that may be potentially distressing. (For guidance on who should seek consent, see Chapter 2, pages 63–64.) The vital importance of communicating effectively with patients, especially in order to enable them to consent to or refuse treatment, is stressed throughout a doctor's undergraduate education, yet junior doctors can find that this importance is diminished in practice when such requests are made of them. In response to this disconnection between theory and practice, the BMA has produced a concise *Consent tool kit*, comprising a series of 'reminder' cards containing frequently asked questions. The fifth edition of this resource was published in 2009.[47]

Consent is only one issue about which newly qualified doctors may encounter pressure to conform to the practice of more senior colleagues. The BMA continues to produce guidance which is designed to support the incorporation of ethical values learnt at medical school into clinical practice, and which is specifically aimed at doctors who are new to practice.[48]

Developing trends in teaching medical ethics

Multi-disciplinary teaching

Medical ethics is increasingly taught on a multi-disciplinary basis. The aims of this approach are to improve patient care by reducing professional compartmentalisation, creating a better understanding of the complementary roles of different professionals in the team and engendering mutual respect between the healthcare professions. In the past, for example, nurses and doctors saw their ethical obligations to patients in rather different terms, with nurses often seeing themselves as the patient's advocate. It was in this context that the report of the public inquiry into children's heart surgery at the Bristol Royal Infirmary (the Bristol Report) made several recommendations about strengthening links between medical schools and schools of nursing 'with a view to providing more joint education between medical and nursing students'.[49]

Reinforcing this process, the development of patient-centred care has led to a softening of traditional boundaries between the various healthcare professions. The professional status and range of responsibilities of nurses and other non-doctors in the medical team has also increased. Awareness of the role of other healthcare professionals is also becoming a core element in the training of doctors. Furthermore, given the general applicability of core ethical issues, such as consent and confidentiality, to all healthcare professionals, it is likely that joint teaching in this area will continue to develop.

Although multi-disciplinary teaching presents administrative and logistical challenges, and its effectiveness needs to be assessed, the BMA nevertheless strongly supports the principle of exploring multi-disciplinary education.

Human rights

The integration of human rights into medical ethics teaching is symptomatic of a growing recognition that human rights are not only of concern in a few specific countries, but that they increasingly relate to the ordinary ethical dilemmas with which health professionals are faced. Policy making in terms of healthcare, for example, frequently raises questions about the rights (and duties) of the individual versus those of society at large, thus echoing one of the central concerns of human rights.[50] In addition, since the Human Rights Act 1998 came into force in the UK, lawyers and ethicists have begun specifically to consider traditional ethical issues, such as the allocation of healthcare resources and the marginalisation of some patient groups, through the prism of human rights discourse. The relationship between medical ethics and human rights is discussed further in the introductory chapter.

Although an awareness of ethical and legal principles is essential for all health professionals, knowledge of the connections between law, ethics and human rights assumes a particular importance for those working in environments that are more likely to generate human rights violations or to bring health workers into contact with evidence of abuse. Forensic physicians, prison doctors (see Chapter 17) and those employed by the armed services (see Chapter 16, pages 679–682) should have training that focuses on their particular dilemmas. Similarly, doctors visiting or working in otherwise 'closed' institutions, such as psychiatric hospitals or children's homes, may need additional training. These doctors work in specialties in which it is easy to become isolated from mainstream practice and to absorb the mindset of other workers, whose dominant concern to maintain order may sometimes be at the expense of concern for the rights, welfare and autonomy of patients or detainees. Their dilemmas are also the ones least addressed in ethical guidelines or training.

Humanitarian and global issues

There is increased recognition that medical students' views on the components to be included in undergraduate teaching should be sought. Medical students' organisations are, however, very conscious of the number of subjects that already have to be compressed into the curriculum. One student organisation active in this sphere is the Medical Students' International Network (MedSIN), which campaigns for the curriculum to be extended to include humanitarian and global health issues and has established links with the BMA Medical Students Committee.[51] In the UK, MedSIN works closely with another organisation, Medact, on education issues. Medact has produced an undergraduate teaching pack with a public health focus, covering:

- social and economic development
- environmental change and pollution
- the health implications of conflict
- the interconnections between poverty, environmental pollution and conflict.[52]

These teaching materials can be used flexibly to suit local needs, either as a complete course or as separate modules. Some UK medical schools have been very responsive to the inclusion of these materials as special study modules in global health. Among the key topics that MedSIN recommends as appropriate for inclusion in the curriculum are: human rights generally; social inequality; migration and refugees; conflict and trauma; and ethics and reproductive health. In addition to its projects on the curriculum, MedSIN undertakes a range of practical community and public health activities to encourage medical student involvement in community and intersectoral work. Such projects complement the theoretical and academic teaching in human rights and may produce a more enduring impact on future doctors' views and attitudes than academic study alone.

Medical humanities

In *Tomorrow's Doctors*, the GMC stresses the importance of developing the cultural sensitivities, imagination and interpretive skills of medical students.[53] The study of medical humanities has been portrayed as one means of achieving this, by relating issues in medicine to those portrayed in art, literature, popular culture, film and theatre.[54] The integration of medical humanities into the teaching of medical ethics has among its key aims to help students to:

- think of themselves as embryonic doctors and promote an understanding of professional identity by reference to cultural images of the profession
- understand the disparity between the reality of medicine and public expectations
- develop analytical and interpretive skills
- come to terms with their own mortality
- enhance and extend their understanding of doctors, medicine and medical practice as perceived from a huge range of different perspectives.

Concerned as they are with imagination and insight, the medical humanities fit closely with a great deal of core ethical discourse. Literature, art and poetry share with medical ethics a preoccupation with the most troubling human questions relating to death, illness, suffering and disability. Some see the subject as a counterbalance to a potentially excessive focus on scientific knowledge alone. Goodwin argues:

> . . . science can tell us nothing about an individual. Science speaks in terms of probabilities, of means and standard deviations, the behaviour of groups of electrons or proteins or people, not of individual entities. Everything that makes an individual an individual, everything that importantly defines an individual's life, is outside the realm of science. The practice of medicine involves only individuals.[55]

Ideally, of course, doctors and other health professionals should be exposed to a wide range of influences that can contribute positively to their personal and professional development and to the manner in which they approach patients.

Distance learning materials

The BMA has long been aware of an international need for teaching packs consisting of basic learning materials in ethics and relevant law. Such packs could either be used as self-teaching tools or as a means of training medical students and others where access to such material is restricted. It has urged that high-quality teaching materials be made available online, so that they can be accessed by doctors and medical students who have no other easy means of increasing their knowledge about medical ethics. Most BMA ethics and law materials are freely available on its website. Clearly, in a competitive market, it may be difficult for academic institutions to disseminate material without charge.

Summary – the teaching of medical ethics and law

- The GMC requires that medical students and graduates behave according to ethical and legal principles.
- Medical ethics and law should form part of the core curriculum for medical undergraduates.
- Medical ethics teaching has two main objectives, ensuring that medical students acquire:
  - a knowledge and understanding of ethical and legal issues relevant to medicine
  - an ability to understand and analyse ethical problems.
- Meeting the objectives of medical teaching will make medical students better doctors and thus improve patient care.
- Good communication skills are essential to the ethical practice of medicine.
- The BMA supports the practice of health professionals making a formal commitment to ethical standards at the beginning of their careers.
- Education and training are continuing processes throughout a doctor's career.
- The teaching of medical ethics has increasingly adopted methods and principles from other disciplines, such as human rights and medical humanities.

Ethical issues raised in teaching medical students

In addition to teaching medical ethics, tutors, supervisors and other doctors also need to ensure that the practice of teaching medical students, including while on clinical placement, is undertaken in an ethical manner. Inevitably, during their training, medical students come into contact with patients and, in some cases, as well as observing, they undertake examinations or procedures. The general ethical principles that guide all medical practice are also central to any contact between patients and medical students. To support medical students in this aspect of their training, a range of guidance, supplementary to *Tomorrow's Doctors,* is produced by the GMC,[56] along with online learning materials which explain how GMC guidance applies in practice.[57] This section considers the issues raised by such encounters and also other aspects of the ethical teaching of medicine.

Consent in the context of teaching

It is essential that medical students develop their clinical skills through steadily increasing involvement with patients, but this should be done only with the knowledge and consent of the patients concerned. In order for this consent to be valid, patients need to be aware of the following:

- who will be present
- why they will be present
- what, if any, involvement they will have with the procedure being undertaken.

Patients must always be able to refuse to consent to students being involved in their treatment, or to their presence during treatment, and should be able to do so without prejudicing their care. (For a detailed discussion of the principles of patient consent, see Chapter 2.) Medical students are sometimes an integral part of the care team and *Tomorrow's Doctors* encourages their incorporation into the team.[58] It should be made clear to patients when this is the case and patients must be given the opportunity to refuse to have students present. Patients should be reassured that their refusal will not in any way affect the care they receive.

These basic principles of consent apply whether training is undertaken in a teaching hospital or in any other clinical setting. All healthcare establishments involved in education and training may find it helpful to draw up protocols about the extent to which medical students and other doctors in training will be present during, and involved with, examination and treatment.

Introducing students

The BMA is sometimes asked how students should be introduced to patients, whether as 'medical students' or 'student doctors', for example. The most important factor is that the patient is left in no doubt about whether the individual is a qualified doctor who is learning new skills or is an undergraduate undergoing his or her initial training. Indeed, GMC and MSC guidance states that, in order for them to demonstrate they are fit to practise, students should accurately represent their position or abilities.[59] The BMA believes that the phrase 'medical student' is the most appropriate and unambiguous term for those who are undergoing their medical training.

Presence of medical students

Even when medical students will not be involved in the consultation and are simply observing the practice of the treating doctor, consent is needed for them to be present; this includes where large numbers of students are present during ward rounds. The doctor who is carrying out the consultation should explain to the patient that one or more observers would like to be present during the consultation, examination or procedure, who they are, and why they wish to observe. Patients should be given the opportunity to refuse the presence of medical students or, if they prefer, to limit the number who will be present. Patients should be reassured that their decision will not affect their treatment. In most circumstances, it is possible and good practice to give patients the option of considering this request prior to the arrival of the students.

Examining patients

Learning to carry out examinations with the necessary degree of technical expertise and appropriate communication skills is an essential part of medical training. As with doctors, any touching of patients by medical students needs consent. When patients are conscious and have capacity, the nature and purpose of the examination should be described, and they should be asked to consent to one or more students examining them. It should be made clear whether the procedure is being undertaken as part of their treatment or for the educational benefit of the examining students. Where procedures or examinations are solely for the purpose of educating students, it is essential that the patient understands this and gives explicit consent for it to take place. If the patient does not give consent, students should not take part in the examination. Patients should be asked for their consent in private and not in the presence of students, as some patients may be unwilling to express their reluctance in front of those whom they wish to exclude.

Students who are present while patients are anaesthetised are sometimes asked to examine the patient or simply to 'have a feel' of the surgeon's findings. In the past, it was common to conduct rectal or vaginal examinations on patients under anaesthesia, often without their consent. Surveys into the quality of the consent sought for intimate examination of anaesthetised patients by students have found that up to one-quarter of intimate examinations on the patients studied did not have adequate consent.[60] Such practice is entirely unacceptable. Doctors must not ask students to be involved in any physical touching or exploration unless the patient has given explicit consent in advance and students should refuse to participate if they are not satisfied that consent has been obtained. In addition to the ethical problems that can arise, the Royal College of Obstetricians and Gynaecologists has questioned the value of pelvic examination under anaesthesia because it does not teach students the 'combination of communication and expert examination that characterise sensitive pelvic examination'.[61] Instead, it recommends that students should learn how to don gloves and handle a vaginal speculum in a classroom, and practise using a mannequin in a clinical skills laboratory. Observation of an awake patient in an outpatient clinic is the next step, before ultimately the student performs pelvic and speculum examination of an awake patient who has capacity, under supervision and with the patient's consent. This model of acquiring technical expertise and observing good practice is important throughout medical training. Whether students are performing the examination or merely observing, explicit consent is required from patients. When consent cannot be obtained, intimate investigations by or in the presence of students should not be undertaken. (For further information on the involvement in teaching of patients who lack capacity, see page 755.)

Carrying out procedures as part of the patient's care

Medical students and doctors in training often carry out procedures that patients need as part of their care, such as taking blood samples. The Department of Health advises that:

> [a]ssuming the student is appropriately trained in the procedure, the fact that it is carried out by a student does not alter the nature and purpose of the procedure. It is therefore not a legal requirement to tell the [patient] that the clinician is a student, although it would always be good practice to do so.[62]

The BMA believes that patients should be told if a student is to undertake the procedure, but they should be reassured that the student has had the necessary training and will be given an appropriate level of supervision. Openness and honesty with patients are key if their consent to the procedure is to be valid.

Responsibility for seeking consent rests with the doctor recommending the procedure, who should tell the patient what the procedure involves, including a discussion of the various treatment options, the alternatives available, the prognosis and the risks associated with the intervention. Although the process of seeking consent may be delegated in certain circumstances (see Chapter 2, pages 63–64), the person seeking consent must always be suitably trained and have sufficient knowledge and understanding of the proposed procedure and any risks involved.

As with qualified doctors, if students are asked during their training to carry out procedures they do not feel competent to perform, they should make their concerns known and ask for additional guidance and supervision. The GMC explicitly states that, in order to demonstrate that they are fit to practise, students should 'recognise and work within the limits of their competence and ask for help when necessary',[63] and are responsible for 'ensuring patient safety by working within the limits of their competence, training and status as medical students' and for 'raising any concerns about patient safety'.[64] All medical schools should have accessible procedures for medical students to express any such concerns. Where students feel they are being asked to act beyond their competence, they can seek further advice from the GMC or BMA.

Children, young people and patients who lack capacity

When the patient is a young child the consent of someone with parental responsibility should be sought. Older children and young people may themselves be competent to consent to being examined by a student, but may also wish to involve their parents. (For information about consent by or on behalf of children and young people see Chapter 4.)

Whenever possible, students should learn their technical skills by working with patients who have capacity and who have given consent. Inevitably, they also need to learn to examine and interact with people who lack capacity. Extreme care needs to be taken before including incapacitated people in teaching, whether they are temporarily incapacitated, as a result of an accident or trauma for example, or have long-term incapacity. This issue can arise in a variety of clinical settings, but will commonly require consideration in the context of mental health, intensive care, geriatric care and surgery. The legal position regarding the involvement of adults who lack capacity in teaching is unclear and the BMA is seeking clarification of the legal status of such involvement under the Mental Capacity Act 2005. Legal advice should therefore be sought before involving incapacitated adults in teaching. (Further guidance is provided by the BMA, via its website. More detailed guidance on capacity and capacity to consent can be found in Chapter 3.)

Confidentiality in the context of teaching

Patients who are involved in teaching do not relinquish their rights to, or their interests in, confidentiality. In the process of seeking consent to the presence or involvement of medical students during consultations (see above), patients should be advised that necessary information will be shared with students as part of that process. Patients should be reassured that medical students have an ethical and legal duty to keep the information confidential.

The amount of information that medical students are given should be judged on the same basis as deciding whether information should be shared within healthcare teams. Information should therefore be limited to those who have a demonstrable 'need to know' as a part of their role in providing care (this is discussed further in Chapter 5). When medical students or doctors in training are providing care to a patient, they should be provided with as much information as they need in order to carry out the procedure safely and effectively. However, when they require information solely for their own education, it is essential that patients are made aware of this and give explicit consent to the sharing of information for that purpose.[65] If patients refuse to consent to this information being released, this must be respected. When patients give consent, the information disclosed should be the minimum necessary to achieve the purpose. If student involvement is limited to teaching on the basis of patient notes, or if students are using the case studies of particular patients for a dissertation or other research project, anonymised information should be used wherever possible. If identifiable information is required, patient consent must be sought, ideally by the responsible tutor, and either a written statement of consent or a record of verbal consent placed in the notes. Further advice is given in the GMC's supplementary guidance on disclosing information for education and training purposes.[66]

The involvement of children who lack the capacity to consent to projects of this kind requires consent from someone with parental responsibility (regarding incapacitated adults, see page 755).

Patient confidentiality and log books

The BMA Junior Doctors Committee currently advises the following in relation to keeping records on patients for training purposes:

> Junior doctors who make personal manual or electronic records of patient data, for example for training logbook purposes, should be aware of the provisions of the Data Protection Act 1998. If patient data are recorded on, for example, personal computers, and that data can identify a patient, then the data must be held subject to the provisions of the Data Protection Act. This would require the doctor to be registered for this purpose. Further information on the Act can be found on the Information Commissioner's website at www.informationcommissioner.gov.uk.
>
> The Information Commissioner enforces and oversees the Data Protection Act 1998, and has a range of duties including the promotion of good information handling and the encouragement of codes of practice for data controllers, that is, anyone who decides how and why personal data (information about identifiable, living individuals) are processed.
>
> The BMA advises junior doctors not to record data that identifies a patient, for example a patient's name, though data which can be matched to a patient only through use of a hospital record system or separate second data set is lawful on an unregistered computer. For example, a hospital number can only identify a patient if cross referred with the hospital records system.
>
> Please consult your medical royal college if you feel you are placed in breach of the Act.[67]

Doctors keeping log books should also be aware of their legal and ethical obligations in relation to keeping patient data secure at all times (see Chapter 6, pages 243–245).

Work observation and experience

Young people who are reaching the end of their secondary education and are considering applying to medical school sometimes ask doctors if they can observe their work (shadowing) in order to gain a clearer picture of the reality of medical practice. During such observation, they may have access to confidential medical information. As with all employees and volunteers, it is the doctor's responsibility to emphasise to those on work experience the importance of patient confidentiality and the doctor retains overall responsibility for any breaches that might occur. Doctors must be satisfied that the observer is sufficiently mature and responsible to understand the principles of confidentiality. It is good practice to obtain a signed commitment that the observer will maintain strict confidentiality concerning all information that might identify any of the patients observed. As with medical students, observers should be present during consultations only if patients have given their consent. Patients should be given time to consider such requests, without the potential observer present, and it must be made clear that a refusal will not in any way adversely influence their treatment.

Handling requests for work observation in clinical settings

The following points should be considered where requests for work observation are received.

- Observers should be present during consultations only if patients have given their express consent, ideally in writing. It should be explained who the observer is and that patients can change their mind at any point without prejudice to their treatment.
- Only those students who are aged 16 or over should be allowed into clinical areas for work observation. It should be made clear to the observers that they will not be able to participate in any clinical work.
- Doctors must emphasise the importance of patient confidentiality to observers before they begin the placement. Doctors retain responsibility for the confidentiality of patients in their care and are therefore responsible for any breaches of confidentiality that occur.
- It is good practice to obtain a signed confidentiality agreement from the observer before the placement goes ahead.
- Work observation should take place outside the observer's immediate locality wherever possible. It would be inappropriate for local observers to sit in on consultations with patients they know.
- The BMA recommends that doctors confirm that work observers are covered in their insurance policy.

Teaching using new technologies

Technological developments have facilitated the use of innovative teaching methods in medical education. For example, the use of live and recorded surgery in the context of teaching and training raises a range of ethical questions. Viewing of real-time surgery by medical audiences is an established practice, but it is now easier than ever to record surgery. Such transmissions and recordings are predominantly used for educational purposes; for example, in its education and training courses, the Royal College of Surgeons of England incorporates footage of surgery recorded live. Recording surgical procedures for educational purposes is valuable, particularly because of the ability to replay and review. The ease of recording, uploading and making such footage universally available does mean, however, that caution must be exercised to ensure that patient confidentiality is respected and valid patient consent is always obtained. Patients should be clear as to whether they will be recognisable from any images captured and this information is a fundamental part of the consent process. Where recordings are broadcast to wider, public audiences, there may be a risk of departing from the purpose of information giving and education, into the realm of sensationalism and entertainment; where recordings are put to an alternative use from that to which the patient originally consented, or where recorded clips are distributed and used out of context, explicit patient consent must be obtained for this alternative use, in line with GMC guidance.[68] (For guidance on the use of audio and visual recordings, see also Chapter 6, pages 247–253.)

Royal College of Surgeons of England and live surgery broadcasts

The Royal College of Surgeons of England (RCS) asserts that when broadcast to an audience of clinicians, the risks of live surgery are outweighed by the educational benefits to such an audience. This established teaching method is directed towards producing better trained surgeons and ultimately improvements in patient safety. The College does not endorse the practice of live surgery broadcasts to public audiences.

> The RCS recommends that, when considering live surgery for the education of clinicians, the three principles listed below should be adhered to in order to ensure the best patient care.
>
> - Professionalism and a fundamental duty of care to the patient must be the sole motivation for all clinical decisions undertaken during live surgery.
> - Assessment, consent and follow up of the patient must pay particular attention to the issues surrounding live transmission of the procedure.
> - The surgeon and surgical team must be willing and prepared to stop interaction with the audience and/or transmission of the operation as necessary.[69]

The 'hidden', 'silent' or 'informal' curriculum

It has long been recognised that students learn not only from their formal teaching, but also from their experiences of observing and working with practising doctors. This aspect of teaching has been referred to as the 'hidden curriculum'.[70] The GMC emphasises that every doctor who comes into contact with medical students should recognise the importance of role models in developing appropriate behaviours towards patients, colleagues and others.[71] Many doctors provide excellent role models and reinforce the lessons and principles that students have learnt throughout their studies. It has been argued, however, that it is in the corridors and cafeteria, and in the methods and manners of their teachers, that medical students absorb a distinctive 'medical morality', a morality that is sometimes at odds with the interests of their patients.[72] The example of how their tutors practice can be a far more powerful influence in the development of ethical, or unethical, practice than the edicts of formal ethics teaching.

This potential for conflict between formal and informal learning underlies the tensions that many medical students, motivated as they are to be 'good doctors', articulate in their response to the teaching of ethics. On the one hand they have strong moral instincts and express considerable interest in ethics, but on the other they aspire to the professionalism and confidence of their senior colleagues, some of whom may seem to pay scant attention to medical ethics in their actual practice. In fact, their senior colleagues may unwittingly give the impression that medical ethics gets in the way of good practice. Anecdotal support for the existence of this tension has been reported to the BMA by its student members, who describe how they learn about ethics in the classrooms of medical schools but sometimes find that some of their senior colleagues appear to ignore ethical and legal precepts.

One possible effect of this tension is the growth of cynicism and the erosion of ethical beliefs and conduct.[73] 'When . . . there is a discrepancy between what students are taught about good ethico-legal practice and what they experience on clinical firms, anger, disillusionment, and cynicism may follow.'[74] Feudtner *et al.* have studied a range of ethical dilemmas faced by medical students in their clinical practice, all of which displayed this tension between the formal and the hidden curricula.[75] When asked why they did not respond when they witnessed unethical behaviour by other, frequently senior, members of medical teams, medical students gave the following reasons:

- wanting to be seen as 'team players'
- concern that if they did not 'toe the line' they would receive negative evaluations from other team members.

The way in which medical students can begin to address this type of situation, given the inevitable imbalance of power, is discussed on pages 762–763. It is essential, however, that all doctors are conscious of the impact of their words and behaviour on those who are learning. In terms of their own practice, as well as their informal role as teachers, doctors should ensure that they always act in accordance with good ethical practice and that they are willing to respond to questions and challenges about their methods and decisions.

The ethical doctor: teaching skills or inculcating virtues?

It has been suggested that part of the response to the problems caused by the 'hidden curriculum' lies in the recognition that ethical principles need to be fully integrated into doctors' professional identities before they can begin to resist unethical practice.[76] Essentially, medical ethics cannot be taught in the same way as science or technical skills, but requires an understanding of the virtues that make a good doctor. Virtue ethics, which is discussed further in the introductory chapter, focuses discussion of medical ethics on the inner moral development of doctors and asks questions about what values doctors have absorbed rather than focusing on the rules and duties that should guide their behaviour and on its consequences. In drawing attention to the centrality of virtues such as caring, concern for others, appreciation of their predicament, a proper sense of humility and the ability to communicate clearly and compassionately with a person while he or she is under a great deal of stress, virtue ethics points to qualities that are 'the heart and soul of good clinical judgment'.[77] Others argue that duty-based, consequence-based and virtue-based approaches to ethics should *all* contribute to medical ethics. It is also argued that apparently irreconcilable distinctions between them can be overcome in practical medical ethics teaching by requiring medical students and doctors to understand widely agreed moral principles and their implications, to consider consequences of their possible actions with a view to optimising those consequences and to integrate these considerations and their outcomes into their habitual attitudes and behaviour.

Creating the necessary distance: professionalism or dehumanisation?

The training and practice of medicine is intellectually and emotionally demanding. An important part of medical training is to help medical students develop the skills required to assist people during some of the most difficult times of their lives, without themselves ceasing to function either as professionals or as human beings.[78] The relative youth and inexperience of the majority of medical students mean that they are frequently unprepared for the experiences of suffering and death they will inevitably encounter.[79] In order to deal with this '[a] kind of emotional hardening has to take place . . . The student must quickly learn ways of coping not only with cadavers, but with the pain, distress, and mutilation associated with serious disease and injury.'[80] A delicate balance is required, however. If the process of 'hardening' is too complete or if too great an emotional distance is established, those who become technically competent may not, in the end, be the best (or even good) doctors. It is during the period of their training, when medical students begin the process of 'detachment', that some of the most important ethical lessons are learnt and habits of feeling towards patients are developed that can persist for a professional lifetime. It is also at this stage that 'the informal curriculum reigns'[81] and the scope for ethical teaching to encourage sensitivity towards patients is at its greatest. Those who teach medical students have a responsibility to show by their words and example that this process of detachment can be achieved without diminishing the respect and dignity due to those who are suffering or who have died. Reports, such as that below, of cadavers being treated merely as objects, reflect outdated attitudes and practices that have no place in the teaching of medical students.

Encountering death

The reality of death is thrust at us as medical students. From the moment we swung through the doors of the dissection room in the first year, we were faced with the immensity of what we will have to cope with during our studies and professional lives... Because we did not and still do not understand death and what it involves, we did not know how to react to the bodies, or deal with the horrific thought that we were cutting up human flesh. During our first session, the anatomy demonstrator casually threw a pile of books down on our group's cadaver, making us flinch: this was the first time that the body was treated as an object in our presence.[82]

Students' experiences of the dissecting room inevitably alter their perceptions of human beings and instil in them the importance of emotional distance. They have been described as the 'first bridge leading us away from the lay public towards the medical world' where patients come to be seen less as people than as 'cases of disease'.[83]

One of the clear and essential contributions that the teaching of ethics and law can have at this point is to demonstrate that the process of detachment is not linear. Medical students move away from lay responses – from squeamishness and fear – in order to return, but to return not to see their patients as elaborate machines that require tinkering with, but as suffering human beings whom, through their professionalism, they can assist.

The healing ethos combines this necessary detachment with a genuine concern for the individual patient, an attitude requiring a degree of empathy and emotional closeness. Only when the medical ethos includes a profound respect for the individuality of each patient will it serve the true purpose of medicine – the health of the patient.[84]

Summary – ethical issues raised in teaching medical students

- Tutors, supervisors and other doctors must ensure that the practice of teaching medical students is undertaken in an ethical manner.
- Medical students should be present during, or involved with, consultations only where appropriate consent has been obtained.
- Medical students should never touch or examine a patient, including those under anaesthetic, without the necessary consent.
- Information should be shared with medical students only with appropriate patient consent.
- All doctors must be aware of students' informal methods of learning by experience and observation; they must always ensure that their behaviour complies with good ethical practice.
- Doctors should always be willing to respond constructively to questions and challenges from medical students about their methods and decisions.

Particular dilemmas of medical students

The question is often raised of whether there are ethical dilemmas that are peculiar to medical students. In order to ensure that this publication addressed the particular needs of medical students, the Medical Ethics Committee asked the BMA Medical Students Committee to draw up a list of common ethical dilemmas faced by medical students. These are listed in the box below.

Ethical dilemmas faced by students

The following are common ethical dilemmas faced by medical students and relevant guidance can be found in this book, as detailed:

- the proper form by which students should be introduced to patients (see page 753)
- patients' consent to student involvement in consultations and treatments (see pages 752–755)
- the sharing of confidential patient information with clinical firms (see pages 755–757)
- inexperience in carrying out procedures (see pages 754–755)
- carrying out intimate examinations on patients while under anaesthetic (see pages 753–754)
- conflicts between medical education and patient care (see pages 752–757)
- witnessing poor practice (see pages 758–759 and pages 762–763)
- how to respond when senior colleagues have impaired judgement (see Chapter 19, page 778 and Chapter 21, pages 878–879)
- physical or verbal assault from patients (see Chapter 1, pages 55–57)
- disclosure from patients that they have been subjected to abuse (see Chapter 5, page 205)
- concealment of mistakes by senior colleagues (see Chapter 1, pages 36–38 and Chapter 21, pages 869–872)
- responding to admissions of criminal behaviour from patients (see Chapter 5, pages 203–204)
- providing medical treatment to family and friends, and medical students treating themselves (see Chapter 1, page 45 and Chapter 21, pages 879–883)
- when questions arise about the competence or behaviour of fellow students (see Chapter 19, page 778 and Chapter 21, pages 878–879)
- students being recruited to take part in the research projects of their teachers (see Chapter 14, page 592)
- conscientious objection to being taught, or involvement in, certain procedures, such as abortion (see Chapter 1, pages 32–33 and Chapter 7, pages 288–289).

Although many of the issues highlighted are similar to those encountered by fully qualified doctors, what is different for medical students is their relationship to those dilemmas and to their professional colleagues. Students do not need to take full responsibility for decision making and should seek the advice of clinical tutors if confronted by some of the situations outlined above. If, for example, patients disclose to a student that they have been subjected to abuse or if they disclose past criminal activity, students should seek advice from a senior colleague or member of the teaching staff who can take the matter forward if necessary.

More difficult are cases where students' concerns relate to the behaviour or performance of a senior colleague or teacher. They often feel unable to speak out, even though they recognise unethical practice, because of the power imbalance in the relationship. Medical students are dependent on their senior colleagues and teachers in order to progress in their medical career; criticising them for practising unethically may seem like a certain path to failure. One medical student, commenting on this power imbalance, said:

[c]linical students walk this ethical tightrope every day – to refuse or object when placed in an unethical situation you have to be brave and tread carefully. It is often the arrogant clinician, with little interest in ethics, who puts the student in this difficult position, and too often it is the same arrogant clinician who grades the student.[85]

The power difference is based on more than just status. There are inevitably and properly very real differences in knowledge and experience, and a respect for this may lead students to question their own perception of poor practice. (For guidance on how to respond to concerns regarding unethical practice, see below.)

Students and tutors: managing inequalities in power

In a profession as complex, demanding and technically refined as medicine, students will always begin their training entirely dependent on the expertise and instruction of tutors and senior colleagues, and it is appropriate that they should defer to them. An inability to take instruction or recognise legitimate authority can be as much of an impediment to becoming a good doctor as obsequiousness and a suppression of critical faculties. Lives may be at stake and the overwhelming majority of senior doctors have arrived at their positions because of their professional excellence, and most students recognise this. Frequently, what is at issue is little more than a disagreement over which of several legitimate approaches is the best. In such cases, it is appropriate that the doctor with overall responsibility for the patient should have the final word, after discussing and considering the views of other members of the team. Students who disobey instructions whenever they feel they have a better idea are likely to harm their patients,[86] but when students have serious concerns that carrying out instructions will significantly compromise patient care, or where the practice they see is seriously at odds with the principles they have been taught, they have a duty to make their concerns known. Initial concerns may be overcome simply by questioning why a particular decision was made, or why one option was chosen over another, and asking the doctor to explain the reasoning behind it. When a satisfactory answer is not received, however, or where there are remaining concerns, further steps may need to be taken despite the huge burden that this can place on the students concerned.

A primary aim of the teaching of medical ethics is to develop within students a questioning, enquiring and analytical mind. This needs to be backed up by a mechanism for students to exercise these qualities without fear of repercussions. It is therefore incumbent upon teaching institutions to devise safe methods for students and staff to discuss such problems as and when they arise, in ways that enhance rather than jeopardise the students' progress. Those involved with teaching students, both in the classroom and on the wards, need to be aware of the impact of their practice on others, and to recognise that, when students raise legitimate concerns or questions, they have a duty to respond.

Questions students should consider if they believe they have witnessed unethical practice

- Is it possible to raise questions about the episode in an enquiring and non-confrontational manner?
- If not, or if this has proved unsatisfactory:
  - are there local protocols for managing problems of this nature?
  - are there personal tutors, mentors or pastoral carers who may be able to advise?
  - are there other senior colleagues who may be able to give advice?
  - would it be useful to discuss the concerns with fellow students to see if they agree?
- If advice on the general ethical issues the dilemma raises is required, would it be helpful to seek independent advice from, for example, the BMA or the GMC?

These problems are not easily resolved, and speaking out can require courage. Singer argues that what is required is a systematic change in the procedures for accountability. Medical schools, he argues, need to develop formal guidelines for ethics in clinical teaching that:

- highlight the responsibility of clinical teaching staff to serve as appropriate role models to medical students and to provide them with an opportunity to discuss ethical challenges
- require university and teaching hospitals to develop processes for reporting ethical concerns
- ensure that medical students and their tutors have access to individuals they can approach with ethical problems
- ensure that when medical students express concern about ethical issues or decline to take part in certain activities for ethical reasons, this will not have any repercussions for them.

Finally, Singer argues that the reporting of ethical problems should model itself upon the 'medical error movement', which seeks to promote a blame-free environment in which errors and difficulties are openly reported and discussed. Instead of apportioning blame, which can lead to evasion and cover up, systematic solutions should be found for the ethical challenges of medical education.[87]

Rights of patients asked to participate in medical education

Students at one medical school developed a policy to underline the rights of patients with capacity who were asked to participate in educational activities that were separate from their clinical care. They argued that, in addition to reminding teachers of their duties as medical educators, such a policy would also help students to question activities they perceived to be unacceptable. The policy included the points listed below.

- Patients must understand that medical students are not qualified doctors.
- Clinical teachers and students must obtain explicit consent from patients before students take their case histories or physically examine them.
- Clinical teachers and students should never perform physical examinations or present cases without the patient's consent.
- Students should never perform any physical examination on a patient who is under general anaesthesia without the patient's prior written consent.
- Clinical teachers should obtain patient consent for students to participate in treatment.
- Students must respect the confidentiality of all information communicated by patients in the course of their treatment or educational activity.
- Patients should understand that students may be obliged to inform a responsible clinician about information relevant to their clinical care.
- Clinical teachers are responsible for ensuring that these guidelines are followed.
- If students are asked by anyone to act contrary to this policy, they must politely refuse, referring to these guidelines.[88]

Medical electives

Medical electives, particularly those undertaken in resource-poor countries, have come under increasing ethical scrutiny in recent years. Such electives can be a rewarding part of an undergraduate medical education, providing valuable opportunities for students to learn about contemporary global health issues, to gain experience of diseases seldom seen in the UK and to develop independence and self-reliance. Resource-poor settings can, however, present medical students with ethical challenges. There can be shortages of highly qualified medical staff and students have reported being asked to undertake procedures that lie beyond their competence, procedures that they would not be permitted to undertake without appropriate supervision in the UK. Additionally, an understanding of what constitutes ethical practice can be subject to cultural variation. In relation to consent and confidentiality, for example, in some cultures, family groups or the heads of families are expected to be much more widely involved in decision making than is the norm in the UK. Gender differences can be more pronounced in certain cultures and some patients may expect to be seen by a doctor of the same gender. More worryingly, there is some evidence to suggest that a small number of students have used electives in order to try to increase their experience by seeking out opportunities to undertake intrusive procedures that they know to be beyond their competence. Such behaviour is clearly unethical and any student acting in such a way risks being reported to their medical school for grossly improper conduct.

Unethical behaviour by a student on a medical elective

In 2009, after receiving a letter from a group of students expressing concern about the behaviour of a student colleague during an elective, the *British Medical Journal* published an analysis of the episode, inviting comment from the GMC, a dean, an ethicist and a lecturer from an African university.[89] The letter referred to a variety of inappropriate activities by the student in question including altering a prescription, photographing patients undergoing invasive procedures without consent and performing an unnecessary lumbar puncture because he 'fancied having a go'. 'The local healthcare professionals', wrote the students, 'sometimes perceived white skin to be synonymous with expertise, placing unprecedented levels of trust in us and allowing us to make decisions and perform procedures that would be unacceptable in the United Kingdom.' As medical students, therefore, they were in a position of considerable responsibility. Although the authors declined to undertake interventions beyond their competence, regarding it as unethical, their colleague viewed it as an opportunity; 'it doesn't matter if we mess up', he was reported as saying, 'no one would know.'

Commenting on the case, there was a general consensus that the students had done as much as they could to tackle grossly unethical behaviour by their colleague. The main points to emerge are listed below.

- Before going on an elective, students should ensure that they have with them contact details of a senior member of their medical school's faculty who can be contacted when problems arise that cannot be resolved locally.
- Although moral relativism can be attractive overseas, respect for human dignity, trust and vulnerability must always be at the centre of medical practice.
- Students and doctors have a professional duty to work within the limits of their competence.

Successful electives: planning in advance

The BMA provides guidance for medical students on both the practical[90] and the ethical[91] aspects of medical electives. Advance planning is a key part of any successful elective. Students need to give consideration to ensuring that, as far as possible, their elective provides an overall benefit to the host country. It is important therefore that students consider factors such as whether they can speak the language of the host country or whether translators may be needed, therefore imposing greater burdens on a health system already restricted in its resources. It is also essential that students find out in advance about the main features of the health system in which they will be working and any significant cultural differences that might impact on the provision of healthcare.

Medical emergencies

The case of unethical behaviour on a medical elective, detailed above, clearly demonstrates that students are under an obligation to work within their competence. There may be circumstances, however, such as in an emergency, when students might be called upon, or might feel that they are obliged, to intervene beyond their ordinary levels of competence. Ethical dilemmas arising as a result of an emergency are clearly not restricted to medical students working overseas – they can arise anywhere. In emergencies and where there are no qualified staff available, students need to act carefully. Where there is a reasonable likelihood that an intervention in an emergency can prevent or mitigate serious harm to a patient, it can be appropriate to assist. In resource-poor settings, situations may routinely occur that would be regarded as emergencies in more developed countries. It is important to stress that students must avoid getting involved in providing routine care that is outside their level of competence. In all other cases where students believe that they are being asked to act beyond their clinical competence, they should politely but firmly decline. (Acting within the limits of competence is also discussed in Chapter 15, pages 642–643.)

Summary – particular dilemmas of medical students

- Many of the dilemmas that arise for medical students are the same as those experienced by fully qualified doctors, although their relationship to such dilemmas is different.
- Students do not need to take full responsibility for decision making and should seek the advice of clinical tutors if confronted by ethical dilemmas involving patients or patient care.
- Difficulties can arise when medical students have concerns about the behaviour or performance of a senior colleague or tutor; these are exacerbated by the imbalance of power within the relationship.
- Medical students who have concerns that carrying out instructions will compromise patient care, or who witness practice that is seriously at odds with the principles they have been taught, have a duty to make their concerns known.
- Those involved with teaching students, both in the classroom and on clinical placements, need to be aware of the impact of their practice on others and to recognise that, when students raise legitimate concerns or questions, they have a duty to respond constructively.
- Teaching institutions have a responsibility to establish mechanisms for students to raise ethical concerns about aspects of their training without fear of repercussions.
- Students undertaking medical electives in resource-poor countries must be aware of their professional duty to work within the limits of their competence. They should plan ahead for their elective and consider in advance the ethical challenges they might face.

The teaching of ethics and the ethics of teaching

Ethics and law training provide a framework, and the skills and awareness, that can help doctors to maintain intellectual independence and to keep sight of accepted moral norms in the face of contrary pressures. One of the objectives of training in ethics is to assist doctors to look beyond the immediate system within which they work and, through analytical reasoning, help them to assess whether the treatment of the patients they see corresponds with professional obligations, public expectations and widely accepted standards. Raising awareness about duties and rights can make a significant difference only if this is accompanied by other practical measures that allow theory to be implemented in daily practice.

Doctors and tutors have a responsibility not only to teach medical ethics but also to teach medicine in an ethical manner. This involves, for example, ensuring that patients have given consent to the presence of, or examination by, students and showing, by example, the respect and dignity owed to patients both during life and after death. Medical students and junior doctors, however, sometimes report discrepancies between the ethical standards they are taught formally and the practices of senior colleagues and teachers. This 'hidden curriculum' needs to be recognised and used to emphasise the role of qualified doctors in the teaching of tomorrow's doctors. Students are taught to have enquiring minds and to challenge unethical practices; those who are responsible for teaching them have a duty to allow them to do so without jeopardising their future careers.

References

1 Department of Health (2010) *Liberating the NHS: Developing the Healthcare Workforce*, DH, London.
2 General Medical Council (2009) *Tomorrow's Doctors: Outcomes and standards for undergraduate medical education*, GMC, London.
3 General Medical Council (2009) *Tomorrow's Doctors: Outcomes and standards for undergraduate medical education*, GMC, London, para 20.
4 General Medical Council (2009) *Tomorrow's Doctors: Outcomes and standards for undergraduate medical education*, GMC, London, para 20(a).
5 General Medical Council (1993) *Tomorrow's doctors: recommendations on undergraduate medical education*, GMC, London, p.5, para 11.
6 General Medical Council (2006), *Good Medical Practice*, GMC, London.
7 General Medical Council (2009) *Tomorrow's Doctors: Outcomes and standards for undergraduate medical education*, GMC, London, para 7.
8 General Medical Council, Postgraduate Medical Education and Training Board (2010) *Final Report of the Education and Training Regulation Policy Review: Recommendations and Options for the Future Regulation of Education and Training*, GMC and PMETB, London.
9 British Medical Association (1995) *Report of the working party on medical education*, BMA, London, p.1.
10 British Medical Association (1995) *Report of the working party on medical education*, BMA, London.
11 See the BMA website at www.bma.org.uk (accessed 7 March 2011) for updates on the work of the Medical Students Committee in relation to this policy.
12 British Medical Association (1999) *Selecting our doctors: A report of a BMA conference on selection for medical school*, BMA, London, p.2.
13 Medical Schools Council (2010) *Guiding principles for the admission of medical students*, MSC, London.
14 General Medical Council (2009) *Tomorrow's Doctors: Outcomes and standards for undergraduate medical education*, GMC, London, para 73.
15 The Panel on Fair Access to the Professions (2009) *Unleashing Aspiration: The Final Report of the Panel on Fair Access to the Professions*, The Panel on Fair Access to the Professions, London, p.49.
16 British Medical Association (2009) *Equality and diversity in UK medical schools*, BMA, London, pp.7–8.
17 General Medical Council (2009) *Tomorrow's Doctors: Outcomes and standards for undergraduate medical education*, GMC, London, para 57.
18 For an overview, see: Preston-Shoot M, McKimm J. (2010) *Teaching, Learning and Assessment of Law in Medical Education: Special Report 11*, The Higher Education Academy, Newcastle.
19 Pond D. (1987) *Report of a working party on the teaching of medical ethics*, Institute of Medical Ethics, London.
20 Consensus statement by teachers of medical ethics and law in UK medical schools (1998) Teaching medical ethics and law within medical education: a model for the UK core curriculum. *J Med Ethics* **24**, 188–92, p.188.
21 Mattick K, Bligh J. (2006) Teaching and assessing medical ethics: where are we now? *J Med Ethics* **32**, 181–5.

22 Institute of Medical Ethics (2006) *Conference on Learning, Teaching and Assessing Medical Ethics, BMA House, London, Wednesday 29 March 2006, Draft Report on the Proceedings*. Available at: www.instituteofmedicalethics.org (accessed 10 March 2011).

23 Institute of Medical Ethics (2008) *Conference on Supporting the Integrated Teaching, Learning and Assessment of Medical Ethics and Law in UK Medical Schools, BMA House, Friday 25 January 2008*. Available at: www.instituteofmedicalethics.org (accessed 10 March 2011).

24 Stirrat GM, Johnston C, Gillon R. *et al.* (2010) Medical ethics and law for doctors of tomorrow: the 1998 Consensus Statement updated. *J Med Ethics* **36**, 55–60.

25 Thanks to Dr Laura Bowater and Dr Mark Wilkinson for providing details and references for this case study.

26 Glasziou P, Chalmers I. (2004) Ethics review roulette: what can we learn? *BMJ* **328**, 121–2. Henderson M. (2007) Constant policing of our research makes us look sinister, say scientists. *The Times* (25 October). Available at: www.timesonline.co.uk (accessed 30 March 2011).

27 Tan SP. (2004) My disappointment with an ethics committee. *BMJ* **329**, 807.

28 McGee R, Almquist J, Keller JL. *et al.* (2008) Teaching and learning responsible research conduct: influences of prior experiences on acceptance of new ideas. *Accountability in Research* **15**, 30–62.

29 For further discussion of the importance of communication skills, see: British Medical Association (2011) *The psychological and social needs of patients*, BMA, London, pp. 5–8. British Medical Association (2004) *Communication skills education for doctors: an update*, BMA, London.

30 General Medical Council (2009) *Tomorrow's Doctors: Outcomes and standards for undergraduate medical education*, GMC, London, para 20.

31 Rennie SC, Rudland JR. (2003) Differences in medical students' attitudes to academic misconduct and reported behaviour across the years: a questionnaire study. *J Med Ethics* **29**, 97–102.

32 British Medical Association (2011) *Using social media: practical and ethical guidance for doctors and medical students*, BMA, London.

33 General Medical Council (2009) *Tomorrow's Doctors: Outcomes and standards for undergraduate medical education*, GMC, London, para 28.

34 General Medical Council, Medical Schools Council (2009) *Medical students: professional values and fitness to practise*, GMC, London, para 3.

35 Reid A. (2010) Identifying medical students at risk of subsequent misconduct. *BMJ* **340**, 1041–2.

36 Yates J, James D. (2010) Risk factors at medical school for subsequent professional misconduct: multicentre retrospective case–control study. *BMJ* **340**, 1073.

37 Stirrat GM, Johnston C, Gillon R. *et al.* (2010) Medical ethics and law for doctors of tomorrow: the 1998 Consensus Statement updated. *J Med Ethics* **36**, 55–60.

38 Stirrat GM, Johnston C, Gillon R. *et al.* (2010) Medical ethics and law for doctors of tomorrow: the 1998 Consensus Statement updated. *J Med Ethics* **36**, 55–60, pp.57–8.

39 Stirrat GM, Johnston C, Gillon R. *et al.* (2010) Medical ethics and law for doctors of tomorrow: the 1998 Consensus Statement updated. *J Med Ethics* **36**, 55–60, p.59.

40 Sritharan K, Russell G, Fritz Z. *et al.* (2001) Medical oaths and declarations: a declaration marks an explicit commitment to ethical behaviour. *BMJ* **323**, 1440–1.

41 See, for example: Gillon R. (2000) White coat ceremonies for new medical students. *J Med Ethics* **26**, 83–4. Veatch RM. (2002) White coat ceremonies: a second opinion. *J Med Ethics* **28**, 5–6. Gillon R. (2002) Commentary: In defence of medical commitment ceremonies. *J Med Ethics* **28**, 7–9. Huber SJ. (2003) The white coat ceremony: a contemporary medical ritual. *J Med Ethics* **29**, 364–6. Glick SM. (2003) White coat ceremonies: another commentary. *J Med Ethics* **29**, 367–8.

42 For further information, see: www.gmc-uk.org (accessed 10 March 2011).

43 See the BMA website: www.bma.org.uk (accessed 10 March 2011) for further information on professional ethics training for doctors new to the UK, provided by the BMA.

44 Slowther A, Lewando Hundt G, Taylor R. *et al.* (2009) *Non UK qualified doctors and Good Medical Practice: The experience of working within a different professional framework*, University of Warwick, Warwick.

45 General Medical Council (2006) *Good Medical Practice*, GMC, London, para 12.

46 See: www.bma.org.uk (accessed 10 March 2011).

47 British Medical Association (2009) *Consent tool kit*, BMA, London.

48 British Medical Association (2010) *Doctors new to practice: an ethical survival kit*, BMA, London. Further ethical guidance is available at: www.bma.org.uk (accessed 10 March 2011).

49 The Bristol Royal Infirmary Inquiry (2001) *The Report of the Public Inquiry into children's heart surgery at the Bristol Royal Infirmary 1984–1995: Learning from Bristol*, The Stationery Office, London, p.446, recommendation 76.

50 This is discussed in several chapters of: British Medical Association (2001) *The medical profession and human rights: handbook for a changing agenda*, Zed Books, London.

51 For further information, see the Medsin website: www.medsin.org (accessed 10 March 2011).

52 Medact (2001) *Global health studies: Proposals for medical and nursing undergraduate teaching*, Medact, London.

53 General Medical Council (2009) *Tomorrow's Doctors: Outcomes and standards for undergraduate medical education*, GMC, London, paras 20–1.

54 See, for example, the journal *Medical Humanities*. Available at: www.mh.bmj.com (accessed 10 March 2011).

55 Goodwin J. (1997) Chaos, and the Limits of Modern Medicine. *JAMA* **278**, 1399–400, p.1399.

56 General Medical Council (2011) *Clinical placements for medical students: Advice supplementary to Tomorrow's Doctors (2009)*, GMC, London. General Medical Council (2011) *Assessment in undergraduate medical education: Advice supplementary to Tomorrow's Doctors (2009)*, GMC, London. At the time of writing, the GMC was due to publish further advice supplementary to *Tomorrow's Doctors*, focusing on 'developing teachers and trainers' and 'involving patients and the public'. See the GMC website at: www.gmc-uk.org (accessed 10 March 2011) for all new publications.

57 The GMC has developed an interactive website for medical students, *Medical students: Professional values in action*. Available at www.gmc-uk.org (accessed 7 March 2011). Users can test their knowledge of the guidance and principles in *Tomorrow's Doctors* through a series of case studies and other activities. Also available via the GMC website is *Good Medical Practice in Action*, which uses interactive scenarios to allow the user to follow a patient journey and choose what the doctor should do at crucial points in the process, and case studies on topics such as confidentiality and end of life care.

58 General Medical Council (2009) *Tomorrow's Doctors: Outcomes and standards for undergraduate medical education*, GMC, London, para 108.

59 General Medical Council, Medical Schools Council (2009) *Medical students: professional values and fitness to practise*, GMC, London, para 16(b).

60 Hicks LK, Lin Y, Robertson DW. *et al.* (2001) Understanding the clinical dilemmas that shape medical students' ethical development: questionnaire survey and focus group study. *BMJ* **322**, 709–10. Coldicott Y, Pope C, Roberts C. (2003) The ethics of intimate examinations: teaching tomorrow's doctors. *BMJ* **326**, 97–101.

61 Royal College of Obstetricians and Gynaecologists (2002) *Gynaecological Examinations: Guidelines for Specialist Practice*, RCOG, London, pp.18–9.

62 Department of Health (2009) *Reference guide to consent for examination or treatment*, 2nd edn. DH, London, p.12. See also: Welsh Assembly Government (2009) *Reference Guide for Consent to Examination or Treatment*, WAG, Cardiff, p.13. Department of Health, Social Services and Public Safety (2003) *Reference Guide to Consent for Examination, Treatment or Care*, DHSSPS, Belfast, pp.5–6.

63 General Medical Council, Medical Schools Council (2009) *Medical students: professional values and fitness to practise*, GMC, London, para 16(a).

64 General Medical Council (2009) *Tomorrow's Doctors: Outcomes and standards for undergraduate medical education*, GMC, London, para 6(b)–(c).

65 General Medical Council (2009) *Confidentiality: disclosing information for education and training purposes*, GMC, London, para 10.

66 General Medical Council (2009) *Confidentiality: disclosing information for education and training purposes*, GMC, London.

67 British Medical Association (2008) *Junior doctors' handbook*, BMA, London, pp.76–7.

68 General Medical Council (2011) *Making and using visual and audio recordings of patients*, GMC, London.

69 Royal College of Surgeons of England (2010) *Live Surgery Broadcasts policy statement, September 2010*, RCS, London.

70 Harden RM. (2005) Curriculum planning and development. In: Dent JA, Harden RM. (eds.) *A practical guide for medical teachers*, 2nd edn, Elsevier Churchill Livingstone, London, p.12. Rhodes R, Cohen DS. (2003) Understanding, being, and doing: medical ethics in medical education. *Camb Q Healthc Ethics* **12**, 39–53. Hafferty FW, Franks R. (1994) The hidden curriculum, ethics teaching, and the structure of medical education. *Acad Med* **69**, 861–71.

71 General Medical Council (2009) *Tomorrow's Doctors: Outcomes and standards for undergraduate medical education*, GMC, London, para 149.

72 Hafferty FW, Franks R. (1994) The hidden curriculum, ethics teaching, and the structure of medical education. *Acad Med* **69**, 861–71.

73 Yamey G, Roach JO. (2001) Witnessing unethical conduct: the effects. *Student BMJ* **9**, 2–3.

74 Doyal L. (2001) Closing the gap between professional teaching and practice. *BMJ* **322**, 685–6, p.685.

75 Feudtner C, Christakis DA, Christakis NA. (1994) Do clinical clerks suffer ethical erosion? students' perceptions of their ethical environment and personal development. *Acad Med* **69**, 670–9.

76 Hafferty FW, Franks R. (1994) The hidden curriculum, ethics teaching, and the structure of medical education. *Acad Med* **69**, 861–71.

77 Campbell A, Gillett G, Jones G. (2005) *Medical ethics*, 4th edn, OUP, Oxford, p.9.

78 Campbell A, Gillett G, Jones G. (2005) *Medical ethics*, 4th edn, OUP, Oxford, p.20.

79 Doyal L. (2001) Closing the gap between professional teaching and practice. *BMJ* **322**, 685–6.

80 Campbell A, Gillett G, Jones G. (2005) *Medical ethics*, 4th edn, OUP, Oxford, p.20.

81 Singer PA. (2003) Intimate examinations and other ethical challenges in medical education: medical schools should develop effective guidelines and implement them. *BMJ* **326**, 62–3, p.63.

82 Finlay SE, Fawzy M. (2001) Becoming a doctor. *Medical Humanities* **27**, 90–2, p.91.

83 Finlay SE, Fawzy M. (2001) Becoming a doctor. *Medical Humanities* **27**, 90–2, p.91.

84 Campbell A, Gillett G, Jones G. (2005) *Medical ethics*, 4th edn, OUP, Oxford, p.20.

85 Woodall A. (2001) Should I do what they say to secure that grade A? *Student BMJ* **9**, 169.

86 Trotter G. (2001) Commentary: Hierarchy and the dynamics of rank. In: Kushner TK, Thomasma DC. (eds.) *Ward ethics: Dilemmas for medical students and doctors in training.* CUP, Cambridge, p.191.

87 Singer PA. (2003) Intimate examinations and other ethical challenges in medical education: medical schools should develop effective guidelines and implement them. *BMJ* **326**, 62–3, p.63.

88 Doyal L. (2001) Closing the gap between professional teaching and practice. *BMJ* **322**, 685–6, p.685.

89 Cohen J, Bowman D, Trowell J. *et al.* (2009) What should you do when you see a fellow student behaving inappropriately? *BMJ* **338**, 204–7.

90 British Medical Association (2009) *Electives for medical students*, BMA, London. For further planning resources and information, see: British Medical Association. *Electives for medical students*. Available at: www.bma.org.uk (accessed 11 March 2011).

91 British Medical Association (2009) *Ethics and medical electives in resource-poor countries: A Tool Kit*, BMA, London.

19: Teamwork, shared care, referral and delegation

The questions covered in this chapter include the following.

- What are the responsibilities of doctors who lead multi-disciplinary teams?
- How should personal health data be made available within teams and to other professionals?
- Is there a different degree of accountability for doctors who refer or delegate treatments to a non-regulated therapist?
- Can patients switch between the care of NHS and private practitioners?

Healthcare is increasingly provided by multi-disciplinary teams, in which collaborative teamwork is highly valued and good communication is vital. This chapter focuses on how doctors work with each other and with other professionals. It covers inter-agency liaison, including cooperation between health and social services, and liaison with alternative and complementary therapy practitioners. It discusses how some patients combine private care with NHS treatment or seek treatment abroad. Also, as the UK develops more public–private partnerships, patient care needs to be well coordinated between public and private healthcare providers, as well as across traditional professional boundaries. Delegation of duties and issues such as who should be ultimately responsible for different facets of care are discussed, as is the role of doctors as managers.

General principles

- In multi-disciplinary care, particular emphasis is given to the need to communicate effectively and ensure that all care is patient-focused. The interests and safety of patients are the primary concerns.
- Consistency is vital when care is shared; consistency both in terms of the clinical activities undertaken and of the information provided to colleagues and patients so that mixed messages are avoided.
- Clear communication is also needed between health and social care professionals. Good coordination of a wide range of services is particularly important for patients who have multiple health and social care needs.
- Patients need to know how widely their personal health information is shared among the different professionals involved in their care.
- Staff working together should respect the autonomy and skills of colleagues and try to ensure that the best use is made of the range of skills and expertise available.
- Delegation of tasks is an important facet of multi-disciplinary care but it should be clear who has ultimate responsibility for each aspect of care.

Medical Ethics Today: The BMA's Handbook of Ethics and Law, Third Edition. Sophie Brannan, Eleanor Chrispin, Martin Davies, Veronica English, Rebecca Mussell, Julian Sheather and Ann Sommerville.
© 2012 BMA Medical Ethics Department. Published 2012 by Blackwell Publishing Ltd.

Working in multi-disciplinary teams

Constructive teamwork

Multi-disciplinary working is commonplace but effective team work does not automatically follow from groups of professionals working together. Teamwork is defined as coordinated action, carried out by two or more individuals jointly, concurrently or sequentially. It implies commonly agreed goals, an awareness of others' roles, supportive cooperative relationships, mutual trust, effective leadership and good communication.[1] It also requires adequate staffing and material resources to achieve the agreed objectives and mechanisms for evaluating and improving the services provided. Mutual respect and commitment to shared goals are essential to ensure that individuals work 'together' rather than simply 'alongside' each other.

Disagreement or conflict within teams can be minimised by effective communication, sharing of information (with due regard to confidentiality), constructive discussion and acknowledgement of the skills, expertise and opinions of other professionals.

Principles for teamwork

- Good communication and mutual respect are key. It should always be made clear who in the team is responsible for passing on information necessary for patient care to others providing it.
- All shared policies and aims should be clear to all team members.
- It should be clear who is ultimately accountable for decision making but there should be opportunities for all team members to contribute their knowledge and expertise.
- All team members have a responsibility for ensuring the team's effective functioning.
- Team members should be supported in their role. They should not be expected to take on tasks beyond their experience and competence but part of their learning experience may involve stretching themselves. This should only be done with appropriate supervision.

The General Medical Council (GMC) highlights the importance of team working emphasising that, in providing a good standard of care, doctors need to interact constructively with other care providers. They 'must act as partners to their colleagues, accepting shared accountability for the service provided to patients. They are expected to offer leadership, and to work with others to change systems when it is necessary for the benefit of patients.'[2] The GMC also stresses that doctors must recognise their own limitations, and be willing to consult colleagues and keep them well informed when sharing the care of patients.[3]

In 2006, the GMC published guidance[4] aimed particularly at doctors in management but which also set out some general duties for all doctors about how they work with others, regardless of their specific role. It began to update this advice in 2011 and published a consultation as a first step.[5] This suggested separating much more distinctly the duties of every doctor and those of doctors who have an additional management responsibilities, while recognising that there would continue to be overlap between the two in terms of their moral obligations. The aim was to emphasise that all doctors should continue to make care of patients their first concern while trying to ensure that resources are used most effectively and appropriately. Those in a management role clearly have enhanced obligations and responsibilities for resource allocation, leadership, team management and overseeing the provision of good quality services. Doctors who have a managerial role also have responsibility for the welfare and safety of patients, even when their contractual duties are non-clinical. They remain accountable to the GMC for their decisions and actions even when the role they fulfil could be done by a non-doctor. At a time of financial stringency, the GMC draft also recognised that all doctors would potentially have more conflicts of interest and face difficult decisions about doing the best for individual patients while working within resource constraints.[6] It noted that some significant changes proposed by the Government in the organisation of the NHS would, if implemented, increase many doctors' managerial responsibilities. The GMC consultation was issued when there was considerable debate about proposals in the Health and Social Care Bill intended, among other things, to change the role of GPs in England in relation to commissioning services. However, it was unclear if these proposed changes would be implemented or modified and the GMC, in its draft advice, provided general principles about the planning, use and management of resources, which are likely to be the same regardless of doctors' roles or where they work in the UK. As a basic principle, it said that all doctors working in an organisation should be prepared to contribute to discussions about resource allocation, priority setting and the commissioning of services.[7]

Doctors working in teams are generally expected to act as a positive role model and to try to motivate colleagues. In its consultation exercise in 2011, the GMC said that all doctors have a responsibility to show 'leadership', whether or not they have a formal role as leader or manager, but it also clarified that leadership does not necessarily mean taking charge of the situation but rather exercising the joint responsibility that all team members have for identifying and solving problems.[8]

Teamwork in primary care

Effective teamwork is crucial in general practice, as in hospital care. As well as providing diagnostic and treatment services, primary care teams have the main responsibility for maintaining patient records, arranging referrals and keeping an overview of care arrangements. They implement vaccination programmes and preventive measures to avoid ill health, coordinate screening programmes and initiatives to encourage patients to adopt healthy habits. In addition to their healthcare role, primary care professionals participate in many social tasks on patients' behalf, such as providing reports for employers, insurers, housing and benefits agencies, certifying fitness to drive or providing reports for people wanting to adopt children, or act as child minders. The wider care team includes district nurses, health visitors and midwives. It may also include specialist nurses, physiotherapists, counsellors, pharmacists and complementary therapists. Nurse practitioners provide various forms of advice and treatment and specialised nurses such as Macmillan nurses work with the primary care team in the community. All these perspectives are important in providing appropriate care to patients and good communication between the care providers is essential. Making the best use of the skills and experience available is part of the rationale for team working. When it works well, it can greatly improve the quality of care for patients and increase their satisfaction.

In addition to other professionals who form part of the primary care team, integrated care also requires good liaison between pharmacists and doctors. The involvement of pharmacists can improve patient care and manage demand, when, for example, patients consult pharmacists rather than their GP for self-limiting illnesses. Pharmacists can also support patients to look after themselves by providing advice on over-the-counter medication and provide advice to patients with complex conditions requiring a number of different medications.

In 2010, the Government proposed that GP-led consortia take a major role in commissioning services within the NHS in England.[9] Some practices already do so and face potential challenges in terms of conflicts of interest. (Referral management and commissioning of services are covered briefly on pages 789–792 and for more information, see the British Medical Association (BMA) website.) Some primary care teams also engage with a very wide range of agencies which are responsible for specific aspects of their patients' physical and psychological welfare, either in hospitals or in the community. This may extend beyond the provision of traditional concepts of health and social care to encompass the provision of support or training in a number of practical areas. Various models have been developed to reflect such involvement with a range of voluntary and professional agencies, across the wider community and one is described below.

The Bromley by Bow model

The Bromley by Bow Centre was established in 1984 through the work of Reverend Andrew Mawson, later Lord Mawson, in Tower Hamlets, East London, one of the UK's most deprived areas. Initially, he offered the church facilities to the local, culturally diverse community which had high unemployment, low incomes, poor health outcomes and overcrowded, substandard housing. The health facilities were added in 1997 and pioneered an outreach model of community development. The health staff aim to encourage a healthy lifestyle in the broadest sense and work with commercial organisations in the area to provide facilities for exercise, leisure and food shopping. The goal is to improve the community's physical and psychological health, not least by helping people to gain practical skills to find work and develop their potential. It represents a model of community regeneration, containing three key elements: accessibility, the provision of integrated services and the creation of progression pathways. Its services are easy to access and facilitate patient involvement, with locally recruited staff who understand the community. The range of services is unusually broad, involving partnerships with other organisations which offer advice, support and training, including in the arts to build self-esteem and help people express their creativity. The Centre also offers its experience to help transform other deprived communities.

Teamwork in secondary care

In addition to qualified professionals in hospital teams, some NHS trusts are teaching hospitals with links to medical schools. Medical students may be part of the team looking after a patient but it is important that patients' views are sought in advance to ensure that they are aware that students may be involved in their care. Patients should have a choice about whether they are willing to participate in bedside presenting with students, for example, and whether they agree to students having access to their health information. (Patient consent as well as some of the dilemmas faced by medical students in such situations are covered in Chapter 18.)

Leading teams

A large and specialised literature exists on leadership and management in healthcare. The two roles are not necessarily the same, as all doctors are deemed to have leadership responsibilities although they may not have a management role. Various organisations such as the NHS Institute for Innovation and Improvement and the National Leadership and Innovations Agency for Healthcare (Wales) provide codes of practice, guidance and training. In this chapter, we only seek to highlight some key points. In order to ensure patient safety and quality of care, team leaders need to check that communication within the team is consistently effective and that responsibilities are clear to everyone. Patients, as well as colleagues, need to understand who is responsible for each facet of care.

The GMC has said that when leading a team:

. . . you should:

- respect the skills and contributions of your colleagues; you must not make unfounded criticisms of colleagues, which can undermine patients' trust in the care provided
- make sure that colleagues understand the professional status and specialty of all team members, their roles and responsibilities in the team, and who is responsible for each aspect of patient care
- make sure that staff are clear about their individual and team objectives, their personal and collective responsibilities for patient and public safety, and for openly and honestly recording and discussing problems
- communicate effectively with colleagues within and outside the team; you should make sure that that arrangements are in place for relevant information to be passed on to the team promptly
- make sure that all team members have an opportunity to contribute to discussions and that they understand and accept the decisions taken
- encourage team members to co-operate and communicate effectively with each other
- make sure that each patient's care is properly co-ordinated and managed, and that patients are given information about whom to contact if they have questions or concerns; this is particularly important when patient care is shared between teams
- set up and maintain systems to identify and manage risks in the team's area of responsibility
- monitor and regularly review the team's performance and take steps to correct deficiencies and improve quality
- deal openly and supportively with problems in the conduct, performance or health of team members through effective and well-publicised procedures
- make sure that your team and the organisation have the opportunity to learn from mistakes.[10]

Within multi-disciplinary teams, all members have responsibility for ensuring the proper functioning of the team but the team leader is ultimately accountable for making certain that the patient's care is properly coordinated and managed. The leader is often, but not always, a doctor. It could be a social worker, a community psychiatric nurse or a health visitor if care is carried out primarily in the community, with the GP as one member of the broader team. Such teams may also include specialists in palliative care, mental health, and optical and dental services. In hospitals, the consultant in charge of the patient's care is assumed to be the team leader unless otherwise designated. Team leaders should ensure that, in difficult ethical situations (as well as in complex clinical scenarios), less experienced staff are not expected to make critical decisions without formal and comprehensive input from a senior colleague. All members of the team have a duty to take steps to avoid errors that could put patients at risk, audit their own professional practice, raise problems for discussion and draw attention to bad practice. Team members who have concerns over the professional practice of a colleague from another profession should bring these to the attention of the leader of that professional group.

Doctors as managers

When doctors have a management role, they still have a duty of care for patients and are accountable to the GMC. They must make the care and safety of patients their first concern and take responsibility for their own work and the performance of the people they manage. They should work with others to create an environment in which individuals can perform well and cooperate in group goals.[11] In addition, they should ensure that systems are in place to investigate complaints promptly, fairly and thoroughly. When they are managers of their own companies, they generally have more control over how the organisation works and should make sure that the GMC's guidance is followed. The GMC's guidance for doctors as managers says that they should do their best

[t]o ensure that:

- systems are in place to enable high quality medical services to be provided
- care is provided and supervised only by staff who have the appropriate skills (including communication skills), experience, training and qualifications
- significant risks to patients, staff and the health of the wider community are identified, assessed and addressed to minimise risk, and that they are reported in line with local and national procedures
- the people you manage (both doctors and other professionals) are aware of and follow the guidance issued by relevant professional and regulatory bodies, and that they are able to fulfil their professional duties so that standards of practice and care are maintained and improved
- systems are in place to identify the educational and training needs of students and staff, including locums, so that the best use is made of the time and resources available for keeping knowledge and skills up to date
- all decisions, working practices and the working environment are lawful, with particular regard to the law on employment, equal opportunities and health and safety
- information and policies on clinical effectiveness and clinical governance are publicised and implemented effectively.[12]

In 2011, when the GMC consulted widely on updating its guidance for managers, it echoed very similar principles to those above from its previous publication but also highlighted managers' responsibilities in terms of:

- staff recruitment based on fair and transparent criteria
- the provision of appropriate training for themselves and others responsible for recruitment
- awareness of equality, diversity and non-discrimination in employment matters
- the importance of providing induction and mentoring, especially for doctors who are new to practice or who trained outside the UK
- their own willingness to take on and fulfil properly a mentoring role, with clear objectives, advice and support.[13]

Example of poor management and teamwork

Dr X appointed matrons to run a nursing home which she owned, and for which she acted as Director. The matrons were designated as 'the person in charge' of day-to-day care in accordance with the accepted guidance but were unable to carry out that role because Dr X constantly interfered with their decisions and did not permit them to use their skills and experience. She did not allow them to assess new patients prior to admission, so that a patient with learning difficulties was inappropriately accepted into the home by Dr X, contrary to the terms of the nursing home licence. A good level of care could not be provided for the patient who was left in a urine-soaked bed where he was unable to reach his food or water. No steps were taken to maintain his nutrition and hydration and he eventually had to be admitted to hospital where he died of range of serious ailments including hypothermia, septicaemia and lung infection. Dr X took over the recruiting of staff, excluding the matrons who would normally have done this, but she failed to employ enough staff to provide nursing care, cleaning and kitchen work. Staff had to do jobs outside their normal duties and there was a very high staff turn over, particularly of nurses. She did not check that people she recruited were suitable for the job, nor did she consider the skill mix that was needed and, having employed some applicants with no previous experience, Dr X did not provide any training or induction. References were not taken up and no effort was made to check that nurses were registered with the Nursing and Midwifery Council. Dr X rationed supplies so that there was inadequate food of acceptable quality for the residents and she instructed staff to re-use incontinence pads. She did not arrange any alternative cover when the matron was absent, so that effectively there was no appropriate person in charge. Some patients received seriously inadequate care, resulting in deep sores or septicaemia. While not providing clinical care herself to the nursing home residents, Dr X undermined the authority of the local GPs who did, by interfering with the decisions they had made. The GMC found Dr X guilty of misconduct, in that her actions fell far short of what was proper in the circumstances.[14]

Doctors in management roles generally have responsibilities to the wider community, the organisation in which they work and their colleagues, as well as to patients. Balancing these different obligations in an ethical manner is a crucial element of their job. The BMA has published specific practical advice for doctors who work as medical directors or as part of a management team.[15] A range of other guidance and training is also available. For example, the Medical Leadership Competency Framework (MLCF)[16] was jointly developed by the Academy of Medical Royal Colleges and the NHS Institute for Innovation and Improvement in conjunction with other stakeholders. The Framework describes the leadership competencies doctors need in order to become more actively involved in the planning, delivery and transformation of health services.

Keeping team support and developing a shared vision with colleagues are seen as key skills for medical managers. Providing leadership, encouraging good communication, demonstrating strategic thinking and enabling improvement are also part of the manager's role. In addition, medical managers have to ensure that agreed services can be delivered within resource constraints. This involves setting objectives that ensure the most effective deployment of resources, consistent with the provision of services to a high standard. Medical managers may also bear the responsibility for promoting the development of information systems for audit and risk management, as well as for patient care. (Risk management and clinical governance are discussed in Chapters 21. Audit and information management are discussed in Chapters 5 and 6.)

Pressures on managers: meeting targets

All doctors have to think about the effective use of resources but this can be a particular area of conflict for doctors who act as managers, where the needs of individual patients and the needs of a population may come into starker conflict. They may also have to make difficult choices between meeting targets so that patients are treated as promptly as possible, and focusing more on providing a high quality of care. Obviously, both aspects should be in balance and strategies, such as partnership programmes which provide interventions earlier and in a community setting, can combine a high level of patient satisfaction with an effective use of resources. It is a fundamental principle of the NHS that the order in which patients are treated should be determined by their clinical priority so that those in greatest need are generally treated first. Resource allocation is an inevitable part of health service management and difficult decisions must be made. Doctors should ensure that their decisions are equitable, supported by sound evidence from research and clinical audit, and can be justified. They should also take account of the priorities set by the government and the NHS, but any pressure, whether explicit or implied, for example to adjust NHS waiting lists inappropriately to meet waiting list targets, must be resisted. Patients should always be prioritised in the first instance according to clinical need, not in order to meet externally imposed targets.

Whistleblowing

In their role as managers, doctors must ensure that measures are in place to identify poor practice or unacceptable behaviour, such as bullying of staff, unfair discrimination and racism. The BMA has published specific advice about whistleblowing in NHS secondary care, which includes the importance of ensuring that staff are not victimised for raising concerns.[17] This also provides advice for doctors in the armed forces who should raise their concerns according to the chain of command. (This is also discussed in Chapter 16.) The steps that should be followed are those set out in the Public Interest Disclosure Act 1998 which deals with raising concerns about some form of wrongdoing in the workplace. The Act covers England, Wales and Scotland. In Northern Ireland, some of the same issues are covered by the Public Interest Disclosure (Northern Ireland) Order 1998. Individuals should start by raising concerns within their team or with their manager or immediate superior. If concerns are not addressed satisfactorily at that level, the correct procedure is to escalate the matter up to a higher level of management or to raise concerns externally. The BMA can provide advice in individual cases. (This is discussed further in Chapter 21.) All NHS organisations should have a policy setting out how concerns should be escalated within the organisation.

Concerns may be raised about systemic problems or the performance of colleagues. The GMC's advice is that steps must be taken without delay, in either case, so that any problems can be properly investigated.[18] In 2011, the GMC published draft guidance on this topic,[19] emphasising the duty to raise concerns when it appears that patient safety may be compromised and suggesting a series of steps to take, such as first alerting a manager or appropriate officer of the employing or contracting body. In various sections of this book, the BMA also makes clear that it is part of doctors' duty to protect patients, colleagues and themselves from unprofessional conduct or acts of clinical negligence (see, for example, Chapter 21).[20] To take appropriate action is a professional obligation and not just a matter of personal conscience. The Association also publishes specific guidance for medical students.[21] Doctors working in a management role may receive information about individuals, practices or resource failings that put patients at risk. They should ensure that systems are in place that provide opportunities for colleagues to raise any such concerns.[22] They have a duty to investigate them and to take appropriate action by establishing the facts as quickly as possible. (For further information on reporting poor performance, whatever its origin, see Chapter 21.)

Conflict in teams

Conflict can arise for a variety of reasons, including personality clashes and poor functioning of some aspect of teamwork. Team leaders need to be able to recognise when some aspect of the team is not functioning well and know where to obtain help to address such problems. Foreseeable potential areas of conflict should be planned for and strategies put in place to address them. The GMC advises doctors to work cooperatively with others to monitor the general quality of care provided and be willing to deal openly and supportively with problems that arise.[23] The team leader needs to ensure that this is possible and that all team members can contribute to discussions so that they understand and accept the reasons for the decisions taken. Part of the leader's role is also to encourage staff to cooperate and communicate with each other.

Summary – working in multi-disciplinary teams

- Safe and good quality care for the patient is the priority. Patient satisfaction and good clinical outcomes require cooperation in teams.
- Effective teamwork relies on good communication and willingness to work constructively with others. It also requires respect for the skills of others, shared objectives and genuinely joint working.
- All members of the team have a duty to ensure it works well and to flag up any problems.
- The team leader has ultimate responsibility for ensuring that the patient's care is properly coordinated and managed.
- Doctors who work as managers have to balance their obligations to patients, employees and often to the wider community.
- Doctors who are managers must ensure that structures are in place to ensure efficiency and quality of care.
- Taking appropriate action when poor care or negligence is suspected is a professional obligation and not just a matter of personal conscience.

Coordination and information sharing among care providers

Sharing information with colleagues

The importance of effective communication with patients and other people caring for them is emphasised throughout this book. Patients and families lose confidence in the service if different messages are given, or contradictory actions proposed, by different team members or different professionals. Lack of good communication can also be a major cause of errors in treatment or failure to recognise when further active treatment would be futile. (This is discussed, in relation to dying patients, in Chapter 10, pages 418–426.) As part of good communication, staff also need to ensure that crucial information about the patient which is in the medical record is passed on to those who need it.

Poor coordination

In September 2004, the Royal Devon and Exeter hospital paid £8,500 compensation in an out-of-court settlement to a renal patient who had been given a blood transfusion 3 years previously. Dialysis and a blood transfusion would have normally been the correct course of action for the condition but in this case the patient was known to be a Jehovah's Witness and had been attending the hospital for treatment for 20 years. As was clearly marked on his medical records, he had previously refused blood transfusions in various life-threatening situations. In 2001, a transfusion was carried out without his consent. The initial error was made by a nurse on night duty. As team leader, the consultant in charge of his care accepted full responsibility for the mistake.[24]

Confidential medical information should be shared on a 'need to know' basis with professionals providing care to the patient, unless the patient has forbidden it.

Generally, patients refuse to share their health information only in exceptional cases and most assume that relevant information about their condition will be made available to other professionals providing them with care or treatment. (This is discussed further in Chapter 5, pages 187–189.) The need to know is an important benchmark, however. In primary care, for example, patients who experience depression, or receive counselling in relation to events in their personal life, do not expect such information to be shared with others for unrelated aspects of treatment.

Where particularly sensitive information is recorded in a shared record, varying levels of access should be integrated into the system so that professionals providing care to the patient have access to the information they need to have without automatically seeing everything. This can be difficult if an old system is in place which may not allow varying levels of access to patient data. It is important that all staff understand the importance of patient confidentiality. The issue of inappropriate access should be dealt with through information governance policies, practice protocols and employment contracts as well as through electronic solutions. In some healthcare settings, multi-disciplinary healthcare records are increasingly commonplace.

The GMC emphasises the importance of sharing relevant information with other healthcare professionals in order to provide safe and effective patient care.[25] It says that doctors referring patients should provide appropriate information, including their medical history and current condition. The patient's GP should also be kept informed about investigations or treatment, unless the patient, after being advised of the benefits of involving the GP, refuses to do so.

Exchange of information should be prompt, coherent and relevant between primary care practitioners, hospitals and other facilities where patients may receive care, including psychiatric facilities, prison health services and centres for asylum seekers. Other community-based services such as palliative care outreach teams and community psychiatric nurses also need to have well-coordinated contact with the primary care team. The team providing care in a hospital setting needs to have access to the information necessary to provide care safely and appropriately. (General issues concerning patient confidentiality, security of data, access, record keeping, and informed consent to disclosure are discussed in Chapters 5 and 6.)

Liaison between NHS and private practitioners

Patients who are eligible to receive NHS care can combine it with private treatment. The requirements for eligibility for free NHS care are complex. Generally, people are eligible if they are 'ordinarily resident' in the UK but there is no clear definition of what that entails.

Good liaison, with patient consent, between NHS and private practitioners is essential for safe and effective care. GPs cannot charge NHS patients for providing relevant information to private doctors at the patient's request. Good communication with patients is also essential so that they know the options available. In the context of NHS care, the initiative for discussing private treatment should rest with patients but if a clinically indicated treatment is *only* available privately, patients should be told that. The priority should be to enable them to make informed choices, without pressure. Private practice codes of conduct in England and Northern Ireland, however, are explicit that, in the course of NHS care, consultants should not initiate discussion about private services.[26]

NHS GPs may be asked to prescribe medication recommended by a private specialist when, for example, patients seek private fertility treatment. Drugs can be prescribed on the NHS if the need arises as part of private care if the GP considers them to be clinically necessary and is willing to take responsibility for them. All doctors must only act within their sphere of competence and providing a prescription makes the prescriber responsible for it, even if it is recommended by a specialist colleague. The same applies to requests from private doctors to NHS staff to undertake diagnostic tests or other procedures within the NHS. Many of the problems that arise in relation to prescribing shared between the private sector and the NHS could be avoided by better communication.

The Department of Health and Scottish Government have issued guidance for health authorities in their respective countries on the circumstances in which it is acceptable for patients to combine NHS and private healthcare services.[27] Patients who opt to supplement their NHS treatment bear the full cost of any private services through 'top up payments' and pay for the delivery and monitoring costs if these can be separated from the NHS care that they receive free. The distinction between different components of care should be achieved by keeping treatment provision in the two sectors separate, with private treatment taking place alongside, but distinct from, NHS treatment. In practice, however, it is difficult to keep a clear idea of which organisation is responsible for the assessment of the patient, the delivery of care and the management of any complications. Nor is it always possible to have treatments separated out and delivered at different locations, or disentangle what is, and what is not, NHS care. Continuity of care is lost if patients have elements of their care delivered by different teams in different settings. (Prescribing decisions generally and top up payments for medication are discussed in Chapter 13).

Liaison when patients seek treatment abroad

Coordination of care can be particularly difficult when patients receive episodes of care from different providers in different countries. The main reasons for people to travel to other countries to receive treatment are that the treatment in question is illegal or simply not available in their own country or is more expensive. Although freedom of movement, for patients and health staff, can have many advantages it can also mean that there is a risk of a serious lack of continuity. Different health systems tend to use different drugs or may employ different procedures to those of the patient's home environment which can make after care problematic. A tragic example of diverse approaches to medication is highlighted by the case of a German doctor who caused a patient's death in the UK by administering a drug unfamiliar to him. In this case, it was the doctor, not the patient who was facing unfamiliar procedures but the principle is the same. (This case is discussed in Chapter 21, page 864.) Dilemmas can also arise if patients who have had treatment such as organ donation or cosmetic surgery abroad suffer ongoing health problems on their return to the UK but lack detailed documentation about the procedures carried out abroad. Planned information sharing, with patient consent, is an important consideration.

In some instances, patients may be eligible to receive planned treatment abroad as part of their ongoing NHS care. Under European Union case law, patients have been recognised as potentially having the right to be treated in another Member State and receive reimbursement of the cost from the NHS under certain conditions. The treatment in question must be offered on the NHS but not be available without 'undue delay'.[28] The case that illustrated some of the complexities of attempting to obtain faster treatment in another jurisdiction was that of Mrs Watts in 2003 (see below). Doctors approached by patients who want treatment in another country should advise them that they need to receive prior approval from the Department of Health and an opinion from an NHS consultant as well as from the relevant commissioning body. They also need to think about effective liaison between the different care providers in terms of pre-treatment investigations and the provision of after care.

The Watts case

Yvonne Watts had osteoarthritis in both hips and rather than wait several months, she enquired about receiving treatment for it abroad. Initially informed that this was not possible on the NHS under existing rules, as the anticipated UK waiting time (2–3 months) was within the Government's target, Mrs Watts arranged a private operation in France. She then claimed reimbursement from the NHS on the grounds that she would have faced 'undue delay' in the UK. The High Court confirmed that undue delay for treatment is not the same as being outside NHS waiting list targets. In assessing what amounts to 'undue delay', the Department of Health has to consider the circumstances of the case including the patient's condition, pain and disabilities. In Mrs Watts' case, Mr Justice Munby held that an 'undue delay' was less than a year but more than 3 months, so Mrs Watts lost her case. She succeeded, however, in demonstrating that the NHS would have to reimburse the cost where there had been undue delay. The Watts case was subsequently heard by the European Court of Justice,[29] which held that patients have the freedom to receive treatment abroad including from a tax-funded health service such as the NHS.

In 2008, a European Directive on cross-border healthcare was issued and this is expected to come into force in 2012–2013 (see Chapter 20, page 840).[30] Following the Watts case, the NHS (Reimbursement of the Cost of EEA Treatment) Regulations were laid before Parliament and came into force in June 2010. They cover England and Wales, amend the NHS Act 2006 and set out the conditions under which the NHS must reimburse patients for health services in another European State. Although the original case concerned hospital treatment, the Regulations also cover non-hospital care.[31] In Scotland, the National Health Service (Reimbursement of the Cost of EEA Treatment) (Scotland) Regulations 2010[32] came into force in July 2010. Under these Regulations, patients can go abroad for treatment within the European Union if they fulfil the criteria or if a commissioning body decides to commission care abroad for its patients.

Liaison with social workers, advocates and other agencies

Healthcare services often need to work closely with social workers, particularly in relation to child protection, the provision of support to people with physical or mental impairments and in the integrated care of older people with multiple health problems. It is vital that inter-agency liaison is well coordinated so that patients receive as seamless a service as possible and that it is tailored to their specific needs. This includes routine liaison to ensure, for example, that patients are not left in hospital when intermediate care or additional support in their own home would better suit their needs. In the past, common causes of delay in discharging older patients were waiting times for a placement in a nursing or residential home, or delays in arranging an assessment of their needs. More recently, great emphasis has been placed on the need of those working across the health and social care sectors to have to meet their patients' requirements.

In 2009, the Secretary of State for Health in England issued a plan for the NHS which focused particularly on good liaison between NHS staff and adult social care services.[33] It was drawn up in the light of the predicted rise in the number of older patients needing social care which could create unsustainable pressure on health services, unless integration between health and social care could be significantly improved and made more preventative in nature. Part of its aim in focusing on preventative care was to enable more people to be treated by GPs and community services, rather than be seen as emergency hospital cases.

Well-integrated care

A pilot programme aimed at better integrating health and social care services was run in Northumbria, Birmingham and Solihull and in Torbay in 2009. By 2010, all the areas had received recognition in national healthcare ratings and national awards. Torbay, in particular, was held out as having demonstrated significant measurable progress in the care of older patients. Fewer patients were admitted to hospital as emergencies as their health could be maintained at home. The hospital had been designated an NHS Beacon, drawing lessons from the USA, which relies less than the NHS on hospitalising older people when they could be well cared for in other ways. This included giving better care to people with long-term conditions earlier in their illness, having recognised pathways of care so that patients could pass smoothly from one part of NHS or social care to another, having rehabilitation facilities to restore their independence and patient education programmes so they could better understand their illness. It involved all of the organisations responsible for delivering health and social care services in the area. All services were designed around the whole needs of patients and clients. Social care and healthcare were integrated and the social care professionals kept closely in touch with the general practices. Patients needed only one point of contact and one care assessment. A team working with the hospital organised patient transfers to nursing homes or other care after a hospital stay. Remote monitoring was used to support people living at home. As a result, by 2010 Torbay had one of the lowest rates of unplanned admissions to hospital in the region and low rates of emergency re-admissions to hospital. Hospital clinicians worked closely with community services and GPs to ensure older people experience good quality care.[34]

The need to support patients effectively across professional boundaries must be balanced with their rights to confidentiality, especially in relation to very sensitive information. Patients with capacity should be made aware of how information is shared within teams and they should be actively involved in deciding who needs to know what.

Liaison in care provision to mentally incapacitated adults

Anyone legally empowered to make decisions on behalf of an incapacitated patient needs to be involved in discussions about that patient's welfare. Patient advocates are increasingly available for hospital patients who are particularly vulnerable. These may be relatives or friends nominated by the patient, or an advocacy service may provide a volunteer. In England and Wales, mentally incapacitated patients may have given lasting power of attorney to someone who can decide for them or the Court of Protection may have appointed a deputy to make health and welfare decisions for the patient. In the absence of anyone being available to speak on behalf of an incapacitated patient, an Independent Mental Capacity Advocate (IMCA) may be appointed. In Scotland, proxy decision makers may be appointed to decide about medical treatment and they will need information to fulfil their duty of care under the Adults with Incapacity (Scotland) Act 2000. The guiding principle should be patients' overall best interests or what would benefit them most, bearing in mind the duty of confidentiality owed to the patient (see Chapter 3, pages 94–95).

Liaison in care provision to families with social problems

Prompt and effective liaison between different agencies is particularly important in relation to the provision of support to families with social problems. These may be households where there is domestic violence, inadequate parenting skills, adults with mental health problems or substance misuse. Good liaison between a range of services and agencies can provide preventative support so that problems can be addressed before reaching a critical stage. When parents exhibit poor parenting or caring skills, the primary care team is often well placed to take the initiative in engaging positively with them to encourage them to improve their skills and stay together. The needs of children and the capacity of parents or other carers to meet those needs should be assessed with a view to developing strategies to help the family and safeguard the children. Health professionals need to understand and recognise the risk factors for children and vulnerable adults. They should try to identify at an early stage those parents who need extra help. They also need to know where to refer the family for such extra support.

Where there are ongoing concerns, social services and the local safeguarding children board (LSCB) are likely to be involved. Overall responsibility for the safety and welfare of children is the responsibility of local authorities, working in partnership with other public organisations, including health providers. Within local authorities, children's social care staff are the main point of contact for children about whom there are welfare concerns. If the problems are serious enough to trigger statutory child protection proceedings, the local authority social care worker takes the lead in supporting and safeguarding the child or children concerned. The Children Act 2004 imposed a duty on local authorities to establish an LSCB which has overall responsibility for deciding how the relevant organisations work together to promote the welfare of children in its area. In the management of suspected cases of abuse or neglect of children, a strategy discussion needs to take place, involving the social care worker, health professionals and the police, as well as any referring agency. The National Society for the Prevention of Cruelty to Children (NSPCC) is a voluntary agency which may also be involved and is authorised to initiate child protection proceedings. Steps should be taken to ensure that families are included in discussions and case conferences whenever this is feasible and appropriate. GPs frequently receive urgent requests from social workers for patients' notes, or a report on a particular patient, without any indication that the patient is aware of the information being sought. The GP should check with the social worker whether it is possible and appropriate to obtain consent for the information to be disclosed. When it is not possible, or it would be inappropriate to do so, for example because it might expose a vulnerable person to risk of serious harm, the GP needs to weigh up whether a breach of confidentiality is justified in the public interest. Doctors recognise that the best interests of vulnerable parties are the paramount concern. (These issues are explored in more detail in Chapter 4, pages 177–178 and Chapter 5, pages 199–202.) Emphasis is placed on the sharing of such information as is necessary, relevant and in the individual's interest, but without disregarding patients' right to confidentiality.

Liaison with other care providers and local organisations

The 2009 NHS 5-year plan focused on the need for health services to work more effectively with national and local partners, including local authorities and the third sector, to make a stronger contribution to promoting health. It pointed out that the NHS would also need to engage with other stakeholders, such as the life sciences industry, to achieve these aims and introduce cost-effective innovations. It called for more reform of provider services and further integration between different provider sectors.[35]

In 2010, the Government proposed that GP-led consortia take a larger role in commissioning services within the NHS in England.[36] In its response to these proposals,[37] the BMA emphasised that high quality and successful commissioning could only be achieved with GPs, secondary and tertiary care consultants, public health doctors and clinical academics working together. Collaboration rather than competition needed to be the focus, with effective multi-professional involvement to achieve seamless and cost-effective patient care. The BMA recommended that consortia should develop local systems and mechanisms to resolve any conflicts that might arise in the course of multi-professional working. (For the most recent BMA advice on this issue, see the BMA website.)

Liaison in nurse-led care

The medical and nursing professions have long worked very closely. Increasingly, some primary care tasks are nurse led, with nurses providing the majority of consultations for some conditions, both face-to-face and by telephone. Appropriately trained nurses carry out aspects of intravenous therapy, counselling, chronic disease management, health education and promotion, and audit. Nurse practitioners also have an important role in the diagnosis, investigation, and treatment of minor injuries and illnesses.

In hospital care too, the expertise and autonomy of nurses is increasingly acknowledged, with the development of specialist nurse practitioners and nurse consultants. Where appropriate, nurses have consultant support but are able to order investigations themselves and provide continuity of care. Specialist nurses may be responsible for interventions such as cardio-pulmonary resuscitation. Patients with some conditions, such as suspected deep vein thrombosis, can be referred to nurse-led services.

Nurses, midwives and health visitors are accountable for their practice and are subject to statutory regulation by the Nursing and Midwifery Council. *The Code: Standards of conduct, performance and ethics for nurses and midwives*[38] sets out the principles they are obliged to follow. It is similar in content to the GMC's guidance for doctors. Nurses, midwives and health visitors, like doctors, have a duty to acknowledge the limitations in their knowledge and to decline to undertake any duties or responsibilities they consider to be beyond their competence or to be inappropriate in the particular circumstances. They are personally accountable for their actions and omissions.

Multi-disciplinary collaboration in integrated care pathways

Integrated care pathways are structured multi-disciplinary care plans which set out the essential steps in the care of patients with a specific clinical problem. They are mentioned here because they specifically articulate a multi-disciplinary approach to care and can be seen to promote and facilitate effective teamworking in hospitals. They can also be a way of encouraging the translation of national guidelines into local protocols and increasingly cover many conditions and procedures. Integrated care pathways are seen as producing increased adherence to national guidelines and best practice statements, and can result in improved standards of documentation. Integrated care pathways describe each stage in the management of the care of patients with a particular condition, but allow scope for variation, where appropriate, in particular cases. They are useful for the management of conditions such as stroke, in which diagnosis is well defined, complex inter-disciplinary inputs are required and there is good evidence on best practice. The use of a single multi-disciplinary integrated care pathway record, which is available to the patient and forms part of the patient's medical record, also leads to improved communication between the different professionals involved with providing care. (This is discussed further in relation to the example of the Liverpool Care Pathway for the Dying Patient in Chapter 10, pages 432–434.) Another advantage of integrated care pathways is the discussion and communication that takes place while they are being drawn up. This enables the views and approaches of professionals from different disciplines to be shared.

Other tools that facilitate multi-disciplinary working include the Common Assessment Framework, which is a generic assessment for children with additional needs.[39] It can be used by practitioners across all children's services in England and aims to help early identification of need, promote coordinated service provision and reduce the number of assessments that some children and young people go through.

Liaison with practitioners of complementary and alternative medicine

Doctors may receive requests from patients for referral to complementary and alternative medicine (CAM) practitioners. Some GPs are trained to provide such therapies themselves and are accountable to the GMC for their competence in those alternative therapies, in the same way as for their orthodox medicine. Or they may choose to employ practitioners in their teams and delegate some aspects of care to them, so that the GP still retains overall responsibility. Alternatively, they may suggest referring patients to a CAM practitioner. Osteopathy and chiropractic are professionally regulated and so health professionals can liaise with such practitioners with confidence that they are competent in the therapies they provide and legally accountable for them. For some time, acupuncture has also been integrated into treatment programmes offered by the NHS, and guidance from the National Institute for Health and Clinical Excellence (NICE) on the treatment of low back pain, for example, supports the use of alternatives such as acupuncture and manual therapy.[40] This reflects growing interest in some complementary therapy, as well as changing attitudes within the medical profession but evidence of benefit for the individual patient remains a key issue.

There has long been debate about the degree to which conventional health professionals should work closely with CAM practitioners or feel confident in referring patients to them. Liaison generally depends on the type of therapy, whether it is regulated by law and whether there is evidence of safety and efficacy. Some other alternative disciplines, such as crystal therapy and iridology, lack any credible evidence base. Another crucial consideration is whether the CAM therapy supplements conventional methods of diagnosis and treatment or claims to provide an alternative to them.

Complementary therapies are often combined with conventional medicine. Among the therapies that are often used by patients to supplement standard orthodox treatments, which do *not* claim to have any diagnostic or therapeutic purpose are aromatherapy, massage, stress therapy, reflexology and hypnotherapy. Practitioners of these therapies can provide supportive care without impeding conventional treatment. Others, such as Chinese herbal medicine, Ayurvedic medicine and homeopathy are not currently regulated but claim to provide diagnosis and treatment and so are seen as an alternative to orthodox medicine. As they are not regulated, this may mean that the practitioner providing the therapy is insufficiently experienced in the treatments to judge whether or not they are dangerous in an individual case. Doctors may also be worried if patients choose these and decline conventional treatments for which there is evidence of benefit. In such cases, they need to talk to the patient about their concerns, while recognising that ultimately patients can choose whichever therapy they want. Dilemmas also arise for the healthcare team if unregulated practitioners request medical tests to be carried out on the NHS on their behalf or ask for test results. Doctors would need to be convinced that such interventions are necessary in the patient's interest before providing them.

In 2009, a public consultation was carried out in the four nations, seeking views from the public and the scientific community about the regulation of complementary therapies. In April 2010, as a result of the consultation, it was announced that new improved safeguards would be introduced for people using herbal medicine, traditional Chinese medicine and acupuncture. The then-Secretary of State for Health said that legislation would be introduced in England in liaison with Ministers in Scotland, Wales and Northern Ireland. This would ensure that all practitioners supplying unlicensed herbal medicine would be registered. The introduction of a register of practitioners would increase public protection without conferring the same sort of professional recognition that doctors have.

The role of some types of complementary and alternative therapies also came under scrutiny in England in 2010 when the House of Commons Science and Technology Committee published a critical report on NHS funding for homeopathy.[41] Focusing on whether Government policy on homeopathy was evidence-based, the Committee found a mismatch between the evidence and policy. Its main conclusion was that the evidence indicates that homeopathy is not efficacious and does not produce results beyond the placebo effect. It recommended that there should be a clear NHS policy on prescribing placebos, including homeopathic medicines. At its annual meeting in 2010, BMA representatives voted in favour of the NHS discontinuing its funding for homeopathy. (Prescribing issues are discussed in Chapter 13.)

An EU directive[42] on herbal medicinal products, in force since 2004, stipulated that traditional herbal medicinal products had to have been in use for 30 years for them to be licensed and available over the counter. It was designed to protect consumers from unlicensed herbal and Chinese medicine. Member States had until April 2011 to implement the necessary enabling legislation but there was also a derogation option in the Directive that allowed the UK to maintain the availability of unlicensed herbal medicines if practitioners were registered. Despite criticism from some pharmacologists, the Coalition Government said that British consumers should still be able to obtain herbal and Chinese medicines once all UK practitioners supplying them were registered with the Health Professions Council (HPC). This UK register of practitioners held by the HPC will come into force in April 2012.

Doctors may be confident in referring patients to CAM therapists who are subject to a statutory regulatory body, such as chiropractors or osteopaths, or if the person carrying out the therapy is a registered doctor or nurse, accountable to their professional body. When GPs employ CAM therapists who are not subject to a statutory regulatory body, they need to be satisfied that the individual is suitably qualified and experienced to undertake the role. Doctors should also be aware that, in such circumstances, they may be held liable for any harm arising to their patients.

Unregulated practice

The issue of regulation for CAM was highlighted by a legal case in 2010. The court heard that a patient, Mrs Booth, became ill apparently as a result of taking Chinese herbal medicine for acne for over 5 years. The products had been advertised as 'safe and natural' but Mrs Booth was subsequently diagnosed with kidney failure and later with cancer of the urinary tract. Both were allegedly caused by the herbal pills. Ying Wu, a traditional Chinese herbalist was given a conditional discharge by the court after admitting selling the pills which contained aristolochic acid. Prior to being banned, aristolochic acid should have been available by prescription only. Ms Wu, who had initially denied the charges, later pleaded guilty to selling prescription-only medicines without authorisation and to selling a banned substance. Aristolochic acid has been a common feature of Chinese medicine but it is unclear at what dosage it begins to build up in the body and causes health problems. There had been incidents of it causing kidney problems and cancer in the past, including 100 incidents of renal disease among patients at a weight-loss clinic in Belgium between 1990 and 1992. Most of those patients required dialysis or transplantation but some died after taking the substance. In the UK case, the judge ruled that, because the sale of Chinese medicines is unregulated, there was no evidence to show that the herbalist was aware of the potential harm of the pills. He called for greater regulation of such therapies. The Register of Chinese Herbal Medicine also called for statutory regulation of all practitioners of herbal medicine to ensure that practitioners are suitably qualified and competent.[43]

The Complementary and Natural Healthcare Council (CNHC) was set up in 2009 as a voluntary regulatory body for CAM therapies. The BMA has argued that all complementary therapies should be regulated to the same standards expected of the medical profession and should be subject to an independent regulatory body. In 2008, it also called for a ban on the use of NHS resources to fund unregulated therapies whose associations are not affiliated to the CNHC. Regulation for such practices is opposed by some organisations, such as the Academy of Medical Royal Colleges, the Medical Schools Council and the Institute of Biomedical Science. They argue that statutory regulation might encourage the erroneous view that practising such therapies involves thorough medical training and that practitioners are on a par with doctors. These bodies argue that regulation alone is not the answer but, rather, greater distinction needs to be made between safe and effective therapies and those that may not be either.

Summary – coordination and information sharing among care providers

- Patient welfare is the first concern.
- Access to confidential medical information should be on a 'need to know' basis.
- When care is shared, patients can be at risk if information necessary for their care is not passed on to others providing care.
- Doctors increasingly need to liaise with colleagues in other disciplines, such as social work, so that all aspects of patient care can be properly integrated. This requires good coordination and the timely sharing of relevant information to ensure good patient care.
- Patient choice in terms of combining private and NHS care, or seeking aspects of treatment in another jurisdiction, is likely to continue. Consideration may need to be given to ensuring adequately coordinated services, such as pre-treatment investigations and post-treatment aftercare when treatment takes place in diverse settings.
- Tools such as integrated care pathways rely on good multi-disciplinary effort.
- Doctors can refer patients with confidence to CAM therapists who are subject to a statutory regulatory body or if the person carrying out the therapy is a registered health professional.

Delegation, referral and second opinions

Delegation and referral

Delegation involves professionals asking other staff to carry out procedures or provide care. When tasks are delegated, the person delegating retains responsibility for the patient's overall care and must ensure that tasks are delegated only to those who are competent to fulfil them. In some circumstances, nurses, midwives and other therapists, as well as doctors, make and receive referrals, admit and discharge patients, order investigations and diagnostic tests, run clinics and prescribe drugs. When a referral is made, responsibility for the patient is transferred, usually to someone with more specialised knowledge to carry out specific procedures, tests or treatment that fall outside the sphere of competence of the referring doctor. Referrals are usually made to another registered health professional. If this is not the case, the referring doctor or the referral management system (see below), should ensure that the professional to whom the patient is referred is accountable to a statutory regulatory body.

GMC guidance on delegation and referral

'Delegation involves asking a colleague to provide treatment or care on your behalf. Although you will not be accountable for the decisions and actions of those to whom you delegate, you will still be responsible for the overall management of the patient, and accountable for your decision to delegate. When you delegate care or treatment you must be satisfied that the person to whom you delegate has the qualifications, experience, knowledge and skills to provide the care or treatment involved. You must always pass on enough information about the patient and the treatment they need.'[44]

'Referral involves transferring some or all of the responsibility for the patient's care, usually temporarily and for a particular purpose, such as additional investigation, care or treatment that is outside your competence. You must be satisfied that any healthcare professional to whom you refer a patient is accountable to a statutory body or employed within a managerial environment. If they are not, the transfer of care will be regarded as delegation, not referral. This means that you remain responsible for the overall management of the patient, and accountable for your decision to delegate.'[45]

Referrals for private treatment

Investigations or treatment should be arranged on the basis of clinical judgement and if specialist assessment is needed, the patient should be referred to an appropriate service. Some patients request referral to a specialist in the private sector and if the care is covered by the patient's health insurance, the insurer may specify how, and to whom, referrals should be made. If patients request referral in the absence of clear clinical need, the underlying reasons should be explored. If the GP does not consider that specialist treatment is appropriate, this needs to be explained to the patient who may still decide to seek private treatment without a referral.

Patients may choose to pay for private investigations to get a diagnosis quickly and then switch back to the NHS for the subsequent treatment. As long as they are entitled to NHS care, such patients can opt into, or out of, NHS care at any stage and be placed onto the NHS waiting list at the same position as if the investigations had taken place within the NHS. Some doctors think it unfair that patients who can afford to pay are able to jump the queue by getting on to the treatment waiting list before those who wait for NHS investigations. Others argue that, as some people obtain a diagnosis privately, this reduces pressure on the NHS so that NHS patients are seen quicker. NHS patients whose clinical need is greater may join the waiting list later but still receive treatment earlier if their condition is urgent.

Referral management and commissioning of services

In the past, GPs traditionally referred patients needing further specialist treatment directly to named consultants. This process changed in England, when referral management schemes were set up in an attempt to manage the rising costs of hospital referrals. One effect of this was to highlight the degree to which some referrals were unnecessary or did not comply with best practice by, for example, not fully involving the patient in the decision. After 2005, when the Department of Health suggested that referral management was the way to deal with inappropriate demand for hospital services,[46] a range of models developed with varying success. These included Referral Management Centres (RMCs), clinical triage and assessment measures, financial incentives for GPs to refer fewer patients, guidelines and feedback from peer review. By 2006, the BMA found that various models of referral management systems had developed, each with advantages, disadvantages and risks.[47] Referrals could be tracked, linked with patient booking services and waiting times could be reduced for uncomplicated cases, by using an alternative service provider. Referral management schemes could also help manage potential conflicts of interest when GPs have financial interests in providing, or are under financial pressure to limit, referrals.

Problems arose, however, if the GP and the referral management scheme disagreed about the referral or if the patient was redirected to an alternative health professional when the GP thought this inappropriate. Relationships between doctors, and between patients and doctors, could also be adversely affected.

By 2007, RMCs and peer review were increasingly used and, at about the same time, practice-based commissioning (PBC) was introduced. The new PBC consortia also used referral management to manage patient demand and control budgets.[48] PBC gave GPs notional budgets and more autonomy to purchase healthcare services but, from an ethics perspective, by linking treatment decisions much more closely to considerations of cost inevitably gave rise to concerns about conflicts of interest between doing what is best for the individual patient and saving money. Not only doctors, but also referral management services could face that particular dilemma, exacerbated if attempts were made to impose financial penalties on them if referrals to secondary care exceeded specified targets.[49] Other conflicts arose if GPs with PBC wished to purchase private services in which they had a financial interest or when they themselves carried out 'triage or provided out-of-hospital services and were therefore able to refer to themselves or members of their practice'.[50] As well as the potential for financial conflict, this also highlighted the possibility of clinical pathways being distorted by, for example, GPs 'offering minor surgery for a condition that might best be managed through conservative non-invasive treatment'.[51] (Conflicts of interest are discussed further in Chapter 16, page 685.)

GMC guidance on conflicts of interest

'If you have a financial or commercial interest in a business case being considered by your Primary Care Trust under Practice Based Commissioning arrangements, you should declare your interest and exclude yourself from related decisions in accordance with the Department of Health and your PCT's guidance.'[52]

In 2007, the BMA published guiding principles for referral management,[53] emphasising that the primary purpose was to improve the patient care pathway and not lengthen or complicate the patient's experience of care. Such schemes, the BMA said, should not cut across patient choice nor weaken the principle of clinician-to-clinician referral where clinically indicated. Doctors involved in the referral management process must act in accordance with GMC guidance and be clear about their own and other people's responsibility and accountability. Patients should be properly informed about the process, with advice about implications for their care. Working at the interface of primary and secondary care, referral management measures should help to integrate rather than separate the two and facilitate collaboration between primary and secondary care clinicians. Any assessment and treatment services provided at this interface should be multi-disciplinary in nature, drawing in expertise already available in the locality.

RMCs gave rise to much debate, not least because they were seen by some GPs as demotivating, an erosion of their clinical autonomy and an intrusion into what would otherwise be close liaison between GPs and hospital consultants. After RMC review, the GP's referral might still be made to a consultant or it could be redirected to a GP with Special Interest (GPSI), specialist nurse or alternative health provider. The aim of RMCs was to divert referrals, where possible, to appropriate but under-used services which could be more cost effective and spread patient demand. Patients could sometimes be treated more quickly, with less cost and closer to home but established clinical relationships between GPs and consultants could become less important and patients might no longer be seen by the specialist who had treated them previously.

Improving quality and ensuring cost-effective use of resources had been the aim but an influential report in 2010 found that referral management schemes were not necessarily doing either.[54] Some undermined quality by misdirecting referrals, based on too little information, or they delayed patients' access to specialists. The report examined evidence about issues such as whether patients had been involved in the decision and were referred without delay when necessary; whether appropriate pre-referral investigations had occurred; whether referral letters contained the relevant information and if all parties understood the purpose and expectations of the referral. It found that, in some cases, one or more of these essential steps had been missed out; appropriate pre-referral investigations had not been done, for example, or the shared understanding of the referral's aim, between the GP, patient and consultant, was frequently lacking. While the evidence suggested that not all referrals to hospital were necessary, and many patients referred to secondary care could be seen elsewhere, some patients genuinely needing a referral did not get one. Other risks included RMCs undertaking clinical triage in the absence of the patient, with limited information about the patient's condition and clinical history. 'Referral management has the capacity both to reduce and exacerbate the clinical risk inherent in any referral process' and, the report suggested that these risks had sometimes not been recognised.[55]

Criteria for good practice in referral and commissioning

Peer review, clear referral criteria, evidence-based guidelines and feedback from hospital consultants were identified by the King's Fund as successful strategies for GPs to avoid inappropriate referrals. Doctors' capacity to refer appropriately would be greatly strengthened by access to decision-support tools, up-to-date information on local services, regular feedback from audit of their referral activity and opportunities to communicate with other clinical professionals, including consultants, by e-mail and telephone. Practice-based commissioning could also reduce inappropriate referrals through primary care practices or consortia analysing and auditing their own and colleagues' referrals. The King's Fund report predicted that all future GP-commissioning consortia would need to look closely at referral management options and pointed out how its analysis of the evidence could help identify which approaches were capable of delivering cost and quality benefits. It said that 'referral management schemes can successfully divert activity away from secondary care. This is not the same as ensuring referrals reach the right destination' and its research provided 'less positive messages about value for money, patient choice and the impact on the relationships between primary and secondary care clinicians'.[56] The report set out a set of principles for commissioners emphasising, for example, the need to understand the context of each referral, rather than considering it in isolation and advising against financial incentives to drive blanket reductions in referral numbers. Also any referral management strategy, it emphasised, needed to include a robust means of managing the inherent risks at the point when clinical responsibility for a patient is handed over from one clinician to another. (Risk management is discussed in Chapter 21.)

At the time of writing, in 2011, the BMA was also finalising guidance on best practice in commissioning. (For further information, see the BMA website.)

Patients' requests for a second opinion

Patients may request a second opinion from a clinician outside the treating team. Patients do not have an automatic right to referral for a further opinion within the NHS but doctors should generally try to accommodate the patient's request, if feasible and reasonable. The GMC says that doctors must respect the patient's right to *seek* a second opinion.[57] Such requests should be handled sensitively and wherever possible dealt with by the consultant with overall responsibility. The patient should not be made to feel a nuisance.

Summary – delegation, referral and second opinions

- Delegation leaves the person delegating with overall responsibility for the patient's care. Doctors who delegate must ensure that tasks are delegated only to those who are competent to fulfil them.
- Referral involves responsibility for the patient being transferred, usually to someone with specialised knowledge.
- Referral and commissioning can involve conflicts of interest for doctors. These need to be minimised or managed carefully, in line with best practice principles.
- In the NHS, patients have no automatic right to a second opinion but requests should be accommodated where reasonable to do so. Private patients have more options in this respect.

Administrative issues in working with others

Partnerships providing services

Doctors increasingly enter into working partnerships to provide patient care with partners, who may be doctors, lay people or other professionals, such as nurses. They can form companies to bid for NHS contracts or they can join together to provide private care. The important points from an ethical perspective are that they give proper attention to patient welfare and have clear policies about who is accountable for what. Doctors sometimes set up limited liability partnerships and limited liability companies: the main advantage over a traditional medical partnership being that members' financial liability is limited (except in cases of negligence by a partner, in which case the assests of the business are used first to settle the claim). Forming a limited liability partnership is more complicated than merely setting up a partnership and entails a number of legal responsibilities. The BMA offers general advice on aspects of partnership arrangements.[58]

Partnership agreements

A formal partnership agreement is useful for setting out the rights and obligations of all the parties. Legal, accountancy and tax advice is needed when drawing up such an agreement. In primary care, the 2004 General Medical Services (GMS) contract made it possible for practice partnerships to include non-clinical members, as long as one of the partners is a doctor. Multi-professional arrangements may include a partnership of doctors, nurses and lay people. When partnership agreements are drawn up between doctors and non-medical partners, it is important to decide at the outset whether some aspects of decision making should be specifically reserved for the health professional partner(s). The BMA's General Practitioners Committee has produced various guidance notes which cover basic information about partnerships, implications of the GMS contract, contractual obligations, discrimination, types of partnership and a standard framework for an agreement.[59]

Informing patients about changes

Separation of patient lists on the dissolution of a partnership is a frequent area of disagreement in primary care if, for example, a partner sets up a separate practice and wants his or her usual patients to move to it. Patients have a choice about which doctor they see and so need to have factual information about changes in the service but restrictive covenants in partnership agreements may determine what happens. Problems also sometimes arise when doctors who are employed by a private company offering elective services, such as weight-loss treatment, feel that those patients (and their records) should transfer with the doctor if he or she moves on. This implies a notion of 'ownership' of patients that does not fit well with modern practice. For doctors working in private companies, much is likely to depend on the contract that the doctor has with the employing company. Again, patients should have a choice about who they see unless they have specifically entered into a contract for services with the private company, in which case their options may be limited. Doctors must not allow false information to circulate, such as rumours that a colleague is intending to retire from practice or move from the area. In this, as in all matters, patients are entitled to receive balanced advice.

Employing other practitioners

Doctors may employ colleagues in private clinics or companies. Also, many primary care practices offer a wide range of health services, such as physiotherapy, chiropody, dietary advice, counselling and acupuncture. A prime consideration is that the safety and welfare of patients be protected by checking the competency and integrity of the employee. For this, they often rely heavily on colleague's references (see page 795).

Recommended health checks for health professionals

Since 2007, it has been recommended that all healthcare workers starting work in the NHS in England and Wales should have standard healthcare clearance checks.[60] Similar rules apply in Scotland and Northern Ireland.[61] New or returning healthcare workers and medical students should be checked for tuberculosis, be offered hepatitis B immunisation and offered tests for hepatitis C and HIV. If their duties include performing exposure-prone procedures, additional healthcare clearance should also be obtained before confirmation of an appointment. This includes testing that staff are non-infectious for HIV, hepatitis B and C. The published guidance provides examples of exposure-prone procedures for each specialty. The BMA has also issued guidance for junior doctors and medical students (see also Chapter 21, pages 879–880).[62]

Vetting and barring

All employers, including GPs and hospital trusts, need to ensure that staff are safe and reliable. Staff working with children or vulnerable adults have long needed to be cleared by a Criminal Records Bureau (CRB) check. In October 2009, a vetting and barring scheme came into force in England, Wales and Northern Ireland to cover everyone working with children, young people under 18 and vulnerable adults. This requires people who work with vulnerable groups to be registered with the Independent Safeguarding Authority (ISA). Patients receiving healthcare are classified as vulnerable. Doctors who employ staff, including other health professionals or who have volunteers who come into contact with children or vulnerable adults in a regulated activity, must ensure that those people are vetted. 'Regulated activity' covers both paid and unpaid work, including any form of healthcare treatment or therapy provided to children or adults. NHS general practice comes under the definition of regulated activity. Any person who is thought to pose a risk should be reported to the ISA. A person who has been barred must not try to obtain work with children or vulnerable adults. The BMA's General Practitioners Committee produced guidance on vetting and barring[63] and in 2009, the Government also published guidance, including a checklist for employers.[64]

In January 2010, the Scottish Government consulted on a similar scheme, proposing that those in regulated work with children or vulnerable adults should join a membership scheme which would indicate that they do not have a known history of harmful behaviour and have not been barred. It replaced the Disclosure Scotland certificates system. Doctors can opt out of membership of the scheme but it is illegal for organisations or individuals to employ someone who has been barred and the only way to check this is via membership of the scheme. People who are self-employed, such as GPs and locums, need to pay for membership for themselves. The BMA Scotland General Practitioners Committee has produced some general guidance.[65]

Such checks have caused delays, however, when specialist staff, such as paediatric surgeons, moved between trusts to cover for colleagues on sick leave at other hospitals. To minimise such delays, it was suggested that NHS staff could be issued with 'passports' so their CRB check from one NHS organisation would be valid in another. Problems have also arisen for junior doctors, who frequently move between posts.

In 2011, the Government announced new recommendations for the future of the vetting and barring scheme and criminal records checks. The Protection of Freedoms Bill was introduced into Parliament in early 2011 with the expectation that it would be finalised by the end of that year. When implemented (scheduled for 2012), it will provide a new legislative framework. Under the revised vetting scheme, doctors will no longer be required to register with the ISA. Other key recommendations included:

- portability of criminal records checks between jobs
- introduction of an online system to allow employers to check if updated information is held on an applicant
- merging of the CRB and ISA
- large reduction of the number of positions requiring checks to just those working most closely and regularly with children and vulnerable adults.

When the new scheme is implemented, criminal records checks will include a check to find out whether an individual is on the Adults' Barred List, the Children's Barred List, or both. Employers will be able to check the status of the potential employee's CRB check online; a new CRB check will only be requested when changes are indicated. The BMA has guidance for doctors in secondary care on vetting and barring.[66]

Providing references

The GMC emphasises that doctors must only provide honest, justifiable and accurate comments when giving references or writing reports about colleagues. They must include all the information relevant to the colleague's competence, performance and conduct.[67] In 2011, the GMC published new draft guidance on this subject,[68] emphasising the duty of referees to take reasonable steps to verify the information they use or provide in a reference. They should avoid comments based on their own personal views where these do not relate to the candidate's suitability. Allowing an inaccurate picture of a prospective employee to be presented could put patients at risk and undermine trust in the profession, as well as leading to the appointment of someone who is not the best candidate (see also Chapter 21, page 872).

Advertising medical services

Traditionally, there were many restrictions on the manner in which medical services could be advertised to the public but most of these are no longer in force. Doctors can make prospective patients aware of their services and can advertise to the public as long as they comply with the brief rules set out by the GMC. These require that information about medical services be factual and verifiable. It must not exploit patients' lack of knowledge, nor put pressure on them by, for example, arousing ill-founded fears about their future health. Doctors are also prohibited from making unjustifiable claims about the quality or outcomes of their service.[69]

In the past, doctors were prohibited from 'canvassing' for patients and were restricted in terms of the type of advertising allowed. A distinction was made between advertising by GPs, which was limited but permitted, and by specialists, which was not. In the late 1980s, a Monopolies and Mergers Commission Inquiry ruled that patients should have ready access to factual information about medical services. After consultation, the GMC decided that all doctors should be able to advertise their services, in order to provide patients with relevant information. The same rules on advertising, mentioned above, now apply to all doctors. The guidance also applies to all advertising, irrespective of the medium, including information provided on the internet, in formal advertisements in newspapers, practice leaflets distributed to residents within a practice area, or an editorial or news piece in a local newspaper. The purpose of doctors' advertising should be to provide factual information about the medical services available to enable patients to make informed decisions.

Summary – administrative issues in working with others

- As a wider range of partnership arrangements occur in the provision of healthcare, thought should be given in advance to administrative matters such as partnership agreements and how patients will be informed of changes.
- All employers must follow the law on vetting and barring and health checks for new NHS staff.
- Doctors must follow the GMC's advice on the provision of references and on advertising.

References

1   World Health Organization Study Group on Multi-professional Education of Health Personnel (1988) *Learning together to work together for health*, WHO, Geneva, p.6.
2   General Medical Council (2009) *Tomorrow's Doctors*, GMC, London, Annex B3.
3   General Medical Council (2006) *Good Medical Practice*, GMC, London, paras 41–55.
4   General Medical Council (2006) *Management for Doctors*, GMC, London.
5   General Medical Council (2011) *Good Management Practice: guidance for all doctors, drafts for consultation*, GMC, London.
6   General Medical Council (2011) *Good Management Practice: guidance for all doctors, drafts for consultation*, GMC, London, para 8.
7   General Medical Council (2011) *Good Management Practice: guidance for all doctors, drafts for consultation*, GMC, London, para 3.
8   General Medical Council (2011) *Good Management Practice: guidance for all doctors, drafts for consultation*, GMC, London, paras 17 and 18.
9   Department of Health (2010) *Equity and excellence: Liberating the NHS*, The Stationery Office, London.
10 General Medical Council (2006) *Management for doctors*, GMC, London, para 50.
11 General Medical Council (2006) *Management for doctors*, GMC, London, para 2.
12 General Medical Council (2006) *Management for doctors*, GMC, London, para 12.
13 General Medical Council (2011) *Good Management Practice: guidance for all doctors, drafts for consultation*, GMC, London, paras 39, 40, 43–5.
14 General Medical Council Fitness to Practise Panel hearing, case number 147.
15 British Medical Association (2007) *Guidance for developing the role of medical directors*, BMA, London. British Medical Association (2009) *Guidance on the role of the Clinical and Divisional Director*, BMA, London.
16 NHS Institute for Innovation and Improvement (2010) *Medical Leadership Competency Framework*, 3rd edn, NIII, London.
17 British Medical Association (2009) *Whistleblowing: advice for BMA members working in NHS secondary care about raising concerns in the workplace*, BMA, London.
18 General Medical Council (2006) *Good Medical Practice*, GMC, London, paras 43–5.
19 General Medical Council (2011) *Raising and acting on concerns about patient safety (draft)*, GMC, London.
20 See, for example: British Medical Association (2009) *Whistleblowing: advice for BMA members working in NHS secondary care about raising concerns in the workplace*, BMA, London.
21 British Medical Association (2008) *Whistle-blowing: guidance from the Medical Students Committee (MSC)*, BMA, London.
22 General Medical Council (2006) *Good Medical Practice*, GMC, London, para 45.
23 General Medical Council (2006) *Good Medical Practice*, GMC, London, paras 41–55.
24 *Patrick McGovern v Royal Devon & Exeter Healthcare NHS Trust* (2004), unreported.
25 General Medical Council (2006) *Good Medical Practice*, GMC, London, paras 50–2.
26 Department of Health (2004) *A code of conduct for private practice: recommended standards of practice for NHS consultants*, DH, London, para 2.9. British Medical Association, Department of Health, Social Services and Public Safety (2003) *A code of conduct for private practice. Recommended standards of practice for HPSS consultants*, DHSSPS, Belfast, para 2.9.
27 Department of Health (2009) *Guidance on NHS patients who wish to pay for additional private care*, DH, London. Scottish Government Health Directorates (2009) *Arrangements for NHS patients receiving healthcare services through private healthcare arrangements*, SGHD, Edinburgh.
28 Department of Health (2007) *Patient mobility: advice to local healthcare commissioners on handling requests for hospital care*, DH, London.
29 *R (on the application of Yvonne Watts) v Bedford Primary Care Trust and Secretary of State for Health* [2006] EUECJ C-372/04.
30 Directive 2008/142/EC of the European Parliament and the Council on the application of patients' rights in cross-border healthcare. Available at: ec.europa.eu (accessed 31 May 2011).
31 National Health Service (Reimbursement of the Cost of EEA Treatment) Regulations 2010. SI 2010/915.
32 National Health Service (Reimbursement of the Cost of EEA Treatment) (Scotland) Regulations 2010. SI 2010/283.
33 Department of Health (2009) *NHS 2010–2015: from good to great. Preventative, people-centred, productive*, DH, London.
34 Ham C. (2010) *Working together for health: achievements and challenges in the Kaiser NHS Beacon Sites Programme*, Health Services Management Centre, University of Birmingham, Birmingham.
35 Department of Health (2009) *NHS 2010–2015: from good to great. Preventative, people-centred, productive*, DH, London.
36 Department of Health (2010) *Equity and excellence: Liberating the NHS*, The Stationery Office, London.

37   British Medical Association (2010) *BMA response to Health Select Committee inquiry on Commissioning*. Available at: www.bma.org.uk (accessed 29 October 2010).
38   Nursing and Midwifery Council (2008) *The Code: Standards of conduct, performance and ethics for nurses and midwives*, NMC, London.
39   Children's Workforce Development Council, *Common Assessment Framework (CAF)*. Available at: www.cwdcouncil.org.uk (accessed 2 June 2011).
40   National Institute for Health and Clinical Excellence (2009) *Management of persistent non-specific low back pain*. Available at: guidance.nice.org.uk (accessed 2 June 2011). All NICE guidance is available at: guidance.nice.org.uk.
41   House of Commons Science and Technology Committee (2010) *Evidence Check 2: Homeopathy, Fourth Report of Session 2009–10*, The Stationery Office, London. Available at: www.parliament.uk (accessed 12 January 2010).
42   Directive 2004/24/EC of the European Parliament and Council of 31 March 2004, amending, as regards traditional herbal medicinal products, Directive 2001/83/EC on the Community code relating to medicinal products for human use.
43   Rose D. (2010) Chinese herbalist's tablets caused 'terrible harm'. *The Times* (18 February). Available at: www.timesonline.co.uk (accessed 3 March 2010).
44   General Medical Council (2006) *Good Medical Practice*, GMC, London, para 54.
45   General Medical Council (2006) *Good Medical Practice*, GMC, London, para 55.
46   Department of Health (2005) *Creating a Patient-Led NHS: Delivering the NHS improvement plan*, DH, London, p.22.
47   British Medical Association (2006) *Referral Management FAQs*. Available at: www.bma.org.uk (accessed 30 March 2011).
48   Imison C, Naylor C. (2010) *Referral management: lessons for success*, King's Fund, London, p.6.
49   Imison C, Naylor C. (2010) *Referral management: lessons for success*, King's Fund, London, p.38.
50   Imison C, Naylor C. (2010) *Referral management: lessons for success*, King's Fund, London, p.37.
51   Imison C, Naylor C. (2010) *Referral management: lessons for success*, King's Fund, London, p.38.
52   General Medical Council (2008) *Conflicts of interest: guidance for doctors*, GMC, London, para 6.
53   British Medical Association (2007) *Referral management principles*. Available at: www.bma.org.uk (accessed 30 March 2011).
54   Imison C, Naylor C. (2010) *Referral management: lessons for success*, King's Fund, London.
55   Imison C, Naylor C. (2010) *Referral management: lessons for success*, King's Fund, London, p.x.
56   Imison C, Naylor C. (2010) *Referral management: lessons for success*, King's Fund, London, p.35.
57   General Medical Council (2006) *Good Medical Practice*, GMC, London, para 3(e).
58   British Medical Association (2010) *Guidance on income tax and partnerships*, BMA, London.
59   See: www.bma.org.uk (accessed 2 June 2011).
60   Department of Health (2007) *Health clearance for tuberculosis, hepatitis B, hepatitis C and HIV: New healthcare workers*, DH, London.
61   Scottish Government (2008) *Health clearance for tuberculosis, hepatitis B, hepatitis C and HIV for new healthcare workers with direct clinical contact with patients*, SG, Edinburgh. Department of Health, Social Services and Public Safety (2009) *Guidance on health clearance for tuberculosis, hepatitis B, hepatitis C and HIV for new healthcare workers with direct clinical contact with patients*, DHSSPS, Belfast.
62   British Medical Association (2008) *Testing for blood borne viruses: BMA guidance for medical staff*, BMA, London.
63   British Medical Association (2009) *Vetting and barring scheme: guidance for GPs*, BMA London. British Medical Association (2010) *Update on DH Vetting and Barring Scheme (VBS) remodelling review*, BMA, London.
64   Home Office, Criminal Records Bureau, Independent Safeguarding Authority, Access Northern Ireland (2009) *The Vetting and Barring Scheme Guidance*. Available at: www.isa.gov.org (accessed 20 May 2011).
65   British Medical Association (2010) *The New Protecting Vulnerable Groups Scheme in Scotland*, BMA Scotland, Edinburgh.
66   British Medical Association (2010) *Vetting and Barring Scheme: ISA Regulations: guidance for doctors in secondary care*, BMA, London.
67   General Medical Council (2006) *Good Medical Practice*, GMC, London, para 19.
68   General Medical Council (2011) *Writing references (draft)*, GMC, London.
69   General Medical Council (2006) *Good Medical Practice*, GMC, London, paras 60–2.

20: Public health dimensions of medical practice

The questions covered in this chapter include the following.

- What do we mean by 'health' and what impact might this definition have on health provision?
- What are the goals of public health practice?
- What are the social determinants of health?
- How coercive should health promotion campaigns be?
- What are the benefits and harms of population screening?
- Should patients be given financial incentives to take up a healthy lifestyle?
- What ethical considerations should be taken into account in priority setting?
- How should the release of information about disease outbreaks be managed?

General principles

Public health is a complex and contested notion, nevertheless from a clinical perspective it is broadly agreed that public health is the branch of medical practice that addresses the health of populations rather than individuals. It is carried out not only by public health specialists, for whom it is their main area of work, but also by many health professionals when they engage in activities such as epidemiology, health advocacy and community involvement or commissioning. Public health practice uses the best available evidence to address the fundamental causes of disease and the requirements for health and well-being, aiming to prevent adverse health outcomes. In undertaking this work, public health practice should:

- promote and protect public health to the greatest extent that is compatible with respecting individual rights
- ensure input from all sections of the community, including those who are unable to speak for themselves
- aim to ensure that the basic resources and conditions necessary for a minimally acceptable level of health are available to all
- seek to prioritise interventions that favour underprivileged sections of society
- seek the best available information for carrying out its role
- provide communities with the information that is required for policy decisions and obtain the agreement of those communities, where appropriate, for their implementation
- act in a timely manner on available information within the resources and the mandate given
- incorporate a variety of approaches that respect the diverse beliefs and values in the community
- implement policies in a manner that promotes the integrity of the physical and social environment
- protect the confidentiality of information where appropriate.[1]

Medical Ethics Today: The BMA's Handbook of Ethics and Law, Third Edition. Sophie Brannan, Eleanor Chrispin, Martin Davies, Veronica English, Rebecca Mussell, Julian Sheather and Ann Sommerville.
© 2012 BMA Medical Ethics Department. Published 2012 by Blackwell Publishing Ltd.

The public health perspective

The focus of medical ethics has ordinarily been on the relationship between a doctor and a patient, and this emphasis can be seen reflected in the majority of chapters in this book. At the centre of this relationship lie the interests of the patient, and key ethical principles include a respect for individual autonomy and, stemming from this, the requirement for consent from the patient or, where the patient lacks capacity, a representative, before treatment can begin. (In the absence of a representative, decisions need to be made on the basis of an assessment of the patient's best interests. For further information see Chapters 2 and 3.) The primary duty of doctors in this relationship is understood to be the well-being of their patients. It is increasingly recognised, however, that this one-to-one relationship exists within a wider context, particularly where health provision is publicly funded. Aspects of this broader context include financial limitations, centrally driven targets, the use of health incentives and the health status of broader communities and populations. It also includes social factors with a significant impact on health outcomes such as social inequalities, employment, education and housing.

Although these broader concerns can be diverse, and at times difficult to specify, they share a focus on groups rather than individuals, whether they are local or wider communities, or indeed whole populations. It is this community or population-based approach that gathers many of these issues under the broad umbrella of public health practice. Public health doctors have particular responsibilities in this area, and many of the topics in this chapter deal with areas of practice with which public health doctors will be engaged. However, there is increasing recognition of the impact of these wider considerations on the practice of a range of clinical disciplines which mean that more and more doctors are both exposed to, and interested in, ethical issues arising in this area. This chapter is therefore aimed at all those whose practice has an impact on, or is informed by that broader public health context, as well as all those doctors who seek a deeper understanding of the complex factors that contribute to health outcomes and of the challenging ethical debates they can give rise to.

Sick individuals and sick populations – the prevention paradox

In a seminal 1985 paper, the epidemiologist Geoffrey Rose distinguished between two possible approaches to understanding the occurrence of illness: one focusing on sick individuals and one focusing on sick populations.[2] He identified two corresponding kinds of aetiological question: one seeking the causes of individual cases of an illness, the other seeking to identify the causes of its population incidence. 'Why do some individuals have hypertension', he writes, 'is a very different question from 'Why do some populations have much hypertension, whilst in others it is rare.'[3] 'The determinants of incidence', he goes on to say, 'are not necessarily the same as the causes of cases.'[4] He also identifies separate prevention strategies for dealing with individual cases and with population incidence. For individual cases he outlines the traditional medical 'high-risk' approach which entails identifying individuals who are at a high risk of developing the illness in question and then intervening accordingly. Benefits include the use of interventions appropriate to the individual, enhanced doctor and patient motivation, a favourable ratio of risk to benefit in relation to the intervention, as well as a cost-effective use of resources. Disadvantages, however, include the costs and potential harms of screening, the fact that it does not seek to identify and change the underlying causes of disease, seeking instead to protect those who are vulnerable and the fact that it can require individuals to step outside persuasive social norms of behaviour.

Against the more patient-focused approach to prevention Rose sets the 'population strategy'. This is characterised by an attempt to identify and control population-wide determinants of incidence. Traditionally it has involved environmental controls. More recently it has focused on encouraging population-wide behavioural change. According to Rose, the benefits of the population approach include the potential to deliver large benefits across a population, and it is 'behaviourally appropriate', in that it aims at changing norms rather than asking people to step outside them. In discussing potential drawbacks to the population approach he reintroduces the 'prevention paradox.' This highlights the fact that measures that may have enormous significance for the population as a whole are likely to offer very little benefit, at least in the short term, to individuals. Given that there is only a small likelihood that any given individual will benefit, even small risks can disturb the cost–benefit ratio. For Rose it is important therefore to distinguish between approaches that remove abnormal exposure, such as smoking cessation, and those that rely on a preventive intervention that may have associated risks, such as jogging or vaccination.

Rose's identification of the paradoxes implicit in an approach to the health of populations, and of the tensions that can arise between individual and population interests, have been enormously influential. Recent work in public health law and ethics has begun to explore some of the ethical and legal challenges raised by these insights.[5]

Public health – a changing practice

Until fairly recently, ethical dilemmas arising in public health have been underrepresented in academic and professional literature, although this has begun to change. There are many reasons for this increasing interest. One important factor is the evolving nature of public health practice itself. The origins of current public health practice lie in the nineteenth century with organised interventions to tackle serious external threats to individual health, such as communicable diseases, poor sanitation and a lack of clean drinking water. More recent examples include the clean air legislation of the 1950s. Many of these early public health interventions proved extremely successful. Between 1841 and 1971, for example, overall mortality rates in England dropped from 23 to 7 per 1,000 for males, and from 21 to less than 5 per 1,000 for females. Life expectancy over a similar period increased from 48 to 80 for women and from 44 to 75 for men.[6] Although the management of these traditional public health threats remains important, and they remain major health threats in the developing world, partly as a result of these early successes, a new generation of public health threats has been identified.

Contemporary public health threats

These include:

- tobacco, drug and alcohol misuse
- obesity
- mental illnesses, such as depression and anxiety
- cancer
- dementia and other forms of age-related cognitive impairment
- climate change.

Contemporary public health threats include diseases associated with ageing, such as cancer and dementia, as well as 'lifestyle' related illnesses resulting from tobacco and drug consumption and alcohol misuse. There are also a new generation of health problems which are thought to be linked in complex ways to wide-ranging social change.

Mental illnesses such as depression, as well as obesity and its associated illnesses, are creating a significant and growing health burden with substantial resource implications for health services. Whereas the more traditional health threats have shown themselves responsive to single interventions, such as vaccinations, or to techniques to deal with individual environmental hazards, the new threats are proving less easy to manage. This new generation of problems have complex origins. Obesity, for example, is influenced by psychological, genetic, social and environmental factors, many of which are resistant to traditional public health tools. In addressing these issues, health professionals and policy experts are increasingly looking at ways to influence individual behaviour, and ethical and political questions arise about the extent to which the state should direct personal lifestyle choices. In the more familiar medical model, it is patients who make the decision to visit doctors in search of remedy for a health problem. In these new areas of public health, the state takes the initiative, actively trying to change people's choices, even where those individuals may not have identified any health problems, and may in fact be highly resistant to state pressures. Live issues here include whether people should be offered incentives to make health-promoting choices, whether patient rights to treatment should be linked to obligations to take responsibility for health, as well as the obligations of large non-health actors, such as fast food or soft drink manufacturers.

'Health' – an evolving concept

Early public health interventions were understandably concerned with reducing overall mortality. More recently, however, along with increased life expectancy has come a concern not only with the length of life, but with the quality of the life that is lived. The provision of direct healthcare has traditionally focused on a clinical model of health, with illnesses being seen as a diversion from ordinary biological functioning, and medicine playing a corrective or remedial role. The increasing understanding of the social, economic and environmental sources of health and well-being has led to a broader, richer and arguably more complex model, a model now somewhat notoriously summed up by the World Health Organization (WHO) definition as 'a state of complete physical, mental and social well-being and not merely the absence of disease or infirmity'.[7] Such an inclusive definition of health, although it acknowledges the multi-factorial origins of human flourishing, presents a number of challenges. Such a broad definition inevitably places responsibility for sustaining and promoting health in areas of policy not ordinarily associated with health departments. These include education, the built environment and transport as well as the regulation of commercial organisations that can have an impact on human health, such as airlines and car manufacturers. 'Health' also ceases to be a matter specifically for health professionals and health budgets, and becomes instead a factor in most private and public endeavours, presenting real challenges for health policy. Normative emphasis on ideas of 'total well-being' also raises questions about the imposition of a single universal concept of human functioning that can sit uneasily alongside more pluralistic accounts of necessary conditions for human thriving.

Such an explicitly aspirational definition of health also raises questions about the scope of more traditional health interventions. To what extent, for example, should medical resources be limited to those with identifiable diseases, or should they extend to preventive interventions aimed at those who may not develop a specific disease for many years, if at all? It also invites questions about whether medical technology has a legitimate role in enhancing health and overall well-being, in the meeting of health 'wants' rather than health 'needs', an issue raised by interventions such as tattoo removal or *in vitro* fertilisation (IVF) treatment for infertility. Decline in cognitive functioning, for example, could be said to be a 'natural' feature of ageing. To what extent therefore should public resources be spent to slow or even to reverse this process? On the other hand, acceptance of a 'natural' decline in functioning can lead to less attention being paid to potentially remediable conditions associated with a longer life. Given that life expectancy and the process of ageing are also subject to significant socioeconomic variation, concepts of health will often raise questions of justice. Further, if pharmaceutical interventions are successful in those groups whose cognitive functioning is declining, should they also be offered to those who show no signs of cognitive decline but whose 'ordinary' functioning could be enhanced?[8] Although a detailed discussion of these topics is outside the scope of this chapter, variations in the definition of health or illness can have a significant impact on the nature and scope of the resources available to health budgets. As the definition of health is an important issue in resource allocation, it follows that health has a political dimension, with a profound effect on the way in which needs are prioritised and collective health goods allocated. Resource allocation is discussed in more detail later in the chapter. The box below gives an outline of some of the main conceptual approaches to health.

What do we mean by health?

Health, illness, disease and sickness

Many commentators draw an interesting distinction between illness and disease.[9] Illness is seen as the subjective experience of ill health in terms of pain or suffering, while disease refers to the presence of a disturbance in biological functioning. According to this view it is possible to feel well while having a serious asymptomatic disease in its early stages, and also to feel ill even where there is no underlying pathology. This distinction has clear relevance in a clinical context, enabling a fuller understanding of both the underlying biology of disease and the subjective experience of illness. Some commentators draw a further distinction and see 'sickness' as the adoption of a changed social role resulting from illness.

Health as the absence of disease

According to this approach, health is defined as an absence of any abnormal biological functioning. An influential proponent of this view is Boorse, who states that a disease can be understood as 'a type of internal state which is either an impairment of normal functional ability, i.e. a reduction of one or more functional abilities below typical efficiency, or a limitation on functional ability caused by environmental agencies.'[10] Boorse links 'normal ability' to ideas of species-typical functioning which is ultimately linked to evolutionary concepts of reproductive fitness.

Health as well-being

According to this view, the most important index of health is the individual's subjective feeling of well-being. Although, as indicated above, disease processes can in their early stages be asymptomatic, they will at some point impact upon the subject's sense of wellness. The goal of health interventions therefore becomes the restoration or maintenance of the subjective experience of well-being. As some critics have noted, however, it can be difficult to distinguish between health as a subjective experience of well-being and happiness, a trap that some believe the WHO has fallen into.[11]

Health as agency

Another influential contemporary approach to health sees it as a necessary condition for the achievement of goals. According to this view a person is healthy in so far as he or she has the ability to do those things that are necessary for his or her well-being. Health is therefore a measure of ability, and disease can be understood as anything that restricts an individual's ability to achieve necessary goals. The difficulty here is identifying those things that are necessary for the individual, as opposed, for example, to those that are merely desirable.

Health as a social description

Doctors are involved in more than the clinical assessment of a patient's health. Decisions made by doctors can have an influence on the provision of a wide range of health and social resources. Entitlement to a range of benefits can be dependent on a medical assessment, as can access to social housing. A psychiatric assessment can lead to the restriction of fundamental freedoms, as well as protection from criminal liability, and certain diagnoses can lead to significant social stigma. Notions of health therefore have an important social dimension that cannot easily be reduced to biological functioning.

Public health – the limits to individualism

Another reason for the growth of interest in ethical issues in this area is the increasing recognition, among health professionals, policy makers and the wider public, that a number of important aspects of health cannot be captured by a sole focus on the needs of individuals. While a respect for the informed choices of patients will always be central to medical treatment, there is a danger that too exclusive a focus on patient autonomy can lead to a neglect of other components of health. Health rights may accrue to individuals, and the decision whether or not to have a particular treatment or intervention is always personal, but this can sometimes obscure the reality that the health of any individual is not an exclusively personal matter. Many conditions that are necessary for individual health, such as a positive environment, lie beyond the direct ability of individuals to change them. These conditions require collective action. Influential work by Sir Michael Marmot[12] and others, for example, on the social determinants of health has provided a strong reminder that health is both a shared good and that the health of individuals is strongly influenced by structural factors such as their position in a social hierarchy. In order to improve both individual and population health outcomes, it follows that such structural factors must be addressed.

The individual and the community

Given that a public health perspective can provide valuable insights into the sources of health and well-being that are wider than the individual, a central ethical issue in this area is the relationship between individual freedom and concepts of the 'public good'. Ordinarily, in a liberal country, the usual justification that is given for limiting individual freedoms is the requirement to prevent direct harm to other identifiable individuals. The idea that individual freedoms should be limited on the basis of an appeal to a community, or a population, is less well developed. Partly in response to this problem, public health professionals have traditionally looked to utilitarian reasoning to support their interventions, arguing that it is appropriate to limit certain individual freedoms in order to maximise health gains across a broad population. Fluoridation of water, for example, may restrict the freedoms of those who do not want fluoride added to their water supply, but it is justified on the basis of the benefits that it brings to the dental health of large numbers of people. Overall benefits outweigh overall harms. Such utilitarian reasoning, however, makes use of a very weak idea of community, which is seen as a mere aggregate of individuals. The benefits and harms are calculated in terms of the numbers of individuals among whom they are distributed. More recent work in public health[13] has argued in favour of a stronger concept of community. According to this view there are social goods that are more than aggregates of individual benefits. Factors seen as vital to well-being, including strong social networks, shared purpose and meaningful activity, cannot be reduced to the sum of the individuals they benefit. This approach sees community less as a necessary negative limit to human freedoms and instead as a fundamental requirement for human flourishing. In this way it becomes possible to speak of individual autonomy and concepts of the public good as being deeply related. Rather than seeing public health interventions in opposition to individual freedoms, they can be seen as complementary, with individual freedom requiring goods held in common. Exploring this relationship presents one of the main challenges for the ethics of public health.

Although the majority of doctors are familiar, through daily examples, with the social gradient in health many will also ask what effect this should or could have on their clinical practice. A doctor's primary focus will be on the presenting health need, and the ability to change underlying structures in people's lives that can undermine health will be limited. Marmot, Wilkinson and others have started to look at the ways in which the social environment impacts on biology to bring about disease. Factors such as insecurity, chronic anxiety, isolation, low self-esteem and a lack of control over work are all identified as operating through biological stress responses in the body to bring about long-term physiological changes that undermine health.[14] In this way, insights from public health can feed directly into clinical practice, enabling doctors to work with individuals who are identified as being at long-term risk of health problems. While underlying structures cannot be easily changed, increased knowledge about their physiological impact can help doctors working with patients to mitigate their impact.

The social determinants of health

In 2003, the WHO published a second edition of *The Solid Facts*, a paper summarising the available evidence relating to the impact of social factors on health. The introduction states:

> Health policy was once thought to be about little more than the provision and funding of medical care: the social determinants of health were discussed only among academics. This is now changing. While medical care can prolong survival and improve prognosis after some serious diseases, more important for the health of the population as a whole are the social and economic conditions that make people in need of medical care in the first place.[15]

The paper identifies 10 key areas in which social factors have a clear impact on health outcomes.

1. *The social gradient:* the lower an individual is in the social hierarchy, the poorer his or her health outcomes.
2. *Stress:* anxiety, insecurity, low self-esteem, social isolation and lack of control over work and home life have a powerful impact on health.
3. *Early life:* many of the foundations of adult health are laid down in early childhood.

4. *Social exclusion:* the longer people live in disadvantage, the more likely they are to develop a range of health problems.
5. *Work:* people who have more control over their work have better health.
6. *Unemployment:* higher rates of unemployment are linked to illness and reduced life expectancy.
7. *Social support:* friendship, good relationships and strong social networks improve health.
8. *Addiction:* alcoholism, illicit drug use and cigarette smoking are all associated with social and economic disadvantage.
9. *Food:* a healthy diet and a secure food supply are necessary for good health.
10. *Transport:* cycling, walking and the use of public transport provide exercise and social contact. They also reduce accidents and improve air quality.

Politics and public health – the challenge of justice

On average, people living in the poorest parts of Glasgow die 12 years before those living in the most affluent.[16] In some American cities, the gulf between the richest and poorest is wider still. Globally, the differences are even starker. In Sierra Leone, life expectancy at birth is 34; in Japan it is 81.9.[17] Although doctors working within the NHS will be familiar with the politicised nature of health delivery in the UK, with its ceaseless restructuring, its centrally driven targets and its rapidly changing agendas, public health, by concerning itself increasingly with the impact of social structure and organisation on population health, is political in a deeper sense. Nor is it a matter of absolute levels of wealth. Cuba has seen little economic growth since the 1950s but has managed to maintain improvements in life expectancy in line with the USA. A glance at these figures, and at the WHO's 10 messages (see box above), clearly demonstrates the link between public health and issues of the social distribution of goods, that is between health and broad concepts of social justice. One of the ways in which public health practitioners approach this issue is through exploring the link between health inequalities and health inequities.[18]

Health inequalities are generally understood as being differences in the comparative health status or health outcomes of individuals or groups. For example, there are widely recognised health inequalities between men and women. Men have higher rates of cardio-vascular disease while women have higher rates of osteoporosis.[19] Inequities in health, by contrast, are said to occur when those inequalities come about as a result of conditions that are seen to be unjust. Health inequalities occurring as a result of genetic makeup, while they can be deeply unfortunate, are naturally occurring and therefore not themselves issues in justice – although the availability or otherwise of treatment and support for individuals with genetic disorders may well be. Health inequalities that arise as a result of poverty, such as those in Glasgow, which are not regarded as natural or inevitable, and arise from social conditions that can be subject to modification, are seen to be unjust and therefore matters of inequity in health.

In 2010, the Department of Health for England published *Fair Society, Healthy Lives*, the report of a strategic review of health inequities in England.[20] The purpose of the review was to propose the most effective strategies for reducing health inequities in England from 2010 onwards. The report corroborated the link in England between social determinants and health outcomes particularly in relation to the impact of social status on infant mortality and life expectancy. The earlier, 2009 'first phase' report that preceded *Fair Society, Healthy Lives* drew an interesting distinction between ideas of 'being well' and 'well-being'. 'Being well' was described as the absence of identifiable physical and mental illness. 'Well-being', however, was described as a far more inclusive concept, referring to an active and positive state of mental, physical and social functioning. Well-being 'is not just the absence of pain, discomfort and incapacity, it requires that basic needs are met, that individuals have a sense of purpose, that they feel able to achieve important goals and participate in society'.[21] A decision to focus on well-being over and above being well will clearly involve addressing the social determinants of ill health, including underlying structural issues such as social inequality. It will ask far-reaching questions about the obligations that society has to its citizens and that citizens have both to each other and to their communities and, ultimately, to the state. Such questions will ensure that public health remains an irreducibly political enterprise.

Summary – the public health perspective

- Public health is primarily concerned with the health status of populations.
- The majority of doctors have some public health obligations.
- Public health practice involves the management of communicable disease, environmental health and risks for non-communicable disease and addresses the underlying conditions for good health, including its social determinants.
- Public health practice seeks a recognition of the alignment of individual and public goods in health.

Legal aspects of public health

In addition to the broader political and ethical aspects of public health discussed in the preceding section, public health broadly conceived is subject to legal articulation and regulation in the UK. This section gives a brief outline of some of the most significant aspects of the law in this area. Acting in unison, these legal instruments set the parameters for the maintenance of public health and the provision of health services in the UK.

Health as a positive right

The UK is a signatory to a number of international human rights treaties or covenants. These treaties set internationally agreed standards of respect for human rights that all signatory states have committed themselves to upholding. Although the extent to which these rights are enforceable within the UK is open to debate, in ratifying them the UK has made a commitment to maintaining a certain minimum set of standards in the areas to which they relate. The UK is a signatory to the International Covenant on Economic Social and Cultural Rights (ICESCR). Article 12 of the Covenant imposes a duty on the state in relation to health broadly conceived. The Article is given below in its entirety:

1. The States Parties to the present Covenant recognize the right of everyone to the enjoyment of the highest attainable standard of physical and mental health.
2. The steps to be taken by the States Parties to the present Covenant to achieve the full realization of this right shall include those necessary for:
    (a) the provision for the reduction of the stillbirth-rate and of infant mortality and for the health development of the child

(b)   the improvement of all aspects of environmental and industrial hygiene

(c)   the prevention, treatment and control of epidemic, endemic, occupational and other diseases

(d)   the creation of conditions which would assure to all medical service and medical attention in the event of sickness.[22]

Article 14 (frequently referred to in shorthand as the 'right to health') by looking beyond healthcare delivery to the underlying conditions of health is clearly relevant to a great deal of public health practice. Although the Article is quite abstract, there has been considerable work on developing an understanding of the concrete content of the right. The United Nations Economic and Social Council has issued an authoritative statement on the meaning of the right, known as 'General Comment 14'. It identifies both 'negative' rights, which relate to freedom from interference, and 'positive' rights, which relate to obligations on the state to provide certain minimal conditions and services for health flourishing. It states, for example, that:

> The right to health is not to be understood as a right to be healthy. The right to health contains both freedoms and entitlements. The freedoms include the right to control one's health and body, including sexual and reproductive freedom, and the right to be free from interference, such as the right to be free from torture, non-consensual medical treatment and experimentation. By contrast, the entitlements include the right to a system of health protection which provides equality of opportunity for people to enjoy the highest attainable level of health.[23]

In 2003, the UN Human Rights Council appointed a human rights expert, known as a special rapporteur, to develop and explore the right to health, and successive post holders have further elaborated the content and meaning of the right. Their work has included the development of sophisticated techniques for measuring the extent to which states are meeting their obligations as well as a focus on practical issues such as the development of drugs for rare conditions. Although the nature and extent of specific health obligations under these treaties are currently underdeveloped, the right to health is becoming increasingly understood as a framework for articulating the responsibilities of states in relation to the health, broadly conceived, of its citizens.

Rights to healthcare

The NHS Act

The legal scope of the services provided by the NHS is defined in the National Health Service Act 1977. In England and Wales, the Act imposes on the Secretary of State an obligation to promote a 'comprehensive health service designed to secure improvements (a) in the physical and mental health of the people of those countries, and (b) in the prevention, diagnosis and treatment of illness'.[24] The Act also states that services must be provided free of charge unless the law expressly permits charges to be made. The duty is to 'promote' a comprehensive health service, not to provide one, and although the Act refers both to personal health services and public health promotion, the duty is phrased in such a way as to make direct enforcement difficult.[25] In Scotland these provisions are given in the National Health Service (Scotland) Act 1978.

NHS constitution

In 2009, the NHS for England published a constitution for the NHS setting out the values and principles on which the NHS is based.[26] In 2010, the incoming administration committed itself to upholding that constitution.[27] Although the constitution relates to England, in 2008, Scotland, Wales and Northern Ireland had signed up to a high-level statement of underlying principles with the intention of affirming that the NHS was committed to the same principles across the UK, even where local needs and circumstances dictated variations in the way care was delivered. The constitution set out a series of patient rights and responsibilities and also made a series of commitments to realising certain aspirations that were not legally binding. The constitution did not introduce any new rights, and the obligations on patients – such as to follow any course of treatment agreed upon, to participate in important public health programmes, such as vaccinations, and to provide accurate health information – were not legally enforceable.

Public health law

Given the earlier discussion about the potential scope of the definition of health, unsurprisingly perhaps the question of what constitutes public health law is itself vexed. It can focus, as Gostin suggests, on the full range of 'legal powers and duties of the state to assure the conditions for people to be healthy ... and the limitations on the power of the state to constrain the autonomy, privacy, liberty, proprietary or other legally protected interests of individuals for the protection or promotion of community health'.[28] This inevitably draws the net very wide. Alternatively, it is possible to focus, as below, on a far smaller patchwork of statutes, statutory instruments and government circulars that are aimed at the control of a range of potential health threats. These include legislation to regulate the quality of air and water, to manage infectious diseases, including sexually transmitted diseases, to limit harms generated by motor vehicles and to control potential threats from contaminants, including threats arising from potential terrorist attacks using chemical, biological or radiological substances.

In 2008, new legislation was introduced separately in Scotland, Northern Ireland and in England and Wales to consolidate and to bring up to date legislation relating to threats from both infectious diseases and environmental contaminants.[29] Earlier legislation had been drawn up to reflect Victorian social conditions and had been adapted piecemeal over the ensuing years. Drawing on the WHO's International Health Regulations, this new legislation takes an 'all hazards' approach. Where earlier legislation was restricted to specific diseases, the new approach includes potential contaminants and is flexible enough to deal with new and emerging threats.[30] Additional statutes that are relevant to public health control of a variety of potential threats include the National Assistance Act 1947 and subsequent amendments, the Environmental Protection Act 1990 and the Environment Act 1995, as well as the Water Industry Act 1991.

Infectious disease reporting

Public health legislation contains a number of powers designed to control the spread of infectious diseases.[31] This includes the power to subject individuals to compulsory medical examination, and to remove people who have a notifiable disease to hospital without their consent, or against a competent refusal if necessary, and to detain them there. Furthermore, people with notifiable diseases can be subject to certain restrictions on their movements and anyone with such a disease is not permitted to use public transport, public libraries or public laundries. Those who exercise these powers must, however, have due regard to the individual rights enshrined in the Human Rights Act 1998.

In England and Wales, doctors are statutorily required to notify the 'proper officer' of their local authority of any patient they believe to have a notifiable disease, which includes conditions such as meningitis, plague, tuberculosis and food poisoning. In Scotland, doctors are required to contact the chief administrative medical officer for the area in which the notifying doctor works. In Northern Ireland, doctors are required to notify the communicable disease surveillance centre.

Infectious disease notification: the current law in England, Wales, Scotland and Northern Ireland

If a registered medical practitioner believes or suspects that a person he or she is attending has a notifiable disease, he or she must send to the proper officer a certificate stating:

- the name, age and sex of the patient and the address of the premises where the patient is residing
- the disease or poisoning from which the patient is, or is suspected to be, suffering and the date, or approximate date, of its onset
- if the premises are a hospital, the day on which the patient was admitted, the address of the premises from which the patient came, and whether or not, in the opinion of the person giving the certificate, the disease or poisoning from which the patient is, or is suspected to be, suffering was contracted in the hospital.

Although consent is not required for the disclosure of this information, the doctor should nevertheless explain to the patient his or her duty to make this report.

Unless consent has been obtained for wider disclosure, only the information required by the legislation should be released. In exceptional cases, the need to prevent the spread of a serious disease may constitute an overriding public interest in disclosure, such that a breach of confidentiality would be justified (see Chapter 5, pages 199–202).

Summary – legal aspects of public health

- The UK is a signatory to a variety of international treaties or covenants that impose obligations relating both to the provision of health services and the maintenance of the underlying conditions for health.
- The NHS is subject to legal requirements to promote both a comprehensive health service and to secure improvements in the underlying conditions of health, but the enforcement of these duties is difficult to achieve.
- New public health legislation in the UK has moved away from specified health targets toward a new 'all hazards' approach based on WHO regulations.
- All doctors have a statutory obligation to provide information to an appropriate person about notifiable diseases.
- The agreement and cooperation of infected individuals should be sought, wherever possible, for both reporting notifiable diseases and contact tracing.

Public health threats – tackling diseases, changing lives

As the introductory section to this chapter makes clear, public health is a dynamic discipline in which there is increasing recognition of the variety of factors that interact to create the background conditions for a population's health. Controlling infectious diseases and identifying non-infectious threats from the environment, while a traditional part of public health practice, require responsiveness both to new organisms and new contaminants or other sources of harm, and strategies have to be adapted to the requirements of each particular threat. Alongside this, changing socioeconomic conditions and the success of earlier public health interventions have, as already indicated, combined to create new and emergent challenges. This section looks at a number of representative current threats to health and at the variety of ethical issues that responding to them raises.

Climate change – opportunities and threats

The scale of some of the most significant contemporary public health threats means that it can be very difficult for individuals, and for individual healthcare practitioners, to identify ways to make a practical contribution. There is a consensus, for example, that climate change presents a very serious potential threat to health, particularly to populations that may already be vulnerable, such as those living in areas exposed to coastal flooding or experiencing very low rainfall. It could also lead to global instability in food and water supplies, to the migration of infectious diseases and to increasing numbers of severe weather events. One way in which public health experts are looking to link these large-scale threats to individual behaviour change is by exploring the potential health co-benefits of action to mitigate or to adapt to climate change. In the UK, for example, physical inactivity and the consumption of excessive amounts of animal fats are leading causes of ill health. As transport and cattle farming are major sources of greenhouse gases, promoting walking and cycling, and encouraging diets with fewer animal products can simultaneously improve health and reduce carbon output. While the evidence is convincing, the big challenge is translating these insights into political activity that can lead to change.[32]

Obesity

According to the Department of Health, obesity represents one of the UK's key health threats.[33] WHO figures suggest that the UK has the highest prevalence of obesity in Europe, with nearly one in four of the adult population having a body mass index (BMI) in excess of 30.[34] In the last 30 years, obesity has trebled in the UK, with projections suggesting that at some point between 2010 and 2015 nearly one-third of the population will be obese.[35] Obesity is an important risk factor for a wide range of chronic diseases including type 2 diabetes, hypertension and coronary heart disease. By 2050, the costs of treating obesity and its health and economic consequences is estimated to be in excess of £10 billion a year.[36] Although the biological causes of individual weight gain are straightforward, resulting from the consumption of calories exceeding expenditure, the underlying factors behind the rapid growth of obesity are far more complex. A recent report by the Nuffield Council on Bioethics points to the influence of a large number factors including:

- the development of more highly calorific and processed foods with increased levels of salt and sugar to make it more palatable

- food becoming cheaper and far more widely available
- increased portion sizes
- changing patterns of home life that have led to a decrease in 'traditional' eating patterns, a loss of cooking skills and a greater reliance on processed and take away foods which often have higher salt, sugar and fat contents
- aggressive marketing of energy-rich foods
- the replacement of walking and cycling with motorised transport
- the increasingly sedentary nature of both work and recreation.[37]

The Government's report *Tackling Obesities – Future Choices* places the responsibility for increasing levels of obesity on the combination of underlying human biology, which has a propensity to store and conserve energy, and an 'obesogenic environment', a combination of sedentary work and leisure patterns and enormously increased availability of energy-rich foods, which has exposed our underlying biological vulnerability.[38] The report groups the factors that regulate our energy balance into four areas: physiology, eating habits, levels of activity and the influence of psychosocial factors. From these it draws the following key determinants of obesity:

- primary appetite control in the brain
- the force of dietary habit
- levels of physical activity
- psychological difficulties in making lifestyle choices.[39]

Earlier in this chapter attention was drawn to those aspects of health that are not easily reducible to questions of personal choice and individual autonomy. Although we are at liberty to make choices about what we eat and how we exercise, environmental factors clearly shape them, inclining some to make healthier choices than others. Obesity has a social gradient and its resulting disease burden contributes to social inequities in health. Doctors and other health professionals can provide advice on diet and exercise, and can address some of the health problems arising from obesity, but the extent to which individuals act upon the information provided will depend upon a variety of factors that have their origins in individual psychology and background. As *Tackling Obesities* points out:

> The encouragement of physical activity in daily life or modifying the nutritional balance of the diet might appear at first glance to be relatively simple to achieve. In fact, the scale of change required to make a significant impact at the population level would need to be very substantial, raising difficult and complex economic and social questions about how public policy can be reshaped across a number of very diverse areas, including food production, food manufacturing, retailing and marketing, healthcare, town planning, transport, education, culture and trade.[40]

Although a successful response to obesity will require widespread change to the 'obesogenic' environment, including changes to transport policy and the built environment, given that benefits stemming from these changes will take considerable time to feed through to individuals, health professionals have also been looking at innovative methods of encouraging behaviour change. While many people may wish to lose weight, dieting frequently has only short-term success and sustaining weight loss can prove difficult. Key issues in promoting behaviour change therefore include inducing people to desire healthy outcomes and, once healthy preferences have been established, encouraging people to sustain them. One approach that is being explored is the use of incentives, either direct financial incentives or incentives in kind, such as free or discounted gym membership, or, in relation to private healthcare, cost reductions contingent upon healthy choices. The use of incentives raises a number of interesting ethical questions. Although at times incentives are said to reinforce the desirability of choices that people would make anyway, they will also involve attempts to induce people to make choices they would not otherwise. In justifying the use of incentives, appeal must therefore be made to ideas of autonomy more complex than the respecting of short-term preferences. The use of incentives in the management of obesity suggests that public health will make use of a more paternalistic practice. A more objective judgement of the conditions for personal flourishing is used as the justification for directing individual choices, choices that are understood to be beneficial not only to the individual, but, through health savings, the wider public. Greater detail about ethical issues arising from the use of specific public health tools is given later in the chapter.

'Libertarian paternalism' – making healthy choices easier

One approach that innovative public health specialists are currently exploring in relation to lifestyle-based health problems such as obesity has been described as 'libertarian', 'soft' or 'asymmetric' paternalism. Sometimes involving techniques referred to as 'nudging', such an approach involves making healthy choices easier – the 'paternalistic' part – while leaving people free to make less-healthy choices should they so wish – the 'libertarian' part. Examples include replacing high-calorie snacks next to tills with fruit, thus reducing the likelihood of 'impulse' purchases of foods with high sugar or fat content. Those who want to buy crisps or chocolate are able to do so, but it supports those who struggle to make choices in their own longer-term interests.

Public health emergencies

Where obesity presents a structural, developing and chronic threat to population health, unpredictable events such as terrorist attacks, natural or man-made disasters and outbreaks of highly infectious diseases, such as influenza pandemics, can make very different demands. As indicated above, tackling lifestyle diseases raises long-term questions about the nature of the relationships between individuals, the state and the public good. In emergencies, the focus is on tackling the immediate threat to health and utilitarian reasoning is often invoked, ensuring that interventions are justified on the basis of ensuring the maximum benefit to the largest number of individuals. When the risk to public health is very high, even apparently draconian measures may be justified. If the level of risk to public health is low, such actions would not be proportionate. In this section we look at some general lessons that have been learnt from the British experience of the H1N1 pandemic in 2009–2010. Fortunately, H1N1 turned out to be far less virulent than feared, but it nevertheless triggered a great deal of ethical reflection, much of which is relevant to a wide range of large-scale public health emergencies, particularly those where health need stemming from the emergency significantly outstrips available resources.

Policy making in the face of future threats

In developing public health policy the usual process is to assess, as accurately as possible, the level and severity of risk to public health and, on the basis of that assessment, to devise a system of public protection that is proportionate to those risks. One of the difficulties that frequently arises in practice, however, is the lack of clear evidence on which to base accurate risk assessment. An important part of the role of those planning public health policies, therefore, is to predict, using the best information available at the time, the likely scale of the problem, so that an appropriate response can be initiated. Given that this will always be a matter of judgement, and that it is often not feasible to wait until more evidence is available, these decisions are often controversial. Planning models for the H1N1 pandemic were based on extrapolations from earlier flu pandemics, the 'Hong Kong flu' of 1968–1969, the 'Asian flu' of 1957 and, by far the most virulent, the 1918 'Spanish flu' which is estimated to have killed between 40 and 50 million people worldwide.[41] In hindsight, given the relative mildness of H1N1, questions were asked about how responses drawn from modelling based on earlier pandemics could be made sufficiently flexible to respond proportionately to more modest threats.

The importance of fair process

In order for any response to a large-scale public health emergency to be ethically defensible, consideration has to be given to questions of procedural ethics – to ensuring that decisions are made openly, accountably, transparently, by appropriate bodies and with full public participation. Public acceptance of rationing decisions, and their cooperation in a health emergency, is more likely if citizens accept the fairness and legitimacy of allocation decisions, and have been informed beforehand of the expected response. Advance discussion of the decision-making process, and of the ethical principles and reasoning upon which decisions are made is likely to lead to greater public acceptance.

The need for proportionality

It is possible that decisions about access to scarce resources that are taken during the course of an emergency will result in some people dying who would, in less extreme circumstances, have been saved. Human rights legislation allows for derogation from fundamental rights where it is both necessary and proportional to the required goal.

Resource allocation

Ordinarily, the provision of health services in the NHS is linked to an assessment of clinical need. Those with the greatest need are given priority and treatment is provided until it becomes futile. Where resources are scarce they are effectively rationed by waiting times. In the face of an emergency, decisions about how to meet individual need can give way to decisions about how to maximise overall benefit. The requirement to meet the needs of the most ill individuals may give way to quantitative decisions based on maximising the overall reduction of mortality and morbidity, and the need to maintain vital social functions. Treatment may also have to be withdrawn from some patients to allow their application to patients with a higher survival probability.

During an emergency, decisions may need to be made about whether treatment should be withdrawn from those already receiving it in favour of other individuals who are more likely to benefit, or to benefit more quickly, so that others can be treated. The fact that a course of treatment has already started need not necessarily be determinative. The morally relevant factor will be to ensure the maximisation of overall health benefit from a given health resource, not the continuation of a treatment procedure that has already commenced.

Triage

Triage is a form of rationing or allocation of scarce resources under critical or emergency circumstances where decisions about who should receive treatment must be made immediately because more individuals have life-threatening conditions than can be treated at once. Triage sorts or grades persons according to their needs and the probable outcomes of intervention. It can also involve identifying those who are so ill or badly injured that even with aggressive treatment they are unlikely to survive and should therefore be set aside for non-treatment. Any system of triage has to be simple enough to be practical in emergency conditions and flexible enough to respond to rapid changes in available resources. In disaster triage, priority will normally be given to those whose conditions are the most urgent, the least complex and who are likely to live the longest, thereby maximising overall benefit in terms of reduced mortality and morbidity.

Medical utility

During an emergency, the main focus of health professionals' attention is on delivering the greatest medical benefit to the greatest number of people. Although the majority of health professionals will be involved in making decisions about individual patients, strategic public health decisions will also need to be made about how best to maximise overall utility. During the critical stages of an emergency, it is unlikely that an initial application of utilitarian principles in clinical decision making will be seriously challenged. The difficulty lies in applying the general principles to a complex, unpredictable and evolving health crisis of uncertain duration and extent. Ethical questions are likely to arise, however, where the requirements of medical utility have been met, but choices between individuals with equal need still have to be made. In these circumstances, consideration may need to be given to an egalitarian approach that ensures a fair distribution of resources.

Social utility

If the public health emergency is severe, decisions about the most beneficial distribution of resources will not be restricted to medical utility alone. Where the emergency results in widespread social and economic disruption, decisions about which groups will have first call on scarce resources will also contain elements of social utility. In addition to delivering maximum direct clinical benefit, priorities during a severe emergency are likely to include:

- limiting social disruption
- ensuring maintenance of healthcare systems
- ensuring integrity of social infrastructure
- limiting economic losses.

Scientific and medical functioning

An important aspect of any coordinated response to an emergency such as a pandemic is the need to protect key individuals who are involved in the production of countermeasures, which could include vaccines, antivirals and other essential health products. Special measures will also need to be introduced to protect those personnel who are involved in the provision of health services, and those involved in protecting public health.

Social functioning and critical infrastructure

In addition to those individuals broadly involved in tackling the health aspects of the emergency, many public and private actors are necessary to ensure both the successful delivery of health interventions and the long-term public safety. These include personnel in the emergency services, security, essential products and services, the maintenance of critical infrastructure such as transportation, utilities, telecommunications and sanitation. Priority will also need to be given to the continued function of governance structures. Consideration will also have to be given to the families of key workers.

Management of risk to health professionals

During public health emergencies it is possible that health professionals may find themselves exposed to risks of serious harm. In its 1988 discussion of the responsibilities of doctors to put themselves at risk in the aftermath of a nuclear attack, the British Medical Association (BMA) stated: 'professional concern for the injured should be tempered with reason, and doctors or nurses should not consider it a duty to risk their lives'.[42]

Although this related to the specific conditions of doctors fatally exposing themselves to fallout to treat patients who would almost certainly die, it is possible to apply these general principles more widely. In *Good Medical Practice*, the General Medical Council (GMC) states: '[y]ou must not refuse to treat a patient because you may be putting yourself at risk. If patients pose a risk to your health or safety you should take reasonable steps to protect yourself before investigating their condition or providing treatment.'[43] Discussing review of this guidance in 2005, the BMA's Medical Ethics Committee argued that there were limits to the risks doctors could be expected to accept as part of their professional responsibilities and there may be situations when a doctor could justify not treating a patient because of the extreme risks involved.

Liability issues

Depending upon the nature of the emergency it may be necessary to 'draft in' retired health professionals. The skills of these professionals may not meet expected standards of fitness to practise, but they may nevertheless be able to make a vital contribution. In extreme circumstances, even untrained staff may be required to undertake some functions. In this context, it may be necessary to consider the development of legislation that would restrict liability to cases of wilful misconduct in an emergency.

Managing threats in the face of uncertainty – the case of CJD

Although Creutzfeldt–Jakob disease (CJD) was first identified in the 1920s, public concern about the disease increased with the identification, in 1996, of a new variant (vCJD) linked to bovine spongiform encephalopathy (BSE), more commonly known as 'mad cow disease', and believed to be transmitted through the consumption of infected beef products. Although CJD is rare, with annual deaths in the UK ranging between 28 and 87,[44] given the numbers of people potentially exposed to vCJD through the food chain, there has been concern that cases might rise significantly and the disease could present a major threat to public health. Although by 2010 these concerns had not been realised, the management of CJD and its variants have presented a number of significant ethical challenges. Since the beginning of 2000, the BMA's Medical Ethics Committee has responded to a number of consultations from government agencies, and this section outlines key ethical questions raised by this evolving public health threat.

CJD – a little understood disease

There is considerable uncertainty surrounding many aspects of the transmissibility of CJD and its variants. It is a rare and ultimately fatal degenerative brain disease, one of a group of diseases called transmissible spongiform encephalopathies (TSEs) which affect both humans and animals. TSEs are thought to be caused by the build up in the brain of an abnormal form of a naturally occuring 'prion' protein, although controversy about its origins remains. The disease comes in several forms, including an inherited form, a naturally occurring 'sporadic' form of unknown origin, iatrogenic forms linked to transmission of the disease during medical treatment and the new variant that is associated – although the link has not been categorically proven – with the consumption of beef products contaminated with the bovine form of the disease. There is no known cure for the disease, nor any currently available prophylaxis, and there is considerable uncertainty about the mode of transmission, the incubation period and the likelihood that exposure to the abnormal prion through food or via medical treatment will result in the development of the disease. Early in 2011 the development of a pre-symptomatic test for vCJD was announced.[45] In the absence of a cure for the disease, such a test can enable infected individuals to make decisions about how to spend the time available to them.

Harmful knowledge

Given the severity of the disease, and given the strong likelihood that it could be passed on via surgical instruments – the abnormal prion is resistant to ordinary sterilisation procedures – and through contaminated blood and tissue products, it was a matter of clear public importance that appropriate precautionary measures were taken to limit transmission as far as possible. Although the removal of potentially contaminated meat products from the food chain was uncontroversial, managing information about people who may have been exposed to the prion in order to minimise secondary transmission was far more challenging.

One of the key ethical questions that needed to be addressed was the extent to which it would be appropriate to inform people that they might have been exposed to CJD.

Informing patients about possible exposure

In August 2002, a patient at Middlesborough General Hospital was unexpectedly diagnosed as having CJD after a brain biopsy. In the period between the biopsy and the diagnosis being received, the same surgical instruments were used in other patients' operations, raising the possibility that they may have been exposed to the risk of transmission of CJD. The Government's advisory group, the CJD Incidents Panel, advised that, of the 34 patients in Middlesborough who were subsequently operated on using the same instruments, 24 should be contacted and informed of their possible exposure, even though at the time there was no test that could confirm their infection and there were no steps that could be taken to prevent or delay the onset of the condition if they had been infected. A subsequent independent review of the incident, carried out for the Department of Health, reported that, after ongoing assessment, it appeared that not all of the patients who were contacted were, in fact, at any real risk of exposure, and for those who were, the risk was described as 'very small'.[46]

In the scenario described in the box above, several interests had to be balanced. Identifying and contacting all individuals who may have been exposed would ensure that future risks from those individuals could, theoretically, be better managed. It could also assist in gathering knowledge about the natural history and progression of the disease and enable researchers to identify potential participants for future studies. Given the lack of a cure or prophylaxis, and the level of uncertainty about what exposure meant in terms of likelihood of contracting the disease, informing people that they had been exposed and might go on to develop the disease clearly involved imparting burdensome information without any direct benefits to the individual. As the independent review demonstrated as well, the risks were in fact very small or non-existent, while the knowledge of exposure presented potential, if unquantifiable, psychological harms. The BMA expressed serious concerns about the potential harm of informing all people who were potentially exposed and argued that an appropriate balance needed to be reached between harms to the individual and broader public health benefits.

Ensuring a safe blood supply

One of the most significant sources of potential transmission for CJD was identified as being the blood supply for transfusion. Again the public health interest in ensuring a safe supply of blood is clearly very significant. Anticipating the development of a blood test for CJD, the Health Protection Agency (HPA), working with the UK Blood Services (UKBS), held an expert seminar on ethical and social issues that might arise should a blood test become available.[47] A key recommendation of the seminar and the subsequent report was that, should a blood test become available, potential donors should be asked to consent for testing for CJD and would be informed of the outcome. If individuals did not want to be informed of the outcome, they would not be able to donate.

Such an approach raised a number of ethical concerns. The primary reason for introducing a test for vCJD on blood donations would be to improve the safety of blood transfusions for patients in the UK. Where a reliable test was available, the most effective way of ensuring public safety would be to test individuals and to inform them of their status. Blood that may have been exposed to the abnormal prions would be removed from the supply, and individuals who have tested positive would be advised not to donate blood, organs or tissue, and to notify surgical teams before any future surgery. Secondary benefits would include the opportunities to enrol individuals in research to improve understanding of the disease, its prevalence and transmissibility, and enable individuals to be contacted should treatments become available. If the test had a fairly low specificity, however, a comparatively large number of false positives could be expected. It would therefore be difficult to assess whether a positive test indicated an individual's true infective status or whether a true positive test meant that the individual would go on to develop the disease.

Given the uncertainty surrounding the test, and its potential for both psychological harm and reducing levels of blood donation, in the BMA's view there were strong arguments for changing the UKBS policy in relation to vCJD and for giving donors the option of not receiving their test results. The blood from donors who tested positive could be used for research so donors would not be able to infer their status. Although the HPA expressed some concern about the legal situation where blood was taken but not used as intended, in the BMA's view, if the donor consents to their blood being used either for donation or research, this should not be an issue. However, there were one or two other problems associated with this approach, including the following.

- The full public health benefits of informing individuals of their test results would not be realised as individuals would not themselves be able to inform health professionals, in relation to future surgical or other interventions, that they might be at risk.
- Opportunities for research, and, potentially, for future treatment or management options may not be available to the patient, although all donors could be contacted at a later stage once more information became available.

In the BMA's view, however, donors should be given the opportunity of not receiving information about their test results.

Summary – public health threats

- Public health interventions need to seek ways to promote individual and public goods.
- Large-scale public health emergencies may require an approach focused on maximising overall health outcomes.
- Where public health threats are characterised by very high degrees of uncertainty, careful consideration may be required when informing individuals of potential risks.

Public health tools

Earlier sections in this chapter sketched out some of the central ethical concerns raised by public health practice and also looked at both established and emerging threats to health. Over the years, public health practice has developed, and is continuing to develop, a range of tools designed to tackle these threats. In addition to the benefits that are sought, each intervention may carry inherent risks or necessitate balancing potential restrictions of individual liberties against benefits that may accrue to the wider community. All public health tools therefore have the potential for controversy and can meet resistance from citizens who may question whether the restrictions or sacrifices that might be involved are justified. Although there are a wide range of such tools, this section focuses on a number of key public health interventions that raise indicative ethical dilemmas: health promotion campaigns as a means of influencing behaviour; initiatives to alter the environment to maximise benefit to the health of communities; population screening for diseases; vaccinations and the use of incentives as a preventative measure against the spread of communicable diseases. The section also looks at the impact of the media on public health initiatives.

Health promotion campaigns

Health promotion is clearly a core function of public health. The WHO defines it broadly as the 'process of enabling people to increase control over their health and its determinants, and thereby improve their health'.[48] This section takes a slightly narrower focus, and looks at targeted campaigns designed to change public attitudes towards unhealthy lifestyle choices and to promote the uptake of healthier lifestyles.

Understood simply as a means of public education, health promotion campaigns are a relatively uncontroversial public health tool, which only those who object to any but the most minimal state intervention would criticise. The dissemination of positive health messages or information about the causes of ill health can empower individuals, enabling them to make informed decisions about lifestyle choices and to improve their access to healthcare. Health campaigns, however, often go beyond public education and actively seek to influence personal choices and change behaviours. These interventions can entail varying degrees of coercion; including legal restrictions, taxation and labelling of risk as well as the active suppression of certain images or messages. This can raise questions over acceptable levels of state interference in the lives of individuals and in the business practices of companies who stand to profit from unhealthy lifestyle choices.

There are numerous examples of campaigns which seek to promote healthy living or better understanding of ill health. Obesity, sexual health and excessive alcohol consumption have all been targeted by health promotion campaigns in recent times. This section focuses on tobacco control, one of the best-established and longest-running health promotion campaigns in the UK and one in which the BMA has been heavily involved.

Tobacco control

The anti-smoking campaign is possibly the most extensive public health intervention of its kind. Since the link between tobacco and ill health was first identified by Sir Richard Doll and Sir Austin Bradford Hill in the 1950s there has been a concerted effort on behalf of the Government to discourage people from smoking and to restrict the freedoms of the tobacco industry. Throughout this time, the BMA was heavily involved in campaigns to raise awareness of the health risks associated with tobacco use and published a number of reports on the social and environmental influences that can normalise smoking behaviour and lead to young people taking up the habit.[49]

Tobacco control encompasses a wide range of interventions entailing various levels of state involvement and coercion. Although the extent of these interventions is perhaps unique to this campaign, many of the tools and strategies that have been developed in this area are now increasingly being applied to other health promotion campaigns – food labelling to help prevent obesity and taxation on alcohol, for example – thereby raising similar ethical questions.

Tobacco control regulation

Control measures include:

- comprehensive ban on advertising and promotion of tobacco products including the sponsorship of sporting events
- restrictions on broadcasting smoking on television and radio to protect young people
- age restrictions on the sale of tobacco to young people
- enforced labelling depicting written health warnings, the disclosure of ingredients, a ban on misleading descriptors like 'light' or 'mild' and images illustrating the negative health consequences of smoking
- duty imposed on purchasing and importing tobacco goods
- ban on smoking in indoor workplaces and indoor public places.

Combined with hard-hitting and emotive mass-media communication campaigns, the measures outlined in the box above represent a concerted effort to influence behaviour change in individuals. Given that people are broadly informed of the health threats posed by tobacco use, it could be argued that, as people have rights that provide them with the opportunity to make unhealthy choices, coercing individuals into behaviour change is an unacceptable and paternalistic extension of the role of the state. Such an argument, however, fails to take into account the huge costs smoking imposes on the NHS and the complex factors contributing to tobacco use. Smoking has both age and social gradients and is also subject to gender variation. The addictive nature of tobacco use, and the fact that many people start at an early age when the full implications of the hazards may not be appreciated, also mean that a simple model of autonomous choice is unlikely to be adequate. Most people will, at times, act in ways that they recognise are not in their best interests and a majority of smokers report that, but for the addiction, they would like to give up smoking altogether.[50] As with many other 'lifestyle' threats, a key challenge is therefore developing methods for encouraging people to act on positive preferences in a sustainable fashion. It could be argued therefore that health promotion campaigns have a role in promoting and reinforcing autonomous choices, rather than restricting them.

Although public health campaigns frequently involve widespread dissemination of information about health threats and how best to make health-promoting choices, decisions to start smoking are often influenced by a wider cultural environment which can promote positive images of smoking. Where films, television programmes, advertising and other influential media outlets show positive representations of smokers and smoking, they can generate resistance to health information campaigns. Part of the long-term goal of public health campaigns can be to bring about a change in this deeper information environment, thereby making unhealthy choices less attractive.

The argument that smoking represents an autonomous choice and should not be subject to state interference is also challenged by the recognition that historically tobacco companies had a significant role in encouraging smoking. Advertisements and positive product placements throughout the media have promoted positive images of smoking, and a key part of the public health response to tobacco use has involved curtailing the influence of the tobacco industry. Restricting access to harmful products, minimum pricing, strict regulations on advertising and enforced labelling of health risks are all strategies that make it more difficult for companies to sell tobacco products. Interventions that restrict the freedoms of businesses can face fierce opposition and legal challenges. Nevertheless they can be regarded as necessary in order to ensure that the information environment is balanced and individuals are not subject to coercive commercial pressures to take up or sustain unhealthy choices.

Health promotion campaigns are not just aimed at discouraging those that regularly make unhealthy choices, but also at preventing or discouraging the uptake of these practices, particularly among young people. Here again we see the limitations of an autonomy-based approach to public health. By and large we acknowledge, as a society, that younger people are more vulnerable to manipulation. Given that around two-thirds of current or former smokers started smoking regularly before the age of 18, young people are clearly an important group to target to reduce uptake of the habit.[51] Although age restrictions exist to prevent access to harmful substances, the prevalence of smoking and smoking-related imagery within society can be attractive to young people and can have a negative influence on the lifestyle decisions they make.[52] Hard-hitting education campaigns and interventions deglamourising smoking can therefore help to dissuade young people from making this unhealthy lifestyle choice and therefore help to protect this vulnerable group against the potential harms.

Discussion of the appropriate limits of state intervention in individual life choices often invokes a principle of third-party harm: that the only justification for the state to restrict an individual's freedom is to prevent harm to another, not to the individual. The protection of the public from the harms of second-hand smoke, for example, was a key motivation in introducing the ban on smoking in indoor public places and work places. As the direct burden of ill-health that stems from smoking falls largely upon the smoker, however, once third-party harms are minimised, arguments for intervention into the personal lives of individuals from this principle are not very strong. The difficulty here is that it is not always easy to identify precisely where harms fall. There may, for example, be considerable indirect harms caused by unhealthy living and policy makers have a duty to consider the cost to the public purse of health-damaging behaviour and to take appropriate action to minimise it. Chronic morbidity associated with smoking places a significant financial burden on state-funded healthcare. The responsibility for meeting these costs falls on all members of society, including those who choose not to participate in unhealthy living. A common argument in defence of tobacco control policies is that some degree of intervention is therefore justified in order to limit these wider harms.

Summary – health promotion campaigns

- Health promotion is a core public health function.
- The dissemination of positive health messages and information about health threats can empower people to make informed choices.
- Key challenges in health promotion include encouraging people to make positive health choices that are sustainable over time.

Changing the environment

A great deal of public health activity is focused on making changes to the overall environment in which populations live. Since the Sanitary Act was introduced in 1866, requiring local authorities to supply running water and to remove sewerage and waste, there have been a number of measures introduced to help secure the environmental conditions conducive to healthy living. The idea of the 'environment' is complex, and ranges from the quality of food, air and water supply, through to the standard of the built environment, the control of traffic, the reduction of noise pollution and the quality of the public service infrastructure. Interventions that alter the environmental conditions in which people live are especially effective public health tools as they enable large numbers of people to benefit but without requiring any significant behaviour change from individuals. By creating or sustaining environments conducive to healthy living, governments can also address the social determinants of ill health and help to tackle inequalities.

Efforts to change environmental conditions can be controversial. The ongoing debate surrounding the fluoridation of the water supply encapsulates both the key motivations for an intervention of this kind and the ethical issues that can arise from its proposed introduction.

Fluoridation of water – state beneficence or individual freedom?

Dental caries (tooth decay) is a major oral health problem in most industrialised countries, with children an especially vulnerable group. In the UK, levels of dental caries vary[53] with children in socially deprived areas more likely to have decayed, missing or filled teeth than those in areas that are more affluent. The benefits of fluoridated water to help combat the problem of dental caries were discovered in the 1930s and there is now a body of evidence to show that the artificial fluoridation of the mains water supply is an effective and economical public health tool for improving the oral health of a particular area.[54] Fluoridation is a redistributive intervention that especially favours children and the underprivileged sections of society that are most at risk of dental caries. Although there are health risks associated with high concentrations of fluoride, the levels permitted within the UK are considered safe. Dental fluorosis, a developmental defect of tooth enamel, is a known adverse effect of exposure to fluoridated water. The severity of the condition can range from barely visible white speckling to staining or pitting of the tooth enamel which can be of aesthetic concern. Where it occurs, the majority of fluorosis cases are mild. Estimates regarding the prevalence of fluorosis of aesthetic concern can vary; some studies[55] estimate it to be 12.5 per cent in areas where the water supply is fluoridated at one part per million, while other research estimates the prevalence to be lower.[56] Studies into fluoridation have not found evidence to substantiate a link between the artificial fluoridation of the water supply and increased incidence of bone fracture, osteoporosis, cancer or other adverse effects.

Despite evidence suggesting that it can improve oral health and help address dental inequalities, fluoridation remains controversial. Only something in the region of 10 per cent of the UK population receive water that is either naturally or artificially fluoridated and there are no artificial schemes in place outside of England.[57] Despite legislation that allows health authorities in England and different bodies within the devolved administrations to fluoridate water supplies after appropriate public consultation, few have taken up the opportunity. The decision of Southampton Primary Care Trust (PCT) in 2009 to fluoridate its water supply was the first decision of its kind in over 25 years.[58]

Objections to the artificial fluoridation of water centre on the belief that it constitutes the forced medication of a population without the consent of individuals in that area, that it restricts their choices about the water they and their children drink and ignores any values they might have, for example on the purity of the water. That these concerns can be decisive in obstructing the implementation of fluoridation schemes, despite their considerable benefits, highlights the tensions that exist between the need to protect what is sometimes claimed as a 'right' of individuals to drink non-fluoridated water and the need to create conditions that benefit some individuals within a specific area, but at small potential cost to others. It would clearly be impossible to obtain individual consent from all citizens within an affected population. Fluoridating a water supply also inevitably restricts individual choice because it is not possible for those living in the targeted area to opt out or choose an alternative water supply once a fluoridation scheme has been implemented. People are able purchase bottled water as an alternative if their water supply is fluoridated; however, the cost of doing so is likely to be prohibitive for many people. Not all areas would be suitable for fluoridated water and only those known to suffer high levels of dental caries would reap the full benefit from its introduction. Even within these areas there will be sections of the local population who have good oral health that would be forced to receive fluoridated water even though they are unlikely to benefit from its introduction. It is imperative within public health medicine that methods are developed to resolve this type of conflict. Large-scale interventions will rarely be unopposed but where there are limited harms resulting from an intervention, the absence of consent from a minority should not ordinarily be sufficient to obstruct the delivery of a genuine benefit to the majority of a population.

In discussing the ethical issues associated with the fluoridation of water supplies the Nuffield Council on Bioethics stated that the key motivations for fluoridating a water supply – tackling health inequalities, reducing harm to children and creating an environment conducive to health – were all consistent with the responsibilities a liberal state has to intervene in the interests of public health.[59] The Council recognised that, despite the evidence of the health benefits of fluoridation, there was a lack of high quality evidence regarding potential harms. Local consultation and adequate dissemination of the pros and cons of fluoridation were seen as imperative to address concerns regarding the absence of individual consent and to enable the public to make informed decisions appropriate to the needs of the local area. The BMA supports the fluoridation of water supplies, after appropriate public consultation, on the grounds of effectiveness, safety and equity.

Summary – changing the environment

- Interventions that alter the environmental conditions in which people live are effective public health tools as large numbers of people can benefit but without requiring any significant behaviour change from individuals.
- Measures which alter people's environment can be controversial as it is often not possible to obtain consent from everyone within a population for the measure to be introduced.
- The debate over the fluoridation of water is an example of the tensions that can exist between the motivations for an intervention of this kind and the ethical issues that can arise from its proposed introduction.

Population screening

Screening involves the systematic testing of a defined, usually asymptomatic, population for a specific disorder with the aim of identifying those requiring further investigation or direct medical intervention. In the UK, screening programmes are employed to help detect cancer, sexually transmitted infections (STIs), vascular disease and diseases in pregnancy, newborn babies and children, although different schemes are in place in each of the devolved nations. In some respects, screening is different from other forms of healthcare. Typically, it is the patient who approaches the health worker in search of relief or treatment for a particular disorder. With screening, however, the health service usually approaches apparently healthy individuals and invites them to undergo a test or survey from which they may derive some benefit. Clearly, in such circumstances those offering a screening programme need to be certain that there is a substantive benefit to health, and that it outweighs any resulting harms. According to the National Screening Committee (UK NSC), 'it is unknown to find a programme that gives 100 per cent benefit'.[60] It is vital, therefore, that an informed judgement is made about the programme's ability to provide a net good for those being screened. Although screening in the private sector is likely to be driven by market forces, the same rigorous standards should apply.

Criteria for introducing a screening programme

There is general consensus about the basic criteria that must be fulfilled prior to the introduction of any new screening programme and the UK NSC publishes its appraisal criteria on its website.[61]

- The problem must be important. This includes conditions that are important because they affect a relatively high proportion of the population as well as conditions that are less common but are very severe.
- A suitable screening test should be available. The test being used must be not only reliable, but also effective at detecting the condition being sought. It must have both a high sensitivity and a high specificity, as well as a high positive predictive value (a high proportion of positive results should be true positives). A high positive predictive

value is not so important if the screening test is being backed up by a 'gold standard' follow-up test.
- The results must provide useful information. There are a number of ways in which the results of screening may be useful. They may, for example:
  - permit early diagnosis followed by effective management of the condition
  - give information that would offer increased choices
  - provide information to permit planning for the future, for both the individual and the health service
  - prevent the spread of disease
  - in the case of prenatal screening, give time to prepare for the birth of a disabled child
  - permit lifestyle changes to minimise the risk of disability or disease
  - give time to adapt one's lifestyle to an impending disability.

  Screening that provides no benefit to the individuals being tested would not meet these criteria but may be helpful for planning the health needs of populations or groups.
- The benefits must outweigh the harms. Benefits would include the provision of curative treatment, the ability to prioritise treatment services effectively, patient well-being and satisfaction, and the promotion of informed decision making. These need to be balanced against any actual or perceived adverse effects, particularly those resulting from false positive or false negative results, the risks of labelling people as 'sick', the social disadvantages of the information being available and the likelihood of increased anxiety. Some form of cost–benefit analysis is also needed because, whenever different disciplines and treatments compete for limited funding, any screening programme must make good use of resources.
- Adequate provision must be made for information, counselling and privacy. Careful consideration should be given to the provision of information about the test and its implications, and the need for and the availability of counselling. Assurances must be provided that the information obtained will remain confidential. Patients should be made aware if information will be used for planning or research purposes in an anonymised form. Information should be provided about the potential uses of the data that will be collected, including the implications for insurance and employment where appropriate.

Benefits and harms

Before a particular type of population screening is recommended, the UK NSC must be satisfied that the benefits, such as those outlined above, outweigh the harms. One of the known harms of screening is the raised levels of anxiety that have been reported in all forms of screening programmes including cervical, breast and general health screening, as well as genetic screening. (For specific information on genetic screening see Chapter 9.) For some people, simply receiving an invitation to participate in screening causes anxiety and some have been found to be more anxious after screening than before, regardless of the result. It should also be remembered that the motivation of those offering the screening may be different from that of the individuals who accept it. The service is provided in order to identify people who are at risk, but most individuals, believing themselves to be healthy, undertake screening for reassurance that they are not at risk. Some people therefore accept screening without properly considering the implications of receiving an unfavourable result; when they do not receive the expected result, their certainty about their health status shifts to uncertainty and this can cause considerable anxiety.[62]

There is little that can be done to counter such reactions except to ensure that individuals are provided with an adequate supply of accurate information in a manner they are able to understand and are given the opportunity to discuss the information and ask questions. It is important that the purpose of any screening programme is clearly explained as part of the process of seeking consent, including being clear about for whose benefit it is being undertaken. Undoubtedly, some of the anxieties that arise from screening are caused by a misunderstanding of the information provided, particularly about the accuracy of the test and the implications of a positive or negative result. Accurate recall of information, in all spheres of medicine, is a problem and it can therefore be helpful to supplement discussion with written material for people to take away with them.

A number of the benefits that can derive from population screening, such as informed decision making or any relief or reassurance from a negative result, will clearly not be available for adults who lack capacity and participation in screening itself may raise levels of anxiety for these patients. These issues raise questions about whether they should be automatically included in such screening. Their exclusion could, however, be perceived as discriminatory and while the patient may not directly benefit from the results, screening could provide useful information about his or her health for carers. Decisions on the merits of screening for these patients therefore, need to be made on a case-by-case basis, weighing up the risks and benefits for the individual and based on the efficacy of the screening for the early identification of disease. (For more information on the provision of care and treatment for adults lacking capacity, see Chapter 3.)

Screening tests can have four possible outcomes: true negative; false negative; true positive; false positive. All tests generate a certain number of false negatives and positives. Those managing such programmes need to aim at finding the right balance between its sensitivity (picking up a very high proportion of positive cases) and its specificity (giving a negative result in a high proportion of negative cases). This balance usually depends on the consequences of making or not making a positive finding. For example, where a positive finding would be particularly associated with anxiety or stigma, then a higher specificity is desirable. Alternatively, where the adverse consequences of a missed positive are considerable, a higher sensitivity would be preferred.

People who are given a false negative or a false positive result are likely to be harmed in some way, although those with a false positive probably less so than those with a false negative, because the former will usually proceed to a definitive test, which will demonstrate that these people are free of the disease. Those with a true positive are normally regarded as enjoying a benefit, because they go on to receive treatment for the condition, but this is not always the case. Some true positives, for example, would not have gone on to develop a debilitating version of the disease – it may have been a slowly developing condition and they would have died of something else – and the screening may therefore not have been beneficial. This issue has been particularly relevant to the prostate specific antigen (PSA) test used to detect prostate cancer. Prostate cancer is a major health problem, which in 2008 caused around 258,000 deaths worldwide.[63] In the UK, the disease is the most common cancer in men, responsible for around 25 per cent of all newly diagnosed cases[64] and there have been calls for screening to be introduced to help combat this problem. PSA testing can help to detect cancer while it is still localised in the prostate; however, the test can also lead to considerable false positives and over-diagnosis of disease that may not have gone on to present serious health risks. Given these problems, and assessing the test against its criteria, the UK NSC does not recommend screening men for the condition, although testing is available on request from individual patients who are offered support in assessing the relative benefits and harms for themselves.[65]

Screening for breast cancer

In many western countries, mammography is routinely offered to women over a certain age, usually 40 or 50. The majority of medical opinion supports such screening, which saves an estimated 1,400 lives a year.[66] However, the screening process can identify small tumours that are growing so slowly that, without treatment, the woman could live her life without ever knowing of the cancer, which would play no part in the cause of her death. Because the screening process is not 100 per cent effective at identifying which cancers will go on to pose a serious health risk, some women may be treated for cancer unnecessarily. Research exists that points to significant over-diagnosis and over-treatment as a result of screening and a number of commentators therefore claim that the benefits of such programmes remain in the balance.[67]

Individuals who receive a true negative result may of course enjoy the welcome benefit of reassurance. Such a result can, however, inspire a false sense of security. With breast screening, for example, a negative result indicates only that the disease was not detectable at the time of the test. For some, this may be interpreted as meaning that they are not at risk of developing the disease, which consequently prevents them from responding to early warning signs should the disease appear later. There is the additional danger that a negative test is interpreted as a 'green light' to continue with unhealthy lifestyle choices. To an extent, these harms can be moderated by the provision of clear health advice at all stages of the screening process.

Summary – population screening

- Those offering screening programmes need to be certain that they offer a net benefit.
- The purpose of a screening programme, including for whose benefit it is being undertaken, needs to be clearly explained, as part of the consent process, to those who participate.
- For any screening programme, the following five criteria must be met:
  - the problem must be important
  - a suitable screening test should be available
  - the results must provide useful information
  - the benefits must outweigh the harms
  - adequate provision must be made for information, counselling and privacy.

Vaccination

Vaccination programmes are among the most widely used and cost-effective public health tools available. It is difficult to exaggerate the contribution of vaccines to the improvement of health in the years since their development. Smallpox, which plagued civilisation for millennia and which only 40 years ago killed 2 million people a year worldwide, is now completely eradicated as a result of a global vaccination programme.[68] Despite success stories like this, infectious disease remains one of the world's leading causes of illness and death which disproportionately affects socially and economically disadvantaged populations worldwide.[69] In helping to tackle this problem, vaccinations serve two of the key goals of public health medicine: they protect the most vulnerable members of society, saving the lives of an estimated 2.5 million children under 5 every year, and remove one of the key obstacles to human development, thereby helping to tackle inequality.[70]

Vaccines are regulated and tested thoroughly but, as with all health interventions, they may still carry small risks for an individual. A person's decision to vaccinate either themselves or their child therefore entails the need to balance these risks against benefits accrued through vaccination. This gives rise to interesting ethical questions around individual patient choice, community responsibility and the role of governments and doctors in maintaining sufficient levels of immunity.

Vaccination, immunisation and population immunity

There is a clear public health justification for the broad deployment of vaccines. If sufficient numbers of people within a population are immunised, there is less chance of people catching and spreading the disease. Given that the risks are relatively small, vaccination can benefit large numbers of people in return for a small degree of risk to individuals. Population immunity against a disease is only achieved, however, if a substantial majority of people opt to vaccinate themselves – from 85 to over 90 per cent, dependent on the infectiousness of the disease.[71] Individual choices not to vaccinate therefore expose others to risk, and if sufficient numbers refuse immunisation the result can be a 'tragedy of the commons'[72]: population immunity collapses and epidemics sweep through the community. Moreover, not all unvaccinated individuals have chosen to put themselves at risk:[73] neonates may not be old enough for vaccination and the ill and those whose immune systems are compromised are not vaccinated for good medical reasons.

In the UK, vaccination is entirely voluntary. However, there are a number of issues that may lead people to question the advantages of being vaccinated. At an individual level, it can be difficult to weigh up the respective costs and benefits of vaccination. Although vaccination is beneficial to the community as a whole, the likelihood of any particular individual benefiting reduces as the percentage of the population vaccinated increases. This is because if sufficient numbers of the population are immunised, there is a dramatic reduction in the likelihood of coming into contact with the disease. Where there is already population immunity – as is the case with a variety of common diseases in the UK – a vaccination's potential harms, such as side-effects, could be more substantial than the harm that follows from a particular individual not being vaccinated. Considered in isolation, therefore, for any particular individual living in an area with population immunity, the risk of vaccination could outweigh the benefits. This holds true only, however, if that individual remains in the community and does not, for example, travel to an area in which population immunity has not been achieved. Unvaccinated individuals living in communities with highly mobile populations, particularly where people travel from countries where immunisation is not widespread, can also be at risk.

Public perceptions regarding the prevalence and severity of a disease can also influence the decision making of individuals. It could be argued that in this respect vaccination programmes have become the victims of their own success. As the mortality and morbidity associated with their target diseases have become so unusual as to fall out of popular memory, so public perception has begun to focus on potential threats from vaccines, which are comparatively minor. Such perceptions can also affect attitudes towards the risks associated with a particular vaccine. The measles, mumps and rubella vaccine (MMR) controversy (see below) highlighted how susceptible public perceptions can be to stories about potential health threats. It also raised several questions regarding the rights of parents to make decisions about the welfare of their children; the lack of public faith in scientific expertise and government advice; and the role of the media in exacerbating health scares through sensationalist and unbalanced coverage (see pages 833–835).

The MMR controversy

In 1998, *The Lancet* published an article in which the authors speculated about a possible link between the combined MMR vaccine and autism and/or inflammatory bowel disease.[74] The link was subsequently refuted by several studies and a Cochrane systematic review conducted in 2005 concluded that there was no credible evidence of a link between the MMR vaccine and autism.[75] However, the article was widely reported in the press, sometimes in a sensationalist way, which had a detrimental effect on parents' confidence in the combined vaccine and led to notable reductions in its uptake. Between 2003 and 2004, the Department of Health reported that vaccination coverage for MMR in England dropped to 80 per cent; 15 per cent lower than the level recommended by the WHO for population immunity.[76] The controversy around MMR also led to distorted perceptions regarding the relative risks of immunisation compared to those of the disease, such that in 2002, almost one-quarter of UK mothers considered MMR a greater risk than the diseases it prevents.[77] Towards the end of the decade the uptake of the MMR vaccine began to rise again, although only slowly, and by 2009 levels in England, at just over 88 per cent[78] were still less than the WHO target for population immunity.

The MMR controversy (see above) is an example of how sensationalist reporting of potential health threats can seriously undermine key public health messages. That the perception that MMR was unsafe persisted for many years, despite overwhelming scientific evidence to the contrary, shows how difficult it is to change attitudes once fragile public confidence in a public health measure has been compromised. The MMR case is also a cautionary illustration of what can happen when levels of immunity within a population drop below the requisite levels to prevent outbreaks. In 1998, when 91 per cent of 2-year-olds were immunised,[79] there were 56 confirmed cases of measles in England and Wales.[80] In 2008, following the drop in uptake of the MMR vaccination, this figure had jumped to 1,370 cases.[81] In 2006, the UK recorded the first death from acute measles in 14 years.[82]

The reduction in uptake of the MMR vaccine coincided with an increase in parents choosing to vaccinate their children with three separate vaccines. This is contrary to the advice from the HPA, which stated not only that the MMR vaccine is safe, but that individual vaccines represent a comparatively untested and inferior alternative.[83] Opting for separate vaccines increases the risk of infection because the vaccinations need to be spread over a period of time. It also increases the likelihood that the course of vaccination will not be completed, thus exposing children, and the population, to risks in the future. There is also the ethical objection that giving children three separate injections, especially when they could be better protected by just one, causes unnecessary harm to the child.

Given the scientific consensus in support of the MMR vaccine, the government is under no obligation to provide separate vaccines for parents who have lost faith in the MMR vaccine. Discussing the issue in the wake of the MMR controversy the BMA's Medical Ethics Committee agreed that parents are accountable both to society and to their children for the decisions they make on their children's behalf and there is a limit to the risk to which parents can expose their children. The Committee maintained, however, that parents were the best people to make decisions for their children and they had general rights to choose inferior treatments both for themselves and within reason for their children. Society though was not under any obligation to fund inferior treatments and governments had a responsibility to make the best use of scarce public resources. Patients should be supported and encouraged to make the correct decision through better communication and education of the relative levels of risk involved.

Compulsory vaccination for patients

The drop in uptake of the MMR vaccine and the subsequent dramatic rise in cases of measles illustrate the potential weaknesses and risks of an entirely voluntary approach to vaccination and has led some to ask if there is a need for a different approach. Morally relevant considerations here extend beyond an assessment of potential risks and benefits to the individual, to include risks to third parties, for example neonates or those in ill health, and population-level benefits and harms. A key factor that proponents for any move away from a voluntary approach to vaccination will therefore have to consider is the point at which potential harms to others stemming from non-vaccination become sufficiently significant to justify placing limits on individual freedoms.

Currently, no country forces its population to be immunised against a particular disease. In its 2007 report on public health ethics, the Nuffield Council on Bioethics highlighted two alternative approaches operating in different jurisdictions worldwide that go beyond the voluntary system that operates in the UK:[84]

- *Quasi-mandatory programmes:* under this approach, individuals are required to be vaccinated unless they qualify for an exemption. If they refuse, they are subject to possible penalties (Belgium, Italy and Poland) or they are prevented from enrolling their child in school (France, Spain and the USA).
- *Incentive-based programmes:* in some countries, parents can be offered certain benefits if their child has appropriate vaccinations (Australia) or payment for ensuring a child completes a vaccination programme (Austria).

Although there is evidence to suggest that these schemes may increase uptake in immunisation for the targeted disease, they both have drawbacks: quasi-mandatory programmes can lead to a lower uptake in voluntary vaccinations while the cost-effectiveness of incentive-based programmes can vary. Cultural, historical and political factors can also affect the viability of any proposed move away from a voluntary approach. In the UK, public health programmes have traditionally been consensual, which has helped ensure positive public approval and uptake of programmes. A quasi-mandatory approach may therefore be seen by the public as confrontational and could lead to public mistrust of government public health interventions and messages more generally.

In 2009, the BMA's Board of Science rejected calls for compulsory vaccination. In discussing the ethical issues associated with compulsory vaccination, the BMA's Medical Ethics Committee also confirmed its overall support for the UK's current voluntary approach to childhood vaccination but felt that greater use should be made of education, publicity and information provision to improve vaccination uptake.

Vaccination for health workers

As we have seen, an individual's decision not to vaccinate himself or herself can contribute to the spread of a disease and put others health at risk. Health professionals, through their close proximity to patients, have an increased likelihood, not only of contracting a disease, but also of transmitting the infection to patients and colleagues. In addition to the potential harm to patients, if sufficient numbers within a healthcare setting are affected this could have a detrimental impact on staffing and put the provision of essential services at risk. Authorities therefore need to balance the liberties of healthcare workers against the need to protect patients and ensure the safe provision of services. In 2007, health departments in England[85] and Wales[86] released guidance recommending health clearance checks for new healthcare workers. Similar guidance was also released in Scotland[87] and Northern Ireland.[88] It is recommended that all new healthcare workers in the NHS, including medical students, undergo standard health clearance checks on appointment, with additional clearance checks for healthcare workers who will perform exposure-prone procedures (EPP). The standard health clearance checks include testing and the offer of vaccination, where appropriate, for tuberculosis and the offer of vaccination against hepatitis B. For posts that require the performance of EPPs additional checks include tests for hepatitis B, hepatitis C and HIV. Failure to agree to testing, or declining the offer of vaccination, may mean that new healthcare workers are not permitted to work in environments where the risk of exposure is high and may be prevented from taking up positions where they would be required to perform EPPs. UK-wide guidance on vaccination and immunisation also recommends that staff involved in direct patient care should be up to date with their routine immunisations including tetanus, diphtheria, polio and MMR.[89] Doctors should consult the relevant occupational health departments for further information on these requirements.

Where no contractual or occupational health requirement exists for a doctor to undergo immunisation, tensions can exist between the rights of individuals to refuse vaccination and the need to manage the potential risk of disease outbreak and ensure the safety of staff and patients alike. The introduction of a vaccine in response to the H1N1 swine flu outbreak in 2009 brought these issues to the fore. Although the Department of Health recommended that frontline staff should be immunised, there were reports that a significant number of health workers would not take up the opportunity, either because they saw it as unnecessary or because they lacked confidence in the safety of the vaccine, despite government assurances to the contrary.[90] The GMC advises that doctors should protect patients, colleagues and themselves by being immunised against common serious communicable diseases where vaccines are available.[91] It does not, however, impose an obligation on doctors to be vaccinated and there is no statutory requirement in place for compulsory vaccination in the event of a pandemic. Ethically, any move towards forced vaccination of healthcare professionals in such cases could be seen to compromise the autonomy of doctors. It could also be argued that such a move would contravene a doctor's right to a private and family life enshrined under Article 8 of the European Convention on Human Rights (ECHR), although the Article does allow for state interference in accordance with the law and when deemed necessary in a democratic society for the protection of health.

Summary – vaccination

- Vaccination programmes are amongst the most widely used and cost-effective public health tools available.
- Doctors need to present the risks and benefits of vaccinations objectively, including the public benefits of maintaining population immunity.
- The BMA supports a voluntary approach to vaccination, backed up by education, information and publicity.
- Doctors should be encouraged to take up vaccinations to protect themselves and their patients, but any such decision is ultimately a personal one.

Incentives

Tackling many of the new public health threats, such as the consequences of poor diet, smoking or drug abuse, involves confronting questions of individual motivation. Why do some people make poor health choices and how can these choices be influenced in a more positive direction? This also extends to the failure of certain groups to take advantage of available healthcare interventions, such as screening or vaccination, something that itself presents a significant public health challenge. The use of incentives, either financial or in kind, to address these psychological dimensions of individual behaviour has received increasing amounts of attention worldwide. Incentive schemes aim to provide an immediate reward for behaviour that will ideally provide health gains in the longer term. Their use draws on empirical research in behavioural psychology that suggests that, for many, a small immediate reward will prove more attractive than a larger but more distant one.[92]

Although a relatively recent public health initiative in the UK, the use of incentives is well established in other countries. Incentives aimed at individuals have been used in the German statutory health insurance scheme since 1989 when individuals who attended for regular dental check ups could reduce their co-payments.[93] Their use has subsequently been expanded to the offer of 'bonuses' in the form of either cash, such as a reduction in insurance contributions, or in kind, such as through gifts of sports equipment. In Latin American countries like Mexico 'conditional cash transfer schemes' (CCTS) offer impoverished families money if mothers attend parenting seminars, infants attend for health checks, and a number of other criteria are met. These schemes have caught the attention of authorities in other jurisdictions. The Opportunity NYC project, piloted in New York, builds on the Mexican CCTS model, offering payment for maintaining subsidised health insurance and attending medical and dental check ups.[94] In the UK, health authorities have offered money or the opportunity to enter a prize draw as incentives to help reach government targets on *Chlamydia* screening.

The use of incentives remains controversial. Although there is evidence to suggest that they can deliver positive outcomes in relation to service uptake, successfully encouraging attendance at clinics for example, evidence of their effectiveness in relation to more complex problems such as obesity or smoking is much weaker.[95] Their use also raises a number of ethical issues. For some, incentives are a coercive measure that undermines the autonomy of individuals. According to this view, individuals are being put under pressure to act in ways that are contrary to their considered choices, even where those choices may not, objectively, be in their long-term health interests. The use of incentives is similarly criticised as paternalistic, as promoting and enforcing choices or lifestyles that are not freely chosen or valued by those at whom they are directed. The idea of 'choice' in this context is not straightforward. As the example of tobacco use indicates, there can often be a stark contrast between how we act, and how, ideally, we would like to act. If incentives can help people align their actual choices with their preferred choices, it could be argued that, using a more developed understanding of the term, they enhance rather than restrict autonomy.

An important issue for the BMA is the extent to which the introduction of financial incentives could change the nature of the doctor–patient relationship, and whether any such change would be desirable. Ideally, the doctor–patient relationship is based upon an open and trusting exchange of information between a professional and a patient. Its goal is to promote the overall interests of the patient. The introduction of explicit monetary concerns may alter this relationship in undesirable ways. It may also undermine the longer term development of personal responsibility in patients, constituting only a short-term solution that fails to address the underlying causes of the problem.

One of the explicit goals of incentive schemes is to tackle health inequities, encouraging and rewarding healthy decision making among groups who traditionally have struggled to make such choices on their own. If incentives prove effective in addressing this fundamental issue in public health medicine then this may counter some of the objections raised above. Research suggests that in some cases incentives may in fact exacerbate health inequalities.[96] People in higher socioeconomic groups may be better placed to take advantage of incentive schemes, which means that those sections of the population least in need may benefit most, further widening the gap in health outcomes. If individuals are being rewarded for making choices they would have made anyway this also raises questions about the cost-effectiveness of incentive schemes. These arguments suggest that schemes targeted at specific groups may be more effective in addressing inequities, but these are not without controversy. Some may argue that it is unfair for individuals to be rewarded for behaviour that others undertake unrewarded, that such a system in effect penalises individuals who choose to live healthier lives. Cash incentive schemes may also stigmatise the groups that the initiative seeks to help, not only by marking off those who require such incentives and those who do not, but also by effectively branding those in need as irresponsible or incapable of making the correct decisions regarding their own welfare.[97]

The debate over the use of incentives requires more detailed research and more conclusive evidence before its value as a public health tool can be properly evaluated. Nevertheless, the continuing interest in incentives shows that public health practitioners are looking at innovative approaches to solving problems that have proved resistant to established public health intervention thus far. Incentives may well have an increasingly important role in public health promotion in the future.

Summary – incentives

- Incentives are designed to address psychological aspects of motivation in order to encourage healthy choices.
- Incentives should be used sensitively to ensure they respect and promote individual choices rather than acting coercively.
- Further research is required to assess the efficacy of incentives in a wide range of settings.

The role of the media

The media can have an important role in the promotion of public health. Its influence and ability to reach large audiences means that it can be an extremely useful tool for disseminating a wide range of information, from general positive health messages to specific details of health risks. The media can also present an emotive, human angle to health stories, making them more accessible than scientific evidence or government health warnings. The effect can sometimes be dramatic. The numbers of women screened for cervical cancer, for example, has twice received a boost from media stories relating to the disease. In 2009, the death of reality television star Jade Goody from cervical cancer was widely reported in the media and the coverage led to an increase of over 10 per cent in the number of all women screened.[98] This increase mirrored the effect in 2002 when, following the death of *Coronation Street* character Alma Sedgewick from the disease, the numbers of women screened nationwide rose and were up as much as 21 per cent on the previous year in the north-west of England where the soap is based.[99] Health reporting in the media can also have an influence on politicians and policy makers. News coverage or public reaction to a story can often provide the motivation for shifts in the prioritisation of funding and changes in public health policy.[100] Although this could have a positive effect, drawing attention and resources to neglected or emerging public health issues, it could also have negative consequences for public health planning, if politicians react impulsively to media coverage without thinking through the overall health implications of their decisions.

Media reporting can also have a detrimental effect on public health. News outlets are keen to maximise their audiences and this can mean that coverage focuses on headline-grabbing stories which may then be reported in a sensationalist way or without appropriate balance and qualification. Although scientific papers or articles may contain carefully modulated and contextualised assessments of public health threats, there is seldom the space in the popular media to provide suitably nuanced comment. The extraction of media friendly 'soundbites' in the search for good headlines can seriously distort evidence and lead to the misreporting of scientific research. These stories are commonplace in the mainstream media and often build up hope over a scientific breakthrough, for example over a new potential cure for cancer, or instil fear in the public with respect to new potential health threats. Public health specialists have complained that media reporting will often favour more exotic or unusual health risks like vCJD, which in reality pose little risk to the general public when compared with more significant and pressing public health threats such as smoking and obesity.[101] There is also a danger that media reporting about conflicting evidence on minor hazards can lead the public to doubt the reality of major health hazards about which there is far wider consensus. Debate about the health benefits of moderate alcohol consumption can, for example, lead to confused messages about excessive consumption, even though the evidence of the potential harms is strong.

The 1998 MMR controversy (see page 829) has become a classic example of how sensationalist reporting, based on imperfect information, can have a detrimental effect on trust in a public health intervention. Despite scientific refutation of the link between MMR and autism, faith in the vaccine was compromised to the extent that parental anxiety over the safety of MMR persisted for over a decade. The story also resurfaced in the media in 2007 when the *Observer* newspaper ran a front page story raising new fears that the vaccine was unsafe, an article which again was shown to be based on misreporting and exaggeration of the facts.[102] This type of story can present difficulties for members of the public who may not have access to the original material or the scientific training to evaluate the evidence presented to them and are therefore unsure whether to take the health threat at face value. Since the MMR scandal, the government has become more aware of the potential impact negative health stories can have on public perceptions of risk. The NHS Choices website has a resource entitled 'Behind the Headlines', which provides independent evidence-based analysis of health and science reporting in the mainstream media and is designed to help both the public and health professionals to assess the validity of scientific evidence and research presented in the media.[103]

When the media becomes interested in a public health issue, and doctors are invited to comment, care must be taken to ensure that only the known facts are disclosed and discussed; speculating about possible dramatic scenarios on the basis of modest information can prove extremely damaging and should be avoided. Care should also be taken to ensure that individuals are not inadvertently identified and, wherever possible, consent should be sought. Nevertheless, there may be health benefits in providing information to the general public when it is not possible to obtain consent about an incident that affects the public health, either to warn about the risks or to provide reassurance about safety. Doctors therefore need to weigh up the benefits of informing the public against the potential risk to the confidentiality of the affected patients. Even if identifying information is not provided, factors such as general location are probably essential and can lead to identification. A case that found its way to the media in 2002, for example, was so unusual as to effectively identify the individual concerned.

Confidentiality and the media – Britain's first case of rabies in a century

In the winter of 2002 a 56-year-old Scottish man contracted European bat lyssavirus, a type of rabies found in several northern European countries.[104] The release of information about the case to the press raised questions about confidentiality. Once it was known, for example, that someone who worked with bats in a specific region of the UK had contracted rabies, it then became quite easy for the media to identify him. In such cases, consideration needs to be given to the extent to which apparently anonymous information can lead to identification. Furthermore, in the absence of consent, disclosure should be restricted to the minimum amount of information necessary to fulfil the aim.

The hospital informed the press that there had been a confirmed case of rabies, and also issued a statement reassuring the public that people were at risk only if they had handled bats or been bitten or scratched by them. It is not known, in this case, whether the man, or his family, were involved in decisions about disclosure to the media.

Before releasing information about public health risks to the media, it is essential to consult with the local public health department in order to assess the nature and level of risk and the need to inform the public. In some circumstances it may also be important to seek advice from press officers, communications managers or lawyers before presenting the information to the media. (For further information on confidentiality and the media see Chapter 5, pages 216–217.)

Summary – the role of the media

- The media can have a positive role in public health promotion but it also has attendant risks.
- When doctors are commenting on public health stories in the media care must be taken to ensure that only the known facts are disclosed.
- Care must be taken to ensure that confidential information is not inappropriately disclosed to the media.
- Before releasing information to the media, advice should be taken from the local public health department and, if appropriate, press officers or communications managers.

Commissioning services – tackling inequities

A key part of public health practice relates to identifying health needs and commissioning services to address those needs. Public health practitioners gather and assess data on relevant health problems and then develop appropriate strategies to respond. These strategies can then be used to approach decisions relating to prioritising, funding, planning and commissioning health services. Three aspects of this broad public health practice raise particular ethical dilemmas. Given that not all health needs can be met from available resources, difficult decisions have to be made about which needs to prioritise, and any such decisions need to be made fairly. In addition, as discussed earlier in this chapter, health inequities are an important focus of interest, because they contribute to poor health outcomes and also because tackling social inequality is a wider political priority. There is also an obligation to use public resources justly. This section gives a brief outline of the main ethical issues that need to be taken into consideration in relation to priority setting. It also looks at clinician involvement in rationing decisions, at the legal context that governs these decisions and at professional guidance for doctors in this area. At the end of the section some practical examples relating to the tackling of health inequities are given.

Priority setting

To ration or to set priorities?

There is disagreement in relation to the terminology used in the area of resource allocation. The term 'rationing' is sometimes thought to be encumbered with negative associations, summoning up images of war-time deprivation, and likely to create resistance and partisan discussion. In its publication on resource allocation, *A rational way forward for the NHS in England*, the BMA states that: 'Priority setting acts at the level of allocating resources to particular services while rationing acts at a lower level in the allocation of resources to individual patients at the point of service delivery.'[105]

Since its inception in 1948, the demand for health services in the NHS has always considerably outstripped available resources. While it has been suggested that greater efficiency in the health service, or the allocation of a greater percentage of the overall domestic budget, would obviate the need for rationing, in recent years need has continued to exceed supply despite significant increases in the overall percentage of UK gross domestic product (GDP) spent on health. Between 1990 and 2010, for example, the percentage of GDP spent on health had risen from 6 to 10.5 per cent. Between 2000 and 2004, the UK also achieved the highest increase in health expenditure as a percentage of GDP, compared with its main European counterparts, and a growth rate three times higher than the EU average.[106] Given that serious shortages remain, it is likely that rationing will continue to be a significant feature of health delivery. In 2007, the BMA called for an open debate about rationing in the NHS. In *A rational way forward* it recommended that there must be explicit recognition of the need to ration services:

> The BMA believes that while the NHS should provide a comprehensive range of services, priority setting, and hence, rationing, is inevitable, if we are to retain an equitable approach within limited resources. This needs to be recognised by politicians so that the right environment will exist for politicians, health professionals and the public to debate and decide upon a process to define a 'core' list of services that will be nationally available. The approach should be national and explicit, setting priorities for the whole service. It should provide an ongoing mechanism to review and change priorities in the NHS, which must include an effective way of incorporating public and patient views.[107]

In order to understand how priority setting works in the UK, a background knowledge of the way health resources are allocated is useful. The structure of publicly funded healthcare is extremely complex and a detailed description is outside the scope of this book. In addition, at the time of writing, the Government has signalled its intention to make wide-ranging changes to the structure of health services in England by means of a new Health and Social Care Bill. Among the many reforms aimed at devolving responsibility away from central government is the proposal to involve GPs far more closely in the commissioning of health services for their patient populations. A brief outline of resource allocation in the NHS is given below.

How are resources allocated in the NHS?

Initially, the Government makes a decision about the percentage of the overall national budget that will be dedicated to healthcare. This is a decision for the Treasury, which is responsible for allocating Government spending to the various departments. Health professionals and their representative bodies, such as the BMA, can and do have an input in this process. They lobby to ensure that health remains a priority, and they can also influence the way in which budgets are allocated through collective bargaining in relation to terms and conditions of service. The initial budget is then devolved down to local commissioning bodies where overall priorities for services within the regions are decided. Although the budgets are to some extent controlled by the commissioning bodies, many priorities are still set centrally in ways that can have a considerable influence on allocation decisions further down the line. Despite recent changes to the structure of health services in England and Wales, the Government retains the power to insist that treatments recommended by the National Institute for Health and Clinical Excellence (NICE) in England and Wales are funded. In Scotland, the responsibility for providing advice to health boards about new and existing interventions falls to Healthcare Improvement Scotland (HIS). Doctors in Scotland are also supported by the Scottish Intercollegiate Guidelines Network (SIGN) which draws up national clinical guidelines. In Northern Ireland, the Department of Health, Social Services and Public Safety assesses guidance produced by NICE to decide whether it is appropriate to introduce it in Northern Ireland. NICE and SIGN are discussed below, as well as in Chapter 13. Guidelines can also be issued by central government in relation to waiting times, and the treatment of specific diseases.[108] Any such directions have an impact on allocation decisions further down the line, and such decisions clearly relate to the rationing of resources. To date the Government has declined to offer a comprehensive framework within which these decisions should be made. Instead, responsibility falls on commissioning bodies to develop local solutions. Although such responses can be flexible, they can also lead to patchy and ad hoc approaches with, at times, inequitable variation in regional supply.

The National Institute for Health and Clinical Excellence (NICE) and Scottish Intercollegiate Guidelines Network (SIGN)

In addition to the rationing processes outlined above, in 1999 the Government set up what was then the National Institute for Clinical Excellence (NICE), which became, in 2004, the National Institute for Health and Clinical Excellence, retaining the same acronym. NICE produces guidance on health technologies and clinical practice for the NHS in England and Wales.[109] Because NICE assesses interventions on the basis of both clinical and economic evidence – cost-effectiveness is taken into account – it is clearly involved in providing an evidence base for possible rationing and priority setting decisions.

The Scottish Intercollegiate Guidelines Network (SIGN) was set up in 1993. Its aim is to improve patient care by reducing variations in practice and outcome. Like NICE, it does this through the development and dissemination of clinical guidelines based upon the best available clinical evidence. (More information on NICE and SIGN can be found in Chapter 13, pages 552–554.)

Clinician involvement in rationing

Although the BMA argues for a 'national and explicit' approach to rationing, the vast majority of rationing decisions in the NHS are made implicitly, without being recognised as such, and often involving health professionals in decisions that have a significant, and often unacknowledged or unrecognised non-clinical aspect. The length of GP appointment times, for example, reflect the reality of limited staff time as much as the requirement for optimal outcomes from a consultation and clearly have an aspect of implicit rationing. Other examples include decisions to restrict the number of marginal investigations or interventions that may only provide small incremental benefits.

The most high-profile rationing cases usually occur where choices have to be made as to whether a specific individual will receive a potentially life-saving intervention. These cases also present healthcare professionals with acute ethical dilemmas, as they attempt to square their duties to provide healthcare on the basis of need, with the recognition that there are simply insufficient resources available. The obligation to act as the advocate of the interests of their patients can therefore conflict with the need to use available resources as efficiently as possible in order to ensure that the acutest needs can be satisfied. Although individual cases can be the subject of extensive media scrutiny, the overwhelming majority of rationing of this kind is implicit rather than explicit:

> [r]ationing in the NHS has never been explicitly organised but has hidden behind each doctor's clinical freedom to act solely in the interests of his individual patient. Any conflict of interest between patients competing for scarce resources has been implicitly resolved by doctors judgments as to their relative needs for care and attention.[110]

One frequently cited example of this is the use of GPs to act as 'gate keepers'. Although many GPs may not think of their activities as explicit rationing, the decisions they make can largely determine the extent to which individuals will have access to health resources.

Judicial review of rationing decisions – a history of court involvement[111]

The National Health Service Act 1977 imposes upon the Secretary of State a general duty to promote a 'comprehensive health service' to those ordinarily resident in the UK. Those bodies upon whom this responsibility is devolved also have an obligation to operate within their allocated budgets. Because limited budgets will inevitably mean that some beneficial treatments cannot be provided, legal questions arise about the lawfulness of the decisions to restrict certain services and treatments. In England and Wales, legal scrutiny of resource allocation decisions is made by judicial review when the Courts examine the propriety of public authority decision making. The focus is usually on the reasonableness of the decision-making process.

Gender identity dysphoria – the need for a consistent approach

In 1999, a case taken by three individuals with gender identity dysphoria raised some interesting questions about the limits to the treatments or interventions that should ordinarily be provided by a publicly financed health service. The trio challenged their health authority's decision to refuse to provide them with gender realignment surgery.

The case is interesting for a number of reasons. In 1995, the authority had decided to allocate a low priority to such surgery, considering it to achieve little in the way of clinical gain. In its 1998 revision of its policy the health authority stated that: '[t]he health authority will not commission drug treatment or surgery that is intended to give patients the physical characteristics of the opposite gender.' The only exception that it would allow was where 'there is evidence (including consultant advice) that the problem is the cause of serious mental illness, which can be expected to be substantially improved if the exception is granted.'[112] The justification for providing treatment was therefore severe – and treatable – mental illness associated with the gender dysphoria, not the condition itself. The case touched upon the question of whether people who felt they were born into the wrong gender were experiencing a health problem and therefore whether they should receive publicly funded health services. Here clinical judgement is central, and gives some indication of the power of clinicians and their professional clinical organisations in deciding whether individuals will be eligible to receive treatment. The trio won their appeal. The Court stated that as the authority accepted that gender dysphoria was a recognisable clinical condition, restrictions that effectively amounted to a complete ban on providing treatment were unacceptable and the authority needed to review its approach. The Court did not comment on whether an authority should make money available for treatment of gender identity dysphoria. Its concern was with the reasonableness of the decision-making process.

In scrutinising decisions, the courts acknowledge the duty of public authorities to balance competing claims upon their finite resources and have traditionally been extremely reluctant to overturn health authority decisions not to fund particular patients' treatments.[113] Where the court does find in favour of the applicant, the health authority is required to make the decision again, but it is not necessarily required to pay for treatment. As long as the decision is made lawfully, for example by the health authority offering reasons for the decision to refuse treatment and assessing the individual circumstances, rather than operating a 'blanket' ban, it is possible that the authority will come to the same decision again and still refuse to fund the applicant's treatment. Court review is not restricted to decisions by health trusts. As outlined in the case below, decisions by NICE have also been subject to legal criticism.

Court of Appeal questions NICE decision in relation to Alzheimer's drug

In May 2008, the decision by NICE to restrict the availability of acetylcholinesterase inhibitors, such as Aricept, for the treatment of Alzheimer disease was held to be procedurally unfair by the Court of Appeal. Overturning an earlier decision at the High Court, the Court of Appeal held that the decision by NICE not to publish the full version of the cost-effectiveness model that it used when reaching the decision was 'procedurally unfair'. The Court held that as NICE discharged a serious public function it was therefore subject to the general principles of procedural fairness. The Court asked NICE to look again at its decision, taking into account the views of the drug companies involved after they had had time to consider the full cost-effectiveness model.[114]

Resource allocation decisions have also been challenged under the Human Rights Act 1998. Although both the European Court of Human Rights and UK domestic courts have been reluctant to interfere with health authority resource allocation decisions, there was a successful case brought against such an authority under Article 2 of the European Convention, protecting the right to life, in 2008. The House of Lords ruled that hospitals and other health organisations have a positive obligation to protect the lives of patients in their care against suicide attempts where there is a known suicide risk.[115]

Legal review of rationing decisions – the current position

In a 2008 judicial review case, in which a patient challenged a PCT's refusal to pay for expensive renal cancer treatment, Mr Justice Burnett laid down the principles to be applied where rationing decisions are brought before the courts.

- When an NHS body makes a decision about whether to fund a treatment in an individual patient's case it is entitled to take into account the financial restraints on its budget as well as the patient's circumstances.
- Decisions about how to allocate scarce resources between patients are ones with which the courts will not usually intervene unless there was irrationality on the part of the decision maker. There are severe limits on the ability of the court to intervene.
- The courts' role is not to express opinions as to the effectiveness of medical treatment or the merits of medical judgement.
- It is lawful for an NHS body to decide to decline to fund treatment save in exceptional circumstances, provided that it is possible to envisage such circumstances arising.[116]

Seeking treatment overseas

In 2003, after being put on a waiting list for a hip replacement, Yvonne Watts travelled to France for the operation and sought reimbursement from Bedford PCT for the cost on her return. In ruling in favour of Ms Watts, the European Court of Justice held that patients seeking treatment overseas must obtain prior authorisation from their PCT or commissioning body. The possible exceptions to this would be where the delay arising from waiting lists would be unacceptable, based upon an objective test of the patient's medical condition.[117] In 2008, the European Union issued a Directive to provide greater clarity on the question of cross-border healthcare provision within Europe. Although it does not seek to enforce a system of prior authorisation, it holds that it would be legitimate for a state to require prior authorisation where it was necessary to avoid disruption to health planning. The Directive is expected to come into force in 2012–2013.[118]

A defined package of healthcare?

One possible approach to rationing is the development of a core bundle of services that will be universally available, an approach recommended by the BMA.[119]

To a limited extent, and in an ad hoc and decentralised fashion, such an approach to the provision of healthcare is already in place. Not all potential services are available everywhere, with certain services, such as tattoo removal or aesthetic plastic surgery, only being available in some areas. Adult dentistry is subsidised by central government, but considerable costs are passed on to the 'consumer'.[120] On the face of it, it is clearly inequitable that one's place of residence should determine whether one can access a particular service and, in this context, calls for centralising a core list can seem attractive, although drawing up such a list can present difficulties. Even if some of the more obviously 'marginal' interventions, such as tattoo removal in the absence of severe psychological stress, are excluded, the impact on overall funding will be negligible. When it comes to the more substantive and expensive services, we come back to the question of the principle or principles that should guide the decision to fund or not to fund.[121] Among other difficulties faced by this approach is its potential for a rigidity that overrides the clinical flexibility to meet genuine need, and a vulnerability to judicial review for excluding the possibility of exceptional cases.[122]

One of the questions raised by the possible introduction of a defined core set or package of healthcare that is made available to all is the tension that inevitably runs through rationing decisions, between decisions made at the centre and the requirement to meet need flexibly at the local level. While a centralised approach would overcome the so-called 'post-code lottery', it can remove the flexibility to deal with geographical variations in health need. The question then becomes how best to steer a path between excessively rigid centralism on the one hand, and ad hoc local solutions that may not be firmly rooted in evidence.

Ethical priorities in resource allocation

The BMA has identified a number of key ethical issues that both public health practitioners and other health professionals need to consider when thinking through resource allocation decisions. These are given in the box below and are discussed in more detail in the section that follows.

> ### Ethical considerations engaged in rationing decisions
>
> These include:
>
> - need
> - welfare maximisation
> - clinical effectiveness
> - relative cost-effectiveness
> - equity
> - individual rights
> - patient choice
> - communication and public involvement
> - transparency and rationality of decision making.

Need

Approaches to priority setting in healthcare require an understanding of the healthcare needs of target populations. Although these are usually approached via health needs assessments, which aim systematically to identify unmet healthcare needs, these in turn necessarily require some prior understanding of what is meant by 'need', and of the difference between 'health' and 'healthcare'. On the face of it, the idea of need may seem straightforward, understood as a health deficit that can benefit from an intervention. Nevertheless, on closer inspection it becomes more problematic, with perceptions of need varying according to what interventions are possible, available and affordable.[123] The understanding of need also varies according to the definition of health employed and whether it is limited to discrete medical conditions or widened to incorporate social determinants of health and well-being. It can also be difficult clearly to distinguish between a health 'need' and a 'want' or a 'desire'. (For further discussion, see pages 802–804.)

Welfare maximisation

At the heart of debate about rationing lies the fundamentally utilitarian goal of managing and providing healthcare in ways that maximise the welfare of those who are using them within the available resources.[124] Although much inevitably depends on the definition of 'welfare', where resources are limited and the welfare of some cannot be increased without reducing the welfare of others, attention must be shifted to maximising the welfare of the population viewed in its entirety.

Clinical effectiveness

Decisions relating to an intervention's effectiveness are based exclusively on clinical criteria (both physical and psychological), unaffected by issues of cost. A treatment is clinically effective if it alters a particular condition for the better. One treatment is more effective than another if it alters the condition more successfully or with fewer side effects or under a wider range of conditions.[125]

Relative cost-effectiveness

Cost-effectiveness combines clinical efficacy and cost, with the aim of achieving the most effective use of the limited resources available. A range of measures of health benefit[126] can be used to determine cost-effectiveness but this is not a straightforward process and there are always considerable practical difficulties. Whatever measure is used, several important issues need to be addressed, including the additional length and quality of life a treatment brings and the contribution particular treatments make to an individual's well-being.

Equity

Equity requires that like cases are treated alike, and unlike cases treated differently. This principle, applied to healthcare, demands that people with the same health needs must be given an equal chance of receiving appropriate treatment of equal quality.[127] In broader public health terms it also means that the same conditions for realising good health are equally available to all members of the population. This can mean that where inequalities exist, goods need to be distributed unequally in order to achieve overall equality.

Individual rights

One of the ways in which the discussion of priority setting has been framed is in terms of individual rights, and the nature and status of these rights have an impact on decisions about resource allocation. The notion of 'rights', incorporating both substantive legal and aspirational moral entitlements, is complex and contentious. However, the NHS is required to ensure that all of its decisions are compatible with the Human Rights Act 1998 and legislation must, as far as possible, be interpreted in ways that are compatible with Convention rights.

Patient choice

There are inevitably recurrent conflicts between centralised rationing decisions and patient choice. Rationing by its nature involves doctors and others in the hard task of denying to some patients interventions from which they could benefit because resources can be more appropriately employed elsewhere. Nevertheless, within this framework, efforts need to be made to maximise patient choice, and a variety of methods for involving patients in decisions about their healthcare choices need to be employed. These include the following:

- when research on the effectiveness of a treatment is being assessed it is important that outcome measures important to patients are used
- where multiple treatments are available within the priority-setting framework, patients should be encouraged to make their own choices
- the priority-setting framework should be suitably flexible to permit legitimate exceptions based on variations between patients
- the impact of choices on carers should also be taken into account.

Patient choice within a public system will not ordinarily extend to procedures that are not regarded as clinically effective.

Truth telling and resources

While truth telling is generally advocated throughout clinical care, some doctors have expressed concern about the implications of telling patients that there are health services available that could potentially help them but which are not available within the NHS or in the area in which they live. In the BMA's view, part of the role of doctors is to ensure that decision making is returned as much as possible to the patient rather than pre-empting the choice by withholding potentially important information. The BMA therefore believes that, as a general rule, patients should be given information about other treatment options that may benefit them, even if the doctor does not believe that the patient could afford to pay for the treatment. There may be rare cases, however, where such information would clearly be unwelcome and, in these cases, doctors should take their cue from the patients as to the amount of information to impart. Where information is to be provided, the manner and timing of its provision will need to be carefully considered and may need to be supported by professional counselling. In cases where the treatment cannot be funded, patients should have access to information about the factors leading to the rationing decision and it should be made clear whether the treatment is unavailable because it is unproven or solely on grounds of cost-effectiveness.

Although it is important to bear all of these ethical considerations in mind when setting priorities for the allocation of resources, it is inevitable that there will be cases in which they come into conflict. Cost-effectiveness can at times work against individual need, for example, and patient choice often runs into conflict with equity. Difficult choices need to be made and must be justified with clear and transparent policies and decisions in individual cases.

The search for equity

Inequalities in health provision – a tale of two cancers

In 2006, the English media picked up on a story about a married couple – one of whom was a journalist on the *Observer* newspaper – who were simultaneously diagnosed as having cancer, the man with prostate cancer, the woman with breast cancer. Somewhere in the region of 42,000 women a year are diagnosed with breast cancer in the UK. It kills around 15,000 patients a year. Nearly 32,000 men are diagnosed with prostate cancer a year and it kills around 10,000 men a year. At the time, breast cancer received 10 times more funding than prostate cancer.[128] Questions were raised in the media about whether clinical factors alone could account for the difference in resources allocated to the two diseases. Commentators pointed to the high profile campaigns supporting breast cancer, the passionate and vociferous supporters of the cause and, consequently, to media interest. Prostate cancer, by contrast, had a much lower media profile. The case highlights the potential in media-driven democracies for public opinion to affect decisions about how resources are allocated. The public furore over Herceptin,[129] for example, resulted in an intervention from the Government and a fast-tracking of NICE approval for its use. However, public opinion can sometimes lead to ethically questionable priorities, routinely favouring the health needs of children over, for example, prisoners or the mentally ill.

One of the biggest challenges in public health is trying to rectify health inequities where equity is understood as the requirement that people in equal positions should be treated equally, and people in unequal positions treated unequally, according to the morally relevant differences between them. In the case of healthcare, the most obvious criterion for discriminating between individuals is clinical need. People with similar clinical need should receive similar treatment, those whose needs require more expensive treatment should receive more. It needs to be recognised here, however, that greater need might not entail greater cost. Some very great health needs can be met inexpensively, other lesser needs might entail far more costly treatment. Waiting lists are often cited as one method of prioritising according to need.

Health inequities arise not only through decisions about allocating resources but also through the broader social, economic and biological factors that affect health. It is therefore not enough to ensure an equitable geographical spread of services. Even if this were to be achieved, rates of uptake would still vary considerably, as would disease variations resulting from genetic and socioeconomic factors. The equity challenge for the provision of comprehensive health services therefore lies far deeper than just the research and assessment of health problems and the commissioning of appropriate services to respond to them. It also entails an understanding of the way social inequities contribute to the development and prevalence of disease, the way different population groups take up health services and respond to health initiatives, and the development of innovative ways to contact different communities and to present the issues in ways that are both meaningful and that invite cooperation.

Non-discrimination

An important aspect of any approach to equity is the elimination of discrimination between individuals on the basis of morally unacceptable criteria. In the provision of publicly funded healthcare in the UK this means that healthcare will ordinarily be provided on the basis of a clinically adjudicated assessment of an individual's clinical need and capacity to benefit. Discrimination will not be permitted, however, on the basis of personal characteristics that have no clinical relevance. These will include factors such as age, gender, sexual orientation, gender identity, race, religion, lifestyle, social position, family or financial status, intelligence, disability, physical or cognitive functioning, where they are not relevant to the clinical decision that needs to be made.

The debate about discrimination is particularly concerned with elderly and disabled patients and with patients from ethnic minorities. Some ethnic minorities, for example, have much lower uptake of some key services, such as palliative care. In 2010, the Equality Act 2010 for England and Wales came into force which prohibits age discrimination against adults in the provision of public services and functions. Subsequently, the Department of

Health issued a consultation document looking at age equality in health and social care in anticipation of the implementation of the equality duty in relation to age which was expected to be in force by 2012. Among the recommendations were:

- a review of any age criteria in use in entitlement for health services, such as breast screening, with the intention of replacing such criteria, where appropriate, with more 'pertinent and individualised evidence'[130]
- a review of the use of quality-adjusted life years (QALYS) and other similar support tools to inform decision making.

Public participation and involvement

There is a tension in resource allocation decisions between centralised policy making, which aims at overall equity, and the requirement to respond flexibly to local variations. It can be just to treat people in the same way, but it can also be just to treat different people differently, depending upon their needs and circumstances. A difficulty that can arise in relation to more central decision making is that it can be based upon poor or inaccurate assumptions of the requirements of local populations. One way of addressing this problem is through public participation. Doctors working in the field of needs assessment have been sensitive to the charges of paternalism that have, from time to time, been directed at their practice, and have used a range of methods for involving populations in their work to ensure that autonomy is eroded to the minimum extent possible. Public involvement requires more than just listening to representatives of 'target' populations, however. At its best it is an ongoing dialogue and involves providing population groups with information about individual policies, the reasons for implementing them and the desired outcome. At times it extends to public participation in the actual decision making itself.

The use of sophisticated methods to involve the public and to maintain an ongoing dialogue can lead to better public understanding and acceptance. Where public involvement has worked well, health initiatives have generally been more successful, particularly among traditionally 'hard to reach' populations.[131] Such measures can also help to overcome the resistance some groups have shown to state initiatives and can enhance the involvement of excluded groups, even when the strategy in question may have some elements of coercion, such as restrictions on smoking in public places. It is important therefore that before policies are introduced and services are offered, a wide range of stakeholders is consulted both to inform the development of the policy and to gain the acceptance and cooperation of the local population. Achieving this is not unproblematic, however. It can be difficult, for example, to identify appropriate representatives and many of the most needy can be so disenfranchised as to be almost silent.[132] Local health professionals in both primary and secondary care have important contributions to make, as do local government and voluntary groups. Listed below are a number of methods that can be used to enhance public involvement.

Methods for public involvement

- *Public consultations:* these are an increasing feature of Government activity and are used to ensure stakeholders have an opportunity to have their voices heard in decision-making processes.
- *Health panels:* these are standing panels of local people who are seen to be representative of the local population. They vary in size and in the frequency with which they meet and members tend to be replaced at frequent intervals.

- *Citizens' juries:* these are made up of local people who sit on a jury for a specified time and debate a variety of health topics presented by health practitioners.
- *Focus groups:* these tend to comprise groups of between 6 and 12 local people and are run by a facilitator who promotes discussion on a variety of local health topics.
- *Interviews:* individuals are selected either at random, or because they are particularly representative, and their views are sought on a variety of issues.
- *Questionnaires:* these enable the gathering of structured information from a variety of target populations.
- *Experimental methods:* these are used by professional researchers such as psychologists and economists to elicit and quantify public preferences.

Although public involvement in decision making should be encouraged, it does not necessarily guarantee an ethically justifiable outcome. Public priorities may be inconsistent, based upon a faulty understanding of complex issues or based on individual prejudices.[133] Attempts to ascertain the public's views about healthcare priorities, for example, have shown a clear preference for the treatment of acute, life-threatening diseases among children over similar treatment for older people, psychiatric services or general health promotion. Considerable support has also been expressed for the notion that those who have contributed to their own illness, through smoking, obesity or drinking for example, should have lower priority for treatment.[134] As we have seen, such views are at odds with the general principles that underpin the NHS. While it is important to be aware of these inherent difficulties, they do not outweigh the value of such exercises and the benefits of achieving the agreement and cooperation of the local population in public health policy.

Learning from past successes – Julian Tudor Hart's 'anticipatory care' approach

Discussion of public health goals and methods can, at times, seem remote, dealing with large populations and with abstract ideas such as 'community' and 'the common good' and with impersonal tools such as epidemiology. Health professionals have, however, developed innovative methods for combining public health approaches with the delivery of individual healthcare to members of target populations. In the 1960s, the British GP Julian Tudor Hart started using routine contact with patients – typically he would see over 90 per cent of his patients over a 5-year period – to assess not only immediate health problems, but also anticipated future health needs. Hart's approach focused on preventing future risks, particularly those associated with high blood pressure, smoking, obesity, diabetes and excess alcohol use. As a result of his approach, compared with neighbouring populations with a similar health profile, premature mortality among his patients dropped by 28 per cent. Aspects of Hart's groundbreaking approach have been adopted, and adapted, throughout the UK, and it remains a powerful example of the productive interface between a public health and an individual health approach to health maximisation.[135]

Summary – commissioning services

- The need for priority setting emerges from the gap between the demand for healthcare and available resources.
- Priority setting is an inevitable part of healthcare provision in the UK and this should be openly acknowledged.
- Decisions must be equitable and comply with the Human Rights Act 1998.
- Decisions must be justified with clear and transparent policies and decisions in individual cases.

- Equity requires that equal people should be treated equally and unequal people treated unequally, according to the morally relevant distinctions between them.
- Equity relates to more than just health need – it also requires addressing the underlying determinants of health.
- Public participation is crucial, although public priorities may not in themselves lead to just or equitable outcomes.

Processing health data for public health management

A great deal of the management of public health takes place at a local level. This obviously includes the implementation of national policies and will often involve the application of some of the tools and strategies outlined above. The day-to-day management of public health incidents also operates at a local level. A central feature of this practice is the gathering and processing of health information. This final section looks at some of the ethical issues raised by this practice.

The use of health information

Public health medicine uses a large amount of health information gathered from a variety of sources, including population registers, birth notification and mortality records, disease registries, health service data banks, national and regional screening or surveillance programmes, data specifically collected through surveys and research, and medical notes. Often the data are linked together, for example information from cancer registries is linked to mortality data, to increase its potential uses. The use of these types of data is crucial to the development of public health strategies, and to the delivery of significant public goods, but the usual rules of confidentiality still apply. Specific information about confidentiality and the use of personal health information is covered in Chapter 5 but the main principles that apply to the use of information for public health purposes are summarised below.

When public health doctors use data or design projects that involve data capture, the following principles should be followed.

- Wherever possible, anonymised data should be used.
- Consent should ordinarily be sought for any use or disclosure of identifiable personal health information.
- Occasionally, when it is not possible to obtain consent, information may be disclosed with strict safeguards (see below).
- Where consent is sought from patients for the use of their information, they must be properly informed about the purpose and nature of its use.
- Where practitioners are not directly involved in the consent process, they should accept data only from reputable sources that have in place appropriate mechanisms for information gathering and handling.
- All processing of identifiable health data must comply with legal requirements and must be fair and lawful.
- Information should not be kept for longer than is necessary to fulfil the purposes for which it was sought.
- Disclosure should be kept to the minimum necessary to achieve the purpose.
- All patient identifiable data must be properly protected against inappropriate or inadvertent disclosure.

- All individuals who come into contact with personal health information in their work must be trained in confidentiality issues.

Where it is not possible to use anonymous information, or to obtain consent, information may be disclosed to comply with a statutory requirement or where there is an overriding public interest (see Chapter 5). In England and Wales, disclosure is also permitted, in some circumstances, under the terms of regulations made under section 251 of the NHS Act 2006 (for more information see Chapter 5, pages 209–211).

Statutory exemptions for communicable diseases and other risks to public health

Regulations under the Health and Social Care Act 2001 have been made to permit confidential patient information to be processed, when it is not possible to obtain consent, for the following purposes:

- diagnosing communicable diseases and other risks to public health
- recognising trends in such diseases and risks
- controlling and preventing the spread of such diseases and risks
- monitoring and managing outbreaks of communicable disease
- incidents of exposure to communicable disease
- the delivery, efficacy and safety of immunisation programmes
- adverse reactions to vaccines and medicines
- risks of infection acquired from food or the environment (including water supplies)
- the giving of information to persons about the diagnosis of communicable disease and risks of acquiring such disease.[136]

At the time of writing, there was no equivalent provision in legislation in Scotland or Northern Ireland, and doctors in those jurisdictions should follow the advice in Chapter 5 and consider whether the public interest overrides the duty of confidentiality. They must also be prepared to justify their decisions.

Looking towards the future

Media and public attention frequently focus on exciting and innovative areas of medicine, such as new advances in surgical techniques or developments in genetics and, as a result, the potential for simple public health techniques to deliver extraordinary communal benefits sometimes goes unremarked. Vaccinations, sanitation, a clean water supply and the recognition of the hazards of tobacco use have contributed, and continue to contribute, incalculable benefits both to the developed and the developing worlds. In the West, however, as one generation of problems has receded, others have come to fill their place.

Whereas some of the original problems, many of which still dominate the health agendas of developing countries, were amenable to simple, cost-effective interventions or improvements, many of the new generation of public health issues, such as attempting to modify individual behaviour, have proved less responsive to public health initiatives. This new generation of problems include the health effects of sedentary lifestyles and poor eating habits; alcohol and tobacco use; the effects of social disintegration, such as violence and depression; the continuing consequences of social inequalities; bioterrorism; and the emergence of new drug resistant versions of older diseases. As public health professionals continue to develop methods to deal with these issues, it is likely that the ethical questions generated by the friction between state beneficence and individual autonomy, and the appropriate balance between benefits and harms, particularly for patients who lack capacity, will be subject to increased scrutiny. As part of this process it is also likely that work will continue on the development of a stronger understanding of the moral goods of community. Where discussion of the ethics of public health practice has traditionally made use of an aggregate understanding of community, the sum of the interests of the individuals who make it up, more communitarian approaches, which will try to articulate a more substantive understanding of the moral importance of shared goods, such as health, will be an increasing feature of reflection on public health.

Public health medicine can provide important ethical insights, insights that can easily be overlooked in the mainstream rights discourse that, at times, dominates discussion of health and healthcare. It reminds us that health is not only a private issue, but also, and inevitably, a shared undertaking.

References

1 Adapted from: Public Health Leadership Society (2002) *Principles of the Ethical Practice of Public Health*. Public Health Leadership Society, New Orleans. Available at: www.apha.org (accessed 16 February 2011).
2 Rose G. (1985) Sick individuals and sick populations. *Int J Epidemiol* **14**, 32–8.
3 Rose G. (1985) Sick individuals and sick populations. *Int J Epidemiol* **14**, 32–8, p.33.
4 Rose G. (1985) Sick individuals and sick populations. *Int J Epidemiol* **14**, 32–8, p.33.
5 Coggon J. (2010) Does public health have a personality (and if so, does it matter if you don't like it)? *Camb Q Healthc Ethics* **19**, 235–48.
6 Montgomery J. (2003) *Health Care Law*, OUP, Oxford, p.24.
7 World Health Organization (1946) *Preamble to the Constitution of the World Health Organization as adopted by the International Health Conference, New York, 19–22 June, 1946; signed on 22 July 1946 by the representatives of 61 States (Official Records of the World Health Organization, no. 2, p.100) and entered into force on 7 April 1948*, WHO, Geneva.
8 See, for example: British Medical Association (2007) *Boosting your brain power: ethical aspects of cognitive enhancement*, BMA, London.
9 Nordenfelt L. (2007) The concepts of health and illness. In: Ashcroft RE, Dawson A, Draper H. *et al*. (eds.) *Principles of Health Care Ethics*, Wiley, Chichester, pp.537–42.
10 Boorse C. (1977) Health as a theoretical concept. *Philosophy of Science* **44**, 542–73, p.567.
11 Nordenfelt L. (2007) The concepts of health and illness. In: Ashcroft RE, Dawson A, Draper H. *et al*. (eds) *Principles of Health Care Ethics*, Wiley, Chichester, p.539.
12 Marmot M, Wilkinson RG. (eds.) (2006) *The Social Determinants of Health*, OUP, Oxford.
13 See, for example: Jennings B. (2007) Community in public health ethics. In: Ashcroft RE, Dawson A, Draper H. *et al*. (eds.) *Principles of Health Care Ethics*, Wiley, Chichester, pp.543–8.
14 Brunner E, Marmot M. (2006) Social organization, stress, and health. In: Marmot M, Wilkinson G. (eds.) *Social Determinants of Health*, OUP, Oxford, pp.6–30.
15 Wilkinson R, Marmot M. (2003) *The solid facts*, 2nd edn, WHO, Geneva, p.7.
16 Marmot M, Wilkinson RG. (eds.) (2006) *The Social Determinants of Health*, OUP, Oxford, p.1.
17 Marmot M. (2005) Social determinants of health inequalities. *Lancet* **365**, 1099.
18 See, for example: Rogers W. (2007) Health inequities and the social determinants of health. In: Ashcroft RE, Dawson A, Draper H. *et al*. (eds.) *Principles of Health Care Ethics*, Wiley, Chichester, pp.585–91.
19 Rogers W. (2007) Health inequities and the social determinants of health. In: Ashcroft RE, Dawson A, Draper H. *et al*. (eds.) *Principles of Health Care Ethics*, Wiley, Chichester, pp.585–91.
20 Department of Health (2010) *Fair Society, Healthy Lives: Strategic review of health inequalities in England post-2010*, DH, London.
21 Department of Health (2009) *Strategic review of health inequalities in England post-2010. Marmot review: first phase report*. DH, London, p.44.
22 United Nations International Covenant on Economic Social and Cultural Rights 1966, art 12.
23 United Nations Economic and Social Council (2000) *The right to the highest attainable standard of health. 11/08/2000. E/C.12/2000/4 (General Comments)*, United Nations, Geneva.
24 National Health Service Act 1977, s1(1).

25 Montgomery J. (2003) *Healthcare Law*, OUP, Oxford, p.53.
26 Department of Health, NHS for England (2009) *The NHS Constitution: the NHS belongs to us all*, DH, London.
27 Department of Health (2010) *Equity and Excellence: Liberating the NHS*, The Stationery Office, London, p.6.
28 Gostin LO. (2002) *Public health law and ethics: a reader*, University of California Press, California, p.8.
29 In England and Wales, the Health and Social Care Act 2008 amended the Public Health (Control of Disease) Act 1984. Scotland introduced the Public Health etc (Scotland) Act 2008. In Northern Ireland the Public Health (Amendment) Act (Northern Ireland) amended the Public Health Act (Northern Ireland) 1967.
30 World Health Organization (2005) *International Health Regulations*, 2nd edn, WHO, Geneva, 2005.
31 In England and Wales, the Health and Social Care Act 2008 amended the Public Health (Control of Disease) Act 1984. Scotland introduced the Public Health etc (Scotland) Act 2008. In Northern Ireland it is the Public Health Act (Northern Ireland) 1967.
32 Roberts I. (2009) Climate change: is public health up to the job? *BMJ* **339**, 1226–8.
33 Department of Health (2011) *Obesity*. Available at: www.dh.gov.uk (accessed 28 February 2011).
34 Nuffield Council on Bioethics (2007) *Public health: ethical issues*, NCB, London, p.83.
35 Department of Health (2006) *Forecasting obesity to 2010*, DH, London.
36 Government Office for Science (2007) *Tackling Obesities: Future Choices – Project Report*, 2nd edn, Government Office for Science, London.
37 Nuffield Council on Bioethics (2007) *Public health: ethical issues*, NCB, London, p.83.
38 Government Office for Science (2007) *Tackling Obesities: Future Choices – Project Report*, 2nd edn. Government Office for Science, London.
39 Government Office for Science (2007) *Tackling Obesities: Future Choices – Project Report*, 2nd edn. Government Office for Science, London, p.8.
40 Government Office for Science (2007) *Tackling Obesities: Future Choices – Project Report*, 2nd edn. Government Office for Science, London, p.124.
41 Potter C. (1998) Chronicle of influenza pandemics. In: Nicholson KG, Webster RG, Hay AJ. (eds.) *Textbook of Influenza*, Blackwell Science, Oxford.
42 British Medical Association (1988) *Nuclear Attack: Ethics and Casualty Selection*, BMA, London, p.48.
43 General Medical Council (2006) *Good Medical Practice*, GMC, London, para 10.
44 The National Creutzfeldt–Jakob Disease Surveillance Unit, *CJD Statistics*. Available at: www.cjd.ed.ac.uk (accessed 28 February 2011).
45 McGilchrist S. (2011) Blood test for vCJD 'could identify carriers.' *BBC News Online* (3 February). Available at: www.bbc.co.uk/news (accessed 28 February 2011).
46 Kirkup B. (2003) *Incident arising in October 2002 from a patient with Creutzfeldt–Jakob disease in Middlesbrough: Report of incident review*, Department of Health, London, para 27.
47 Populus, Health Protection Agency (2007) *Opinion former attitudes towards the possible introduction of a vCJD test for blood donations: qualitative and quantitative research report*, Populus, HPA, London.
48 World Health Organization (2009) Bangkok Charter for Health Promotion in a Globalised World. In: World Health Organization *Milestones in Health Promotion: Statements from Global Conferences*, WHO, Geneva, p.25.
49 See, for example, British Medical Association (2007) *Breaking the cycle of children's exposure to tobacco smoke*, BMA, London; British Medical Association (2008) *Forever cool: the influence of smoking imagery on young people*, BMA, London.
50 Robinson S, Harris H. (2011) *Smoking and drinking among adults 2009*. Office for National Statistics, London, p.14.
51 Robinson S, Harris H. (2011) *Smoking and drinking among adults 2009*. Office for National Statistics, London, p.13.
52 British Medical Association (2008) *Forever cool: the influence of smoking imagery on young people*, BMA, London, pp.9–10.
53 British Association for the Study of Community Dentistry (2007) *The Caries Experience of 5-year-old children in Great Britain (2005/06)*. Available at: www.bascd.org (accessed 28 February 2011).
54 McDonagh M, Whiting P, Bradley M. *et al*. (2000) *A Systematic Review of Public Water Fluoridation*, University NHS Centre for Reviews and Dissemination, University of York. See also: Medical Research Council (2002) *Water Fluoridation and Health*, MRC, London.
55 McDonagh M, Whiting P, Bradley M. *et al.* (2000) *A Systematic Review of Public Water Fluoridation*, NHS Centre for Reviews and Dissemination, University of York, p.45.
56 Medical Research Council (2002) *Water Fluoridation and Health*, MRC, London, p.20.
57 Jones S, Lennon K. (2004) *One in a Million: the facts about water fluoridation*, 2nd edn, British Fluoridation Society, UK Public Health Association, British Dental Association, Faculty of Public Health, London, p.55. This figure does not include the numbers resulting from Southampton PCT's decision to fluoridate the water supplies in 2009.

58 Meikle J. (2009) Fluoridation scheme could go England-wide. *The Guardian* (27 February). Available at: www.guardian.co.uk (accessed 4 February 2010).

59 Nuffield Council on Bioethics (2009) *Public Health: Ethical Issues*, NCB, London, p.139.

60 UK National Screening Committee (1998) *First report of the National Screening Committee*, DH, London, p.14.

61 UK National Screening Committee. *Programme appraisal criteria*. Available at: www.screening.nhs.uk (accessed 6 January 2010).

62 Marteau TM. (2005) Towards an understanding of the psychological consequences of screening. In: Croyle RT (ed.) *Psychosocial effects of screening for disease prevention and detection*, OUP, Oxford, p.187.

63 Cancer Research UK (2011) *CancerStats Key Facts: prostate cancer*. Available at: info.cancerresearchuk.org (accessed 22 February 2011).

64 Cancer Research UK (2011) *CancerStats Key Facts: prostate cancer*. Available at: info.cancerresearchuk.org (accessed 22 February 2011).

65 UK National Screening Committee (2011) *The UK NSC policy on Prostate cancer screening/PSA testing in men over the age of 50*. Available at: www.screening.nhs.uk (accessed 22 February 2011).

66 NHS Breast Screening Programme (2010) *Annual Review 2010*. Available at: www.cancerscreening. nhs.uk (accessed 22 February 2011), p.2.

67 Gøtzsche PC, Nielsen M. (2009) Overdiagnosis in publicly organised mammography screening programmes: systematic review of incidence trends. *BMJ* **33**, b2587.

68 Barquet N, Domingo P. (1997) Smallpox: the triumph over the most terrible of the ministers of death. *Ann Intern Med* **127**, 635–42.

69 Nuffield Council on Bioethics (2007) *Public Health: the ethical issues*, NCB, London, p.51.

70 World Health Organization, UNICEF, World Bank (2009) *State of the world's vaccines and immunization*, 3rd edn, WHO, Geneva, p.4.

71 Nuffield Council on Bioethics (2007) *Public Health: the ethical issues*, NCB, London, p.54.

72 Hardin G. (2002) The tragedy of the commons. In: Gostin LO (ed.) *Public health law and ethics: a reader*, University of California Press, Berkeley, p.383.

73 Dawson A. (2002) Vaccination ethics. In: Ashcroft RE, Dawson A, Draper H. *et al.* (eds.) *Principles of Health Care Ethics*, Wiley, Chichester, p.618.

74 Wakefield AJ, Murch SH, Anthony A. *et al.* (1998) Ileal-lymphoid-nodular hyperplasia, non-specific colitis, and pervasive developmental disorder in children. *Lancet* **351**, 637–41.

75 Demicheli V, Jefferson T, Rivetti A. *et al.* (2005) Vaccines for measles, mumps and rubella in children. *Cochrane Database Syst Rev* **4**, CD004407. DOI: 10.1002/14651858.CD004407.pub2.

76 Department of Health (2004) *NHS Immunisation Statistics, England: 2003–04*. Available at: www.dh.gov.uk (accessed 1 March 2011).

77 Quoted in: McIntyre P, Leask J. (2008) Improving the uptake of MMR vaccine. *BMJ* **336**, 729–30, p.729.

78 The NHS Information Centre (2010) *NHS Immunisation Statistics, England 2009–10*. Available at: www.ic.nhs.uk (accessed 22 February 2011), p.5.

79 Department of Health (1998) *NHS Immunisation Statistics, England: 1997–98*. Available at: www.dh.gov.uk (accessed 1 March 2011).

80 Health Protection Agency (2011) *Confirmed cases of measles by region and age: 1996–2010*. Available at: www.hpa.org.uk (accessed 1 March 2011).

81 Health Protection Agency (2011) *Confirmed cases of measles by region and age: 1996–2010*. Available at: www.hpa.org.uk (accessed 1 March 2011).

82 Health Protection Agency (2010) *Measles deaths: England and Wales, by age group, 1980–2007*. Available at: www.hpa.org.uk (accessed 4 January 2010).

83 Heath Protection Agency (2011) *Why is MMR preferable to single vaccines?* Available at: www.hpa.org.uk (accessed 1 June 2011).

84 Nuffield Council on Bioethics (2007) *Public Health: the ethical issues*, NCB, London, p.58.

85 Department of Health (2007) *Health clearance for tuberculosis, hepatitis B, hepatitis C and HIV: New healthcare workers*, DH, London.

86 Welsh Assembly Government (2007) *Health Clearance for Tuberculosis, Hepatitis B, Hepatitis C and HIV: New Health Care Workers (HCWs)*, WAG, Cardiff.

87 Scottish Government (2008) *Health Clearance for Tuberculosis, Hepatitis B, Hepatitis C and HIV for New Healthcare Workers with Direct Clinical Contact with Patients*, SG, Edinburgh.

88 Department for Health, Social Services and Public Safety (2009) *Guidance on Health Clearance for Tuberculosis, Hepatitis B, Hepatitis C and HIV for New Healthcare Workers with Direct Clinical Contact with Patients*, DHSSPS, Belfast.

89 Department of Health (2006) *Immunisation against infectious disease (the 'Green Book')*, The Stationery Office, London.

90 Campbell D. (2009) Swine flu fears grow as NHS staff shun vaccine. *The Guardian* (11 October). Available at: www.guardian.co.uk (accessed 1 June 2011).

91   General Medical Council (2006) *Good Medical Practice*, GMC, London, para 78.
92   Marteau M, Ashcroft RE, Oliver A. (2009) Using financial incentives to achieve healthy behaviour. *BMJ* **338**, b1415.
93   Gerber H, Schmidt H, Stock S. (2009) What can we learn from German health incentive schemes? *BMJ* **339**, b3504.
94   McColl K. (2008) New York's Road to Health. *BMJ* **337**, a673.
95   Marteau M, Ashcroft RE, Oliver A. (2009) Using financial incentives to achieve healthy behaviour. *BMJ* **338**, b1415.
96   Gerber H, Schmidt H, Stock S. (2009) What can we learn from German health incentive schemes? *BMJ* **339**, b3504.
97   Popay J. (2008) Head to head: should disadvantaged people be paid to take care of their healthcare? No. *BMJ* **337**, a594.
98   NHS Information Centre (2009) *Cervical Screening Programme England 2008–2009*, NHS IC, London, p.5.
99   Howe A, Owen Smith V, Richardson J. (2002) The impact of a television soap opera on the NHS cervical screening programme in the north west of England. *J Public Health Med* **24**, 299–304.
100 Harrabin R, Coote A, Allen J. (2003) *Health in the News: risk reporting and media influence (summary)*, King's Fund, London.
101 Harrabin R, Coote A, Allen J. (2003) *Health in the News: risk reporting and media influence (summary)*, King's Fund, London.
102 Goldacre B. (2007) MMR: the scare stories are back. *BMJ* **335**, 126–7.
103 NHS Choices, *Behind the Headlines*. Available at: www.nhs.uk (accessed 31 May 2011).
104 Anon. (2002) Rabies confirmed in bat worker. *BBC News Online* (24 November). Available at: www.bbc.co.uk/news (accessed 1 March 2011).
105 British Medical Association (2007) *A rational way forward for the NHS in England: a discussion paper outlining an alternative approach to health reform*, BMA, London, p.10.
106 Office of Health Economics (2007) *How UK NHS expenditure and staffing has changed*. Press release, 26 February.
107 British Medical Association (2007) *A rational way forward for the NHS in England: a discussion paper outlining an alternative approach to health reform*, BMA, London.
108 Newdick C. (2006) *Who should we treat? Rights, rationing, and resources in the NHS*, OUP, Oxford, p.46.
109 National Institute for Health and Clinical Excellence (2005) *A guide to NICE*, NICE, London, p.6.
110 Cooper M. (1975) *Rationing Health Care*, Croom Helm, London, p.59. Quoted in: Newdick C. (2006) *Who should we treat? Rights, rationing, and resources in the NHS*, OUP, Oxford, p.19.
111 Jackson E. (2010) *Medical Law: Text, Cases and Materials*, 2nd edn. OUP, Oxford, pp.77–89.
112 *R v North West Lancashire Health Authority, ex parte A and Others* [2000] 1 WLR 977: 984.
113 *Re J (a minor) (wardship: medical treatment)* [1992] 4 All ER 614.
114 *Eisai Ltd v NICE* [2008] EWCA Civ 438.
115 *Savage v South Essex Partnership NHS Foundation Trust* [2008] UKHL 74.
116 *R (on the application of Murphy) v Salford Primary Care Trust* [2008] EWHC 1908 (Admin).
117 *R (on the application of Watts) v Bedford Primary Care Trust and another* [2004] EWCA Civ 166.
118 Directive 2008/142/EC of the European Parliament and the Council on the application of patients' rights in cross-border healthcare. Available at: ec.europa.eu (accessed 31 May 2011).
119 British Medical Association (2007) *A rational way forward for the NHS in England: a discussion paper outlining an alternative approach to health reform*, BMA, London, p.45.
120 New B. (2007) Defining a package of healthcare services the NHS is responsible for. In: New B. (ed.) *Rationing: talk and action in health care*, BMJ Publishing Group, London, pp.79–84.
121 Newdick C. (2006) *Who should we treat? Rights, rationing, and resources in the NHS*, OUP, Oxford, p.13.
122 Newdick C. (2006) *Who should we treat? Rights, rationing, and resources in the NHS*, OUP, Oxford, p.14.
123 Butler J. (1999) *The ethics of healthcare rationing*, Cassell, London, p.132.
124 Butler J. (1999) *The ethics of healthcare rationing*, Cassell, London, p.133.
125 This is taken from: Cochrane AL. (1972) *Effectiveness and efficiency*, The Nuffield Provincial Hospitals Trust, London. Quoted in: Butler J. (1999) *The ethics of health care rationing*, Cassell, London, p.32.
126 See, for example, information on quality adjusted life years (QALYs) in Butler J. (1999) *The ethics of health care rationing*, Cassell, London, p.135.
127 Gutman A. (2002) For and against equal access to health care. In: Gostin LO. (ed.) *Public health law and ethics: a reader*, University of California Press, Berkeley, p.256.
128 Revil J. (2006) Both have cancer. But why can't one get the best care? *The Observer* (9 July). Available at: www.guardian.co.uk (accessed 31 May 2011).
129 See, for example: Abelson J, Collins P. (2009). Media hyping and the "Herceptin access story": an analysis of Canadian and UK newspaper coverage. *Healthc Policy* **4**(3), e113–28.
130 Department of Health (2009) *Age Equality in health and Social Care*, DH, London, para 5.17.

131   Pencheon D, Guest C, Melzer D. *et al*. (eds.) (2001) *Oxford handbook of public health practice*, OUP, Oxford, pp.229–30.

132   For a discussion of the concept of 'community' see: Heginbotham C. (1999) Return to community: the ethics of exclusion and inclusion. In: Parker M. (ed.) *Ethics and community in the health care professions*, Routledge, London, pp.47–61.

133   For further discussion of these issues, see: Doyal L. (1993) The role of the public in health care rationing. *Critical Public Health* **4**, 49–52. Doyal L. (1997) The moral boundaries of public and patient involvement. In: New B. (ed.) *Rationing: talk and action in health care*, BMJ Publishing Group, London, pp.171–80.

134   Bowling A. (1996) Health care rationing: the public's debate. *BMJ* **312**, 670–4.

135   Hart JT. (1974) Milroy Lecture: the marriage of primary care and epidemiology: continuous anticipatory care of whole populations in a state medical service. *J R Coll Physicians Lond* **8**, 299–314.

136   The Health Service (Control of Patient Information) Regulations 2002. SI 2002/1438, s 1(a–d).

21: Reducing risk, clinical error and poor performance

The questions covered in this chapter include the following.

- What is the role of individual doctors in minimising risk and improving quality?
- Why is reporting of adverse events and near misses crucial to improving care?
- What support is available for doctors who are struggling to cope?
- What legal protection is available for doctors who blow the whistle on substandard care?

This chapter focuses on doctors' duties to try to ensure patient safety, minimise risks and improve quality of care. The emphasis is on doctors working within their competence, auditing performance, keeping their skills up to date, admitting errors and learning from them. The benchmark legal cases featured in this chapter are mainly about medical mistakes but some indicate how prompt action, once the error is realised, can rectify the situation and exonerate the doctor from blame. The cases also illustrate how poor performance can inadvertently result from well-intentioned actions, particularly when doctors are inexperienced or insufficiently supported. The chapter mentions various measures to capture information about how aspects of practice can be improved and some such measures are also covered in other parts of the book (see, for example, Chapter 12, page 511). Whistleblowing is discussed here, including the duty to take action if the care provided by colleagues or by institutions appears inadequate. This chapter also covers the care and management of sick doctors.

The duty to protect patients

Patient safety and quality of care are key concerns for everyone providing or receiving health services. Medicine is about providing net health benefit with minimum harm and all doctors have an important role in improving quality of care while addressing indicators of possible harm. They have obligations to monitor their own conduct, performance and health and those of colleagues with whom they work. Mistakes have profound effects on patient trust so that the uptake of beneficial procedures can be adversely affected. Errors cause suffering, stress and lost resources, especially if litigation results. Having safeguards in place to minimise mistakes and adverse incidents is crucial.

The monitoring of doctors' performance and guidance around issues such as adverse event reporting developed considerably after the publication in 2001 of the report of the Inquiry into paediatric surgery at the Bristol Royal Infirmary (see page 867).[1] The period following the Bristol Report saw significant development in clinical governance, including risk management, evidence-based practice, audit, the monitoring of outcomes of care and the promotion of lifelong learning among health professionals. Such measures contributed greatly to the development of a strong ethical framework for reducing risk. Examples of

Medical Ethics Today: The BMA's Handbook of Ethics and Law, Third Edition. Sophie Brannan, Eleanor Chrispin, Martin Davies, Veronica English, Rebecca Mussell, Julian Sheather and Ann Sommerville.
© 2012 BMA Medical Ethics Department. Published 2012 by Blackwell Publishing Ltd.

poor quality care still occur, however, despite wide recognition of the importance of identifying adverse events and continually improving standards.

Causes of poor practice include health professionals under stress, particularly if they are working long or unsocial hours, with insufficient support. Repeated investigations within the NHS have identified problems such as inexperienced doctors being expected to tackle complex procedures without adequate supervision. Error and substandard care need to be addressed by managers implementing good governance procedures with which all staff are familiar, including the following:

- the setting and monitoring of clear quality standards
- open discussion of errors and situations in which mistakes were narrowly averted
- efforts to dismantle the blame culture to allow such discussion
- appropriate systems to rectify the consequences of any error
- measures to provide people who suffer harm with an explanation and compensation
- support for healthcare staff who acknowledge their own mistakes and limitations
- supportive systems for doctors and other health professionals who are themselves sick.

Despite the very positive growth in safeguards and professional awareness of risk management, litigation against the NHS has increased for a number of reasons. These include the social climate which 'encourages expectations of cure. When these are not met, the culture of consumerism – fuelled by a press eager to disclose wrongdoing – advocates the allocation of blame and the seeking of compensation.'[2] The National Health Service Litigation Authority (NHSLA) handles claims against the NHS. In 2009–2010, 6,652 claims of clinical negligence and 4,074 claims of non-clinical negligence against NHS bodies were received by the Authority. This was an increase from 6,088 claims of clinical negligence and 3,743 claims of non-clinical negligence in the previous year. The NHSLA reports that £787 million was paid in connection with clinical negligence claims during 2009–2010, up from £769 million in 2008–2009.[3] Only a small percentage of claims received by the NHSLA reach court, however, and the majority that do so fail, but the entire process is extremely stressful for both patients and doctors, as well as being costly. This is one of the reasons why the British Medical Association (BMA) supports alternative measures such as mediation and a system of no-fault compensation. (These are discussed below on pages 868–869.)

Professionalism

The nature and content of medical professionalism have been the subject of much debate as the context of healthcare has changed (see also the introductory chapter, pages 4–6). Some traditional aspects of professionalism, including the freedom that doctors once enjoyed to define standards of care and to control the organisation of their work, have long been under pressure due to factors such as the courts increasingly arbitrating on standards of good practice. (Some of the key legal cases in terms of defining negligence, for example, are set out on pages 858–861.) Despite changes in notions of professionalism, ensuring patient safety has long been seen as a crucial part of it:

[t]he first duty of a doctor must be to ensure the wellbeing of patients and to protect them from harm – this responsibility lies at the heart of medical professionalism. Patients expect doctors to be technically competent, open and honest, and to show them respect. By demonstrating these qualities, doctors earn the trust that makes their professional status and privileges possible.[4]

New interpretations of professionalism also place a duty on doctors to engage in improving services but, in the past, doctors have sometimes been alienated and marginalised from organisational governance and improvement. Implementing governance measures is primarily a managerial task but clearly healthcare staff need to engage with them. A key comment of the Healthcare Commission's 2009 report into the failures at the Mid Staffordshire NHS Trust (discussed on page 874) was that governance systems must not only appear persuasive on paper but must actually work in practice. The Commission found that staff who were marginalised or were left feeling disillusioned gave up expressing their views on what was going wrong. 'Worryingly, many consultants considered that governance was something that was done to them, rather than being a key part of a clinical activity in which they had a major part to play.'[5] For this to happen, they need opportunities to be heard and have their views taken seriously.

General principles

There is a large body of literature on clinical governance and the setting of quality markers in primary, secondary and specialised areas of healthcare, such as palliative care. Our aim is not to reproduce it but to focus on the fundamental obligation of all doctors to provide safe and effective care. In particular, the General Medical Council (GMC) requires that doctors:

- make care of patients their first concern
- protect and promote the health of patients and the public
- provide a good standard of practice and care
- keep their knowledge and skills up to date throughout their working life
- recognise and work within the limits of their professional competence
- work with colleagues in ways that best serve patients' interests
- observe and keep up to date with the laws and statutory codes of practice that affect their work
- take part in regular and systematic medical and clinical audit and respond appropriately to the outcomes of any review, assessment or appraisal of performance
- be willing to take action if they have reason to think patient safety is compromised by inadequate premises, equipment, resources, policies or systems
- be aware of the performance of colleagues and be willing to address problems identified.[6]

Standard setting

Standards are set by a range of professional bodies, including the GMC, and by the law – both statute and case law. Clinical standards are also set by professional guidelines or protocols. The legal and professional standards in relation to specific areas of practice are discussed in each chapter of this book. When a doctor's failure or error results in harm for a patient, the case may be heard before the GMC as one of fitness to practise, or in the courts either as negligence or gross negligence.

The NHSLA also has a role in setting some standards, as part of its remit is to contribute to incentives for reducing the number of negligent or preventable incidents. It aims to do this through an extensive risk-management programme. NHS organisations are assessed against its risk-management standards, developed to reflect issues that have arisen in the negligence claims reported to the NHSLA.

In legal cases of alleged negligence, patients have to establish that they are owed a duty of care by the defendant who breached that duty, causing them injury. (Duty of care is discussed in Chapter 1, pages 29–31.) As a yardstick, the courts measure the doctor's action against the practice accepted as reasonable by a responsible body of medical opinion, provided that the opinion withstands logical analysis (see page 859). If doctors do something which no reasonable practitioner in that situation would do, they attract blame and may be subject to disciplinary procedures, the criminal courts or civil litigation. In law, they are deemed negligent if they allow harm to occur by failing to take reasonable action; what is 'reasonable' depends on the facts and circumstances. Health professionals should be aware of good practice, as established by professional bodies. Normally, this is an indicator of what is 'reasonable' but doctors also need to know when to deviate from the accepted standard. Failure to adapt to circumstances when they require a deviation from accepted rules is likely to be criticised. The Scottish case of *Hunter v Hanley* and the English cases of *Bolam* and *Bolitho* established key legal benchmarks in negligence cases, emphasising that the standards expected of doctors reflect those set by their peers within the specialty in question but their decisions must also be shown to be reasonable.

Hunter v Hanley

This Scottish case was important in establishing the concept that a doctor's conduct should be in line with the standards of other similar doctors. Mrs Hunter brought an action against her GP, Dr Hanley, after being injured in 1951 as a result of a hypodermic needle breaking as she was given a penicillin injection. Part of the needle remained in her body, requiring hospital treatment. She alleged the injury was due to Dr Hanley's negligence and claimed that 'any doctor possessing fair and average knowledge of his profession' would not use this type of needle for an intramuscular injection. In the first trial, the jury found in favour of Dr Hanley, having been directed by the judge that a doctor would not be negligent unless he had departed very significantly from usual practice. Mrs Hunter challenged the judge's view and the case was heard again before the First Division where the President, Lord Clyde, pointed out that progress in medicine depends upon doctors being able to deviate from ordinary practice in some circumstances. The relevant test, he said, is not how much or how little a doctor deviates from normal practice but whether the deviation is one which no other careful doctor would have chosen. He said that:

> In the realm of diagnosis and treatment there is ample scope for genuine difference of opinion, and one man clearly is not negligent merely because his conclusion differs from that of other professional men, nor because he has displayed less skill or knowledge than others would have shown. The true test for establishing negligence in diagnosis or treatment on the part of a doctor is whether he has been proved to be guilty of such failure as no doctor of ordinary skill would be guilty of if acting with ordinary care.[7]

> To establish liability by a doctor where deviation from normal practice is alleged, three facts require to be established. First of all it must be proved that there is a usual and normal practice; secondly it must be proved that the defender has not adopted that practice; and thirdly (and this is of crucial importance) it must be established that the course the doctor adopted is one which no professional man of ordinary skill would have taken if he had been acting with ordinary care.[8]

Lord Clyde's dictum in the Hanley case was later quoted approvingly by Mr Justice McNair in the English case of *Bolam v Friern Hospital Management Committee.*

Bolam v Friern Hospital Management Committee

In this case, the High Court considered the fracture sustained by a mentally ill patient during electroconvulsive therapy (ECT). The patient had signed a consent form but had not been warned of the risk of fracture, which was estimated at 1 in 10,000. Nor had he been given a muscle relaxant and he was not physically restrained during the treatment. He sustained a fractured hip and brought an action for damages for negligence.

There were two schools of medical opinion about the management of patients undergoing ECT: one favoured routinely using relaxant drugs and the other said that medication increased the risks for patients and should be used only in exceptional cases. There were also differing views on whether patients should be warned of the risks of fracture. The judge directed the jury that: (1) doctors were not negligent if they acted in accordance with a practice accepted as proper by a responsible body of medical opinion, even if another body of medical opinion took another view; and (2) the patient seeking to prove negligence had to show not only that the non-disclosure was negligent but also that he would not have consented to the treatment had he been informed of the risk. The effect of the case was to emphasise that doctors must be judged by the standards of care expected of professionals in that particular specialty.[9]

In the *Bolitho* case in 1997, the House of Lords revisited the implications of the *Bolam* test. It also made clear that the courts were increasingly the arbiters of good practice.

Bolitho v City and Hackney Health Authority

Patrick Bolitho, a 2-year-old child, had a brain injury after being admitted to hospital with breathing difficulties. He had a cardiac arrest which led to brain damage and his death. Intubation might have prevented the respiratory failure but it also had risks. The paediatric registrar on duty had not seen the child but said that even if she had done, she would not have intubated him. Expert witnesses expressed opposing views as to whether intubation would have been reasonable. The initial trial judge thought it should have been provided but when the case went to the Lords, they noted that a responsible body of medical opinion supported non-intubation. The House of Lords adopted a revised version of the test of negligence, saying that not only should doctors' actions be measured against responsible medical opinion, but also that, if the expert opinion did not stand up to logical analysis, judges could reject it. The Bolitho family lost the case. The Lords' decision was a strong affirmation that the courts should set standards and, in some cases, would decide that negligence had occurred even if some medical experts agreed with the defendant's actions. Lord Browne-Wilkinson said:

> In the vast majority of cases the fact that distinguished experts in the field are of a particular opinion will demonstrate the reasonableness of that opinion. In particular, where there are questions of assessment of the relative risks and benefits of adopting a particular medical practice, a reasonable view necessarily presupposes that the relative risks and benefits have been weighed by the experts in forming their opinions. But if, in a rare case, it can be demonstrated that the professional opinion is not capable of withstanding logical analysis, the judge is entitled to hold that the body of opinion is not reasonable or responsible.[10]

The effect of these cases is to emphasise that, throughout their careers, doctors should be aware of current professional opinion within their own area of practice and that adherence to such opinion must be demonstrably logical. Consultants are not judged to be negligent if they act in accordance with the standards expected of consultants and junior doctors must generally comply with what is reasonably expected of their peer group and take advice when uncertain. There can be some ambiguity, however, when doctors are inexperienced in the tasks delegated to them. The paradigm case illustrating this was the *Wilsher* case.

Wilsher v Essex Area Health Authority

A junior doctor mistakenly inserted a catheter into a premature baby's vein rather than an artery and the baby was deprived of oxygen and became virtually blind, although there were also other possible causes of his condition.[11] Lawyers acting for the doctor argued that the standard of care expected of a junior doctor was not the same as would be expected from a more experienced colleague as it was unavoidable that staff had to learn on the job. The case was went on to be heard in the Appeal Court and the House of Lords and, although he made a mistake in inserting the catheter and a second mistake in not recognising the signs that he had done so on the X-ray, the junior doctor was ultimately judged to have acted reasonably. He had done what he thought was right and then asked a senior registrar to check.

This conclusion was not as straightforward as it might at first seem as the views expressed in the Appeal Court, were 'not free of ambiguity'.[12] The majority of judges said that the public should expect a reasonable standard of competence from doctors and held that the standard of care should not be lower for inexperienced doctors. On the other hand, the point was made by one judge that the expected standard should be defined in accordance with the post the doctor filled – in this case a junior one. The conclusion most often cited as indicative of the judges' final view is that of Lord Justice Glidewell who argued that the standard should be objective rather than taking account of the doctor's inexperience. He said that the law required trainees to be judged by the same standard as more experienced colleagues but mitigated this when he went on to say:

> If this test appears unduly harsh in relation to the inexperienced, I should add that, in my view, the inexperienced doctor called on to exercise a specialist skill will, as part of that skill, seek the advice and help of his superiors when he does or may need it. If he does seek such help, he will often have satisfied the test, even though he may himself have made a mistake.[13]

Therefore, the fact that the junior doctor had promptly asked a senior colleague to check what he done exonerated him.

Mason and Laurie conclude that the implications of the Wilsher case set:

> [a] standard of care test which is based on the doctor of similar experience irrespective of the post in which he operates. Conversely, however, an experienced doctor occupying a junior post would be judged according to his actual knowledge rather than by the lower standard of the reasonably competent occupant of that post – the rationale being that, by reason of his superior expertise, he would be more able to foresee the damage likely to arise from any negligent acts or omissions.[14]

Harm might be caused to the patient if a GP fails to diagnose the patient's condition correctly but this would not necessarily be negligent, even though a specialist's failure to make an accurate diagnosis in the same patient would be unacceptable. So when cases are heard in court, an expert report is required from a practitioner in the same area of practice as the defendant, rather than from a doctor who is an expert in the patient's actual condition. A GP, for example, cannot necessarily be expected to have identified symptoms that might be obvious to a specialist in a particular condition although the GP might well be expected to identify that the patient needed further specialist investigation.

When harm is thought to have been caused by a mistake in treatment, the courts have to look closely at the evidence rather than assume that an error was the trigger, especially if there could possibly be another cause. This was one of the issues raised in the *Wilsher* case and was also illustrated by the Scottish case of *Kay's Tutor v Ayrshire and Arran Health Board*.

Kay's Tutor v Ayrshire and Arran Health Board

A child was treated with oral ampicillin by his GP for a respiratory infection but the boy vomited, diminishing the effect. He remained seriously ill and was taken to hospital where benzyl penicillin was given intravenously and he was diagnosed with pneumococcal meningitis. A consultant paediatrician instructed that 10,000 units of penicillin be injected intrathecally (by lumbar puncture) but the senior house officer mistakenly gave the patient 30 times too much – 300,000 units of penicillin. The child went into convulsions and developed temporary paralysis on one side of his body. The senior house officer quickly realised the mistake and successfully initiated measures to save the child's life but, when discharged from hospital, the child was profoundly deaf. Meningitis can cause deafness but the parents argued that, in this case, the overdose caused or contributed to the child's deafness. A neurosurgeon supported that view, putting forward the theory that pencillin injected intrathecally could damage the auditory nerve. The court of first instance found in favour of the family but this was overturned on appeal when it was held that where two potential causes of damage exist, it cannot be presumed that the doctor's mistake was responsible. There must be clear factual evidence to support the claim that the error caused the damage. In this case, an expert in antibiotics said that there was simply no evidence to support the theory that the penicillin overdose could have caused deafness, as no single case of this happening had previously been recorded.[15]

All doctors must work within their competence and so embarking on an inherently difficult procedure might be rash and negligent if done by a GP, but quite acceptable if undertaken by an experienced specialist.

Failure to meet expected professional standards

A GP was struck off the medical register by the GMC after being found guilty of 42 counts of serious professional misconduct. Over 2 years, he had undertaken 100 private liposuction operations. He was an experienced GP but had no training in surgery or anaesthesia. One patient was given an unsuitable local anaesthetic and two others woke up during the operation. The doctor was accused of giving inadequate anaesthetic, failing to monitor sedated patients, not carrying out a proper physical examination and failing to explain the risks of the procedure. Giving evidence to the GMC, he acknowledged that the treatment he provided fell short of what was required.[16]

Both the law and professional standards emphasise the importance of discussing with patients the risks as well as the anticipated benefits of any proposed intervention and informing them about reasonable alternatives. Failure to do so may invalidate any consent or refusal the patient gives. (This is discussed further below and in Chapter 2, pages 64–72.)

The duty to explain reasonable alternatives

Mrs Birch agreed to a catheter angiography after being warned that there was a 1 per cent risk of a stroke as a result of the procedure. She was not informed that a magnetic resonance imaging (MRI) scan would be an alternative diagnostic technique which was slightly less exact but carried no stroke risk. Mrs Birch had a stroke and, while acknowledging that the doctor had informed her of the risk associated with the catheter angiogram, argued that he had breached his duty of care by failing to explain the comparative risks of the two procedures. The judge agreed that the doctor had a duty not only to tell the patient about the risks of the procedure he proposed, but also to explain that there were fewer, or no risks, associated with an alternative procedure. Without this information, the patient could not give properly informed consent and the failure to provide it was in breach of the doctor's duty.[17]

Standards of practice

Standards can be established by court judgments which illustrate the law's, as well as the GMC's, expectation that doctors should recognise their limitations and not undertake procedures for which they lack training or supervision. Emergency situations may be an exception as the GMC requires doctors to offer assistance in such cases while taking account of their own safety, competence and the availability of other options for the patient's care (see Chapter 15, pages 642–644).[18] Various legal cases show how doctors have little defence if they deliberately work beyond their capability, and if the patient dies the doctor may face a manslaughter charge. In terms of criminal negligence, a distinction may be drawn in terms of medical actions that deliberately or recklessly expose a patient to risk of harm and those in which the (often inexperienced) doctor was simply unaware of the risks. In particular, if a doctor knowingly and recklessly puts a patient at risk so that death results, the action may be judged to be criminal. 'Such prosecutions used to be rare; their increase points to heightened interest in the external regulation of medicine and to a diminution in the professional immunity which doctors may previously have enjoyed.'[19] This is a cause of regret to some legal experts as well as to doctors, who acknowledge that all professionals should be accountable for their failures but 'what is more dubious is that the criminal law and particularly manslaughter prosecutions, should be the instrument chosen to perform that task'.[20]

Hospital practice

Junior doctors can be particularly vulnerable in terms of being expected to perform, without appropriate supervision, tasks for which they lack expertise. The BMA publishes a brief 'ethical survival kit' for doctors new to practice and those who are simply new to working in the UK.[21] If asked to take on tasks with which they are unfamiliar, doctors need to acknowledge if they are out of their depth and talk to senior colleagues. Pressure to handle things without calling senior staff should be resisted. BMA members can also contact the BMA for advice.

Unsupervised junior doctors

A teenaged patient with leukaemia was admitted to hospital for his monthly treatment with cytotoxic drugs. Under the supervision of a senior house officer, a pre-registration house officer injected vincristine (which should be given intravenously) into the patient's cerebrospinal fluid instead of methotrexate. There had been a failure of communication and the more senior doctor thought that he was supervising only the lumbar puncture but the less experienced colleague thought that the whole procedure was being supervised. The patient died. The judge summing up in the subsequent legal case said: 'you could have been helped more than you were helped' and 'you are good men who contrary to your normal behaviour were guilty of momentary recklessness'.[22] Both doctors were convicted of manslaughter and given suspended prison sentences. The case caused great concern within the medical profession as the mistake was not perceived as reckless or without concern for the patient. The convictions were overturned on appeal.[23]

A similar case occurred at Great Ormond Street Hospital for Children when a 12-year-old was given vincristine, but charges against the two junior doctors were withdrawn because it was acknowledged that the hospital system had contributed significantly to the error. The vincristine was wrongly sent to the operating theatre by a nurse, contrary to hospital rules, and was administered by the junior doctor after being advised by telephone by a registrar in haematology to administer the drugs that had been sent. A notable feature in both cases was that no member of the hospital's management was held liable even though aspects of the system in which the doctors were working had clearly contributed to the errors.[24]

In cases such as these, the risks for future patients are not necessarily reduced if individuals alone are blamed for errors, rather than lessons being learned about how to address the chain of events which led to them.

R v Misra

In 2003, two junior doctors were found guilty of manslaughter after having ignored warnings from nursing staff that a patient had become seriously ill. After a routine knee operation on a damaged ligament, the patient developed a rapid pulse, raised temperature and low blood pressure. Toxic shock syndrome developed. Although this is a relatively uncommon condition, it was argued in court that the doctors should have noticed that the patient's condition was significantly abnormal and sought help but they were reluctant to admit they were out of their depth and did not call a senior colleague. Nor did they take the patient's blood pressure or carry out tests. The toxic shock syndrome led to kidney failure and, by the time senior doctors were called, the patient was beyond help. He was transferred to the intensive care department but died. The two junior doctors were convicted of manslaughter by gross negligence and given a suspended prison sentence. Their appeal against conviction was dismissed.[25]

Specialists may also be tempted to act outside their normal sphere of treatment rather than referring a patient on to a colleague. This can involve various risks, including the fact that doctors working outside their area of expertise may fail to give the patient all the information about risks and side effects that someone routinely carrying out the same procedure would do.

A specialist working outside his sphere of expertise

While examining a patient who was consulting him for advice on hormone replacement therapy, a specialist in gynaecology noticed several unsightly skin lesions. He asked the patient whether they had changed or bled. She said some had expanded and agreed to have them removed under a general anaesthetic but was given no warning about possible scarring. The gynaecologist carried out the procedure himself, excising nine senile keratoses but, when the sutures were later removed, some of the wounds gaped and Steristrips were applied. No follow-up treatment had been planned or given. The patient developed keloid scarring and successfully sued the gynaecologist. Following the case, the Medical Protection Society emphasised the importance of doctors not acting outside their area of professional practice but of referring patients to a colleague in the relevant specialty.[26]

Primary care

As with all doctors, GPs should ensure that they maintain an awareness of best practice standards and keep their skills up to date. This includes ensuring that specialist advice is sought in a timely manner when there is some evidence that the patient needs to be referred on.

Diagnostic error

A GP was found guilty of serious professional misconduct by the GMC when he failed to diagnose early signs of breast cancer in two women who later died of the disease. He was told that he should have referred the two patients to a specialist when they showed signs of cancer. His work had to be supervised for a year and he underwent additional training in cancer care prior to being allowed to resume unsupervised work.[27]

In addition to monitoring their own performance, GPs (and all other doctors who employ staff) also have clear responsibilities for the reliability of the people they employ. Ensuring patient safety not only involves checking staff competency, but also carrying out criminal record checks. (This is discussed in Chapter 1, pages 49–50 and Chapter 19, pages 794–795.)

Locums, out-of-hours services and arranging medical cover

The GMC tells doctors that when off duty, they must be satisfied that suitable arrangements have been made for patient care. The arrangements should include effective hand-over procedures and good communication beforehand with colleagues. If the cover arrangements appear inadequate to ensure patient safety, the doctor has a duty to either put the matter right or draw it to the attention of the employing or contracting body.[28] Employers must ensure that the staff they employ are competent and properly supported by a thorough induction if the setting is unfamiliar to them. Inexperienced doctors and those new to the UK should not be left facing decisions beyond their clinical competence. Following the implementation of the European Working Time Directive in 2009 there was increased demand for locums at a time when some employers found it difficult to find doctors who were familiar with NHS practice. In 2010, there was considerable media debate about the potential risks posed by some overseas doctors working as locums in the NHS where the work was different to their usual practice.

Ubani case

In February 2008, Daniel Ubani, a German doctor providing out-of-hours cover, administered 10 times the clinically indicated dose of diamorphine to David Gray who died as a result. Dr Ubani said he was tired, stressed and unfamiliar with the drug. Errors were also made in the treatment of two other patients in the same shift. The GMC later said there had been wide-ranging, serious and persistent failings in his basic competence. Dr Ubani had only undergone a brief induction and the assessor had warned that there was insufficient time for a full appraisal. Dr Ubani said that the fatal mistake derived from a confusion between two drugs, one of which was not used by on-call services in Germany. Other German doctors had also been in difficulties with the same drug. Dr Ubani was given a 9-month suspended prison sentence in Germany for negligence. In Britain, he was struck off in June 2010 by the GMC which said that he had shown a persistent lack of insight into the seriousness of his actions and had not attempted to improve his skills. The GMC also called for EU doctors to be tested on their clinical skills and language abilities. It is primarily up to employers, however, to ensure doctors are competent.[29]

Following the Ubani case, the BMA's annual representatives meeting in 2010 echoed the GMC in insisting that any doctor practising in the UK should demonstrably have a good command of English, equivalent breadth of clinical skills, training and knowledge as would normally be associated with their specialty and understand the operation of the NHS, as well as being subject to UK regulatory processes.

Locums, like all other doctors, must ensure their own competence and are directly accountable to the GMC. Agencies and employers also have responsibility for checking their performance. They should ensure that pre-employment checks have been properly carried out. Dealing with poor performance by locum or deputising doctors can be problematic as there is seldom an ongoing relationship but, if problems remain unresolved, the doctor may pose a threat to patient safety elsewhere. (See pages 869–870 on appraisal and page 872 on writing references.) If it is not possible to resolve problems with locums through standard local procedures it may be necessary to contact the GMC directly for advice. Doctors employing locums whose performance is a matter of doubt have a responsibility to inform the locum agency and they may also need to discuss the possibility of issuing an alert letter (see page 875). Employers should only use agencies that have reliable quality control systems in place.

Summary – standard setting

- Doctors should be familiar with professional standards relevant to their area of practice.
- They must follow GMC advice and ensure that they work within their limitations.
- Junior doctors should insist on appropriate support.
- Doctors should avoid embarking on medical procedures or providing advice in specialties outside their own area of expertise, other than in emergency situations where a more experienced professional is not available.

Duties of doctors to monitor quality and performance

Duties regarding risk

All health professionals should audit their own performance and participate in processes such as revalidation and appraisal. The risk of errors and adverse events can be categorised in a way that helps to clarify the duties of individual doctors in different situations.

- Clinical errors affect the doctor–patient relationship and are a significant cause of stress to all parties. Doctors should obviously do their best to minimise them by taking proportionate action. Misdiagnosis is one of the most common errors in primary care but is not entirely avoidable in a necessarily uncertain process. Misdiagnosis could be reduced if over-referral were the norm but this would result in many pointless referrals, with unjustified anxiety for many patients, as well as wasting resources. Over-referral, therefore, is not the answer and would cause delays in the treatment of patients with a clear diagnosis if all others about whom there is any uncertainty are slotted into the queue. Traditionally, the proportionate response has been that GPs refer promptly when signs of a potentially serious condition are detected while accepting the uncertainties and possibility of misdiagnosis.
- Risks can be a symptom of systems failure. Errors are often rooted in a series of interrelated situations and events. The systems within which doctors work can give rise to conditions in which errors are more likely to occur. Part of risk management – with which all health professionals need to cooperate – involves the identification and remedying of such situations.

- Risks may be imposed by cost constraints. Shortage of staff and other resources create pressure, reduce safety margins and affect the capacity of healthcare systems to cope with unexpected challenges. (See also the box on the Mid Staffordshire Inquiry on page 874.) Health staff have obligations to whistleblow if, for example, standard internal notifications have no effect (see also pages 878–879).
- Risks are also inherent in clinical procedures. Even if all other risks could be eliminated, patients receiving treatment would still be subject to the inherent risks of the actual procedures they undergo. These vary according to factors such as gender, age, co-morbidity and lifestyle, which affect individuals' ability to cope with medical interventions and recover from them.

Analysing risks in terms of these categories can help to define the means of managing them in each case. It also helps to identify whose responsibility it is to manage the different levels of risk. Clinicians are accountable for their own decisions but not for the levels of risk over which they have no influence. The BMA believes that 'if the distinction between different categories of risk can be made explicit, it should be possible for each party to acknowledge and bear the risks which are properly their responsibility. This bargaining process should not be left implicit.'[30]

The duty to discuss risks with patients

Patients' perception of risk affects their willingness to accept treatment and they often have unrealistic expectations. Doctors need good communication skills and meaningful data to help patients make realistic assessments of the risk involved. Explaining risk in a meaningful way is notoriously difficult, not least because there is often uncertainty about the likely outcome. Trust and openness can help patients make a decision that is right for them, even in the face of uncertainty. Chapter 2 sets out the kind of information that patients need in order to make a valid decision. It mentions that, in law, the known risks associated with a specific medical procedure need to be explained to patients facing that intervention. An action in negligence may arise if the patient is not told of a risk which then occurs if, for example, the patient would not have undergone the procedure if aware of the risk (see Chapter 2, pages 66–70).

Patients also need to understand that no medical interventions are entirely risk free but that they are only recommended when the anticipated benefits are reasonably expected to exceed the foreseeable harms. The more invasive the procedure, the more likely it is to disrupt the body's natural functions but may offer a patient a better chance of recovery. The anticipated trade-off between risk and benefit should be discussed with patients. Patients need to be aware about any risks associated with their own situation and lifestyle and how age, gender, co-morbidity, obesity, smoking or alcohol consumption can affect outcomes. They should be aware of factors within their control that could help to minimise risks.

Doctors monitoring their own performance

Poor practice is often the result of many factors, including high patient demand and inadequate support but some extreme behaviour is the result of doctors exploiting vulnerable patients (see Chapter 1, pages 50–51).

In other cases, doctors sincerely intend to act in patients' interests but fail to seek their views. They may believe that their opinion is more important or better informed than what the patient would choose. They may make a deliberate decision to circumvent usual professional standards. Even if they believe it is for a good reason, making life and death decisions without considering the patient's viewpoint is always likely to be unacceptable.

Dr Martin

Dr Howard Martin was arrested in 2004 in County Durham after relatives of an elderly patient raised concerns with the police. He was charged with, and acquitted of, the murder of three patients whose bodies were exhumed. He said, however, that he had helped two patients to die 'not because they wanted to die but because they had dreadful suffering'.[31] In July 2010, the GMC looked at his case and struck him off the medical register. Dr Martin admitted giving fatal doses of painkillers to seriously ill patients without their consent. The GMC disciplinary panel ruled that he was guilty of serious professional misconduct for administering excessively high doses of morphine to 18 vulnerable elderly people without consent between 1994 and 2004. The panel said his actions were not negligent but down to an autocratic attitude in which he believed he was always right and showed no remorse. The GMC hearing was told that while some of the 18 patients may have had only days or hours to live, at least one patient might have recovered from oesophageal cancer had Dr Martin not administered 200 mg diamorphine.[32]

Crucial benchmarks in the awareness of doctors' duty to monitor their performance and abide by peer group standards came with the interim and then the 2001 final report of the public inquiry into children's heart surgery at the Bristol Royal Infirmary (the Bristol Report).[33] This disclosed in a very high profile way many of the problems associated with doctors' under-performance, failure to acknowledge problems and the silencing of whistleblowers, as well as issues related to poor management. The report also brought together much of the thinking within the profession itself about practical ways to measure and improve performance.

Impact of the Bristol Royal Infirmary case

The Bristol Royal Infirmary had been designated as a supra-regional centre for paediatric heart surgery but from 1988 to 1994 the mortality rate was roughly double that elsewhere. This could not be accounted for solely by the case mix, nor by the high-risk procedures carried out. Concerns began to be expressed by health professionals from the mid-1980s but these were portrayed by the surgeons involved as a campaign of vilification. Even when higher mortality rates were acknowledged, it was claimed that these were due to the complex procedures carried out. A pattern of poor outcomes was emerging. An anaesthetist, Stephen Bolsin, repeatedly attempted to draw attention to the mortality rates but was rebuffed. In 1995 an operation on Joshua Loveday was the catalyst for intervention when the child died after staff had attempted to prevent the operation. A review was instituted and two of the cardiac surgeons and the Trust's chief executive were found guilty of serious professional misconduct by the GMC in 1998. The surgeons' decision to persist with the operations in the face of mounting evidence of unacceptable outcomes sparked disciplinary proceedings against them by the GMC.

Addressing the blame culture

When harm occurs, there is often a sense that someone must be responsible and individuals may be blamed for institutional failures or unforeseeable accidents. It has long been recognised that this is counter-productive and that the blame culture contributes to the occurrence of more medical errors. By focusing on individuals, investigations can fail to identify the systemic deficiencies that create situations in which error is likely to occur and also makes health professionals reluctant to admit to mistakes. The 2001 Bristol Report strongly urged that more effort be made to abolish the culture of blame, which it saw as undermining patient safety by inhibiting open discussion of adverse events. The report emphasised that a concern for safety can only flourish in a non-punitive environment in which health professionals talk frankly.

Much debate has focused on improving care by redesigning systems, particularly management structure and the reporting systems for capturing errors. A blame culture is more likely to occur in healthcare organisations with rigid hierarchical management systems and occurs less where there is greater employee involvement in decision making.[34] It has been suggested that 'health care organisations need to develop a culture that harnesses the ideas and ingenuity of health care professionals by employing a commitment-based management philosophy rather than strangling them by over-regulating their behaviours using a control-based philosophy'.[35] On the other hand, it might be argued that by focusing attention entirely on the multiple factors underpinning common errors in a 'blame-free' approach, the accountability of individual health professionals is diminished. Clearly, a balance is required. When the systems within which they work contribute to the risk of harm, doctors should persist in engaging with managers to have those risks addressed. This requires a culture in which open discussion and reflection can occur. (For monitoring quality through mechanisms such as random case review, see page 876.)

Mediation

In the UK, one hindrance to eliminating the blame culture and encouraging health staff to speak openly about errors is the clinical negligence system (discussed above in relation to the *Bolam* and *Bolitho* cases). It is often criticised as inefficient, costly and an inappropriate way of dealing with medical mistakes. It can drive medical practice in an overly cautious direction and fosters a blame culture which inhibits improvement and learning from errors.

The BMA has long supported the use of mediation to try to resolve cases through discussion and a system of no-fault compensation which would provide redress for patients without having to prove that someone had been at fault. Making a complaint or claim is often disruptive to the doctor–patient relationship and often seriously impedes meaningful communication between doctor and patient during a process which can last years. The BMA's Medico-Legal Committee has drawn attention to the potential benefits in mediation for both claimants and the healthcare professionals:[36]

- it can be set up speedily and is confidential and without prejudice, so it is largely risk-free even if the claim is not settled
- non-threatening surroundings enable claimant and clinician to re-establish communication in a direct and positive way, far more akin to doctor–patient than defendant–claimant
- the process is informal yet managed by a neutral mediator/facilitator, who takes responsibility and control of the process but only to enable the parties to craft their own solutions if they so wish, as the mediator makes no finding or recommendation
- it is not always essential for a defendant lawyer to attend, although claimants may need to be legally represented to ensure a properly binding settlement is reached

- claimants have the opportunity of being heard and of venting their feelings – if they can do this, and be heard respectfully, this can be very positive
- clinicians can explain what they did and why, express regret and offer an apology (if appropriate) without any necessary or consequent admission of negligence or causation of injury, and contribute directly to any debate between the parties and expert witnesses.

No-fault compensation

An alternative to the established system of alleged medical negligence is that of no-fault compensation which has operated in some other countries, such as New Zealand. The scheme allows injured patients to obtain compensation without having to prove fault by health professionals. In the New Zealand version of the scheme, patients need to demonstrate that the injury resulted from a medical or surgical misadventure. The BMA has long supported such a system, which seems to fit well with the goals of getting justice for patients while minimising the blame culture for health professionals.[37] Under the scheme proposed by the BMA, patients would be entitled to compensation for injury resulting from medical intervention, apart from any injuries that are unavoidable through the exercise of reasonable care. Under such a scheme, 'the concept of negligence is effectively preserved, although it would undoubtedly be easier to establish; moreover there would be no inference of "fault" of quite the same nature as arises in a tort-based system'.[38] Other medical bodies, such as the Royal College of Physicians, have also supported such as system, as did the Bristol report (see page 867), but as yet the Government has rejected this reform option on cost grounds.[39]

Recognising and dealing with poor performance

The inevitability of some error must be accepted and single incidents may not constitute poor performance by doctors. Various definitions of impaired performance exist, including activities that expose patients to an unjustifiable level of risk or which, without good cause, deviate from professional standards and guidelines. Various indicators of poor clinical performance have been identified:

- errors or delays in diagnosis
- use of outmoded tests or treatments
- failure to act on the results of monitoring or testing
- technical errors in the performance of a procedure
- uncooperative attitude and behaviour
- inability to work as a member of a team
- poor communication with patients.

Stress and fatigue can result in decreased concentration, inadequate patient care and potentially serious clinical mistakes. The provision of appropriate support, particularly for junior doctors, needs to be better recognised as does the fact that the professional culture sometimes inhibits doctors from using formal support services, even when they are available.

Appraisals and revalidation

Appraisal and revalidation are among the responses to the problem of under performance. They require that doctors periodically demonstrate that their clinical skills are up to date and they are fit to practise. As a regular part of medical practice, appraisal must be done honestly, with opportunities to discuss any instances where the wrong decision was made. The GMC says 'you must be honest and objective when appraising or assessing the performance of colleagues, including locums and students. Patients may be put at risk if you describe as competent someone who has not reached or maintained a satisfactory standard of practice.'[40] Although it has debated with the GMC about how revalidation procedures can best be implemented, the BMA supports the principle of successful completion of revalidation as a prerequisite for doctors' continued licence to practise.

Addressing poor performance by colleagues

When doctors experience difficulties, early intervention is generally beneficial both for the doctor and for patients but there is often reluctance on the part of colleagues to intervene or appear to criticise. An awareness of patterns of poor performance also takes time to develop. Doctors who have concerns about the performance of colleagues or about the impact of substandard services on patient care should, where possible, establish the facts. This does not mean that doctors have to take on the role of detective but audit, random case note reviews and the results of patient experience surveys can help identify problems and patterns of poor care. Patient confidentiality needs to be taken into account. Unless they are treating the patient, doctors do not have rights of access to identifiable patient data without patient consent but the same restrictions do not apply to anonymised data. Depending on the circumstances, there may be a public interest justification in breaching confidentiality in order to prevent harm occurring (see Chapter 5).

Random case note review using anonymised cases of deceased patients is also discussed later in this chapter. Doctors should discuss their concerns with those in authority so that, if appropriate, a formal audit can be carried out. Regulatory bodies, such as the GMC, have some statutory powers to access patient information as part of an investigation. Whenever possible, doctors should discuss the matter with senior or experienced colleagues before deciding on a course of action. Further advice is available from the BMA and medical indemnity organisations.

Clearly, any system of monitoring must be consistent, fair and equitable. This is a particular concern for overseas trained doctors who may experience complaints, not necessarily due to lesser skills but because of factors such as cultural differences, communication problems or patient prejudice. Transparent and well-structured approaches to measuring performance should ensure consistency.

Using local procedures

Problems should be addressed as early as possible, either through informal discussion with the person concerned or through local mechanisms. It is generally preferable to try to attend to problems as close as possible to their source but they still need to be addressed robustly and not 'brushed under the carpet'. Local policies and procedures for dealing with poor practice vary across the UK, as do the exact roles and responsibilities of the individuals involved but where there is a pattern of poor outcomes or an apparent threat to patient safety, action must be taken. The GMC emphasises that appropriate steps must be taken without delay which may involve discussing the matter with the employing or contracting body, or seeking advice from the GMC itself.[41]

General Medical Council procedures

Ultimate responsibility for investigating and monitoring the performance and behaviour of doctors lies with the GMC and if there is a risk to patients that cannot be resolved locally, referral to the GMC is the appropriate course of action. It carries out an investigation to decide whether there is evidence of impaired fitness to practise. This may occur, for example, if doctors have not kept their medical knowledge and skills up to date or if they have exploited a vulnerable patient in some way (see Chapter 1, pages 50–51). Even if the GMC finds that a doctor's fitness to work is not impaired but there has been a serious deviation from GMC guidance and the standards expected, a warning may be issued to the doctor. In some cases, the doctor may be sick and unable to work safely (see pages 879–883). In 2004, the GMC reformed its procedures, introducing a single set of rules and fitness to practise panels that examine a range of concerns relating to doctors' health, conduct and performance. It also moved to the civil standard of proof in adjudication, which means that the standard that must be satisfied is 'the balance of probability' rather than the standard used in criminal proceedings of 'beyond reasonable doubt'. In 2007, it was proposed that the GMC's adjudication function be transferred to a new body called the Office of the Health Professions Adjudicator (OHPA).[42] Provisions to establish the OHPA were included in the Health and Social Care Act 2008 but, by 2011, the idea of establishing the OHPA had been dropped and repeal of the relevant section of the 2008 Act was pursued in the Health and Social Care Bill 2011.

When the GMC investigates a case, it decides on one of four outcomes:

- the case is concluded with or without the doctor being given specific advice
- a warning may be issued to the doctor
- a formal agreement is set up between the doctor and the GMC, under which the doctor accepts various undertakings and the agreement is published online in the list of registered doctors
- the case may be referred for a public hearing before a fitness to practise panel, which can set conditions on the doctor's registration for up to 3 years, suspend the doctor's registration for up to a year or erase the doctor's name from the medical register so that the doctor cannot practise.

In March 2011, the GMC consulted on proposals to further reform its procedures, including the final step of passing the case to one of its fitness to practise panels.[43] Its aim was to establish a new tribunal service, the Medical Practitioners Tribunal Service (MPTS), operationally separate from the GMC's role in investigating fitness to practise concerns about doctors and bringing proceedings. This would reinforce the distinction between investigation and adjudication. The new independent tribunal would be led by a chair with judicial experience, and report directly to Parliament on an annual basis. The proposals came at a time when the GMC said that there had been significant change in the environment in which it operates: many more cases were being referred for adjudication and the time taken by hearings had also increased. The proposed changes were designed to speed up the hearing process and reduce the stress and anxiety of the experience for the doctors and witnesses involved.

Writing references for colleagues

When doctors write references for colleagues, they must give an honest and factual appraisal of performance. Bland references should not be given in order to encourage the mobility of under-performing colleagues.

Providing honest references

A consultant anaesthetist was found guilty of serious professional misconduct by the GMC for an opinion he had provided. He had been asked by a colleague for advice about the professional performance of a locum doctor in order to write a reference but failed to disclose that the locum had been involved in a serious incident that was the subject of a pending inquiry. The GMC said that doctors who have reason to believe that a colleague's conduct or professional performance poses a danger to patients must act to ensure patient safety. Before taking action, they should do their best to establish the facts. Where there is doubt, it is unethical for a doctor to give a reference about a colleague, particularly if it may result in the employment of that doctor elsewhere. References about colleagues must be carefully considered; comments made in them must be justifiable, offered in good faith and intended to promote the best interests of patients.[44]

Acknowledging error to patients

One of the problems arising from the under-reporting of adverse events and near misses is that patients are often unaware of them, even when their health has been affected. When a mistake has occurred, it is important to talk to the patient, providing as full an explanation as possible of the facts and their implications (see Chapter 1, pages 36–38). Patients who have suffered harm need appropriate help and compensation, for which they need access to information about precisely what has occurred. Doctors should ensure that the patient is supported if the information is likely to be distressing. Who should tell patients of past errors or substandard care is a matter to be decided within the relevant health team.

Summary – duties of doctors to monitor quality and performance

- Doctors need to be aware of the main causes of error, including problems that arise if they ignore the limits of their own experience or continue to practise when they themselves are sick.
- Identifying poor performance can be complex and its causes multi-factorial.
- Successful risk management depends on developing a culture in which mistakes and errors can be openly reported and analysed.
- Systems managers have a duty to take all reasonable steps to avoid situations of foreseeable risk or the repetition of errors.
- There must also be appropriate support in place for health professionals who are still learning.
- When problems are identified, local procedures should be the first avenue to be tried, followed by a formal audit or investigation if problems cannot be resolved.

Poorly performing systems and poor management

Doctors who find themselves working in poorly performing systems cannot necessarily resolve the problems but nor should they ignore them and, as the GMC makes clear, they should take steps to have them addressed by those with the authority to do so.[45] This can be immensely frustrating if employing organisations appear unresponsive. Some doctors are employed as managers and they need to address actively any concerns that arise about workplace practices and ensure that the work environment implements safeguards to minimise mistakes. Events at the Bristol Royal Infirmary highlighted a mixture of failings on multiple levels, including by medical managers. The case illustrated that:

- the doctors at fault were dedicated but lacked insight and their behaviour was flawed
- staff failed to communicate and work together – open review and discussion among the staff were discouraged
- leadership and teamwork were lacking
- management failed to listen to the concerns of junior staff
- doctors were caught up in poor working systems, poor organisation and staff shortages
- there were no agreed means of assessing quality of care
- there was no systematic monitoring of doctors' or hospitals' clinical performance, nor any independent external surveillance to review patterns of performance over time
- a 'club culture' existed in which power and control were in the hands of a few individuals
- there was no requirement for doctors to keep their skills and knowledge up to date and senior doctors could introduce new techniques as they wished.

Following the events at Bristol (see page 867), there was widespread agreement about the need for better surveillance of standards. The term 'clinical governance' became widely used in health care, centring on the importance of maintaining high standards of care, accountability for ensuring standards, transparency and a continuing drive for improvement. Measures such as a system of appraisal of doctors, an emphasis on continuing professional development, agreed pathways and shared standards of clinical care were developed. The need continually to monitor clinical performance and introduce revalidation were widely discussed.

Promoting safety by reporting adverse events

Internationally, institutional structures and processes to improve quality and minimise unfair discrepancies in care were introduced in the early years of the twenty-first century. In the UK, the National Patient Safety Agency (NPSA) was established in 2003 to improve safety by developing a national framework for the reporting and analysis of serious adverse incidents in the NHS.[46] Its aim was to promote a culture in which reporting was a normal response to evidence of harm. Attributing blame was not the central issue. Health staff were encouraged to report incidents without fear, learn from the event and initiate preventative steps to avoid recurrence of it. Nevertheless, its work was dogged by problems of under-reporting, partly because some doctors thought it was not part of medical culture to report or they were worried about potentially incriminating themselves or colleagues. In some cases, doctors said that they were unsure what actually merited reporting because they had not seen clear guidance. In others, the reasons for non-reporting were relatively trivial and practical such as not knowing how to access the reporting mechanisms or concern that the staff who gave out the reporting forms were the ones involved in the adverse event.[47] So, despite the encouragement given to discussion of adverse events, the health service found it hard to embed that into daily practice. From April 2010, as part of the requirements of registration with the Care Quality Commission (CQC),[48] English NHS trusts had to report serious patient safety incidents, deaths or events that may indicate risks to ongoing compliance with registration requirements.[49] Such reports have usually been made via the NPSA which forwards the information to the CQC. In 2010, however, it was proposed that the NPSA be abolished as part of the Government's plan to reduce the number of arms-length bodies.[50] (Up-to-date information is available on the BMA website.)

Although there was considerable change in governance structure and the management of risk in the years following the Bristol Report, some health organisations still failed to monitor untoward incidents in a systematic manner. A clinical governance review at the Mid Staffordshire Foundation Trust in 2002, for example, called for an open culture to be developed so that staff concerns could be discussed and resolved. This was in line with the recommendations from the Bristol report but lack of openness, bullying of staff and failure to address problems continued in the Trust for the following 5 years.[51]

The Mid Staffordshire NHS Foundation Trust

Through its programme of analysis of hospital data and 'alerts', the Commission for Healthcare, Audit and Inspection (Healthcare Commission) noted particularly high mortality rates for patients admitted as emergencies from 2005/6 to 2007/8 at the Mid Staffordshire NHS Foundation Trust. The Trust had a poor history of recording data about its services and did not monitor clinical outcomes. It lacked clear protocols and pathways for managing emergency patients and the accident and emergency department was understaffed and poorly equipped. Over 150 posts were cut and staffing problems were left unaddressed, even when the Trust declared a financial surplus in 2006/7. This left insufficient consultants and middle grade doctors, especially out of hours, and acute physicians were expected to cover emergency cases outside their professional competence. Junior doctors were inadequately supervised, demoralised, lacked support and not given feedback about their performance but were put under pressure to make decisions quickly to meet targets. Receptionists without clinical knowledge carried out immediate assessments of patients due to the lack of nurses. Leadership was weak, communication between staff poor and the unit was often chaotic. Record keeping was also poor which led to inadequate care and patients being given the wrong medication. Provision of pain relief and other medication was delayed. Some nursing staff lacked the skills or training needed and were not shown, for example, how to read the hospital's cardiac monitors. Infection control was poor. Patient care and general cleanliness were judged to be unacceptable. Patients were left in soiled sheets in dirty wards and were not given help with food or drink. Requests for help were ignored and many patients developed pressure sores. There was no system for prioritising emergency surgery cases and postoperative care was inadequate. The Trust was secretive in not acknowledging the high rates of *Clostridium difficile* in 2006. In all, the Trust was judged poor at recognising errors, reporting serious incidents and learning lessons.[52]

Following the investigation into emergency care at the Mid Staffordshire NHS Foundation Trust, the Healthcare Commission urged that:

- trusts should be able to have prompt and reliable data on comparative mortality rates and other outcomes
- they should identify when the quality of patient care falls below acceptable standards – target setting and managing elective work should not interfere with the quality of emergency care which must be available 24 hours a day, 7 days a week
- preoccupation with finances and strategic objectives should not cause insufficient attention to be given to patient care
- governance systems that appear persuasive on paper must actually work in practice
- senior clinical staff should be personally involved in managing vulnerable patients and training junior staff

- shortcomings in matters such as hygiene, provision of medication, nutrition and hydration and use of equipment should be identified and resolved
- failures of compassion, empathy and communication need to be addressed
- there needs to be an open, learning culture within which detailed information is collected, risks to patients identified and mitigated and errors reported; lessons must be learned from serious incidents, near misses and complaints, and improvements made
- handovers need special attention when reorganisations occur in the NHS
- those commissioning care need to ensure that they have effective ways of finding out about the experience of patients.

Implementing the findings from adverse event reporting

Under-reporting and failure to inform patients has remained a problem but reporting has little impact if organisations do not then act upon the information provided. Even when presented with clear information about risks to patient safety, some health organisations have still failed to implement the recommendations stemming from the adverse event reporting of other organisations. From 2004 in England and Wales, the NPSA regularly issued patient safety alerts highlighting known problems that repeatedly harmed patients or caused avoidable deaths. The alerts contain recommended actions that health organisations should implement within a defined timescale. Some particularly serious problems needing urgent action were sent in this way but, in August 2010, it was disclosed that over 200 NHS organisations had failed to comply with patient safety alerts issued by the NPSA.[53] Many care providers had not complied with the most serious alerts prompted by the death or serious injury of patients and over 100 had not implemented recommendations on measures such as the safe use of oxygen with patients or the safe administration of drugs known to have caused deaths.

Failure to implement safety alerts

In July 2007, Paul Richards died in Birmingham's Heartlands Hospital as a result of a massive overdose of the drug amphotericin. His death was caused by confusion over two different types of the drug. A patient safety alert, 'Promoting the Safer Use of Injectable Medicines', issued by the NPSA 4 months earlier might have saved his life but had not been implemented. Following his death, the NPSA issued a further urgent 'rapid response alert' to NHS trusts on the safer use of amphotericin. Two years later, however, over 100 trusts had not implemented the recommendations and 67 trusts had still not implemented the earlier alert of March 2007.[54]

Some such errors are generated by organisational delays. Doctors working as medical managers are likely to be better placed to address these than other clinicians. Complex technological systems, centralised decision making and competing political demands can contribute to such problems. Scarce resources coupled with high patient demand, shortage of time and managerial systems undergoing repeated change can also impose pressure. These essentially managerial and resource problems need to be addressed by managers in a position to effect stability and improvement within the system. Audit of performance and outcomes not only flag up poor performance and provide opportunities for doctors to consider positive measures to improve their skills, but also help to identify any practical obstacles to best practice, such as avoidable delays in implementing recommendations.

Monitoring quality

Institutional mechanisms to improve quality of care include the National Institute for Health and Clinical Excellence (NICE) and the Scottish Intercollegiate Guidelines Network (SIGN) which advise on effective treatments (for the scope and relationship of these bodies see Chapter 13, page 553 and Chapter 20, page 837), as well as the CQC in England and Wales. Although not mandatory throughout the UK, advice from NICE is generally seen as reflecting 'best practice', in particular for quality purposes. Healthcare Improvement Scotland (previously known as the NHS Quality Improvement Scotland) provides guidance on effective practice, sets standards and supports their implementation. It also assesses and reports on NHS performance. The Regulation and Quality Improvement Authority (RQIA) is the independent health and social care regulatory body for Northern Ireland.

Evidence-based national service frameworks set out what patients can expect to receive in major care areas or disease groups and quality markers exist for a wide range of services. Measures such as the NHS performance assessment framework and national surveys of patient and user experience also enable quality to be monitored. Case note review, using various methodologies for logging and categorising trigger situations, has long been another method for improving safety and quality of care. Clearly, issues of patient confidentiality need to be considered and, in some situations, patients can be asked in advance for permission to use their data.

There is also a role for gathering and analysing aggregate anonymised data. This should be the preferred approach if identifiable information is not essential and consent is not possible. Where information cannot be anonymised and obtaining consent is not a practical option, there may be a strong public interest in disclosure if avoidable deaths can be minimised (see Chapter 5, pages 193–194 and 199–202).

Random case note review

In 2003, two Medical Directors at the Luton and Dunstable Hospital looked at post-procedure deaths and found 'alarming vignettes of care failures'.[55] They presented anonymised and undated patient stories to staff in a Grand Round, illustrating the harmful events that occurred to 15 patients who died. The hospital subsequently became part of a patient safety initiative which involved regularly reviewing sets of patient case notes to look for 'triggers' and harm events. Case notes from deceased patients were categorised into several groups, the most significant being those who had not been expected to die when initially admitted to hospital but who had unexpectedly deteriorated and died. Some were affected by adverse drug reactions or poor monitoring. For some, their care had not been appropriately escalated as their condition changed. The data also provided information about deaths from methicillin-resistant *Staphylococcus aureus* (MRSA) and *Clostridium difficile*. Improvements were made on the basis of the data, including the creation of an outreach intensive treatment unit team which reduced cardiac arrest rates. New observation charts were introduced and staff trained to observe patients in a different way. They were increasingly able to recognise the physiological changes requiring an escalation of treatment and felt empowered to initiate it. Such training had to be ongoing to meet newly arising challenges. The move towards electronic patient records, for example, with electronic laboratory and imaging tests, changed the way that case notes were reviewed, bringing both some advantages and some new failures in the process of results being checked and actioned. The hospital recognised the need to address such practical changes to continually improve safety.

Improving care with the Quality and Outcomes Framework

In primary care, the development of the Quality and Outcomes Framework (QOF) was one of the measures introduced UK-wide in 2004 to improve quality, using evidence-based indicators that are shown to have worked particularly well. It is a voluntary incentive scheme for primary care practices, rewarding them in proportion to the increased quality of patient care. The aim is to encourage improvements in health outcomes and reduce premature deaths. Primary care practices score points according to their level of achievement against indicators in several domains: clinical, organisational, patient experience and additional services. QOF gives an indication of the quality of care provided in specific areas and also allows linkage payments to reward breadth of achievement.

Quality in relation to commissioning services

In 2010, the Government proposed that 'GP-led consortia' (commissioning groups) take a major role in commissioning services within the NHS in England.[56] The BMA emphasised that high quality and successful commissioning could only be achieved with GPs, secondary and tertiary care consultants, public health doctors and clinical academics working together. Collaboration rather than competition needed to be the focus, with effective multi-professional involvement to achieve seamless and cost-effective patient care. The BMA saw it as essential that any new system should maintain patient trust, protect professional values and be transparent. It strongly supported greater clinical involvement in the design and management of clinical services and said that consortia would have to develop local systems and mechanisms to resolve any conflicts that might arise in the course of multi-professional working. It also warned that commissioning groups would only be able to commission effectively if the relevant information were to hand: data to suport commissioning decisions would need to be accurate, timely, quality-checked and validated. Data sets should include information on expenditure, referrals, prescribing and clinical performance across secondary and community care. The BMA's General Practice Committee drew up some guidance, emphasising the principles set out by the GMCin *Good Medical Practice*, and also the Nolan Committee's seven principles of public life: selflessness, integrity, objectivity, accountability, openness, honesty and leadership. (For up-to-date information about changes to NHS commissioning, see the BMA's website.)

Risks to doctors' health and patient safety in the workplace

Doctors' health problems are discussed in detail below but they can also be an indicator of a poorly functioning system. Traditionally, doctors were routinely expected to work long shifts and unsocial hours when training, working on-call and providing out-of-hours care or emergency care, but maximum hours for all workers were cut to meet the European Union employment directives. The UK's Working Time Regulations encompass the European Working Time Directive and limit the working week to 48 hours. Shift working and unsocial hours, however, remain common features for professions where a 24-hour service is required. Cutting the number of hours doctors were allowed to work increased the need within the NHS for variable shift patterns. The BMA has produced a number of reports on the problems for patient and personal safety related to shift work.[57] In 2010, it looked at the adverse health effects for doctors of such shift working, including the impact on mental health.[58] It pointed out that shift working is associated with higher levels of burnout, emotional exhaustion, depression and stress as well as physical health problems. It can contribute to behaviour change, such as indecisiveness, and impact on doctors' performance in terms of lower concentration, impaired memory, reduced problem-solving and decision-making skills and slower reaction times.[59] This can have an adverse impact on patient safety and doctors' own safety. A number of studies found that tired junior doctors have more attention failures and make more clinical errors and shift workers are also less able to judge their own performance accurately.

Whistleblowing

GMC advice on raising concerns about patient safety

'If you have good reason to think that patient safety is or may be seriously compromised by inadequate premises, equipment or other resources, policies or systems, you should put the matter right if that is possible. In all other cases you should draw the matter to the attention of your employing or contracting body. If they do not take adequate action, you should take independent advice on how to take the matter further. You must record your concerns and the steps you have taken to try to resolve them.'[60]

In cases in which it is essential to draw attention to dangerous practice or substandard conditions, health professionals who have exhausted local remedies should consider raising the issues more widely. In July 1999, the Public Interest Disclosure Act 1998 came into force in England, Wales and Scotland. This legislation was designed to encourage people to raise concerns about malpractice in the workplace by protecting whistleblowers in a variety of circumstances. In Northern Ireland, some of the features of this legislation are covered by the Public Interest Disclosure (Northern Ireland) Order 1998. These regulations apply to people at work who raise concerns about crime, civil offences (including negligence), danger to health and safety or any attempt to cover these up. They apply whether or not the information is confidential and extend to malpractice occurring overseas. The legislation also applies to trainees and is therefore relevant to medical students who are undertaking clinical training. It protects whistleblowers who disclose information in good faith to a manager or employer. Within the NHS, disclosure in good faith direct to the Department of Health is protected in the same way as internal disclosure. The provision of information to the police, media or MPs, for example, is protected, as long as this is 'reasonable', not made for personal gain and meets one of three conditions:

- whistleblowers reasonably believe they would be victimised if they raised the matter internally or with a prescribed regulator
- they believe a cover-up is likely and there is no prescribed regulator
- they have already raised the matter internally or with a prescribed regulator.

If, as a result of their activities, whistleblowers are victimised, they can bring a claim to an employment tribunal for compensation. If sacked, they can apply for an interim order to keep their job. So-called 'gagging clauses' in employment contracts are void in so far as they conflict with the legislation. As a separate issue, the terms and conditions of hospital doctors also contain a provision allowing them 'without prior consent of the employing authority, to publish books or articles and to deliver any lecture or speak', including on matters relating to their hospital service.

In 2011, the BMA urged that policies relating to whistleblowing be strengthened so that NHS trusts cannot pressure staff who report concerns. Responding to a Department of Health consultation on the subject,[61] the Association emphasised that staff should be encouraged to report concerns about patient care, safety, risks or malpractice. It called on the Government to ban gagging clauses by law and urged the clearer regulation of whistleblowing policies, which are left for NHS trusts to manage. It said that incident forms and patient safety software could be used to safeguard those who raise concerns but a change in attitudes and behaviour is needed to protect their reputations.

Summary – poorly performing systems and poor management

- Responsibility for minimising risk lies with everyone, but doctors have special duties to address problems within their own direct sphere of control.
- Health staff must do all in their power to minimise the risks of individual or corporate failure. This can be particularly difficult if employing organisations appear unresponsive but should still be addressed in line with GMC guidance.
- Doctors should engage with mechanisms for monitoring quality of care, bearing in mind patient confidentiality.
- The importance of implementing the findings from adverse event reporting cannot be overemphasised.

Identifying and addressing doctors' health problems

It is widely recognised that doctors often overlook their own health needs, either from a lack of insight or as a response to the culture in which they work. Long-established taboos and anxiety about stretched resources often leave them fearful to disclose illness and reluctant to take time off to recover. Frequently, there is an unspoken pressure for health professionals not to take sick leave but work through their illness. Failure to take time off when necessary weakens doctors' ability to cope with stress, delays their recovery from illness and can endanger patients, but a culture of guilt about taking sick leave remains. The BMA emphasises the importance of doctors with health problems being able to access confidential and non-judgemental sources of help.

Conditions relating to stress and mental health problems leave staff most fearful of discrimination or stigma. Historically, the types of disorders experienced by doctors are perceived as depression, anxiety, drug use disorders and alcoholism, none of which are easy to resolve but all of which are treatable. Commonly reported problems include a sense of isolation, confusion about where to seek help and stress relating to drawn-out complaints procedures. Some health problems, particularly addiction and mental illness, attract stigma but, with a structured approach to treatment, including long-term support, doctors have very good outcomes. Many return to safe and effective clinical practice but support mechanisms need to be available.

Employment and pre-employment health checks

New healthcare workers in the NHS should have standard health clearance checks for tuberculosis and be offered hepatitis B immunisation and tests for hepatitis C and

HIV, but they are not obliged to accept hepatitis C or HIV testing or be immunised against hepatitis B if they do not carry out exposure-prone procedures (EPPs). Additional healthcare clearance should be obtained if they will perform EPPs, and they need to be free from hepatitis B, hepatitis C, HIV and tuberculosis before appointment. This does not apply to staff who already do EPPs and change jobs within the NHS.[62]

Clear guidance should be available for healthcare staff and for medical students on how to protect themselves against infection. Students may wish to be tested for serious communicable diseases if they may have been exposed to infection, as early diagnosis of hepatitis B or C allows for treatment and possible clearance of the disease, still giving the individual an opportunity to pursue a career that involves EPPs.

Doctors with infectious conditions

Doctors who think that they may have infectious conditions such as hepatitis B or HIV should follow advice from a suitably qualified doctor, such as a consultant in occupational health, infectious diseases or public health. The GMC says that they must obtain specialist advice on whether and to what extent they can continue their professional practice.[63] They must act upon the advice given, which may be not to practise, or to limit their practice in certain ways. Doctors should not continue in clinical practice merely on the basis of their own assessment of the risk to patients.

If a doctor is treating a colleague with a serious communicable disease who refuses to modify his or her professional practice in order to safeguard patients, the treating doctor has a duty to inform an appropriate body. Wherever possible, the infected doctor should be informed before information is passed on to an employer or regulatory body. The GMC can take action to limit the practice of such doctors or to suspend their registration.

Exposure to health risks

Doctors are routinely exposed to health risks in the course of their work, including exposure to infection, needle-stick injuries and possible attacks by violent or mentally ill patients. They can experience health problems associated with their routine working patterns. Long hours, workload pressures, dealing with organisational change and coping with patients' anxieties take a toll. Many doctors also feel that such factors cause problems in their personal or family life. Stress can also contribute to clinical mistakes and, unfortunately, some doctors deal with this by self-prescribing or by consulting colleagues informally rather than seeing their GP.

Self-treatment

Health professionals sometimes fear that there would be career risks in acknowledging health problems, particularly psychological illness and substance misuse. Some doctors self-medicate, are reluctant to seek outside help or only do so at a late stage. Among their anxieties is often a fear of the stigma associated with illness. In the past, they assumed that they could treat themselves, their friends and families but the GMC now cautions strongly against it. In an emergency, there may be no choice but, as a general rule, self-treatment should be avoided, as should the informal treatment of colleagues, friends or family.

GMC advice on self-treatment

'Wherever possible, you should avoid providing medical care to anyone with whom you have a close personal relationship.'[64]

'You should be registered with a GP outside your family to ensure that you have access to independent and objective medical care. You should not treat yourself. You should protect your patients, your colleagues and yourself by being immunised against common serious communicable diseases where vaccines are available. If you know that you have, or think that you might have, a serious condition that you could pass on to patients, or if your judgement or performance could be affected by a condition or its treatment, you must consult a suitably qualified colleague. You must ask for and follow their advice about investigations, treatment and changes to your practice that they consider necessary. You must not rely on your own assessment of the risk you pose to patients.'[65]

In the past, few doctors registered with a GP. Although more do so now, many tend not to consult their GP when problems arise. Unease about adopting the role of a patient and worries about confidentiality can lead to self-treatment. The hazards of self-diagnosis are many (see Chapter 1) but particular concerns include the temptation to extend oneself beyond one's competence and the ever-present possibility of denial about the true nature or extent of the condition.

Responsibility for colleagues

Doctors have a responsibility to ensure that their health does not adversely affect their care of patients. In some cases, however, insight into the need for help and treatment is diminished. The doctor's colleagues then have a duty to take action, in the interests both of patient care and of the doctor's health. Not to intervene risks patient safety and can lead to further deterioration in the doctor's health and performance. Colleagues, particularly junior staff, are sometimes reluctant to speak out due to loyalty or for fear of damaging their own careers. However, the GMC emphasises the duty of all doctors to prevent risks to patients, including those arising from the ill health of colleagues. Early recognition and treatment considerably increase the chances of successful rehabilitation for the sick doctor. Colluding with the doctor does not help patients or the doctor.

GMC guidance on colleagues' performance

'You must protect patients from risk of harm posed by another colleague's conduct, performance or health. The safety of patients must come first at all times. If you have concerns that a colleague may not be fit to practise, you must take appropriate steps without delay, so that the concerns are investigated and patients protected where necessary. This means you must give an honest explanation of your concerns to an appropriate person from your employing or contracting body and follow their procedures.'

'If there are no appropriate local systems, or local systems do not resolve the problem, and you are still concerned about the safety of patients, you should inform the relevant regulatory body. If you are not sure what to do, discuss your concerns with an impartial colleague or contact your defence body, a professional organisation, or the GMC for advice.'

'If you have management responsibilities you should make sure that systems are in place through which colleagues can raise concerns about risks to patients, and you must follow the guidance in the GMC's *Management for doctors*.'[66]

GMC sick doctors procedure

The GMC's fitness to practise procedures are part of a wider system of healthcare regulation. The Council recommends that, if a medical professional has concerns about a colleague, this should normally first be dealt with at a local level. If reported to the GMC, an assessment is made which may be that the concerns are more appropriate to be considered locally. The fact that a health problem is referred to the GMC for consideration does not necessarily lead to the doctor being suspended from practice. In many cases, doctors can continue if they follow an agreed treatment regime and are suitably supervised. Although the GMC lets employers know when doctors have been given a warning through its fitness to practise procedure, a warning is not given where the concerns relate to the doctor's physical or mental health. The GMC emphasises that doctors who suspect or know that they have a health problem should not rely on their own judgement of their ability to continue working but seek expert assessment.[67]

BMA services

For help, counselling and personal support, doctors and medical students who are BMA members can call a special BMA service and choose to speak to a counsellor or an advisor who is a doctor.[68]

The Counselling Service is staffed by professional counsellors, 24 hours a day, 7 days a week. All counsellors are members of the British Association for Counselling and Psychotherapy and are bound by strict codes of confidentiality. They advise on work stress, mental health issues and issues such as drug misuse, as well as providing information about other specialist resources. BMA Counselling is confidential and callers can choose to remain anonymous. Ongoing counselling is available and doctors can arrange regular appointments.

For those who prefer to talk in confidence to a doctor, the Doctor Advisor Service is available to doctors and medical students in difficulty. The service is not intended to be an emergency medical service and when an emergency arises, callers should contact their own GP or usual medical adviser. The aim of the Doctor Advisor Service is to help callers to gain insight into their problems, supporting and helping them to move on. A wide range of problems is dealt with including drug and alcohol problems, bullying at work and mental health issues, as well as the problems of doctors who have been referred to the GMC or the National Clinical Assessment Service (NCAS).

Treating patients who are doctors

Confidentiality

Doctors who are patients are entitled to the same high standards of care and confidentiality. Unless the patient consents, health professionals must not share information with others not directly concerned with his or her treatment. Sick doctors, particularly those with mental health and addictive problems, are often reluctant to seek medical advice due to concerns about confidentiality in the small world of the medical profession. These fears are not entirely unfounded, not least because the treating doctor must also take action if the sick doctor might be a risk to others. Worries about whether their confidentiality will be protected deter some doctors from seeking help. Generally, they should be reassured that their confidentiality will be as closely protected as that of any other patient. Out-of-area referrals may be an option in cases where sick doctors have particular worries about confidentiality or fears that they are likely to be formally treated by colleagues who are acquaintances, which may lead to inadvertent disclosure of their information.

Treatment providers need to ensure that the confidentiality of all patients – including health professionals who are undergoing care – is properly protected. Medical and nursing staff have clear professional duties in this respect. Auxiliary and administrative staff must also understand their contractual duties of confidentiality. As with all other patients, however, doctors' rights to confidentiality are not absolute and action needs to be taken where their health poses a threat to other people. Wherever possible, this should be discussed by the treating doctor with the sick doctor prior to disclosure.

Treating the doctor as a patient

Treating a fellow health professional can be challenging. Doctors providing care for other health professionals need to treat them as their patients, avoiding short cuts and unjustified assumptions. Doctor patients should be offered proper explanations of what is involved in the investigation and management of their condition. They may already be well aware of such information but should be allowed the opportunity to be the patient and be offered advice and support, if they want that, as other patients would be. They may be much better informed than most other patients and their special knowledge should be recognised, without assumptions being made about the amount of information and detail they want. They should be reassured that seeking formal medical care is the right decision, rather than relying on their own interpretation of their condition. They should be encouraged to develop a continuing relationship with their doctor, including where appropriate routine recall for follow up.

Summary – identifying and addressing doctors' health problems

- All doctors should be registered with a GP and act promptly on any early warning signs, especially where they have a suspicion that their health is affecting their performance.
- Informal or 'corridor' consultations with colleagues should be avoided.
- Doctors need to monitor their own health and also take action if colleagues' health gives cause for concern.
- Doctors are entitled to the same strict rules of confidentiality as other patients.
- Doctors should seek and follow advice from a suitably qualified practitioner if they may have been exposed to a serious communicable disease.

References

1   The Bristol Royal Infirmary Inquiry (2001) *Learning from Bristol: the report of the public inquiry into children's heart surgery at the Bristol Royal Infirmary 1984–1995* (Cm 5207 (I)), The Stationery Office, London.
2   Mason JK, Laurie GT. (2011) *Mason & McCall Smith's Law and Medical Ethics*, 8th edn, OUP, Oxford, p.122.
3   National Health Service Litigation Authority, *Key facts about our work*. Available at: www.nhsla.com (accessed 24 May 2011).
4   Rosen R, Dewar S. (2004) *On Being a Doctor*, King's Fund, London, pp.1–2.
5   Healthcare Commission (2009) *Investigation into Mid Staffordshire NHS Foundation Trust*, HC, London, p.131.

6   General Medical Council (2006) *The duties of a doctor registered with the General Medical Council*. Available at: www.gmc-uk.org (accessed 2 June 2011).
7   *Hunter v Hanley* [1955] SLT 213: 217.
8   *Hunter v Hanley* [1955] SC 200: 206.
9   *Bolam v Friern Hospital Management Committee* [1957] 2 All ER 118.
10 *Bolitho v City and Hackney Health Authority* [1997] 4 All ER 771.
11 *Wilsher v Essex Area Health Authority* [1987] 1 QB 730; [1988] AC 1074; [1988] 1 All ER 871, HL.
12 Mason JK, Laurie GT. (2006) *Mason & McCall Smith's Law and Medical Ethics*, 7th edn, OUP, Oxford, p.323.
13 *Wilsher v Essex Area Health Authority* [1986] 3 All ER 801: 831.
14 Mason JK, Laurie GT. (2006) *Mason & McCall Smith's Law and Medical Ethics*, 7th edn, OUP, Oxford, p.323.
15 *Kay's Tutor v Ayrshire & Arran Health Board* [1987] 2 All ER 417; (1987) SC 145; (1987) SLT 588.
16 General Medical Council Professional Conduct Committee hearing, 20–23 August 2001.
17 *Birch v UCL Hospital NHS Foundation Trust* [2008] 104 BMLR 168.
18 General Medical Council (2006) *Good Medical Practice*, GMC, London, para 11.
19 This is discussed in detail in: Mason JK, Laurie GT. (2011) *Mason & McCall Smith's Law and Medical Ethics*, 8th edn, OUP, Oxford, ch 5.
20 Mason JK, Laurie GT. (2011) *Mason & McCall Smith's Law and Medical Ethics*, 8th edn, OUP, Oxford, p.167.
21 British Medical Association (2010) *Doctors new to practice: an ethical survival kit*, BMA, London.
22 *R v Prentice* [1993] 3 WLR 927.
23 Dyer C. (1993) Manslaughter verdict quashed on junior doctors. *BMJ* **306**, 1432.
24 Merry A, McCall Smith A. (2001) *Errors, medicine and the law*, CUP, Cambridge, p.19.
25 *R v Misra* [2004] EWCA Crim 2375.
26 Medical Protection Society (1999) Act within the limits of your expertise. *UK Casebook* **13**, 12.
27 General Medical Council Professional Conduct Committee hearing, 16–17 October 2001.
28 General Medical Council (2006) *Good Medical Practice*, GMC, London, paras 6 and 48.
29 General Medical Council Fitness to Practise Panel, 2–18 June 2010.
30 British Medical Association (2002) *Patient safety and clinical risk*, BMA, London, p.9.
31 Anon. (2011) Former GP will not face new charges. *BMJ* **342**, 406.
32 Batty D. (2010) I helped patients to die, says doctor cleared of murder. *The Guardian* (19 June). Available at: www.guardian.co.uk (accessed 24 May 2011).
33 Bristol Royal Infirmary Inquiry (2001) *Learning from Bristol: the report of the public inquiry into children's heart surgery at the Bristol Royal Infirmary 1984–1995* (Cm 5207 (I)), The Stationery Office, London.
34 Khatri N, Brown GD, Hicks LL. (2009) From a blame culture to a just culture in health care. *Health Care Manage Rev* **34**(4), 312–22.
35 Khatri N, Brown GD, Hicks LL. (2009) From a blame culture to a just culture in health care. *Health Care Manage Rev* **34**(4), 312–22.
36 British Medical Association (2007) *Mediation, clinical negligence claims and the medical profession: policy paper*. Available at: www.bma.org.uk (accessed 24 May 2011).
37 British Medical Association (1987) *Report of the BMA No Fault Compensation Working Party*, BMA, London. British Medical Association (2003) *Funding No Fault Compensation for Medical Injuries*, BMA, London.
38 Mason JK, Laurie GT. (2011) *Mason & McCall Smith's Law and Medical Ethics*, 8th edn, OUP, Oxford, p.125.
39 For a detailed discussion of this subject, see Mason JK, Laurie GT. (2011) *Mason & McCall Smith's Law and Medical Ethics*, 8th edn, OUP, Oxford, ch 5.
40 General Medical Council (2006) *Good Medical Practice*, GMC, London, para 18.
41 General Medical Council (2006) *Good Medical Practice*, GMC, London, paras 43–4.
42 Department of Health (2007) *Trust, Assurance and Safety: the Regulation of the Health Professions in the 21st Century*, DH, London.
43 General Medical Council (2011) *Reform of the fitness to practise procedures of the GMC: a paper for consultation*, GMC, London.
44 General Medical Council Professional Conduct Committee hearing, 14–18 March 1994.
45 General Medical Council (2006) *Good Medical Practice*, GMC, London, para 6.
46 National Reporting and Learning Service (2010) *National Patient Safety Agency: National Framework for Reporting and Learning from Serious Incidents Requiring Investigation*, NPSA, London.
47 Sharma A, Ray B, Jain P. *et al.* (2006) Adverse incidents in NHS still under-reported, BMJ rapid response (14 July) to: O'Dowd A. (2006) Adverse incidents in NHS still under-reported. *BMJ* **333**, 59.
48 Registration with the Care Quality Commission by all NHS trusts is a requirement under the Health and Social Care Act 2008.

49 Care Quality Commission (2010) *Essential Standards of Quality and Safety: The Care Quality Registration Regulations*, CQC, London.
50 Department of Health (2010) *Liberating the NHS: report of the arms-length bodies review*, DH, London.
51 Healthcare Commission (2009) *Investigation into Mid Staffordshire NHS Foundation Trust*, HC, London, p.133.
52 Healthcare Commission (2009) *Investigation into Mid Staffordshire NHS Foundation Trust*, HC, London.
53 Action Against Medical Accidents (2010) *Implementation of patient safety alerts*, AvMA, Croydon.
54 Action Against Medical Accidents (2010) *Implementation of patient safety alerts*, AvMA, Croydon.
55 Carter M. (2010) Measuring harm levels with the Global Trigger Tool. *Clinical Risk* **16**, 122–126, p.122.
56 Department of Health (2010) *Equity and excellence: Liberating the NHS*, The Stationery Office, London.
57 British Medical Association (2006) *Implications for health and safety of junior doctors' working arrangements, Sleep deprivation – effect on doctors*. Available at: www.bma.org.uk (accessed 24 May 2011). British Medical Association (2009) *Shift and resident working – guidance for consultants: maintaining the continuity and quality of care*, BMA, London. British Medical Association (2010) *Shift work, Rest and Sleep: minimising the risks discussion paper*, BMA, London.
58 British Medical Association (2010) *Health effects of working unsocial hours and shift work*, BMA, London.
59 British Medical Association (2010) *Health effects of working unsocial hours and shift work*, BMA, London, p.13.
60 General Medical Council (2006) *Good Medical Practice*, GMC, London, para 6.
61 Department of Health (2011) *The NHS Constitution: The Introduction of New Expectations and Commitments Around Whistleblowing*, DH, London.
62 Department of Health (2007) *Health clearance for tuberculosis, hepatitis B, hepatitis C and HIV: New healthcare workers*, DH, London.
63 General Medical Council (2006) *Good Medical Practice*, GMC, London, para 79.
64 General Medical Council (2006) *Good Medical Practice*, GMC, London, para 5.
65 General Medical Council (2006) *Good Medical Practice*, GMC, London, paras 77–9.
66 General Medical Council (2006) *Good Medical Practice*, GMC, London, paras 43–5.
67 General Medical Council (2006) *Good Medical Practice*, GMC, London, para 79.
68 The BMA Counselling Service can be contacted on 08459 200 169.

Appendix a

The Hippocratic Oath

The methods and details of medical practice change with the passage of time and the advance of knowledge. Some fundamental principles of professional behaviour have, however, remained unaltered throughout the recorded history of medicine, including some of those enunciated in the Hippocratic Oath. This was probably written in the fifth century BC and was intended to be affirmed by each doctor on entry to the medical profession. In translation (this by Francis Adams, London, 1849) it reads as follows.

> I swear by Apollo the physician, and Aesculapius and Health, and All-heal, and all the gods and goddesses, that, according to my ability and judgement, I will keep this Oath and this stipulation – to reckon him who taught me this Art equally dear to me as my parents, to share my substance with him, and relieve his necessities if required; to look upon his offspring in the same footing as my own brothers, and to teach them this Art, if they shall wish to learn it, without fee or stipulation; and that by precept, lecture and every other mode of instruction, I will impart a knowledge of the Art to my own sons, and those of my teachers, and to disciples bound by a stipulation and oath according to the law of medicine, but to none other. I will follow that system of regimen which, according to my ability and judgement, I consider for the benefit of my patients, and abstain from whatever is deleterious and mischievous. I will give no deadly medicine to anyone if asked, nor suggest any such counsel; and in like manner I will not give to a woman a pessary to produce abortion. With purity and with holiness I will pass my life and practise my Art. I will not cut persons labouring under the stone, but will leave this to be done by men who are practitioners of this work. Into whatever houses I enter, I will go into them for the benefit of the sick, and will abstain from every voluntary act of mischief and corruption; and, further, from the seduction of females, or males, of freemen or slaves. Whatever, in connection with my professional practice, not in connection with it, I see or hear, in the life of men, which ought not to be spoken of abroad, I will not divulge, as reckoning that all such should be kept secret. While I continue to keep this Oath unviolated, may it be granted to me to enjoy life and the practice of the Art, respected by all men, in all times. But should I trespass and violate this Oath, may the reverse be my lot.

Medical Ethics Today: The BMA's Handbook of Ethics and Law, Third Edition. Sophie Brannan, Eleanor Chrispin, Martin Davies, Veronica English, Rebecca Mussell, Julian Sheather and Ann Sommerville.
© 2012 BMA Medical Ethics Department. Published 2012 by Blackwell Publishing Ltd.

Appendix b

Declaration of Geneva

Adopted by the 2nd General Assembly of the World Medical Association, Geneva, Switzerland, September 1948

and amended by the 22nd World Medical Assembly, Sydney, Australia, August 1968

and the 35th World Medical Assembly, Venice, Italy, October 1983

and the 46th WMA General Assembly, Stockholm, Sweden, September 1994

AT THE TIME OF BEING ADMITTED AS A MEMBER OF THE MEDICAL PROFESSION:

I SOLEMNLY PLEDGE myself to consecrate my life to the service of humanity;

I WILL GIVE to my teachers the respect and gratitude which is their due;

I WILL PRACTISE my profession with conscience and dignity;

THE HEALTH OF MY PATIENT will be my first consideration;

I WILL RESPECT the secrets which are confided in me, even after the patient has died;

I WILL MAINTAIN by all the means in my power, the honour and the noble traditions of the medical profession;

MY COLLEAGUES will be my sisters and brothers;

I WILL NOT PERMIT considerations of age, disease or disability, creed, ethnic origin, gender, nationality, political affiliation, race, sexual orientation, or social standing to intervene between my duty and my patient;

I WILL MAINTAIN the utmost respect for human life from its beginning even under threat and I will not use my medical knowledge contrary to the laws of humanity;

I MAKE THESE PROMISES solemnly, freely and upon my honour.

Medical Ethics Today: The BMA's Handbook of Ethics and Law, Third Edition. Sophie Brannan, Eleanor Chrispin, Martin Davies, Veronica English, Rebecca Mussell, Julian Sheather and Ann Sommerville.
© 2012 BMA Medical Ethics Department. Published 2012 by Blackwell Publishing Ltd.

Appendix c

Declaration of a new doctor, as devised by Imperial College School of Medicine graduating year of 2001[1]

Now, as a new doctor, I solemnly promise that I will to the best of my ability serve humanity – caring for the sick, promoting good health, and alleviating pain and suffering.

I recognise that the practice of medicine is a privilege with which comes considerable responsibility and I will not abuse my position.

I will practise medicine with integrity, humility, honesty, and compassion – working with my fellow doctors and other colleagues to meet the needs of my patients.

I shall never intentionally do or administer anything to the overall harm of my patients.

I will not permit considerations of gender, race, religion, political affiliation, sexual orientation, nationality, or social standing to influence my duty of care.

I will oppose policies in breach of human rights and will not participate in them. I will strive to change laws that are contrary to my profession's ethics and will work towards a fairer distribution of health resources.

I will assist my patients to make informed decisions that coincide with their own values and beliefs and will uphold patient confidentiality.

I will recognise the limits of my knowledge and seek to maintain and increase my understanding and skills throughout my professional life. I will acknowledge and try to remedy my own mistakes and honestly assess and respond to those of others.

I will seek to promote the advancement of medical knowledge through teaching and research.

I make this declaration solemnly, freely, and upon my honour.

Reference

1   Sritharan K, Russell G, Fritz Z. *et al.* (2009) Medical oaths and declarations: a declaration marks an explicit commitment to ethical behaviour. *BMJ* **323**, 1440–1441, p.1441.

Medical Ethics Today: The BMA's Handbook of Ethics and Law, Third Edition. Sophie Brannan, Eleanor Chrispin, Martin Davies, Veronica English, Rebecca Mussell, Julian Sheather and Ann Sommerville.
© 2012 BMA Medical Ethics Department. Published 2012 by Blackwell Publishing Ltd.

Index

Abortion (Scotland) Regulations 1991 (SI
     1991/460) 225
Abortion Act 1967 276, 277, 283, 290, 293
  calls for reform 290–1
Abortion Regulations 1991 (SI 1991/499) 195
abortion
  see also reproductive ethics
  background to abortion debate 281
    arguments against abortion 282
    arguments supporting abortion in some
       circumstances 282–3
    arguments supporting wide availability
       281–2
  BMA policy 281
  consent
    incapacitated adults 293–4
    involvement of father 294
    young people 292–3
  difference from emergency hormonal
     contraception 276–7
  law in England, Scotland and Wales 283
    Abortion Act, calls for reform 290–1
    abortion of healthy twin 287
    abortion on grounds of fetal sex 287–8
    conscientious objection to abortion 288–9
    early medical abortion 285–6
    late gestation abortion 284
    national data 284
    questions about abortion in job
       applications 290
    selective reduction of multiple pregnancy
       286–7
    serious handicap 283–4
  law in Northern Ireland 291–2
    conscientious objection 292
abuse and domestic violence 205
abuse perpetrators
  emergency treatment 637
    child abuse or neglect 640–1
    domestic violence 640
abuse victims
  emergency treatment 637
    child abuse or neglect 640–1
    domestic violence 640

abusive behaviour by health professionals 50–1
Access to Health Records (Northern Ireland)
     Order 1993 222, 256, 259, 527, 660
Access to Health Records Act 1990 222, 256,
     259, 527, 660
Access to Medical Reports Act 1988 27, 256,
     260, 653, 655
Access to Personal Files and Medical Reports
     (Northern Ireland) Order 1991 256,
     260
accident sites 644
  dealing with stress and trauma 645–6
  patients refusing to attend hospital 645
  teamwork 645
  triage 644
addicts
  prescribing for 566
adherence of patients to medicines 539–40
administering medication 572
  adverse drug reactions 573–4
  covert administration 573
  special safeguards 572–3
adoption
  health records 234
Adult Support and Protection (Scotland) Act
     2007 49
Adults with Incapacity (Conditions and
     Circumstances Applicable to Three
     Year Medical Treatment Certificates)
     (Scotland) Regulations 2007 (SI
     2007/100) 142
Adults with Incapacity (Requirements for
     Signing Medical Treatment Certificates)
     (Scotland) Regulations 2007 (SI
     2007/105) 126
Adults with Incapacity (Scotland) Act 2000 62,
     122, 123, 124, 219, 371, 400, 442, 595,
     614, 630, 660, 694, 783
  advance decisions 128–9
  areas of incapacity 126–7
  assessment 124
    definition of incapacity 124–5
  basic principles 123
  benefit 123

Medical Ethics Today: The BMA's Handbook of Ethics and Law, Third Edition. Sophie Brannan, Eleanor Chrispin,
Martin Davies, Veronica English, Rebecca Mussell, Julian Sheather and Ann Sommerville.
© 2012 BMA Medical Ethics Department. Published 2012 by Blackwell Publishing Ltd.

Adults with Incapacity (Scotland) Act 2000
(*Continued*)
   consultation of relevant others 123–4
   encouragement to exercise residual
     capacity 124
   minimum necessary intervention 123
   taking account of wishes 123
  certificate of incapacity 127
  dispute resolution 133
   appeal to Court of Session 134
  exceptions to general authority to treat 131
   covert medication 133
   special safeguards 131–2
   use of force or detention 132–3
  intervention orders and welfare guardianship
   130
  outline 123
  proxies 129–30
  research 614
  taking account of patient views 128
  taking account of views of those close to
   patient 129
  treatment plan approach 127–8
  treatment, definition of 127
  welfare attorneys 130
  withdrawing and withholding treatment
   131
Adults with Incapacity (Specified Medical
  Treatments) (Scotland) Regulations
  2002 (SI 2002/275) 143
advance care planning (ACP) 428–31
advance decisions refusing treatment (ADRT)
  96
  pregnancy 299
  suicide and self-harm 631–3
  unusual requests 520
advance requests for end of life treatment
  GMC guidance 430–1
adverse drug reactions 573–4
  implementing findings 875
  reporting 872–3
advertising medical services 795
Age of Legal Capacity (Scotland) Act 1991 149,
  159
Age of Majority Act (Northern Ireland) 1969
  180
aggressive patients 55–7
  health records 233
alcohol
  blood alcohol tests of incapacitated drivers
   637–8
Alder Hey Hospital 495

'alien limbs' 85
Alport's syndrome 82
alternative medicine *see* complementary and
  alternative medicine (CAM)
altruistic organ donations 81
  expanding pool of donors 83–4
  independent assessors report 83
  non-directed donations 84
  safeguards 82–3
  special case of kidney donations 84–5
amputation of healthy limbs 85–8
  ethical issues 87–8
  legal issues 86–7
  UK practice 86
amputee identity disorder 85
Anatomy (Northern Ireland) Order 1992 522
Anatomy Act 1984 522, 526
anonymised information 193–4
  definition 184
anonymity of gamete or embryo donors 330–3
  arguments for and against 331–3
armed forces, doctors in 679–80
  boxing 681
  confidentiality 680
  consent 681
  disciplinary or forensic procedures 681
Assessment, Care in Custody and Teamwork
  (ACCT) 707
Assisted Dying for the Terminally Ill Bill 2005
  467–8
assisted reproduction
  access to treatment
   NHS funding 318–19
   right to assistance 316–18
   welfare of the child 319–23
  consent to storage of gametes and embryos
   324
   storage and use following withdrawal of
    consent 326–7
   storage and use without effective consent
    324–5
  donated gametes or embryos 327–8
   donor anonymity 330–3
   donor payments 333–7
   informing children of their conception
    329–30
   psychological studies of children from
    donations 328–9
  duties to 'hypothetical people' 316
  general principles 312
  monitoring outcomes 314–16
  preimplantation genetic testing

diagnosis (PGD) 337–9
    embryo selection on tissue type
      compatibility 342–5
    exclusion testing 340–2
    revealing additional information 339–40
    screening (PGS) 342
prisoners' rights 706
regulation 312
    future of HFEA 314
    Human Fertilisation and Embryology Act
      2008 313–14
    Human Fertilisation and Embryology
      Authority (HFEA) 312–13
    regulated activities 312–13
    role of HFEA 314
    Warnock Committee 312
sex selection 345–6
    BMA view 347
    consultation and debate 346–7
surrogacy 348
    doctors' duties 354–5
    future directions 357
    regulatory framework 348–9
      enforcement of arrangement 350
    review of law 349–51
    seeking treatment in other countries 355–7
    society's ambivalence 351–4
assisted suicide 465
    see also physician assisted suicide
    legal definition 472–5
Association of Anaesthetists of Great Britain
    and Ireland
    pre-operative assessments 65
Association of British Pharmaceutical Industry
    (ABPI) 554–5
asylum seekers
    see also immigration removal centres
    doctors' discretion on registration 28
    examination of 667
      expert assessment 667–8
      language services 668
audit
    definition 585–6
autonomy 2
    doctor–patient relationship 22
autopsy *see* post mortem
autosomal recessive disorders 390–1
Avastin 537

bad news, communicating 35–6
behaviour genetics 405
beneficence 11

benefit 2
bequests 53–4
bereavement 455
    support for healthcare team 456
    support for those close to patient 456
bioethics 1
birth *see* childbirth
blame culture, addressing 867–8
blood supplies, ensuring safety 818–19
body dysmorphic disorder (BDD) 85
body integrity identity disorder (BIID) 80, 85
    treatment 88
Body Mass Index (BMI) 811
bovine spongiform encephalopathy (BSE) 816
boxing
    armed forces 681
breast cancer screening 827
British Medical Association (BMA) 1
    abortion 281
    approach to medical ethics
      arguments to justify decisions 16–17
      critical analysis of dilemma 16
      identification of component parts 15
      information gathering 15
      legal/professional guidance 15–16
      recognition of ethical issue 14–15
      theory and practice 13–17
    assisted dying 469
    breakdown of doctor–patient relationship
      43–4
    characteristics of a 'good' doctor 23
    cloning 407–8
    consent to intimate body searches 730
    direct-to-consumer genetic testing 394–6
    doctor–patient relationship
      duties 27, 30
    doctors' health problems 882
    doctors' moral views 33
    doctors working in prisons 690
    education and training 741
    genetics 368
    health records 233
    mistakes by doctors 37
    organ and tissue donation 514–15
    payments to research participants 591
    sex selection of embryos 347
    surrogacy 348, 350
    *Withholding and Withdrawing Life-Prolonging
      Treatment* 131
British National Formulary (BNF) 534
British National Formulary for Children (BNFC)
    544, 601

British Pregnancy Advisory Service (BPAS) 285–6
business interests of doctors 685

caesarean section
refusal of 268–9, 304–6
requests for 302–4
cafeteria medicine 24
capacity *see* mental capacity
cardio-pulmonary resuscitation (CPR) 24–5
end of life 447
discussion with patients 447–9
when to attempt CPR 450
care at a distance 23–4
care homes
discussion with patients 449
Care Quality Commission (CQC) 192, 196, 605
prison healthcare 690
Care Quality Commission (Registration) Regulations 2009 (SI 2009/3112) 529
Care Record Guarantee 239
carrier testing for recessive or X-linked conditions 368, 378–9
adults lacking capacity 379
children 379–82
casuistry 12
Central Office for Research Ethics Committees (COREC) 608
chaperones for patients 47–9
children and young people 156
GMC guidance 48
Charter for the Rights of Older People in Clinical Trials 596
child abuse or neglect 640–1
young offender institutions 723
peer mentoring 723–4
self-harm and suicide risk 723
Child Support (Pensions and Social Security) Act 2000 412
Child Support, Pensions and Social Security Act (Northern Ireland) 2000 412
childbirth 301
caesarean section refusals 304–6, 302–4
home births and role of GPs 302
pain relief 306
Children (Northern Ireland) Order 1995 145
Children (Scotland) Act 1995 145
Children Act 1989 145, 723
refusal of medical or psychiatric examination 178–80
Children Act 2004 176, 784

children and young people
see also young offender institutions
abortion, consent for 292–3
chaperones 47
child protection issues 174–7
confidentiality and disclosure about abuse or neglect 177–8
refusal of medical or psychiatric examination 178–80
combining autonomy with best interests 145–6
confidentiality
children who are competent 220–1
children who lack competence 220
research and innovative treatment 606
Scotland 221
conjoined twins 173–4
consent
examination by forensic physicians 730
teaching of medical students 755
court involvement 165–6
covert video surveillance (CVS) 41–2
cultural practices
female genital mutilation 171–3
male circumcision 170–1
decision-making by competent young people 154–5
advance decisions 159–60
chaperones 156
child donors 156–7
consent 155–6
refusal 157–9
effect of human rights legislation 146–7
emergencies 154
end of life care 451–2
communication with parents 451–2
communication with young patients 451
disagreement 452–3
palliative care 453–4
general principles 147
assessing competence 151–2
best interests 152–3
communication 147–8
competency to make decisions 149–50
confidentiality and involving parents 152
growth of competence 150–1
involving children 148–9
preventing harm 153–4
genetic testing
carrier testing for recessive or X-linked conditions 379–82
predictive genetic testing 386

health records
   access to 258–9
   adoption 234
   child protection case notes 233
immigration removal centres (IRCs) 726–7
prescribing for 543–4
recordings
   as part of patient care 249
   for research, teaching, training and other
     healthcare-related reasons 250
   for widely accessible public media 251
refusal of blood by Jehovah's Witnesses
   166–8
research and innovative treatment 599–600
   confidentiality 606
   consent 602
   paediatric formulary 600–1
teenage contraception
   consent and confidentiality 273–4
   individuals with learning difficulties
     275
   law on sexual offences in Northern
     Ireland 275
   public policy 271–2
treatment against patient wishes 168
   detention 169
   restraint, use of 168–9
welfare of children from assisted
    reproduction 319
   enquiries to GPs 322–3
   individual assessments 321
   informing children of their conception
     329–30
   non-traditional families 322
   postmenopausal women 321
   psychological studies 328–9
   review of difficult cases 323
   supportive parenting 320–1
   threshold for concern 320
   tissue donors 344–5
choice
   doctor–patient relationship 22
   patients choosing doctors and hospitals
     28–9
cigarette smoking 820–2
circumcision 170–1
Civil Partnership Act 2004 181
climate change 811
clinical freedom
   official guidance 552
     National Institute for Health and Clinical
      Excellence (NICE) 552–3

Scotland, Wales and Northern Ireland
   553–4
   resources 549–50
clinical trials of investigational medicinal
    products (CTIMPs) 599
   children and young people 600
cloning 407–8
cognitive enhancement drugs 548–9
colleagues, checking reliability 49–51
Committee on Publication Ethics (COPE)
   622–3
Common Assessment Framework (CAF) 211
communicable disease
   detention settings 708–10
   testing deceased patients 517–18
communication
   providing information 65–71
   test results 31
communitarian ethics 10
comparative genomic hybridisation (CGH) 342
compassion 5
competence *see* mental capacity
complaints 44
   disclosure of patient information 214–15
complementary and alternative medicine
    (CAM)
   end of life
     communicating with therapists 425
   prescribing 563–4
   shared care 786–8
   shared prescribing 561–2
Complementary and Natural Healthcare
    Council (CNHC) 788
compulsory vaccination 830
Computer Misuse Act 1990 192
concordance in decision making 540
   older patients 542
condoms
   provision in prisons 709
Confidential Enquiry into Maternal and Child
    Health (CEMACH)
   post-mortem examinations 509
confidentiality 2, 31
   anonymous information 193–4
   armed forces 680
   children and young people
     children who are competent 220–1
     children who lack competence 220
     Scotland 221
   conflict of moral rights 8
   contacting patients 186–7
    by text message 187

confidentiality (*Continued*)
  deceased patients 221–2, 498–9
    benefit and harm 499–500
    entitlement of relatives to medical records
      222
    information disclosure to coroner or
      procurator fiscal 500
    information on death certificates 500–1
    other circumstances for disclosures 223
  definition of terms 183–4
  detention settings 696–8
    prisoners' medical correspondence 697–8
  disclosure in the public interest 199–201
    abuse and domestic violence 205
    balancing benefits and harms 201
    examples 202
    gunshot and knife wounds 204
    health 202
    informing sexual contacts 202–3
    involving the individual 201
    making the disclosure 201–2
    patients lacking capacity 206
    public safety 203
    serious crime and national security 203–4
    urgency of disclosure 201
    workplace safety 204–5
  dual obligations 652–3
  duty of confidentiality 184
  emergency situations 633
    after death 633
    disclosure to police 639
    sharing information with healthcare team
      633
  forensic physicians 731–2
    information on police records 732
  general principles 184–5
  genetic testing 374–7
    use of information by clinics 377–8
  GMC guidance 192
  health records 234–5
  immigration removal centres (IRCs) 727–8
  implied consent for information disclosure
    187–8
    clinical audit 188–9
  incapacitated (incompetent) patients 218–19
    proxy decision makers 219–20
    sharing information with relatives, carers
      and friends 219
  information that should not be disclosed
    256–7
  information to be kept confidential 185–6

  legal issues 189
    common law 189–90
    Computer Misuse Act 1990 192
    Data Protection Act 1998 190–1
    Human Rights Act 1998 191
    NHS Act 2006 191–2
  NHS Care Record Guarantee 192–3
  non-healthcare reasons for disclosure 216
    employers, insurance and other affairs
      217–18
    media (the press, etc.) 216–17
    spiritual care 216
  occupational health physicians 674–6
  pseudonymous information 194
  research and innovative treatment 604
    children and young people 606
    publication 606
    records-based searches 604–6
  secondary uses of patient information
    complaints 214–15
    financial audit and other management
      purposes 213–14
    healthcare provision 207
    medical research 207–9
    NHS Act 2006 209–11
    public health 211–12
    social care 211
    teaching 212–13
  statutory and legal disclosures 194–5
    all citizens 195
    courts, tribunals and regulatory bodies
      196–7
    police, social services and partner
      organisations 197–8
    solicitors 197
  statutory restrictions on disclosure 198–9
  teaching medical students 755–6
    log books 756
    work observation and experience 756–7
  teenage contraception 273–4
  violent patients 56
Congenital Disability (Civil Liability) Act 1976
  309
conjoined twins 173–4
conscientious objection 32–3
consent 31
  abortion
    incapacitated adults 293–4
    involvement of father 294
    young people 292–3
  armed forces 681

capacity to consent and refuse 100–1
children and young people
  research and innovative treatment 602
adults with capacity 59–88
detention settings 693
emergency situations 629–30
  suicide attempts and self-harm 630–3
general principles 60
genetic testing 369
  adults lacking capacity 370–2
  information and counselling 369–70
Human Tissue Act 2004 523–4
immigration removal centres (IRCs) 727
incapacitated (incompetent) patients 93–141
limits to individual choices 80–8
  amputation of healthy limbs 85–8
  procedures to benefit others 80–5
nature and purpose 59–60
occupational health physicians 676
pre-employment testing 670–1
pressures on consent 74–5
refusal of treatment 75–80
  benefit to others 77
  continuing care 78
  documenting refusal 78
  failure to respect 79
  informed refusal 77–8
  right to refuse 75–7
research and innovative treatment 587
  children and young people 602
  detainees 592
  discussing risk 588
  donation of bodily material and payment 591–2
  financial incentives 589–91
  obligation to participate 592–3
  people in a dependent situation 592
  placebos and patient preferences 593
scope of consent 73–4
  duration 73
  exceeding consent 73–4
seeking consent 61
  accessibility of information 64–5
  amount of information 66–70
  capacity 61–2
  documentation 72–3
  duty to warn about risks 67
  failure to warn of risks of surgery 68–9
  providing information 64–71
  refusing to receive information 70–1
  type of information 66

  who should seek 63–4
  withholding information 70
standards and good practice 60–1
sterilisation 278
storage of gametes and embryos 324
  storage and use following withdrawal of consent 326–7
  storage and use without effective consent 324–5
teaching medical students
  carrying out procedures 754–5
  children, young people and patients lacking capacity 755
  examining patients 753–4
  introducing students 753
  presence of students 753
teenage contraception 273–4
young offender institutions 722–3
consequentialist ethics 10
consultants
  duty of care 30
contextualism 12
continuous deep sedation 436, 466
contraception 271
  see also reproductive ethics
  conscientious objection to 277
  doctors' moral views 32
  emergency hormonal contraception 276
    difference from abortion 276–7
  teenagers
    consent and confidentiality 273–4
    individuals with learning difficulties 275
    law on sexual offences in Northern Ireland 275
    public policy 271–2
controlled drugs, prescribing 565–6
  addicts 566
coroners 500
  post-mortem examinations 506–7
  referring a death to 502–3
Coroners (Amendment) Rules 2005 (SI 2005/420) 529
Coroners (Amendment) Rules 2008 (SI 2008/1652) 528
Coroners Act (Northern Ireland) 1959 506
Coroners Act 1988 526
Coroners and Justice Act 2009 500–1, 511, 526, 469, 470
corporate responsibility 5
Counter Fraud and Security Management Service (CFSMS) 196

Court of Protection 118
covert medication 39–40
covert video surveillance (CVS) 41–2
cremation, removal of medical devices 504
Cremation (England and Wales) Regulations
    2008 (SI 2008/2841) 498, 528
Cremation (Scotland) Regulations 1935 506
Cremation Act 1902 506
Cremation Act 1952 506
cremation certificates 504
Creutzfeldt–Jakob disease (CJD) 816–17
    ensuring safe blood supply 818–19
    harmful knowledge 817–18
    informing patients about possible exposure
        817
    poorly understood 817
Crime and Disorder Act 1998 197
crime victims
    consent
        examination by forensic physicians 729
    emergency treatment 637
    forensic testing 637
Criminal Attempts Act 1981 469
Criminal Justice (Northern Ireland) Act 1966
    470
Criminal Justice (Northern Ireland) Order 1998
    737
Criminal Justice (Northern Ireland) Order 2005
    638, 730, 731
Criminal Justice Act 2003 401, 467
Criminal Justice and Police Act 2001 401
Criminal Procedure and Investigations Act
    1996 731
Criminal Records Bureau (CRB) 49, 794–5
criminals
    emergency treatment 637
        blood alcohol tests of incapacitated
            drivers 637–8
        detained people 638
        disclosure of information in public
            interest 639–41
cryonics 520
cultural and religious sensibilities 34
    chaperones 47
    circumcision 170–1
    consent to treatment
        Jehovah's Witnesses 74–5, 78–9, 166–8
    disclosure of patient information 216
    end of life care 439–40
    genital mutilation of females 171–3
    prescriptions 544–5
    treatment of body following death 492–3

Data Protection (Miscellaneous Subject Access
    Exemptions) Order 2000 (SI 2000/419)
    264
Data Protection (Processing of Sensitive
    Personal Data) (Elected
    Representatives) Order 2002 (SI
    2002/2905) 215
Data Protection (Processing of Sensitive
    Personal Data) Order 2000 (SI
    2000/417) 191
Data Protection Act 1998 190–1, 214, 234, 239,
    240, 244–5, 253, 256, 527, 604, 614,
    655, 669, 728, 756
    research 614–15
death
    encountering during medical training 760
    in hospitals 416
    preparing for 426–7
death certificates 500–1
    England and Wales 503
        cremation certificates 504
        independent scrutiny by medical examiner
            503–4
        removal of medical devices 504
        role of medical examiner 505
        stillbirths 505
    Northern Ireland 505–6
    Scotland 506
Death with Dignity Act 1994, Oregon
    (DWDA) 477, 479, 484–5
deceased patients
    confidentiality 221–2
        entitlement of relatives to medical records
            222
        other circumstances for disclosures 223
    health records
        access to 259–60
    insurance medical reports 660
    recordings 252
deceased patients, responsibilities to after death
    489–90
    anatomical examination 516
    attitudes to
        health professionals 494
        public dissection 493–4
        treatment of the body 492–3
        wishes of the dead 491–2
    certifying and confirming death 501–2
        England and Wales 503–5
        referring death to coroner or procurator
            fiscal 502–3
    confidentiality 498–9

benefit and harm 499–500
   information disclosure to coroner or
      procurator fiscal 500
   information on death certificates 500–1
dealing with unusual requests 520
duties
   to patient 496–7
   to patient's relatives 497–8
general principles 490
law
   Access to Health Records Act 1990 527
   Anatomy Act 1984 526
   Coroners and Justice Act 2009 526
   Human Tissue (Scotland) Act 2006 524–6
   Human Tissue Act 2004 522–4
law reform 494–6
   Alder Hey Hospital 495
organ and tissue donation for research and
     teaching 515–16
organ and tissue transplantation 512
   increasing number of donors 512–15
post-mortem examinations 506
   concern for justice and public good
     510–11
   coroner or procurator fiscal examinations
     506–7
   discussing with families 507
   hospital examinations 507
   importance 508–10
   minimally invasive autopsies 511
   retention and use of organs 507–8
   testing DNA 518–19
   testing for communicable diseases 517–18
practicing procedures on newly deceased 520
skeletons for private study 517
terminology
   consent and authority 490–1
   next of kin 491
trade in body parts and tissues 521
   legal situation 522
use of bodies or body parts for display
   516–17
decision-making, sharing with patients 22
Declaration of Geneva 889
declaration of new doctor, Imperial College
     School of Medicine (2001) 891
deep sedation
   appropriate 437
   inappropriate 439
delegation 788–9
deontological ethics 10–11
Deprivation of Liberty Safeguards (DOLS) 113

Detention Centre Rules 2001 (SI 2001/238)
   726, 727
detention settings, treatment within
   consent, confidentiality and choice 692
     advance decisions and suicide attempts
     696
     assessing capacity 694–5
     choice 695–6
     choice of doctor 700
     disclosures connected with crime 698–9
     respecting confidentiality 696–8
     respecting refusal 695
     seeking consent 693
     translation and interpretation 699–700
   doctors' duties 689–91
   general principles 691–2
   immigration removal centres (IRCs) 724
     confidentiality 727–8
     consent 727
     duty of care 724–6
     welfare of children 726–7
   police stations 728
     confidentiality 731–2
     consent 729–31
     detainees held without charge 732–3
   practical issues common to various settings
     701–2
     assessment of potential of self-harm
     706–8
     communicable diseases 708–10
     communications with other health
       professionals 703–4
     communications with patients 703
     emergency attention 707
     ensuring access to appropriate care 704–6
     hunger strikes 713–16
     restraint and control 711–13
     rights to assisted reproduction 706
     solitary confinement, segregation and
       separation 710–11
     treatment under human rights legislation
     705
   prison healthcare 716–17
     challenges 716
     diversion from prison 721–2
     independence of health professionals 720
     mental health services 717–18
     pregnancy and childcare 718–20
     substance misuse services 718
   young offender institutions 722
     child protection 723–4
     consent and refusal of treatment 722–3

diagnostic error 864

diagnostic genetic testing 368, 378

Dignitas 473

Dignity in Dying 472–3

dignity of patients 23

direct-to-consumer genetic testing 393–6
  common framework 394

disaster sites 644
  dealing with stress and trauma 645–6
  patients refusing to attend hospital 645
  teamwork 645
  triage 644

discharge summaries 562–3

disclosure
  children and young people
    children who are competent 220–1
    children who lack competence 220
    Scotland 221
  deceased patients 221–2
    entitlement of relatives to medical records
      222
    other circumstances for disclosures
      223
  definition 183
  disclosure in the public interest 199–201
    abuse and domestic violence 205
    balancing benefits and harms 201
    examples 202
    gunshot and knife wounds 204
    health 202
    informing sexual contacts 202–3
    involving the individual 201
    making the disclosure 201–2
    patients lacking capacity 206
    public safety 203
    serious crime and national security 203–4
    urgency of disclosure 201
    workplace safety 204–5
  incapacitated (incompetent) patients 218–19
    proxy decision makers 219–20
    sharing information with relatives, carers
      and friends 219
  non-healthcare reasons for disclosure 216
    employers, insurance and other affairs
      217–18
    media (the press, etc.) 216–17
    spiritual care 216
  secondary uses of patient information
    complaints 214–15
    financial audit and other management
      purposes 213–14
    healthcare provision 207

medical research 207–9
  public health 211–12
  social care 211
  teaching 212–13
  statutory and legal duties 194–5
    all citizens 195
    courts, tribunals and regulatory bodies
      196–7
    police, social services and partner
      organisations 197–8
    solicitors 197
  statutory restrictions on disclosure 198–9

discrimination
  doctors' moral views 32

DNA samples, retention of 402–3

doctor(s)
  dual obligations 649
    access to reports 653
    armed forces 679–82
    asylum seekers, examination of 667–8
    business interests of doctors 685
    circumstances 651
    confidentiality 652–3
    expert witnesses 661–3
    general principles 651
    implications 649–50
    media doctors 684–5
    medical reports for insurance 654–61
    occupational health physicians 673–9
    pre-employment reports and testing
      669–73
    providing reports for third parties 651
    refereeing firearms licences 663–6
    sports doctors 682–4
    truthfulness 653
  duties
    GMC framework 6–7
    to speak out when necessary 720
  duties towards commissioning agent 27
  duties towards patients 27
  duty to acknowledge mistakes 36–8
  duty to help
    accident and disaster sites 644–6
    emergency situations outside of healthcare
      establishments 642–4
  employment disputes 38
  health problems 879
    BMA services 882
    employment and pre-employment health
      checks 879–80
    exposure to health risks 880
    GMC sick doctors procedure 882

responsibility for colleagues 881
self-treatment 880–1
treating patients who are doctors 882–3
monitoring own performance 866–7
addressing blame culture 867–8
moral outlook 17–18, 32–3
personal beliefs 26
self-diagnosis 45
surrogacy, duty in 354–5
treatment as patients
confidentiality 882–3
doctor–patient relationship 21–57
assisted dying 478–9
balanced relationships 31–3
breakdown 43–4
complaints 44
changing expectations 22–3
background to 24–5
patient-centred and personalised care 25–6
telemedicine and care at a distance 23–4
choice and duty 28–31
doctors 29
duty of care 29–31
patients 28–9
communication 33–9
concordance 34
duty to acknowledge mistakes 36–8
interpretation and translation 38–9, 65
patient refusal 34–5
truth telling by doctors 35–8
truth telling by patients 38
concordance 34, 541
older patients 542
general principles 21–2
GMC guidance 25
patient expectations 546
patients' responsibilities
aggression 55–7
health service 54–5
responsibilisation 54
violence 55–7
responsibilities and boundaries 45–54
chaperones 47–9
colleagues' reliability 49–51
emotionally close patients 45
managing patient expectations 46–7
personal relationships with patients 51–4
self-diagnosis 45
staff as patients 45–6
trust and reciprocity
covert medication 39–40
financial interests 42

recording of consultations by doctors 41–2
recording of consultations by patients 40–1
second opinions 42–3
types of relationship 27
dual obligations 27–8
independent assessors 27
therapeutic 27
domestic violence 205, 640
domino transplants 81
donations *see* organ donations
do-not-attempt-CPR (DNACPR) decisions 447, 448
do-not-attempt-resuscitation (DNAR) decisions 415
double effect 434–5
drinking water, fluoridation of 822–4
Drug Rehabilitation Requirements (DRRs) 721
drugs
controlled
prescribing 565–6
prescribing to addicts 566
in sport 683–4
lifestyle drugs 22
off-label
prescribing 536–7
supply to UK 575
parallel trading 575–6
testing, random 676–7
treatment and testing orders (DTTOs) 721
unlicensed
prescribing 536–7
drunk drivers
blood alcohol tests 637–8
dual obligations 649
armed forces 679–80
boxing 681
confidentiality 680
consent 681
disciplinary or forensic procedures 681
asylum seekers, examination of 667
expert assessment 667–8
language services 668
business interests of doctors 685
expert witnesses 661–3
reforming delivery of expert opinion 663
general principles 651
implications 649–50, 651
media doctors 684–5
medical reports for insurance 654

dual obligations (*Continued*)
    adults lacking capacity 660
    collection 654
    content for disclosure 656
    content of report 657–9
    deceased patients 660
    evidence to verify claim 659–60
    explanations 659
    family history information 659
    genetic information 658
    GP reports (GPR) 655–6
    HIV, hepatitis B and C 657–8
    independent medical reports 656
    lifestyle questions 658
    sexually transmitted infections (STIs) 657
    occupational health physicians 673–4
    confidentiality 674–6
    consent 676
    health records 678–9
    liaison with colleagues 679
    pre-employment assessment 674
    random drug testing 676–7
    sickness absence 677–8
    pre-employment reports and testing 669
    consent 670–1
    genetic screening 672–3
    GP involvement 671–2
    HIV, drugs and alcohol 670
    information on occupational hazards 673
    providing reports for third parties 651
    access to reports 653
    confidentiality 652–3
    truthfulness 653
    refereeing firearms licences 663–4
    applicants who may present a risk 666
    current legal situation 664
    issues for concern 655
    medical information 664
    objections to signing 666
    role of referee or countersignatory 655
    tagging medical records 666
    sports doctors 682–3
    drugs and sport 683–4
Duchenne muscular dystrophy 392
duration of consent 73
duty of care 29–31
duty to acknowledge mistakes 36–8
duty to pursue 30–1

education and training
    changing situation 740–1
    medical school selection 741–2

dilemmas of medical students 761–2
    emergencies 765
    medical electives 763–5
    patient rights 763
    student and tutor inequalities 762–3
    witnessing unethical behaviour 762
ethical issues from teaching medical students 752
    confidentiality in teaching context 755–7
    consent in teaching context 752–5
    encountering death 760
    hidden, silent or informal curriculum 758–9
    professionalism vs dehumanisation 759–60
    teaching using new technologies 757–8
ethical practice 739
general principles 739–40
medical ethics and law 742–3
    academic and professional misconduct 746
    core curriculum 746–7
    distance learning materials 751–2
    goals and objectives 744–5
    graduation oaths 747–8
    human rights 750
    humanitarian and global issues 750–1
    medical humanities 751
    multi-disciplinary teaching 749–50
    postgraduate training 748–9
    theory to practice 749
    trends 749–52
teaching of ethics and ethics of teaching 765–6
elder abuse 543
Electronic Care Record (ECR) 241
embryos and fetuses
    see also abortion
    assisted reproduction
        embryo selection on tissue type compatibility 342–5
    legal rights 269–70
    sex selection 345–6
        BMA view 347
        consultation and debate 346–7
    research
        human admixed embryos 619–20
        stem cell research 617–19
Emergency Care Record (ECR) 242
Emergency Care Summary (ECS) 241, 242
emergency research 599
    children and babies 603

emergency situations 629
  confidentiality 633
    after death 633
    sharing information with healthcare team 633
  consent and refusal 629–30
    suicide attempts and self-harm 630–3
  detention settings 707
  duties to families 634
    organ and tissue donations 636
    research and education 636
    witnessed resuscitation 634–5
  general principles 629
  medical students 765
  outside healthcare establishments
    accident and disaster sites 644–6
    duty to help 642–4
  public health considerations 813
    fair process 814
    liability issues 816
    medical utility 815
    policy making for future threats 813–14
    proportionality 814
    resource allocation 814
    risk to health professionals 816
    scientific and medical functioning 815
    social functioning and infrastructure 816
    social utility 815
    triage 815
  recognising skill and competence levels 641–2
    acting within limits of competence 642
  victims or perpetrators of crime or abuse 637
    blood alcohol tests of incapacitated drivers 637–8
    disclosure of information in public interest 639–41
    treating detained people 638
employers of patients
  disclosure of patient information 217–18
employing other practitioners 793
  health checks 793
  providing references 795
  vetting and barring 794
employment disputes 38
  genetic testing 398
Encryption Code of Practice 246
end of life 415–17
  after patient death 455
    bereavement support for those close to patient 456

    last offices 455
    support for healthcare team 456
  cardio-pulmonary resuscitation (CPR) 447
    discussion with patients 447–9
    when to attempt CPR 450
  children and young people 451–2
    communication with parents 451–2
    communication with young patients 451
    disagreement 452–3
    palliative care 453–4
  communication 418
    adults lacking capacity 424
    among care professionals 424–5
    complementary therapists 425
    GMC guidance 420
    information provision 418–19
    level of detail 422–3
    listening to patient 419–20
    patients in denial 420–2
    sharing information with those close to patient 423–4
  definition 415–16
  denial and collusion 420–1
  diagnosis and preparing for death 426–7
    advance care planning (ACP) 428–31
    communication after assessment 428
    Liverpool Care Pathway for the Dying Patient (LCP) 432–4
    pain and symptom relief 434–5
    palliative care 431–3
    quality markers 432
    sedation 435–9
    spiritual and pastoral care 439–40
  general principles 417–18
  hope and positive attitudes 421–2
  training
    non-specialists 456–8
  withholding or withdrawing life-prolonging treatment 440–1
    adults lacking capacity 442–3
    adults with capacity 441–2
    conventional treatment 443
    definition 466
    disagreements about treatment withdrawal 446
    discussion within healthcare team 443
    nutrition and hydration 444–6
End of Life Care Strategy 416
ending professional relationship with a patient 43–4
entitlement rights 8
Environment Act 1995 809

Environmental Protection Act 1990 809
epigenetics 404–5
equity in health care provision 2, 842
  inequalities 843–4
  non-discrimination 844–5
  public participation and involvement 845–6
error
  acknowledging to patients 872
  diagnostic 864
ethical behaviour 5
ethical priorities in resource allocation 841
  clinical effectiveness 842
  equity 842
  individual rights 842
  need 841
  patient choice 842–3
  relative cost-effectiveness 842
  truth telling 843
  welfare maximisation 841–2
ethics 1
  amputation of healthy limbs 87–8
  communitarian ethics 10
  consequentialist ethics 10
  deontological ethics 10–11
  dilemmas of medical students 761–2
  education and training in 742–3
    academic and professional misconduct
      746
    core curriculum 746–7
    distance learning materials 751–2
    goals and objectives 744–5
    graduation oaths 747–8
    human rights 750
    humanitarian and global issues 750–1
    medical humanities 751
    multi-disciplinary teaching 749–50
    postgraduate training 748–9
    research ethics 744
    theory to practice 749
    trends 749–52
  ethical issues from teaching medical students
    752
    confidentiality in teaching context 755–7
    consent in teaching context 752–5
    encountering death 760
    hidden, silent or informal curriculum
      758–9
    professionalism vs dehumanisation
      759–60
    teaching using new technologies 757–8
  ethical practice of medicine 739
  four principles approach 11

genetics 366–7
  ethical framework 368
narrative ethics 11
relationship with law 7
reproductive ethics 267–8, 306
teaching of ethics and ethics of teaching
  765–6
value of varied approaches 12
virtue ethics 12
European Association for Palliative Care 438
European Committee for the Prevention of
      Torture and Inhuman or Degrading
      Treatment or Punishment (CPT)
      711
  force and restraint 712
European Convention for the Protection of
      Human Rights and Fundamental
      Freedoms 9
European Medicines Agency (EMA) 536
European Working Time Directive 23
euthanasia 463–4
  general principles 464
  terms and definitions 464–7
examinations, intimate 47–9
exceeding consent 73–4
existential suffering 437–8
expert witnesses 661–3
  reforming delivery of expert opinion 663
explicit (express) consent 61
exposure-prone procedures (EPPs) 831
express consent
  definition 183

Faculty of Forensic and Legal Medicine
      (FFLM) 728
  intimate body searches 730
fairness 2
Family Law Reform (Northern Ireland) Order
      1977 412
Family Law Reform Act 1969 412
Family Planning Association (FPA) 292
Fatal Accidents and Sudden Deaths Inquiry
      (Scotland) Act 1976 735
feeding, forcible 714
female genital mutilation 171–3
Female Genital Mutilation Act 2003 172
feminist ethics 12
fertility see reproductive ethics
fetuses see embryos and fetuses
financial audits
  disclosure of patient information 213–14
financial interests of doctors 42

Firearms (Northern Ireland) Order 1981 686
Firearms (Scotland) Rules 1989 (SI 1989/889) 686
Firearms Acts 1968 to 1997 665
firearms licences, refereeing 663–4
  applicants who may present a risk 666
  current legal situation 664
  issues for concern 655
  medical information 664
  objections to signing 666
  role of referee or countersignatory 655
  tagging medical records 666
Firearms Rules 1998 (SI 1998/1941) 686
fluctuating capacity 100
fluorescent *in situ* hydribisation (FISH) 342
fluoridation of water 822–4
forcible feeding 714
forensic physicians 728
  confidentiality 731–2
    information on police records 732
  consent
    acting without consent 730–1
    examination of incapacitated detainees 730
    examination of those held in custody 729–30
    examination of victims of crime 729
    minors 730
  detainees held without charge 732–3
forensic testing
  crime victims 637
forensic use of genetic testing 401–2
  developments in genetic analysis by criminal justice system 403–4
  involvement of doctors 402–3
Freedom of Information (Scotland) Act 2002 222, 259
Freedom of Information Act 2000 221, 259, 660
future prospects of medical ethics 3–4

gamete interfallopian transfer (GIFT) 313
gender identity dysphoria 838–9
Gender Recognition Act 2004 188, 198, 237
gene therapy 405–6, 621
Gene Therapy Advisory Committee (GTAC) 406
General Medical Council (GMC) 1
  abortion, conscientious objection to 289
  abusive behaviour 51
  chaperones 48
  colleagues' performance 881

communicating with children and young people 148
confidentiality 192
  disclosure for medical research 208
conflicts of interest 790
cultural sensitivities 34
delegation and referral 789
doctor–patient relationship 25
doctors' personal beliefs 26
dual obligations
  confidentiality and medical reports 652
  report writing 654
education and training 740–1
  Tomorrow's Doctors 740, 742, 751
  ethical and legal principles 745
emergency treatment
  gunshot and knife wounds 639
end of life
  adults lacking capacity 424
  advance care planning (ACP) 430
  advance requests 430–1
  cardio-pulmonary resuscitation (CPR) 448
  children and young people 454
  communicating with patient 420
  confidentiality after death 498–500
  definition 415–16
  persistent vegetative state (PVS) 446
family members as patients 45
good practice framework 6–7
  doctors' duties 6–7
health records 231–2
intimate examination 47–8
mistakes by doctors 36–7
Personal Beliefs and Medical Practice 33
poor performance, recognising and dealing with 871
prescriptions
  best interests of patients 541
  errors 538
  off-label or unlicensed drugs 536
research and innovative treatments
  disclosure in public interest 605
  discussing risks 588
  information giving 587
research regulation 611
seeking consent 63
  documentation 72
  withholding information 70
self-treatment 45, 881
sexualised behaviour 50–1
sick doctors procedure 882
teamwork 772–3

General Practitioners (GPs)
  doctor–patient relationship
    balanced relationships 31–3
    changing expectations 22–6
    doctor choice 29
    duties 27
    duty of care 29–31
    patient choice 28
  medical reports for insurance (GPR)
      655–6
  pre-employment reports and testing 671–2
  role in home births 302
  standards 863–5
    diagnostic error 864
    locums, out-of-hours services and medical
        cover 864–5
  teamwork 773–4
  transmission of patient records 246–7
generic prescribing 574
  drug switching 574–5
Genetic Information Non-discrimination Act
    2008 (USA) 413
genetic screening
  pre-employment reports and testing 672–3
genetic testing
  carrier testing for recessive or X-linked
      conditions 378–9
    adults lacking capacity 379
    children 379–82
  confidentiality within families 374–7
    use of information by clinics 377–8
  consent 369
    adults lacking capacity 370–2
    information and counselling 369–70
  controversial uses 396
    employment 398
    forensic use 401–4
    insurance 396–8
    paternity testing 398–401
  diagnostic testing 378
  family history of genetic disease 368–9
  impact on others 375
  incidental findings 389–90
  law and regulation 408–9
  non-consensual testing 372
    exceptions to offence of non-consensual
        DNA testing 373
    qualifying consent 372
  other developments
    behaviour genetics 405
    cloning 407–8
    epigenetics 404–5

gene therapy 405–6
    whole genome testing 404
  population genetic screening 390
    autosomal recessive disorder carriers
        390–1
    neonatal screening 391–2
    predisposition to common disorders
        392–3
  predictive of presymptomatic testing 383–5
    adults lacking capacity 385
    children 386–8
    young people 386
  susceptibility testing 388–9
  tests supplied direct to consumers 393–6
genetics
  ethical dilemmas 12
  ethical issues 366–7
    ethical framework 368
  general principles 366
  impact of development 365–6
  research 620–1
genital mutilation of females 171–3
gifts 53–4
  from pharmaceutical companies 554–6
Good Medical Practice 12
good practice framework
  ethics and law 7
  GMC 6–7
    doctors' duties 6–7
  medical ethics and human rights 7–9
green bag scheme 563
Groningen Protocol 480–3
gunshot and knife wounds 204, 639

H1N1 swine flu 535, 813, 814, 831
handicap
  abortion for serious cases 283–4
harm 2
health
  as a right 807–8
  definitions 803–4
  rights to healthcare
    NHS Act 1977 808
    NHS constitution 809
  social determinants 805–6
Health and Social Care Act 2001 53, 209, 848
Health and Social Care Act 2008 196, 871
health information, use of 847–8
  statutory exceptions for communicable
      diseases 848
health promotion campaigns 819–20
  tobacco control 820–2

Health Protection (Notification) (Wales)
    Regulations 2010 (SI 2010/1546) 224
Health Protection (Notification) Regulations
    2010 (SI 2010/659) 224
health records
    access
        by patients 255–8
        medical reports 260–1
        to records of children and young people
            258–9
        to records of deceased patients 259–60
        to records of incapacitated adults 259
    content of health records 231–2
        adoption 234
        aggressive behaviour 233
        altering records 232
        child protection case notes 233
        level of detail 233
    disposal 255
    documenting patient views about
        confidentiality 234–5
    electronic records 239
        national summary records 241–2
        online patient portals 242–3
        removing information 237
        shared detail care records 239–41
    facilitating access to records 234
    future directions 261–2
    general principles 230–1
    importance of health information 229–30
    omitting information 235
    ownership 253
    private records 255
    recordings 247
        adult patients who lack capacity 248–9
        as part of patient care 247–8
        children and young people 249
        deceased patients 252
        for research, teaching, training and other
            healthcare-related reasons 249–50
        for widely accessible public media 250–1
        storing and disposing of 252
        telephone and other audio recordings
            251–2
    records and record keeping 230
    removing information 235–6
        disputes over accuracy 237–8
        electronic records 237
        transsexualism 237
    retention 253–5
    security 243–5
        sending patient information abroad 245

tagging records 238–9
transmission 246
    GP records 246–7
Health Research Agency (HRA) 609–10
Health Service (Control of Patient
    Information) Regulations 2002 (SI
    2002/1438) 185, 188, 195, 210, 604
healthcare ethics 1
healthcare team
    definition 183
heel-prick test 392
Her Majesty's Inspectorate of Prisons (HMIP)
    690
Hippocratic Oath and values 1, 11, 748,
    887
historical development of medical ethics 3
HIV/AIDS
    detention settings 708
        condoms in prisons 709
        needle exchange 709–10
    medical reports for insurance 657–8
    pre-employment reports 670
homelessness 29
homeopathic treatment 564
honest brokers 209
honesty 2
hospitality from pharmaceutical companies
    554–6
hospitals
    post-mortem examinations 507
Howard League for Penal Reform 719
human admixed embryos 619–20
human embryo research
    stem cell research 617–19
Human Fertilisation and Embryology
    (Deceased Fathers) Act 2003 325
Human Fertilisation and Embryology
    (Disclosure of Donor Information)
    Regulations 2004 (SI 2004/1511) 360
Human Fertilisation and Embryology
    (Disclosure of Information for
    Research Purposes) Regulations 2010
    (SI 2010/995) 199
Human Fertilisation and Embryology (Parental
    Orders) Regulations 2010 (SI
    2010/985) 360
Human Fertilisation and Embryology (Quality
    and Standards) Regulations 2007 (SI
    2007/1522) 360
Human Fertilisation and Embryology
    (Research Purposes) Regulations 2001
    (SI 2001/188) 626

Human Fertilisation and Embryology
(Statutory Storage Period for Embryos
and Gametes) Regulations 2009 (SI
2009/1582) 359
Human Fertilisation and Embryology Act 1990
72, 199, 286, 312, 313–14, 616
Human Fertilisation and Embryology Act 2008
199, 290, 313, 325, 348, 619
Human Fertilisation and Embryology
Authority (HFEA) 312–13
future 314
monitoring outcomes 314–16
role 314
Human Genetics Commission 408, 409
human leucocyte antigen (HLA) 343–4
Human Organ and Tissue Live Transplants
(Scotland) Regulations 2006 (SI
2006/390) 532
Human Organ Transplants (Northern Ireland)
Order 1989 522
Human Organ Transplants Act 1989 84,
522
Human Reproductive Cloning Act 2001 407,
618
human rights
assisted dying 477–8
education and training in medical ethis and
law 750
European Convention for the Protection of
Human Rights and Fundamental
Freedoms 9
Human Rights Act 1998 8–9
medical ethics 7–9
treatment in prison 705
United Nations' Universal Declaration of
Human Rights (1948) 8
Human Rights Act 1998 8–9, 29, 132, 160, 676,
704, 750, 810, 842
DNA sample retention 402
refusal of treatment 75
research 614
Human Tissue (Quality and Safety for Human
Application) Regulations 2007 (SI
2007/1523) 523
Human Tissue (Scotland) Act 2006 524
authorisation 524–6
organ donations 82
Human Tissue (Scotland) Act 2006 489
Human Tissue Act 1961 522
Human Tissue Act 2004 522–3
consent 523–4
organ donations 82

organ retention following post-mortem 508
retention of organs after port mortem 490–1
Human Tissue Act 2004 (Persons who lack
capacity to consent and transplants)
Regulations 2006 (SI 2006/1659) 91
Human Tissue Act (Northern Ireland) 1962 522
Human Tissue Authority (HTA) 82
hunger strikes 713–16
advance decisions 714–15
doctor–patient discussion 714
forcible feeding 714
respecting treatment refusal 715–16
Huntingdon disease
genetic tests 394
hydration
withdrawal at end of life
patients with low awareness or vegetative
state 445–6
when patient is nearing death 444
when patient is not nearing death 444–5
hysterectomy
for severe menstrual bleeding 280–1

identifiable information
definition 183
Immigration and Asylum Act 1999 727
immigration removal centres (IRCs) 724
confidentiality 727–8
consent 727
duty of care 724–6
children 726–7
immunisation 828
implied consent 61
definition 183
information disclosure 187–8
incapacitated (incompetent) patients 93–141
abortion, consent for 293–4
assessment of decision-making capacity
98–102
capacity to consent and refuse 100–1
definition of capacity 98–9
fluctuating capacity 100
unwise decisions 101
children and young people
confidentiality 220
confidentiality 218–19
proxy decision makers 219–20
sharing information with relatives, carers
and friends 219
consent and alternatives 93–7
advance decisions refusing treatment 96
balancing freedom with protection 95

emergency treatment 95–6
mental health legislation 96–7
proxy decision making 94–5
consent
teaching of medical students 755
detention settings 694–5
end of life
communication 424
withholding or withdrawing
life-prolonging treatment 442–3
general principles 97–8
genetic testing 370–2
carrier testing for recessive or X-linked
conditions 379
predictive genetic testing 385
health records
access to 259
insurance medical reports 660
providing treatment
England and Wales 102–22
Northern Ireland 134–139
Scotland 122–34
recordings
as part of patient care 248–9
for research, teaching, training and other
healthcare-related reasons 250
for widely accessible public media 251
research and innovative treatment 102
fluctuating capacity and dementia research
598–9
incentive-based vaccination programmes 830
incentives for public health 832–3
indecent assault 47
independent mental capacity advocates
(IMCAs) 119, 219, 443
appointment 120
scope of powers 120–1
serious medical treatment 120
Independent Review Group on Retention of
Organs at Post Mortem 490
Individual Health Record (IHR) 242
individual responses to drugs 576–7
Infant Life (Preservation) Act 1929 291
infectious disease notification 809–10
in-flight emergencies 643–4
informal discussions 185
Information Commissioner
advice on violent patients 56
data loss 245
information for patients
accessibility 64–5
amount 66–70

refusal to receive 70–1
type 66
withholding 70
Information Governance Toolkit 244
innovative treatment 583
confidentiality 604
children and young people 606
publication 606
records-based searches 604–6
definitions 585
audit 586
benefit, harm and risk 586–7
fraud and misconduct 621–2
Committee on Publication Ethics (COPE)
622–3
whistleblowing 622
general principles 587
consent 587–93
inclusiveness 596–7
proportionate safeguards 596
truth telling and effective communication
594–6
welfare of individuals 593–4
people who cannot consent 597–8
adults lacking capacity 598–9
children and young people 599–604
Institute for Medical Ethics (IME) 743
insurance industry
disclosure of patient information 217–18
insurance medical reports 654
adults lacking capacity 660
collection 654
content for disclosure 656
content of report 657–9
deceased patients 660
evidence to verify claim 659–60
explanations 659
family history information 659
genetic information 658
GP reports (GPR) 655–6
HIV, hepatitis B and C 657–8
independent medical reports 656
lifestyle questions 658
sexually transmitted infections (STIs)
657
insurance, personal
genetic testing 396–8
integrated care pathways 785–6
integrity 2
intention 467
International Covenant on Economic Social
and Cultural Rights (ICESCR) 807

interpreting patients' communications 38–9
  detention settings 699–700
intimate body searches 730
intimate examinations 47–9
intuitionism 12
in vitro fertilisation (IVF) 311
Ionising Radiation Regulations 1999 (SI
  1999/3232) 686

Jehovah's Witness
  refusal of blood products 74–5, 78–9
    children and young people 166–8
Joint Inspection of Children's Services and
    Inspections of Social Work Services
    (Scotland) Act 2006 221
junior doctors, unsupervised 862–3

Kant, Immanuel 10–11
karyomapping 339
Key Information Summary (KIS) 242
kidney donations 81–5
King's Fund
  report on professionalism (2004) 5
knife wounds 204, 639

Lasting Powers of Attorney (LPA) 115–16
  confidentiality 218
  consent 74
  creating an LPA 116
  registering health and welfare LPA 116
  scope and extent 116–17
late gestation abortion 284
law
  education and training in 742–3
    academic and professional misconduct
      746
    core curriculum 746–7
    goals and objectives 744–5
    graduation oaths 747–8
  public health 807, 809
    health as a positive right 807–8
    infectious disease reporting 809–10
  relationship with ethics 7
Law Reform (Miscellaneous Provisions)
    (Scotland) Act 1990 412
leadership 774–5
learning difficulties, young people with
  sterilisation
    as contraceptive 279–80
    hysterectomy for severe menstrual
      bleeding 280–1
  teenage contraception 275

legal documents, witnessing 46–7
liberalism 12
libertarian paternalism 813
liberty rights 8
life-prolonging treatment
  refusal 114–15
    anorexia nervosa treatment refused by
      16-year-old 157
    heart transplant refused by 12-year-old
      158
    heart transplant refused by 15-year-old
      150
    hunger strikes 715–16
    hypothetical case 17–18
lifestyle drugs 22, 547–9
Liverpool Care Pathway for the Dying Patient
    (LCP) 417, 427, 428, 432–4
living organ donation 81–5
  expanding pool of donors 83–4
  independent assessors report 83
  safeguards 82–3
  special case of kidney donations 84–5
Local Research Ethics Committees (LRECs)
    608
locums 864–5
log books and patient confidentiality 756
Lucentis 537

male circumcision 170–1
market-based operation of healthcare services
    concerns about 6
media (the press, etc.)
  disclosure of patient information 216–17
  responding to criticism 216–17
media doctors 684–5
media role in public health 833–5
mediation 868–9
Medical Act 1983 196
Medical Certificate of Cause of Death (MCCD)
    500–1, 503
  independent scrutiny by medical examiner
    503–4
  Northern Ireland 505–6
  Scotland 506
medical cover 864–5
medical electives 763–4
  advance planning 764–5
  student unethical behaviour 764
medical ethics
  BMA approach
    theory and practice 13–17
  definition 1–6

development 3
future directions 3–4
human rights 7–9
key concepts 2
life-sustaining treatment
    anorexia nervosa treatment refused by
        16-year-old 157
    heart transplant refused by 12-year-old
        158
    heart transplant refused by 15-year-old
        150
    hypothetical refusal case 17–18
    refusal 114–15
theoretical and philosophical background
    9–13
    communitarian ethics 10
    consequentialist ethics 10
    deontological ethics 10–11
    four principles approach 11
    narrative ethics 11
    value of varied approaches 12
    virtue ethics 12
Medical Ethics 3, 24
Medical Ethics Committee (MEC) of the BMA
    professionalism 5
medical examiners
    role 505
    scrutiny of death certificates 503–4
medical reports
    confidentiality 652
        access to reports 653
        truthfulness 653
    GMC advice 654
medical reports for insurance 654
    adults lacking capacity 660
    collection 654
    content for disclosure 656
    content of report 657–9
    deceased patients 660
    evidence to verify claim 659–60
    explanations 659
    family history information 659
    genetic information 658
    GP reports (GPR) 655–6
    HIV, hepatitis B and C 657–8
    independent medical reports 656
    lifestyle questions 658
    sexually transmitted infections (STIs) 657
Medical Research Council (MRC)
    research and innovative treatment
        children and young people 602
medical schools, selection for 741–2

Medical Schools Council (MSC) 742
medication, covert 39–40
medication, prescribing and administering
    adverse drug reactions 573–4
    at a distance
        internet, email or telephone 567–9
        patients in other countries 569–70
        prescription-only medication on internet
            570–1, 572
    challenges and dilemmas 533–4
    clinical freedom and official guidance 552
        National Institute for Health and Clinical
            Excellence (NICE) 552–3
        Scotland, Wales and Northern Ireland
            553–4
    complementary and alternative medicine
        (CAM) 563–4
    conflicts of interest 554
        financial involvements in external
            health-related services 556
        gifts or hospitality from pharmaceutical
            companies 554–6
        ownership of pharmacies 557
        participation in market research 556–7
        payments for meeting pharmaceutical
            representatives 556
    controlled drugs 565–6
        addicts 566
    covert administration 573
    employer pressure 549
        clinical freedom and resources 549–50
        truth telling and resources 550–1
    general principles 534
    generic prescribing 574
        drug switching 574–5
    patient groups
        children 543–4
        older people 542–3
        religion and belief 544–5
    patient pressure 545
        dealing with expectations 546
        repeat prescriptions 547
        request to continue with medication
            547
        requests for lifestyle drugs 547–9
        requests for particular medications 545–6
    pharmacogenetics 576–7
    placebos 564–5
    providing information to patients 539
        adherence and concordance 539–42
    referrals and discharge summaries 562–3
    responsibility for prescribing 534–6

medication, prescribing and administering
  (*Continued*)
    errors 537–8
    failings 535–6
    off-label and unlicensed drugs 536–7
  self-prescribing or for family members 567
  shared prescribing 557–8
    complementary therapists 561–2
    GPs and hospital doctors 558–9
    patient group directions (PGDs) 560
    private sector and NHS 559–60
    supplementary prescribing and
      independent non-medical prescribing
      560–1
  special safeguards 572–3
  supply of drugs to UK 575
    parallel trading 575–6
Medicines (Advertising) Regulations 1994 (SI
    1994/1932) 554
Medicines (Marketing Authorisations etc.)
    Amendment Regulations 2005 (SI
    2005/2759) Mental Capacity Act 2005
    554
Medicines and Healthcare Products Regulatory
    Agency (MHRA) 536, 611
Medicines for Human Use (Clinical Trials) and
    Blood Safety and Quality (Amendment)
    Regulations 2008 (SI 2008/941) 603
Medicines for Human Use (Clinical Trials)
    Regulations 2004 (SI 2004/1031) 599,
    602, 612–13
Medicines for Human Use (Marketing
    Authorisations etc.) Regulations 1994
    (SI 1994/3144) 581
Medicines for Human Use (Manufacturing,
    Wholesale Dealing and Miscellaneous
    Amendments) Regulations 2005 (SI
    2005/2789) 581
Mendelian single gene disorders 365
Mental Capacity Act 2005 61–2, 103
  advance decisions refusing treatment 114–15
    definition 114
    life-sustaining treatment 114–15
    making advance decisions 114
    under compulsory mental health powers
      115
  appropriate regime 121–2
  assessing capacity
    definition of lacking capacity 105
    enhancing capacity 106
    method of assessment 105–6
    refusal to be assessed 107

    uncertainties about capacity 106–7
    who should assess capacity 105
  basic principles 104
    best interests 104
    freedom to make unwise decisions 104
    less restrictive alternative 105
    maximising decision-making 104
    presumption of capacity 104
  best interests 107
    challenges 109
    checklist 108
    exceptions 109
    factors to be taken into account 108
  care and/or treatment 109–10
    court approval 110–11
    extent of powers 110
  courts and deputies
    Court of Protection 118
    court-appointed deputies 119
  dispute resolution 117
  independent mental capacity advocates
    (IMCAs) 119
    appointment 120
    scope of powers 120–1
    serious medical treatment 120
  interface between capacity and legislation
    122
  lasting powers of attorney (LPA) 115–16
    creating an LPA 116
    scope and extent 116–17
  relationship with mental health legislation
    121
  research 613–14
  restraint or deprivation of liberty 111
    authorisation 113
    denial of liberty 112
    Deprivation of Liberty Safeguards
      (DOLS) 113
    differentiation 112–13
    lawful restraint 111
  scope and extent
    importance of good communication 118
    mediation 118
Mental Capacity Act 2005 (Independent Mental
    Capacity Advocates) (General)
    Regulations 2006 (SI 2006/1832) 142
Mental Capacity Act 2005 (Loss of Capacity
    During Research Project) (England)
    Regulations 2007 (SI 2004/679) 626
Mental Capacity Act 2005 (Loss of Capacity
    During Research Project) (Wales)
    Regulations 2007 (SI 2007/837) 626

mental capacity of patients
  capacity to consent and refuse 100–1
  consent
    adults with capacity 59–88
    definition 98–9
    fluctuating capacity 100
    medication 39–40
Mental Health (Care and Treatment) (Scotland)
    Act 2003 124, 130, 694, 717
  treatment 131
Mental Health (Northern Ireland) Order 1986
    694
Mental Health (Scotland) Act 1984
    159
Mental Health Act 1983 117, 121–2, 305, 502,
    694, 714
mental health legislation
  consent from vulnerable adults
    96–7
mental health services
  prisons 717–18
minimally invasive autopsies 511
misconduct, professional 746
mistakes
  duty to acknowledge 36–8
MMR controversy 829
moral questions 7
morals 1
  doctors' personal views 32–3
motivation 467
Multi-centre Research Ethics Committees
    (MRECs) 608

narrative ethics 11
National Assistance Act 1947 809
National Encryption Framework 246
National Health Service (General Medical
    Services Contracts) (Prescription of
    Drugs etc.) Regulations 2004
    (SI 2004/629) 579
National Health Service (General Medical
    Services Contracts) Regulations 2004
    (SI 2004/291) 579
National Health Service (NHS)
  Care Record Guarantee 192–3
  central tenets 4
  constitution 809
  patient choice 28–9
  proposed restructuring from 2010 onwards
    3–4
  rationing of medications 550
  resource allocation 837–8

clinician involvement in rationing 838
  NICE and SIGN 837
  unfunded treatments 36
National Health Service (Primary Medical
    Services) (Miscellaneous Amendments)
    Regulations 2010 (SI 2010/578) 228
National Health Service (Reimbursement of the
    Cost of EEA Treatment) Regulations
    2010 (SI 2010/915) 782
National Health Service (Venereal Disease)
    Regulations 1974 (SI 1974/29) 198-9
National Health Service (Scotland) Act 1978
    808
National Health Service Act 1977 808
National Health Service Act 2006 188,191, 209,
    212, 216, 782, 848
National Health Service Litigation Agency
    (NHSLA) 85
National Institute for Health and Clinical
    Excellence (NICE) 546, 552–3, 837
  Alzheimer's drug decision 839
National Institute for Health Research 609
National Pandemic Flu Service (NPFS) 535
National Patient Safety Agency (NPSA) 511,
    537–8, 873
National Research Ethics Service (NRES) 406,
    610–11
  General Medical Council (GMC) 611
  guidance from other UK bodies 611–12
  Medicines and Healthcare Products
    Regulatory Agency 611
  specialist bodies 611
needle exchange 709–10
neonates
  assisted dying 481–3
  stillbirths
    certification 505
next of kin
  deceased patients 491
NHS Blood and Transplant (NHSBT) 518
NHSmail 246
no-fault compensation 869
non-discrimination 5
Northern Ireland provision for adults lacking
    capacity 134
  advance decisions refusing treatment 137–8
    format of advance decisions 138–9
    scope and nature of advance decisions
      138
    storage of decisions before treatment 139
  assessing capacity 136–7
  best interests and necessity 135

Northern Ireland provision for adults lacking
capacity (*Continued*)
common law test of capacity 135–6
control, restraint and deprivation of liberty
140
emergency treatment 135
factors affecting capacity 137
presumption of capacity 134
proposals for legal reform 140–1
treatments requiring special safeguards
139–40
Nuffield Council on Bioethics 26, 394
nurse-led care 785
nursing homes
cardio-pulmonary resuscitation (CPR)
discussion with patients 449
nutrition
withdrawal at end of life
patients with low awareness or vegetative
state 445–6
when patient is nearing death 444
when patient is not nearing death 444–5

obesity 811–13
libertarian paternalism 813
occupational health physicians 673–4
confidentiality 674–6
consent 676
liaison with colleagues 679
pre-employment assessment 674
random drug testing 676–7
sickness absence 677–8
occupational health records 678
transfer of records 678–9
Offences Against the Person Act 1861 277
off-label drug prescriptions 536
economic reasons 536–7
older patients
prescribing for
challenges 541–2
concordance 542
elder abuse and over-medication 543
research and innovative treatment
fluctuating capacity and dementia research
598–9
opioids
end of life use 434–5
organ and tissue donations
emergency situations 636
for research and teaching 515–16
organ and tissue transplantation 512
increasing number of donors 512–13

opt in or opt out system 513–15
organ donation taskforce 513
living donors
consent
expanding pool of donors 83–4
independent assessors report 83
safeguards 82–3
special case of kidney donations
84–5
Organ Donor Register 512
organs, retention of after post mortem 490–1,
507–8
Alder Hey Hospital 495
existing holdings 508
out-of-hours services 864–5
over-medication 543

paediatric formulary 600–1
paediatric investigation plan (PIP) 601
pain relief
childbirth 306
paired organ donations 83–4
palliative care 419, 431–3
children and young people 453–4
pandemic flu
prescribing 535
parental responsibility 160–1
parents
decision-making on behalf of offspring
consent 161–3
disagreement between parents 164
parental responsibility 160–1
refusal 163–4
pastoral care 439–40
paternalism 24
paternity testing 398–401
ethical obligations 400–1
legal issues 399–400
pathology
examination of deceased patients 517–18
Patient Administration Systems (PAS) 239
patient expectations 46–7
patient group directions (PGDs) 560
Patient Information Leaflets (PILs) 545
patient information
NHS Act 2006 158
patient-centred care 25–6
patient's own drug (POD) scheme 563
patients
access to health records 255–6
copies of letters 257
disproportionate effort 256

electronic records 257–8
  information that should not be disclosed 256–7
balanced relationships with doctors 31–3
  rights to non-judgemental care 32–3
choice
  doctors and hospitals 28–9
  treatments 36
communication with doctors 33–9
  concordance 34
  interpretation and translation 38–9, 65
  patient refusal 34–5
  truth telling by doctors 35–8
  truth telling by patients 38
complying with wishes 17–18
dignity 23
duties of doctors 27
expectations of doctors 22–3
failure to take up treatment 30–1
pressure to prescribe 545
  dealing with expectations 546
  repeat prescriptions 547
  request to continue with medication 547
  requests for lifestyle drugs 547–9
  requests for particular medications 545–6
prudent patient 68
recording of consultations 40–1
requests for second opinions 42–3
responsibilities
  health service 54–5
  responsibilisation 54
  violence 55–7
uneconomic 29
who are doctors
  confidentiality 882–3
payments for referrals or recommendations 42
Percival, Thomas 3, 24
persistent vegetative state (PVS) 445–6
Personal Beliefs and Medical Practice 33
personal information
  definition 183
personal relationships with patients 51–4
personalisation 25
personalised care 25–6
pharmacies
  ownership of 557
pharmacists
  communication with patients 34
pharmacogenetics 576–7
pharmaceutical industry
  gifts or hospitality 554–6
  payments for meeting representatives 556

phenylketouria (PKU) 391
philosophy of medical ethics 9–13
  communitarian ethics 10
  consequentialist ethics 10
  deontological ethics 10–11
  four principles approach 11
  narrative ethics 11
  value of varied approaches 12
  virtue ethics 12
phobia
  refusal of treatment 99–100
physician assisted suicide 463–4
  general principles 464
  law
    attempts to change 470–1
    definition of assisting suicide 472–5
    England and Wales 469–71
    Northern Ireland 470
    policy for prosecutors 474
    Scotland 470, 471
  moral, legal and pragmatic arguments 476
    autonomy, human rights and impact on others 477–8
    available alternatives 483–4
    Death with Dignity Act 1994, Oregon (DWDA) 484–5
    doctor–patient relationship 478–9
    opposed to assisted dying 476–7
    slippery slope 479–83
    support for assisted dying 476
  opinions upon
    BMA policy 469
    doctors 467–8
    public 468–9
  terms and definitions 464–7
placebo effect 546
placebos
  prescribing 564–5
  research and innovative treatment 593
poaching patients 29
Police and Criminal Evidence (Northern Ireland) Order 1989 738
Police and Criminal Evidence Act 1984 700
Police Reform Act 2002 730
police stations 728
  confidentiality 731–2
  consent
    acting without consent 730–1
    examination of incapacitated detainees 730
    examination of those held in custody 729–30

police stations (*Continued*)
   examination of victims of crime 729
     minors 730
   detainees held without charge 732–3
police
   disclosure to during emergency treatment
     639
politics of public health 806–7
pooled organ donations 83–4
poor performance, recognising and dealing
     with 869
   acknowledging error to patients 872
   appraisals and revalidation 869–70
   poor performance by colleagues 870
   using local procedures 870–1
     GMC procedures 871
   writing references for colleagues 872–3
poorly performing systems and poor
     management
   implementing findings 875
   monitoring quality 876
   Quality and Outcomes Framework (QOF)
     877
   quality in relation to commissioning services
     877
   reporting adverse events 872–3
   risks to doctors' health and patient safety in
     the workplace 877–8
   whistleblowing 878–9
population genetic screening 390
   autosomal recessive disorder carriers 390–1
   neonatal screening 391–2
   predisposition to common disorders 392–3
population immunity 828
population screening 824
   benefits and harms 825–6
   breast cancer 827
   introduction criteria 824–5
post code lottery 36
Postgraduate Medical Examination and
     Training Board (PMETB) 740
posthumous use of gametes 324
postmenopausal women and assisted
     reproduction 321
post-mortem examinations 506
   concern for justice and public good 510–11
   evidence in legal cases 510
   coroner or procurator fiscal examinations
     506–7
   discussing with families 507
   importance 508–10
   minimally invasive autopsies 511

retention and use of organs 490–1, 507–8
   Alder Hey Hospital 495
   existing holdings 508
   law reform 494–6
   testing DNA 518–19
   testing for communicable disease 517–18
practical support to patients 26
practice standards 862
   hospital practice 862–3
     specialist working outside area of expertise
       863
     unsupervised junior doctors 862–3
   primary care 863–5
     diagnostic error 864
     locums, out-of-hours services and medical
       cover 864–5
practice-based commissioning (PBC) 790
pragmatism 12
predictive genetic testing 369, 383–5
   adults lacking capacity 385
   children 386–8
   young people 386
pre-employment reports and testing 669
   consent 670–1
   doctors 879–80
   genetic screening 672–3
   GP involvement 671–2
   HIV, drugs and alcohol 670
   information on occupational hazards 673
   occupational health physicians 674
Preferred Priorities for Care (PPC) 431
pregnancy
   prisons 718–20
   protecting fetus from harm 298–9
     making fetus a Ward of Court 298
   providing life support to woman for benefit
     of fetus 299–300
   routine screening 299
   selective reduction of multiple pregnancy
     286–7
preimplantation genetic screening (PGS) 342
preimplantation genetic testing
   diagnosis (PGD) 327–9
     non-disclosure 340–2
   exclusion testing 340–2
   revealing additional information 339–40
   selecting embryos on tissue type
     compatibility 342–5
preimplantation haplotyping (PGH) 339
prenatal diagnosis 296
   setting boundaries 297
   social implications 296–7

prenatal genetic testing 295–6
prescribing medication
  at a distance
    generic prescribing 574
    internet, email or telephone 567–9
    patients in other countries 569–70
    prescription-only medication on internet
      570–1
  clinical freedom and official guidance
    552
    National Institute for Health and Clinical
      Excellence (NICE) 552–3
    Scotland, Wales and Northern Ireland
      553–4
  complementary and alternative medicine
    (CAM) 563–4
  conflicts of interest 554
    financial involvements in external
      health-related services 556
    gifts or hospitality from pharmaceutical
      companies 554–6
    ownership of pharmacies 557
    participation in market research 556–7
    payments for meeting pharmaceutical
      representatives 556
  controlled drugs 565–6
    addicts 566
  employer pressure 549
    clinical freedom and resources 549–50
    truth telling and resources 550–1
  generic prescribing
    drug switching 574–5
  patient groups
    children 543–4
    older people 542–3
    religion and belief 544–5
  patient pressure 545
    dealing with expectations 546
    repeat prescriptions 547
    request to continue with medication 547
    requests for lifestyle drugs 547–9
    requests for particular medications 545–6
  pharmacogenetics 576–7
  placebos 564–5
  referrals and discharge summaries 562–3
  responsibility for 534–6
    adherence and concordance 539–42
    errors 537–8
    failings 535–6
    off-label and unlicensed drugs 536–7
    providing information to patients 539
  self-prescribing or for family members 567

shared prescribing 557–8
  complementary therapists 561–2
  GPs and hospital doctors 558–9
  patient group directions (PGDs) 560
  private sector and NHS 559–60
  supplementary prescribing and
    independent non-medical prescribing
    560–1
supply of drugs to UK 575
  parallel trading 575–6
Prescription Only Medicines (Human Use)
  Amendment (No. 3) Order 2000 (SI
  2000/3231) 307
prescription-only medication on internet 570–1
prison healthcare 716–17
  challenges 716
  diversion from prison 721–2
  independence of health professionals 720
  mental health services 717–18
  pregnancy and childcare 718–20
  substance misuse services 718
prisoners
  see also detention settings, treatment within
  assisted reproduction 706
  choice of GP 28
  communicable diseases 708–10
    condom provision 709
    needle exchange 709–10
  confidentiality 696–8
    disclosures connected with crime 698–9
    medical correspondence 697–8
  emergency attention 707
  hunger strikes 713–16
    advance decisions 714–15
    doctor–patient discussion 714
    forcible feeding 714
    respecting treatment refusal 715–16
  medical student's perspective 701–2
  national prison healthcare IT system 697
  prison healthcare 690
  restraint and control 711–13
    in transit 713
    NHS facilities 712
  self-harm 706–8
  solitary confinement, segregation and
    separation 710–11
  suicides 702
private health screening 25–6
private healthcare 36
procurator fiscal 500
  post-mortem examinations 506–7
  referring a death to 502–3

Professional and Linguistics Assessment Board
(PLAB) 748
professional conscience 5
professionalism 4–6, 856–7
core elements 5
Prohibition of Female Genital Mutilation Act
2005 172
prolonging life 23
property in a corpse 521
Protection of Vulnerable Groups (Scotland)
Act 2007 49
proxy decision makers 94–5
disclosure of patient information
219–20
prudent patient 68
pseudonymised information 194
definition 184
psychological suffering 437–8
psychological support to patients 26
public dissection of bodies 493–4
public health
commissioning services 835–6
defined package of healthcare 840–1
ethical priorities in resource allocation
841–3
judicial review in rationing decisions
838–40
priority setting 836–7
resource allocation to NHS 837–8
searching for equity 843–6
seeking treatment overseas 840
disclosure of patient information 211–12
future directions 848–9
general principles 799
legal aspects 807
health as a positive right 807–8
public health law 809–10
rights to healthcare 808–9
processing health data 847
use of health information 847–8
public health perspective 800–1
changing practice 801–2
evolving concepts 802–4
individuals and communities 804–5
limits to individualism 804–6
politics and justice 806–7
social determinants of health 805–6
threats to 811
climate change 811
emergencies 813–16
obesity 811–13
uncertainty 816–19

tools 819
changing environment 822–4
health promotion campaigns 819–22
incentives 832–3
media 833–5
population screening 824–7
vaccination 827–31
Public Health (Control of Disease) Act 1984
850
Public Health (Infectious Diseases) Regulations
1988 (SI 1988/1546) 224
Public Health Act (Northern Ireland) 1967 850
Public Health etc (Scotland) Act 2008 850
Public Interest Disclosure (Northern Ireland)
Order 1998 778
Public Interest Disclosure Act 1998 778
public interest disclosures 199–201
abuse and domestic violence 205
balancing benefits and harms 201
definition 183–4
examples 202
gunshot and knife wounds 204
health 202
informing sexual contacts 202–3
involving the individual 201
making the disclosure 201–2
patients lacking capacity 206
public safety 203
serious crime and national security 203–4
urgency of disclosure 201
workplace safety 204–5
public service ethos 6
Public Services Reform (Scotland) Act 2010 221

Quality and Outcomes Framework (QOF) 877
quasi-mandatory vaccination programmes 830

random drug testing 676–7
randomised controlled trials (RCTs)
consent 593
patient preferences 593
placebos 593
rationing of medication in NHS 550
recording of consultations by doctors 41–2
recording of consultations by patients 40–1
records *see* health records
refereeing firearms licences 663–4
applicants who may present a risk 666
current legal situation 664
issues for concern 655
medical information 664
objections to signing 666

role of referee or countersignatory 655
tagging medical records 666
referral 562–3, 788–9
  commissioning of services 789–91
    good practice 791–2
  private treatment 789
Referral Management Centres (RMCs) 30,
    790–1
refractory symptoms 435
Registration of Births, Deaths and Marriages
    (Scotland) Act 1965 506
Regulation of Investigatory Powers (Scotland)
    Act 2000 58
Regulation of Investigatory Powers Act 2000 41
relativism 12
religion *see* cultural and religious sensibilities
repeat prescriptions 547
Reporting of Injuries, Diseases and Dangerous
    Occurrences Regulations 1995 (SI
    1995/3163) 195
reproduction, assisted *see* assisted reproduction
reproductive ethics 267–8, 306
  autonomy, rights and duties
    autonomy of pregnant women 268–9
    duties towards fetuses 270
    legal rights of fetus 269–70
    right to reproduction 271
  contraception 271
    teenagers 271–5
  general principles 268
research 583
  centralised bodies involved in regulation and
    governance
    Health Research Agency (HRA) 609–10
    National Institute for Health Research 609
    UK Ethics Committee Authority
      (UKECA) 609
  confidentiality 604
    children and young people 606
    publication 606
    records-based searches 604–6
  definitions 583–4
    audit 586
    benefit, harm and risk 586–7
    therapeutic and non-therapeutic research
      584–5
  fraud and misconduct 621–2, 746
    Committee on Publication Ethics (COPE)
      622–3
    whistleblowing 622
  general principles 587
    consent 587–93

  inclusiveness 596–7
  proportionate safeguards 596
  truth telling and effective communication
    594–6
  welfare of individuals 593–4
governance 607
  background to regulation 607–8
  role of ethics committees 608–9
international guidance 612
law and regulation
  Adults with Incapacity (Scotland) Act
    2000 614
  Data Protection Act 1998 614–15
  Human Rights Act 1998 614
  Medicines for Human Use (Clinical Trials)
    Regulations 2004 612–13
  Mental Capacity Act 2005 613–14
National Research Ethics Service (NRES)
    610–11
  General Medical Council (GMC) 611
  guidance from other UK bodies 611–12
  Medicines and Healthcare Products
    Regulatory Agency 611
  specialist bodies 611
people who cannot consent 597–8
  adults lacking capacity 598–9
  children and young people 599–604
specialised areas 616
  fetuses or fetal material 620
  gene therapy 621
  genetic research 620–1
  human admixed embryos 619–20
  human embryo research 616–20
research ethics 744
research ethics committees (RECs)
  research governance 608–9
responsibilisation 54
restraint and control within detention settings
    711–13
  in transit 713
  NHS facilities 712
resuscitation
  witnessed resuscitation 635
right to found a family 317
'rights' as a concept 7–8
risk reduction 855
  doctors' health problems 879
    BMA services 882
    employment and pre-employment health
      checks 879–80
    exposure to health risks 880
    GMC sick doctors procedure 882

risk reduction (*Continued*)
    responsibility for colleagues 881
    self-treatment 880–1
    treating patients who are doctors 882–3
    duty to protect patients 855–6
    professionalism 856–7
    general principles 857
    monitoring quality and performance
        discussing risks with patients 866
        doctors monitoring own performance
            866–8
        duties regarding risk 865–6
        mediation 868–9
        no-fault compensation 869
        recognising and dealing with poor
            performance 869–72
    poorly performing systems and poor
            management
        implementing findings 875
        monitoring quality 876
        Quality and Outcomes Framework (QOF)
            877
        quality in relation to commissioning
            services 877
        reporting adverse events 872–3
        risks to doctors' health and patient safety
            in the workplace 877–8
        whistleblowing 878–9
    standard setting 857–62
        practice standards 862–5
risks
    duty to warn patients 67
    failure to warn in surgery 68–9
Road Traffic Act 1988 195
Royal College of Anaesthetists
    patient information leaflets 65
Royal College of Obstetricians and
            Gynaecologists (RCOG)
    chaperones 48
Royal College of Paediatrics and Child Health
            (RCPCH)
    covert video surveillance (CVS) 41–2
Royal College of Physicians (RCP)
    report on professionalism (2005) 5
Royal College of Surgeons
    live surgery broadcasts 757–6

safe havens 209
Safeguarding Vulnerable Groups Act 2006
    49
Sanitary Act 1866 822

schizophrenia
    refusal of treatment 99
Scottish Information Store (SCI) 241
Scottish Intercollegiate Guidelines Network
            (SIGN) 837
second opinions 42–3, 792
sedation
    end of life 435
        intention of doctor and patient 438–9
        international debate 436–7
        psychological or existential suffering
            437–8
        terminology 435–6
self-determination 2
self-diagnosis 45
self-harm
    assessing prisoners 706–8
    consent 630–1
        advance decisions refusing treatment
            (ADRT) 632–3
    young offender institutions 723
self-treatment 880–1
serious adverse events (SAEs) 607
serious crime and national security 203–4
sex offenders' register 47
sex selection of embryos 345–6
    BMA view 347
    consultation and debate 346–7
Sexual Offences (Northern Ireland) Order
        2008 275
Sexual Offences Act 2003 198, 273
sexual offences
    Northern Ireland 275
sexualised behaviour 50–1
sexually transmitted infections (STIs)
    medical reports 657
shared care
    complementary and alternative therapists
        786–8
    families with social problems 783–4
    information sharing 779–80
    integrated care pathways 785–6
    liaison between NHS and private
        practitioners 780–1
    liaison for treatment abroad 781–2
    mentally incapacitated adults 783
    nurse-led care 785
    other care providers and local authorities
        784–5
    poor coordination 779
    social workers 782–4

shared prescribing 557–8
  complementary therapists 561–2
  GPs and hospital doctors 558–9
  patient group directions (PGDs) 560
  private sector and NHS 559–60
  supplementary prescribing and independent
    non-medical prescribing 560–1
Shipman, Harold 496
sick doctors procedure 882
sickness absence
  occupational physicians 677–8
side effects of medications
  informing patients 539
skeletons for private study 517
'slippery slope' argument against assisted dying
    467, 479–83
smoking 820–2
social care
  disclosure of patient information 211
social determinants of health 805–6
Social Exclusion Unit 271
social media, use by doctors 52–3
social workers 782–4
spiritual support to patients *see* cultural and
    religious sensibilities
sports doctors 682–3
  drugs and sport 683–4
staff who are also patients 45–6
stem cell research 617–19
sterilisation 277–8
  consent 278
  people with learning difficulties
    as a contraceptive 279–80
    hysterectomy for severe menstrual
      bleeding 280–1
stillbirths
  certification 505
substance misuse services
  prisons 718
suffering, psychological or existential 437–8
suicide
  refusal of treatment following attempt 77
  young offender institutions 723
  prisoners 702
suicide, assisted *see* physician assisted suicide
Suicide Act 1961 470, 473, 496
suicide attempts
  consent 630–1
    advance decisions refusing treatment
      (ADRT) 632–3
Summary Care Record (SCR) 241–2

surgery
  amputation of healthy limbs 85–8
  consent
    refusal by surgeon 82
  risks
    failure to warn patients 68–9
surrogacy 348
  doctors' duties 354–5
  future directions 357
  regulatory framework 348–9
    enforcement of arrangement 350
    review of law 349–51
  seeking treatment in other countries 355–7
  society's ambivalence 351–2
    concepts of motherhood 353–4
    exploitation 353
    legacy of informal surrogacy 354
    payments 352
    risk of psychological harm to all parties
      353
    validity of consent 352–3
Surrogacy Arrangements Act 1985 313, 348,
    349
susceptibility genetic testing 369, 388–9
suspected unexpected serious adverse reactions
    (SUSARs) 586, 607
swine flu (H1N1) 535, 813, 814, 831

tampering with health records 232
Tay–Sachs disease 390
teaching
  disclosure of patient information 212–13
teamwork 771
  administrative issues
    advertising medical services 795
    employing other practitioners 793–5
    informing patients about changes 793
    partnership agreements 792–3
    partnerships providing services 792–3
  delegation and referral 788–9
    commissioning of services 789–91
    good practice 791–2
    private treatment 789
    second opinions 792
  general principles 771
  multi-disciplinary teams
    Bromley by Bow model 774
    conflict within teams 778–9
    constructive teamwork 772–3
    doctors as managers 775–9
    leadership 774–5

teamwork (*Continued*)
    meeting targets 777–8
    poor management and teamwork 776–7
    primary care 773–4
    principles 772–3
    secondary care 774
    whistleblowing 778
    shared care
        complementary and alternative therapists 786–8
        families with social problems 783–4
        information sharing 779–80
        integrated care pathways 785–6
        liaison between NHS and private practitioners 780–1
        liaison for treatment abroad 781–2
        mentally incapacitated adults 783
        nurse-led care 785
        other care providers and local authorities 784–5
        poor coordination 779
        social workers 782–4
Teenage Pregnancy Unit 272
Telecommunications Act 1984 251
telemedicine 23–4
telephone messages 186–7
    recordings 251–2
terminal illness *see* end of life
terminal sedation 436
Termination of Life on Request and Assisted Suicide (Review Procedures) Act 2001 (The Netherlands) 480
terminations
    doctors' moral views 32
Terrorism Act 2000 195
Terrorism Act 2006 732
test results
    young people 31
text (SMS) messages 187
TGN1412 incident 588–9
time-delayed telemedicine 24
tobacco control 820–2
Tomorrow's Doctors 740, 742, 751
tooth decay and water fluoridation 822–4
top up fees 551
trade in body parts and tissues 521
    legal situation 522
training *see* education and training
translation of patients' communications 38–9, 65
    detention settings 699–700

transsexualism
    health records 237
treatment
    emergency
        incapacitated (incompetent) adults 95–6
    incapacitated (incompetent) patients
        England and Wales 102–22
        Northern Ireland 134–139
        Scotland 122–34
    limits to individual choices 80–8
        amputation of healthy limbs 85–8
        procedures to benefit others 80–5
    refusal 75–80, 114–15
        advance decisions 96
        anorexia nervosa treatment refused by 16-year-old 157
        benefit to others 77
        caesarean section 268–9, 304–6
        continuing care 78
        documenting refusal 78
        failure to respect 79
        heart transplant refused by 15-year-old 150
        hunger strikes 715–16
        hypothetical case 17–18
        informed refusal 77–8
        phobia 99–100
        psychotic illness treatment refused by 15-year-old 159
        right to refuse 75–7
        schizophrenia 99
treatments
    covert medication 39–40
    financial interest by doctors 42
    unfunded 36
triage
    accident and disaster sites 644
truth telling and resources 550–1
    top up fees 551
tuberculosis 708–9
twins
    abortion of healthy twin 287
    conjoined 173–4
tyranny of normality 296

UK Border Agency 724
UK Ethics Committee Authority (UKECA) 609
UK National DNA Database 401
    familial searching 403
uneconomic patients 29
unfunded treatments 36

United Nations' Universal Declaration of
    Human Rights (1948) 8
unlicensed drug prescriptions 536
    economic reasons 536–7
Unrelated Live Transplants Regulatory
    Authority (ULTRA) 82
unsupervised junior doctors 862–3
USB memory sticks and data security 245

vaccination 827–8
    compulsory vaccination 830
    health workers 830–1
    immunisation and population immunity
        828
    MMR controversy 829
vegetative state
    withdrawal of nutrition or hydration 445–6
Vetting and Barring Scheme 49
victims of crime or abuse
    consent
        examination by forensic physicians 729
    emergency treatment 637
        child abuse or neglect 640–1
        domestic violence 640
video and picture messages as records 247
violent patients 55–7
virtue ethics 12
Voluntary Euthanasia Society (VES) 470,
    472–3
vulnerable adults
    balancing freedom with protection 95

Warnock Committee 312
water fluoridation 822–4
Water Industry Act 1991 809
welfare of individuals participating in research
    593–4
welfare rights 8
Welsh Clinical Portal 241
whistleblowing
    multi-disciplinary teams 778
    poorly performing systems and poor
        management 878–9
    research fraud and misconduct 622
    witnessing unethical behaviour 762
whole genome testing 404
whole-person care 25–6
wills, witnessing 46–7
*Withholding and Withdrawing Life-Prolonging
    Treatment* 131
witnessed resuscitation 634–5
witnessing wills and legal documents 46–7
workplace safety 204–5
wounds from firearms or knives 204

Yellow Card Scheme 573–4
young offender institutions 722
    see also detention settings; prisons
    child protection 723
        peer mentoring 723–4
        self-harm and suicide risk 723
    consent and refusal of treatment 722–3
young people *see* children and young people